SCANDINAVIAN JOURNAL

OF

Infectious Diseases

Vol. 27, 1995

INDEX

No. 1

Articles

P. Sangfelt, O. Reichard, K. Lidman, M. von Sydow and M. Forsgren: Prevention of hepatitis B by immunization of the newborn infant – a long-term follow-up study in Stockholm, Sweden 3

P. Coursaget, D. Leboulleux, Y. Gharbi, N. Enogat, M.-A. Ndao, A. M. Coll-Seck and R. Kastally: Etiology of acute sporadic hepatitis in adults in Senegal and Tunisia 9

R. D'Amelio, T. Stroffolini, P. M. Matricardi, R. Nisini, M. E. Tosti, M. Trematerra, U. Villano, M. Rapicetta and A. Mele: Low prevalence of anti-HCV antibodies among Italian Air Force recruits 12

D. Prokopowicz, E. Bobrowska, M. Bobrowski and A. Grzesczuk: Prevalence of antibodies against tick-borne encephalitis among residents of north-eastern Poland 15

P. Carlson, S. Kontianinen, O.-V. Renkonen, A. Sivonen and R. Visakorpi: Arcanobacterium haemolyticum and streptococcal pharyngitis in army conscripts 17

H. C. Schønheyder, A. Gottschau, A. Friland and V. T. Rosdahl: Mortality rate and magnitude of Staphylococcus aureus bacteremia as assessed by a semiquantitative blood culture system 19

C. Farina, P. Boiron, A. Goglio, F. Provost and the Northern Italy Collaborative Group on Nocardiosis: Human nocardiosis in northern Italy from 1982 to 1992 23

Treatment of louse-borne relapsing fever with low dose penicillin and tetracycline: a clinical trial: T. Seboxa and S. I. Rahlenbeck 29

J. Hedlund, L.-O. Hansson and Å. Örtqvist: Short- and long-term prognosis for middle-aged and elderly patients hospitalized with community-acquired pneumonia: impact of nutritional and inflammatory factors 32

E. Rintala, K. Pulkki, J. Mertsola, T. Nevalainen and J. Nikoskelainen: Endotoxin, interleukin-6 and phospholipase-A2 as markers of sepsis in patients with hematological malignancies 39

R. Manninen, E. Eerola and P. Huovinen: Disk diffusion susceptibility tests: need for laboratory-specific breakpoints 45

A. Nissinen, H. Seppälä, P. Huovinen and the Finnish Study Group for Antimicrobial Resistance (FiRe): Detecting erythromycin resistance in Streptococcus pyogenes: reliability of the disk diffusion method and the breakpoint susceptibility testing method 52

A. Nissinen, E. Herva, M.-L. Katila, S. Kontiainen, O. Liimatainen, S. Oinonen, A. K. Takala and P. Huovinen: Antimicrobial resistance in Haemophilus influenzae isolated from blood, cerebrospinal fluid, middle ear fluid and throat samples of children. A nationwide study in Finland in 1988–1990 57

S. Hugosson, S.-A. Silfverdal, Ö. Garpenholt, E. Esbjörner, B. Lindquist, T. Vikerfors, B. Werner and P. Olcén: Invasive Haemophilus influenzae disease: epidemiology and clinical spectrum before large-scale H. influenzae type b vaccination 63

M. Tanyüksel, H. Gün and L. Doğanci: Prevalence of Cryptosporidium sp. in patients with neoplasia and diarrhea 69

H. Albrecht, J. Skörde, K. Arasteh, W. Heise, H.-J. Stellbrink, G. Grosse and M. L'Age: Disseminated toxoplasmosis in AIDS patients – report of 16 cases 71

Case Reports

C.-H. Chiu, T.-Y. Lin and Y.-C. Huang: Cranial nerve palsies and cerebral infarction in a young infant with meningococcal meningitis 75

R. S. Crausman, W. T. Pluss and C. A. Jennings: Acute epiglottitis in the adult caused by neisseria meningitidis 77

H. M. L. Oh and L. Tay: Bacteraemia caused by Rahnella aquatilis: report of two cases and review 79

Å. Melhus, T. Holmdahl and I. Tjernberg: First documented case of Bacteremia with Vibrio vulnificus in Sweden 81

P. M. Landsaat, H. van der. Lelie, G. Bongaerts and E. J. Kuijper: Fusobacterium nucleatum, a new invasive pathogen in neutropenic patients? 83

S. Yamada, T. Maruoka, K. Nagai, N. Tsumura, T. Yamada, Y. Sakata, K. Tominaga, T. Motohiro, H. Kato, K. Makimura and H. Yamaguchi: Catheter-related infections by Hansenula anomala in children 85

R. Colebunders, K. van den Abbeele, E. Hauben, T. Verstraeten, T. Heremans, J. van den Ende and E. van Marck: Histoplasma capsulatum infection in three AIDS patients living in Africa 89

X. Corbella, M. Vadillo, C. Cabellos, P. Fernandez-Viladrich and G. Rufi: Hypersensitivity hepatitis due to pyrazinamide 93

Letters to the Editors

P. Domingo, M. Puig, R. Pericas, B. Mirelis and G. Prats: Moraxella catarrhalis bacteræmia in an immunocompetent adult 95

A. Cabíe, S. Matheron, M.-A. Khuong, O. Bouchaud, A. G. Saimot and J.-P. Couland: Dapsone as prophylaxis for disseminated Mycobacterium avium complex infection 96

No. 2

Articles

S. Shev, S. Hermodsson, A. Lindholm, E. Malm, A. Widell and G. Norkrans: Risk factor exposure among hepatitis C virus RNA positive Swedish blood donors – the role of parenteral and sexual transmission 99

P-G. Babu, T. Ishida, J. Nesadoss and T. J. John: Prevalence of HTLV-I/II antibodies in HIV seropositive and HIV seronegative STD patients in Vellore region in southern India 105

K. Ekdahl, L. Truedsson, A. G. Sjöholm and J. H. Braconier: Complement analysis in adult patients with a history of bacteremic pneumococcal infections or recurrent pneumonia 111

A. Österlund and L. Engstrand: DNA fingerprinting of Streptococcus pyogenes from patients with recurrent pharyngotonsillitis by means of random amplified polymorphic DNA analysis 119

A. Norrby-Teglund, K. Pauksens, M. Norgren and S. E. Holm: Correlation between serum TNFα and IL6 levels and severity of group A streptococcal infections 125

A. Österlund: Are penicillin treatment failures in Arcanobacterium haemolyticum pharyngotonsillitis caused by intracellularly residing bacteria? 131

M. Doğanay, S. Çalangu, H. Turgut, M. Bakir and B. Aygen: Treatment of tuberculous meningitis in Turkey 135

O. Admoni, P. Yagupsky, A. Golan, Y. Kenes, G. Schifroni and I. Horowitz: Epidemiological, clinical and microbiological features of shigellosis among hospitalized children in northern Israel 139

H. C. Schønheyder, P. Søgaard and W. Frederiksen: A survey of campylobacter bacteremia in three Danish counties, 1989 to 1994 145

N. Banatvala, Y. Abdi, L. Clements, A-M. Herbert, J. Davies, J. Bagg, J. P. Shepherd, R. A. Feldman and J. M. Hardie: Helicobacter pylori infection in dentists – a case-control study 149

B. Kristensen, H. C. Schønheyder, N. A. Peterslund, S. Rosthøj, N. Clausen and W. Frederiksen: Capnocytophaga (Capnocytophaga ochracea group) bacteremia in hematological patients with profound granulocytopenia 153

M. E. Ellis, D. Spence, A. Bouchama, J. Antonius, M. Bazarbashi, F. Khougeer, E. B. De Vol and the Fungal Study Group: Open lung biopsy provides a higher and more specific diagnostic yield compared to broncho-alveolar lavage in immunocompromised patients 157

J. Logar, Ž. Novak-Antolič and A. Zore: Serological screening for toxoplasmosis in pregnancy in Slovenia 163

Case Reports

A. Salazar, D. Podzamczer, R. Reñe, M. Santin, J. L. Perez, I. Ferrer, P. Fernandez-Viladrich and F. Gudiol: Cytomegalovirus ventriculoencephalitis in AIDS patients 165

J. C. Graham, P. J. Moss, M. W. McKendrick: Primary group A streptococcal peritonitis 171

C. Mussini, F. Trenti, G. Manicardi, N. Mongiardo, M. Codeluppi, L. D'Andrea, G. Guaraldi, F. Squadrini and B. De Rienzo: Non-typhoid salmonella subdural empyema in a patient with AIDS 173

A. Gutiérrez, R. Teira, M. Varona, S. González de Etxabarri and J. M. Santamaría: Recurrent Salmonella enteritidis meningitis in patient with AIDS 177

G. Falck, L. Heyman, J. Gnarpe and H. Gnarpe: Chlamydia pneumoniae and chronic pharyngitis 179

A. K. Al-Kassab, E. Habte-Gabr, W. F. Mueller and Q. Azher: Fulminant disseminated toxoplasmosis in an HIV patient 183

Letter to the Editors

G-B. Lindblom, E. Sjögren, J. Hansson-Westerberg and B. Kaijser: Campylobacter upsaliensis, C. Sputorum sputorum and C. concisus as common causes of diarrhoea in Swedish children 187

No. 3

Articles

H. L. Hansen, P. L. Anderson, L. Brandt and O. Broløs: Antibodies against hepatitis viruses in merchant seamen 191

K. Persson, A. Månsson, E. Jönsson and E. Nordenfelt: Decline of herpes simplex virus type 2 and Chlamydia trachomatis infections from 1970 to 1993 indicated by a similar change in antibody pattern 195

P. Moine, J. B. Vercken, S. Chevret, P. Gajdos and The French Study Group of Community-Acquired Pneumonia in ICU: Severe community-acquired pneumococcal pneumonia 201

H. Rautelin, A. Sivonen, A. Kuikka, O-V. Renkonen, V. Valtonen, H. Lehti, A. Kahanpää and T. U. Kosunen: Role of Aeromonas isolated from feces of Finnish patients 207

V. H. San Joaquin, J. C. Griffis, C. Lee and C. L. Sears: Association of Bacteroides fragilis with childhood diarrhea 211

T. L. Nielsen, B. N. Jensen, S. Nelsing, L. R. Mathiesen, P. Skinhöj and J. O. Nielsen: Randomized study of sulfamethoxazole-trimethoprim versus aerosolized pentamidine for secondary prophylaxis of Pneumocystis carinii pneumonia in patients with AIDS 217

S. Holm, C. Henning, E. Grahn, H. Lomberg and H. Staley: Is penicillin the appropriate treatment for recurrent tonsillopharyngitis? Results from a comparative randomized blind study of cefuroxime axetil and phenoxymethylpenicillin in children 221

C. von Sydow, S. Savolainen and A. Söderqvist: Treatment of acute maxillary sinusitis – comparing cefpodoxime proxetil with amoxicillin 229

A. Ammassari, A. Linzalone, R. Murri, G. Marasca, G. Morace and A. Antinori: Fluconazole for primary prophylaxis of AIDS-associated cryptococcosis: a case-control study 235

N. Gürses, S. Uysal, F. Çetinkaya, İ. İşlek and A. G. Kalayci: Intravenous immunoglobulin treatment in children with Guillain-Barre syndrome 241

M. Arpi, J. Renneberg, H-K. Andersen, B. Nielsen and S. O. Larsen: Bacteremia at a Danish university hospital during a twenty-five-year period (1968–1992) 245

B. Olesen, H. J. Kolmos, F. Ørskov, I. Ørskov and A. Gottschau: Bacteraemia due to Escherichia coli in a Danish university hospital, 1986–1990 253

M. Lebech and E. Petersen: Detection by Enzyme Immunosorbent Assay of Toxoplasma gondii IgG antibodies in dried blood spots on PKU-filter paper from newborns 259

M. Lappalainen, H. Sintonen, M. Koskiniemi, K. Hedman, V. Hiilesmaa, P. Ämmälä, K. Teramo and P. Koskela: Cost-benefit analysis of screening for toxoplasmosis during pregnancy 265

J. Isacson, B. Trollfors, G. Hedvall, J. Taranger and G. Zackrisson: Response and decline of serum IgG antibodies to pertussis toxin, filamentous hemagglutinin and pertactin in children with pertussis 273

S. A. Halperin, B. Eastwood, L. Barreto, E. Mills, M. Blatter, K. Reisinger, G. Bader, H. Keyserling, E. A. Roberts, R. Guasparini, L. Medd and G. Humphreys: Safety and immunogenicity of two acellular pertussis vaccines with different pertussis toxoid and filamentous hemagglutinin content in infants 2–6 months old 279

Case Reports

A-C. Chen, C-C. Liu, W-J. Yao, C-T. Chen and J-Y. Wang: Actinobacillus actinomycetemcomitans pneumonia with chest wall and subphrenic abscess 289

J. C. O'Driscoll, G. S. Keene, M. J. Weinbren, A. P. Johnson, M-F. Palepou and R. C. George: Haemophilus aphrophilus discitis and vertebral osteomyelitis 291

T. Hur, K-C. Cheng and J-M. Hsieh: Aeromonas hydrophila lung abscess in a previously healthy man 295

M. O. McBride, M. Fisher, C. J. Skinner, R. Golden and J. Main: An unusual gastrointestinal presentation of leishmaniasis 297

Short Communications

T. O. Linglöf: Hepatitis B in parts of former USSR 299

No. 4

Review Article

A. Samuelson, S. Borrelli, R. Gustafson, L. Hammarström, C. I. E. Smith, J. Jonasson and A. A. Lindberg: Characterization of Haemophilus influenzae isolates from the respiratory tract of patients with primary antibody deficiencies: evidence for persistent colonizations 303

Articles

A. Andersson-Ellström, B. Svennerholm and L. Forssman: Prevalence of antibodies to herpes simplex virus types 1 and 2, Epstein–Barr virus and cytomegalovirus in teenage girls 315

O. Weiland, M. Chen, G. Lindh, L. Mattsson, R. Schvarcz, A. Sönnerborg, M. Wahl, R. Wejstål, A. Widell and G. Norkrans: Efficacy of human leucocyte alpha-interferon treatment for chronic hepatitis C virus infection 319

J. H. Braconier, O. Paulsen, K. Engman and A. Widell: Combined alpha-interferon and ribavirin treatment in chronic hepatitis C: a pilot study 325

K. Stark, E. Schreier, R. Müller, D. Wirth, G. Driesel and U. Bienzle: Prevalence and determinants of anti-HCV seropositivity and of HCV genotype among intravenous drug users in Berlin 331

Y. A. Al-Eissa: Clinical and therapeutic features of childhood neurobrucellosis 339
M. Montes, G. Cilla, J. M. Marimon, J. L. Diaz de Tuesta and E. Pérez-Trallero: Coxiella burnetii infection in subjects with HIV infection and HIV infection in patients with Q fever 344
H. Nielsen and L. P. Andersen: Activation of phagocytes by Helicobacter pylori correlates with the clinical presentation of the gastric infection 347
S. Nelsing, B. N. Jensen and V. Backer: Persistent reduction in lung function after Pneumocystis carinii pneumonia in AIDS patients 351
F. Moonens, C. Liesnard, F. Brancart, J. P. Van Vooren and E. Serruys: Rapid simple and nested polymerase chain reaction for the diagnosis of Pneumocystis carinii pneumonia 358
J. Skøt, A. G. Lerche, H. J. Kolmos, J. O. Nielsen, L. R. Mathiesen and J. D. Lundgren: Pneumocystis carinii in bronchoalveolar lavage and induced sputum: detection with a nested polymerase chain reaction 363
G. Müns, I. Rubínstein and K.-C. Bergmann: Phagocytosis and oxidative burst of blood phagocytes in chronic obstructive airway disease 369
B. Söderquist, K.-G. Sundqvist, I. Jones, H. Holmberg and T. Vikerfors: Interleukin-6, C-reactive protein, lactoferrin and white blood cell count in patients with S. aureus septicemia 375
M. Antonelli, G. M. Raponi, P. Martino, G. Rosa, G. Conti, J. Jalouk and A. Gasparetto: High IL-6 serum levels are associated with septic shock and mortality in septic patients with severe leukopenia due to hematological malignancies 381
G. Heresi, F. Pizarro, M. Olivares, M. Cayazzo, E. Hertrampf, T. Walter, J. R. Murphy and A. Stekel: Effect of supplementation with an iron-fortified milk on incidence of diarrhea and respiratory infection in urban-resident infants 385
E. Chryssanthou, J. Torssander and B. Petrini: Oral Candida albicans isolates with reduced susceptibility to fluconazole in Swedish HIV-infected patients 391

Case Reports

S. Lund-Tønnesen: Liver abscess: an unusual manifestation of pneumococcal infection 397
R. A. Doedens, C. J. Miedema, S. B. Oetomo and J. L. L. Kimpen: Atypical cellulitis due to Group B streptococcus 399
S. J. Antony, P. Matherin and C. Stratton: Increased bactericidal activity as documented by serum bactericidal titers for a triple combination of cell wall active agents against gentamicin-resistant enterococci 401
R. Manfredi, A. Mazzoni, G. Marinacci, A. Nanetti and F. Chiodo: Progressive intractable actinomycosis in patients with AIDS 405
L. Coppens, B. Sztern, D. Korman and F. Lustman: Yersinia enterolitica bacteremia with intracranial extension 409
S. J. Antony and D. W. Haas: Tuberculous pericarditis in an HIV-infected patient 411
R.-J. Ben, T. Young and H.-S. Lee: Hepatobiliary tuberculosis presenting as a gall bladder tumor 415
J. O. Jarløv, P. Born and B. Bruun: Candida albicans meningitis in a 27 weeks premature infant treated with liposomal amphotericin-B (AmBisome[R]) 419
L. Jahnson, E. Chryssanthou, B. Petrini and T. Vikerfors: Fluconazole failure in two cases of disseminated candidosis 421

Short Communications

L. Doğanci, H. Gün, M. Baysallar, A. Albay, E. Çinar and T. Haznedaroğlu: Short-term quinolones for successful eradication of multiply resistant Vibrio cholerae in adult patients 425
M. Čobeljić, Z. Lepšanović and S. Velimirović: Infrequent finding of verotoxin-producing Escherichia coli in diarrheal stools in Belgrade, Serbia 427

No. 5

Review Article

A. Lauritsen and B. Øberg: Adjunctive corticosteroid therapy in bacterial meningitis 431

Articles

I. Hökeberg, B. Zweygberg-Wirgart, B. M. Eriksson, G. Tufvesson, E. Olding-Stenkvist and L. Grillner: Diagnostic markers and risk factors of cytomegalovirus infection and disease in renal allograft recipients 435
A. Mele, R. Corona, M. E. Tosti, F. Palumbo, A. Moiraghi, F. Novaco, C. Galanti, R. Bernacchia and P. Ferraro: Beauty treatments and risk of parenterally transmitted hepatitis: Results from the hepatitis surveillance system in Italy 441
S. Nelsing, P. Wantzin, J. Skøt, E. Krarup, T. L. Nielsen, H. B. Krarup and J. O. Nielsen: The seroprevalence of hepatitis B and C in hospitalized Danish patients 445
R. Norda, A.-S. Duberg, A. Sönnerborg and P. Olcén: Transmission of hepatitis C virus by transfusion in Örebro County, Sweden, 1990–1992 449
P. H. P. Groeneveld, P. Colson, K. M. C. Kwappenberg and J. Clement: Increased production of nitric oxide in patients infected with the European variant of hantavirus 453
Å. Örtqvist, J. Hedlund, B. Wretlind, A. Carlström and M. Kalin: Diagnostic and prognostic value of interleukin-6 and C-reactive protein in community-acquired pneumonia 457
S. Cronberg, S. Banke. A.-M. Bruno, M. Carlsson, H. Elmrud, S. Elowsson, K. Josefsson, A.-C. Lindholm, H. Montelius, R. Neringer, B. Ode, G. Stenlund, B. Svanteson, A. Thorén, M. Walder and E. Wallmark: Ampicillin + mecillinam vs. cefotaxime/cefadroxil treatment of patients with severe pneumonia or pyelonephritis: A double-blind multicentre study evaluated by intention-to-treat analysis 463
F. Fuentes Martinez, M. M. Martín Caminero, J. Izquierdo Izquierdo, M. L. Gomez-Lus Centelles and J. Prieto Prieto: In vivo and in vitro study of several pharmacodynamic effects of meropenem 469
P. Kotilainen, J. Hyvärinen, H. Järvinen, L. Linko, E. Eerola, O.-P. Lehtonen, A. Sivonen, P. Huovinen and J. Vuopio-Varkila: Testing of methicillin resistance by in vitro susceptibility and the presence of the mecA gene in clinical Staphylococcus aureus isolates in Finland 475
M. Faber, N. Frimodt-Møller, F. Espersen, P. Skinhøj and V. Rosdahl: Staphylococcus aureus endocarditis in Danish intravenous drug users: High proportion of left-sided endocarditis 483
E. Kihlström and B. Normann: Occurrence of pneumococci with resistance or decreased susceptibility to penicillin in southeast Sweden 489
H. Rautelin, A. Sivonen, A. Kuikka, O.-V. Renkonen, V. Valtonen and T. U. Kosunen: Enteric Plesiomonas shigelloides infections in Finnish patients 495
J. Wüst, R. Frei, H. Günthard and M. Altwegg: Analysis of restriction fragment length polymorphism and ribotyping of multiresistant Stenotrophomonas maltophilia isolated from persisting lung infection in a cystic fibrosis patient 499
I. Kuzman, I. Soldo, S. Schönwald and J. Čulig: Azithromycin for treatment of community acquired pneumonia caused by Legionella pneumophila: A retrospective study 503

S. K. Schepetiuk, R. Norton and T. W. Kok: Rapid diagnosis of chlamydial respiratory infection in children 507
J. Gascon, M. Corachan, J. A. Bombi, M. E. Valls and J. M. Bordes: Cyclospora in patients with traveller's diarrhea 511

Case Reports

M. Valtonen, M. Kauppila, P. Kotilainen, J. Lähdevirta, C.-M. Svartbäck, O. Kosunen, J. Nurminen, H. Sarkkinen and M. Brummer-Korvenkontio: Four fatal cases of nephropathia epidemica 515
R. Khatib, M. C. Thirumoorthi, B. Kelly and K. J. Grady: Severe psittacosis during pregnancy and suppression of antibody response with early therapy 519
J. López-Contreras, J. Ris, P. Domingo, M. Puig, N. Rabella and J. Nolla: Disseminated cytomegalovirus infection in an immunocompetent adult successfully treated with ganciclovir 523
R. P. Young, M. Ip and D. C. J. Bassett: Fatal rickettsial meningitis in Hong Kong: A need for rapid laboratory diagnosis 527
R. Khatib, K. M. Riederer, M. Held and H. Aljundi: Protracted and recurrent methicillin-resistant Staphylococcus aureus bacteremia despite defervescence with vancomycin therapy 529
M. Valtonen, J. Lommi, S. Pohjola-Sintonen, P. Ljungberg, M. Hynninen and M. Vaara: Low levels of cytokines and endotoxin in a fatal case of myocardial depression and septic shock due to Yersinia pseudotuberculosis 533

Short Communication

P. Olcén, P.-G. Lantz, A. Bäckman and P. Rådström: Rapid diagnosis of bacterial meningitis by a seminested PCR strategy 537

No. 6

Articles

P. J. H. Johansson, I. K. Mushahwar, G. Norkrans, O. Weiland and E. Nordenfelt: Hepatitis E virus infections in patients with acute hepatitis non-A–D in Sweden 543
S. Andersson, A. Krook, K. Käll, I. Julander, R. Thorstensson and G. Biberfeld: HTVL infections among Swedish intravenous drug users in 1992 547
J. R. Kerr, M. D. Curran, J. E. Moore and P. G. Murphy: Parvovirus B19 infection – persistence and genetic variation 551
M. Shinkai and S. A. Spector: Quantitation of human cytomegalovirus (HCMV) DNA in cerebrospinal fluid by competitive PCR AIDS patients with different HCMV central nervous system diseases 559
R. Skov, A. Gottchau, P. Skinhøj, N. Frimodt-Møller, V. T. Rosdahl and F. Espersen: Staphylococcus aureus bacteremia: a 14-year nationwide study in hematological patients with malignant disease or agranulocytosis 563
A. Lerche, N. Rasmussen, J. H. Wandall and V. A. Bohr: Staphylococcus aureus meningitis: a review of 28 consecutive community-acquired cases 569
O. Lyytikäinen, V. Valtonen, A. Sivonen, R. Ryhänen and J. Vuopio-Varkila: Molecular epidemiology of Staphylococcus epidermidis isolates in a hematological unit during a 4-month survey 575
J van der Lelie, M. Leverstein-Van Hall, M. Mertens, H. C. T. van Zaanen, M. H. van Oers, L. L. M. Thomas, A. E. G. Kr. von dem Borne and E. J. Kuijper: Corynebacterium CDC group JK (Corynebacterium jeikeium) sepsis in haematological patients: A report of three cases and a systematic literature review 581
A. Dalsgaard, O. Serichantalergs and P. Echeverria: Restriction fragment length polymorphisms (RFLP) of cholera toxin genes in Vibrio cholerae O139 recovered from patients in Thailand, India, and Bangladesh 585
G.-B. Lindblom, C. Åhrén, J. Changalucha, R. Gabone, B. Kaijser, L.-Å. Nilsson, E. Sjögren, A.-M. Svennerholm and M. Temu: Campylobacter jejuni/coli and enterotoxigenic Eschericia coli (ETEC) in faeces from children and adults in Tanzania 589
R. Gustafson, T. G. T. Jaenson, A. Gardulf, H. Mejlon and B. Svenungsson: Prevalence of Borrelia burgdorferi sensu lato infection in Ixodes ricinus in Sweden 597
B. E. B. Claesson, S. Filipsson and D. E. W. Holmlund: Dipslide culture in colonic surgery: A tool for assessment of surgical performance and a guide to antibiotic use 603
G. Barbaro, G. Barbarini and G. Di Lorenzo: Fluconazole compared with itraconazole in the treatment of esophageal candidiasis in AIDS patients: A double-blind, randomized, controlled clinical study 613
I. Brook: Pneumonia in mechanically ventilated children 619
P. Bernhard and N. Obel: Chronic ulcerating acyclovir-resistant varicella zoster lesions in an AIDS patient 623
F. T. Hufert, T. Diebold, B. Ermisch, D. Von Laer, U. Meyer-König and D. Neumann-Haefelin: Liver failure due to disseminated HSV-1 infection in a newborn twin 627
E. D. Heegaard, N. A. Peterslund and A. Hornsleth: Parvovirus B19 infection associated with encephalitis in a patient suffering from malignant lymphoma 631
S. Yildiz, H. Y. Yildiz, I. Çetin and D. H. Uçar: Total knee arthroplasty complicated by Corynebacterium jeikeium infection 635
R. S. Dykhuizen, G. Douglas, J. Weir and I. M. Gould: Corynebacterium afermentans subsp. lipophilum: Multiple abscess formation in brain and liver 637
R. Schvarcz, J. Svedenhag and K. Rådegran: A case of Brucella melitensis endocarditis successfully treated by a combination of surgical resection and antibiotics 641
I. Mohammedi, B. Gachot, M. Grossin, C. Marche, M. Wolff and F. Vachon: Overwhelming myocarditis due to Fusarium oxysporum following bone marrow transplantation 643
M. Ip, N. Leung and A. F. Cheng: Acute clonorchiasis 645

Scandinavian Journal of

INFECTIOUS DISEASES

Vol. 27, no. 1, 1995
pp. 1–96

SCANDINAVIAN
UNIVERSITY PRESS

Oslo - Copenhagen -
Stockholm - Boston

Scand J Infect Dis 27: 3–7, 1995 ORIGINAL ARTICLE

Prevention of Hepatitis B by immunization of the Newborn Infant – a Long-term Follow-up Study in Stockholm, Sweden

PER SANGFELT[1], OLLE REICHARD[1], KNUT LIDMAN[1], MADELEINE VON SYDOW[2] and MARIANNE FORSGREN[3]

From the Departments of [1]Infectious Diseases, Karolinska Institute, Danderyd Hospital, [2]Virology, Karolinska Hospital and [3]Clinical Virology, Huddinge Hospital, Huddinge, Sweden

In order to assess the present hepatitis B immunization program in Stockholm, Sweden, 212 children of HBsAg carrier mothers were followed up 2–9 years after birth. In babies of HBeAg-positive mothers a combined passive and active immunization schedule with hepatitis B immunoglobulin (HBIG) and hepatitis B vaccine was used. Among 25 children to such mothers, 1 HBsAg carrier and 5 children with asymptomatic seroconversion were found. To newborns of HBeAg-negative/anti-HBe-negative mothers, only vaccine was given. Among 15 such children, no HBsAg carrier (but 1 child with an asymptomatic seroconversion) was found. In babies of HBeAg-negative/anti-HBe-positive mothers, immunization was withheld between 1983 and 1987. Among 90 such children, 1 HBsAg carrier and 8 asymptomatic seroconversions were detected. After 1987, newborns in this group were vaccinated whereafter 3 asymptomatic seroconversions were found among 82 children. We conclude that in low prevalence areas a screening program for HBsAg should be offered to pregnant women originating from hepatitis B endemic regions, since immunoprophylaxis gave long-term protection to most children at risk. Children born to HBeAg-positive mothers should receive vaccine in combination with HBIg, whereas for children of mothers lacking HBeAg, vaccination only seems sufficient, at least if a rapid vaccination schedule is used.

P. Sangfelt, MD, Department of Internal Medicine, Enköping Hospital, S-745 25 Enköping, Sweden

INTRODUCTION

Vertical transmission of hepatitis B virus (HBV) is an important factor in perpetuating a reservoir of HBV infection, since up to 90% of children of HBsAg carrier mothers with HBeAg will become chronic carriers (1, 2). Babies of HBeAg-negative/anti-HBe-negative mothers also run a certain risk of infection (3). Babies infected perinatally may develop liver cirrhosis or hepatocellular carcinoma later in life (4, 5). It is therefore important to prevent early transmission of HBV.

Hepatitis B immunoprophylaxis of newborns is highly effective in preventing a chronic carrier state (6). The protective efficacy rate of hepatitis B immunoglobulin (HBIg) and vaccine, both alone and in combination, is estimated to be 70 and 95%, respectively (6–8). Perinatal infection of infants born to HBeAg-negative/anti-HBe-positive mothers is considered rare, even without immunization. Nevertheless a risk of later horizontal infection exists (9), and acute fulminant cases of hepatitis B have been reported among such infants (10–12). In the County of Stockholm, Sweden, pregnant women originating from endemic countries have been screened for HBsAg since 1983. Should a mother react positively to HBsAg screening, the child will be treated prophylactically according to maternal HBeAg/anti-HBe status. This immunization program has previously been assessed after short-term follow-up (13). In the present study, data from long-term follow-up 2–9 years after birth are presented for 212 children.

MATERIALS AND METHODS

Screening and immunization program

In the County of Stockholm, all pregnant women originating from Asia, Africa and South America have been screened for HBsAg since 1983. In 1987, women from the Mediterranean area were also included in the screening program. A total of 10,519 women were screened and 416 (4%) HBsAg carriers were identified. A positive HBsAg result was followed by analyses of HBeAg, anti-HBe and anti-HBc. The HBsAg-positive mothers were divided into three groups according to the HBe-antigen status; HBeAg-positive ($n = 58$), HBeAg-negative/anti-HBe-negative ($n = 27$) and HBeAg-negative/anti-HBe-positive ($n = 331$). The immunization program is described in Table 1. 10 newborns of HBeAg-negative/anti-HBe-positive mothers born after 1987 missed their vaccination and 4 born before 1987 were vaccinated. These children have been included in the non-vaccinated and vaccinated group, respectively. Plasma-derived HBV vaccine 0.5 ml (10 μg/ml; HB-Vax MSD), later replaced by recombinant produced vaccine (10 μg/ml; H-B-

Table I. *Maternal HBV markers and immunization schedules in their off-spring*

Maternal category	At birth	3 weeks	2 months
HBeAg pos	HBIg + Vaccine	Vaccine	Vaccine
HBeAg neg/anti-HBe neg	Vaccine	Vaccine	Vaccine
HBeAg neg/anti-HBe pos (1983–1987)	–	–	–
HBeAg neg/anti-HBe pos (1987–1989)	Vaccine	Vaccine	Vaccine

 ISSN 0036-5548

Table II. *Geographical origin of the HBsAg-positive mothers*

Region	HBeAg-pos	HBeAg-neg/ anti-HBe neg	HBeAg-neg/ anti-HBe pos (no vaccine)	HBeAg-neg/ anti-HBe pos (vaccine)	Total
East	10	12	61	41	124
(Turkey)	(10)	(12)	(59)	(38)	(119)
Middle East	4	1	16	22	43
Far-East	9	2	3	4	18
Africa	2	0	2	4	8
North Africa*	0	0	8	9	17
South Europe	0	0	0	2	2
Total	25	15	90	82	212

* Includes Algeria, Morocco and Tunisia.

Vax N MSD), was administered i.m., alone or combined with 5 ml HBIg (Aunativ, Kabi Vitrum), within the first hours of life.

Serological tests

Commercially available RIA or ELISA tests were used for HBsAg, HBeAg, anti-HBe, anti-HBc and anti-HBs (MEIA) determinations (Abbott Laboratories, North Carolina, IL, USA). All tests were performed according to the manufacturer's instructions.

Patients and design of the follow-up study

In 1991, mothers found positive for HBsAg in the screening program during 1983–89 were contacted and serological follow-up of their children was offered. 373 of 416 (90%) mothers were traced. Among these 373 women, 415 pregnancies were recorded, whereof 47 did not go to term, due to abortion (spontaneous or induced). Among the remaining 368 children, 156 were lost to follow-up as they declined to participate ($n = 45$), did not answer repeated requests ($n = 56$), had left from the County of Stockholm ($n = 46$), were not vaccinated according to the study schedule ($n = 7$) or were not alive ($n = 2$ deaths unrelated to hepatitis B). Thus, altogether 212 children born in 1983–89 were included in the serological follow-up. Their geographical origin is presented in Table II.

Each child was tested for anti-HBc and anti-HBs. If anti-HBc proved positive and anti-HBs negative, HBsAg was analysed; and if HBsAg was positive, HBeAg/antiHBe was also analysed. If anti-HBs was positive, at a level >10 mIU/ml, and anti-HBc was negative, the child was considered to have protective immunity after vaccination. If both anti-HBc and anti-HBs were positive, an asymptomatic seroconversion was diagnosed. An isolated positive anti-HBc was also regarded as an asymptomatic seroconversion. If HBsAg was positive and persisted for more than 6 months, a chronic HBsAg-carrier state was diagnosed.

The study was approved by the Medical Ethics Committee at the Karolinska Institute.

Statistical analyses were made with the Mann-Whitney U-test on a Macintosh computer using the Statview Se + Graphics TM program.

RESULTS

Children born to HBeAg-positive mothers

25 children with a mean follow-up time of 4 years (range 28 months–8 years) were tested (Table III). One child, 5 years of age, was positive for HBsAg, anti-HBc (IgG) and HBeAg. This child was HBsAg-positive (in capillary blood) already at birth. Five children were both anti-HBs and anti-HBc-positive, and 19 were anti-HBs-positive only, whereof 3 with values <10 mIU/ml (Table III).

Children born to HBeAg-negative/anti-HBe-negative mothers

15 children with a mean follow-up time of 5 years (range 30 months–8 years) were tested. One child was positive for both anti-HBs and anti-HBc, and 14 were anti-HBs-positive only, whereof 1 with a value <10 mIU/ml (Table III).

Children born to HBeAg-negative/anti-HBe-positive mothers

Results were obtained from 172 children divided into 2 subgroups.

Non vaccinated: 90 children with a mean follow-up time of 5 years (range 24 months–9 years) were tested (Table III). One child, a 6-year-old girl of Turkish origin, was positive for HBsAg, anti-HBc (IgG) and HBeAg. This girl was HBsAg-negative at 6 months of age. One child was positive for anti-HBc (IgG) only, and 7 were positive for anti-HBs and anti-HBc.

Vaccinated: 82 children with a mean follow-up time of 3 years (range 24 months–5 years) were tested (Table III). No chronic carrier was found. Three children were both anti-HBs and anti-HBc positive, and 2 were negative for all HBV markers in spite of vaccination. 77 children were anti-HBs-positive, whereof 4 with values <10 MIU/ml.

Persistence of anti-HBs titres

Anti-HBs titres were available from all vaccinated children. Children positive for anti-HBc were excluded. The overall persistence of anti-HBs, and the geometric mean titre (GMT) in the different age groups are presented in Fig. 1. The rate of detectable anti-HBs activity was 110/112 (98%), and the number with an anti-HBs titre ≥ 10 mIU/ml was 102/112 (91%). The GMT for children 2 years of age was higher than for 3-year-olds, 124 vs. 66 mIU/ml, a difference, however, which did not reach statistical signifi-

Table III. *Hepatitis B virus markers at follow-up in 212 children recruited in the immunization program in Stockholm, Sweden*

Maternal category	No. (%)	HBsAg-pos	HBeAg-pos	Anti-HBc-pos	Anti-HBs-pos/ anti-HBc-pos	Anti-HBs-pos	No marker
HBeAg-pos	25 (12)	1[a]	1[a]	1[a]	5	19[b]	0
HBeAg-neg/anti-HBe-neg	15 (7)	0	0	0	1	14[c]	0
HBeAg-neg/anti-HBe-pos (not vaccinated)	90 (43)	1[d]	1[d]	2[d,e]	7	0	81
HBeAg-neg/anti-HBe-pos (vaccinated)	82 (38)	0	0	0	3	77[f]	2
Total	212 (100)	2[a,d]	2[a,d]	3[a,d,e]	16	110	83

[a] The same child.
[b] Three children had anti-HBs levels below 10 mIU/ml; (7, 8, 5 mIU/ml respectively).
[c] One child had anti-HBs levels below 10 mIU/ml; (7 mIU/ml).
[d] The same child.
[e] One child with only anti-HBc.
[f] Four children had anti-HBs levels below 10 MIU/ml; (8, 7, 4 and 3 mIU/ml respectively).

cance ($p = 0.07$). A significantly higher GMT was observed for the children who received only vaccination at birth, compared with that in children who received both vaccination and HBIg, 84 vs. 43 mIU/ml, respectively ($p < 0.05$).

DISCUSSION

The result of our immunoprophylaxis regimen was satisfactory, since only 2 out of 212 children became chronic HBsAg carriers. Furthermore, none was judged to be infected at birth. Thus, the preventive measures of vaccination in combination with HBIg to children of HBeAg-positive mothers gave protection to nearly all. Only 1 out of 25 children (4%) became a chronic carrier. The mother of this child had high levels of HBV DNA during pregnancy, and the child was probably infected in utero, as HBsAg was positive in a capillary blood sample drawn at birth, as previously reported (13). In addition, 5 children (20%) had signs of asymptomatic seroconversion. This is in accordance with previous observations that some mothers with high level viremia will transmit HBV infection to their offspring even if immediate immunoprophylaxis is given to the newborn (14).

In our study, the dosage of HBIg was very high, and a vaccine schedule was used with booster doses given after

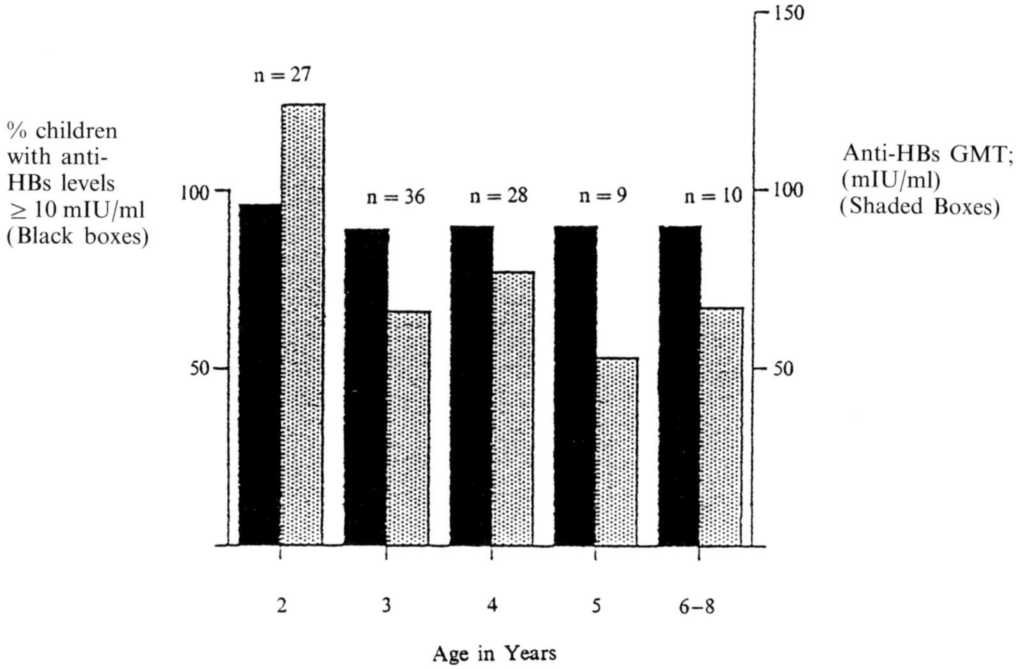

Fig. 1. Anti-HBs geometric mean titre (GMT; mIU/ml) in hepatitis B vaccinated children and % children with anti-HBs titres ≥ 10 mIU/ml according to age. ■ = % children with anti-HBs levels ⩾10 mIU/ml. ▨ = Anti-HBs Geometric mean titre (GMT).

only 3 weeks and 2 months. This schedule was introduced with the aim of rapidly establishing a protective anti-HBs level. HBIg administration is generally believed not to interfere with the vaccine response (5, 15, 16) although this has been suggested in some reports (6, 17). We found a significantly lower mean anti-HBs titre among 'our' children who received both vaccination and HBIg, compared with those who received vaccine only. This finding may have been due to the very high doses of HBIg used. However, all children had demonstrable anti-HBs activity at follow-up, and only few at very low levels.

There is evidence of an increased risk of HBV transmission to children whose anti-HBs levels are not kept sufficiently high (5, 18). This has been shown in high endemic situations where only HBIg was given (9). A report from Senegal indicated an increased risk of horizontal transmission also when the vaccine-induced anti-HBs level wears off (19). Senegal has, however, a fairly high HBV mutant prevalence and these late infections may have originated from a mutant virus. In our study, 9 children contracted a transient subclinical infection. However, whether these asymptomatic seroconversions were related to low anti-HBs titres or not, cannot be concluded from the present material.

The anti-HBs GMT tended to be higher in children 2 years of age as compared with older children, although the difference did not reach statistical significance ($p = 0.07$). In agreement with studies by Poovorawan et al. (20) and Lieming et al. (21), the GMT did not decrease markedly after 3 years of age (Fig. 1). A probable explanation for this maintenance of anti-HBs could be natural boosters in this population.

The vast majority of chronic carrier mothers in Sweden belong to the HBeAg-negative/anti-HBe-positive group. Opinions have differed regarding the need to immunize children born to these mothers (22–24). When the immunization program started in 1983, the risks of giving plasma-derived products were not fully elucidated and in the light of the increasing epidemic of HIV/AIDS it was decided to withhold vaccination from these children. A previous follow-up study in the County of Stockholm, of 43 such children, born in 1983–86, revealed no chronic carriers. However, in the present study 1 non-vaccinated child became a chronic carrier and 8 non-vaccinated children seroconverted asymptomatically. This illustrates the risk of horizontal transmission of hepatitis B, further emphasizing that immunization is clearly indicated. In late 1987, the safety of the vaccine had been established and recombinant vaccines had been developed. By then it also had become evident that children of anti-HBe positive mothers would occasionally develop fulminant hepatitis (10–12).

We conclude that our screening program and immunoprophylaxis scheme resulted in protection of most children. Newborns of HBeAg-positive mothers should be given vaccine in combination with HBIg, whereas for children born of HBeAg-negative mothers, vaccination alone seems to be sufficient – at least if a rapid vaccine schedule is used. In selective screening programs there is always a considerable risk for drop-outs. A general childhood vaccination program avoids such pitfalls. Since the vaccine is safe and offers good protection in children, such a program may be considered if the cost of the vaccine is kept low (25).

ACKNOWLEDGEMENTS

We thank the staff of the Child Welfare Centres in Stockholm and nurse Yvonne Greitz at the Department of Infectious Diseases, Danderyd, Sweden. Merck, Sharp and Dohme, Kabi Vitrium and Department of Environmental Health and Infectious Control, Stockholm County Council are thanked for financial support.

REFERENCES

1. Stevens CE, Beasley RP, Julia T, Wy-Chan L. Vertical transmission of hepatitis B antigen in Taiwan. N Engl J Med 229: 771–774, 1975.
2. Zanetti AR, Ferroni P, Magliano EM, Pirovano P, Lavarini C, Massaro AL, Gavinelli R, Fabris C, Rizzetto M. Perinatal transmission of the hepatitis B virus and of the HBV-associated delta agent from mothers to offspring in northern Italy. J Med Virol 9: 139–148, 1982.
3. Okada K, Kamiyama I, Inomata M, Imai M, Miyakawa M, Mayumi M. E-antigen and anti-e in the asymptomatic carrier mothers as indicators of positive and negative transmission of hepatitis B virus to their infants. N Engl J Med 294: 746–749, 1976.
4. Beasley RP, Hwang L-Y, Lin C-C, Chien C-S. Hepatocellular carcinoma and hepatitis B virus: A prospective study of 22,707 men in Taiwan. Lencet 2: 1129–1133, 1981.
5. Bortolotti F, Calzia R, Giacchini R, Ciravegna B, Armigliato M, Piscopo R, Realdi G. Liver cirrhosis associated with chronic hepatitis B virus infection in childhood. J Pediatr 108: 224–227, 1986.
6. Beasley RP, Hwang L-Y, Lee C-Y-G, Lan C-C, Roan C-H, Huang F-Y, Chen C-L. Prevention of perinatally transmitted hepatitis B virus infections with hepatitis B immune globulin and hepatitis B vaccine. Lancet 2: 1099–1102, 1983.
7. Wong VCW, Reesink HW, Reerink-Brongers EE, Yeung CY, Henrietta M, Ip H, Lelie PN, Ma HK. Prevention of the HBsAg carrier state in newborn infants of mothers who are carriers of HBsAg and HbeAg by administration of hepatitis B vaccine and hepatitis B immunoglobulin. Lancet 1: 921–926, 1984.
8. Ip HM, Lelie PN, Wong VCW, Kuhns MC, Reesink HW. Prevention of hepatitis B virus carrier state in infants according to maternal serum levels of HBV DNA. Lancet 406–410, 1989.
9. Beasley RP, Hwang LY. Postnatal infectivity of hepatitis B surface antigen-carrier mothers. J Infect Dis 147: 185–190, 1983.
10. Shiraki K, Yoshihara N, Sakurai M, Eto T, Kawana T. Acute hepatitis B in infants born to carrier mothers with the antibody to hepatitis B e-antigen. J Pediatr 97: 768–770, 1980.
11. Sinatra FR, Shah P, Weisman JY, Thomas DW, Merritt RJ, Tong MY. Perinatal transmitted acute icteric hepatitis B in infants born to hepatitis B surface antigen-positive and anti-hepatitis Be-positive carrier mothers. Pediatrics 70: 557–559, 1982.

12. Tong M, Sinatra F, Thomas D, Nair P, Merritt R, Wang D. Need for immunoprophylaxis in infants born to HBsAg positive carrier mothers who are HBeAg negative. J Pediatr 105: 945–947, 1984.
13. Reichard O, von Sydow M, Dennerstam L, Norder H, Magnius L, Berglund O, Enocksson E, Ginsburg BE, Grillner L, Lidman K, Forsgren M. Prevention by immunisation of hepatitis B in the newborn infant in Stockholm, Sweden. In: Zuckermann AJ, ed. Viral Hepatitis and Liver Disease. Alan R Liss Inc, 989–991, 1988.
14. Lee SD, Loo KJ, Wu JC, Tsai Y-T, Wang JY, Ting L-P, Tong MJ. Prevention of maternal-infant hepatitis B virus transmission by immunisation: The role of serum hepatitis B virus DNA. Hepatology 6: 369–373, 1986.
15. Szmunness W, Stevens CE, Oleszko WR, Goodman A. Passive-active immunisation against hepatitis B: Immunogenicity studies in adult Americans. Lancet 1: 575–577, 1981.
16. Gonzalez ML, Gonzalez JB, Salva F, Lardinois R. A 7-year follow-up of newborns vaccinated against hepatitis B. Vaccine 11: 1033–1036, 1993.
17. Esteban JE, Genesca J, Esteban JM, Hernandez G, Seijo M, Buti M, Muniz R, Guardia J. Immunoprophylaxis of perinatal transmission of the hepatitis B virus: Efficacy of hepatitis B immune globulin and hepatitis B vaccine in a low-prevalence area. J Med Virol 18: 381–391, 1986.
18. Stevens CE, Taylor P, Tong M, Toy P, Vyas G, Nair P, Weissman J, Krugman S. Yeast-recombinant hepatitis B vaccine. Efficacy with hepatitis B immune globulin in prevention of perinatal hepatitis B virus transmission. JAMA 257: 2612–2616, 1987.
19. Coursaget P, Yvonnet B, Chotard J, Sarr M, Vincelot P, N'doye R, Diop-Mar I, Chiron JP. Seven-year study of hepatitis B vaccine efficacy in infants from an endemic area (Senegal). Lancet 2: 1143–1145, 1986.
20. Poovorawan Y, Sanpavat S, Pongpunglert W, Chumdermpadetsuk S, Sentrakul P, Vandepapeliere P, Safary A. Long-term efficacy of hepatitis B vaccine in infants born to hepatitis B e antigen-positive mothers. Pediatr Infect Dis J 11: 816–821, 1992.
21. Lieming D, Mintai Z, Yinfu W, Shaochon Z, Weiqin K, Smego RA. A 9-year follow-up study of the immunogenicity and long-term efficacy of plasma-derived hepatitis B vaccine in high-risk Chinese neonates. Clin Infect Dis 17: 475–479, 1993.
22. Rosendal C, Kochen MM, Kretchmer R, Wegscheider K, Kaiser D. Avoidance of perinatal transmission of hepatitis B virus: Is passive immunisation always necessary? Lancet 1: 1127–1129, 1983.
23. Barbara J, Howell DR, Contreras M, Tedder RS, Briggs M, Sanderson PJ, Wood J, Bevan G. Indications for hepatitis B immunoglobulin for neonates of HBsAg carrier mothers. BMJ 289: 880, 1984.
24. ACIP. Hepatitis B and perinatal exposure and recommendations. MMWR 39: 17–19, 1990.
25. World Health Organization. Expanded programme on immunisation. Programme report 1992.

Submitted August 2, 1994; accepted October 10, 1994

Etiology of Acute Sporadic Hepatitis in Adults in Senegal and Tunisia

PIERRE COURSAGET[1], DIDIER LEBOULLEUX[2], YOUSSEF GHARBI[3], NATHALIE ENOGAT[1], MARIE-AWA NDAO[2], AWA MARIE COLL-SECK[2] and RADHIA KASTALLY[3]

From the [1]Institut de Virologie de Tours, Faculté de Pharmacie, Tours, France, [2]Service des Maladies Infectieuses, Faculté de Médecine et de Pharmacie, Dakar-Fann, Sénégal and [3]The Service des Laboratoires, Hôpital H. Thameur, Tunis, Tunisia

Markers for acute hepatitis A, B, C and E virus infections were examined in the sera of 72 patients suffering from acute hepatitis in Senegal and Tunisia. Hepatitis B was responsible for 36% and hepatitis C for 21% of the cases. Acute hepatitis A was not diagnosed. HEV infection was not observed in Senegal and represents only 4% of the acute hepatitis cases in Tunisia.

P. Coursaget, MD, Faculté de Pharmacie, 31 avenue Monge, F-37200 Tours, France

INTRODUCTION

It is a rarity in Africa that patients with acute hepatitis receive care in hospital and the exact prevalence of acute hepatitis is uncertain, due mostly to the fact that acute hepatitis is known to be treated by traditional medicine men or at home without the knowledge of public health officials. Accordingly, little is known regarding the etiology of acute hepatitis in Africa. In the great majority of African countries, hepatitis A virus (HAV) and hepatitis B virus (HBV) infections are endemic and more than 90% of the adult population have evidence of past infection by both forms. Consequently, it is generally believed that few cases of acute hepatitis in adults are caused by these viruses. However, the few published studies on the etiology of acute hepatitis in Africa report figures in the range 40–70% due to HBV and 2–10% due to HAV (1–4).

With the advent of sensitive methods for the detection of hepatitis A, B, C and E, it has now become possible to determine the relative incidence of each type of viral hepatitis. Hepatitis E virus (HEV) infection cases have been identified in many African countries (5–9). On the other hand, the prevalence of antibodies to hepatitis C virus (anti-HCV) observed in Africa is in the range 0.3 to 4% (10–13). It is also evident that African countries such as Rwanda (14) and Egypt (15) must have a high incidence of HCV infection, since 10–22% of the adult population have anti-HCV antibodies. However, little is known concerning the etiological role of HCV in acute hepatitis in these countries.

We report here the results of a study on the prevalence of HBV, HAV, HCV and HEV in patients with acute hepatitis in an African country with a high incidence of HBV infection (Senegal) and in another with a moderate incidence of HBV infection (Tunisia).

MATERIALS AND METHODS

Sera were collected from patients hospitalized at the Fann Dakar Hospital, Senegal due to acute hepatitis and also at the H. Thameur Hospital in Tunis, Tunisia. Acute viral hepatitis was defined as the sudden onset of clinical symptoms compatible with viral hepatitis, an increase in serum aminotransferase concentration in excess of 2.5 times the upper normal limit and the absence of other liver toxic agents. Serum specimens collected at the time of hospitalization were retrospectively studied to establish the viral etiology of the disease. Serum samples obtained from control groups were also investigated for hepatitis serological markers.

A total of 27 Senegalese patients in the age range 15 to 48 years (mean 28 years) (7 women and 20 males, M/F ratio = 2.9) were diagnosed as having acute viral hepatitis and were enrolled in the study. A control group was formed of 61 Senegalese adults aged 18 to 50 years (means 35 years) (14 females and 47 males, M/F ratio = 3.4). The control group included 39 patients hospitalized for non-hepatic diseases and 30 individuals from the general population.

In Tunisia, 45 patients (27F, 22M) aged 16 to 70 years (mean 36 years) were diagnosed as having acute hepatitis. A control group was formed of 45 blood donors (23M, 22F) aged 18–53 years (mean 29 years).

Commercially available ELISA test kits were used for the detection of serological markers of hepatitis A (anti-HAV IgM, Diagnostic Pasteur, Marnes la Coquette, France), hepatitis B (HBsAg, Abbott, North Chicago, IL, USA or Diagnostic Pasteur, Marnes la Coquette, France), and hepatitis C (Diagnostic Pasteur, Marnes la Coquette, France; or Abbott Diagnostika, Wiesbaden-Delkenheim, RFA). HBsAg-positive sera were also investigated for IgM anti-HBc (Corzyme-M, Abbott, North Chicago, IL). All sera from the patients and controls were also tested for IgG antibodies to hepatitis E virus using an ELISA designed to detect antibodies to the protein encoded by the ORF3 of HEV (16). Within this test, anti-HEV antibodies are detected only during the acute phase of the disease and the subsequent months. Thus a positive result with this test is indicative of a recent infection with HEV.

Comparisons of proportions were performed with the χ^2-test. Significance was set at the 0.05 level.

Table I. *Serological markers of hepatitis A virus (HAV), hepatitis B virus (HBV), hepatitis C virus (HCV) and hepatitis E virus (HEV) in acute hepatitis patients and controls from Senegal and Tunisia*

			Number (%) with				
Country	Group	Nos tested	IgM anti-HAV	HBsAg	IgM anti-HBc	anti-HCV	anti-HEV
Senegal	Acute hepatitis	27	0 (0%)	14 (52%)	11 (41%)	7 (26%)	0 (0%)
	Controls	69	1 (1.5%)	10 (14%)	0 (0%)	2 (2.9%)	0 (0%)
Tunisia	Acute hepatitis	45	0 (0%)	21 (47%)	15 (33%)	8 (18%)	2 (4.4%)
	Controls	45	0 (0%)	3 (6.7%)	0 (0%)	1 (2.2%)	0 (0%)

RESULTS

Anti-HAV IgM antibodies were not detected in the 72 sporadic hepatitis cases from Senegal and Tunisia, but in 1 of the 106 controls. HBsAg was detected in 6.7% and 14% of the control groups from Tunisia and Senegal respectively, and in 47% and 52% of the acute hepatitis patient groups from Tunisia (21/45) and Senegal (14/27) ($p < 0.0001$, and $p < 0.001$ respectively). Evidence of acute HBV infection was based on the detection of IgM anti-HBc which was not observed in any of the controls. Anti-HBc IgM was detected in 33% of the hepatitis cases in Tunisia (15/45) and in 41% in Senegal (11/27) ($p < 0.0001$ and $p < 0.000\,001$ respectively). Anti-HCV antibodies were detected in 2.2% (1/45) of the controls from Tunisia, in 2.9% (2/69) of the controls from Senegal, and in 18% (8/45) and 26% (7/27) of the patients from Tunisia and Senegal respectively ($p < 0.05$ and $p < 0.01$ respectively). Anti-HEV antibodies were not detected among patients and controls from Senegal. In Tunisia, HEV antibodies were observed in only 2 of the 45 acute cases tested (4.4%).

DISCUSSION

The testing of anti-HAV IgM confirmed that HAV is associated with very few acute hepatitis cases in African adults. The figure observed in this study is lower than those observed by Bassily et al. (1) in Egypt and Greenfield et al. (3) in Kenya. However, HBsAg was present in half of the patients with acute hepatitis compared with only 6.7%–15% of the controls in Tunisia and in Senegal, respectively. Moreover, no anti-HBc IgM was detected among the HBsAg-positive controls, but in 74% (26/35) of HBsAg-positive acute hepatitis cases, indicating that HBV was responsible for a considerable proportion (33–41%) of the acute viral hepatitis cases, as observed previously in Africa by others (2–4). One-third of the acute hepatitis cases were thus due to HBV in our study with no obvious difference between a country with a high incidence of HBV infection (Senegal) and a country with a moderate incidence (Tunisia).

Hepatitis C virus also seems to play an important role in the etiology of acute hepatitis, since some 19–26% of the patients had anti-HCV antibodies, compared with only 2–3% in the control groups. It must be noted that the HCV prevalence observed in the control groups is overestimated as a result of the small number of patients tested. A lower prevalence has been observed in larger epidemiologic studies, viz. 0–1.5% in Senegal (11, 13) and 0.5–1% in Tunisia (unpublished data). The causal relationship of HCV with the acute viral hepatitis cases, on the other hand, is probably underestimated, since anti-HCV seroconversion often occurs weeks after the appearance of clinical signs of hepatitis and because only acute-phase sera were tested in this study. However, since no follow-up of the patients was performed, the HCV-positive cases diagnosed could constitute chronic HCV infections with an exacerbation, accompanied by clinical signs of hepatitis. It should be noted that in 4 Senegalese patients anti-HCV, HBsAg and IgM anti-HBc antibodies were detected concomitantly. Moreover, 1 other patient was anti-HCV and HBsAg positive but lacked IgM anti-HBc. These data can be interpreted as a reactivation of the HBV infection in a chronic HBsAg carrier or as a superimposed HCV infection on a chronic HBV infection.

Surprisingly, no sporadic cases of HEV were identified in Senegal. However, HEV infection was observed in 2 patients from Tunisia, indicative of the low but steady presence of HEV in Tunisia. Although HEV does not seem to be a major health problem in the countries tested, the occurrence of sporadic HEV cases and the frequent migration of people between different African countries can lead to a rise in sporadic cases in the future, due to poor sanitary conditions. Further investigations are necessary to learn the epidemiology of HEV in Africa. A test is also needed which can detect antibodies HEV years after the acute infection, in order to accurately assess the prevalence of HEV in these countries.

REFERENCES

1. Bassily S, Boctor FN, Farid Z, Fanous A, Yassinmy Wallace CK. Acute hepatitis non-A, non-B in Cairo residents. Trans R Soc Trop Med Hyg 77: 382–383, 1983.
2. Crocchiolo PR, Caredda F, D'Arminio Monfork A, Lencioni R, Ragni MC, Cenzuales S, Farci P, Lavarini C, Latif AS. The

etiology of acute hepatitis in Zimbabwe. Trans R Soc Trop Med Hyg 78: 514–518, 1984.
3. Greenfield C, Karayiannis P, Wankya BM, Shah MV, Tukei P, Galpin S, Jowett TP, Thomas HC. Aetiology of acute sporadic hepatitis in adults in Kenya. J Med Virol 14: 367–362, 1984.
4. Nouasaria B, Trepo C, Larouze B, Saimot G, Aouati A. Non-A, non-B acute hepatitis in Eastern Algerian adults. Trans R Soc Trop Med Hyg 78: 137–138, 1984.
5. Tsega E, Krawczynski K, Hansson BG, Nordenfelt E, Negusse Y, Alemu W, Bahru Y. Outbreak of acute hepatitis E virus infection among military personnel in Northern Ethiopia. J Med Virol 34: 232–236, 1991.
6. Goldsmith R, Yarbourgh PO, Reyes GR, Fry KE, Gabor KA, Kamel M, Zakaria S, Amer S, Gaffar Y. Enzyme-linked immunosorbent assay for diagnosis of acute sporadic hepatitis E in Egyptian children. Lancet 339: 328–331, 1992.
7. Hyams KC, Purdy MA, Kaur M, McCarthy MC, Hussain MAM, El-Tigani A, Krawczynski K, Bradley DW, Carl M. Acute sporadic hepatitis E in Sudanese children: analysis based on a new western blot assay. J Infect Dis 165: 1001–1005, 1992.
8. Coursaget P, Krawczynski K, Buisson Y, Nizou C, Molinié C. Hepatitis E and hepatitis C virus infections among French soldiers suffering from non-A, non-B hepatitis. J Med Virol 39: 163–166, 1993.
9. Mushahwar IK, Dawson GJ, Bile KM, Magnius LO. Serological studies of an enterically transmitted non-A, non-B hepatitis in Somalia. J Med Virol 40: 218–221, 1993.
10 Jackson JB, Guay L, Goldfarb J, Olness K, Ndugwa C, Mmiro F, Kataaha P, Allain JP. Hepatitis C virus antibody in HIV-1 infected Ugandan mothers. Lancet 337: 551, 1991.
11. Coursaget P, Leboulleux D, Le Cann P, Bao O, Coll-Seck AM. Hepatitis C virus infection in cirrhosis and primary hepatocellular carcinoma in Senegal. Trans R Soc Trop Med Hyg 86: 552–553, 1992.
12. Develoux M, Meynard D, Delaporte E. Low rate of hepatitis C virus antibodies in blood donors and pregnant women in Niger. Trans R Soc Trop Med Hyg 86: 553, 1992.
13. Denis F, Aussel L, Ranger S, Martin P, Itoua-Ngaporo A, Frommel D, Teckle-Haimanot, Sangare A, Mboup S, Millan J, al Qubati Y. Prevalence of antibodies to hepatitis C virus among patients with leprosy in several African countries and the Yemen. J Med Virol 43: 1–4, 1994.
14. Mets T, Smitz J, Ngendahayo P, Sabbe L, Bigilimana I, Ngirabatware B. Hepatitis C virus infection in African patients with liver cirrhosis or primary hepatocellular carcinoma. Scand J Gastroenterol 28: 331–334, 1993.
15. Darwish MA, Raouf TA, Rushdy P, Constantine NT, Rao MR, Edelman R. Risk factors associated with a high seroprevalence of hepatitis C virus infection in Egyptian blood donors. Am J Trop Med Hyg 49: 440–447, 1993.
16. Coursaget P, Depril N, Buisson Y, Molinié C, Roué R. Hepatitis type E in a French population: detection of anti-HEV by a synthetic peptide-based enzyme-linked immunosorbent assay. Res Virol 145: 51–57, 1994.

Submitted September 12, 1994; accepted November 20, 1994

Low Prevalence of anti-HCV Antibodies among Italian Air Force Recruits

RAFFAELE D'AMELIO[1], TOMMASO STROFFOLINI[2], PAOLO MARIA MATRICARDI[1], ROBERTO NISINI[1], MARIA ELENA TOSTI[3], MICHELE TREMATERRA[4], UMBERTINA VILLANO[4], MARIA RAPICETTA[4] and ALFONSO MELE[3]

From the Laboratorio di Immunologia, Divisione Aerea, Studi, Ricerche e Sperimentazione, Aereonautica Militare, Rome, [2]Divisione Medicina, Ospedale Montefiascone, [3]Laboratorio di Epidemiologia, Istituto Superiore di Sanità, [4]Laboratorio di Virologia, Istituto Superiore di Sanità, Rome, Italy

In 1990, the prevalence of antibodies to hepatitis C virus (anti-HCV) was assessed among 4,978 Air Force recruits aged 18–26 years coming from all regions of Italy. Positivity to anti-HCV was found by both IIIrd generation EIA and RIBA in 24 (0.48%) study participants. The prevalence was twice as high in Southern Italy and the islands as in Northern and Central Italy (0.76% vs. 0.35%), a difference which was not statistically significant. The results of multiple logistic regression showed that no sociodemographic variable (region of birth, father's years of education, number of siblings) was associated with anti-HCV positivity. No anti-HCV-positive individual was positive for HBsAg. Anti-HCV positivity was found in 0.8% (2/236) of the participants who were positive for anti-HBc and in 0.5% (22/4742) of those who were anti-HBc negative, also a difference which was not statistically significant. Thus no association was found between HCV and HBV infections. These findings indicate that in Italy, HCV infection is an uncommon event among young adult males.

T. Stroffolini, MD, Laboratory of Epidemiology, I.S.S. Viale Regina Elena 229, I-00161 Rome, Italy

INTRODUCTION

Surveys conducted among the general population in different countries on the prevalence of antibodies to hepatitis C virus infection (anti-HCV) have generally used a target population consisting of voluntary or paid blood donors. However, these populations usually have special characteristics regarding age, socio-economic level, and selective procedures, so that they are not representative of the general population.

Very few studies conducted among the general population have used valid sampling procedures (1–3). In Italy, a recent population-based survey among children and teenagers recruited by systematic cluster sampling showed an anti-HCV prevalence as low as 0.4%; no child was reported to have been infected before 6 years of age (4).

We recently conducted a sero-epidemiological study on a national sample of Air Force recruits from all parts of Italy to assess the prevalence of hepatitis B virus (HBV) infection (5). This cohort also seemed to be a valid target population for assessing the prevalence of anti-HCV infection among young Italian adults, for whom these figures are currently lacking.

MATERIALS AND METHODS

Military service in Italy is compulsory. Selection of subjects applying for air force assignment does not differ from that of subjects applying for army or naval service. A small proportion in each year's cohort are excluded from recruitment due to unfitness. There are no recruits of foreign origin.

All Italian men aged 18–26 years must report to recruitment centres. There are many such centers throughout Italy; however, recruits to the surveillance corps of the Italian Air Force all report to a single centre, located in Viterbo (close to Rome). Between September 1989 and June 1990, all recruits (4,978) aged 18–26 years and residents of all Italian regions who had been accepted for Air Force military service in Viterbo were included in this study. The recruits represented all 21 regions of Italy.

A standard precoded questionnaire was designed to collect information on date of birth, place of birth and residence, father's years of education, number of siblings and risk factors of parenteral HCV exposure (previous blood transfusion, history of intravenous drug abuse, major surgical intervention). Questions were asked in the same sequence and in the same style as questions routinely asked by military personnel during the examination. In addition to the blood routinely drawn as part of the standard military procedure, an additional 8 ml of blood was taken at the time of examination and centrifuged at the local Air Force laboratories; sera were then stored in 3 aliquots of 1 ml each at −30°C until tested.

The study was approved by the Medical Ethics Committee.

Laboratory tests

Serum samples were tested for anti-HCV antibodies by means of a IIIrd generation ELISA test (Ortho Diagnostic, Raritan, NY). Repeatedly reactive sera were further assayed by IIIrd generation RIBA (RIBA III, Ortho Diagnostic).

Anti-HCV ELISA reactive sera that showed ≥2 bands in the RIBA assay (24/29) were considered anti-HCV positive. Sera that showed 1 band (1/29) or no bands (4/29) were considered anti-HCV negative.

Statistical analyses

Differences in proportions were evaluated by χ^2-test. A P-value <0.05 was considered to be significant. The associations (Odds Ratios) between anti-HCV prevalence and socio-demographic variables (place of birth, father's years of education, and number of siblings) were calculated by multiple logistic regression (6). Thus the Odds Ratio (O.R.)-for each variable was adjusted for the confounding effect of all other variables considered.

For each variable, the reference category for O.R. estimates was that at the most favourable level of exposure (birth in the North, highest number of father's years of education, and lowest number of siblings, respectively).

RESULTS

Of the 4,978 individuals examined, 24 (0.48%) were found to be repeatedly positive for anti-HCV antibodies by EIA and RIBA. The prevalence was twice as high in Southern Italy and the Islands as in Northern and Central Italy (0.76% vs. 0.35%), a difference which was not statistically significant (Table I). All of these subjects were previously unaware of their HCV carrier state. None of them reported risk factors for parenteral exposure (blood transfusion, i.v. drug use, major surgical intervention).

The results of multiple logistic regression showed that no socio-demographic variable was associated with anti-HCV positivity, as the O.R. confidence limits include units (Table II).

In this population, we have previously estimated the prevalence of HBV markers (5). The percentage who were HBsAg and anti-HBc positive were 1.6% and 5.8%, respectively.

No anti-HCV-positive subject was positive for HBsAg. Anti-HCV positivity was found in 0.8% (2/236) of the anti-HBc-positive subjects and in 0.5% (22/4742) of those who were anti-HBc negative; this difference was not statistically significant. Thus no association was found between HCV and HBV infections.

DISCUSSION

The Air Force recruits came from all parts of Italy. Military service is compulsory for all Italian men aged 18–26 years, and selective procedures are not used for enrolment. Air Force recruits thus represent a valid sample of the young adult general population of Italy, even if confined to the male sex only.

There are no data from other European countries to compare with those reported here.

This population-based survey shows an overall anti-HCV positivity rate of 0.48%, similar to that of 0.4% recently found among a national sample of children and teenagers (4) using 2nd generation ELISA tests, and slightly lower than the 0.87% found among an urban population aged 30–60 years in Central Italy (3), and lower than the 1.3% found among Italian blood donors (7). In the latter two studies a 1st generation ELISA test was used.

The low prevalence of anti-HCV among Italian young people is also supported by a family study showing no or very little serological evidence of HCV infection among subjects below 15 years of age (8).

In spite of the low circulation of HCV among younger generations, Italy is a country with a rather large number of adult patients with chronic HCV infection (7). A possible explanation is that exposure to HCV may occur mainly during adult life or that most elderly HCV-positive persons acquired their infection some decades earlier, when the spread of infection may have been greater than in recent years. Prevalence of anti-HCV was twice as high in the South as in the North. This pattern, similar to that observed for HBV (5, 9) and HDV (10) infections, may reflect the poorer hygienic and socio-economic conditions which have affected the southern regions during recent decades.

Despite the fact that HCV and HBV infections have several modes of transmission in common, though at different degrees of virulence (usually greater for HBV infection), we failed to find an association between these viral infections. The most likely explanation may be the fact that in a population with a low overall incidence of both viruses, the risk of people being co-infected with both viruses may be very low.

These findings indicate that in Italy, HCV infection is uncommon in young people.

Table I. *Prevalence of anti-HCV according to area of residence, in a national sample of Air Force recruits in Italy, 1990*

Area of residence	Total no. tested	anti-HCV positive no	anti-HCV positive %
Northern and Central Italy	3392	12	0.35
Southern Italy and the Islands	1586	12	0.76
Total	4978	24	0.48

Table II. *Variables associated with presence of anti-HCV in Air Force recruits in Italy, 1990*

Variables	Logistic regression odds ratios (C.I. 95%)
Region of birth	2.50
(South or the Islands/North or Center)	(1.08–5.80)
Father's education	0.68
(elementary/ > elementary)	(0.29–1.62)
No. of siblings	0.83
(≥3/<3)	(0.35–1.95)

The Odds Ratios for each variable are adjusted for all other variables in the table.

REFERENCES

1. Ngatchu T, Stroffolini T, Rapicetta M, Chionne P, Lantum D, Chiaramonte M. Seroprevalence of anti-HCV in an urban child population: a pilot survey in a developing area, Cameroon J Trop Hyg 95: 57–61, 1992.
2. Alfaleh FZ, Ayoola EA, Aljeffry M, Ahashed R, Almofarreh M, Arif M, Rannia S, Alkarawi M. Prevalence of antibody to hepatitis C virus among Saudi Arabian children: a community based study. Hepatology 14: 215–218, 1991.
3. Rapicetta M, Attili AF, Mele A, De Santis A, Chionne P, Cristiano K, Spada E, Giuliani E, Carli L, Goffredo F, Capocaccia L. Prevalence of hepatatis C virus antibodies and hepatitis C virus RNA in an urban population. J Med Virol 37: 87–92, 1992.
4. Romanò L, Azara A, Chiaramonte M, De Mattia D, Giammanco A, Moschen ME, Scarpa B, Stroffolini T, Zanetti

AR. Low prevalence of anti-HCV antibody among Italian children. Infection 22: 350–351, 1994.
5. D'Amelio R, Matricardi PM, Biselli R, Stroffolini T, Mele A, Spada E, Chionne P, Rapicetta M, Ferrigno L, Pasquini P. Changing epidemiology of hepatitis B in Italy: Public health implications. Am J Epidemiol 135: 1012–1018, 1992.
6. Hosmer DW, Lemeshow S. Applied logistic regression. New York: John Wiley and Sons, 1990.
7. Chiaramonte M, Stroffolini T, Caporaso N, Coppola R, Craxì A, Gaeta GB, Sagnelli E, Zanetti AR. Hepatitis C virus infection in Italy: a multicentric sero-epidemiological study. Ital J Gastroenterol 23: 555–558, 1991.
8. Chiaramonte M, Lorenzoni V, Ntakirutimana E, Stroffolini T. Household clusters of anti-HCV positive subjects: family transmission or common exposure to the same risk factors? Ital J Gastroenterol 25: 473, 1993.
9. Stroffolini T, Chiaramonte M, Craxì A, Franco E, Rapicetta M, Crivello R, De Mattia D, Mura I, Giammanco A, Rigo G, Scarpa B. Baseline sero-epidemiology of hepatitis B virus in children and teenagers in Italy. A survey before mass hepatitis B vaccination. J Infect 22: 191–199, 1991.
10. Sagnelli E, Stroffolini T, Ascione A, Bonino F, Chiaramonte M, Colombo M, Craxì A, Giusti G. The epidemiology of hepatitis Delta infection in Italy. J Hepatol 16: 350–363, 1992.

Submitted July 21, 1994; accepted September 21, 1994

Scand J Infect Dis 27: 15–16, 1995 ORIGINAL ARTICLE

Prevalence of Antibodies against Tick-borne Encephalitis among Residents of North-Eastern Poland

DANUTA PROKOPOWICZ[1], ELŻBIETA BOBROWSKA[1], MIROSŁAW BOBROWSKI[2] and ANNA GRZESZCZUK[1]

From the Departments of [1]Infectious Diseases, Medical University, and of [2]Sanitary Biology, Technical University, Białystok, Poland

In 37 out of 613 (6%) residents of north eastern Poland, IgG antibodies to tick-borne encephalitis virus (TBEV) were detected at levels exceeding the diagnostic value of 60 VIEU/ml. The prevalence of the antibodies was not related to sex or place or residence. However, significantly higher antibody levels were found in the group of forest workers than in individuals not professionally connected with forestry.

D. Prokopowicz, MD, Department of Infectious Diseases, Żurawia 14, 15-540 Białystok, Poland

INTRODUCTION

The increase in tick-borne encephalitis (TBE) morbidity in Poland is confined mainly to north eastern Poland (1). In 1993, 30 times more cases were registered than in 1992. Among 249 patients, 111 were inhabitants of Białystok voivodeship and 91 others were from neighbouring voivodeships (1).

The observed increase in sick rate forced us to investigate the presence of specific protective antibodies in healthy persons who have not been infected with TBE but are living in endemic areas.

MATERIALS AND METHODS

The study was conducted in a group of 613 healthy individuals, 262 females and 351 males, aged 16 to 68 years, residents of Białowieża and other forest areas of the Białystok region, as well as of 2 cities: Białystok and Giżycko.

After the record epidemiological anamneses and making of routine medical examinations, the subjects agreed to blood tests. The titre of IgG antibodies to TBE virus (TBEV) was measured using an ELISA test, Immunozym® FSME-IgG, manufactured by Immuno AG, Vienna (Austria). A titre of 60 VIEU/ml was considered diagnostic, according to the manufacturer's instructions.

Statistical analyses were performed with the χ^2-test.

RESULTS

Of the subjects examined, 37/613 (6%) had specific IgG class antibodies against TBEV at a titre of $\geq$60 VIEU/ml.

Fig. 1 presents the proportions of seropositive individuals in various tested groups. The highest proportion (13.7%) was detected in forestry workers, whereas the lowest (1.5%) was found in the group who spend some leisure time in the forest.

Data from the subgroups (Table I) showed no statistically significant difference between males and females among non-forest workers (F1 and F2), nor between parallel subgroups of urban and rural populations (U1 and R1). Lack of statistically significant differences was also noted in the subgroups of exclusively forest workers (F2 and M2, U2 and R2). Thus neither the sex of the people examined, nor their residence had any bearing on the occurrence of anti-TBEV antibodies.

Numbers and percentages of seropositive people in the different age groups are shown in Table II. The prevalence of anti-TBEV antibodies increased with age. The highest proportion of seropositive people (12.7%) was found in those 51–60 years old.

DISCUSSION

Prevalence studies on TBE antibodies have been conducted in many European countries (2, 3). The lowest percentages (1.5%) were found in Italy (4), Switzerland (5) and Denmark (2). Higher figures (11.6%) have been found in Sweden (6) and the highest (above 30%) in Czechoslovakia (2, 7) and the former Soviet Union (2, 8).

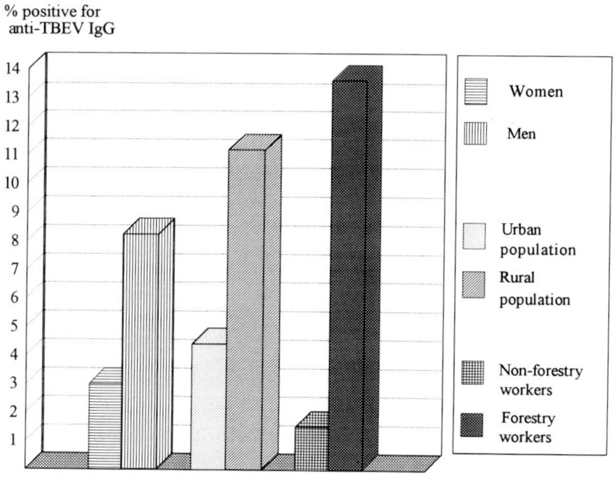

Fig. 1. Prevalence of IgG antibodies against tick-borne encephalitis virus in various subgroups of healthy individuals from the Białystok region.

 ISSN 0036-5548

Table I. *Prevalence of antibodies against Tick-borne encephalitis virus (anti-TBEV) in healthy individuals from the Bialystok region, as related to sex and place of living*

Subgroup	Number of subjects tested	Subjects with anti-TBEV n (%)	Subgroups compared	χ^2 value	P-value
F1	243	4 (1.6)	F1 vs F2	22.4	<0.001
F2	19	4 (21.1)	M1 vs M2	15.0	<0.001
M1	143	2 (1.4)	F1 vs M1	0.04	NS
M2	208	27 (13.0)	F2 vs M2	0.96	NS
U1	346	5 (1.4)	U1 vs U2	28.3	<0.001
U2	114	15 (13.2)	R1 vs R2	4.0	0.04
R1	40	1 (2.5)	U1 vs R1	0.26	NS
R2	113	16 (14.2)	U2 vs R2	0.05	NS

F1 = women not working in forestry; M1 = men not working in forestry.
F2 = women working in forestry; M2 = men working in forestry.
U1 = urban population not working in forestry; U2 = urban population working in forestry.
R1 = Rural population not working in forestry; R2 = rural population working in forestry.
NS = not significant.

Table II. *Prevalance of antibodies to tick-borne encephalitis virus (anti-TBEV) in healthy individuals from the Bialystok region, related to age*

Age group (years)	Number of subjects tested	Subjects with anti-TBEV n (%)
<21	47	0 (0.0)
21–30	192	7 (3.6)
31–40	176	11 (6.3)
41–50	114	9 (7.9)
51–60	71	9 (12.7)
>60	13	1 (7.7)

Our studies have confirmed the presence of TBEV, responsible for severe illness in the North-Eastern part of Poland (9–11). In the present study we found that the prevalence of antibodies to TBEV was the same in males and females as well as in urban and rural populations, and that it is highest in the elderly and in forestry workers.

The high proportion of seropositive subjects among forestry workers indicates that people who are recruited for such work should be vaccinated.

REFERENCES

1. Żabicka J. Tick borne encephalitis in Poland [in Polish]. Przegl Epidemiol 48: 197–203, 1994.
2. Acermann R, Rehse-Küpper B. Die Zentraleuropäische Enzephalitis in der Bundesrepublik Deutschland. Fortschr Neurol Psychiatr 47: 103–122, 1979.
3. Kunz Ch. Tick-borne encephalitis in Europe. Acta Leiden 60: 1–14, 1992.
4. Verani P, Ciufolini M, Nicoletti L, Lopes MC, Amaducci L, Fratiglioni L, Paci P, Leoncini F, Balducci M. Circulation of TBE virus in Italy: Sero-epidemiological and ecovirological studies. Tick-borne encephalitis, International Symposium, Baden/Vienna, 1979. Wien: Facultas-Ferlag, 265–272, 1981.
5. Wyler R, Schmidtke W, Kunz C, Radda A, Henn V, Meyer V. Zeckenenzephalitis in der Region Schaffhausen: Isolierung des Virus aus Zecken und serologische Untersuchungen. Schweiz Med Wochenschr 103: 1487–1492, 1973.
6. Gustafson R, Svenungsson B, Forsgren M, Gardulf A, Granström M. Two year survey of the incidence of Lyme borreliosis and tick-borne encephalitis in a high-risk population in Sweden. Eur J Clin Microbiol Infect Dis 11: 894–900, 1992.
7. Blaskovic D. Tick-borne encephalitis in Czechoslovakia. Arch Environ Health 21: 453–461, 1970.
8. Kunz Ch. Arbovirus-B-Infektionen. In: Die Infektionskrankheiten des Menschen und ihre Erreger. Stuttgart: Thieme-Verlag, vol Bd II, 1595–1629, 1969.
9. Wróblewska-Mularczykowa Z, Żabicka J, Nawrocka E, Olkowska D, Taytsch-Kaputkin FZ. Occurrence of arbovirus antibodies in foresters in Poland in 1971–1972. Acta Microbiol Pol 5: 123–129, 1973.
10. Bobrowska E, Prokopowicz D, Pytel B. Prevalence of tick borne encephalitis antibodies among residents of north-eastern Poland [in Polish]. Przegl Epidemiol 46: 11–16, 1993.
11. Jeżyna Cz, Zając W, Ciesielski T, Pancewicz S. Epidemiologische und klinische Untersuchungen von Kranken mit Zecken-Encephalitis aus Nord-OstPolen. Zentralbl Bakteriol [B]. Abt. I. Orig. B 178: 510–521, 1984.

Submitted July 22, 1994; accepted November 20, 1994

Scand J Infect Dis 27: 17–18, 1995 ORIGINAL ARTICLE

Arcanobacterium haemolyticum and Streptococcal Pharyngitis in Army Conscripts

PETTERI CARLSON[1], SIRKKA KONTIANINEN[1,2], OLLI-VEIKKO RENKONEN[2], AULIKKI SIVONEN[2] and RISTO VISAKORPI[3]

From the [1]Department of Medical Microbiology, Aurora Hospital, the [2]Department of Bacteriology and Immunology, University of Helsinki, and [3]the Research Institute of Military Medicine, Helsinki, Finland

Arcanobacterium haemolyticum was found in 1.4% and β-haemolytic streptococci in 23% of throat cultures from army conscripts with sore throat ($n = 498$). 38% of the β-haemolytic streptococci were of group A. Patients culture-positive for A. haemolyticum or β-haemolytic streptococci had pharyngeal exudate, cervical lymphadenopathy and ear ache significantly more often – but cough less often – than culture-negative patients. The pharyngeal colonization rate of healthy conscripts ($n = 232$) by A. haemolyticum was 0.4% and by β-haemolytic streptococci, 6.5%.

S. Kontiainen, MD, Department of Medical Microbiology, Aurora Hospital, Nordenskiöldinkatu 20, FIN-00250 Helsinki, Finland

INTRODUCTION

Sore throat is a common complaint among army conscripts. The most common causative agents are respiratory viruses and β-haemolytic streptococci (1, 2), but other agents may also be involved (2–4). Arcanobacterium haemolyticum (formerly Corynebacterium haemolyticum), first reported in 1946 in infections of nasopharynx and skin of natives and American soldiers evacuated from tropical islands of the Pacific (5), causes pharyngitis resembling that caused by Streptococcus pyogenes (6). It has been reported in up to 2% of 15–25-year-old patients with pharyngitis (6, 7). Since 1946 there have been no reports on A. haemolyticum as a cause of pharyngitis in soldiers. We performed cultures on throat swabs from army conscripts seeking medical attention because of sore throat, to ascertain the frequency with which A. haemolyticum could be isolated, and now report the results of the study.

MATERIALS AND METHODS

Subjects. During a 10-month period (Dec. 1991–Sep. 1992) 730 conscripts were studied. Of these, 498 complained of sore throat; 232 others were controls. The mean age of the patients was 20.4 ± 1.5 years and that of controls 20.4 ± 1.4 years.

Microbiology. Throat swabs were transported to the microbiological laboratory in Stuart transport tubes (Transpocult[R], Orion Diagnostica, Espoo, Finland). Cultures were performed and A. haemolyticum and beta-haemolytic streptococci identified as previously described (7).

Clinics. Clinical data were collected by doctors and nurses in charge of the patients.

Statistics. The χ^2-test was used.

RESULTS

All pharyngitis cases were sporadic. A. haemolyticum was isolated from 7 (1.4%) and β-haemolytic streptococci from 112 (22.5%) of the 498 patients with sore throat, and from

Table I. *Bacteria isolated from patients with acute pharyngitis and from healthy controls*

	Number (%) of	
Bacterium	Patients ($n = 498$)	Controls ($n = 323$)
A. haemolyticum	7 (1.4)	1 (0.4)
Streptococci, all	112 (22.5)***	15 (6.5)
Group A	42 (8.4)***	4 (1.7)
Non-group A, all	70 (14.1)***	11 (4.7)
Group B	13 (2.6)*	1 (0.4)
Group C	20 (4.0)**	1 (0.4)
Group G	37 (7.4)	9 (3.9)

***$p < 0.001$, **$p < 0.01$ and *$p < 0.05$ by χ^2-test.

1 (0.4%) and 15 (6.5%), respectively, of the 232 controls (Table I). Group A streptococci were isolated from 8.4% of the patients and 1.7% of the controls ($p < 0.001$) and non-group A (see Table I) streptococci from 14.1% vs. 4.7% ($p < 0.001$). Three of the 7 patients (43%) with A. haemolyticum also had group G beta-haemolytic streptococci in the throat. No secondary cases of A. haemolyticum pharyngitis or symptomless carriers were detected by throat cultures performed on conscripts sharing accommodation with the index cases.

Clinical symptoms and the frequency with which they occurred were similar in patients with A. haemolyticum and beta-haemolytic streptococci (Table II). Patients culture-positive for A. haemolyticum and/or beta-haemolytic streptococci had tonsillar exudate, cervical lymphadenopathy and ear ache significantly more often and cough significantly less often than culture-negative patients. 31% of the culture-positive patients had a high temperature (≥ 38°C), but none had skin rash. Clinical (not culture confirmed) pharyngitis during the preceding 6 months was reported by 16% of the culture-positive patients, by 21% of the culture-

 ISSN 0036-5548

Table II. *Clinical features of patients culture positive and negative for β-haemolytic streptococci and* A. haemolyticum

	Throat culture		
Symptoms	Streptococci	A. haemolyticum	Negative
Pharyngeal exudate	36/99 (36.0)[a]	3/7 (42.9)	89/339 (26.2)*
Lymphadenopathy	57/112 (56.4)	3/6 (50.0)	159/354 (44.9)*
Cough	36/112 (32.1)	2/7 (28.6)	238/381 (62.5)***
Ear ache	20/112 (17.9)	0/7 (0)	40/381 (10.5)*

[a] Number (%) positive for the symptom/number studied.
***$p < 0.001$, **$p < 0.01$ and *$p < 0.05$ by χ^2-test; culture-positive for streptococci, and/or A. haemolyticum and culture-negative compared.

negative patients (p = NS), and by one of the patients culture-positive for A. haemolyticum (14%).

DISCUSSION

Although most cases of pharyngitis are of viral origin, finding and treatment of patients with bacterial pharyngitis is important. In this study, A. haemolyticum was isolated from 1.4% of army conscripts with pharyngitis. This frequency is similar to that found at the same time in similarly aged civilians (6, 7). As expected, beta-haemolytic streptococci were isolated about 20 times more often than A. haemolyticum, in one-fifth of the patients with pharyngitis. In agreement with a previous study on army conscripts, the majority of the beta-haemolytic streptococci, 38%, were of group A (2), but in contrast to that report we found non-A beta-haemolytic streptococci significantly more frequently in patient than in controls. The difference may be due to different methods used in the culture and identification of the streptococci.

Patients with A. haemolyticum had fever, pharyngeal exudate and cervical lymphadenopathy as often as patients with beta-haemolytic streptococci. The army patients with A. haemolyticum, however, had these symptoms less often than civilians (7). Thus 30% vs. 80% had fever, 50% vs. 67% lymhadenopathy and 43% vs. 69% pharyngeal exudate. None of the conscripts had skin rash, which was detected in a quarter of the civilians. The reason(s) for the differences in the frequency of symptoms are not known, but may be due to army conscripts seeking medical attention earlier than the civilians.

Patients with A. haemolyticum did not report pharyngitis in the preceding 6 months more often than patients with beta-haemolytic streptococci. This, together with the similarity of symptoms in these patients and in patients with beta-haemolytic streptococci, makes it unlikely that A. haemolyticum was associated with a more complicated disease, as has been suggested (6).

A. haemolyticum is usually susceptible to antimicrobial agents used to treat streptococcal tonsillitis, viz. penicillin, erythromycin, clindamycin and oral cephalosporins (8). Reports on the efficacy of penicillin therapy in A. haemolyticum pharyngitis are contradictory, however (6, 7, 9, 10) and tolerance to penicillin has been described (11). Controlled studies of the treatment are therefore required.

A. haemolyticum can thus be isolated in sporadic cases of pharyngitis in army conscripts. Family outbreaks have been described (9, 10), but any evidence of possible epidemics caused by A. haemolyticum is still lacking.

REFERENCES

1. Gwaltney JM. Pharyngitis. In: Mandel GL, Douglas RG, Bennet JE, eds. Principles and practice of infectious diseases, 3rd edn. New York: Churchill Livingstone, 493–498, 1990.
2. Ylikoski J, Karjalainen J. Acute tonsillitis in young men: etiological agents and their differentiation. Scand J Infect Dis 21: 169–174, 1989.
3. Huovinen P, Lahtonen R, Ziegler T, Meurman O, Hakkarainen K, Miettinen A, Arstila P, Eskola J, Saikku P. Pharyngitis in adults: the presence and coexistence of viruses and bacterial organisms. Ann Intern Med 110: 612–616, 1989.
4. Sloss JM, Faithfull-Davies DN. Non-toxigenic Corynebacterium diphtheriae in military personnel. Lancet 341: 1021, 1993.
5. MacLean PD, Liebow AA, Rosenberg AA. A hemolytic corynebacterium resembling Corynebacterium ovis and Corynebacterium pyogenes in man. J Infect Dis 79: 69–90, 1946.
6. Banck G, Nyman M. Tonsillitis and rash associated with Corynebacterium haemolyticum. J Infect Dis 154: 1037–1040, 1986.
7. Carlson P, Renkonen OV, Kontiainen S. Arcanobacterium haemolyticum and streptococcal pharyngitis. Scand J Infect Dis 26: 283–287, 1994.
8. Carlson P, Kontiainen S, Renkonen OV. Antimicrobial susceptibility of Arcanobacterium haemolyticum. Antimicrob Agents Chemother 38: 142–143, 1994.
9. Miller RA, Brancato F, Holmes KK. Corynebacterium haemolyticum as a cause of pharyngitis and scarlatiniform rash in young adults. Ann Intern Med 105: 867–872, 1986.
10. Fell HWK, Nagington J, Naylor GRE. Corynebacterium haemolyticum infections in Cambridgeshire. J Hyg 79: 269–274, 1977.
11. Nyman M, Banck G, Thore M. Penicillin tolerance in Arcanobacterium haemolyticum. J Infect Dis 161: 261–265, 1990.

Submitted July 26, 1994; accepted October 10, 1994

Scand J Infect Dis 27: 19–21, 1995 ORIGINAL ARTICLE

Mortality Rate and Magnitude of Staphylococcus aureus Bacteremia as Assessed by a Semiquantitative Blood Culture System

HENRIK C. SCHØNHEYDER[1], ADAM GOTTSCHAU[2], ANNE FRILAND[3] and VIBEKE THAMDRUP ROSDAHL[3]

From the Departments of [1]Clinical Microbiology, Aalborg Hospital, Aalborg, [2]Biostatistics, Statens Seruminstitut, Copenhagen S, and [3]Hospital Infections and Antibiotics, Statens Seruminstitut, Copenhagen S, Denmark

A 4-year retrospective study ascertained the relation between the magnitude of Staphylococcus aureus bacteremia and mortality. 253 episodes of S. aureus bacteremia diagnosed in a Danish regional Department of Clinical Microbiology were included. Blood cultures were routinely done by inoculation of aseptically drawn blood into multiple tubes of bacteriological media. The rate of positive tubes was assumed to distinguish high- from low-grade bacteremia without providing an absolute count of colony forming units. The median number of tubes inoculated was 18 (range 6–48) with approximately 0.5–1 ml of blood per tube. The rate of positive tubes was related neither to the source of infection, i.e. whether the S. aureus infection was nosocomially or community-acquired, nor to the portal of entry. However, mortality increased with increasing rate: it was 18% for rates <0.30, 23% for 0.30–0.69, 30% for 0.70–0.99, and 37% for a rate of 1.0. Thus, for S. aureus infections the magnitude of bacteremia seems to be a prognostic factor with possible bearings on clinical and therapeutic decisions.

H. C. Schønheyder, Department of Clinical Microbiology, Aalborg Hospital, P.O. Box 365, DK-9100 Aalborg, Denmark

INTRODUCTION

Recent developments of blood culture systems have focused on broth culture systems and laboratory automation (1, 2). The volume of blood processed is a determinant factor for detection of bacteremia (3–5) and inoculation of sets of broth culture bottles increases the amount of blood and allows for varying culture conditions. However, high- and low-grade bacteremia is not easily distinguished. Only limited attention is currently being given to quantitative aspects of bacteremia, although the number of colony forming units may be assessed, e.g. by pour-plate and centrifugation techniques (6, 7). A blood culture system with multiple tubes of bacteriological media was commonly used in Denmark until the system was replaced by broth culture (8–11). We have undertaken a retrospective analysis of the quantitative aspect of Staphylococcus aureus bacteremia in a Danish county during a 4-year period 1986–89. The aim was to assess to what extent the magnitude of S. aureus bacteremia is clinically significant.

MATERIAL AND METHODS

14 hospitals in the County of Northern Jutland (population approximately 500,000 inhabitants) were served by the regional Department of Clinical Microbiology at Aalborg Hospital. The study conformed with the rules of the regional Scientific Ethics Committee concerning use of registered medical data.

Patients

Patients with S. aureus bacteremia during the 4-year period 1986 to 1989 were identified by manual survey of laboratory records. Patients were included only once and were excluded in case of polymicrobial bacteremia. Patients were also excluded if the volume of blood did not suffice for inoculation of more than 5 tubes of bacteriological media.

Blood cultures

Two samples of nominally 8 ml of blood each were recommended for adult patients (Vacutainer^R) (5). From children, smaller amounts of blood were accepted. It was advised that blood cultures be obtained prior to antibiotic chemotherapy, and sampling from vascular catheters was not permitted.

Specimens drawn between 8 a.m. and 6 p.m. were normally transported to the Department of Clinical Microbiology and processed without delay, whereas specimens taken during evening and night shifts were transferred and processed the following morning. Aliquots of blood were inoculated on a 10% (vol/vol) basis into glass tubes with enriched broth medium, semisolid agar, and semisolid thioglycollate broth (Statens Seruminstitut, Copenhagen) (5, 8). Normally, 4 tubes of each medium type were inoculated (0.5–1 ml), thus providing 12 tubes per sample.

Inspections for growth were carried out once or twice daily for 1 week. In the case of macroscopically visible growth at least 1 tube of each medium type was examined by direct microscopy and subcultured on appropriate plate media. Isolates of S. aureus were identified on the basis of Gram stain, colony morphology on 5% horse blood agar, and tube coagulase test with horse citrate plasma incubated for 24 h. Phage-typing of S. aureus isolates was carried out according to Blair & Williams (12).

If serial blood cultures were obtained, only samples taken within 24 h of the first positive sample were included in the analysis. Numbers of positive tubes (no. of pos.) and numbers of tubes inoculated (no. inoc.) were tabulated from the laboratory records, and the rate of positive tubes (no. of pos./no. inoc.) was calculated as a measure of the grade of bacteremia.

Mortality and origin of infection

A national register of S. aureus bacteremia at Statens Seruminstitut, Copenhagen, has been a basis for continuous surveillance of S. aureus epidemiology since 1956. The definition of nosocomial-versus community-acquisition ('source') of bacteremia accorded with the guidelines suggested by CDC (13). The likely portal of entry was identified on the basis of both microbiological and clinical data as obtained from attending physicians. Mortality associated with S. aureus bacteremia was taken to include both death as a direct consequence of the staphylococcal infection and death that occurred before signs of septicemia had remitted. The register did not include antibiotic therapy or the nature of the underlying disease.

Statistical methods

Logistic regression analysis was used to assess the effect on mortality of source of infection and rate of positive tubes. The rate of positive tubes was scored as follows, 1 (<0.30), 2 (0.30–0.69), 3 (0.70–0.99), and 4 (1.00). The χ^2-test was used to test the association between rate of positive tubes and phage type and source of infection.

RESULTS

Over the 4-year period, S. aureus bacteremia was recorded in 253 patients. 120 patients were admitted to departments of medicine, 69 to departments of surgery, 15 to intensive care units, and 14 to departments of pediatrics. 35 patients were admitted to non-specialized local units. Of the 120 patients in medical departments, 19 were in hematological or oncological units. The median age of patients was 65 years, range 0–88 years. The male/female ratio was 157/96. 61 bacteremias were community-acquired, 151 were nosocomial, and 32 were of indeterminate origin; data were missing for 9 patients.

A primary infection was located to the skin in 21 and the lungs in 17 patients, 17 patients had endocarditis and 25 osteomyelitis or arthritis. The entry was related to invasive procedures in 59 patients. The mortality for S. aureus bacteremia was 28%, and this was slightly above the national average for the same period (26%), but the difference did not reach statistical significance. The median number of tubes inoculated was 18 (range 6 to 48). The episodes were distributed into 4 groups of fairly equal size, according to the rate of positive tubes (Table I). A statistical analysis showed that the mortality increased with increasing rate, and the association was statistically significant (χ^2 for trend $= 6.72$, DF $= 1$, $p = 0.0095$). In a logistic regression model, neither source of infection nor phage-type was found to be significant. Likewise, the rate was not related to portal of entry.

Table I. *The relation between mortality and magnitude of bacteremia in 253 episodes of S. aureus bacteremia by a multiple-tube blood culture system in the Danish County of Northern Jutland 1986 to 1989*

Magnitude of bacteremia[a]	Number of episodes	Mortality[b] (%)
<0.30	62	18
0.30–0.69	49	23
0.70–0.99	59	30
1.00	83	37
All	253	28

[a] The magnitude of bacteremia was assessed by rate of positive tubes, i.e. the number of tubes growing S. aureus divided by the number of tubes inoculated with blood. For further explanation, see main text.

[b] Mortality was directly related to magnitude of bacteremia (χ^2 for trend $= 6.72$, DF $= 1$, $p = 0.0095$).

The impact of phage-type was ascertained separately. It was observed that staphylococcal bacteremias with strains belonging to the 83A and the 94, 96 complexes as well as non-typable strains tended to have the highest rate of positive tubes, but the overall impact of phage-type on rates was marginal ($\chi^2 = 35.7$, DF $= 24$, $p = 0.058$).

DISCUSSION

Recent changes in blood culture practices toward widespread use of broth culture systems have been beneficial in terms of sensitivity and speed of detection (1, 2, 15, 16). However, the inoculation of culture flasks with several millilitres of blood tends to obscure the distinction between low- and high-grade bacteremia, and hence information on the magnitude of bacteremia is not routinely obtainable. The current retrospective study of 253 episodes of S. aureus bacteremias supports the notion that the magnitude of bacteremia is of clinical importance, as the rate of positive blood culture tubes was directly related to mortality. In fact, the mortality of patients with low-grade bacteremia (rate less than 0.3) was half the mortality of patients with high-grade bacteremia (rate $= 1.0$) (Table I). In addition to the possible prognostic value, quantitative aspects of staphylococcal growth in blood cultures have previously been useful for distinguishing contaminants from isolates of clinical significance (5, 10, 14). The rate of positive tubes must not be taken as a direct measure of colony forming units (cfu) as the actual sample volume was not measured and, e.g., transport time was not monitored. Arpi et al. (5) has previously studied the 12-tube blood culture system and observed that doubling of the blood sample volume increased the yield of S. aureus by 26% and by inference this gain was equated to 1–2 cfu per nominal volume of 8 ml. In our laboratory a rate of 1.0 (Table I) may cautiously be equated with ≥ 1–2 cfu per ml as the amount of blood inoculated per tube was ~ 0.5–1 ml. S. aureus bacteremia of a similar order of magnitude was reported by Dorn et al. (6) who found <1 cfu/ml in 5 cases and 1–10 cfu/ml in another 5 cases by a centrifugation technique.

The clinical data were retrieved from a national register of S. aureus bacteremias, which has been continuously updated for epidemiological and scientific studies since 1956. Therefore the assessment of patients was highly standardized. Neither predisposing nor concomitant diseases or previous antibiotic therapy were available for analysis. However, our patients represented a broad group admitted to both primary and secondary hospital care. Whimbey et al. (7) made an observation similar to ours for S. aureus bacteremia in a group of patients admitted to a cancer centre using a quantitative lysis-centrifugation technique. There was a trend toward higher mortality with higher counts: 8 (27%) of 30 cases with ≤ 10 cfu/ml died, compared with 4 (36%) of 11 cases with ≥ 100 cfu/ml. Our larger study confirms that the relationship observed by Whimbey et al. (7) pertains to patients with S. aureus bacteremia in general. From a biological point of view, high-grade bacteremia may reflect a fulminating primary infection or per se carry an increased risk of serious metastatic infections, e.g., endocarditis or abscess formation.

S. aureus bacteremia still carries a high mortality and information on the magnitude of bacteremia could help to delineate groups who should be treated most vigorously. Moreover, quantitative aspects of S. aureus bacteremia could be relevant to clinical and therapeutic decisions, although this remains to be confirmed by prospective study.

REFERENCES

1. Washington JA & International Collaborative Blood Culture Study Group. An international multicenter study of blood culture practices. Eur J Clin Microbiol Infect Dis 11: 1115–1128, 1992.
2. Brown DFJ, Perry SF. Methods used in the United Kingdom for the culture of micro-organisms from blood. J Clin Pathol 45: 468–474, 1992.
3. Hall MM, Ilstrup DM, Washington JA. Effect of volume of blood cultured on detection of bacteremia. J Clin Microbiol 3: 643–645, 1976.
4. Tenney JH, Reller LB, Mirrett S, Wang W-LL, Weinstein MP. Controlled evaluation of the volume of blood cultured in detection of bacteremia and fungemia. J Clin Microbiol 15: 558–561, 1982.
5. Arpi M, Bentzon MW, Jensen J, Frederiksen W. Importance of blood volume cultured in the detection of bacteremia. Eur J Clin Microbiol Infect Dis 8: 838–842, 1989.
6. Dorn GL, Burson GG, Haynes JR. Blood culture techniques based on centrifugation: clinical evaluation. J Clin Microbiol 3: 258–263, 1976.
7. Whimbey E, Kiehn TE, Brannon P, Benezra D, Armstrong D. Clinical significance of colony counts in immunocompromised patients with Staphylococcus aureus bacteremia. J Infect Dis 155: 1328–1330, 1987.
8. Henrichsen J. Recent trends of isolates from cases of bacteremia in Denmark. Scand J Infect Dis 6: 145–151, 1974.
9. Bruun B, Sloth K, Bentzon MW, Frederiksen W. A study of bacteremias in Denmark from 1977–1978. Acta Pathol Microbiol Immunol Scand Sect B 90: 309–317, 1982.
10. Gahrn-Hansen B. Etiologic importance of coagulase-negative Micrococcaceae isolated from blood cultures. Acta Pathol Microbiol Immunol Scand Sect B 93: 1–6, 1985.
11. Bergman O. Oral infections and septicemia in immunocompromised patients with hematologic malignancies. J Clin Microbiol 26: 2105–2109, 1988.
12. Blair JE, Williams REO. Phage typing of staphylococci. Bull World Health Organ 24: 771–784, 1961.
13. Garner JS, Jarvis WR, Emori TG, Horan TC, Hughes JM. CDC definitions for nosocomial infections, 1988. J Infect Control 16: 128–140, 1988.
14. Siboni K. Clinical evaluation of blood cultures. Ugeskr Læger 124: 464–467, 1962 [in Danish].
15. Prag J, Jensen J, Lebech K. Colorbact, a visually read blood culture system using darkening of haemoglobin in aerobic blood cultures as an early growth indicator, compared with Bactec 6A and 7A. APMIS 99: 1089–1095, 1991.
16. Wilson ML, Weinstein MP, Reimer LG, Mirrett S, Reller LB. Controlled comparison of the BacT/Alert and BACTEC 660/730 nonradiometric blood culture systems. J Clin Microbiol 30: 323–329, 1992.

Submitted June 30, 1994; accepted September 12, 1994

Scand J Infect Dis 27: 23–27, 1995 ORIGINAL ARTICLE

Human Nocardiosis in Northern Italy from 1982 to 1992

CLAUDIO FARINA[1], PATRICK BOIRON[2], ANTONIO GOGLIO[1], FRÉDÉRIQUE PROVOST[2] and the NORTHERN ITALY COLLABORATIVE GROUP ON NOCARDIOSIS

From the [1]Microbiology Institute, Ospedali Riuniti, Bergamo, Italy and the [2]Mycology Unit, Pasteur Institute, Paris, France

We conducted a retrospective survey of nocardiosis in 9 city hospitals in northern Italy from 1982 to 1992. The medical records of 30 patients with documented nocardiosis were reviewed. Microbiological data included morphology, biochemical characteristics, serology and in vitro susceptibility testing. The 29 isolates (1 case was diagnosed on the basis of serological results) were Nocardia asteroides ($n = 25$) and Nocardia farcinica ($n = 4$). Predisposing factors included immunosuppression for organ transplant rejection prophylaxis, lung disease (silicotuberculosis and pulmonary fibrosis), solid tumours and hematological malignancies, and AIDS. Three patients had no identified risk factors. 20 cases of pulmonary nocardiosis were observed. Sites of infection in patients without previous pulmonary involvement were: brain abscesses, soft tissues, pericardium, blood, and cerebrospinal fluid. Most strains tested were susceptible to amikacin and imipenem. Resistance to several antimicrobial agents was found, particularly erythromycin, fosfomycin, pefloxacin, sulphonamides and trimethoprim. Antimicrobial chemotherapy included sulphonamides, amikacin, ceftriaxone, imipenem and minocycline. 21 patients survived, although 2 relapsed transiently. Nocardiosis appears to be more common than generally realised by physicians in northern Italy. The local species distribution and disease spectrum are similar to those described elsewhere. Nocardiosis should be part of the differential diagnosis in patients with pulmonary infiltrates or brain abscess, particularly those with predisposing factors.

C. Farina, MD, Microbiology Institute, Ospedali Riuniti, 1, Largo Barozzi, I-24128 Bergamo, Italy

INTRODUCTION

Nocardia spp. are ubiquitous, soil-borne, aerobic, very fine and branching Gram-positive and weakly acid-fast filamentous actinomycetes with a tendency to fragment into bacillary and coccoid forms (1).

Systemic nocardiosis is a rare but life-threatening infection, which complicates immunosuppression caused by anticancer chemotherapy, anti-rejection regimens and steroid therapy, as well as underlying diseases such as solid and hematological malignancies, alcoholism, chronic lung disease (e.g., pulmonary alveolar proteinosis and chronic obstructive pulmonary disease), and AIDS. Nocardiosis can also occur in otherwise healthy subjects (2). We carried out a retrospective survey to determine the presenting signs and symptoms and outcome of nocardial infection in northern Italy over an 11-year period.

Members of the Northern Italy Collaborative Group on Nocardiosis: Eliseo Minola, Infectious Diseases Institute, Ospedali Riuniti, Bergamo; Fredy Suter, Infectious Diseases Institute, Ospedale Civile, Busto Arsizio; Nicoletta Marinoni, Microbiology Institute, Ospedale Civile, Legnano; Anna Maria Tortorano, Institute of Hygiene and Preventive Medicine, University of Milan; Claudio Bonato, Microbiology Institute, Ospedale H San Raffaele, Milan; Chiara Casolari, Microbiology Institute, University of Modena, Modena; Paolo Grossi, Lorenzo Minoli, Infectious Diseases Institute, Policlinico S. Matteo, University of Pavia, Pavia; Giovanna Marchiaro, Microbiology Institute, Ospedale San Giovanni Battista, Le Molinette, Turin; Claudio Scarparo, Microbiology Institute, Ospedale Civile, Vicenza.

 ISSN 0036-5548

MATERIALS AND METHODS

We reviewed the records of 9 hospital microbiology laboratories in 8 northern Italian cities from 1982 to 1992. The isolates, which had been stored at −70°C, were sent to the Microbiology Institute of the Ospedali Riuniti (Bergamo, Italy) and then to the French National Reference Centre for Mycosis and Antifungal Agents (NRC) (Pasteur Institute, Paris, France) for further testings.

Medical and epidemiological data

We examined the medical records of 30 patients with documented nocardial infection. The following data were recorded: age, sex, drug abuse, underlying conditions, and antimicrobial, steroid and cytotoxic chemotherapy. Clinical data included sites of infection, physical examination and imaging studies (radiographs, scintigraphy, computerized tomography (CT) and ultrasonography).

Microbiological methods

Microbiological data included morphology, biochemical characteristics (3), serological test results (4), and in vitro antimicrobial susceptibility data (5). Specimens were sent to the local microbiology laboratory for routine bacteriological and mycological evaluation.

Pus, cerebrospinal fluid and pulmonary specimens were examined directly after Gram staining and Kinyoun acid-fast staining for actinomycetes. Blood was cultured in Bactec 6A and 7A bottles (Becton, Dickinson and Co., Paramus, N.J., USA) or the Isolator system (DuPont Co., Wilmington, DE, USA).

All suspected Nocardia isolates were stained by the partial acid-fast method. Each organism was subcultured on trypticase broth (Difco Laboratories, Detroit, MI, USA), blood agar and Sabouraud dextrose agar, and sent to the Microbiology Institute of Ospedali Riuniti (Bergamo).

Identification was based on a battery of physiological tests, viz., the capacity to hydrolyse caseine, xanthine, hypoxanthine, tyrosine, adenine, uric acid, Tween 20 and esculin, and urease activity on Christensen urea agar (Sanofi Diagnostics Pasteur, Marnes la Coquette, France) (3). Isolates were also tested for acid production from mannitol and sorbitol after 4 weeks of incubation at 35°C. Most (23/29) were sent to the NRC of the Pasteur Institute (Paris, France) for thin-layer chromatographic analysis, according to Staneck & Roberts (6) and Minnikin et al. (7), and further physiological investigations.

Serodiagnosis of nocardiosis was performed at the NRC by Western blot (immunoblot) assay using a 54-kilodalton immunodominant antigen (4), in comparison with known negative and positive nocardiosis sera.

Disc susceptibility testing on Mueller Hinton agar (Difco Laboratories) was performed according to Boiron and Provost (5). The results were read after 24 h of incubation at 37°C according to the recommendations of the Antibiogram Committee of the French Society for Microbiology (8).

RESULTS

Gram-positive, partially acid-fast, branching, filamentous Nocardia spp. were isolated from 29 patients. In 1 additional case (case 26), identification was based on serological testing of 3 samples collected when the patient was taking antibacterial and antifungal drugs.

Table I summarizes the epidemiological and medical data, sites of infection and outcome.

Medical and epidemiological data

11 cases of nocardiosis (36.7%) occurred between 1982 and 1987 and the remaining 63.3% between 1988 and 1992 (Table 1).

21 patients were men (sex ratio, 2.3:1). The patients' ages ranged from 11 to 70 years (average 41.8 years). Underlying conditions were present in 90% of the patients (27/30). Seven patients (23.3%) were heroin addicts, whereof 6 were seropositive for HIV. Immunosuppressive therapy for organ rejection prophylaxis was a common predisposing factor. Nosocomial infection was documented in 2 cases. There was no identified underlying disease in 3 patients (cases 28 to 30).

There were 20 (66.7%) cases of pulmonary nocardiosis. Seven of these patients had only a solitary lung nodule or diffuse infiltrates; 13 initially developed pulmonary infection which later spread to the brain (6 cases), soft tissues (2 cases) or liver (1 case), or to various sites, including the bloodstream (4 cases). No previous pulmonary involvement was found in 10 of the 30 cases.

In 7 cases, physical examination revealed soft-tissue infection in the thigh (cases 1 and 22), abdomen (cases 17 and 18), shoulder (cases 5 and 19) and arm (case 14). In 1

Table I. *Nocardia infections observed in a multicentre study in northern Italy (1982–1992)*

Patient	Sex	Age	Underlying condition	Site	Outcome	Microbiology
1	F	44	Kidney transplant	Lung/soft tissues	Cured	N. asteroides
2	M	41	Kidney transplant	Lung/liver	Cured	N. asteroides
3	F	58	Kidney transplant	Lung/brain	Cured	N. asteroides
4	M	40	Heart transplant	Lung/brain	Cured	N. asteroides
5	M	54	Heart transplant	Soft tissues	Cured	N. asteroides
6	M	50	Heart transplant	Lung/brain	Dead	N. asteroides
7	M	57	Heart transplant	Lung	Cured	N. asteroides
8	M	23	AIDS, i.v. drug abuse	Lung	Cured	N. asteroides
9	M	35	AIDS, i.v. drug abuse	Lung	Cured	N. asteroides
10	F	40	AIDS, i.v. drug abuse	Lung/sepsis	Dead	N. farcinica
11	M	32	AIDS, i.v. drug abuse	Lung	Cured	N. asteroides
12	M	29	HIV+, i.v.drug abuse	Brain	Dead	N. farcinica
13	F	35	HIV+, i.v. drug abuse	Lung	Cured	N. farcinica
14	M	30	i.v. drug abuse	Soft tissues	Cured	N. asteroides
15	M	38	Lymphoma	Lung/sepsis	Dead	N. asteroides
16	M	61	Lymphoma	Lung/sepsis	Dead	N. asteroides
17	M	50	Lymphoma	Lung/soft tissues	Dead	N. asteroides
18	M	50	Lymphoma	Soft tissues	Cured	N. asteroides
19	M	29	Lymphoma	Lung/brain/soft tissues	Cured	N. asteroides
20	M	11	Astrocytoma	Brain/sepsis	Cured	N. farcinica
21	M	58	Pulmonary carcinoma	Lung/brain	Cured	N. asteroides
22	M	70	Silicotuberculosis	Soft tissues	Dead*	N. asteroides
23	F	67	Pulmonary fibrosis	Lung	Cured	N. asteroides
24	F	47	Pericardiocentesis	Pericardium	Cured	N. asteroides
25	F	45	Diabetes	Brain	Dead	N. asteroides
26	F	16	SLE	Lung/brain	Cured	Serology
27	M	28	Nephrotic syndrome	Brain	Dead	N. asteroides
28	M	20	None	Lung/brain	Cured	N. asteroides
29	M	52	None	Brain	Relapse/cured	N. asteroides
30	F	42	Unknown	Lung	Cured	N. asteroides

* = No evidence of nocardial infection at autopsy.
SLE = Systemic lupus erythematosus.

case, a bone radiogram revealed a vertebral erosion, confirmed by scintigraphy (case 22). Brain CT revealed intracerebral abscesses in 14 of 30 cases and pulmonary CT or magnetic resonance imaging confirmed the radiographic findings in 2 cases (cases 4 and 19). Abdominal CT revealed infection of the bladder and liver (case 2) and peritoneum (case 6). In 1 case, echocardiography showed a severe pericardial effusion (case 24). In 26 of the 30 cases, nocardiosis was diagnosed before death, while in cases 10, 15, 16 and 25, blood cultures yielded a Nocardia sp. after the patient's death.

19 of the 30 patients survived (63.3%). 13 with extra-pulmonary nocardiosis underwent drainage and recovered; these included patient no. 22, who died of other causes and had no evidence of nocardial infection at autopsy. One of the 20 patients treated by means of surgical excision and minocycline therapy relapsed (case 29) but further neurosurgery was successful. Five patients recovered after antimicrobial chemotherapy alone, although 1 had a cerebral relapse (case 4). All the patients with isolated pulmonary infection responded to medical therapy alone.

Microbiological findings

Respiratory tract specimens yielded Gram-positive branching bacilli in 11 cases; these included 3 sputum cultures, 3 bronchial washing or transbronchial biopsy specimens, 4 transthoracic biopsy specimens, 1 from a patient with a positive pus culture from the thigh; and 1 open-lung biopsy specimen. Cerebrospinal fluid culture was positive in 2 patients, 1 of whom also had a positive blood culture. Blood was the only specimen that yielded a Nocardia sp. in 1 patient. Soft tissue, brain and visceral pus cultures were positive in the remaining patients. Four positive pus specimens were obtained from superficial lesions: 1 thigh fistula, shoulder abscess, abdominal and arm-skin each. Invasive procedures were necessary in 6 cases, and included arthrocentesis, pericardiocentesis, brain biopsy or brain abscess excision. All specimens obtained from patient 21 by non-invasive (sputum) and invasive (bronchial washing, transbronchial biopsy, genyantrum biopsy) procedures were negative, although a brain abscess was not sampled; the diagnosis was made by Western blotting of sera.

Of the 29 isolates identified in local laboratories as Nocardia spp., 25 were N. asteroides and 4 N. farcinica.

In all cases, identification was based on the failure to hydrolyse caseine, xanthine, hypoxanthine, tyrosine, adenine, uric acid and Tween 20, but not esculin. All but 1 (case 16) of the 25 isolates tested were urease-positive; the negative strain did not produce acid from mannitol or sorbitol after 4 weeks of incubation, that differentiated N. carnea from N. asteroides (9). N. farcinica and N. asteroides were separated by the ability of the former to grow at 45°C, to grow on rhamnose, 2,3-butylene glycol and 1,2-propylene glycol as a sole carbon source, and to use acetamide as nitrogen and carbon source (3).

Thin-layer chromatography showed that all the isolates identified as Nocardia spp. contained the meso-isomer of diaminopimelic acid, as well as galactose, arabinose and nocardomycolic acid.

All 18 isolates tested for antimicrobial susceptibility proved susceptible to amikacin, and 16 were susceptible to imipenem. Ampicillin, chloramphenicol, erythromycin, fosfomycin, pefloxacin, sulphonamide, trimethoprim, and trimethoprim plus sulphonamide were inactive. Susceptibility ranged from 5.6% of strains (kanamycin) to 66.7% (amoxicillin plus clavulanic acid).

Sulphonamides alone were rarely (11.8%) chosen as first-line therapy, other drugs being combined in 41.2% of cases (amikacin, ceftriaxone, imipenem and minocycline). The choice of sulphonamides was never based on in vitro test results. One-third of the patients underwent surgical excision or drainage before receiving antimicrobial therapy.

DISCUSSION

Pathogenic species of Nocardia are universally present in the soil. Infection of humans and other animals is rare, complicating both immunosuppression and pre-existing diseases. A survey of pathogenic Actinomycetales in soil from some areas of Italy confirmed that Nocardia spp. are common in the Italian environment, where they exist as saprophytes (10). However, few clinical infections were reported in Italy during the 1970s and 1980s (11–13).

On the basis of an epidemiological survey, Beaman et al. estimated that about 500–1,000 cases of nocardiosis were diagnosed every year in the USA during the 1970s (14). Boiron et al. estimated that 150 to 250 cases of nocardiosis occurred yearly in France (15). It is not possible to estimate the number of Italian cases, because nocardiosis is not a notifiable disease and because Nocardia strains are not collected by a National Reference Centre.

N. asteroides was the most common species in this series (86.2%, 25/29). No clinically relevant differences were observed between urease-positive and urease-negative strains (16). N. farcinica was identified in 4 cases (13.8%) and exhibited a specific drug resistance pattern (17). The prevalence of this species was lower than in other European series (France, 27.1%, Germany, 58.6%) (15, 18). N. carnea and N. brasiliensis were not recovered from these patients, probably because they are rarely found in soil in temperate areas. No significant clinically relevant differences were noticed between infections due to N. asteroides and N. farcinica, but the number of the latter was low.

Pediatric nocardiosis is uncommon (19), as reflected by the fact that all but 1 case in this series involved adults. Because of the ubiquitous habitat of Nocardia in soil and dust inhabitants, 2 cases were probably hospital-acquired (20).

Purulent pericarditis caused by Nocardia is extremely rare. The literature describes 14 cases of nocardial pericarditis, but there have only been 6 reports of Nocardia isolation from cultures of pericardial fluid or from the pericardium (21). The relevant patient in this series (case 5) had nosocomial nocardiosis following pericardiocentesis to drain a pericardial effusion, probably of viral origin. Central nervous system (CNS) involvement during nocardial infection is well known. 10 of the 30 patients had an intracranial space-occupying lesion. Although Nocardia is an uncommon cause of meningitis (22), it must be borne in mind not only in patients with depressed cell-mediated immunity but also in people with CNS trauma or undergoing invasive CNS procedures.

The association between nocardial infection and cancer (especially solid tumours) is well documented (23), particularly in patients who have received cytotoxic therapy or steroids. Nocardia infection has also been described in splenectomized patients (24) and in heart or kidney transplant recipients, in whom it can be life-threatening (25).

Nocardiosis was recently described in drug addicts, sometimes in association with other pulmonary pathogens. Nocardial infection has so far rarely been described in AIDS patients (26).

It is important to detect all pulmonary lesions and to suspect nocardiosis in patients who develop pulmonary infiltrates, which may be associated with skin, brain or intra-abdominal abscesses. Pulmonary infection may be missed, particularly in AIDS patients with other pulmonary infections, such as Pneumocystis carinii, Mycobacterium spp., Legionella spp. and cytomegalovirus pneumonia (27). Pulmonary infection can only be documented by biopsy and appropriate incubation in some cases. We isolated a Nocardia sp. from broncho-alveolar fluid on selective Legionella medium. Because of detection of Nocardia sepsis, blood cultures should be performed systematically (28).

Although effective antimicrobial therapy is available, opportunistic nocardial infections remain life-threatening in the immunocompromised host. Considerable differences in susceptibility were observed between N. asteroides and N. farcinica. In particular, N. farcinica was regularly resistant to cephalosporins (cefuroxime and cefotaxime), aminoglycosides (gentamicin and kanamycin) and tetracyclines, whereas N. asteroides presented a heterogeneous pattern of sensitivity to the same drugs. An interesting finding is the inactivity of the sulphonamides, trimethoprim and trimethoprim plus sulphonamide in vitro against all the isolates, although this is generally considered the reference treatment for nocardiosis. Our data suggest that the most effective drugs against both Nocardia species are imipenem and amikacin, in agreement with other authors (29).

All the cases were difficult to diagnose. Systemic nocardiosis is no longer a differential clinical diagnosis in Italy because it is considered to be extremely rare. However, physicians should be aware of the fact that Nocardia is far from rare in some categories of patients (cancer patients, organ transplant recipients and AIDS patients). Close collaboration between clinicians and medical microbiologists is required for early diagnosis and therapy.

ACKNOWLEDGEMENT

Maurizio Parea, MD, Microbiology Institute, Ospedali Riuniti, Bergamo, helped to prepare the manuscript.

REFERENCES

1. Goodfellow M, Lechevalier MP, Genus Nocardia Trevisan 1889, 9AL. In: Williams ST, Sharpe ME, Holt JG, eds. Bergey's manual of systematic bacteriology, vol. 4. Baltimore: Williams and Wilkins, 2350–2361, 1989.
2. Beaman BL, Beaman L. Nocardia species: host-parasite relationships. Clin Microbiol Rev 7: 213–264, 1994.
3. Boiron P, Provost F, Dupont B. Laboratory methods for the diagnosis of nocardiosis. Paris: Institut Pasteur, 188, 1993.
4. Boiron P, Provost F. Use of partially purified 54-kilodalton antigen for diagnosis of nocardiosis by Western blot (immunoblot) assay. J Clin Microbiol 28: 238–231, 1990.
5. Boiron P, Provost F. Characterization of Nocardia, Rhodococcus and Gordona species by in vitro susceptibility testing. Zbl Bakt 274: 203–213, 1990.
6. Staneck JL, Roberts GD. Simplified approach to identification of aerobic actinomycetes by thin-layer chromatography. Appl Microbiol 28: 226–231, 1974.
7. Minnikin DE, Alshamaony L, Goodfellow M. Differentiation of Mycobacterium, Nocardia and related taxa by thin-layer chromatographic analysis of whole-organism methanolysates. J Gen Microbiol 88: 200–204, 1975.
8. Acar J, Begogne-Bérézin E, Brogard JM, Chabbert Y, Cluzel R, Courvalin P, Dabernat H, Drugeon H, Dubreuil L, Duval J, Flandrois JP, Fleurette J, Goldstein F, Meyran M, Morel Cl, Philippon A, Sirot J, Soussy CJ, Thabaut A, Veron M. 1993 Statement of the Antibiogram Committee of the French Society for Microbiology. Pathol Biol 41: 741–748, 1993.
9. Gordon RE, Mishra SK, Barnett DA. Some bits and pieces of the genus Nocardia: N carnea, N vaccinii, N. transvalensis, N. orientalis and N. aerocolonigenes. J Gen Microbiol 109: 69–72, 1978.
10. Polonelli L, Morace B, Barcaioli M, Cossu LA. Survey of pathogenic actinomycetes and fungi in soil from Rome and other Italian areas. Mycopathologia 73: 161–167, 1981.
11. Amato G, Bocchetti M, Cerbo M, Gargiulo F, Piccirillo MM. Nocardia asteroides: un caso di ascesso sottocutaneo. G Batteriol Virol Immunol 82: 64–69, 1989.
12. Bianchi L, Fazia Mercadante NF, Caretta G. Un caso di nocardiosi localizzata alla regione sopraioidea (studio clinico, istopatologico e microbiologico). Boll Ist Sieroter Milan 67: 165–172, 1988.
13. Pesce CM, Quaglia AC. Nocardia lung infection with hematogenous spread in a woman with adrenal cortical hyperfunction. Eur J Respirat Dis 64: 613–615, 1984.
14. Beaman BL, Burnside J, Edwards B, Causey W. Nocardial infections in the United States, 1972–1974. J Infect Dis 134: 286–289, 1976.
15. Boiron P, Provost F, Chevrier G, Dupont B. Review of nocardial infections in France 1987 to 1990. Eur J Clin Microbiol Infect Dis 11: 709–714, 1992.
16. Boiron P, Provost F. Urease-negative Nocardia asteroides causing cutaneous nocardiosis. J Clin Microbiol 28: 801–802, 1990.
17. Wallace RJ Jr, Tsukamura M, Brown BA, Brown J, Steingrube VA, Zhang Y, Nash Dr. Cefotaxime-resistant Nocardia asteroides strains are isolates of the controversial species Nocardia farcinica. J Clin Microbiol 28: 2726–2732, 1990.

18. Schaal KP. Actinomycetes as human pathogens. In: Okami Y, Beppu T, Ogawara H, eds. Biology of actinomycetes. Tokyo: Japan Scientific Societies Press, 277–282, 1988.
19. Law BJ, Marks MI. Pediatric nocardiosis. Pediatrics 70: 560–565, 1982.
20. Smeal WE, Schenfeld LA. Nocardiosis in the community hospital. Report of three cases. Postgrad Med 79: 77–82, 1986.
21. Poland GA, Jorgensen CR, Sarosi GA. Nocardia asteroides pericarditis: report of a case and review of the literature. Mayo Clin Proc 64: 819–824, 1990.
22. Bross JE, Gordon G. Nocardial meningitis: case reports and reviews. Rev Infect Dis 13: 160–165, 1991.
23. Berkey P, Bodey GP. Nocardial infection in patients with neoplastic disease. Rev Infect Dis 11: 407–412, 1989.
24. Abdi EA, Ding JC, Cooper IA. Nocardia infection in splenectomized patients: case report and a review of the literature. Postgrad Med J 63: 455–458, 1987.
25. Wilson JP, Turner HR, Kirchner KA, Chapman SW. Nocardial infections in renal transplant recipients. Medicine 68: 38–57, 1989.
26. Uttamchandani RB, Daikos GL, Reyes RR, Fischl MA, Dickinson GM, Yamaguchi E, Kramer MR. Nocardiosis in 30 patients with advanced Human Immunodeficiency Virus infection: clinical features and outcome. Clin Infect Dis 18: 348–353, 1994.
27. Lynn W, Whyte M, Weber J. Nocardia, Mycobacteria and AIDS. AIDS 3: 766–767, 1989.
28. Kasten MJ, Telenti A, Keating MR, Roberts GD. Nocardemia: clinical characteristics and significance. In: Proceedings XI I.S.H.A.M. Congress, PS 2.72, Montreal, Canada, 108, 1991.
29. Beaman BL, Boiron P, Beaman L, Brownell GH, Schaal K, Gombert ME. Nocardia and nocardiosis. J Med Vet Mycol 30 (suppl 1): 317–331, 1992.

Submitted August 24, 1994; accepted October 19, 1994

Scand J Infect Dis 27: 29–31, 1995

Treatment of Louse-borne Relapsing Fever with Low Dose Penicillin or Tetracycline: A Clinical Trial

TESHALE SEBOXA and SIBYLLE I. RAHLENBECK

From the Department of Internal Medicine, Gondar College of Medical Sciences, Addis Abeba University, Gondar, Ethiopia

A clinical trial was conducted in order to evaluate the efficacy of procaine penicillin and tetracycline, respectively, in the treatment of louse-borne relapsing fever. 184 patients (160 men, 24 women) admitted to the Gondar hospital during the rainy season 1992 were assigned to 1 of 4 treatment groups: procaine penicillin 100,000 (PP100), 200,000 (PP200) or 400,000 (PP400) international units (IU) intramuscularly (i.m.), or tetracycline 250 mg per os (TTC, p.o.). All drugs were given as single doses. The overall case fatality rate was 3.3%. Frequency of relapses, Jarisch-Herxheimer-like reactions (JHR) and deaths were significantly different between patients treated with TTC and those treated with PP100. Relapses occurred most often in the group receiving the lowest dose of penicillin (46%), and decreased with increasing dosage of penicillin; none of the patients treated with TTC had a relapse. Occurrence of JHR showed the opposite pattern: whilst 2 (5%) patients treated with PP100 developed a JHR, 16 (29%) in the PP200 group, 10 (31%) in the PP400 group, and 27 (47%) in the TTC group developed a JHR. As mortality is linked to severe JHR, and most relapses are clinically mild and easily treated, these results speak in favour of using low-dose penicillin to initiate the treatment of relapsing fever.

T. Seboxa, MD, Gondar College of Medical Sciences, P.O. Box 196, Gondar, Ethiopia

INTRODUCTION

Louse-borne relapsing fever (LBRF) is an acute febrile disease caused by an infection with Borrelia recurrentis, a spirochetal organism that is transmitted to humans by the infected human body louse, Pedunculus humanus. Outbreaks of the disease are related to poor hygiene and crowding, and occur mainly during wars and periods of famine. The disease is endemic in Northeast Africa, South America and East Asia (1–7). In Ethiopia, more than 10,000 cases occur each year (4). If untreated, the case-fatality rate ranges from 30 to 70% (1). Antibiotic treatment has reduced mortality to 2–6% (3, 8, 9).

A variety of antibiotic drugs have been used in the treatment and have been proved to be efficient in removing spirochetes, for example tetracyclines including doxycycline, erythromycin, chloramphenicol, and penicillin. Clinicians favour a single dose or multiple doses of tetracyclines (8–11), low dose penicillins (3), or a combination of both (7) for treatment of adults. The clearance of borreliae is often accompanied by a Jarisch-Herxheimer-like reaction (JHR), characterized by a sudden rise in fever, blood pressure, and respiratory rate, being followed by a severe hypotonic phase. It has been shown that highly efficient drugs such as tetracyclines are associated with the highest rate of JHR. Drugs that are more slowly combatting the infection, for example slow-release penicillins, induce JHRs not only at a lower rate, but also less severely (1). Deaths during the shock phase of a JHR have been reported, with a case-fatality rate of up to 4% in patients treated with penicillins (5), and up to 6% in those receiving tetracyclines (1, 2, 7).

Clinical trials so far conducted have not resulted in a consensus as to the optimal drug, dose, and route of administration for the treatment of LBRF. Often, the trials included only low numbers of patients (5, 9, 11, 12), had a high percentage of lost-to-follow-ups (1, 8), and/or were not conducted as controlled clinical trials (8, 10).

The purpose of our study was to conduct a controlled clinical trial comparing single doses of the most commonly recommended drugs, tetracycline and penicillin, the latter one at different dose levels.

PATIENTS AND METHODS

During the rainy season (June–September) 1992, 255 patients with LBRF were admitted to the medical wards of the Gondar College of Medical Sciences in Gondar, Ethiopia. The diagnosis was verified microscopically by identifying the spirochetes in the patients peripheral blood smears. Patients in serious condition on admission (systolic blood pressure below 75 mmHg, coma, anuria, severe jaundice and/or acute heart failure with pulmonary edema), children below age 15 years, and those with a history of allergy to penicillin or tetracycline were not included in the study. All others were eligible for the study and consent was obtained from 184 patients, 160 men and 24 women. These were assigned to one of the following 4 treatment groups:

- procaine penicillin, 100,000 IU i.m. (PP100): 39 patients;
- procaine penicillin, 200,000 IU i.m. (PP200): 55 patients;
- procaine penicillin, 400,000 IU i.m. (PP400): 32 patients;
- tetracycline, 250 mg, p.o. (TTC): 58 patients.

The assignment of a patient's drug regimen was chosen by drawing a card labeled with the drug and dose to be given. Out of 300 cards prepared, 30% were labeled PP200, 30% TTC, and 20% each were prepared for PP100 and PP400. PP200 and TTC were the treatments of choice at the clinic, and were therefore overrepresentated. All drugs were given as a single dose after i.v. fluid installment. Both antibiotics were from Epharm Co., Addis Abeba, Ethiopia. Patients were monitored closely for one week for the development of signs of JHR and/or relapses. A JHR was defined

 ISSN 0036-5548

as an increase in body temperature (>1°C) combined with tachycardia (pulse rate >100 min^{-1}), occurring within 4 h after treatment, followed by a drop in systolic and diastolic blood pressure greater than 10 mmHg. A relapse was recorded for those patients who suffered a further fever attack with positive blood smear at least 2 days after the first attack. The study was approved by the Ethics Committee in Gondar, Ethiopia.

Differences in the proportion of JHR and relapse among groups were tested using the Cochran-Mantel-Haenszel statistics, controlling for gender and age group. Age groups were set up as follows: 15–19, 20–29, 30–39, ≥40 years. Because of the low number of patients, all those above 30 years (n = 37) were included in 1 group when analyzing age as a risk factor for the development of JHRs and relapses. Logistic regression analysis was used to study the effect of clinical parameters on mortality, relapse and JHR incidence. Independent variables included in these models were: age, sex, drug, jaundice, cardiac gallop rhythm, blood pressure, and duration of symptoms before admission. All data analyses were performed using the SAS statistical analysis software (SAS Institute, Cary, NC).

RESULTS

Epidemiological characteristics

The patients' age ranged from 15 to 56 years with a mean of 23.4 years; 98 patients (53%) were in the age group from 20 to 30 years. The male : female ratio was 6.7 : 1. Of the male patients, 38 (23.8%) were soldiers or ex-soldiers, 30 (18.7%) students, 14 (8.8%) prisoners, 30 (18.7%) daily labourers or unemployed, and 12 (7.5%) farmers.

Clinical symptoms and signs

The average duration of symptoms before admission was 4.5 days (range 1–21 days). The most prominent symptoms reported were fever (100%), general malaise (82%), and headache (76%). Myalgia occurred in 104 patients (66%), arthralgia in 75 (41%), cough in 22 (12%), and diarrheoa in 21 patients (11%). On admission, all patients were febrile with a mean axillary temperature of 38.5°C. Jaundice was noticed in 45% of the patients, abdominal tenderness, hepatomegaly or splenomegaly or both were less common findings, occurring in 18.5%. The average blood pressure was 103/69 mmHg.

Fatalities

Out of the 184 patients 6 (3.3%) died after development of a JHR; no death occurred in the PP100 group, 1 in the PP200, 2 in the PP400, and 3 in the TTC group. The case fatality rate between PP100 and TTC was significantly different ($p = 0.03$). Mortality was significantly associated with the occurrence of a JHR ($p = 0.009$), but was unrelated to relapses, jaundice, cardiac gallop rhythm, age, gender, blood pressure, and length of symptoms prior to admission.

Relapses

Overall, 30 patients (16.3%) developed a relapse. Relapses occurred in nearly one-half ($n = 18$; 46.2%) of the patients in the PP100 group, and decreased in number with increasing dosage of penicillin. No relapse was noted in patients receiving TTC (Fig. 1). The differences between TTC and PP100 and PP200 were highly significant ($p = 0.001$). Relapses tended to occur at a higher rate in younger patients: 12 (26.7%) patients aged below 20 ys, 16 (16.3%) of those aged between 20 and 30 ys, and 2 patients (5.4%) aged above 30 years developed a relapse. When controlled for sex and drug, this trend was not significant (Table I).

Table I. *Adjusted odds ratios and 95% confidence intervals for the development of Jarisch-Herxheimer-like reactions and relapses in patients with louse-borne relapsing fever, Gondar, Ethiopia, 1992*

Age (years)	Number	JHR OR[a]	JHR 95% CI	Relapse OR[a]	Relapse 95% CI
15–19	49	1.00		1.00	
20–29	98	0.56	0.25–1.24	0.82	0.31–2.14
≥30	37	0.32	0.11–0.95	0.23	0.04–1.34

[a] adjusted for drug and gender

Jarisch-Herxheimer-like-reactions

In contrast to what was observed for relapses, JHR occurred in about half of the patients treated with tetracycline (46.6%), and in about one-third (31.3%) of those receiving PP400. The JHR-rate decreased with decreasing dosage of penicillin: 15 patients (27.8%) in the PP200 group and only 2 (5%) of the patients in the PP100 group developed a JHR (Fig. 1). When controlling for age and gender, the difference in this regard between TTC and PP100 treatment was significant ($p = 0.005$), but not between TTC and PP200 or PP400, respectively.

Development of a JHR was significantly less frequent in patients above 30 years than in those aged below 20 years (Table I). Gender was unrelated to the occurrence of JHR, and none of the other variables were associated with an increased rate of development of JHR at a significant level.

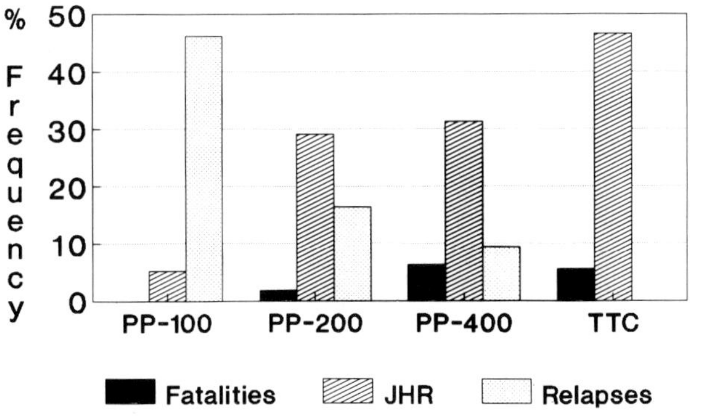

Fig. 1. Frequency of relapses, Jarisch-Herxheimer-like reactions (JHR), and fatalities in patients with louse-borne relapsing fever treated with penicillin or tetracycline, June–September 1992, Gondar, Ethiopia.

DISCUSSION

We found an increasing rate of JHRs with increasing dose of penicillin, from 5.1% (PP100) to 31.1% (PP400). Penicillin clears the blood of spirochetes more slowly than do other relevant antibiotics, and accordingly induces JHRs later, at a lower rate and with less severity. Combined treatment using PP400, followed by 2 g of TTC a day later, has resulted in a JHR-rate of 13% (7). 47% of our patients receiving tetracycline developed a JHR. All but 1 (8) previous studies reported the development of JHR in all patients receiving tetracycline (1, 5, 9, 11, 12). These studies included severely ill patients – who in our study were excluded. Moreover, criteria for JHR were not clearly defined in those studies, so that a comparison with our results is hampered.

Low age was found to be a risk factor for the development of a JHR. A possible explanation is that younger individuals are likely to be of lower weight than older ones, thus receiving a higher drug dose per kg body mass. Unfortunately, the weight of patients was not recorded, and it can not be established if this association is spurious or real. More likely, the difference reflects a partial immunity to Borrelia and borrelia toxins in patients aged 30 years or more. When comparing our results to reports from other countries the high prevalence of malnutrition in our region has to be taken into consideration. Lack of data on body mass index unabled us to evaluate the effect that malnutrition could have on the incidence of JHR and/or relapses.

We noticed an overall case fatality rate of 3.3%. Deaths were significantly associated with the occurrence of JHRs. The different mortality rates between patients treated with PP100 and TTC are likely to reflect the different rates of JHRs.

The relapse rate in our study decreased with increasing dose of penicillin from 45.0% (PP100) over 16.7% (PP200) to 9.4% (PP400). Relapse rates of 1.2% have been reported for combined penicillin-tetracycline treatment (7), and 1.8% for PP400 administered twice (2). None of our patients treated with TTC showed a relapse, a finding consistent with previous reports (1, 5, 8, 11, 12).

In conclusion, it appears that treatment of LBRF should be initiated with low dose penicillin rather than the common use of tetracycline. A low dose of penicillin obviously reduces the rate of JHR, and thus mortality. Further clinical trials are needed to establish the optimal dose, or possibly combinations of doses or drugs for the treatment of this disease.

ACKNOWLEDGEMENTS

We thank the medical and nursing staff at the Gondar College of Medical Sciences for their help in the study.

REFERENCES

1. Bryceson AD, Parry EH, Perine PL, Warrell DA, Vukotich D, Leithead CS. Louse-borne relapsing fever. A clinical and laboratory study of 62 cases in Ethiopia and a reconsideration of the literature. Q J Med 153: 129–170, 1970.
2. Borgnolo G, Hailu B, Ciancarelli A, Almaviva M, Woldemariam T. Louse-borne relapsing fever. Trop Geogr Med 45: 66–69, 1993.
3. Borgnolo G, Denku B, Chiabrera F, Hailu B. Louse-borne relapsing fever in Ethiopian children: a clinical study. Ann Trop Paediatr 13: 165–171, 1993.
4. Hodes R. Relapsing Fever. In: Zein AZ & Kloos H, eds. The Ecology of Health and Disease in Ethiopia. Addis Abeba: Ministry of Health, 177–183, 1988.
5. Perine PL, Teklu B. Antibiotic treatment of louse-borne relapsing fever in Ethiopia: A report of 377 cases. Am J Trop Med Hyg 32: 1096–1100, 1983.
6. Salih SY, Mustafa D, Abdel Wahah S, Ahmed MA, Omer A. Louse-borne relapsing fever: I. A clinical and laboratory study of 363 cases in the Sudan. Trans R Soc Trop Med Hyg 71: 43–48, 1977.
7. Salih SY, Mustafa D. Louse-borne relapsing fever: II. Combined penicillin and tetracycline therapy in 160 Sudanese patients. Trans R Soc Trop Med Hyg 71: 49–51, 1977.
8. Gebrehiwot T, Fiseha A. Tetracycline versus penicillin in the treatment of louse-borne relapsing fever. Ethiop Med J 30: 175–178, 1992.
9. Warrell DA, Perine P, Krause D, Bing D, MacDougal S. Pathophysiology and immunology of the Jarisch-Herxheimer-like reaction in louse-borne relapsing fever: comparison of tetracycline and slow-release penicillin. J Infect Dis 147: 898–909, 1983.
10. Sundenes KO, Haimonot AT. Epidemic of louse-borne relapsing fever in Ethiopia. Lancet 342: 1213–1215, 1993.
11. Butler T, Jones PK, Wallace CK. Borrelia recurrentis infection: single-dose antibiotic regimens and the management of the Jarisch-Herxheimer reaction. J Infect Dis 147: 898–909, 1983.
12. Teklu B, Habte-Michael A, Warrell DA, White NJ, Wright DM. Meptazinol diminishes the Jarisch-Herxheimer reaction of relapsing fever. Lancet 311: 837–839, 1983.
13. Butler T. Relapsing fever. New lessons about antibiotic action. Ann Intern Med 102: 397–399, 1985.

Submitted April 28, 1994; accepted October 17, 1994

Scand J Infect Dis 27: 32–37, 1995 ORIGINAL ARTICLE

Short- and Long-Term Prognosis for Middle-Aged and Elderly Patients Hospitalized with Community-Acquired Pneumonia: Impact of Nutritional and Inflammatory Factors

JONAS HEDLUND[1], LARS-OLOF HANSSON[2] and ÅKE ÖRTQVIST[1]

From the Departments of [1]Infectious Diseases, Karolinska Institutet, Danderyd Hospital, and [2]Clinical Chemistry, Karolinska Hospital, Karolinska Institutet, Stockholm, Sweden

To investigate the impact of nutritional and inflammatory factors on short- and long-term prognosis for patients hospitalized for community-acquired pneumonia (CAP), 97 patients, 50–85 years old, admitted to the Department of Infectious Diseases at Danderyd Hospital were enrolled in a prospective study. 13 enrolment variables were examined for association with 6 outcome variables. Serum orosomucoid concentration, acute physiology and chronic health evaluation (APACHE) II score, body mass index (BMI) and triceps skinfold (TSF) were each associated with duration of hospital stay. A low TSF and BMI, and a high APACHE II score were all associated with death. A high APACHE II score and a high TSF were both associated with readmission within 6 months of discharge. The alfa-1-antitrypsin concentration was the most closely correlated with duration of fever. We conclude that the admission concentrations of alfa-1-antitrypsin and orosomucoid are better predictors of hospital morbidity than the more commonly used albumin and C-reactive protein (CRP) levels. Measurement of APACHE II and TSF on admission may give additional prognostic information on the interval from admission to 6 months after discharge.

J. Hedlund, MD, Department of Infectious Diseases, Karolinska Institute, Danderyd Hospital, S-182 88 Danderyd, Stockholm, Sweden

INTRODUCTION

Several risk factors have been associated with increased mortality during an acute episode of community-acquired pneumonia (CAP) (1–5). In a previous study (1) we found that a low serum albumin concentration was the only independent factor that on admission was significantly correlated with a higher case fatality rate. Furthermore, a low serum albumin concentration on primary admission seems to be a negative prognostic factor also for the outcome during subsequent pneumonia recurrences (6).

It is not clear why low serum albumin concentrations are correlated with a less favourable prognosis in CAP. Serum albumin is considered to be an indicator of nutritional status (7–9). At the same time, experimental (10, 11) and clinical (9) data indicate that in inflammatory disorders, synthesis of acute-phase proteins occurs at the expense of albumin. Thus, low serum albumin concentrations in patients treated in hospital for CAP could be caused both by malnutrition and by the phlogistic reaction per se.

The concentration of serum albumin is included in 2 scoring systems devised to predict morbidity and mortality in hospital-treated patients. The 'Prognostic Nutritional Index' (PNI) was developed from an analysis of the outcomes of non-emergency general surgical patients (12). The most important predictive variables found were serum albumin, transferrin, triceps skinfold, and delayed hypersensitivity. Calculated PNI is the percentage likelihood of a complication occurring in an individual patient. A modified PNI (in which the skin test has been replaced by total lymphocyte count) has since been used in studies on bacterial colonization in the lower respiratory tract (13, 14).

The 'Prognostic Inflammatory and Nutritional Index' (PINI) was devised in order to focus on both the phlogistic and the nutritional aspects of the stress reaction (15). The PINI is based on C-reactive protein (CRP), orosomucoid, albumin and transthyretin (formerly called prealbumin) which, in an analysis of blood markers of the phlogistic reaction and of nutritional status in patients with surgical and medical disorders, was most closely correlated with complications and death.

Another way to predict in-hospital mortality is the 'Acute physiology and chronic health evaluation' (APACHE II) (16). This severity-of-disease classification system has been shown to correctly predict those patients requiring intensive care treatment (16). However, to our knowledge, no prospective study on the usefulness of APACHE II as a prognostic instrument in moderately severe pneumonia has been published previously.

Our purpose was to assess the prognostic value of serum albumin in middle-aged or older patients with CAP, compared with the prognostic accuracy of: (*a*) the above-mentioned scoring systems; (*b*) other serum proteins, including acute-phase proteins; (*c*) clinical nutritional measurements.

 ISSN 0036-5548

PATIENTS AND METHODS

Patients

Danderyd Hospital is a university hospital at which the Department of Infectious Diseases serves approximately 750,000 inhabitants in Stockholm County.

All patients, 50–85 years old with CAP, admitted to the Department, from January 14th, 1992 to January 10th, 1993 were reviewed for inclusion. No immunocompromized patients, i.e. patients with HIV infection, active malignant disease, immunoglobulin deficiency, aspleni or those receiving cytostatic or dialysis treatment were included in the study, nor were patients incapable of following the study instructions. All enrolled patients gave their informed consent.

CAP was defined by the following criteria: 1) symptoms of an acute lower respiratory tract disease, i.e. cough, tachypnea or chest pain; and 2) fever before admission to hospital; and 3) radiological signs of acute pneumonia, i.e. pulmonary infiltrates proved by previous and/or later X-ray to be new, or to diminish with clinical improvement.

A total of 97 patients were included for analysis. The patients were followed during hospitalization and were seen at follow-up visits 8 weeks ($n = 71$) and 6 months ($n = 63$) after discharge from hospital. For patients who did not return for follow-up visits, data on new hospital admissions and on hospital mortality from the time of discharge until 6 months later were obtained from the central computerized data register of Stockholm County Council. This register maintains data and diagnoses for all inpatients treated at any hospital in the Stockholm area. Data on causes of death outside hospital were obtained from the National Central Bureau of Statistics, Sweden.

Protocol

Data were collected on specially-designed forms. On enrolment, the medical history, anthropometrics, and a modified APACHE II score (see below) were recorded. On the follow-up visits, 8 weeks and 6 months after discharge, anthropometrics and the extent of chest X-ray resolution were recorded. Furthermore, the patients were asked whether (or not, i.e. delayed recovery) they had returned to normal daily activities.

Nutritional assessment

After admission (in most cases within 24 h), the patient's nutritional status was assessed by one of the authors, (J.H. or Å.Ö). The nutritional assessment included weight, history of weight loss, body mass index (BMI) and triceps skinfold (TSF). BMI was calculated as weight (kg) divided by height squared (m^2). Measurements of weight and TSF were repeated at the follow-up visits. The same scale and instrument for measurement of TSF was used for all patients on all occasions.

Blood chemistry

From all enrolled patients, venous blood samples were drawn within 24 h of admission (day 0). The laboratory measurements included the serum proteins albumin, transthyretin and transferrin, as well as the acute-phase proteins alfa-1-antitrypsin, orosomucoid, haptoglobin and CRP.

All serum proteins were measured using Behring Nephelometer Analyzer (Behring, Marburg, Germany) using antisera and calibrations from DAKO a/s (Glostrup, Denmark).

Assessment of severity of disease

Assessment of severity of disease was performed with 24 h after admission using the APACHE II severity of disease classification system (16). APACHE II is based upon initial values of age, previous health status and 12 routine physiological measurements and the Glasgow coma score. In our modified version we did not include oxygenation of arterial pH, nor hematocrit which was replaced by hemoglobin. In accordance with Daley et al. (17) we used the first data collected during the first 24 h to get a measure of risk that is independent of early treatment.

Prognostic indices

PNI was calculated according to the formula of Niederman et al. (13):

$$\text{PNI} = 158 - 16.6 \times \text{serum albumin(g/l)} - 0.78 \times \text{TSF(mm)}$$
$$- 0.2 \times \text{serum transferrin(mg/dl)} - 5.8\text{(lymphocyte score)}$$

where lymphocyte score is measured on a scale of 0 to 2, in which $0 = <1000$, $1 = 1000$ to 2000, and $2 = >2000$/ml total lymphocytes.

PINI was calculated as the ratio between the product of the serum proteins CRP (mg/l) and orosomucoid (mg/l) and the product of albumin (g/l) and transthyretin (mg/l) (15).

Etiology of pneumonia

A complete etiological investigation was not performed as this was not the primary aim of our study. On admission, blood samples for culture were obtained from 70 patients, and culturing from sputum was performed in 37 patients. Paired sera from 71 patients were examined for antibodies to: pneumococcal haemolysin (pneumolysin), Legionella spp, Chlamydia pneumoniae and C. psittaci, Mycoplasma pneumoniae and respiratory tract viruses (respiratory syncytial virus, para-influenza 1-3, influenza A and B virus and adenovirus). The same diagnostic criteria as in an earlier report (1) were applied, with the exception that no single antibody titre was used as a diagnostic criterion. An etiological diagnosis was established in 37 patients (38%). S. pneumoniae was the predominant pathogen, accounting for 25 (26%) of the cases. No other pathogen was found in >4% of the cases.

Statistical analysis

Data on blood chemistry, nutritional evaluation and APACHE II score, altogether 13 variables (Table II), were examined for association with 6 outcome variables: death during hospitalization or during the 6-month follow-up period, duration of hospital stay, duration of fever, delayed recovery, delayed X-ray resolution and readmission within 6 months after discharge from hospital. For univariate analysis of categorical variables, the χ^2-test was used. For variables with small expected values, Fisher's exact test (2-tailed) was used. Continuous variables were analysed with Student's t-test or by linear regression. For the continuous outcome variables 'duration of hospital stay' and 'duration of fever', all 13 variables were used in a stepwise multiple regression analysis, and logarithmic transformations were performed as necessary. For the outcome variable 'readmission' a logistic regression analysis was employed including all 13 variables (Table IV). All analyses were performed with the JMP statistical computer program (SAS Institute, Cary, North Carolina, USA). A p-value of <0.05 was deemed significant.

The study was approved by the Ethics Committee of Karolinska Institutet, Stockholm, Sweden.

RESULTS

Demographic data

A total of 97 patients were included, 50 men and 47 women, ranging in age from 50 to 84 years (mean, 69.6 years). 17 patients were smokers, 1 a known alcoholic and 55 had a chronic disease of which the most serious were chronic obstructive pulmonary disease ($n = 19$), congestive heart failure ($n = 16$) and diabetes mellitus ($n = 7$). None of the patients had a pre-existing severe liver disease.

On admission

The median duration of illness prior to admission was 4 days (range <1–25 days). A respiratory rate of ≥30 per minute was registered in 28/79 patients (35%), and 18/95 patients (19%) had a diastolic blood pressure of ≤60 mmHg. Seven patients had both a high respiratory rate and a low blood pressure. Two patients were confused on admission. The mean scores were 9.2 (range 3–16) for APACHE II, 49.7 for PNI (−2.7–80.5) and 124.8 for PINI (2.6–1040.1). The patients' mean weight was 68.2 kg (38.2–117.2 kg), the mean TSF was 13.6 mm (range 5–31 mm) and the mean BMI was 23.5 (range 0–37.5). A history of weight loss within 6 months of admission, averaging 6.3% was reported from 21/93 patients. The mean values and ranges of the investigated serum proteins are shown in Table I.

Table I. *Serum proteins on admission – mean values and range (n = 97)*

Serum protein	Mean value	Range	Reference values
Albumin (g/l)	33.9	15.2–49.3	37–52
Transthyretin (mg/l)	135.9	49.0–240.0	200–400
Transferrin (g/l)	1.86	0.95–3.61	1.5–2.7
Alfa-1-antitrypsin (g/l)	2.44	1.26–6.23	0.9–1.8
Orosomucoid (g/l)	2.27	0.74–4.91	0.5–1.0
Haptoglobin (g/l)	4.92	0.60–9.77	0.4–2.5
CRP (mg/l)[a]	172.6	12.0–367.0	<10

[a] CRP = C-reactive protein.

Clinical course during hospitalisation

Only 1 of the 97 patients required treatment in the intensive care unit. This was 1 of the 2 patients who died during the hospital stay. The duration of hospital stay for the 95 surviving patients was 8.7 days on average (median 7 days). Admission data significantly associated with a longer hospitalization in the univariate analysis were high APACHE II score, high PNI and PINI, low serum albumin and transthyretin, and high levels of the serum acute phase proteins (Table II). The surviving patients' body temperature had normalized (a stable level below 37.5°C) after 3.8 days on average (median 3 days). Low admission levels of serum albumin and transferrin were significantly associated with longer duration of fever, as were high admission levels of serum haptoglobin, alfa-1-antitrypsin, orosomucoid and a high PNI (Table II), while a high PINI was just below the significance level ($p = 0.06$).

Deaths

Pneumonia was the direct cause of death in the 2 patients who died in hospital. Four others died during the 6-month follow-up period: 2 patients before the first follow-up visit and 2 between 8 weeks and 6 months after discharge from hospital. The primary cause of death in these cases was congestive heart failure ($n = 3$) and an ovarian neoplasm ($n = 1$). The neoplasm was unknown when the patient was enrolled in the study. Admission data significantly associated with a fatal outcome during the study period were a low TSF value, a low BMI, and a high APACHE II score (Table II). The mean APACHE II score in the patients who subsequently died was 12.2 compared with 9.0 in the surviving patients. The patients who died had a mean TSF of 8.8 mm and a mean BMI of 20.35, to be compared with

Table II. *Significant results in univariate analysis concerning outcome in 97 patients hospitalized because of community-acquired pneumonia*

Variable	Outcome: Death within 6 months	Length of hospital stay	Duration of fever	Readmission
History of weight loss	–	–	–	–
TSF	*(−)	–	–	*
BMI	*(−)	–	–	–
APACHE II	*	**	–	**
PINI	–	***	–	–
PNI	–	**	*	–
Albumin	–	**(−)	**(−)	–
Transthyretin	–	*(−)	–	–
Transferrin	–	–	**(−)	*
CRP	–	**	–	–
Haptoglobin	–	*	**	–
Alfa-1-Antitrypsin	–	***	***	–
Orosomucoid	–	****	**	–

****$p < 0.0001$; ***$p < 0.001$; **$p < 0.01$; *$p < 0.05$.
–: NS; (−) = negative correlation.

TSF 13.9 and BMI 23.7, respectively, in the patients who survived the study period.

Course after discharge

21 of the 95 discharged patients (22%) were readmitted within 6 months. A high APACHE II score on admission was significantly correlated with readmittance, with a mean score of 11.0, compared with 8.6 in the patients not readmitted. To a lesser degree, a high TSF value and a high serum transferrin level were also found to be correlated with readmission (Table II). Three of the patients were readmitted because of malignancies. In all cases the malignant disease was unknown when the patient was enrolled in the study. The patients primary reason for readmittance is shown in Table III.

At follow-up, 8 weeks after discharge from hospital, 71 patients (76% of the patients alive at the time of the visit) were clinically examined and, of these, 78% had returned to their normal daily activities. The 26 patients who were not seen at the follow-up visit included 4 who died before the visit, 3 who were hospitalized, 7 who visited other physicians not involved in the study, and 12 patients who were unwilling to participate further in the study. At the follow-up visit 6 months after discharge, 63 patients were examined and, of these, 87% had returned to normal daily activities.

Chest X-ray 8 weeks after discharge showed complete (or nearly complete) resolution of infiltrates in 64/71 patients. All 7 patients with delayed X-ray resolution had an underlying chronic disease. In 5/7 patients with delayed X-ray resolution, subsequent radiography showed complete (or nearly complete) resolution. In the 2 remaining patients with delayed X-ray resolution, a bronchial carcinoma was later diagnosed in 1, while the other was lost to follow-up. No significant correlation between delayed recovery and delayed X-ray resolution was found for any of the 13 variables investigated.

Multivariate analysis of outcome

Admission data independently associated with a longer hospitalization were: high serum orosomucoid, high APACHE II score, high TSF, and a low BMI (Table IV). The mathematical model generated in the multivariate analysis predicted the time spent in hospital as follows:

$$\text{Predicted length of hospital stay (days)} = e^{0.35} \times \text{orosomucoid} - 0.04 \times \text{BMI} + 0.03 \times \text{TSF} + 0.06 \times \text{APACHE II score.}$$

When the serum acute-phase proteins were included one at a time in a mathematical model containing BMI, TSF and APACHE II, a significant correlation with length of hospital stay was found for all parameters except haptoglobin. The correlation was strongest for orosomucoid ($p < 0.0001$) and alfa-1-antitrypsin ($p < 0.0001$), but was also strong for CRP ($p = 0.01$).

Table III. *Primary reason for readmittance within 6 months in 21 patients discharged after hospitalization because of community-acquired pneumonia*

Diagnosis	Number of patients	Number of readmittances
Vascular diseases	5	8
Respiratory tract infections	5	5
Malignancies	3	5
Chronic obstructive pulmonary disease	1	3
Diabetes mellitus	1	2
Rheumatoid arthritis	1	2
Other	5	5

Table IV. *Summary of significant results in multivariate analysis concerning outcome in 97 patients hospitalized because of community-acquired pneumonia*

Independent variable	Outcome: Log length of hospital stay	Duration of fever	Readmission
TSF	**	*	*
BMI	* (−)	−	−
APACHE II	***	−	**
Log Alfa-1-Antitrypsin	−	***	−
Orosomucoid	****	−	−

****$p < 0.0001$; ***$p < 0.001$; **$p < 0.01$; *$p < 0.05$.
−: NS; (−) = negative correlation.

High admission levels of alfa-1-antitrypsin were closely associated with longer duration of fever and a weak association was also found between TSF and this outcome variable ($p = 0.0497$). In a mathematical model containing TSF and including one of the serum acute-phase proteins at a time, a significant correlation was found for alfa-1-antitrypsin ($p = 0.0001$) and orosomucoid ($p = 0.01$), but not for CRP or haptoglobin.

Patients with high APACHE II score and TSF on admission were more likely to be readmitted within 6 months after discharge. Six of 14 patients (43%) with both an APACHE II score and a TSF above the median level (8 for APACHE II score and 13 for TSF) were readmitted, compared with 0/20 for those with an APACHE II score and TSF at or below the median level. In patients with an APACHE II score or a TSF above the median level, 28% and 24%, respectively, were readmitted. There were too few deaths to include this outcome variable in the multivariate analysis. Neither were the outcome variables 'delayed recovery' or 'delayed X-ray resolution' included due to the complete lack of correlation for any of the 13 variables investigated in the univariate analysis.

DISCUSSION

This is, to our knowledge, the first attempt to analyse the impact of nutritional and inflammatory factors on the prognosis for middle-aged and elderly patients hospitalized because of CAP. Of the investigated serum proteins, only alfa-1-antitrypsin and orosomucoid were independently associated with hospital morbidity, measured as length of hospital stay and duration of fever. APACHE II score was also found to be predictive for days spent in hospital, as well as for mortality and readmission. There was no absolute discriminatory level that separated surviving patients from those who were destined to die within 6 months, but all patients with an APACHE II score of ≤ 8 survived.

TSF and BMI are documented as measures of nutritional status in clinical and epidemiological studies (18, 19). In agreement with earlier studies (20) we found that malnutrition, reflected by low TSF and BMI values, was correlated with death. In the multivariate analysis however, TSF was positively correlated with all three outcome variables (fever, length of stay, readmission), whereas BMI was negatively correlated with length of hospital stay. These conflicting observations could perhaps be explained by the fact that, although mutually correlated (18), TSF is a measure of body fat, while BMI measures both body fat and muscle mass. The prognostic importance of high TSF values may thus speak in favour of a greater morbidity in patients with excess body fat.

PNI and PINI both correlated significantly, or almost significantly, with the same end-points as albumin: length of hospital stay and duration of fever. No correlation was found between these indices and other investigated end-points, i.e. they offered no extra prognostic information, in comparison with albumin. For PNI, this is in accordance with earlier findings, where albumin was found to be the most important of the four nutritional markers included in the index (21). In the PINI, albumin, orosomucoid and transthyretin have a rather narrow distribution range, around 1 : 2–1 : 4, while CRP can rise several hundred-fold (8, 22). Accordingly, CRP has been shown to be the principal determinant of the PINI values in conditions with a pronounced phlogistic reaction (23). However, in the present study neither CRP nor PINI was independently correlated to any of the outcome variables. A possible explanation for this is the difference in turnover rate between the acute-phase proteins. The half-life for CRP is 4–6 h, compared with 5–7 days for orosomucoid and alfa-1-antitrypsin (23). The patients entered our study after a median illness duration of 4 days, and some patients had already received antibiotics before admission. Possibly the patient's CRP concentrations may already have been declining from a peak before admission, while orosomucoid and alfa-1-antitrypsin better reflected the actual state of inflammation at admission in the individual patient.

The largest report on the prognosis of CAP patients admitted to hospital is a study from the British Thoracic Society (BTS) (3). In that study, the 3 most predictive features for death were a respiratory rate of ≥ 30/min, a diastolic blood pressure of ≤ 60 mmHg, and confusion. Patients with at least 2 of these 3 risk factors ran a 10-fold higher mortality risk. In the present study, none of the patients had all 3, but 8 patients had 2 of the risk factors. Only 1 of these 8 patients died (after discharge) during the 6-month study period.

In the BTS study, as reported by others (1, 7, 24–26), patients with hypoalbuminemia on admission had a higher morbidity. This finding was also confirmed in the present study. In the univariate analysis, patients with low serum concentrations on admission had a significantly longer hospital stay, and significantly more days spent with fever after admission. In contrast to our earlier findings (1) the albumin level on admission in the present study was not correlated with mortality. A possible explanation for this could be the low number of fatal cases with a subsequent risk for 'false-negative' results (type II, or beta, errors).

At our Department, serum albumin and CRP are routinely measured in all patients on admission. In this study, serum albumin and CRP were both associated with hospital morbidity measured as duration of fever and days spent in hospital. However, the most significant association with these two outcome variables was found for alfa-1-antitrypsin and orosomucoid. When measuring alfa-1-antitrypsin and orosomucoid the same technique is used as when measuring CRP, and the cost of the analysis is the same. Perhaps measurement of serum levels of alfa-1-antitrypsin and orosomucoid on admission should be considered in order to better predict hospital morbidity in this patient category. Our findings do not support the use of the prognostic indices PNI and PINI in this category, as they are more complicated to calculate and prognostically are no more informative than the serum albumin level. However, measurement of APACHE II and TSF on admission may give additional prognostic information on the interval from admission to 6 months after discharge.

ACKNOWLEDGEMENTS

This project was supported by grants from the Swedish Heart-Lung Foundation and Karolinska Institutet. We thank Ragna Lindberger, Kabi Pharmacia AB, Sweden for kindly providing the TSF measuring instrument.

REFERENCES

1. Örtqvist Å, Hedlund J, Grillner L, Jalonen E, Kallings I, Leinonen M, Kalin M. Aetiology, outcome and prognostic factors in community-acquired pneumonia requiring hospitalisation. Eur Respir J 3: 1105–1113, 1990.
2. Marrie TJ, Durant H, Yates L. Community-acquired pneumonia requiring hospitalisation: 5-year prospective study. Rev Infect Dis 11: 586–599, 1989.

3. Harrison BDW, Farr BM, Pugh S, Selkon JB. Community-acquired pneumonia in adults in British hospitals in 1982–1983: a survey of aetiology, mortality, prognostic factors and outcome. Q J Med 62: 195–220, 1987.
4. Sullivan RJ, Dowdle WR, Marine WM, Hierholzer JC. Adult pneumonia in a general hospital. Arch Intern Med 129: 935–942, 1972.
5. Venkatesan P, Gladman J, Macfarlane JT, Barer D, Berman P, Kinnear W, RG Finch. A hospital study of community acquired pneumonia in the elderly. Thorax 45: 254–258, 1990.
6. Hedlund UJ, Örtqvist ÅB, Kalin ME, Granath F. Factors of importance for the long term prognosis after hospital treated pneumonia. Thorax 48: 785–789, 1993.
7. Randle NW, Hubert-Hartmann K, Mulheran LC. Serum albumin levels: Relationship to length of hospital stay. Hosp Pharm 19: 802–805, 1984.
8. Pressac M, Vignoli L, Aymard P, Ingenbleek Y. Usefulness of a prognostic inflammatory and nutritional index in paediatric clinical practice. Clin Chim Acta 188: 129–136, 1990.
9. Ingenbleek Y. Usefulness of prealbumin as nutritional indicator. In: Allen RC, Bienvenu J, Laurent P, Suskind RM, eds. Marker proteins in inflammation, vol. 1. Berlin: Walter de Gruyter, 405–414, 1982.
10. Birch HE, Schreiber G. Transcriptional regulation of plasma protein synthesis during inflammation. J Biol Chem 261: 8077–8080, 1986.
11. Moshage HJ, Janssen JAM, Franssen JH, Hafkenscheid JCM, Yap SH. Study of the molecular mechanism of decreased liver synthesis of albumin in inflammation. J Clin Invest 79: 165–1641, 1987.
12. Mullen JL, Buzby GP, Waldman M, Gertner MH, Hobbs CL, Rosato EF. Prediction of operative morbidity and mortality by preoperative nutritional assessment. Surg Forum 30: 80–82, 1979.
13. Niederman MS, Merrill WW, Ferranti RD, Pagano KM, Palmer LB, Reynolds HY. Nutritional status and bacterial binding in the lower respiratory tract in patients with chronic tracheostomy. Ann Intern Med 100: 795–800, 1984.
14. Niederman MS, Mantovani R, Schoch P, Papas J, Fein AM. Patterns and routes of tracheobronchial colonisation in mechanically ventilated patients. Chest 95: 155–161, 1989,
15. Ingenbleek Y, Carpentier YA. A prognostic inflammatory and nutritional index scoring critically ill patients. Int J Vitam Nutr Res 55: 91–101, 1985.
16. Knaus WA, Draper EA, Wagner DP, Zimmerman JE. APACHE II: A severity of disease classification system. Crit Care Med 13: 818–829, 1985.
17. Daley J, Jencks S, Draper D, Lenhart G, Thomas N, Walker J. Predicting hospital-associated mortality for medicare patients. JAMA 260: 3617–3624, 1988.
18. Must A, Dallal GE, Dietz WH. Reference data for obesity: 85th and 95th percentiles of body mass index (wt/ht^2) and triceps skinfold thickness. Am J Clin Nutr 53: 839–846, 1991.
19. Menotti A, Descovich GC, Lanti M, Spagnolo A, Dormi A, Seccareccia F. Indexes of obesity and all-causes mortality in Italian epidemiological data. Prev Med 22; 293–303, 1993.
20. Salive ME, Satterfield S, Ostfeld AM, Wallace RB, Havlik RJ. Disability and cognitive impairment are risk factors for pneumonia-related mortality in older adults. Public Health Rep 108: 314–322, 1993.
21. Buzby GP, Mullen JL, Matthews DC, Hobbs CL, Rosato EF. Prognostic nutritional index in gastrointestinal surgery. Am J Surg 139: 160–167, 1980.
22. Kushner I. The phenomenon of the acute phase response. Ann NY Acad Sci 389: 39–48, 1982.
23. Vehe KL, Brown RO, Kuhl DA. The prognostic inflammatory and nutritional index in traumatized patients receiving enteral nutrition support. J Am Coll Nutr 10: 355–363, 1991.
24. Herrmann FR, Safran C, Levkoff SE, Minaker KL. Serum albumin level on admission as a predictor of death, length of stay and readmission. Arch Intern Med 152: 125–130, 1992.
25. Andersson CF, Wochos DN. The utility of serum albumin values in the nutritional assessment of hospitalised patients. Mayo Clin Proc 57: 181–184, 1982.
26. Warnold I, Lundholm K. Clinical significance of preoperative nutritional status in 215 noncancer patients. Ann Surg 199: 299–305, 1984.

Submitted September 13, 1994; accepted November 13, 1994

Scand J Infect Dis 27: 39–43, 1995 ORIGINAL ARTICLE

Endotoxin, Interleukin-6 and Phospholipase-A2 as Markers of Sepsis in Patients with Hematological Malignancies

ESA RINTALA,[1] KARI PULKKI,[2] JUSSI MERTSOLA,[3] TIMO NEVALAINEN[4] and JUKKA NIKOSKELAINEN[1]

From the Departments of [1]Medicine, [2]Clinical Chemistry and [4]Pathology, University of Turku, and the [3]National Health Institute, and Department of Pediatrics, Turku University Central Hospital, Turku, Finland

The concentrations of endotoxin, interleukin-6 (IL-6) and group II phospholipase-A2 (PLA2-II) were measured in serum or plasma during cytotoxic chemotherapy, fever of unknown origin and sepsis in 56 patients with hematological malignancies and during sepsis and viral infections in 22 non-hematological patients. High concentrations of IL-6, PLA2-II and endotoxin were detected in sepsis, the levels being similarly elevated in hematological and non-hematological patients. The levels of IL-6 and PLA2-II correlated closely with that of C-reactive protein (CRP). The levels of PLA2-II and IL-6 declined earlier than the level of CRP during the course of antimicrobial treatment. The levels of IL-6 also rose earlier than the level of CRP. The ability of IL-6 and PLA2-II and endotoxin to discriminate between sepsis and other causes of fever was comparable to that of CRP. IL-6 and PLA2-II are, together with CRP, valuable tools for the detection of sepsis in patients with hematological malignancies who undergo cytotoxic medication. Endotoxin is not suitable for routine laboratory diagnosis of sepsis.

E. Rintala, MD, Department of Medicine, University of Turku, FIN-20520 Turku, Finland

INTRODUCTION

C-reactive protein (CRP) has proved to be an early and reliable indicator of sepsis in patients with hematological malignancies (1). Inflammatory mediators such as interleukin-6 (IL-6) and group II phospholipase-A2 (PLA2-II) have been shown to be correlated with infection-related manifestations, e.g. fever and the acute-phase reaction, the severity of sepsis and the outcome in both hematological and non-hematological patients (2–5). Endotoxin has also been used for detecting sepsis (6).

To our knowledge, there are no published reports in which endotoxin, IL-6 and PLA2-II have been compared with CRP for the detection of sepsis in patients with hematological malignancies.

The aims of the present study were: 1) to determine the levels of circulating IL-6, PLA2-II and endotoxin in hematological patients during cytotoxic chemotherapy, fever and sepsis and in non-hematological patients during sepsis and viral infections; 2) to examine the relationship between the levels of IL-6, PLA2-II, endotoxin and CRP, and 3) to assess the clinical usefulness of endotoxin, IL-6 and PLA2-II for the diagnosis of sepsis and in the follow-up of antimicrobial treatment in patients with hematological malignancies.

MATERIAL AND METHODS

Endotoxin, IL-6, PLA2-II and CRP were analysed in 34 patients with hematological malignancies and in 22 non-hematological patients admitted to the Departments of Medicine and Infectious Diseases at Turku University Central Hospital and to Turku Military Hospital. In addition, endotoxin, IL-6, PLA2-II and CRP were analysed in 22 afebrile patients with hematological malignancies who received cytotoxic chemotherapy at the Department of Medicine at Turku University Central Hospital. For control purposes, endotoxin, IL-6 and PLA2-II levels were determined in 35 healthy blood donors. The inclusion criteria for the patients with infections were: an axillary temperature of at least 38°C >12 h, and the presence of a microbiologically documented bacterial or viral infection, or a suspicion of such an infection.

The afebrile patients with hematological malignancies who underwent cytotoxic treatment and the febrile hematological patients all received intravenous cytotoxic treatment capable of inducing neutropenia (neutrophil count $<1.0 \times 10^9$/l). 32 patients (57%) with hematological malignancies were neutropenic. Table I lists the diagnoses of the hematological patients and the number in each patient category.

Ten non-hematological patients had a viral infection and 12 had a blood culture positive sepsis. In the group with viral infections, 4 patients had a respiratory tract infection caused by Influenza A virus, 3 had tonsillitis caused by Epstein-Barr virus and 3 had chickenpox. Table II shows the bacterial isolates in sepsis. The underlying disease was known in 8/12 non-hematological patients with sepsis. One patient had anorexia nervosa, 1 had duodenal cancer, 1 had diabetes mellitus, 1 had pernicious anemia and 1 had partial complement defect. Of the 3 patients who had sepsis caused by Candida sp., 1 had colorectal cancer (not operated), 1 had nosocomial sepsis in the intensive care unit and 1 had a hypopharyngeal carcinoma (operated).

Of the 56 patients with hematological malignancies, 33 were male and 23 female, mean age 54 yrs (range 17–76 yrs). Of the 22 non-hematological patients, 12 were male and 10 female, age 47 yrs (17–82 yrs). Of the 35 healthy control patients, 21 were male and 14 female, age 43 yrs (19–71 yrs).

 ISSN 0036-5548

Table I. *The diagnoses of the patients in each patient category*

Diagnosis	Cytotoxic treatment *n*	Fever of unknown origin *n*	Sepsis *n*
Acute myeloblastic leukemia (M1–5)	6	7	4
Malignant lymphoma	7	3	3
Multiple myeloma	5	8	1
Acute lymphoblastic leukemia	3	5	1
Aplastic anemia	1		
Chronic myelocytic leukemia		1	
Myelodysplastic syndrome			1
Total	22	24	10

Table II. *Blood culture isolates and numbers of patients*

Isolate	Patients with hematological malignancies *n*	Patients without hematological malignancies *n*
Escherichia coli	4	4
Candida albicans		3
Coagulase-negative staphylococci	2	
Streptococcus viridans	2	
Staphylococcus aureus		2
Pseudomonas sp.	1	
Streptococcus pneumoniae	1	1
Enterobacter sp.		1
Haemophilus influenzae		1
Total	10	12

Antimicrobial treatment was initiated after taking the first blood sample for culture and biochemical analyses. Subsequent samples were taken after 12, 24 and 48 h. The first blood samples from the afebrile hematological patients undergoing cytotoxic treatment were taken just before the initiation of a new cytotoxic treatment cycle and 3, 7 and 14 days thereafter. Blood samples for bacterial culture were taken simultaneously from febrile patients.

The medians and ranges of the intervals between the onset of fever and the initiation of blood sampling were as follows: 1.5 days (0.5–6 days) in the group with fever of unknown origin, 2 d (1–14 d) in the hematological sepsis group, 2 d (1–20 d) in the non-hematological sepsis group and 3.5 d (1–9 d) in the viral infections group.

The concentration of IL-6 in plasma was determined by a sandwich-type of ELISA (Quantikine[R], Research & Diagnostic Systems Inc., Minneapolis, MN, USA) according to manufacturer's instructions. The detection limit was 0.4 ng/l. The concentration of PLA2-II in serum was determined by a time-resolved fluoro-immunoassay (7), whose detection limit was 0.65 μg/l. The concentration of endotoxin in plasma was determined by a chromogenic Limulus assay using a microtitre modification (Coatest[R], Chromogenix AB, Mölndal, Sweden) (8); detection limit 5 ng/l. The concentration of C-reactive protein (CRP) in serum was determined by immunoturbidimetry. The upper limit of the reference interval was 10 mg/l.

Statistical analyses

Correlations were measured by Spearman's rank correlation coefficient. The IL-6 and endotoxin levels in subgroups were compared with the Kruskal-Wallis test. The means of PLA2-II in the subgroups were compared with one-way analysis of variance. All analyses were done with the SAS[TM] statistical analysis software (SAS Institute Inc., Cary, NC, USA).

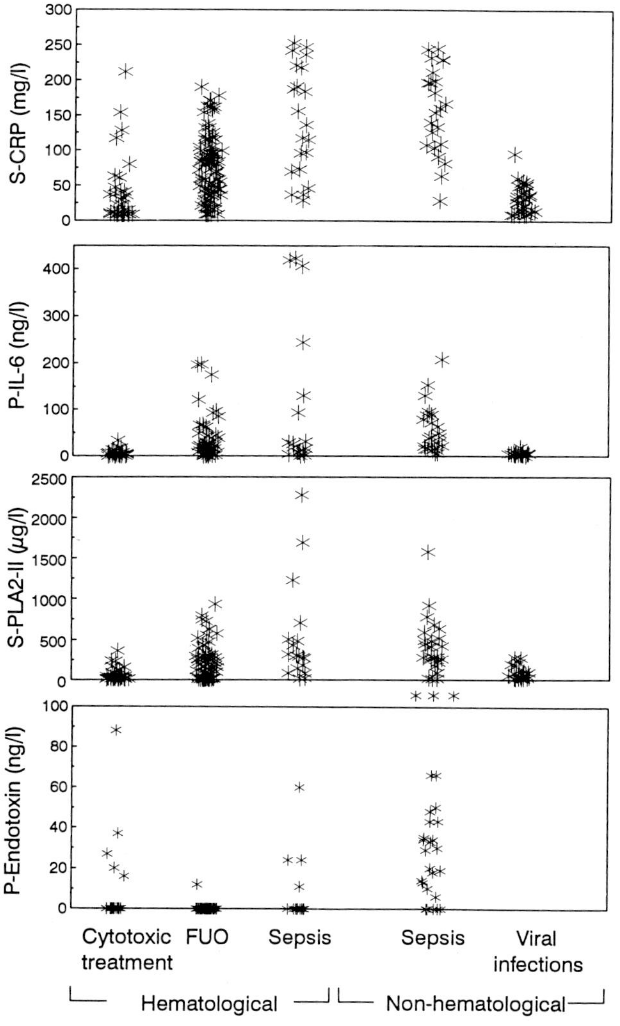

Fig. 1. The concentrations of CRP endotoxin, IL-6 and PLA2-II in each patient group. FUO = fever of unknown origin.

RESULTS

The median concentration of IL-6 in the plasma of 35 healthy blood donors was 1.4 ng/l (range <0.4–3.2 ng/l). The median concentration of PLA2-II in serum of controls was 3.6 μg/l (95% reference interval, 1.3–10.8 μg/l) (7). The concentration of endotoxin in the plasma was below the detection limit in all controls.

Fig. 1 shows the concentrations of CRP, endotoxin, IL-6 and PLA2-II in each patient group. Fig. 2 shows the concentrations of CRP, IL-6, PLA2-II and endotoxin in each patient as a function of time.

IL-6, PLA2-II, endotoxin and CRP were detectable in afebrile patients undergoing cytotoxic chemotherapy, although there were no signs of infection in any of these patients. CRP was elevated (>10 mg/l) in 84% of the patients with normal IL-6 and in 75% of the patients with normal PLA2-II.

The concentrations of IL-6, PLA2-II and endotoxin did not differ significantly in sepsis between patients with vs. without hematological malignancies ($p = 0.231$, 0.721, 0.786 and 0.214, for IL-6, PLA2-II, endotoxin and CRP, respectively). The concentrations of each analyte declined during the course of antimicrobial treatment.

The concentration of IL-6 was correlated significantly with the concentration of CRP ($p < 0.001$). The concentration of PLA2-II correlated significantly with the concentration of CRP ($p < 0.001$) and IL-6 ($p < 0.001$). Fig. 3 shows that the relative concentrations of PLA2-II and IL-6 were significantly lower than the concentration of CRP at 24 h and 48 h in the group with fever of unknown origin and at 48 h in the sepsis group. The relative concentration of IL-6 was significantly higher than the concentration of CRP at 0 h and 12 h in the 'fever of unknown origin' group.

The diagnostic sensitivities and specificities of the concentrations of IL-6, PLA2-II, endotoxin and CRP in the first blood samples obtained at admission were plotted on the ROC curve (Fig. 4). The sensitivity of CRP was 100% at the cut-off levels between <10 and 61 mg/l. The sensitivity of each analyte declined with the increase specificity. The area under the ROC curve (AUC) was 0.698 for CRP, 0.690 for IL-6, 0.783 for PLA2-II and 0.807 for endotoxin.

DISCUSSION

As shown in Fig. 1, a remarkable overlapping was found in the concentrations of CRP between the cytotoxic chemotherapy group and the sepsis group; CRP was increased up to 200 mg/l in non-infected patients receiving cytotoxic chemotherapy. CRP was elevated in 84% of the patients with normal IL-6 and in 75% of those with normal PLA2-II. Much less overlapping was noted regarding the concentrations of IL-6 and PLA2-II between the cytotoxic treatment group and the sepsis group. Because the concentrations of IL-6 and PLA2-II were seemingly not unspecifically elevated by cytotoxic chemotherapy, they can obviously be used more reliably than CRP as markers of viral infection on the one hand and sepsis on the other, in patients receiving cytotoxic chemotherapy.

A distinct rise in the level of each analyte took place in 'fever of unknown origin'. The concentrations of IL-6 and PLA2-II were much lower in viral infections than in

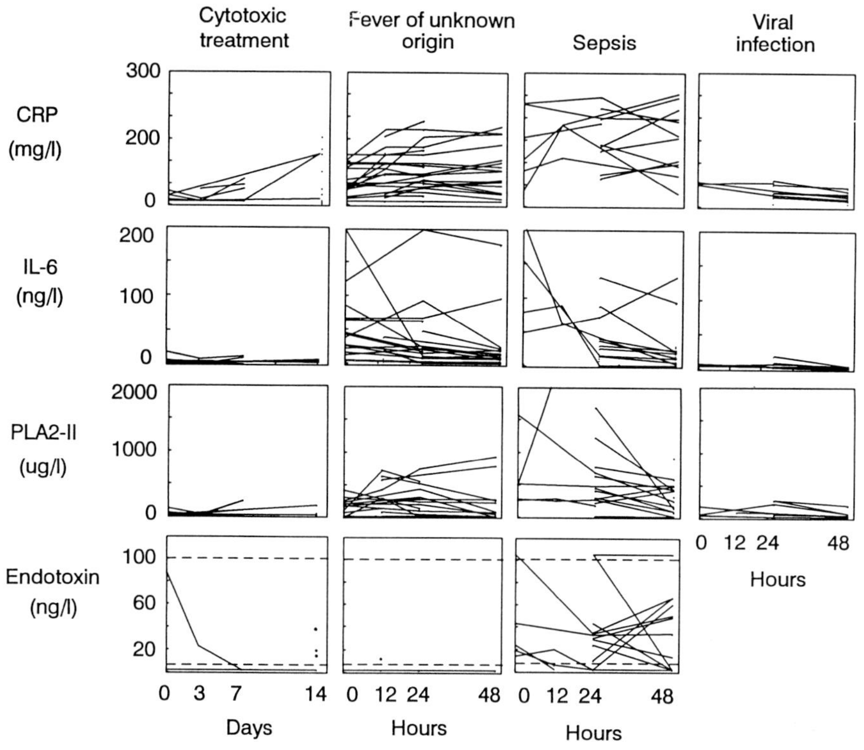

Fig. 2. The concentrations of CRP, IL-6, PLA2-II and endotoxin in each patient as a function of time. The detection limits of the Limulus assay for endotoxin (5 and 100 mg/l) are marked with dotted lines. Zero indicates the day when the cytotoxic treatment cycle was started ('Cytotoxic treatment') or the day when the patient was admitted to hospital ('Fever of unknown origin', 'Sepsis' and 'Viral infection') and the antimicrobial treatment was begun (FUO and 'Sepsis').

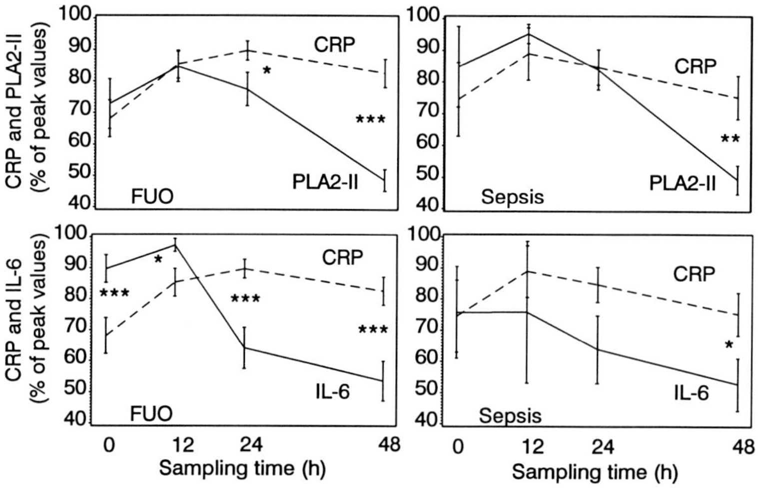

Fig. 3. The relative concentrations of PLA2-II and IL-6 compared with the relative concentration of CRP. The statistical significances between the relative concentrations are marked with asterisks (*$p = 0.05$, **$p = 0.01$, ***$p \leq 0.001$).

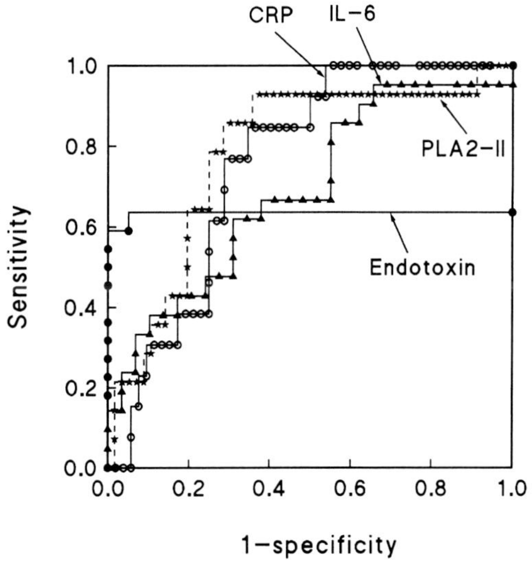

Fig. 4. The receiver operating characteristic (ROC) curves for the variables CRP, PLA2-II, endotoxin and IL-6 in the distinction between sepsis and other causes of fever. Sensitivity (true positive rate, i.e. number of the patients with sepsis who have an elevated concentration of a variable/total number of patients with sepsis) and one minus specificity (false-positive rate, i.e. number of non-septic patients who have an elevated concentration of a variable/ total number of non-septic patients) of each analyte were calculated at each level (cut-off points) obtained from the first blood samples taken on admission. The values were plotted to form a curve. The discriminatory power of each variable can be compared by estimating the area under the curve. The curve that extends close to the upper left corner of the diagram (i.e. the area under the curve is close to 1.0) denotes high discrimination of sepsis by that variable.

fever of unknown origin. These findings indicate that, in most cases, fever of unknown origin was due to bacterial infection. The decline in the concentrations of these analytes during antimicrobial treatment further supports this conclusion.

The concentrations of IL-6, PLA2-II and CRP were high in sepsis and declined during the antimicrobial treatment. The levels of IL-6, PLA2-II and CRP did not differ significantly between hematological and non-hematological patients. It seems obvious, therefore, that patients with hematological malignancies who undergo cytotoxic chemotherapy are able to respond to sepsis in a way similar to patients without hematological malignancy.

A close agreement between the concentrations of IL-6 and PLA2-II on the one hand and between the concentrations of IL-6 and CRP on the other is a logical consequence of the physiological relationship between IL-6 and the acute phase reaction (4). This association was evident in patients with hematological malignancies as well as in non-hematological patients.

According to contemporary literature, it is obvious that IL-6 and PLA2-II reflect earlier biological events in the chain of inflammatory reactions than does CRP (3–5, 9, 10). In the present study, the concentrations of PLA2-II and IL-6 declined more quickly than that of CRP, both in the 'fever of unknown origin' group and in the sepsis group. Moreover, the concentration of IL-6 in the former group was initially higher than that of CRP. Therefore, IL-6 and PLA2-II can be used as earlier indicators of the resolution of inflammatory reaction than CRP, IL-6 can even be used as an earlier indicator of the onset of infection than CRP.

As shown in the ROC curve, the maximum sensitivity of CRP was 100% (at cut-off levels ranging between 10–61 mg/l). The maximum sensitivity of IL-6 and PLA2-II was less than that of CRP. However, sensitivity was achieved at the expense of specificity: the maximum specificities of CRP, IL-6 and PLA2-II were at most 60% or lower when the sensitivities exceeded 80%.

No striking differences were noted between the AUCs of each analyte. Therefore, the discriminative powers of IL-6 and PLA2-II were at least comparable to that of CRP.

Furthermore, PLA2 carries out specific tasks in the host defence against bacterial infections (5, 11). It plays an essential role in the neutrophil and macrophage function and in the degradation of the bacterial membranes (11). The levels of PLA2 in serum are associated with the severity of sepsis and septic shock (5). Therefore PLA2-II can be regarded as a specific, acute-phase reactant against bacterial infections, and is also involved in the pathogenesis of sepsis and septic shock.

For these reasons, IL-6 and PLA2-II are valuable indicators of septic inflammation and have kinetic and biochemical properties superior to those of CRP. They can be used in addition to CRP or even instead of it, for the rapid diagnosis of sepsis in hematological patients and when following up the effect of antimicrobial treatment. Endotoxin had a sensitivity of 60% but was highly specific for sepsis. However, the laborious analytical techniques needed, due to the high risk of endotoxin contamination and its low diagnostic sensitivity, reduce the usefulness of the Limulus assay for routine laboratory diagnosis of sepsis.

In conclusion: septic patients had high concentrations of IL-6, PLA2-II and CRP. Cytotoxic chemotherapy neither reduced nor enhanced the response of IL-6 and PLA2-II in sepsis. Although the maximum diagnostic sensitivities of IL-6 and PLA2-II did not exceed that of CRP, IL-6 and PLA2-II had discriminatory power comparable to that of CRP in sepsis. Furthermore, their biological and kinetic properties favour the use of IL-6 and PLA2-II vis-à-vis CRP for the detection of sepsis in hematological malignancies. Endotoxin had no apparent advantages in this context.

ACKNOWLEDGEMENTS

The authors thank Ms. Birgitta Aittanen and Ms. Sinikka Kollanus for skilful technical assistance, and the staff of the Department of Infectious Diseases, Turku University Central Hospital and the Turku Military Hospital for, cooperation.

REFERENCES

1. Deodhar S. C-reactive protein: clinical applications in monitoring disease activity. Clin Immunol Newsletter 11: 138–143, 1991.
2. Waage A, Steinshamn S. Cytokine mediators of septic infections in the normal and granulocytopenic host. Eur J Haematol 50: 243–249, 1993.
3. Rintala E, Nevalainen T. Synovial-type (group II) phospholipase A2 in serum of febrile patients with haematological malignancy. Eur J Haematol 50: 11–16, 1993.
4. Whicher J, Evans S. Cytokines in disease. Clin Chem 36: 1269–1281, 1990.
5. Pruzanski W, Vadas P. Phospholipase A2 - a mediator between proximal and distal effectors of inflammation. Immunol Today 12: 143–146, 1991.
6. Bayston KF, Cohen J. Bacterial endotoxin and current concepts in the diagnosis and treatment of endotoxaemia. J Med Microbiol 311: 73–83, 1990.
7. Nevalainen T, Kortesuo P, Rintala E, Märki F. Immunochemical detection of group I and group II phospholipases A2 in human serum. Clin Chem 38: 1824–1829, 1992.
8. Mertsola J, Cope L, Munford R, McCracken G Jr, Hansen E. Detection of experimental Haemophilus influenzae type b bacteremia and endotoxemia by means of an immunolimulus assay. J Infect Dis 164: 353–358, 1991.
9. Söderquist B, Sundqvist K-G, Vikefors T. Kinetics of serum levels of interleukin–6 in Staphylococcus aureus septicemia. Scand J Infect Dis 24: 607–612, 1992.
10. Crowl R, Stoller T, Conroy R, Stoner C. Induction of phospholipase A2 gene expression in human hepatoma cells by mediators of the acute phase response. J Biol Chem 266: 2647–2651, 1991.
11. Elsbach P, Weiss J. Phagocytosis of bacteria and phospholipid degradation. Biochim Biophys Acta 947: 29–52, 1988.

Submitted May 18, 1994; accepted October 27, 1994

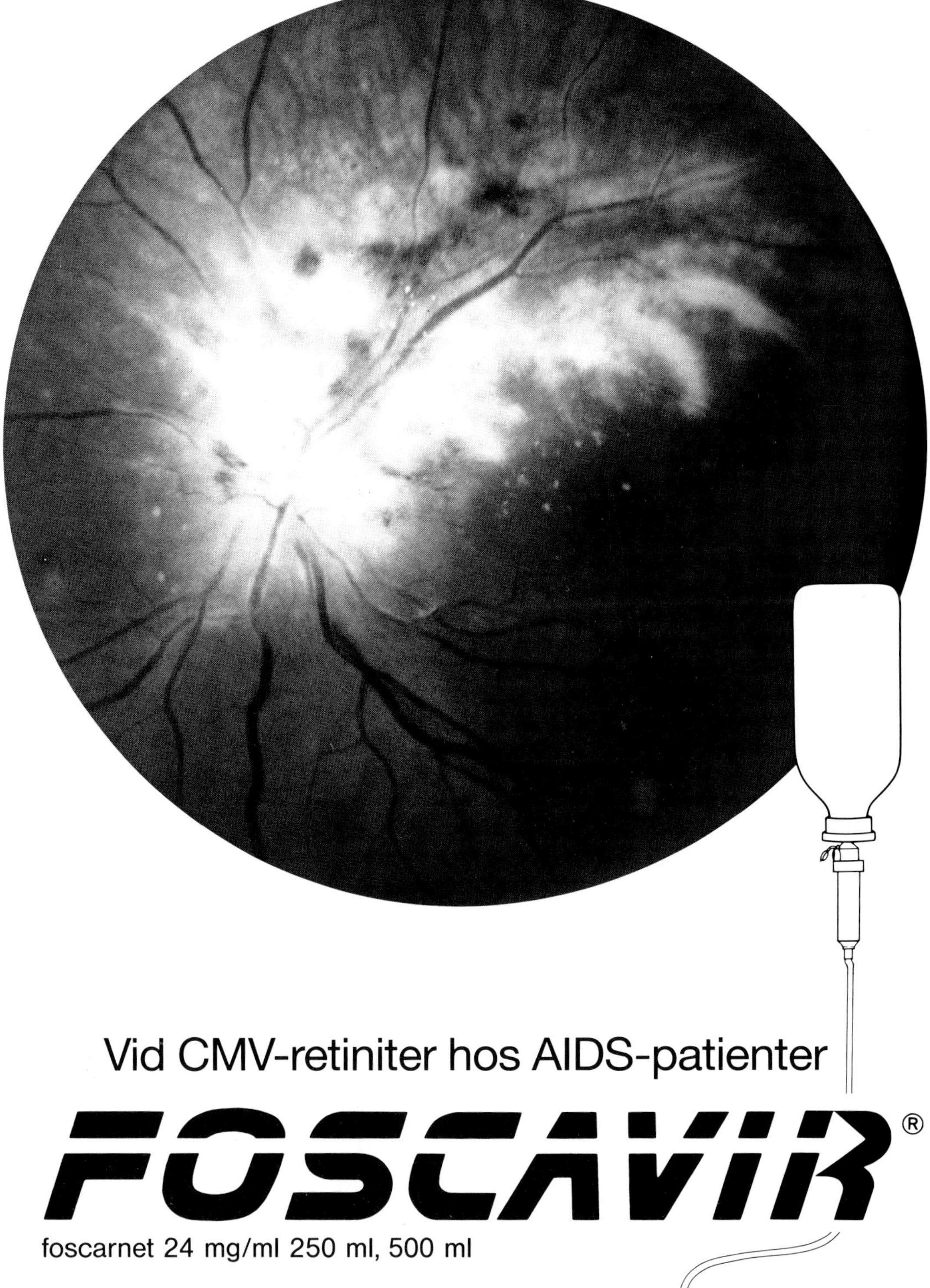
Vid CMV-retiniter hos AIDS-patienter
FOSCAVIR®
foscarnet 24 mg/ml 250 ml, 500 ml
Astra Läkemedel
S-151 85 Södertälje

Scand J Infect Dis 27: 45–49, 1995 ORIGINAL ARTICLE

Disk Diffusion Susceptibility Tests: Need for Laboratory-Specific Breakpoints

RAIJA MANNINEN[1], ERKKI EEROLA[2] and PENTTI HUOVINEN[1]

[1]From the Antimicrobial Research Laboratory, National Public Health Institute, and the [2]Department of Medical Microbiology, Turku University, Turku, Finland

Significant changes were observed in the measured resistance levels of Escherichia coli and Staphylococcus aureus when the Biodisk® disk susceptibility test method used in 1992 was replaced with another commercial method, Oxoid®. For example, when non-species-specific breakpoints were used, the frequency of cephalotin-resistant E. coli was 12% of all isolates in 1992 but only 4% in 1993; the corresponding figures for the intermediately resistant isolates were 84% and 8%. The population distribution histograms were however, practically unchanged. Thus, the resistance percentages apparently did not reflect the real development of resistance. Similar findings were also made for several other antimicrobials. Susceptibility test breakpoints should therefore be examined separately for all bacterial species in each laboratory, and the application of adjusted laboratory-specific breakpoints should be considered. For this purpose, the WHONET computer program provides excellent assistance.

R. Manninen, MD, Antimicrobial Research Laboratory, National Public Health Institute, Kiinamyllynkatu 13, FIN-20520 Turku, Finland

INTRODUCTION

Susceptibility tests are usually carried out in clinical microbiological laboratories by using commercial disk diffusion methods. The interpretation of zone sizes and conversion to SIR-classes follow the guidelines provided by the manufacturers. Despite attempts to standardize these methods, there is a wide variation in the performance of different laboratories (1–3).

Shared breakpoints were formerly used for all aerobic bacterial species. However, although species-specific breakpoints are those currently generally accepted, there is still a need for laboratory-specific breakpoints (2–5).

The minimal inhibitory concentration (MIC) breakpoints are based on 3 factors: bacterial population distribution, the antibiotic concentration attainable in blood or tissues, and the clinical response in infection caused by bacteria with known MICs (6). The zone breakpoints are calculated from the regression line between the MIC for bacterial isolates and the corresponding inhibition zone diameters around the antibiotic disk. In addition, the distribution of zone sizes of a series of bacterial isolates may be determined and the breakpoints selected on the basis of the distribution of susceptible and resistant populations (2, 7).

We found striking differences in the resistance figures of several bacterial species when we changed the commercial disk susceptibility test system. Nevertheless, the distributions of zone diameters changed only slightly. This study compares how the results of two different disk susceptibility test methods fell into the S, I and R categories.

MATERIALS AND METHODS

The Department of Medical Microbiology of the University of Turku receives clinical samples for diagnostic bacterial culture from regional hospitals and health centers. The laboratory changed the supplier of susceptibility disks and medium in November 1992 from Biodisk® (Ab Biodisk, Solna, Sweden) to Oxoid® (Unipath Ltd., Basingstoke, England). The material was selected so that Biodisk® was used for strains in 1992 and Oxoid® for strains in 1993. The numbers of bacterial strains in 1992 and 1993 were: 499 and 3,047 for Escherichia coli, 1,951 and 1,705 for Staphylococcus aureus, 564 and 993 for Enterococcus sp., 542 and 751 for Pseudomonas aeruginosa, 323 and 275 for Streptococcus pneumoniae, 242 and 224 for Haemophilus influenzae, 141 and 174 for Moraxella catarrhalis.

Some antimicrobials were chosen for closer examination. In 1992, the ampicillin susceptibility of 499 and the cephalothin susceptibility of 484 isolates of Escherichia coli was tested. In 1993, the respective numbers were 357 and 3,045. 109 isolates of Staphylococcus aureus were tested for susceptibility to cefaclor in 1992 and 129 in 1993.

Susceptibility tests were carried out according to the guidelines provided by the local representatives of the manufacturers of both tests. The susceptibility results were based on the zone diameters, determined with a caliper rule.

The validity of the species-specific breakpoints for seven common pathogens was evaluated visually from the histograms. The main point determined was whether or not the breakpoints split a homogeneous population. General breakpoints were used for M. catarrhalis because species-specific breakpoints were not available.

The breakpoints selected for closer examination were studied in 2 phases:

Phase I. Susceptibility was determined according to the breakpoints routinely used (Table I). The breakpoints for Biodisk® were not species-specific in 1992 (8), but in 1993 the breakpoints of Oxoid® partially followed the NCCLS standards for species specificity (9).

Phase II. The proportion of resistant strains was calculated by using species-specific breakpoints (Table I), as defined by *Referensgrupp for antibiotikafrågor* in Sweden (RAF) for Biodisk® (10) and Oxoid® (11).

Analysis of the histograms was performed by using the WHONET computer program (12). The WHONET project was established to monitor the patterns of bacterial resistance in clinical microbiology laboratories. The program is freely available to laboratories participating in the WHONET project.

 ISSN 0036-5548

Table I. *Breakpoints for Biodisk® and Oxoid® disk diffusion test methods*

I, General breakpoints for all bacterial species. II, Species-specific breakpoints for the bacteria studied.

Antimicrobial content (μg)	Inhibition zone diameter (mm) Biodisk® R	I	S	Oxoid® R	I	S
Ampicillin 10						
I	≤11	12–24	≥25	≤13	14–16	≥17
II	≤11	12–24	≥25	≤11	12–24	≥25
Cephalothin 30						
I	≤17	18–29	≥30	≤14	15–17	≥18
II	≤13	14-26	≥27	≤13	14–26	≥27
Cefaclor 30						
I	≤19	20–32	≥33	≤14	15–17	≥18
II		[a]			[a]	

[a] Oxacillin-resistant strains are reported as resistant.

The results of the susceptibility tests were saved in the UNIX/MUMPS database and stored in a minicomputer. The data on bacterial isolates were transformed to WHONET files with a data conversion program. The diameters of the inhibition zones in the disk diffusion tests were plotted as histograms, with the frequency of the strains as the ordinate and the grouped zone diameter values as the abscissa.

The means and standard deviations of the main, homogeneous populations were calculated. Student's t-test was used to determine the significance of transition of the zone diameter distribution. In addition, differences in the frequency of totally resistant (no inhibition zone; shown as diameter 6 mm) strains in consecutive years was evaluated by using the χ^2-test. The level of statistical significance for rejecting the null hypothesis was $p < 0.05$.

RESULTS

Validity of breakpoints

27 antimicrobial susceptibility histograms of 7 common pathogens were determined (Table II). The breakpoint split a homogeneous population in 25/90 cases with Biodisk® and in 16/84 cases with Oxoid®.

Ampicillin, Escherichia coli

Phase I. In 1992, the frequency of ampicillin-resistant strains was 25% and that of intermediately resistant strains, 61% (Table III). In 1993, the corresponding rates with the Oxoid® method were 18% and 1%. In 1992, the breakpoints were apparently inappropriate, because they split the homogeneous main population (Fig. 1). The difference in the frequency of totally resistant strains (zone 6 mm), 25% in 1992 vs. 18% in 1993, was statistically significant.

Phase II. The species-specific breakpoints provided by RAF for Biodisk® were the same as in Phase I in 1992. In 1993, the frequency of ampicillin-resistant strains was 18% and that of intermediately resistant strains, 43%, calculated according to species-specific breakpoints. In this case, the general breakpoints were more appropriate, because the species-specific breakpoint was in the middle of the main population.

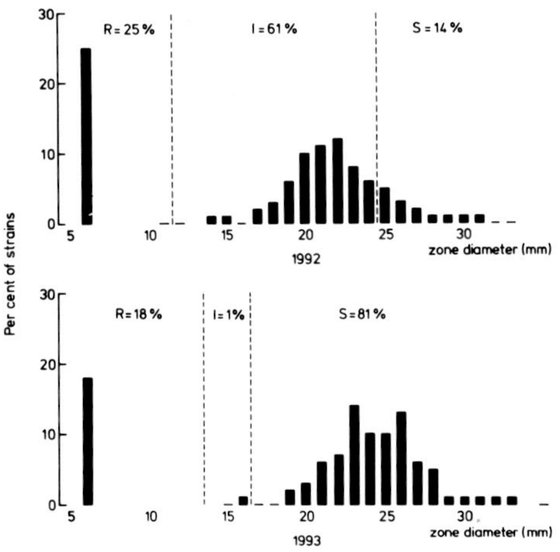

Fig. 1. Histograms of ampicillin inhibition zone diameters of Escherichia coli, determined in 1992 with the Biodisk® method and in 1993 with the Oxoid® method.

Cephalothin, E. coli

Phase I. The frequencies of cephalothin-resistant and intermediately resistant strains in 1992 were 12% and 84%, respectively (Fig. 2). In 1993, the corresponding frequencies were 4% and 8%. The frequency of totally resistant strains did not change significantly from 1992 to 1993.

Phase II. In 1992, when species-specific breakpoints were used, the frequency of cephalothin-resistant strains was 3%, and that of intermediately resistant strains was 86%. In 1993, 3% of the strains were resistant and 92% were intermediately resistant.

Cefaclor, Staphylococcus aureus

Phase I. In 1992, 1% of the S. aureus isolates were resistant to cefaclor and 75% were intermediately resistant (Fig. 3). The following year, all isolates were susceptible.

Phase II. According to species-specific breakpoints, an isolate was regarded as cefaclor-resistant if it was oxacillin-

Table II. *Validity of breakpoints with 2 susceptibility disk methods*

X: Breakpoints split the homogeneous histogram distribution; 0: Breakpoints are properly set; –: Insufficient number of isolates tested; A: Oxacillin-resistant strains reported as resistant. Species-specific breakpoints were used, except for Moraxella catarrhalis.

	Haemophilus influenzae		Moraxella catarrhalis		Staphylococcus aureus		Enterococcus sp.		Streptococcus pneumoniae		Escherichia coli		Pseudomonas aeruginosa	
Antimicrobial agent	1992 (n = 242)	1993 (n = 224)	1992 (n = 141)	1993 (n = 174)	1992 (n = 1951)	1993 (n = 1705)	1992 (n = 564)	1993 (n = 993)	1992 (n = 323)	1993 (n = 275)	1992 (n = 499)	1993 (n = 3047)	1992 (n = 542)	1993 (n = 751)
Amikacin			0	–	X	–					0	0	0	0
Amox/Clav		0	–	0	–	X	–	0	–	0	–	0		
Ampicillin	X	X					0	0	0	0	X	X		
Aztreonam	X	–	–	–							0	0	X	X
Cefaclor	X	X	X	0	A	A			0	0	–	X		
Cefotaxime	X	–	0	–	A	–			0	0	0	0		
Cefoxitin		–	–	–	A	–			–	–	0	–		
Ceftazidime	X	–	0	–	A	–			0	–	0	X		
Cefuroxime	X	0	0	0	A	A			0	0	0	0		
Cephalothin			X	0	A	A			0	0	X	X		
Chloramphenicol	0	0	0	0	0	0	0	0	0	0	0	0		
Ciprofloxacin	X	–	0	–	X	X	0	0	0	0	0	0	X	0
Clindamycin					0	0			0	0				
Erythromycin	X	X	0	0	0	0			0	0				
Fusidic acid					0	0								
Gentamicin			0	–	0	0					0	0	0	0
Imipenem	0	–	0	–	A	A	0	0	0	0	0	0	0	0
Mecillinam											X	0		
Netilmicin			0	–	X	X					0	0	X	–
Norfloxacin					–	0	–	X			–	0	–	0
Oxacillin					X	0								
Penicillin									0	0				
Piperacillin							0	0	0	0	X	X	0	0
Sulfa/Trim	X	0	0	0	0	0	0	0	0	X	0	0		
Sulfonamides			0	0	0	0					0	0		
Tetracycline	0	0	X	0	0	X	X	–	0	0	X	X		
Tobramycin			0	0	0	0					0	0	0	0
No. of valid breakpoints	3	5	13	10	9	10	6	7	15	14	14	15	5	7
No. of erroneous breakpoints	9	3	3	0	4	4	1	1	0	1	5	6	3	1

Table III. *Comparison of susceptibility grouping with different breakpoints*

I, breakpoints common for all species. II, species-specific breakpoints. Tests were performed in 1992 by using the Biodisk® and 1993 by using the Oxoid® method

Species, Antibiotic	Percentage strains 1992 R	I	S	1993 R	I	S
E. coli, Ampicillin						
I	25[a]	61	14	18	1	81
II	25	61	14	18	43	39
E. coli, Cephalothin						
I	12	84	4	4	8	88
II	3	86	11	3	92	5
S. aureus, Cefaclor						
I	1	75	24	0	0	100
II	0	3	97	0	0	100

[a] Percentage of strains in each susceptibility category.

resistant. In 1992, there were 3 strains intermediately resistant to oxacillin. In the histogram, one of them was in a separate peak (Fig. 3) and 2 in the main population.

Shift in inhibition zone distribution

The main populations of the 3 examples described above (excluding the 6 mm zones) shifted statistically significantly as a result of changing the test methods. In the case of ampicillin, the main population shifted to the right. The mean value was 22 mm (SD 3.4) in 1992 and 24 mm (SD 2.9) in 1993. In the case of cephalothin and cefaclor, the main population shifted to the left. The mean values of cephalothin were 22 mm (SD 3.7) in 1992 and 21 mm (SD 3.3) in 1993. The mean values of cefaclor were 30 mm (SD 4.5) and 27 mm (SD 4.3).

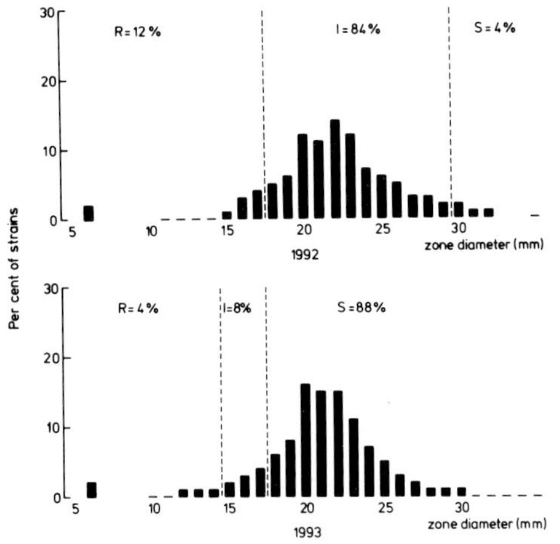

Fig. 2. Distribution of cephalothin inhibition zone sizes of Escherichia coli, determined in 1992 with the Biodisk® method and in 1993 with the Oxoid® method.

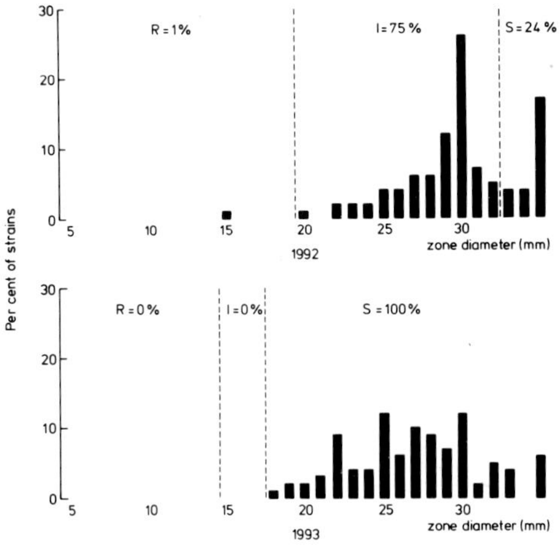

Fig. 3. Distribution of cefaclor inhibition zone diameters of Staphylococcus aureus, determined in 1992 with the Biodisk® method and in 1993 with the Oxoid® method. All zones over 34 mm are shown as 35 mm.

DISCUSSION

Even after standardization of the disk diffusion testing procedure and setting of species-specific breakpoints, there is still a need for local adjustment of the breakpoints. All laboratories should review all antimicrobials with respect to all bacterial species. Without these revisions, one cannot draw reliable conclusions about the true occurrence of resistance.

This study contains a summary of breakpoint validity and some detailed examples concerning some important pathogens. Using the species-specific breakpoints, the ampicillin susceptibility rate of Escherichia coli changed from 14% to 39% and the susceptibility to cephalothin from 11% to 5%. The frequency of cefaclor-susceptible Staphylococcus aureus changed from 97% to 100%. When species-specific breakpoints were not used, the differences were more striking (Fig. 1, 2, and 3).

Despite species-specific breakpoints, the main population was split in about one-fourth of the cases. As reported earlier, the accuracy of susceptibility testing of Haemophilus influenzae was poor (2–4).

Inhibition zone size histograms are the simplest way to compare results obtained with different methods and breakpoints, since they provide all the variables necessary for adequate interpretation of results. Histograms are also valuable when the prevalence of resistance in different laboratories is compared (1).

Compared with MIC determination, the disk diffusion test has certain advantages. The disk diffusion method can detect smaller variations in resistance levels. If the MIC method is used, slight changes in resistance cannot be detected because of the sparse scale. If changes in the resistance levels take place, the shape of the histogram changes. If the whole population shifts on the horizontal axis, this may be due to changes in the testing procedure. In the present study, no notable changes were observed in the shape of the histograms.

When the breakpoints for antimicrobial resistance are established in individual laboratories, the MIC limits issued by reference authorities are used as reference values. The strains classified as susceptible according to MIC values should also be susceptible according to the laboratory-specific breakpoints (9). Homogeneous populations should belong mainly to the same resistance category. If a breakpoint divides a homogeneous population, the breakpoint should be adjusted. If the population distribution is not clearly divided into resistant and susceptible populations, the breakpoints should be set with caution and preferably on the basis of some resistance mechanism, such as beta-lactamase activity (13).

The WHONET computer program may be used in 2 ways to select laboratory-specific breakpoints. First, the distribution of zone sizes of a single species can be studied, and this may then be used as a basis for establishing the breakpoints. Secondly, WHONET can be used to determine breakpoints by regression analysis of MIC and the corresponding zone diameter (14).

There is no generally accepted method for selecting breakpoints on the basis of histograms. Ringertz calculated the breakpoint for susceptible species so that the breakpoint between intermediate and susceptible groups was 2 SD below the mean zone size of the main population, and one additional SD set the breakpoint between resistant and intermediate group (2). We selected the laboratory-specific breakpoints on the basis of the shape of the histograms. For example, when the susceptibility of E. coli to ampicillin is tested, the breakpoints $R \leq 13$ and $S \geq 17$ in 1992 and $R \leq 15$ and $S \geq 19$ in 1993 are suggested (Fig. 1). There was more variation in the cephalothin inhibition zones, making the decision more problematical; breakpoints $R \leq 14$ and $S \geq 17$ in 1992 and $R \leq 13$ and $S \geq 16$ in 1993 are suggested (Fig. 2).

In this study the accuracy of susceptibility testing was unacceptably low, when the recommended zone breakpoints were used. It is difficult to assess the development of resistance, because different breakpoints were used in 1992 and 1993. Histograms are a good aid when susceptibility data obtained with different methods are compared. Adjusted breakpoints for susceptibility and resistance in each individual laboratory would improve the accuracy of susceptibility reporting.

REFERENCES

1. O'Brien TF and the Members of Task Force 2. Resistance of bacteria to antibacterial agents: Report of Task Force 2. Rev Infect Dis 9 (Suppl 3): S244–S259, 1987.
2. Ringertz S, Olsson-Liljequist B, Kronvall G. Antimicrobial susceptibility testing of Haemophilus influenzae. Improvement of accuracy of the disc diffusion test. J Antimicrob Chemother 26: 479–489, 1990.
3. Kronvall G, Ringertz S, Karlsson I, Göransson E, Dornbusch K. Laboratory- and species-specific interpretive breakpoints for disk diffusion tests of chloramphenicol susceptibility of Haemophilus influenzae. Antimicrob Agents Chemother 32: 1484–1489, 1988.
4. Ringertz S, Kronvall G. On the theory of the disk diffusion test. APMIS 96: 484–490, 1988.
5. Björklind A, Ringertz S, Kronvall G. Types of interpretive errors in susceptibility testing. Zone breakpoints for norfloxacin disk diffusion testing. APMIS 97: 941–948, 1989.
6. Acar JF, Goldstein FW. Disk susceptibility test. In: Lorian V, ed. Antibiotics in laboratory medicine. Baltimore: Williams & Wilkins, 1991; 17–52.
7. Williams JD. Prospects for standardisation of methods and guidelines for disc susceptibility testing. Eur J Clin Microbiol Infect Dis 9: 496–501, 1990.
8. PDM Interpretive Chart II. Ab Biodisk, Solna, Sweden, 1990.
9. National Committee for Clinical Laboratory Standards: Performance standards for antimicrobial disk susceptibility test, 4th ed. Villanova: NCCLS, 1990.
10. Komplettering av RAF: s referens- och metodbok, Mars 1991. MIC-gränser & zonbrytpunkter, RAF-M, 1991. [in Swedish]
11. Scandinavian zone diameter breakpoints for isosensitest agar (Oxoid®) and Oxoid® disks. Distributed by Berner Oy Oxoid®-sale. RAF/RAF-M, 1991.
12. WHONET2 [computer program]. Available from O'Brien T, Stelling J. Brigham and Women's Hospital, 75 Francis Street, Boston, MA 02115, USA, 1992.
13. Arstila T, Huovinen S, Huovinen P. Problems in interpretation of piperacillin susceptibility of TEM-1 producing Escherichia coli in the disk diffusion test. Eur J Clin Microbiol Infect Dis 10: 1066–1067, 1991.
14. Whonet2 [computer manual]. O'Brien T, Stelling J. Boston: Brigham and Women's Hospital, 1992.

Submitted June 9, 1994; accepted November 20, 1994

Scand J Infect Dis 27: 52–56, 1995

Detecting Erythromycin Resistance in Streptococcus pyogenes: Reliability of the Disk Diffusion Method and the Breakpoint Susceptibility Testing Method

ANTTI NISSINEN, HELENA SEPPÄLÄ, PENTTI HUOVINEN and the FINNISH STUDY GROUP FOR ANTIMICROBIAL RESISTANCE (FIRE)[1]

From the Antimicrobial Research Laboratory, National Public Health Institute, Turku, Finland

Erythromycin susceptibility of clinical Streptococcus pyogenes isolates was determined at 19 Finnish clinical microbiology laboratories by their routine disk diffusion method and by a screening method adapted from the breakpoint susceptibility testing method. Results obtained at 12 laboratories using 4 major variants of the disk method were further evaluated. From these laboratories, 286 consecutive resistant and 349 consecutive susceptible isolates were sent to the Antimicrobial Research Laboratory, Turku where the MIC of erythromycin was determined. 96% and 97% of the disk results were correct, as compared with MIC results, when general and laboratory-specific breakpoints, respectively, were used. The results of the screening method were comparable to those of the disk method.

A. Nissinen, MSc, Microbiology Laboratory, Central Hospital of Middle Finland, FIN-40620 Jyväskylä, Finland

INTRODUCTION

Detection of acquired antimicrobial resistance by pathogenic bacteria is one of the major tasks of clinical microbiology laboratories. The disk diffusion method is preferred because of its flexibility and ease of performance. This method is reliable for testing antimicrobial susceptibility of rapidly growing bacterial species without growth requirements, e.g. staphylococci and enterobacteria. However, erroneous results, both false resistance and false susceptibility, have been reported when fastidious organisms, e.g. streptococci (1–4) and Haemophilus influenzae (5–8) were tested with this method. Recently, interlaboratory variation of disk diffusion results has been found to cause such false interpretations (8, 9). Consequently, the use of general interpretative breakpoints for resistance and susceptibility have been questioned and the use of laboratory-specific breakpoints have been proposed (8, 9).

One way to overcome the problems of the disk diffusion method is to use a simplified agar dilution method, a so-called breakpoint susceptibility testing method (10).

The emergence of erythromycin-resistant Streptococcus pyogenes in Finland (11) raised the question of the ability of the routine disk diffusion methods used by Finnish laboratories to detect the resistance. The aim of the present study was to assess the reliability of the disk diffusion method, using both laboratory-specific and general breakpoints, and also the reliability of the breakpoint susceptibility testing method. Both methods are used in clinical microbiology laboratories in this country.

---

[1] Ahonen, E., Department of Clinical Microbiology, Central Hospital of Kainuu, Kajaani; Brander, M., Department of Clinical Microbiology, Central Hospital of Etelä-Saimaa, Lappeenranta; Eerola, E., Department of Medical Microbiology, Turku University, Turku; Eskola, J., Department of Clinical Microbiology, Aurora Hospital, Helsinki; Herva, E., National Public Health Institute, Oulu Division, Oulu; Jägerroos, H., Department of Clinical Microbiology, Central Hospital of Lappi, Rovaniemi; Hirvonen, P., Department of Clinical Microbiology, Central Hospital of Keski-Suomi, Jyväskylä; Katila, M.-L., Department of Clinical Microbiology, Kuopio University Hospital, Kuopio; Klossner, M.-L., Department of Clinical Microbiology, Central Hospital of Satakunta, Pori; Kontiainen, S., Department of Clinical Microbiology, Aurora Hospital, Helsinki, Korpela, J., Department of Clinical Microbiology, Central Hospital of Päijät-Häme, Lahti; Koskela, M., Department of Clinical Microbiology, Oulu University Hospital, Oulu; Kostiala-Thompson, A., Department of Clinical Microbiology, Jorvi Hospital, Espoo; Kärkkäinen, P., Department of Clinical Microbiology, Central Hospital of Mikkeli, Mikkeli; Kärkkäinen, P., Clinical Laboratory, Central Hospital of Savonlinna, Savonlinna; Järvinen, H., National Public Health Institute, Department in Turku, Turku; Lantto, K., Deaconess Institution of Oulu, Oulu; Larinkari, U., Department of Clinical Microbiology, Central Hospital of Kymenlaakso, Kotka; Lehtonen, O.-P., Department of Clinical Microbiology, Turku University Hospital, Turku; Liimataine, O., Department of Clinical Microbiology, Tampere University Hospital, Tampere; Oinonen, S., Department of Clinical Microbiology, Central Hospital of Seinäjoki, Seinäjoki; Renkonen, O.-V., Department of Serology and Bacteriology, Helsinki University, Helsinki; Ruuska, P., Department of Medical Microbiology, Oulu University, Oulu; Sarkkinen, H., Department of Clinical Microbiology, Central Hospital of Pohjois-Karjala, Joensuu; Vikberg, V., Department of Clinical Microbiology, Central Hospital of Etelä-Häme, Hämeenlinna.

MATERIAL AND METHODS

The bacteria

19 clinical microbiology laboratories in Finland tested all S. pyogenes strains isolated from throat and pus samples during February–May 1992 for erythromycin resistance, using their routine disk diffusion method and the breakpoint susceptibility testing method (designated as screening method in this paper). Each laboratory was asked to submit, according to the results of the screening method, all resistant and 50 consecutive susceptible S. pyogenes strains and the corresponding disk and screening results, to the Antimicrobial Research Laboratory, National Public Health Institute, Turku, Finland (ARL), giving a detailed description of the routine disk method used. At ARL, the strains were stored deep frozen until further analysis.

S. pyogenes were identified in the isolating laboratories by β-hemolysis on a sheep or horse blood agar plate and the presence of Lancefield group A antigen, tested with a commercial latex agglutination reagent (various manufacturers).

Methods used to detect erythromycin resistance

Disk diffusion methods. Seven variants of the disk diffusion method were used at the 19 laboratories participating in the study. While differing reliability of different variants could be expected, laboratories using a certain variant were grouped. Four of these variants, designated A, B, C, and D (Table I) in this paper, were used at 14 laboratories, 12 of which (3 using each of the 4 variants) were included in the study. Two disk method standards (12, 13) were applied in these 12 laboratories. Either a complex medium, i.e. Mueller-Hinton medium (variants B, C) or a semisynthetic medium, e.g. PDM antibiotic sensitivity medium or Iso-Sensitest medium (variants A, C) supplemented with 5% blood was used. Inoculum from overnight plate culture for either confluent (variant B) or semiconfluent (variants A, C, D) growth was prepared in saline following the instructions of the National Committee for Clinical Laboratory Standards (NCCLS) (12) or the Swedish Reference Group for Antibiotics (SRGA) (13), respectively. Plates were inoculated by swabbing. Paper disks (AB Biodisk, Solna, Sweden) containing 15 μg (variant A) or disks (AS Rosco, Taastrup, Denmark) containing a diffusible amount of 78 μg (variants B, C, D) or erythromycin were placed on the inoculated plates (Table I). Plates were incubated in 5% CO_2 at 35°C for 18 h. The diameter of the zone of inhibition was measured with calipers and the result was recorded in mm. Zone interpretative breakpoints for resistance recommended by the disk manufacturers, based on MIC interpretative breakpoints by SRGA (variants A, C, D) and NCCLS (variant B) were used.

Screening method. The screening method was introduced at all the participating laboratories for the duration of the study. S. pyogenes colonies were cultured by streaking on Mueller-Hinton agar (Becton Dickinson Microbiology Systems, Cockeysville, MD, USA) supplemented with 5% sheep blood and 2 μg/ml erythromycin (Sigma, St Louis, MO, USA) and the plates were incubated in 5% CO_2 at 35°C overnight. In our experience, S. pyogenes strains can be better classified as resistant or susceptible in such an atmosphere, because the difference between susceptible and resistant populations of organisms at their minimal inhibitory concentration (MIC) is greater and more distinct in CO_2 than in ambient air (data not shown). Erythromycin resistance was indicated by growth on the plate with an erythromycin concentration of 2 μg/ml. When cultures are incubated in 5% CO_2, this cut-off point correlates well with an MIC of 0.5 μg/ml on incubation in ambient air; this concentration is recommended as the cut-off point between the susceptible and moderately susceptible bacteria by the NCCLS (14). A similar difference of 2 twofold concentration increments between erythromycin MICs obtained in ambient air and 5% CO_2 was noted also by others (15).

Testing the reliability of the detection method

MIC testing. MICs were performed by the agar dilution method on Mueller-Hinton agar supplemented with 5% sheep blood according to the criteria of NCCLS (14). A series of plates containing doubling dilutions of erythromycin ranging from 0.0625 to 128 μg/ml, were inoculated and incubated in air at 35°C for 18 h. MIC breakpoint for resistance was ≥1 μg/ml (14). S. pyogenes ATCC 10389, Enterococcus faecalis ATCC 29212, and Staphylococcus aureus ATCC 29213 were used as controls.

Histogram analysis. Inhibition zone diameters of the disk diffusion tests from each of the 12 laboratories were plotted as histograms with the number of strains on the y-axis and zone diameter values on the x-axis. Laboratory-specific zone interpretative breakpoints for the disk diffusion method were defined by choosing a zone size value in the middle of the gap between the resistant and susceptible histogram subpopulations. The gap was defined as an area between the 2 histogram subpopulations with a maximum of a single inhibition zone diameter result located ≥2 mm apart from the edge of the subpopulations.

Table I. *Characteristics of 4 major variants of the disk diffusion method used for susceptibility testing of Streptococcus pyogenes in Finnish clinical microbiology laboratories*

Variant of disk method	Agar base[a]	Inoculum[b]	Disk[c]	Resistance breakpoint[d] According to	≤(mm)
A	PDM	Semi-confluent	Biodisk	SRGA	24
B	M-H	Confluent	Rosco	NCCLS	26
C	M-H	Semi-confluent	Rosco	SRGA	29
D	PDM/IS	Semi-confluent	Rosco	SRGA	29/27

[a] PDM, PDM Antibiotic Sensitivity Medium, AB Biodisk, Solna, Sweden; M-H, Mueller-Hinton agar, different manufacturers; IS, Iso-Sensitest agar, Unipath Ltd., Basingstoke, Hants, England.

[b] Semi-confluent, according to ICS (13); confluent, according to Kirby-Bauer (12).

[c] Biodisk, 6 mm paper disk with 15 μg erythromycin, AB Biodisk, Solna, Sweden; Rosco, 9 mm tablet with 78 μg (diffusible amount) erythromycin, AS Rosco, Taastrup, Denmark.

[d] SRGA, Swedish Reference Group for Antibiotics (13); NCCLS, National Committee for Clinical Laboratory Standards (12), breakpoints adapted for 78 μg erythromycin tablets by AS Rosco (17). Intermediate results are interpreted as resistant.

RESULTS

The reliability of the disk method and the screening method was evaluated by comparing results classified susceptible or resistant obtained by these methods at individual laboratories with those obtained by MIC testing at the Antimicrobial Research Laboratory (ARL).

At ARL, MIC was determined for 635 S. pyogenes strains, 286 of which had been classified as resistant and 349 susceptible according to the screening test at the 12 clinical laboratories included in the study. Among these 635 strains, 2 distinct subpopulations, resistant (MIC 1– >32 μg/ml) and susceptible (MIC ≤ 0.06–0.12 μg/ml), were observed. Less than 2% of the strains had MICs between these populations, i.e. 0.25–0.5 μg/ml. The populations at all 12 laboratories were alike (data not shown), thus allowing interlaboratory comparisons of the disk and screening results.

Disk diffusion results. The disk method was evaluated by using general interpretative breakpoints for resistance recommended by the disk manufacturer and laboratory-specific breakpoints based on the inhibition zone histograms of the results of individual laboratories. The ideal position of the zone interpretative breakpoint for resistance/susceptibility is in the middle of the gap separating resistant from susceptible populations. According to this principle, laboratory-specific breakpoints for each of the 12 laboratories were defined by choosing the median inhibition zone diameter value between the 2 histogram subpopulations (Fig. 1). Disk diffusion results were available from 624/635 strains submitted to the ARL.

The laboratory-specific breakpoint at half of the 12 laboratories was equal to that or only slightly (±1 mm) different from that recommended by the disk manufacturer (Fig. 1). Deviations of −2 to −3 mm were observed at three laboratories and still larger, −4 to −5 mm, in three others.

When general breakpoints recommended by the disk manufacturer were used, erroneous disk results (false resistant or false susceptible; open and solid squares on the 'wrong' side of the breakpoint in Fig. 1) were reported in 4% (24/624) of the strains. The number of erroneous results was somewhat less when laboratory-specific breakpoints were used (3%, 19/624). The improvement was due mainly to changes in the interpretation of results from three laboratories where the breakpoint recommended by the disk manufacturer transected the normal (susceptible) population (Fig. 1).

By using the laboratory-specific breakpoints, fewer false results were obtained at laboratories using the variant A of the disk method (1/169) than at those using the other three variants (B, 5/158; C, 9/153; D, 4/144; Fig. 1), but the difference was not statistically significant (χ^2-test).

Screening results. 37 (12.9%) of the 286 strains reported resistant by screening and six (1.7%) of the 349 reported

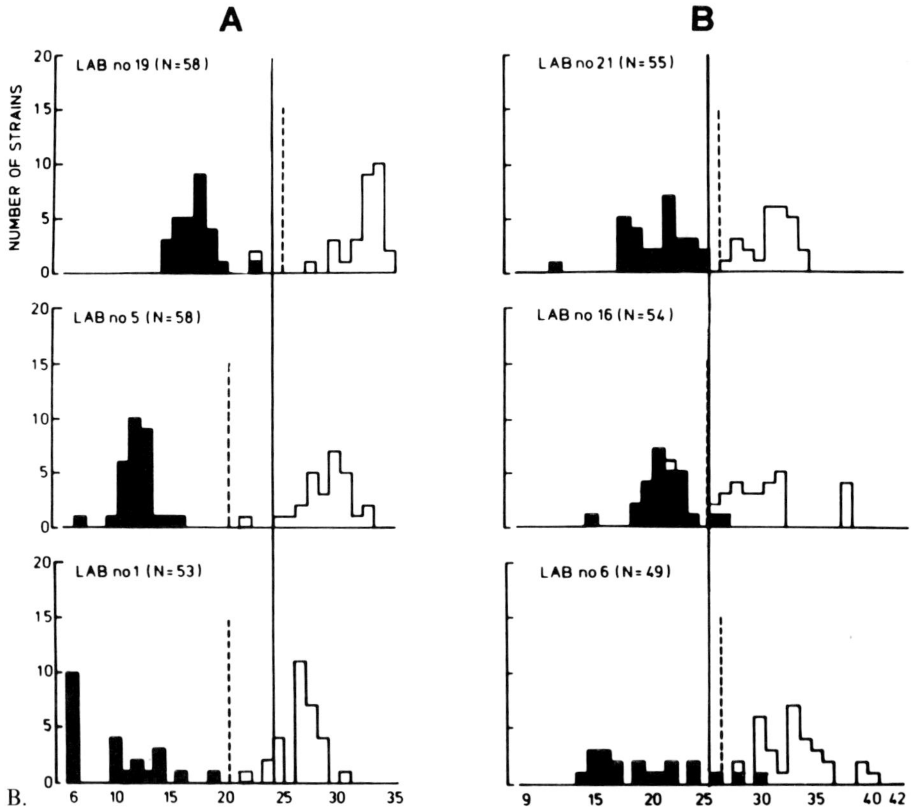

Fig. 1. A, B.

Table II. *Erythromycin MIC of 635 Streptococcus pyogenes strains classified as resistant (286 strains) or susceptible (349 strains) according to the breakpoint (screening) method*

Screening result[a]	Number of strains with MIC (μg/ml) of ≤0.06	0.12	0.25	0.5[b]	1	2	4	8	16	>16
Resistant	36[c]		1	4	34	74	84	40	9	2
Susceptible	311	30	2	3	1		2			

[a] Breakpoint concentration of 2 μg/ml in 5% CO_2, corresponding to a concentration of 0.5 μg/ml in air; see main text.
[b] Breakpoint concentration according to NCCLS (14).
[c] 33/36 results from three laboratories; see main text.

susceptible were interpreted incorrectly, as compared with the MIC (Table II). A majority (8/12) of the laboratories performed well, producing no (5 laboratories) or a single (3 laboratories) false result. Most (33/36) of the highly discrepant screening results came from 3 laboratories reporting resistance by screening, although the MIC was ≤0.06 μg/ml. After interviewing the staff at these laboratories, it became evident that some of the workers had interpreted β-hemolysis caused by the inoculum on the screening plate as growth.

DISCUSSION

The reliability of the disk results was related to the relative resolution of the variant of the method. The SRGA standard method (variant A) using low erythromycin content paper disks and semiconfluent growth had the best relative resolution, whereas a very low relative resolution and, consequently, slightly overlapping resistant and susceptible subpopulations were observed in laboratories using disks with a high erythromycin content and confluent growth (variant B). The lower resolution of the variants B, C, and D of the disk method is probably due to the relatively high erythromycin content of the disks used. A high antimicrobial content of the disk leads to a steep gradient of the drug in the agar (16) and pushing of the resistant and susceptible bacterial populations closer to each other on the plate, thus impairing the resolution of the method. This phenomenon is intensified by a dense inoculum, as used in variant B of the disk method in order to get confluent growth.

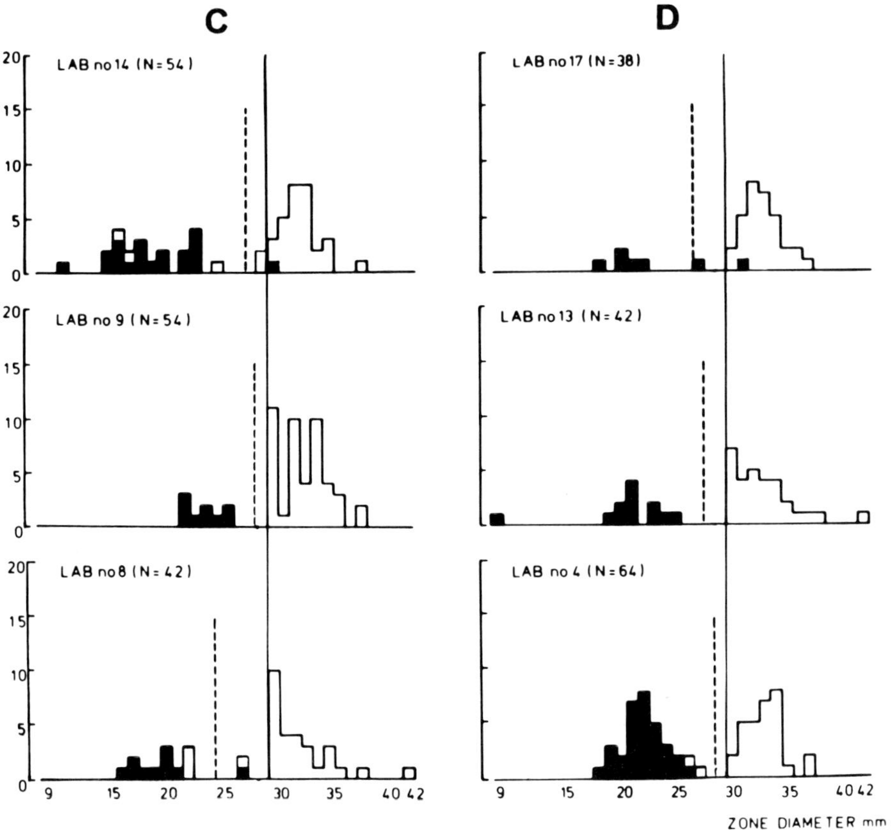

Fig. 1. Histograms of inhibition zone diameters of 4 disk diffusion method variants (Table I) used for erythromycin susceptibility testing of 624 Streptococcus pyogenes strains at 12 laboratories. Variant A was used at laboratories 1, 5, and 19; B at laboratories 6, 16, and 21; C at laboratories 8, 9, and 14; D at laboratories 4, 13, and 17. Symbols: □, susceptible; ■, resistant (interpretations according to MIC). The interpretative breakpoints recommended by the disk manufacturers are indicated by solid lines and laboratory-specific by broken lines.

Interestingly, albeit the most reliable results within one laboratory were obtained by variant A of the disk method, the largest interlaboratory variation was observed by using the same method. This phenomenon has been reported also by others (4, 8). In the study by Kronvall et al. (8), 0–36% false results of resistance to chloramphenicol were observed at 6 laboratories when the SRGA method was used to test the susceptibility of H. influenzae. Whether the SRGA standard method is actually more prone to interlaboratory variation than variants using more dense inoculum or/and high content antimicrobial disks remains to be studied.

The number of variants of the disk diffusion method used at clinical microbiology laboratories in Finland is astonishingly large. Acceptance of a common methodology within the country would minimize the false interpretations and help to obtain comparable results. According to the data presented here, the SRGA method using laboratory-specific interpretative breakpoints would be the most promising candidate for such a common methodology.

Breakpoint susceptibility testing method proved to be a practical and reliable screening method for detecting erythromycin resistance in S. pyogenes; in spite of the non-standard inoculum, most laboratories made very few misinterpretations when using this test. This kind of a screening method could be a useful tool in situations when the disk method has proved unreliable, e.g. susceptibility testing of slow-growing bacterial species.

In conclusion, a standard disk diffusion method, using a laboratory-specific interpretative breakpoint, is a reliable method for detection of S. pyogenes resistant to erythromycin. When screening for antimicrobial resistance in a fastidious bacterial species, the breakpoint susceptibility testing method is a good alternative to the disk diffusion method. However, the findings are a reminder of the high susceptibility of a new methodology for interpretative errors.

ACKNOWLEDGEMENTS

We are indebted to Professor Helena Mäkelä for valuable advice, to Erkki Nieminen, Anne Nurmi, Marja-Liisa Lindman and Heli Espilä for expert technical assistance and to all the staff members at the participating laboratories for their assistance in this collaborative project.

This work was supported by grants from the Sigrid Juselius Foundation (H.S. and P.H.), the Turku University Foundation (H.S.), the Finnish Academy (H.S.) and the Maud Kuistila Foundation (H.S.).

REFERENCES

1. Snell JJS, George RC, Perry SF, Erdman YJ. Antimicrobial susceptibility testing of Streptococcus pneumoniae: quality assessment results. J Clin Pathol 41: 384–387, 1988.
2. Nair P. Incidence of decreased penicillin sensitivity of Streptococcus pneumoniae from clinical isolates. J Clin Pathol 41: 720–721, 1988.
3. Figueiredo AMS, Connor JD, Severin A, Vaz Pato MV, Tomasz A. A pneumococcal clinical isolate with high-level resistance to cefotaxime and ceftriaxone. Antimicrob Agents Chemother 36: 886–889, 1992.
4. Olsson-Liljequist B, Burman LG, Kallings I, and the Swedish respiratory tract study group. Antibiotic susceptibility of upper respiratory tract pathogens in Sweden: a seven year follow-up study including Loracarbef. Scand J Infect Dis 24: 485–493, 1992.
5. Snell JJS, Brown DFJ, Phue TJ. Antimicrobial susceptibility testing of Haemophilus influenzae: trial organized as part of United Kingdom national external quality assessment scheme for microbiology. J Clin Pathol 39: 1006–1012, 1986.
6. Mendelman PM, Chaffin DO, Clausen C, Stull TL, Needham C, Williams JD, Smith AL. Failure to detect ampicillin-resistant, non-β-lactamase-producing Haemophilus influenzae by standard disk susceptibility testing. Antimicrob Agents Chemother 30: 274–280, 1986.
7. Ramos OM, Cepero AE, Resnick TJ. Failure to detect chloramphenicol-resistant Haemophilus influenzae by routine susceptibility testing. Pediatr Infect Dis J 6: 420–421, 1987.
8. Kronvall G, Ringertz S, Karlsson I, Göransson E, Dornbusch, K. Laboratory- and species-specific interpretative breakpoints for disk diffusion tests of chloramphenicol susceptibility of Haemophilus influenzae. Antimicrob Agents Chemother 4: 1484–1489, 1988.
9. Ringertz S, Olsson-Liljequist B, Kronvall G. Antimicrobial susceptibility testing of Haemophilus influenzae. Improvement of accuracy of the disk diffusion method. J Antimicrob Chemother 26: 479–489, 1990.
10. Doern GV. Breakpoint susceptibility testing. Clinical Microbiology Newsletter 9: 81–84, 1987.
11. Seppälä H, Nissinen A, Järvinen H, Huovinen S, Henriksson T, Herva E, Holm SE, Jahkola M, Katila M-L, Klaukka T, Kontiainen S, Liimatainen O, Oinonen S, Passi-Metsomaa L, Huovinen P. Resistance to erythromycin in group A streptococci. N Engl J Med 326: 292–297, 1992.
12. National Committee for Clinical Laboratory Standards. Performance standards for antimicrobial disk susceptibility tests. NCCLS Document M2-A4. Philadelphia: NCCLS, 1990.
13. The Swedish Reference Group for Antibiotics. Antimicrobial Susceptibility Testing of Bacteria – A Reference and a Methodology Manual. Stockholm: The Swedish Medical Society and Statens Bakteriologiska Laboratorium, 1990.
14. National Committee for Clinical Laboratory Standards. Methods for dilution antimicrobial susceptibility tests for bacteria that grow aerobically. NCCLS document M7-A2. Philadelphia: NCCLS, 1990.
15. Dibb WL, Digranes A, Bottolfsen KL. Effects of carbon dioxide upon the in vitro activity of erythromycin. Acta Pathol Microbiol Immunol Scand Sect B 94: 173–176, 1986.
16. Barry AL. The antimicrobial susceptibility test: principles and practices. Philadelphia: Lea & Febinger, 1976, 196–207.
17. Casals JB, Pringler N. Antibacterial and antifungal susceptibility testing using Neo Sensitabs, 9th edn., Taastrup, Denmark: Rosco Diagnostica, 1991.

Submitted August 26, 1994; accepted November 20, 1994

Scand J Infect Dis 27: 57–61, 1995

ORIGINAL ARTICLE

Antimicrobial Resistance in Haemophilus influenzae Isolated from Blood, Cerebrospinal Fluid, Middle Ear Fluid and Throat Samples of Children. A nationwide study in Finland in 1988–1990

ANTTI NISSINEN[1], ELJA HERVA[2], MARJA-LEENA KATILA[3], SIRKKA KONTIAINEN[4], OILI LIIMATAINEN[5], SINIKKA OINONEN[6], AINO K. TAKALA[7] and PENTTI HUOVINEN[1]

From the [1]Antimicrobial Research Laboratory, National Public Health Institute, Turku, [2]Oulu Department, National Public Health Institute, Oulu, the [3]Microbiology Laboratory, Kuopio University Hospital, Kuopio, the [4]Division of Bacteriology, Department of Medical Microbiology, Aurora Hospital, Helsinki, the [5]Microbiology Laboratory, Tampere University Hospital, Tampere, [6]Microbiology Laboratory, Seinäjoki Central Hospital, Seinäjoki, and the [7]National Public Health Institute, Helsinki, Finland

A nation-wide survey of the prevalence of antimicrobial resistance in Haemophilus influenzae was conducted on isolates collected in 1988–90 from middle ear fluid (MEF), blood, or cerebrospinal fluid (CSF) in infected children or throat samples of healthy children. Altogether 885 strains were examined regarding capsular type b, β-lactamase production and the minimal inhibitory concentration (MIC) of ampicillin, cefaclor, erythromycin, tetracycline, chloramphenicol, trimethoprim and trimethoprim-sulfamethoxazole for these strains was determined by the agar dilution method. 99% (578/585) of MEF isolates, 93% (112/121) of throat isolates, but only 6% (10/179) of blood/CSF isolates were *not* of type b (Hib). The rate of β-lactamase production was 11.4% among Hib strains, 8.0% among non-type b MEF isolates, and 4.5% among non-type b throat isolates. No increase in the prevalence of β-lactamase production in H. influenzae has taken place in Finland since the early 1980s. Resistance to ampicillin among strains that lacked β-lactamase activity was rare (0.2%). Of the non-type b MEF and throat isolates, 5.9% and 2.7%, respectively, were resistant to trimethoprim and 3.6% and 2.7%, respectively, to trimethoprim-sulfamethoxazole. Resistance to other drugs was rare (<2%) in all isolate groups.

A. Nissinen, MSc, Central Hospital of Middle Finland, Microbiology laboratory FIN-40620 Jyväskylä, Finland

INTRODUCTION

Haemophilus influenzae is a major cause of severe systemic infection in childhood (1). It is also the second most common etiological agent, after the pneumococci, in acute otitis media in children below school age (2). The systemic infections are almost invariably caused by encapsulated H. influenzae of type b (Hib), otitis media by non-capsulated strains. Both encapsulated and non-capsulated H. influenzae are normal inhabitants of the mucous membranes of the human oropharynx (3).

Apart from β-lactamase production and consequent resistance to penicillins, H. influenzae has remained relatively susceptible. However, increasing resistance to various antimicrobials was reported in the late 1980s (4, 5). β-lactamase-producing strains are more common in children than in adults (6–8); the same may be true of resistance to other antimicrobial agents (9). In addition, strains associated with infections more often produce β-lactamase than do strains from healthy children (7, 10–12).

There is little information on other than β-lactamase-mediated resistance in pediatric H. influenzae isolates. In addition, the use of different resistance breakpoints in these studies often makes comparison impossible (10, 11, 13). We report here the prevalence of antimicrobial resistance in both Hib and non-type b H. influenzae strains isolated from non-invasive and invasive pediatric infections and from the oropharynx of healthy children determined in a nation-wide survey in Finland in 1988–90.

MATERIAL AND METHODS

Bacterial strains. During 3 autumns (November–December) in 1988, 1989 and 1990, 6 Finnish clinical microbiology laboratories in different parts of the country submitted all consecutive H. influenzae strains isolated from middle ear fluid (MEF) of children <6 years with acute otitis media to the National Public Health Institute (KTL) in Helsinki.

In 1985–90, as a part of a Hib vaccination study, throat samples from 3-year-old children had been collected during a regular 'well-child' visit at 7 geographically scattered child health centres, sent to KTL and cultured for H. influenzae as described elsewhere (3). The strains obtained in 1988–90 were included in this study.

As another part of the Hib vaccination study the clinical microbiology laboratories sent all H. influenzae strains isolated from blood and cerebrospinal fluid (CSF) of children <16 to KTL. Strains from the period 1988–90 were included in this study.

At the KTL, the presence of type b capsule was assessed with a commercial latex agglutination test (Wellcome Diagnostics, Kent, England) or on the Levinthal-bacitracin agar containing type b antiserum (14). The pure cultures were stored in skim milk at −70°C until further analyses.

Antimicrobial susceptibility testing. β-lactamase production of the strains was determined by the chromogenic cephalosporin nitrocefin method (15) using commercial nitrocefin disks (Ab Biodisk, Solna, Sweden).

The minimal inhibitory concentrations (MIC) of different antimicrobial agents was determined by the agar dilution method (16) on the Haemophilus Test Medium (17) containing one of the following antimicrobials in 2-fold dilutions (range in μg/ml): ampicillin (0.06–8), cefaclor (0.12–16), erythromycin (0.25–16), tetracycline (0.25–32), chloramphenicol (0.12–16), trimethoprim (0.06–16) or trimethoprim-sulfamethoxazole (1 : 19, trimethoprim conc.: 0.03–4). Thymidine phosphorylase (0.2 IU/ml) was added to plates containing trimethoprim or trimethoprim-sulfamethoxazole. According to the NCCLS criteria (16) the organisms were considered resistant/susceptible if the MICs were $\geq / \leq$ (μg/ml) 4/1 for ampicillin, 32/8 for cefaclor, 8/0.5 for erythromycin, 8/2 for tetracycline, 8/2 for chloramphenicol and 4/0.5 (trimethoprim concentration) for trimethoprim-sulfamethoxazole. The NCCLS does not give SIR interpretative breakpoints for trimethoprim for bacteria isolated from sources other than urine. We therefore chose breakpoints according to the observed population distribution (data not shown), S: ≤ 0.5 and $R \geq 4$. These limits are close to the S/R-breakpoint of 2 μg/ml used by Powell et al. (18) and Howard and Williams (19).

E. coli ATCC 25922, H. influenzae ATCC 49247, H. influenzae PHLS 1139 (20), and H. influenzae PHLS 1141 (20) were used as controls.

Cefaclor was a gift from Eli Lilly Finland Ltd, Vantaa, Finland and the other antimicrobial agents by Orion Ltd, Espoo, Finland.

Statistical analysis was done with χ^2-test for independence in 2 × 2 tables.

RESULTS

885 H. influenzae strains were studied; 185 were of type b (Hib) and 700 of non-type b (Table I). The rate of β-lactamase production was slightly higher among Hib strains (11.4%) than among non-type b strains (7.4%) (p = NS, Table I). Likewise, a slight but non-significant difference was observed between the rates of β-lactamase production among non-type isolates from MEF (8.0%) and among those from healthy children (4.5%) (Table I). The overall prevalence of ampicillin resistance closely paralleled β-lactamase production: 73/75 resistant strains were β-lactamase producers.

Table I. *β-lactamase production by* H. influenzae *type b (Hib) and non-type b strains isolated from middle ear fluid (MEF), throat, blood and cerebrospinal fluid (CSF) samples of children*

	Non-type b		Hib	
Source	No. of strains tested	No. (%) of β-lactamase positive	No. of strains tested	No. (%) of β-lactamase positive
MEF	578	46 (8.0[a])	7	2
Throat	112	5 (4.5[a])	9	2
Blood/CSF	10	1	169	17 (10.0)
All	700	52 (7.4[b])	185	21 (11.4[b])

[a] Not significant, $p = 0.19$.
[b] Not significant, $p = 0.085$.

Resistance to cefaclor was rare, <1%; in addition, 2.6–7.6% of the strains fell in the intermediate category (Table II). A majority of the strains were of intermediate resistance to erythromycin; <2% were resistant and only 2% fully susceptible (Table II). More than 99% and 98% of the strains were susceptible to chloramphenicol and tetracycline, respectively.

The non-type b strains were more often resistant to trimethoprim than were Hib strains (5.4% vs. 1.1%, $p = 0.01$). Of the non-type b MEF or throat isolates, 5.9% or 2.7%, respectively, were resistant to trimethoprim (p = NS) and 3.6% or 2.7%, respectively, to trimethoprim-sulfamethoxazole (p = NS) (Table II).

Of the 73 β-lactamase-producing – i.e. ampicillin-resistant – strains 66 were resistant to ampicillin only and 3 were multiply resistant (resistant to ≥3 unrelated drugs) (Table III).

Two ampicillin-resistant β-lactamase-negative strains were found; both were from MEF and of non-type b. Both were also resistant to cefaclor. In addition, 3 cefaclor resistant β-lactamase-producing strains were detected, 2 from blood (1 non-type b and 1 Hib) and 1 from CSF (Hib) (Table III).

Of the 40 trimethoprim-resistant isolates, 27 were also resistant to co-trimoxazole and only 4 also to other drugs (Table III).

DISCUSSION

Ampicillin resistance mediated by β-lactamase was the most common form of resistance encountered. The prevalence of β-lactamase-producing strains among Hib (11.4%) and non-type b (7.4%) isolates is close to the European average (10.5% and 8.6%, respectively) (21) and significantly lower than reported from USA for the same time period (29.5% and 15.0%, respectively) (5).

In Finland the first β-lactamase-producing H. influenzae was isolated in 1975 from MEF (22) and in 1977 from CSF (23). The prevalence of β-lactamase-producing MEF isolates increased rapidly to reach a level of 15% in 1981 (24). However, this frequency was significantly dependent on the type of otitis media: while the prevalence was 12% in all cases (1978), it was only 8% in primary cases but 17% in recurrent cases and 22% among strains isolated from patients in whom treatment had failed (24). The design of the present study did not permit a separation of these 3 types of acute otitis media. Tympanocentesis is usually not done in all cases of AOM and not all MEF samples are sent for bacteriological analysis; thus complicated cases (treatment failures, recurrent episodes) are overrepresented among the samples sent for culture. This potential bias notwithstanding, it is clear that β-lactamase-producing H. influenzae strains have not continued to increase in prevalence since 1981.

Non-β-lactamase-mediated ampicillin resistance was rare (only 2 instances detected) among the H. influenzae strains

Table II. *Prevalence of susceptibility and resistance among* H. influenzae *strains isolated from throat samples of healthy children, middle ear fluid (MEF) of children with otitis media or from blood or cerebrospinal fluid of children with invasive infection*

Serotype and source of the strains	Proportion of strains showing susceptibility (S) and resistance (R)[a] to													
	Ampicillin		Cefaclor		Erythromycin		Chloram-phenicol		Tetracycline		Trimethoprim		Co-trimoxazole	
	S	R	S	R	S	R	S	R	S	R	S	R	S	R
Non-type b														
Throat ($N = 112$)	95.5	4.5	97.3	0	21.4	1.8	100	0	100	0	97.3	2.7	97.3	2.7
MEF ($N = 578$)	91.7	8.3	95.2	0.5	11.6	0.7	99.7	0.2	99.2	0.4	93.6	5.9	93.8	3.6
Type-b														
Any source[b] ($N = 185$)	88.6	11.4	91.3	1.1	7.0	1.1	99.5	0	98.4	1.6	94.1	1.1	98.9	1.1

[a] Breakpoints according to NCCLS, see main text.
[b] MEF, 7; throat, 9; blood, 111; and cerebrospinal fluid, 58 strains.

Table III. *Resistance patterns of* H. influenzae *non-type b and non-type b (Hib) strains isolated from different sources*

Resistance pattern[a]	Number (%) of resistant strains: Non-type b, Blood/CSF[b] (10[e])	Non-type b, MEF[c] (578[e])	Non-type b, Throat (112[e])	Type b, All[d] (186[e])
AMP(Bla+)		44 (7.6)	5 (4.5)	17 (9.1)
AMP(Bla+), TET				1 (0.6)
AMP(Bla+), TMP		1 (0.2)		
AMP(Bla+), CCL	1			1 (0.6)
AMP(Bla+), TET, CHL, TMP, SXT		1 (0.2)		
AMP(Bla+), TET, TMP, SXT				1 (0.6)
AMP(Bla+), CCL, TMP, SXT				1 (0.6)
AMP(Bla−), CCL		2 (0.9)		
TET		1 (0.2)		2 (1.1)
TMP		12 (2.1)		
TMP, SXT	1	20 (3.4)	3 (2.5)	

[a] AMP, ampicillin; Bla, β-lactamase; CCL, cefaclor; CHL, chloramphenicol; TET, tetracycline; TMP, trimethoprim; SXT, trimethoprim-sulfamethoxazole.
[b] CSF, cerebrospinal fluid.
[c] MEF, middle ear fluid.
[d] All, CSF; blood; MEF; and throat.
[e] Number of strains tested.

studied. This is in agreement with the prevalence in both the USA and Europe (5, 21). It has been postulated that the low, not increasing (5, 7, 12, 21) prevalence of this chromosomal resistance associated with altered penicillin-binding proteins (PBP) might be due to a lower virulence of strains with abnormal PBPs (25, 26). Although the chromosomal resistance to ampicillin is rare, it is important to detect it because of the concomitant resistance to I and II generation cephalosporins (27, 28), though not to third generation cephalosporins or carbapenems (29).

Only 0.6% of the strains were resistant to cefaclor ($MIC \geq 32$ μg/ml). This figure must, however, be regarded with caution, for 2 reasons. First, the normal H. influenzae population ($MIC_{50} = 4$ μg/ml, $MIC_{90} = 8$ μg/ml; data not shown) lies close to the I/R breakpoint (≥ 32 μg/ml) and second, the MIC seems to be easily affected by the composition of the medium and the lability of the drugs (5, 27). The Swedish reference group for antimicrobial agents (SRGA) recently reallocated the S/I breakpoint for cefaclor in H. influenzae downward to ≤ 1 μg/ml (30). The corresponding recommendation of NCCLS is ≤ 8 μg/ml. Most of the H. influenzae strains normally have their MICs for cefaclor between these concentrations. Consequently the laboratories following the SRGA recommendations will rank most of the H. influenzae strains into the intermediate category, whereas laboratories following the NCCLS interpretation find them susceptible. This has led to a confusing situation in Finland and other Scandinavian countries where different laboratories apply one or the other of these recommendations.

Erythromycin has only a marginal effect on H. influenzae and there was no indication of acquired resistance to this drug. This lack of resistance makes the new, more potent macrolides, e.g. azithromycin (31), potentially promising candidates for the treatment of infections caused by H. influenzae.

Tetracycline is not used as a therapeutic agent in young children. This might be one of the reasons why resistance to this drug in the pediatric H. influenzae isolates studied was rare. Resistance to chloramphenicol was even more rare, consistent with the fact that third generation cephalosporins have largely replaced it as the first-line treatment for invasive H. influenzae infections (4, 5, 21).

Resistance to trimethoprim and trimethoprim-sulfamethoxazole was the second most common acquired antimicrobial resistance in H. influenzae in our material. As reported by Collignon et al. (32) in Australia, strains from invasive infections were less often resistant to these agents than strains from localized infections.

We can conclude that acquired antimicrobial resistance in Haemophilus influenzae in the Finnish pediatric population continues to be low. The increase of β-lactamase production, which started in the late 1970s, has halted at a level of approximately 10%.

ACKNOWLEDGMENTS

We thank Ritva Scotford, Hannele Mattila, Kaija Myyryläinen and Anna-Liisa Manninen for technical assistance.

This study was supported by a grant from Eli Lilly Finland Ltd, Vantaa, Finland and the Sigrid Juselius Foundation (P. H.).

REFERENCES

1. Cochi SL, Broome CV, Hightower AW. Immunization of U.S. children with Haemophilus influenzae type b polysaccharide vaccine. A costeffectiveness model of strategy assessment. JAMA 253: 521–529, 1985.
2. Bluestone CD, Stephenson JM, Martin LM. Ten-year review of otitis media pathogens. Pediatr Infect Dis J 11: S7–S11, 1992.
3. Takala AK, Eskola J, Leinonen M, Käyhty H, Nissinen A, Pekkanen E, Mäkelä PH. Reduction of oropharyngeal carriage of Haemophilus influenzae type b (Hib) in children immunized with an Hib conjugate vaccine. J Infect Dis 164: 982–986, 1991.
4. Powell M, Fah YS, Seymor A, Yuan M, Williams JD. Antimicrobial resistance in Haemophilus influenzae from England and Scotland in 1991. J Antimicrob Chemother 29: 547–554, 1992.
5. Jorgensen JH, Doern GV, Maher LA, Howell AW, Redding JS. Antimicrobial resistance among respiratory isolates of Haemophilus influenzae, Moraxella catarrhalis and Streptococcus pneumoniae in the United States. Antimicrob Agents Chemother 34: 2075–2080, 1990.
6. Doern GV, Jorgensen JH, Thornsberry C, Preston DA, and the Haemophilus influenzae Surveillance Group. Prevalence of antimicrobial resistance among clinical isolates of Haemophilus influenzae: a collaborative study. Diagn Microbiol Infect Dis 4: 95–107, 1986.
7. Machka K, Braveny I, Dabernat H, Dornbush K, Van Dyck E, Kayser FH, Van Klingeren B, Mittermayer H, Perea E, Powell M. Distribution and resistance patterns of Haemophilus influenzae: A European cooperative study. Eur J Clin Microbiol Infect Dis 7: 14–24, 1988.
8. Tremblay LD, L'Ecuyer J, Provencher P, Bergeron MG, and the Canadian Study Group. Susceptibility of Haemophilus influenzae to antimicrobial agents in Canada. Can Med Assoc J 143: 895–901, 1990.
9. Garlashi ML, Rusconi F, Colombo R, Conio F, Sideri S, Varotto F, Arghittu M, Passerini C, Sala A. Antimicrobial resistance among clinical isolates of Haemophilus influenzae in northern Italy. Collaborative study on pediatric infectious diseases. Eur J Epidemiol 9: 64–69, 1993.
10. George MJ, Kitch B, Henderson FW, Gilligan PH. In vitro activity of orally administered antimicrobial agents against Haemophilus influenzae recovered from children monitored longitudinally in a group day-care center. Antimicrob Agents Chemother 35: 1960–1964, 1991.
11. Howard AJ, Dunkin KT, Williams GW. Nasopharyngeal carriage and antibiotic resistance of Haemophilus influenzae in healthy children. Epidem Infect 100: 193–203, 1988.
12. Doern GV, Jorgensen JH, Thornsberry C, Preston DA, Tubert T, Redding JS, Maher LA. National collaborative study of the prevalence of antimicrobial resistance among clinical isolates of Haemophilus influenzae. Antimicrob Agents Chemother 32: 180–185, 1988.
13. Kumar A, Kelly KJ. In vitro activity of Cefixime (CL284635) and other antimicrobial agents against Haemophilus influenzae isolates from pediatric patients. Chemotherapy 34: 30–35, 1988.
14. Michaels RH, Stonebaker FE. Use of antiserum agar for detection of Haemophilus influenzae type b in the pharynx. Pediatr Res 9: 513–516, 1975.
15. Bryan LE, Godfrey AJ. Assays for β-lactamase. In: Lorian V, ed. Antibiotics in Laboratory Medicine, 3rd edn., Baltimore: The Williams & Wilkins Co., 643–650, 1991.
16. National Committee for Clinical Laboratory Standards (NCCLS). Methods for dilution antimicrobial susceptibility tests for bacteria that grow aerobically. Approved standard M7-A. Villanova, Pa: National Committee for Clinical Laboratory Standards. 1985.
17. Jorgensen JH, Redding JS, Maher LA, Howell AW. Improved medium for antimicrobial susceptibility testing of Haemophilus influenzae. J Clin Microbiol 25: 2105–2113, 1987.
18. Powell M, Koutsia-Carouzou C, Voutsinas D, Williams A, Williams JD. Resistance of clinical isolates of Haemophilus influenzae in United Kingdom 1986. BMJ 295: 176–179, 1987.
19. Howard AJ, Williams HM. The prevalence of antibiotic resistance in Haemophilus influenzae in Ireland. J Antimicrob Chemother 24: 963–971, 1989.
20. Snell JJS, Brown DFJ, Phua TJ. Antimicrobial susceptibility testing of Haemophilus influenzae: trial organized as part of United Kingdom national external quality assessment scheme for microbiology. J Clin Pathol 39: 1006–1012, 1986.
21. Kayser FH, Morenzoni G, Santanam P. The second European collaborative study on the frequency of antimicrobial resis-

tance in Haemophilus influenzae. Eur J Microbiol Infect Dis 9: 810–817, 1990.
22. Grönroos P, Hällström O, Pitkäjärvi T, Korhonen R, Lehto J. Propagation of a β-lactamase producing strain of gonococcus in Finland [in Finnish]. Finnish Medical Journal 33: 1053–1055, 1978.
23. Siitonen A, Klossner ML, Niemi E, Rantanen P. Meningitis caused by ampicillin-resistant Haemophilus influenzae type b [in Finnish]. Finnish Medical Journal 32: 2282–2285, 1977.
24. Karma P, Luotonen J, Pukander J, Sipilä M, Herva E, Grönroos P. Haemophilus influenzae in acute otitis media. Acta Otolaryngol (Stockh) 95: 105–110, 1983.
25. Clairoux N, Picard M, Brochu A, Rousseau N, Gourde P, Beauchamp D, Parr TR Jr, Bergeron MG, Malouin F. Molecular basis of the non-β-lactamase-mediated resistance to β-lactam antibiotics in strains of Haemophilus influenzae isolated in Canada. Antimicrob Agents Chemother 36: 1504–1513, 1992.
26. Rubin LG, Mendelman PM, Rakita RM, Rosen H. Virulence of non-β-lactamase-mediated ampicillin-resistant Haemophilus influenzae. FEMS Microbiol Letters 84: 27–32, 1991.
27. Powell M, Williams JD. In vitro activity of Cafaclor, Cephalexin and Ampicillin against 2458 clinical isolates of Haemophilus influenzae. J Antimicrob Chemother 21: 27–31, 1988.
28. Mendelman PM, Chaffin DO, Krilov LR, Kataitzoglou G, Serfass DA, Önay O, Wiley EA, Overturf GD, Rubin LG. Cefuroxime treatment failure of nontypable Haemophilus influenzae meningitis associated with alteration of penicillin-binding proteins. J Infect Dis 162: 1118–1123, 1990.
29. Powell M, Livermore DM. Selection and transformation of non-β-lactamase-mediated insusceptibility to β-lactams in Haemophilus influenzae: lack of cross resistance between carbapenems and other agents. J Antimicrob Chemother 26: 741–747, 1990.
30. The Swedish Reference Group for Antibiotics (SRGA). Antimicrobial susceptibility testing of bacteria; Reference and methodology manual [in Swedish]. Stockholm: The Swedish Medical Association and Statens Bakteriologiska Laboratorium, 1990.
31. Goldstein FW, Emirian MF, Coutrot A, Acar JF. Bacteriostatic and bactericidal activity of Azithromycin against Haemophilus influenzae. J Antimicrob Chemother Suppl A: 25–28, 1990.
32. Collignon PJ, Bell JM, MacInnes SJ, Gilbert GL, Toohey M, and the Australian Group for Antimicrobial Resistance (AGAR). A national collaborative study of resistance to antimicrobial agents in Haemophilus influenzae in Australian hospitals. J Antimicrob Chemother 30: 153–163, 1992.

Submitted June 30, 1994; accepted October 3, 1994

Scand J Infect Dis 27: 63–67, 1995

ORIGINAL ARTICLE

Invasive Haemophilus influenzae Disease: Epidemiology and Clinical Spectrum Before Large-scale H. influenzae Type b Vaccination

SVANTE HUGOSSON[1], SVEN-ARNE SILFVERDAL[2], ÖRJAN GARPENHOLT[3], ELISABETH ESBJÖRNER[2], BO LINDQUIST[2], THOMAS VIKERFORS[4], BO WERNER[5] and PER OLCÉN[3]

From the Departments of [1]Otorhinolaryngology, [2]Paediatrics, [3]Clinical Microbiology and Immunology, [4]Infectious Diseases and [5]Community Medicine and Public Health, Örebro Medical Center Hospital, Örebro, Sweden

In a prospective study between January 1987 and December 1992, 103 patients with invasive Haemophilus influenzae (Hi) infection were identified in a well-defined population before large-scale Haemophilus influenzae type b (Hib) vaccination was introduced. The incidence (cases/100,000/year) of invasive Hi infection was 5.9 for the whole population, 55 for children 0–4 years old and as high as 2.8 for adults. Hib was the predominant cause of the infection (83 cases) in children but, in adults, 13/39 (30%) cases were caused by non-typable Hi and 6/39 (19%) by Hi serotype f. Three patients (3%) died and 6 (5.8%) suffered a permanent sequel from the infection. All patients with such a sequel had invasive Hib infection. No significant difference between patients 0–6 years old and matched controls regarding the frequency of subnormal serum levels of immunoglobulins was found.

S. Hugosson, MD, Department of Otorhinolaryngology, Örebro Medical Center Hospital, S-701 85 Örebro, Sweden

INTRODUCTION

Acute meningitis and acute epiglottitis are the commonest and most serious manifestations of invasive Haemophilus influenzae (Hi) disease. Both of these infections are associated with significant morbidity, mortality and residual sequelae in survivors (1–7). H. influenzae type b (Hib) is the predominant serotype causing invasive disease, but other serotypes and non-typable Hi are also prevalent in these severe infections (8, 9).

The most susceptible group for contracting invasive Hi infection are children younger than 5 years. However, immunocompromised adults also risk contracting diseases such as epiglottitis, pneumonia, and septicemia (8, 10, 11). In Örebro County, Sweden, a significantly increased incidence of Hib meningitis was observed during the 1970s and the incidence early in the 1980s was higher than in other populations in the western world (5).

The aim of the present study was to investigate the incidence of invasive Hi disease among children and adults in the well-defined population of Örebro County, Sweden. The introduction of large-scale Hib vaccination of infants on 1st January 1993 in this County made a natural demarcation in the study. The results of other investigations have shown that such vaccination programs have significantly reduced the incidence of invasive Hib disease in the pediatric population (12–14). The clinical manifestations and serotype distribution of invasive Hi disease were documented and deaths and residual sequelae in survivors analysed. Serum levels of immunoglobulins (IgG, A, M and IgG subclasses) were assayed. The possible changes in clinical presentation of invasive Hi disease following the introduction of large-scale vaccination are discussed.

MATERIALS AND METHODS

Örebro County in Sweden had a mean population of 271,491 during the study period. The study design was prospective and all patients were included if they had been diagnosed in Örebro County, Sweden between 1st January 1987 and 31st December 1992 and had a positive culture for Hi from a normally sterile location. All patients with meningitis, epiglottitis, pleuropneumonia, osteitis or arthritis and peritonitis, or with a gynecological infection, had a positive blood culture or a positive culture from the cerebrospinal fluid (CSF), joint fluid, or peritoneum. The initiation of the study led to an increased awareness of the importance of obtained cultures, e.g. blood cultures from febrile patients, in order to establish a correct microbiological diagnosis. For the incidence calculations, only patients residing in Örebro County were considered.

Information about the case history and the clinical course of the disease was obtained and recorded by one of the physicians in our group, after obtaining informed consent.

Bacterial cultures were performed according to standard procedures. For serotyping, agglutination was tested with hyperimmune serum from rabbits immunized with freshly cultivated bacteria. The immunization procedure has been described previously (15). The prevalence of β-lactamase-producing Hi and the pattern of antibiotic resistance were analysed.

Serum from patients was collected in the late convalescent phase of the infection (after approximately 10 weeks) for assays of immunoglobulins (Ig) and IgG subclasses, using Mancini's immunodiffusion technique. For the Ig assays of children 0–6 years old, a control group was recruited. The controls were matched for age, sex and residence. The reference intervals of Stiehm and Fudenberg (16) and of Oxelius (17) were used. All subnormal values were reassessed.

All patients with meningitis made a follow-up visit, when neurological function (physical examination) was assessed and behaviour audiometry was performed on at least 2 occasions after the acute illness. Children with a suspected hearing impairment were tested several times.

For statistical analysis of data, student's *t*-test was used.

The study was approved by Örebro County Council's Ethics Committee.

RESULTS

All 103 patients (59 females and 44 males) diagnosed with invasive Hi infection in Örebro County between 1987 and 1992 were included in the study. Of these, 62% were children <15 years old (29 girls and 35 boys) and 38% were adults. 96 patients were residents in Örebro County and 7 were visitors. The vast majority of patients (98/103) had no known complicating condition. However, 1 adult patient had aplastic anemia and 3 adults and 1 child were treated with steroids and/or chemotherapy for neoplastic diseases when they contracted the invasive Hi infection. No patient had been immunized against Hib infections prior to onset of the disease. All were treated with intravenous antibiotics directly after bacterial cultures had been obtained. No patient with Hib meningitis was treated with steroids.

The incidence of invasive Hi-disease during the period studied was 5.9/100,000/year. The age-specific incidence rates of all invasive Hi disease, invasive Hib disease, Hi meningitis and Hi epiglottitis are shown in Table I. No patient had a recurrence of invasive Hi infection during the study period. There was no clustering or obvious social connection between the cases. The age distributions of the population and the study patients living in Örebro County are shown in Fig. 1. The clinical manifestations of invasive Hi disease are shown in Table II.

Three patients, two children and one adult, died (2.9%). Six (5.8%) patients (all children) suffered a permanent sequel from the infection; of these, 2 developed a severe central nervous lesion with focal seizures, 2 severe unilateral hearing-loss after meningitis, and 2 children unilateral deafness. Of those who had Hi meningitis the mortality rate was 3%; severe brain lesions with mental retardation occurred in 3% and sensorineural hearing-loss or unilateral deafness in 11%. Patient's delay was the same for patients who suffered a permanent sequel as for those who recovered fully. All strains causing sequelae were of serotype b.

In 83 of the 103 cases (81%) the disease was caused by Hib. Hi serotype f was the cause of the disease in 7 cases and non-typable Hi in 13. One non-compromised child (5 months) had a Hi serotype f meningitis, whereas the other

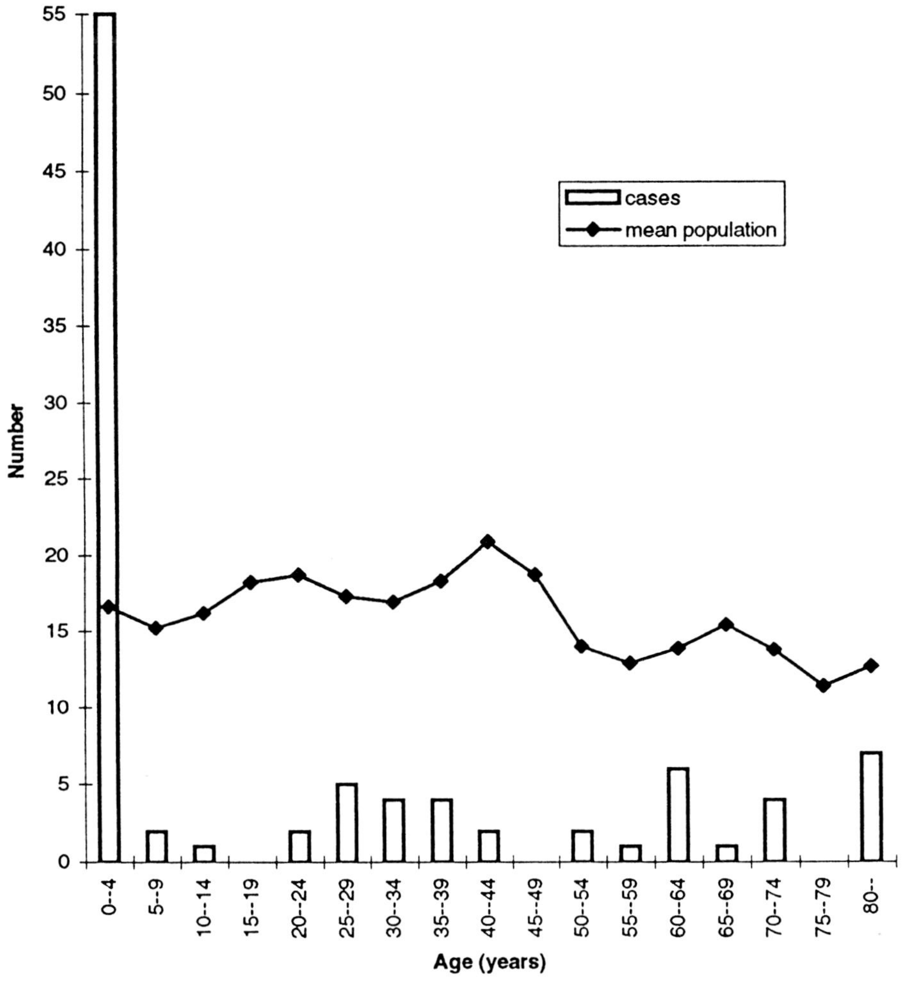

Fig. 1. The number of patients living in Örebro County, Sweden, with invasive H. influenzae disease and their age-distribution, 1987–92. Each age group's mean population × 10^3 is also shown on the *y*-axis. The mean population in the groups ranges between 10,000 and 22,000.

Table I. *Number of cases and age-specific incidence (cases/100,000/year) in children and adults for all cases of invasive H. influenzae (Hi) disease, invasive Hi type b disease, Hi meningitis and Hi epiglottitis in Örebro County, Sweden, 1987–92*

	Number of cases		Incidence	
Age (years)	Hi	Hib	Hi	Hib
Invasive Hi disease				
0–4	55	54	55	54
0–14	58	57	20	20
>14	38	19	2.8	1.5
Total	96	76	5.9	4.7
Hi meningitis				
0–4	31		31	
0–14	31		11	
>14	0		0	
Total	35		1.9	
Hi epiglottitis				
0–4	15		15	
0–14	17		5.9	
>14	9		0.67	
Total	26		1.6	

19 non-Hib cases were adults, 3 of whom had a compromising illness. Resistance to penicillins due to β-lactamase production was found in 7 (6.8%) Hi-strains (all serotype b) which were all isolated from children <4 years of age. Chloramphenicol resistance was found in 1 Hib strain that also produced β-lactamase. This strain was isolated from CSF in a child who arrived from Calcutta, India, only a few days prior to onset of the disease.

Table II. *Clinical manifestations and microbiological isolates of invasive H. influenzae disease in Örebro County, Sweden, 1987–92*

	Microbiological isolate		
Clinical manifestation	Hib	Hi-non-typable	Hif
Meningitis	34		1
Epiglottitis	26		
Pleuropneumonia	6	6	2
Bacteremia/sepsis	6	3	3
Arthritis	5		
Osteitis	1		
Peritonitis		1	1
Salpingitis		2	
Septic abortion		1	
Epiglottitis and pleuropneumonia	2		
Epiglottitis and arthritis	1		
Bacteremia and phlegmone	2		
Total number of patients	83	13	7

Among children 0–6 years old, 36 patients and 107 controls were examined concerning serum titres of IgA, IgG, IgM and IgG subclasses. The geometric mean of each fraction of Ig did not differ significantly between the 2 groups. One patient (2.8%) had a subnormal titre of total-IgG, compared with 6 in the control group (5.6%). In children older than 6 years and adults, serum for Ig assays was collected from 32 patients, 2 of whom had been treated with steroids and chemotherapy for systemic diseases and both had subnormal IgG titres. Among the other non-compromised patients, 1 had a subnormal titre of total IgG (3.3%) due mainly to a low IgG1 fraction, while 5 had an isolated IgG3 deficiency (17%). No patient had an IgA or IgM deficiency.

DISCUSSION

The incidence of invasive Hi disease in children was about the same in the present study as in earlier publications involving Caucasians (1, 18, 19).

Hi meningitis in children also remained at the same level as previously described in Örebro County, viz. 13.5 between 1971 and 1980 (5), 13.8, 1981–86 (unpublished data) and 11.0/100.000/year in the present study, 1987–92. However, the incidence of invasive Hi infection in adults was higher than previously described (8, 10, 11). One reason for this may be that the number of elderly in our population was proportionally high. 10% of the adults in our study had a major illness with or without treatment, which probably made them more susceptible to infections.

The true incidence rates were probably somewhat higher than presented here, since the calculations did not consider residents falling ill outside the county.

The clinical spectrum of invasive Hi disease in our study is consistent with the results of other studies (10, 11, 20). however, a case with simultaneously occurring septic arthritis and epiglottitis has not, to our knowledge, been reported elsewhere.

The distribution of Hi serotypes shows a predominance for serotype b among children. However, the impact of non-b Hi as a cause of invasive disease in adults is substantial. In our study, all non-b Hi strains except 1 were isolated from adults, of which 19/39 (49%) were infected by non-b Hi. The importance of non-typable Hi as a cause of invasive disease has been described both in infants and in adults (9, 11). Patients with invasive non-b Hi infection seem to have a less severe disease course and in the present study all patients with a permanent sequel were infected with Hib.

In estimating hearing in infants following meningitis, behaviour audiometry has limitations in accuracy depending on variations in the child's cooperability and attention. However, these children were investigated several times before a decision was made as to whether hearing had been affected or not. All 4 children with a permanent hearing loss or deafness were followed up rigorously and the last audiometry was performed at the age of 3 years or more.

The finding of subnormal concentrations of IgG3 in uncompromised adults is noteworthy, though interlaboratory variations can affect the validity of the reference values. IgG3 and IgG4 are described as the least important IgG subclasses in host defence against capsulated bacteria (21, 22) and there is probably no clinical importance of such an isolated IgG subclass deficiency as a predisposing factor for invasive Hi disease (21). In children and in adults, the antibody response to the Hib polysaccharide antigen comprises mainly IgG1 and IgG2 subclasses (21, 22).

In the present study we could not verify that a low serum level of an Ig fraction is a risk factor for invasive Hi infection in the most susceptible age group, viz. 0–6 years.

The pattern of change in incidence, of Hib epiglottitis and adult Hib disease, can in the future serve as a functional measure of the effect on Hib carriage in the upper respiratory tract and the transmission of Hib in a population with large-scale vaccination of infants (23). The impact of non-b Hi as invasive organisms may become greater after large-scale Hib vaccination because of the possibility of less competition from Hib, following reduced colonization in the nasopharynx (24). The high incidence of invasive Hib disease among non-compromised and previously healthy adults in our study indicates that the natural acquisition of immunity to Hib can fail, or immunity may become defective with ageing. Hib vaccination failures among children have been reported (25), whereas vaccination failures that are detected later in life have yet to be sought. We believe that invasive Hi disease should still be considered a clinical reality and in adults the incidence may remain unchanged despite successful Hib vaccination in childhood. Further investigations are presently being conducted to follow the effects of vaccination on the incidence, clinical spectrum and age distribution of invasive Hi disease.

ACKNOWLEDGEMENTS

We wish to thank Lars Wranne, Lars Åhman and Ulla Hammar, Dept. of Paediatrics; Hans Fredlund and Eva Törnqvist, Dept. of Clinical Microbiology and Immunology; Lennart Bodin, Dept. of Environmental Medicine; Örebro Medical Center Hospital, Örebro; and Teresa Lagergård, Dept. of Microbiology, University of Gothenburg, Sweden and also The Research Committee of Örebro County Council.

REFERENCES

1. Peltola H, Rod TO, Jonsdottir K, Böttiger M, Coolidge JA. Life-threatening Haemophilus influenzae infections in Scandinavia: a five-country analysis of the incidence and the main clinical and bacteriologic characteristics. Rev Infect Dis 12: 708–715, 1990.
2. Trollfors B, Claesson B, Strangert KH. H. influenzae meningitis in Sweden 1981–83. Arch Dis Child 62: 1220–1223, 1987.
3. Trollfors B, Nylén O, Strangert KH. Acute epiglottitis in children and adults in Sweden 1981–3. Arch Dis Child 65: 491–494, 1990.
4. Gonzales C, Gartner JC, Casselbrant ML, Kenna MA. Complication of acute epiglottitis. Int J Pediatr Otorhinolaryngol 11: 67–71, 1986.
5. Salwén KM, Vikerfors T, Olcén P. Increased incidence of childhood bacterial meningitis. A 25-year study in a defined population in Sweden. Scand J Infect Dis 19: 1–11, 1987.
6. MayoSmith MF, Hirsch PJ, Wodzinski SF, Schiffman FJ. Acute epiglottitis in adults. N Engl J Med 324: 1133–1139, 1986
7. Taylor HG, Mills EL, Ciampi A, du Berger R, Watters GV, Gold R, MacDonald N, Michaels RH. The sequelae of Haemophilus influenzae menningitis in school-age children. N Engl J Med 323: 1657–1663, 1990.
8. Farley MM, Stephens DS, Brachman Jr PS, Harvey RC, Smith JD, Wenger JD. Invasive Haemophilus influenzae disease in adults. A prospective, population-based surveillance. CDC Meningitis Surveillance Group. Ann Intern Med 116: 806–812, 1992.
9. Falla TJ, Dobson SR, Crook DW, Kraak WA, Nichols WW, Anderson EC, Jordens JZ, Slack MP, Mayon-White D, Moxon ER. Population-based study of non-typable Haemophilus influenzae invasive disease in children and neonates. Lancet 341: 851–854, 1993.
10. Takala AK, Eskola J, van Alphen L. Spectrum of invasive Haemophilus influenzae type b disease in adults. Arch Intern Med 150: 2573–2576, 1990.
11. Trollfors B, Claesson B, Lagergård T, Sandberg T. Incidence, predisposing factors and manifestations of invasive Haemophilus influenzae infections in adults. Eur J Clin Microbiol 3: 180–184, 1984.
12. Peltola H, Kilpi T, Anttila M. Rapid disappearance of Haemophilus influenzae type b meningitis after routine childhood immunisation with conjugate vaccines. Lancet 340: 592–594, 1992.
13. Adams WG, Deaver KA, Cochi SL, Plikaytis BD, Zell ER, Broome CV, Wenger JD. Decline of childhood Haemophilus influenzae type b (Hib) disease in the Hib vaccine era. JAMA 269: 221–226, 1993.
14. Kessler A, Wetmore RF, Marsh RR. Childhood epiglottitis in recent years. Int J Pediatr Otorhinolaryngol 25: 155–162, 1993.
15. Dahlberg T, Branefors P. Enzyme-linked immunosorbent assay for titration of Haemophilus influenzae capsular and O antigen antibodies. J Clin Microbiol 12: 185–192, 1980.
16. Stiehm ER, Fudenberg HH. Serum levels of immune globulins in health and disease: A survey. Pediatrics 37: 715–727, 1966.
17. Oxelius V. IgG subclass levels in infancy and childhood. Acta Paediatr Scand 68: 23–27, 1979.
18. Gervaix A, Suter S. Epidemiology of invasive Haemophilus influenzae type b infections in Geneva, Switzerland, 1976 to 1989. Pediatr Infect Dis J 10: 370–374, 1991.
19. McGregor AR, Bell JM, Abdool IM, Collignon PJ. Invasive Haemophilus influenzae infection in the Australian Capital Territory region. Med J Aust 156: 569–572, 1992.
20. Takala AK, Eskola J, Peltola H, Mäkelä PH. Epidemiology of invasive Haemophilus influenzae type b disease among children in Finland before vaccination with Haemophilus influenzae type b conjugate vaccine. Pediatr Infect Dis J 8: 297–302, 1989.
21. Shackelford PG, Granoff DM, Polmar SH, Scott MG,

Goskowicz MC, Madassery JV, Nahm MH. Subnormal serum concentrations of IgG2 in children with frequent infections associated with varied patterns of immunologic dysfunction. J Pediatr 116: 529–538, 1990.
22. Amir J, Scott MG, Nahm MH, Granoff DM. Bactericidal and opsonic activity of IgG1 and IgG2 anticapsular antibodies to Haemophilus influenzae type b. J Infect Dis 162: 163–171, 1990.
23. Takala AK, Eskola J, Leinonen M, Käyhty H, Nissinen A, Pekkanen E, Mäkelä PH. Reduction of oropharyngeal carriage of Haemophilus influenzae type b (Hib) in children immunized with an Hib conjugate vaccine. J Infect Dis 164: 982–986, 1991.
24. Shapiro ED. Infections caused by Haemophilus influenzae type b. The beginning of the end? JAMA 269: 264–266, 1993.
25. Holmes SJ, Lucas AH, Osterholm MT, Froeschle JE, Granoff DM. Immunoglobulin deficiency and idiotype expression in children developing Haemophilus influenzae type b disease after vaccination with conjugate vaccine. The Collaborative Study Group. JAMA 266: 1960–1965, 1991.

Submitted April 27, 1994; accepted October 24, 1994

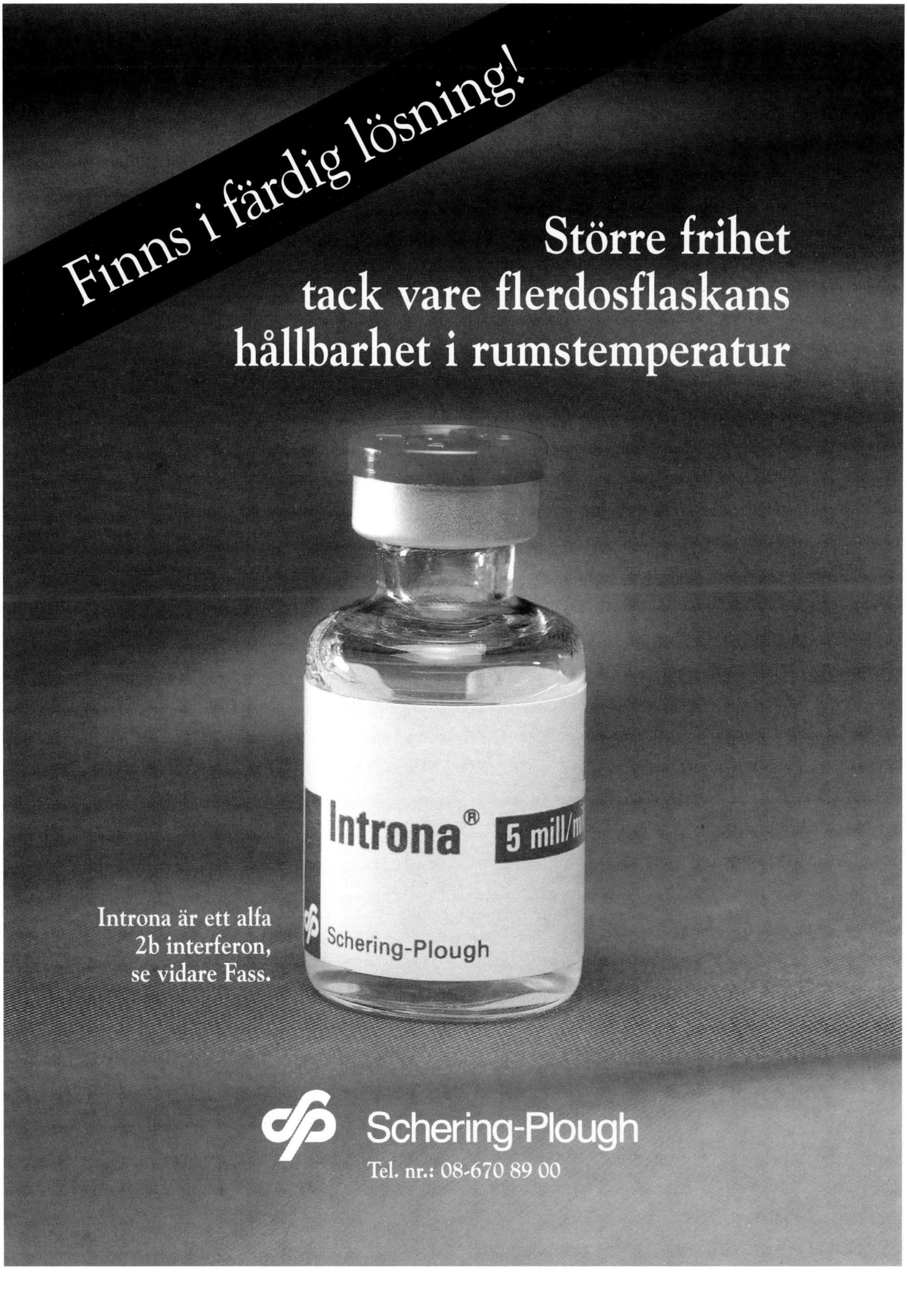
Finns i färdig lösning!
Större frihet
tack vare flerdosflaskans
hållbarhet i rumstemperatur
Introna®
5 mill/m
Schering-Plough
Introna är ett alfa
2b interferon,
se vidare Fass.
Schering-Plough
Tel. nr.: 08-670 89 00

Scand J Infect Dis 27: 69–70, 1995 ORIGINAL ARTICLE

Prevalence of Cryptosporidium sp. in Patients with Neoplasia and Diarrhea

MEHMET TANYÜKSEL, HÜSEYİN GÜN and LEVENT DOĞANCI

From the Department of Microbiology and Clinical Microbiology, Gülhane Military Medical Academy, Etlik, Ankara, Turkey

The prevalence of Cryptosporidium sp. was investigated in fecal specimens from 106 patients with neoplasia and diarrhea (74 females, 32 males) by using Ziehl-Neelsen and Giemsa stains. Oocystic forms of Cryptosporidium sp. were found in 18 (17%) of these patients. No oocystic form of Cryptosporidium sp. was detected in the control group of 60 patients with neoplasia (37 females, 23 males) but without diarrhea. The frequent findings of Cryptosporidium sp. in patients with neoplasia and diarrhea who are undergoing chemotherapy indicates that a search for this organism is justified.

M. Tanyüksel, MD, Department of Microbiology and Clinical Microbiology, Gülhane Military Medical Academy, 06018 Etlik, Ankara, Turkey

INTRODUCTION

Cryptosporidium sp. is a coccidian protozoan which differs from other coccidia. Preliminary prospective studies have indicated the importance of the parasite as a cause of acute, sporadic gastroenteritis in otherwise healthy subjects, particularly children, in both developed (1) and underdeveloped countries (2), and in travellers, most of whom were adults (3). Cryptosporidiosis as an opportunistic infection is also a disease of infants and persons with poor immunity. Our purpose was to investigate the prevalence of Cryptosporidiosis in patients with various forms of neoplasia who had concomitant diarrheal disease.

MATERIALS AND METHODS

Cases of neoplasia with diarrhea diagnosed between March and July 1992 at the Ankara Oncology Hospital were investigated. All patients in the study group either received chemotherapy and/or radiotherapy or surgery. Fecal specimens from 106 patients (74/32, females/males) were investigated with light microscopy for Cryptosporidium sp. The patients in the study group had had neoplasia and diarrheal disease for ≥10 days. Fecal specimens were collected on the 7th, 8th and 10th days of diarrhea. Abdominal pain, subfebrility and watery stools were present in all patients. The 60 patients in the control group (37/23, females/males) had neoplasia without diarrhea. The Giemsa and Ziehl Neelsen Staining methods were used for staining of fecal slides and these preparations were examined with light microscopy (4).

RESULTS

Oocysts of Cryptosporidium sp. were found in 18 (17%) of 106 specimens from the study group [11 (14.8%) of 74 females and 7 (21.8%) of 32 males]. No pathogenic bacteria were isolated in this study group and no protozoal pathogens such as Entamoeba histolytica or Giardia intestinalis were seen by light microscopy. All patients were anti-HIV negative (EIA BioMérioux, France). In the control group, no oocystic form of Cryptosporidium was seen. There was no correlation between the diarrheal illness caused by Cryptosporidium and the type of neoplasia (Table I).

Table I. *Prevalence of Cryptosporidium sp. in faeces in patients with neoplasia undergoing chemotherapy who have diarrhea (Study group) and in a control group with neoplasia without diarrhea*

	No with Cryptosporidium sp./ Total no	
Type of neoplasm	Study group	Control group
Colon carcinoma	4/22	0/8
Breast carcinoma	3/16	0/21
Thyroid carcinoma (papillary)	3/17	0/4
Malignant melanoma	3/16	0/3
Gastric carcinoma	1/6	0/13
Leiomyosarcoma	1/5	0/4
Basal cell carsinoma	1/6	0/3
Squamous cell ca. (bladder)	1/8	0/3
Liposarcoma	1/10	0/1
Total	18/106 (17%)	0/60 (0%)

DISCUSSION

Cryptosporidium sp. is a well known cause of infant diarrhea and occasionally also in adults (3). It causes chronic diarrhea in immunocompromized adults and has since 1980 been recognized as an agent causing gastroenteritius. In some Scandinavian countries, it occurs mainly in adults. Most acquire the infection abroad (especially in Russia), or as a result of occupational exposure (5). In the USA, Cryptosporidium sp. was identified in 1.1% of 5,256 patients who visited the Oregon Public Health Service between 1985 and 1988 (6). The parasite was identified in 2.6% of 735 patients, with acute diarrhea in the Philippines (7), in 13.1% of patients with acute diarrhea in India (8), in 6.4% of 750 with acute diarrhea in Chile and in 0.2% of 455 persons >15 years old in Bangladesh (9). The prevalence was noted to increase when the temperature and humidity were high.

In our study, no Cryptosporidium sp. was isolated in the control group, whereas the prevalence was 16.9% in the

 ISSN 0036-5548

study group. This shows that Cryptosporidium sp. may cause diarrheal illness in persons at high risk. Activation of Cryptosporidium sp. following anti-neoplastic treatment may trigger diarrheal illness. A possible mechanism for this activation may be related to impaired T-cell function which is important for the prevention of diarrhea.

When the immune system is suppressed by the tumour cells, it synthesizes several factors that can lead to impaired defence against parasites (10). The mechanisms of host defence responsible for the control of Cryptosporidium sp. infections are also poorly understood. Infection by Cryptosporidium sp. does not invariably result in diarrhea. The symptoms may include mild epigastric pain, nausea, vomiting and anorexia with or without mild fever. The humoral immunity contributes to the elimination of the infection but whether or not protective humoral immunity against reinfection exists remains unclear. The complex mechanisms of the immunopathogenesis of Cryptosporidium infection have not yet been clarified. Our findings suggest that patients with neoplasia and receiving chemotherapy, who have diarrhea should be screened for Cryptosporidium sp.

REFERENCES

1. Tzipori S, Smith M, Birch C, Barnes G, Bishop R. Cryptosporidiosis in hospital patients with gastroenteritis. Am J Trop Med Hyg 32: 931–934, 1983.
2. Bogaerts J, Lepage P, Rouvroy D, Vandepitte J. Cryptosporidium spp. a frequent cause of diarrhea in central Africa. J Clin Microbiol 20: 874–876, 1984.
3. Holten-Andersen W, Gerstoft J, Henriksen SA, Pedersen NS. Prevalence of Cryptosporidium among patients with acute enteric infection. J Infect 9: 277–282, 1984.
4. Baron EJ, Finegold SM. Diagnostic Microbiology, 8th edn. St. Louis: Mosby Company, 1990, 70–72.
5. Jokipii L, Pohjola S, Jokipii AMM. Cryptosporidiosis associated with travelling and giardiasis. Gastroenterology 89: 838–842, 1985.
6. Skeels MR, Sokolow R, Vance Hubbard C, Andrus JK, Baisch J. Cryptosporidium infection in Oregon Public Health Clinic patients 1985–1988: The value of statewide laboratory surveillance. AJPH 80: 305–308, 1990.
7. Cross JH, Alcantara A, Alquiza L, Zaraspe G, Ranoa C. Cryptosporidiosis in Philippine children. Southeast Asian J Trop Med Public Health 16: 257–260, 1985.
8. Naqash HV, Waltal C. Cryptosporidiosis in Kashmir. Trans R Soc Trop Med Hyg 82: 335, 1988.
9. Shepherd RC, Sinha PG, Reed LC, Russel EF. Cryptosporidiosis in the west of Scotland. Scott Med J 39: 365–368, 1988.
10. Herlyn M, Menrad A, Koprowski H. Structure, function and clinical significance of human tumour antigens. J Natl Cancer Inst 82; 1883–1889, 1990.

Submitted June 20, 1994; accepted October 1, 1994

Scand J Infect Dis 27: 71–74, 1995 ORIGINAL ARTICLE

Disseminated Toxoplasmosis in AIDS Patients – Report of 16 Cases

HELMUT ALBRECHT[1], JÜRGEN SKÖRDE[2], KEIKAWUS ARASTEH[2], WALTER HEISE[2], HANS-JÜRGEN STELLBRINK[1], GERNOT GROSSE[3] and MANFRED L'AGE[2]

From the Departments of [1]Internal Medicine, University Clinic Eppendorf, Hamburg, [2]Gastroenterology and Infectious Diseases and [3]Pathology, Auguste Viktoria Hospital Berlin-Schöneberg, Germany

Between June 1986 and October 1992, disseminated toxoplasmosis was diagnosed in 16 AIDS patients. 13 cases were diagnosed at autopsy where multiple organ involvement was documented in all 13. Three patients were diagnosed intra vitam. All 3 survived with appropriate treatment. Clinical features indicative of disseminated toxoplasmosis were: fever of unknown origin between 39° and 40°C in 16 cases, clinical signs suggestive of sepsis or septic shock in 15, with progression to multiorgan failure in 10, disseminated intravascular coagulopathy in 6, confusion, desorientation or apathy in 13 and lack of a systemic pneumocystis carinii prophylaxis in all 16. Typical laboratory markers were: CD4 cell counts below 100×10^6/l in 16 cases, elevation of serum lactic dehydrogenase in 16 and creatine phosphokinase (in 4/6), normal or only slightly elevated C-reactive protein (in 9/11), positive Toxoplasma gondii IgG antibodies in 15/16 and negative IgM antibodies in all 16. Lesions indicative of cerebral toxoplasmosis were visualized on cranial computerized tomography in only 3/10 evaluated patients. In patients with advanced HIV infection presenting with a systemic illness, including the clinical and laboratory features described above, systemic Toxoplasma gondii infection must be included in the differential diagnosis. In these patients, specific and if warranted, invasive diagnostic procedures followed by early vigorous therapeutic intervention should be considered.

H. Albrecht, MD, University Clinic Eppendorf, Pav 33 Infe, Martinistr. 52, D-20246 Hamburg, Germany

INTRODUCTION

Toxoplasma gondii (TG) infection presenting as encephalitis with cerebral abscess formation is a commonly encountered opportunistic infection in patients with AIDS, especially in Europe (1). Extraneural toxoplasmosis is a well documented, albeit rare entity (2–10). Diagnosis is almost always first made at autopsy. Because most of the case reports have stemmed from autopsies, few reports have documented the clinical features associated with disseminated Toxoplasma gondii infection. We reviewed the clinical data and autopsy material of 13 patients who at autopsy were diagnosed to suffer from disseminated Toxoplasma gondii infection. Three further patients benefitted from the accumulated data and a subsequently higher index of clinical suspicion. Extracerebral toxoplasmosis in these 3 patients was diagnosed intra vitam and treated successfully. Clinical and laboratory data of all 16 patients are presented and clinical implications are discussed.

MATERIAL AND METHODS

Of 1,335 HIV-infected patients admitted to the Auguste-Viktoria-Hospital in Berlin and the University Clinic Eppendorf in Hamburg between 1986 and 1991, 6 patients at autopsy were diagnosed as having died of disseminated toxoplasmosis. Sepsis of unknown origin had been the clinically suspected cause of death in 5 of these patients. This prompted a review of the autopsy material from 14 other patients who had died with a diagnosis of fever or sepsis of unknown origin. Routine staining was performed with hematoxylin and eosin (H&E), Giemsa, PAS, Grocott, methylgreen pyronin and trichrome Goldner. Additionally a specific immunohistochemical detection method for Toxoplasma gondii, using polyclonal rabbit anti-toxoplasma antibodies, was applied to stored samples. The method of this test and examples of its use have been published in a previous report (11).

Three further patients benefitted from the accumulated data and were diagnosed intra vitam. Details of one of these patients who was diagnosed as suffering from isolated cardiac toxoplasmosis, have been presented prior to this report (11). Because this patient's clinical presentation was remarkably similar to the course observed in the other patients, he was included in this report despite the fact that Toxoplasma gondii was only isolated from the myocardium. Details of another patient diagnosed at autopsy, including a description of the use of PCR for the diagnosis of toxoplasmosis, have also been published previously (12). The charts of all 16 patients, 2 women and 14 men with a mean age of 39.7 years (range 24 to 55 years), were reviewed for this report.

RESULTS

The analysis of the clinical data of the 16 patients with disseminated toxoplasmosis led to the recognition of characteristic features encountered in a majority of them. Sustained or intermittent fever of unknown origin between 39° and 40°C was present in all 16. 15/16 patients had clinical signs suggestive of sepsis or septic shock, i.e. hypotension as defined by a systolic blood pressure <90 mmHg or a reduction of >40 mmHg from baseline in the absence of other causes, peripheral cyanosis, oliguria, prostration, tachycardia, tachypnea. 10 patients progressed to multiorgan failure, often with cardiac decompensation and respiratory failure.

Addison's syndrome cannot have been responsible for the observed clinical picture, as involvement of the adrenal glands was documented in only 4 patients, no characteristic

 ISSN 0036-5548

changes in electrolytes were observed and steroids alone did not halt the continuous clinical deterioration. A cardiogenic etiology of shock is also less likely because not all patients with myocardial involvement presented with or progressed to shock. Furthermore, the creatinine phosphokinase (CPK)-MB fraction was normal in all patients assessed, central venous pressure was elevated in only 1/6 patients evaluated, and clinically, peripheral vasodilation was reported much more frequently than vasoconstriction. Disseminated intravascular coagulopathy with elevated fibrin split products and marked reduction of fibrinogen was observed in 6/16. 10 patients showed signs of confusion, desorientation and/or apathy. CD4-counts were below 100×10^6/l in all 16 patients. Serum lactic dehydrogenase (LDH) was elevated in all patients. The average LDH concentration was 726 U/l (range 297–2,100 U/l, normal <240 U/l). CPK was found to be elevated in 4/6 patients tested, with an average of 181 U/l (range 50–576 U/l, normal <80 U/l). The CPK-MB fraction was not elevated in any patient. C-reactive protein (CRP) was assessed in 11 patients and normal results (<6 mg/l) were found in 5 and minimal elevation (6–20 mg/l) in 3. Only 1 patient had a CRP greater than 100 mg/l. Even though leukopenia and mild thrombocytopenia were common, no consistent changes were observed in electrolytes, white blood count and differential or platelet counts. Anemia was present in all cases, but was usually mild.

At autopsy, multiple organ involvement was found in all 13 patients. The most commonly affected organs were brain (12/13 cases), heart (10/13) and lung (10/13). Involvement of spleen, liver, bone marrow, lymph nodes, adrenal glands, skeletal muscle and pancreas was also documented.

In the 3 patients diagnosed intra vitam, Toxoplasma gondii was isolated from the blood of one patient, from blood and lung tissue of another patient, and from heart tissue in the third patient. Prior to the diagnosis of extracerebral toxoplasmosis, all 3 received broad-spectrum antibiotics. Two patients had additionally been treated with steroids and antifungal medication, but without improvement. All 3 showed dramatic improvement after therapy with sulfadiazine, clindamycin and pyrimethamine (plus dapsone in 1 patient) was begun.

Whereas autopsy revealed concomitant cerebral toxoplasmosis in 12/13 patients, cerebral computerized tomography (CCT) had revealed the characteristic lesions indicative of cerebral toxoplasmosis in only 3 of 10 patients evaluated. In 1 patient a magnetic resonance image (MRI) failed to detect focal lesions, but showed a pattern of diffuse infiltration suggestive of progressive multifocal leukoencephalopathy (PML). At autopsy, atypical miliary T. gondii infection of the brain without abscess formation was diagnosed.

Only 1 patient, an intravenous drug user, had previously experienced an episode of cerebral toxoplasmosis. He was non-compliant, did not take his prescribed medication for secondary prophylaxis and relapsed with disseminated and fatal disease. None of the other patients received systemic prophylaxis for the prevention of pneumocystis carinii pneumonia (PcP). Patients were either treated with monthly pentamidine inhalations (12/15) or did not receive any form of prophylaxis (3/15).

Toxoplasma IgM antibodies were undetectable in all 16 patients. With the exception of case 1, specific Toxoplasma gondii IgG antibodies were detected in 15/16 patients. A polymerase chain reaction (PCR) test for T. gondii DNA in blood, currently being evaluated at 1 of our centres, gave strong positive results in the last 2 patients in our study.

DISCUSSION

Toxoplasmosis has become one of the most frequent AIDS-related infections in many European countries, especially France, Switzerland and Germany. Encephalitis with cerebral abscess formation is the most common manifestation in AIDS patients. Disseminated Toxoplasma gondii infection, however, is a rare complication of the infection with HIV (2–10).

Since June 1986 we have diagnosed systemic toxoplasmosis in 16 of our AIDS patients. In 13 patients, diagnosis was first confirmed by autopsy. The analysis of the clinical data of these and 3 other patients who were diagnosed intra vitam showed similar characteristics: sustained or intermittent fever between 39° and 40°C, clinical signs suggestive of sepsis or septic shock, confusion, desorientation and/or apathy, disseminated intravascular coagulopathy, and multiorgan failure. Cardiopulmonary decompensation was observed frequently, resulting in an initial tentative diagnosis of PcP in some cases.

15 of 16 patients fulfilled the criteria of sepsis and 10 of 16 patients presented with or progressed to a clinical picture of septic shock as defined in a recent consensus paper by the American College of Chest Physicians and the Society of Critical Care Medicine (13). Sepsis and septic shock including hemodynamic confirmation have been documented not only in patients with bacteremia but also in patients with disseminated mycobacterial (14) and fungal (15) infections. Septic shock has also been reported in patients with disseminated toxoplasmosis admitted to an intensive care unit (16). Toxoplasma gondii does not produce toxins, but it is conceivable that disseminated infection with the parasite may trigger a cascade of cytokines similar to other infections, resulting in a clinical picture indistinguishable from sepsis or septic shock. All our patients presented with advanced HIV-infection and in the majority of cases intensive care treatment and hemodynamic monitoring was not initiated. We agree that it is difficult or probably even impossible to make a formal diagnosis of sepsis or septic shock without adequate hemodynamic monitoring. For clinical purposes, however, it is helpful to remember that most of our patients clearly 'appeared toxic' and that sepsis or septic shock was the clinical diagnosis in most of our patients.

CD4-cell counts below 100×10^6/l significantly elevated LDH and CPK levels and normal or only slightly increased CRP were typically encountered laboratory markers. Patients suffering from bacterial sepsis usually present with a markedly increased CRP which might be helpful to distinguish these two conditions.

Because serologic tests are rarely of diagnostic value, alternative and specific non-invasive tests have to be instituted to facilitate the diagnosis of systemic Toxoplasma gondii infection (17–20). In a recent report, Pugin et al. suggested measurement of LDH as a sensitive, and in their experience specific test to distinguish disseminated toxoplasmosis from other AIDS-related disorders such as PcP or cerebral toxoplasmosis (6). The mean value for serum LDH in our patients was 726 IU/l (range 297 to 2,110 IU/l). In patients with disseminated toxoplasmosis in which the disease is diagnosed early enough to institute successful treatment, LDH may only be mildly elevated. Disseminated toxoplasmosis should therefore be included in the list of differential diagnoses also in symptomatic patients at risk who do not present with grossly elevated LDH.

Cell culture systems that allow isolation of the parasite from the blood of patients have recently been developed (18). This method, however, requires sophisticated laboratory facilities and is not commonly available for routine diagnostic purposes.

The peroxidase-antiperoxidase method employing monoclonal T. gondii antibodies that was used in some of our patients seems to be a very sensitive test to visualize Toxoplasma antigen in biopsy specimens (11, 17).

Preliminary data on the use of the PCR technique to diagnose T. gondii in the blood and tissue of infected patients are promising and may also be of help in the management of these patients (12, 19, 20). The PCR test gave strong results in the 2 patients tested in this series.

CCT was of minor diagnostic help in our survey. Nevertheless early CCT or MRI is certainly indicated. The question whether MRI is more sensitive in demonstrating small lesions in these patients remains to be answered.

Inhalative pentamidine is currently the most commonly used measure for primary PcP prophylaxis in Germany. With a rising incidence of cerebral toxoplasmosis (21) and the substantial mortality caused by the septic course of systemic T. gondii infection we reported, systemic PcP prophylaxis that is also protective against T. gondii should be considered for all patients with serologic evidence of latent toxoplasma infection.

Our experience suggests that in HIV-infected patients developing a septic illness of unknown origin, presenting with the clinical and laboratory characteristics described above, disseminated toxoplasmosis must be considered.

As outlined above, the new, specific tests may facilitate the establishment of a definite diagnosis of extracerebral toxoplasmosis in these patients.

Because most of these tests are not yet routinely available and are still undergoing clinical evaluation, specific empiric therapy should be considered when initial microbiological assessment fails to reveal another causative pathogen in patients presenting with a septic illness with the clinical and laboratory features outlined.

Untreated disseminated Toxoplasma gondii infection is lethal. Systemic toxoplasmosis, however, is a potentially treatable disease and we hope that awareness of the clinical presentation will reverse the grave prognosis of this infection.

ACKNOWLEDGEMENT

The authors wish to thank Dr David Brewster for his critical review of the manuscript and helpful suggestions.

REFERENCES

1. Luft BJ, Remington JS. Toxoplasmosis of the central nervous system. In: Remington JS, Swartz MN, eds. Current topics in infectious disease, vol. 6. New York: McGraw-Hill, 1985.
2. Derouin F, Sarfati C, Beauvais B, Garin YJF, Larivière M. Prevalence of pulmonary toxoplasmosis in HIV-infected patients. AIDS 4: 1036, 1990.
3. Oksenhendler MD, Cadranel J, Sarfati C, Katlama C, Datry A, Marche C, Wolf M, Roux P, Derouin F, Clauvel JP. Toxoplasma gondii pneumonia in patients with the acquired immunodeficiency syndrome. Am J Med 88: 18N–21N, 1990.
4. Catterall JR, Hofflin JM, Remington JS. Pulmonary toxoplasmosis. Am Rev Respir Dis 133: 704–705, 1986.
5. Israelski DM, Skowron G, Leventhal JP, Long I, Blankenship CF, Barrio GW, Prince JB, Araujo FG, Remington JS. Toxoplasma peritonitis in a patient with acquired immunodeficiency syndrome. Arch Intern Med 148: 1655–1657, 1988.
6. Pugin J, Vanhems P, Hirschel B, Chave JP, Flepp M. Extreme elevations of serum lactic dehydrogenase differentiating pulmonary toxoplasmosis from pneumocystis pneumonia. NEJM 326: 1226, 1992.
7. Garcia LH, Hemphill RB, Marasco HA, Ciano PS. Acquired immunodeficiency syndrome with disseminated toxoplasmosis presenting as an acute pulmonary and gastrointestinal illness. Arch Pathol Lab Med 130: 459–463, 1991.
8. Haskell L, Fusco MJ, Ares L, Sublay B. Disseminated toxoplasmosis presenting as symptomatic orchitis and nephrotic syndrome. Am J Med Sci 198: 185–190, 1989.
9. Tschirrhart D, Klatt ED. Disseminated toxoplasmosis in the acquired immunodeficiency syndrome. Arch Pathol Lab Med 112: 1237–1241, 1988.
10. Matturri L, Quattrone P, Varesi C, Rossi L. Cardiac toxoplasmosis in pathology of acquired immunodeficiency syndrome. Panminerva Med 32: 194–196, 1990.
11. Albrecht H, Stellbrink HJ, Fenske S, Schäfer H, Greten H. Successful treatment of Toxoplasma gondii myocarditis in an AIDS patient. Eur J Clin Microbiol 13: 500–504, 1994.
12. Buhr M, Heise W, Arasteh K, Strathmann M, Grosse M, L'Age M. Disseminated toxoplasmosis with sepsis in AIDS. Clin Invest 70: 1079–1081, 1992.
13. American College of Chest Physicians/Society of Critical Care Medicine Consensus Conference: Definitions for sepsis and organ failure and guidelines for the use of innovative therapies in sepsis. Crit Care Med 20: 864–874, 1992.
14. Ahuja SS, Ahuja SK, Phelps KR, Thelmo W, Hill AR. Hemodynamic confirmation of septic shock in disseminated tuberculosis. Crit Care Med 20: 901–903, 1992.

15. Wiles JB, Cerra FB, Siegal JH, Broder JR. The systemic septic response: Does the organism really matter? Crit Care Med 8: 55–60, 1980.
16. Holliman RE, Johnson JD, Gillespie SH, Johnson MA, Squire SB, Savva D. New methods in the diagnosis and management of cerebral toxoplasmosis associated with the acquired immune deficiency syndrome. J Infect 22: 281–285, 1991.
17. Tirard V, Niel G, Rosenheim M, Katlama C, Ciceron L, Ocunkolade W, Danis M, Gentilini M. Diagnosis of toxoplasmosis in patients with AIDS by isolation of the parasite from the blood. NEJM 324: 634, 1991.
18. Dupouy-Camet J, de Souza SL, Maslo C, Paugam A, Saimot AG, Benarous R, Tourte-Schaefer C, Derouin F. Detection of Toxoplasma gondii in venous blood from AIDS patients by polymerase chain reaction. J Clin Microbiol 31: 1866–1869, 1993.
19. Roth A, Roth B, Hoeffken G, Steuber S, Khalifa KI, Janitschke K. Application of the polymerase chain reaction in the diagnosis of pulmonary toxoplasmosis in immunocompromised patients. Eur J Clin Microbiol Infect Dis 11: 1177–1181, 1992.
20. Lucet JC, Bailly MP, Bedos JP, Wolff M, Gachot B, Vachon F. Septic shock due to toxoplasmosis in patients infected with the human immunodeficiency virus. Chest 104: 1054–1058, 1993.
21. Stellbrink HJ, Führer-Burow R, Raedler A, Albrecht H, Fenske S. Risk factors for severe disease due to Toxoplasma gondii in HIV-positive patients. Eur J Epidemiol 9: 633–637, 1993.

Submitted September 1, 1994; accepted November 27, 1994

Scand J Infect Dis 27: 75–76, 1995

Cranial Nerve Palsies and Cerebral Infarction in a Young Infant with Meningococcal Meningitis

CHENG-HSUN CHIU, TZOU-YIEN LIN and YHU-CHERING HUANG

From the Section of Pediatric Infectious Diseases, Department of Pediatrics, Chang Gung Children's Hospital, Taoyuan, Taiwan

A previously healthy 30-day-old male infant became ill with fever, poor activity, and refusal to feed for 2 days. A cerebrospinal fluid examination revealed 7.15 × 10^8 leukocytes/l with 72% neutrophils, protein 4.6g/l, and glucose 7 mg/dl. Neisseria meningitidis was isolated from the blood and cerebrospinal fluid. On the fourth day of hospitalization, the baby was found to have left oculomotor and facial palsies, which resolved gradually. He was treated with intravenous penicillin for 2 weeks. A repeat CSF examination revealed a high persisting protein level of 2.9 g/l and a computerized tomographic brain scan revealed a cerebral infarction in the bilateral frontal lobes. The treatment was extended to 4 weeks. No relapse of the infection was noted. This is the first case report of an infant with meningococcal meningitis complicated by cranial nerve palsies and cerebral infarction. This and previous reports, show that meningococcal meningitis at an extremely young age is associated with a greater risk of developing neurological complications.

C.-H. Chiu, MD, Department of Pediatrics, Chang Gung Children's Hospital, No. 5, Fu-Shin Street, Kweishan 333, Taoyuan, Taiwan

INTRODUCTION

Meningitis caused by Neisseria meningitidis rarely occurs in very young infants. Only 38 neonatal cases had been reported in the English literature by 1992 (1, 2), but there has never been a report on any case complicated by cerebral infarction. Cranial nerve palsies are common in tuberculous meningitis but relatively uncommon (3–5) in nontuberculous bacterial meningitis. We describe a young infant with meningococcal meningitis complicated by multiple cranial nerve palsies and cerebral infarction.

CASE REPORT

A full-term 30-day-old male neonate was admitted because of fever and poor activity for 2 days. Physical examination disclosed a poorly active newborn with mild respiratory distress and a bulging anterior fontanelle. There was no skin rash. The leukocyte count of the blood was 2.7 × 10^{10}/l (13% segmented neutrophils, 6% band neutrophils, 61% lymphocytes, 19% monocytes and 1% myelocytes). The C-reactive protein concentration was 1.2 g/l. The CSF examination revealed 7.15 × 10^8 leukocytes/l, with 72% neutrophils, a protein concentration of 4.6 g/l and a glucose concentration of 70 mg/l, while that of blood was 620 mg/l. Gram staining of CSF demonstrated intracellular Gram-negative cocci. Both blood and CSF cultures subsequently grew Neisseria meningitidis Group B. Simultaneous ampicillin (200 mg/kg/day) and cefotaxime (200 mg/kg/day) were given, and then replaced by aqueous benzyl penicillin (180 mg/kg/day) once the culture result was known. Clinical improvement was noted after initiation of the antibiotic therapy. Another CSF examination after 3 days showed 4.7 × 10^8 leukocytes/l with 37% neutrophils and 63% lymphocytes, a protein concentration of 6.5 g/l, and a glucose concentration of 11 mg/dl. The culture was now sterile. Four days after admission, the patient developed seizures, which were controlled by anticonvulsant therapy. In the meantime, the patient was found to have ptosis of the left eyelid and a left facial palsy. Physical examination revealed dilatation of the left pupil, which reacted poorly to light. The motion of the left eye was limited. There was no abducens palsy. The Moro reflex was active and symmetric.

All the neurologic signs gradually improved following treatment. The patient received a 14-day course of intravenous penicillin. At the end of the treatment, a repeat CSF examination yielded 1.05 × 10^8 leukocytes/l with 16% neutrophils and 84% lymphocytes, a protein concentration of 2.9 g/l and a glucose concentration of 37 mg/dl. The CSF was sterile. A brain sonography showed subdural fluid collection with increased meningeal echogenicity and a cerebral infarction at the bilateral frontal lobes was suspected. A computerized tomography (CT) scan of the brain was arranged and demonstrated hypodense areas in the bilateral frontal lobes, suggesting cerebral infarction (Fig. 1).

Another 14-day course of intravenous penicillin was given. There was no recurrence of fever or the neurologic signs. A follow-up CT of the brain showed encephalomalacia and atrophy of the bilateral frontal lobes. After discharge, the patient was regularly followed up in the outpatient department. Severe postmeningitic neurologic handicaps were observed in this case.

DISCUSSION

Focal neurologic deficits occur in as many as 15% of infants with meningitis (6). They are more frequently noted in patients with Haemophilus influenzae type b and pneumococcal meningitis than in those with meningococcal infection (6). Seizures, blindness, deafness, and hemiparesis or quadriparesis are the most common clinical manifestations in such cases (6). The underlying pathology is believed to be occlusive vasculitis and thrombosis of the cortical veins with resultant cerebral infarction and necrosis. However, cranial nerve palsies are not the usual presentation (3–5). The most commonly damaged cranial nerve in meningococcal meningitis is the cochlear nerve. If ophthalmoplegia occurs, it is usually caused by abducent palsy. Oculomotor nerve palsy following meningococcal meningitis has

 ISSN 0036-5548

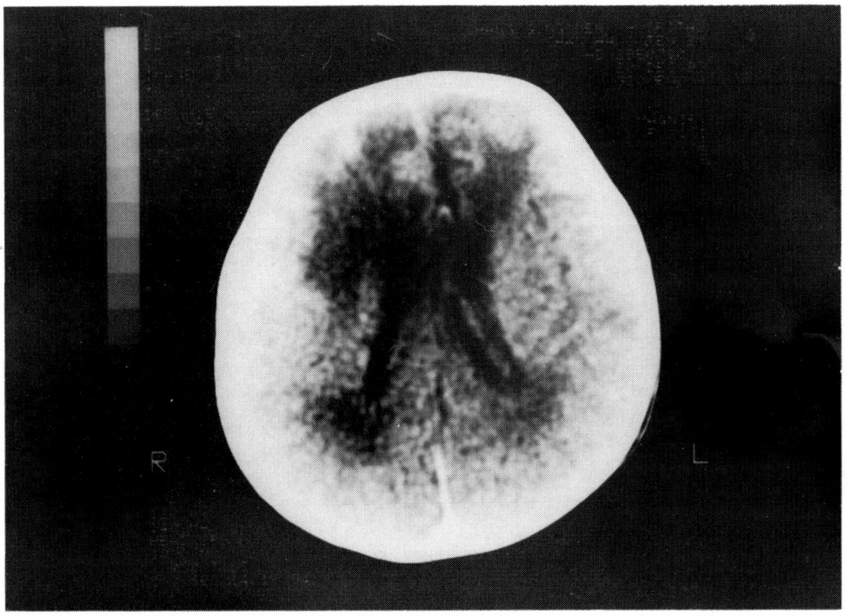

Fig. 1. Computerized tomograph of the brain showing bilateral frontal low density areas, suggesting cerebral infarction.

not been reported (4–6). A 3% incidence of facial palsy in meningococcal meningitis was reported in the early antibiotic era (4), and was described as invariably occurring during the recovery phase of meningitis (4, 5). Our patient had left oculomotor and facial palsies, suggesting an inflammatory infiltration of the meninges of the brainstem. The high initial protein level in the CSF and its rise at 3 days to 6.5 g/l, indicative of a severe inflammatory response, may have been a feature contributing to the unusual manifestations of this case. The clinical resolution of cranial nerve palsies in non-tuberculous bacterial meningitis is usually rapid after commencing therapy (3–5), and this was also observed in our case.

Intravenous penicillin for 7 days is the preferred treatment for uncomplicated meningococcal meningitis in children (6). However, there is no consensus concerning the duration of antibiotic therapy for newborn or young infants. Of the 24 neonatal cases reported in the antibiotic era, at least 9 survived, of whom 8 were treated with different combinations of antibiotics, including penicillin, for periods varying between 7 and 14 days (1, 2). In 1988, a case of meningococcal meningitis in a 3-day-old neonate was complicated by brain abscess, ventriculitis, and hydrocephalus, although penicillin had been given for 30 days, as reported by Chugh et al. (1). The death of this patient was probably due to inadequate antibiotic treatment, resulting in the subsequent development of fatal complications. In our case, we chose to extend the treatment persistently because of the severity of the infection, as indicated by a high CSF protein level of 2.9 g/l after 3 weeks and the presumed resolving cerebritis in the CT scan.

Neurologic complications following meningitis in children are rare in meningococcal infection (6). However, an extremely young age is noted to be independently associated with a greater risk of development of these complications. Hydrocephalus and ventriculitis have been observed in 4/14 neonates who survived meningococcal meningitis in the pre-antibiotic era (1). Even in the antibiotic era, the morbidity rate is high. Of the 24 cases reported (1, 2), 1 developed subarachnoid hemorrhage, 2 adrenal hemorrhage, and another died of brain abscess. This case report shows that meningococcal meningitis in young infancy may be complicated by cerebral infarction and that this is associated with long-term neurological handicaps.

REFERENCES

1. Chugh K, Bhalla CK, Joshi KK. Meningococcal brain abscess and meningitis in a neonate. Pediatr Infect Dis J 7: 136–137, 1988.
2. Ellis M, Weindling AM, Davidson DC, Ho N, Damjanovic V. Neonatal meningococcal conjunctivitis associated with meningococcal meningitis. Arch Dis Child 67: 1219–1220, 1992.
3. Chu MLY, Litman N, Kaufman DM, Shinnar S. Cranial nerve palsies in Streptococcus pneumoniae meningitis. Pediatr Neurol 6: 209–210, 1990.
4. Farmer TW. Neurologic complications during meningococcic meningitis treated with sulfonamide drugs. Arch Intern Med 76: 201–209, 1945.
5. Steven NM, Nathwani D. Facial palsy, meningococcal meningitis, and reactivation of herpes simplex virus. Clin Infect Dis 16: 181, 1993.
6. Feigin RD: Bacterial meningitis beyond the neonatal period. In: Feigin RD, Cherry JD, eds. Textbook of pediatric infectious diseases. Philadelphia: WB Saunders, 401–428, 1992.

Submitted August 29, 1994; accepted October 13, 1994

Scand J Infect Dis 27: 77–78, 1995 CASE REPORT

Acute Epiglottitis in the Adult Caused By Neisseria meningitidis

ROBERT S. CRAUSMAN, WILLIAM T. PLUSS and CONSTANCE A. JENNINGS

From the Division of Pulmonary Sciences and Critical Care Medicine, University of Colorado Health Sciences Center and the National Jewish Center for Immunology and Respiratory Medicine, Denver, Colorado USA

Acute epiglottitis is being increasingly encountered in the adult population. While it has many similarities to its pediatric counterpart, the presentation and associated pathogens are distinct. In addition, although the recent literature has suggested that acute epiglottitis in the adult follows a benign course this is not always the case. Here we describe a case of acute, fulminant epiglottitis in an immunocompetent host, caused by Neisseria meningitidis.

R. S. Crausman, MD, Pulmonary Physiology Unit, National Jewish Center for Immunology and Respiratory Medicine, 1400 Jackson Street, Denver, CO, 80206, USA

INTRODUCTION

Acute epiglottitis or supraglottitis can be a fulminant, life threatening disease in the adult as well as in children (1–4). Although first described in adults, epiglottitis was regarded as primarily a pediatric disease until the 1970s (3). There are now over 400 adult cases documented in the literature, and it is clearly established as a disorder that affects all age groups. In the adult it has a more varied clinical presentation and microbiological spectrum (2, 5, 6). This case report illustrates this variability.

CASE REPORT

The patient was a 54-year-old white male high school teacher who was in his normal state of good health until 2 days before admission when he developed a crusty discharge around his right eye and mild fatigue. Over the ensuing 24 h he developed dysphagia with a sore throat, fever to 39°C and shaking chills. At midnight on the day of admission he came to the emergency ward with acute dyspnea and audible inspiratory stridor.

On physical examination he was in acute respiratory distress, sitting upright and drooling. He had clear breath sounds bilaterally and normal heart sounds. Auscultation over his neck revealed prominent inspiratory stridor. He had neither cutaneous rash nor signs of meningeal irritation and the remainder of his physical examination was unremarkable. A lateral neck X-ray film was obtained, revealing findings consistent with acute epiglottitis (Fig. 1).

The patient deteriorated rapidly while still on the emergency ward and an urgent tracheotomy was performed. He was then admitted to the medical intensive care unit for further management and treated with intravenous steroids and ampicillin/sulbactam.

The laboratory evaluation revealed an elevated white blood cell count of 22,000/µl with 90% PMNs, a normal hematocrit and normal platelet count. Electrolytes, urea nitrogen, creatinine and glucose were also normal. An HIV ELISA proved negative.

On the second hospital day, blood cultures drawn on admission and throat culture grew Neisseria meningiditis (serogroup B). At this time the patient was no longer febrile and was much improved. No lumbar puncture was performed. He continued to recover uneventfully over the next week and his tracheostomy tube was removed. Subsequent blood and throat cultures taken 48 h after his course of antibiotics proved negative. He has since recovered satisfactorily.

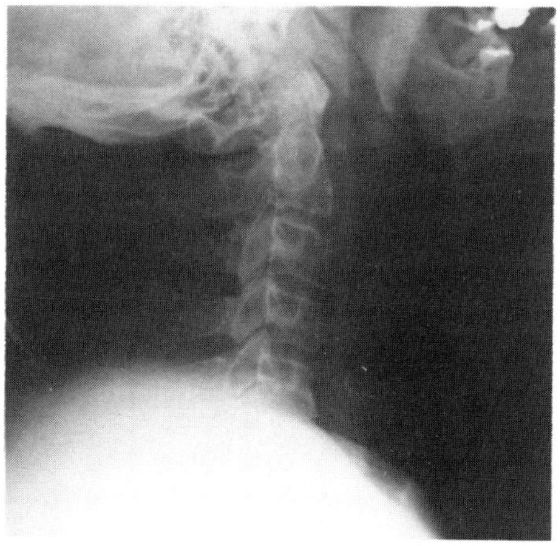

Fig. 1. Lateral neck radiograph demonstrating an enlarged epiglottis with swollen supraglottic structures and a ballooning hypopharynx.

Hospital staff who were directly involved with the placement of his tracheostomy tube on the emergency ward were empirically treated with a course of prophylactic rifampicin.

DISCUSSION

Most adult presentations of acute epiglottitis are less apparent than in this patient. The classic triad of fever, stridor and drooling need not be present in order for a patient to be at serious risk for morbidity. The rapid progression of upper airway obstruction in this patient serves as a reminder that epiglottitis in adults can be life threatening despite epidemiologic evidence favoring a more benign course in this age group (1–9).

The pathogens associated with adult epiglottitis differ markedly from the pediatric form in that only 25% of adult cases are associated with Haemophilus influenzae, compared with over 90% in children (1, 5, 6, 9–11). The potential role of bacterial agents such as Staphylococcus aureus, Streptococcus pyogones, Streptococcus pneumoniae and Haemophilus parainfluenzae has led to the practice of

 ISSN 0036-5548

empiric treatment with β-lactamase-resistant cephalosporins and extended spectrum penicillins (6, 7, 10–14). In most adult cases, an organism is not identified, suggesting a viral or atypical bacterial pathogenesis (7).

N. meningiditis is a well described pathogen that probably spreads via the respiratory route (15). Miningococcal disease causes a wide spectrum of illness including meningitis, meningoencephalitis, meningococcemia with or without sepsis, and pneumonia (16). It may be associated with a petechial rash and can precipitate disseminated intravascular coagulation. The carrier state is common and may be facilitated by coincident viral infection (15). N. meningiditis would seem to be an unusual pathogen in epiglottitis but given its predilection for the upper respiratory tract, we speculate that the association may in fact be underestimated. Additionally, given this patients' rapidly progressing clinical course, we wonder whether it produces a more virulent form of epiglottitis in a manner similar to the precipitous course seen in meningococcal meningeal infections. Although an antibiotic regimen directed against H. influenzae would also be effective against N. meningitidis, screening for this pathogen in adults with epiglottitis may be warranted for diagnostic purposes as there may be public health concerns (17, 18).

REFERENCES

1. Barrow H, Vastola A, Wang R. Adult supraglottitis. Otolaryngol – Head Neck Surg 109: 474–477, 1993.
2. Holbrook PR. Issues in airway management – 1988. Crit Care Clin 4: 789–803, 1988.
3. Shih L, Hawkins DB, Stanley RB. Acute epiglottitis in adults. Ann Oto Rhinol Laryngol 97: 527–529, 1988.
4. Warner J, Finlay W. Fulminating epiglottitis in adults. Report of three cases and review of the literature. Anaesthesia 40: 348–352, 1985.
5. Fontanorosa PB, Polsky SS, Goldman GE. Adult epiglottitis. J Emerg Med 7: 223–231, 1989.
6. Raphael J. Adult epiglottitis. Causative organism may be elusive. BMJ 308: 719, 1994.
7. Tveteras K, Kristensen S. Adult epiglottitis in adults: bacteriology and therapeutic principles. Clin Otolaryngol 12: 337–343, 1987.
8. Kass E, McFadden E, Jacobson S, Toohill R. Acute epiglottitis in the adult: experience with a seasonal presentation. Laryngoscope 103: 841–844, 1993.
9. Devita M, Wagner I. Acute epiglottitis in the adult. Crit Care Med 14: 1082–1083, 1986.
10. Ryan M, Hunt M, Snowberger T. A changing pattern of epiglottitis. Clin Pediatr 31: 532–535, 1992.
11. Carenfelt C. Etiology of acute infectious epiglottitis in adults: septic vs. local infection. Scand J Infect Dis 21: 53–57, 1989.
12. Shapiro J, Eavey R, Baker A. Adult supraglottitis. A prospective analysis. JAMA 259: 563–567, 1988.
13. Rydberg J, White P. Pasteurella multocida as a cause of acute epiglottitis. Lancet 341: 381, 1993.
14. Ridgeway N, Perlman P, Verghese A, Berk S. Epiglottic abscess due to group B Streptococcus. Communication. Ann Otol Rhinol Laryngol 93: 277–278, 1984.
15. Olcen P, Kjellander J, Danielsson D. Epidemiology of Neisseria meningitidis prevalence and symptoms with meningococcal disease. Scand J Infect Dis 13: 105–109, 1981.
16. Berkmen Y. Uncommon acute bacterial pneumonias. Semin Roentgenol 15: 17–24, 1980.
17. Klein N, Heyderman R, Levin M. Management of meningococcal infections. Br J Hosp Med 50: 42–49, 1993.
18. Trollfors B. Invasive Haemophilus influenzae infections in household contacts of patients with Haemophilus influenzae meningitidis and epiglottitis. Acta Paediatr Scand 80: 795–797, 1991.

Submitted July 4, 1994; accepted September 13, 1994

Scand J Infect Dis 27: 79–80, 1995

Bacteraemia Caused by Rahnella aquatilis: Report of Two Cases and Review

HELEN M. L. OH[1] and LENG TAY[2]

From the [1]Department of Infectious Diseases, Communicable Disease Centre, Moulmein Road, and the [2]Department of Pathology, Singapore General Hospital, Singapore

Rahnella aquatilis, a rare Gram-negative rod, usually found in fresh water, was isolated from blood of a diabetic patient and a patient with laryngeal carcinoma. Both recovered from the infection after treatment with parenteral antibiotics including gentamicin.

H. M. L. Oh MD, Department of Infectious Diseases, Communicable Disease Centre, Moulmein Road, Singapore 1130

INTRODUCTION

Rahnella aquatilis, a rare Gram-negative rod, is a member of the family Enterobacteriaceae. The organism's natural habitat is water, from which most isolates have been recovered (1).

Very few human infections due to Rahnella aquatilis have been reported in the literature (2–6). In this report, we describe 2 cases of bacteraemia caused by R. aquatilis, one in a diabetic patient, the other in an immunocompromised patient.

CASE REPORTS

Case 1

A 48-year-old Chinese man was admitted with colicky para-umbilical abdominal pain plus fever and chills, lasting 6 days, and vomiting for 1 day. He had been a diabetic for 2 years and had also been treated for pulmonary tuberculosis with rifampicin, ethambutol and isoniazid for 18 months.

Physical examination revealed a mildly dehydrated patient with a temperature of 38.2°C. The abdomen was soft but tender at the right iliac fossa without any rebound tenderness or guarding. The rest of the examination was unremarkable.

The white cell count was 12,300/μl, with normal differential, serum urea 10.6 mmol/l, and creatinine 182 mmol/l. Chest X-ray showed left upper lobe fibrosis. Sputum smear for acid-fast bacilli gave negative results.

The initial diagnosis was appendicular abscess. He was initially treated intravenously with ampicillin 1 g/6 h; gentamicin, 60 mg/8 h; and oral metronidazole, 400 mg/8 h. Two blood cultures yielded Rahnella aquatilis sensitive to chloramphenicol, ciprofloxacin, co-trimoxazole, amoxicillin-clavulanate, piperacillin, ceftazidime, imipenem, netilmicin, tetracycline and gentamicin. The isolate was moderately sensitive to ceftriaxone, but resistant to ampicillin and cephalothin. A CT scan of the abdomen revealed a small abscess lying medial and adjacent to the ascending colon.

The antibiotic regimen was changed to i.v. amoxicillin-clavulanate, 1.2 g/8 h and gentamicin, 60 mg/8 h. A laparoscopic-assisted limited right hemicolectomy was performed on the 14th hospital day. An abscess enclosing the ileocecal junction and a retrocaecal abscess were found. Pus from the ileocaecal abscess grew Escherichia coli, Acinetobacter baumanii and A. lwoffi. Anaerobic culture was inadvertently omitted.

The patient improved on the 20th hospital day after 14 days on amoxicillin-clavulanate, 19 on gentamicin and 11 days on metronidazole. He was discharged 25 days after admission, but readmitted 3 weeks later with a mild abdominal wound infection which resolved with daily dressings.

Case 2

A 57-year-old Malay man was admitted after 2 months of exertional breathlessness, orthopnoea, stridor, hoarseness and weight loss. He was a chronic smoker and had a history of chronic obstructive lung disease for several years.

On admission, he was afebrile. A fixed left vocal cord with underlying subglottic tumor was detected. No significant cervical lymphadenopathy was detected. Upper airway sounds were transmitted on auscultation of the chest. The rest of his examination was normal.

Investigation revealed a normal full blood count, renal function and chest X-ray. CT scan of larynx and neck revealed an extensive laryngeal carcinoma on the right, extending down to the subglottic region and crossing the midline with erosion of thyroid laminae.

An emergency tracheostomy was performed on the third hospital day and a total laryngectomy on the 25th hospital day. He developed fever on the second post-operative day.

Further investigations revealed haemoglobin, 11 g/dl and a white cell count of 12,000/μl. A repeat chest X-ray was normal. Two blood cultures yielded Rahnella aquatilis sensitive to aztreonam and gentamicin, moderately sensitive to ceftriaxone, but resistant to ampicillin and cephalothin. Anaerobe blood cultures proved negative.

Empirical antimicrobial treatment was started daily intravenously with metronidazole, 500 mg/8 h and ceftriaxone, 1 g for 7 days. This treatment was later changed to daily i.v. gentamicin, 60 mg/8 h for 5 days. The patient was discharged on the 15th day of hospitalization.

He received outpatient irradiation to the laryngeal bed, neck and superior mediastinum and was well when last seen, 3 months after the laryngectomy.

Bacteriology

Cultures of blood from both patients revealed a Gram-negative rod with good growth on sheep blood agar after overnight incubation at 35°C. Colonies were greyish, 1–2 mm in diameter, with no haemolysis. The following reactions were exhibited by the organism: positive citrate and malonate utilization, nitrate reduction to nitrite, Voges-Proskauer test, O-nitrophenyl-B-D-galactopyranoside and esculin hydrolysis. Triple sugar iron agar showed an acid reaction with gas. The sugars that fermented included lactose, sucrose, D-mannitol, salicin, inositol, arabinose, raffinose, maltose, D-xylose, trehalose, D-mannose and D-sorbitol. Motility was noted at 25°C and yellow pigment production was absent. Negative tests were: oxidase, indole production, hydrogen sulphide

 ISSN 0036-5548

Table I. *Features in 8 patients with Rahnella aquatilis*

Patient no.	Age/Sex	Underlying medical condition	Site of isolation	Outcome	Reference
1	42/F	Acute lymphocytic leukaemia, diabetes mellitus, asthma	Blood	Cure*	3
2	79/M	Chronic lymphocytic leukaemia, emphysema, chest infection	Sputum and bronchial aspirate	Cure	2
3	NA	Burn		Burn wound	NA1
4	37/M	AIDS and chest infection	Bronchial	Cure washing	4
5	40/M	Post-renal transplant, hypertension	Urine	Cure*	5
6	16/M	Neuroblastoma	Blood	Cure*	6
7	48/M	Diabetes mellitus, ileocaecal abscess	Blood	Cure	PR
8	57/M	Laryngeal carcinoma	Blood	Cure*	PR

AIDS = acquired immunodeficiency syndrome, PR = present report, NA = not available, * = proven clinical significance.

production, urea hydrolysis, arginine dehydrolase, ornithine decarboxylase, and lysine decarboxylase.

DISCUSSION

On the basis of 11 isolates recovered from water in France in 1976, Gavini et al. (7) defined a new group in the family Enterobacteriaceae which they named "Group H2". Izard et al. (8) showed by DNA-DNA hybridization that the strains of group H2 were only remotely related to other members of the Enterobacteriaceae. Hence, they proposed the new genus Rahnella (in honour of the German-American microbiologist Otto Rahn), with 1 species, Rahnella aquatilis.

R. aquatilis has no single distinguishing characteristic to differentiate it from other Enterobacteriaceae (1). The R. aquatilis was initially identified with the API 20E system. Conventional biochemical tests confirmed the initial identification and differentiated this isolate from the Enterobacter agglomerans–Erwinia herbicola complex which it closely resembles (1). The identification was confirmed at the Tokyo Metropolitan Research Laboratory of Public Health, Japan.

Only a few human infections due to R. aquatilis have been reported. It is noteworthy that one of the isolates described here and those previously reported were all from immunocompromised patients. Because R. aquatilis was found in the blood culture, but not in the pus from the ileocaecal abscess of the first patient, its clinical significance is unclear. The patient had an apparent clinical improvement with gentamicin and amoxicillin-clavulanate, to which the organism was susceptible. Whereas the first 2 reported cases of bacteraemia due to R. aquatilis were related to Hickman catheters (3, 6), our 2 cases of R. aquatilis bacteraemia were not line-related. To our knowledge, the isolates reported here represent the third and fourth isolates from blood and the first in a diabetic patient (Table I). Our results of antimicrobial susceptibility testing are in agreement with reports of susceptibility of R. aquatilis to aminoglycosides, β-lactam and quinolones (3–6). Thus there are several antimicrobial agents available for effective treatment of infections caused by R. aquatilis.

ACKNOWLEDGEMENT

We thank Dr Y. Kudoh, Director, Division of Microbiology, Tokyo Metropolitan Research Laboratory of Public Health, Japan, for confirming the identification results of our isolates.

REFERENCES

1. Farmer, JJ III, Davis BR, Hickman-Brenner FW, McWorther A, Huntley-Carter GP, Asbury MA, Riddle C, Wathen-Grady HG, Elias C, Fanning GR, Steigerwalt AG, O'Hara CM, Morris GK, Smith PB, Brenner DJ. Biochemical identification of new species and biogroups of Enterobacteriaceae isolated from clinical specimens. J Clin Microbiol 21: 46–76, 1985.
2. Christiaens E, Hansen W, Moinet J. Isolement des expectorations d'un patient attaint de leucémie lymphoide chronique et de bronco-emphysème d'une Enterobactericeae nouvellement decrite: Rahnella aquatilis. Med Malad Infect 17: 732–734, 1987.
3. Goubou P, Van Aelst F, Verhaegen J, Boogaerts M. Septicaemia caused by Rahnella aquatilis in an immunocompromised patient. Eur J Clin Microbiol Infect Dis 7: 679–699, 1988.
4. Harrel LJ, Cameron ML, O'Hara CM. Rahnella aquatilis, an unusual gram-negative rod isolated from the bronchial washing of a patient with acquired immunodeficiency syndrome. J Clin Microbiol 27: 1671–1672, 1989.
5. Alballaa SR, Qadri SMH, Al-Furaigh O, Al-Qatary K. Urinary tract infection due to Rahnella aquatilis in a renal transplant patient. J Clin Microbiol 30: 2948–2950, 1992.
6. Hoppe JE, Herter M, Aleksic S, Klingebiel T, Niethammer D. Catheter-related Rahnella aquatilis bacteraemia in a paediatric bone marrow transplant recipient. J Clin Microbiol 31: 1911–1912, 1993.
7. Gavini F, Ferragut C, Lefebvre B, Boogaerts M. E'tude taxonomique d'enterobacteries appartenant ou appararentées an genre Enterobacter. Ann Microbiol (Inst. Pasteur) 127B: 317–335, 1976.
8. Izard D, Gavini F, Trinel PA, Leclerc H. Rahnella aquatilis, membres de la famille des Enterobacteriaceae. Ann Microbiol (Inst. Pasteur) 130A: 163–177, 1979.

Submitted July 25, 1994; accepted October 10, 1994

Scand J Infect Dis 27: 81–82, 1995

First Documented Case of Bacteremia with Vibrio vulnificus in Sweden

ÅSA MELHUS[1], TORSTEN HOLMDAHL[2] and INGELA TJERNBERG[1]

From the Departments of [1]Medical Microbiology and [2]Infectious Diseases, Lund University, Malmö General Hospital, Malmö, Sweden

A few days after a mild trauma to a toe, a 90-year-old woman presented with fever, malaise and cellulitis. On suspicion of erysipelas the patient was initially treated with benzylpenicillin and cefuroxime. Her general condition improved rapidly, but there was local progression with numerous necrotic areas with surrounding bullae. Vibrio vulnificus was isolated from the blood. After susceptibility testing, the patient was finally treated with ciprofloxacin and pivampicillin, and recovered slowly. To our knowledge, this is the first reported case of bacteremia with V. vulnificus in Sweden.

Å. Melhus, MD, Department of Medical Microbiology, Malmö General Hospital, S-214 01 Malmö, Sweden

INTRODUCTION

The genus Vibrio is widespread in the aquatic environment, but the clinical importance of Vibrio species other than V. cholerae has only recently been appreciated. In 1976, Hollis and co-workers described V. vulnificus (1), a particularly virulent bacterium that causes either primary septicemia after consumption of seafood, or wound infections after exposure to seawater or handling of seafood. A high mortality rate is associated with septic infections (40–60%), but wound infections too can be fatal (20%) (2). Although V. vulnificus infections are well known worldwide, only a few cases have been reported in Europe (3–5). The source of the infection has in about half of these cases been contaminated eels (5). The present report describes V. vulnificus bacteremia secondary to a wound infection in an elderly female patient.

CASE REPORT

On August 5, 1994, a 90-year-old woman, previously healthy except for minor heart problems, was admitted to hospital. On the night before admission the patient became acutely ill with high fever, chills and malaise. There were also a throbbing pain and a feeling of rigidity in the right foot and leg. Only a few days earlier, the patient had received a small wound on a toe of the right foot, caused by a mild trauma. The wound did not stop the patient from swimming daily in the sea.

On admission, the patient was subfebrile and in good health. Physical examination revealed a systolic murmur over the heart, a slightly irregular pulse and a blood pressure of 100/60 mmHg. Above the ankle of the right foot there was a tender area with erythema and edema. Results of laboratory tests included a hemoglobin level of 130 g/l, a leukocyte count of 19.6×10^9/l and a C-reactive protein level of 40 mg/l.

The working diagnosis was erysipelas. Cultures were obtained from the blood and the wound, and intravenous treatment with benzylpenicillin was started. Despite antibiotic therapy there was local progression the day after admission, with development of pustular lesions and bullae in the previously erythematous area, and the C-reactive level had increased to 117 mg/μl. Gram staining of the positive blood cultures revealed Gram-negative rods, while cultures of the skin lesion showed only growth of commensals. Antibiotic therapy was changed to cefuroxime and to ciprofloxacin and pivampicillin, after susceptibility testing. The Gram-negative rod was identified as V. vulnificus. 10 days after admission, the patient was discharged. Her recovery has been slow.

Bacteriology

Blood was cultured in a set of blood culture bottles (BactAlert, Organon Teknika, Turnhout, Belgium). After overnight incubation, growth appeared in both the aerobic and the anaerobic bottle. Subculture to blood agar aerobically and anaerobically yielded growth of grey colonies with hemolysis after 48 h. Growth on enteric-selective plating media was poor, while thiosulfate-citrate-bile-sucrose (TCBS) agar, a Vibrio selective medium, yielded growth of green colonies. Catalase and oxidase reactions were positive, as also were lysine and ornithine decarboxylase. The bacteria were motile, indole-positive and could reduce nitrate. Lactose and salicin were rapidly fermented. The Rapid NF Plus System (Innovative Diagnostic Systems, Inc., Atlanta, GA, USA) gave inconclusive results. Identification was confirmed with Biolog MicroStation™ System, Release 3.50, (Biolog, Inc., Hayward, CA, USA) with Bio-number: 1761-3727-3123-0150-0101-3177-0014-3417. Antibiotic susceptibility was determined by the E-test (Biodisk AB, Solna, Sweden). The strain was susceptible to ampicillin, cefuroxime, cefotaxime, tetracycline, gentamicin, netilmicin and ciprofloxacin, but resistant to benzylpenicillin. Resistance to colistin was demonstrated by disk diffusion test.

DISCUSSION

V. vulnificus is a halophilic marine bacterium that can be differentiated from other similar Vibrios by its ability to ferment lactose and by its lower tolerance for sodium chloride (1, 6). It is the most virulent of the non-cholera Vibrios but, unlike most other bacteria of this genus, it seldom causes symptoms from the gastrointestinal tract. The species is associated with 2 categories of infection, primary septicemia, and wound infections (1, 6, 7). Primary septicemia usually has an abrupt onset, with fever, chills, and nausea. The symptoms typically develop within 48 h after ingestion of raw oysters, and a majority of the patients have secondary cutaneous lesions consisting of numerous necrotic areas with surrounding bullae, or a maculopapular rash on the trunk or extremities. The infection progresses rapidly and has a high mortality rate. Most patients have an underlying hepatic disorder, or are not immunologically competent. Patients with wound infections acquire the disease through mild-to-severe trauma to infected sites, and contact with seawater or shellfish is a prerequisite. These patients can also have fever and chills, and the bacterium can occasionally be isolated from blood and skin lesions. The wound infection most commonly presents itself as a cellullitis, sometimes with pustules and bullae, and it may rapidly progress to myositis and deep necrotic ulcers. Recovery is often uneventful, unless accompanied by secondary bacteremia or underlying chronic disease. V. vulnificus infections usually require immediate and appropriate antibiotic treatment, with early surgical intervention if needed. Although tetracycline, often in combination with an aminoglycoside, has in most studies been the preferred drug, ciprofloxacin has been used successfully for the treatment of wound infections (8).

A striking feature of V. vulnificus infections is their seasonal distribution. Most episodes occur during the summer months, and Tilton et al. have shown a direct correlation between water temperature and the isolation rate of the organism from water and seafood (9). A minimum temperature of approximately +17°C is needed for isolation, a temperature seldom reached in Scandinavian seawaters. However, this summer (1994) was extremely hot, and the water temperatures were well above +17°C. In Denmark, 3 cases of serious V. vulnificus infection were reported (SSI, Copenhagen), and even if this bacteremic case in Sweden is a rarity, it is well known that eels in these waters can be contaminated (10, 11). It is possible that minor wound infections go unrecognized due to incorrect identification at the bacteriology laboratory. The organism can easily be mistaken for a Pseudomonas, Aeromonas, Plesiomonas, Serratia or even a contamination of the specimen. In this investigation, V. vulnificus was isolated from a set of blood culture bottles, and it is unlikely that the bottles had become contaminated from the patient's skin or from the hospital environment. The anamnesis, clinical picture and bacteriological findings fit well together. Although the patient had no predisposing diseases and adequate treatment was begun almost immediately, the course was protracted.

With this case report we would like to draw attention to this rare but potentially exceedingly serious infection. Physicians should consider and ask the laboratory for Vibrio species in patients with wound infections or primary septicemia with cutaneous lesions who have recently been exposed to warm seawater, shellfish or eels. An early diagnosis, and adequate antibiotic therapy and surgical treatment are critical for a successful outcome.

REFERENCES

1. Hollis D, Weaver R, Baker C, Thornsberry C. Halophilic Vibrio species isolated from blood cultures. J Clin Microbiol 3: 425–431, 1976.
2. Blake P, Weaver R, Hollis D. Disease caused by a marine vibrio: clinical characteristics and epidemiology. N Engl J Med 300: 1–5, 1979.
3. Mertens A, Nagler J, Hansen W, Gepts-Friedenreich E. Halophilic, lactose-positive Vibrio in a case of fatal septicemia. J Clin Microbiol 9: 233–235, 1979.
4. Mehtar S, Bangham L, Kalmanovitch D, Wren M. Adult epiglottis due to Vibrio vulnificus. BMJ 296: 827–828, 1988.
5. Veenstra J, Rietra P, Stoutenbeek C, Coster J, de Gier H, Dirks-Go S. Infection by an indole-negative variant of Vibrio vulnificus transmitted by eels. J Infect Dis 166: 209–210, 1992.
6. Janda M, Powers C, Bryant R, Abbot S. Current perspectives on the epidemiology and pathogenesis of clinically significant Vibrio spp. Clin Microbiol Rev 1: 245–267, 1988.
7. Ratner H. Topics in clinical microbiology: Vibrio vulnificus. Infect Control 8: 430–433, 1987.
8. Meadors M, Pankey G. Vibrio vulnificus wound infection treated successfully with oral ciprofloxacin. J Infect 20: 88–89, 1990.
9. Tilton R, Ryan R. Clinical and ecological characteristics of Vibrio vulnificus in the northeastern United States. Diagn Microbiol Infect Dis 6: 109–117, 1987.
10. Krovacek K, Baloda S, Dumontet S, Månsson I. Detection of potential virulence markers of Vibrio vulnificus strains isolated from fish in Sweden. Comp Immunol Microbiol Infect Dis 17: 63–70, 1994.
11. Andersen H-K. Vibrio vulnificus. Ugeskr Laeger 153: 2361–2362, 1991.

Submitted September 5, 1994; accepted October 13, 1994

Scand J Infect Dis 27: 83–84, 1995 CASE REPORT

Fusobacterium Nucleatum, a New Invasive Pathogen in Neutropenic Patients?

PETER M. LANDSAAT[1], HANS VAN DER LELIE[1], GER BONGAERTS[3] and ED J. KUIJPER[2]

From the [1]Department of Internal Medicine and Hematology, and the [2]Department of Medical Microbiology, Academic Medical Centre, Amsterdam; and the [3]Department of Medical Microbiology, University Hospital, Nijmegen, The Netherlands

Three chemotherapy-induced neutropenic hematologic patients with severe systemic infection caused by Fusobacterium nucleatum, a Gram-negative anaerobic rod, are described. Anaerobic infections are not very common in this patient category, but in a short period of time, several such patients were seen. The infection was considered to be caused by a combination of chemotherapy-induced mucositis, which served as a portal of entry for the systemic infection, and the antibiotic regime used in these patients. This is a serious infection with a high mortality. In hematological neutropenic patients suffering from severe mucositis and fever, antibiotic therapy should cover anaerobic bacteria.

P. M. Landsaat, MD, F4-119, Academic Medical Center, Meibergdreef 9, 1105 AZ Amsterdam-ZO, The Netherlands

INTRODUCTION

Anaerobic bacteria infrequently cause systemic infection in hematological patients with neutropenia following chemotherapy (1). Recently 3 neutropenic patients with severe oropharyngeal mucositis developed systemic infection caused by Fusobacterium nucleatum, a Gram-negative anaerobic rod.

CASE REPORTS

Case 1

Patient A, a 44-year-old female, underwent an autologous bone marrow transplantation as a consolidation treatment for a refractory anemia with blast excess. Myelo-ablative chemotherapy consisted of etoposide and dimethylbusulphan. As standard infection prophylaxis, oral ciprofloxacin 2×500 mg, oral amphotericin-B 4×500 mg and benzylpenicillin 4×10^6 IU i.v. was given, the latter to prevent streptococcal septicemia. On day 12, mucositis grade 4 on the WHO scale developed. On day 14, penicillin was replaced by vancomycin because of high fever and the suspicion of a central venous catheter associated infection. On day 29, an inspiratory stridor developed and intubation was necessary. Blood cultures were positive for F. nucleatum. Antibiotic therapy was changed to metronidazole and cephalothin. Mucosal damage progressed and a pulmonary infiltrate developed. The bone marrow remained aplastic. On the 36th day after transplantation the patient succumbed. Post-mortem examination revealed a damaged and necrotic mucosa of the throat and the upper respiratory tract, which contained many fusiform Gram-negative rods.

Case 2

Patient B was a 29-year-old female with a myelodysplastic syndrome requiring a large number of blood transfusions, and severe thrombocytopenia. Chemotherapy consisted of idarubicin, ara-c and etoposide. Standard infection prophylaxis was given. On the 16th day, she developed fever with grade 3 mucositis and swelling of the neck. The neutrophil count at that time was $<0.1 \times 10^9$/l. Blood cultures revealed only Staphylococcus epidermidis and vancomycin was given. The fever abated and the general condition of the patient improved, although the mucositis and bone marrow aplasia persisted. On the 46th day she again developed higher fever. Blood cultures revealed F. nucleatum for which clindamycin 4×600 mg i.v. was added. Fever and bone marrow hypoplasia persisted and she developed pulmonary infiltrates for which treatment was started with amphotericin-B i.v. She died on the 77th day. Postmortem examination revealed pulmonary aspergillosis.

Case 3

Patient C was a 44-year-old man with a secondary myelodysplastic syndrome after treatment for Hodgkin's disease. Chemotherapy consisted of idarubicin, etoposide and Ara-C. He received standard infection prophylaxis, but because of penicillin allergy, vancomycin was given. On the 16th day, grade 4 mucositis (WHO) developed, followed by high fever. Blood cultures revealed F. nucleatum for which he was treated with cephalothin. After 5 days the temperature normalized and his mucositis and neutrophils recovered. He achieved complete remission.

Microbiological data

F. nucleatum was identified by conventional bacteriological methods and by gas-liquid chromatography. The strains were susceptible to benzyl penicillin, cephalothin, clindamycin and metronidazole, but resistant to ciprofloxacin and erythromycin. They were all β-lactamase-negative.

DISCUSSION

Three patients with systemic infection caused by F. nucleatum are described. All had severe chemotherapy-induced neutropenia and high fever. In the only patient surviving the infection, bone marrow recovery was probably a significant factor. There is resemblance to post-anginal septicemia (Lemierre's Syndrome, 2) described in 1936 in healthy young adults, usually caused by F. necrophorum.

F. nucleatum is a strictly anaerobic Gram-negative rod normally found in the gastrointestinal, genito-urinary and respiratory tracts. We have no reason to assume that this sudden increase is due to better culture methods, to transmission by personal contact, or to contaminated food.

All 3 patients received our standard infection prophylaxis. For various reasons, penicillin was replaced by vancomycin to prevent endogenic streptococcal infections. This

 ISSN 0036-5548

infection prophylaxis is not active against F. nucleatum and may have resulted in a selection and overgrowth of it.

All patients received very intensive chemotherapy leading to a severe mucositis. F. nucleatum might have exacerbated an oropharyngeal mucositis that could serve as a portal of entry for the systemic infection.

In patients with fever and severe mucositis, early treatment with antibiotics directed at anaerobes should be considered.

REFERENCES

1. van der Lelie H, van Ketel RJ, Borne von dem AEGK, van Oers RHJ, Thomas BLM, Goudsmit R. Incidence and clinical epidemiology of streptococcal septicemia during treatment of acute myeloid leukemia. Scand J Infect Dis 23: 163–168, 1991.
2. Lemierre A. On certain septicemias due to anaerobic mechanisms. Lancet 1: 701–703, 1936.
3. Seidenfeld SM, Sutker WL, Luby JP. Fusobacterium necrophorum septicemia following oropharyngeal infection. JAMA 248: 1348–1350, 1982.

Submitted September 21, 1994; accepted November 20, 1994

Scand J Infect Dis 27: 85–87, 1995 CASE REPORT

Catheter-related Infections by Hansenula anomala in Children

SHUJI YAMADA[1], TAKAYUKI MARUOKA[1], KENSUKE NAGAI[1], NAOKI TSUMURA[1], TAKASHI YAMADA[1], YASUTAKA SAKATA[1], KAORU TOMINAGA[1], TAKASHI MOTOHIRO[1], HIROHISA KATO[1], KOICHI MAKIMURA[2] and HIDEYO YAMAGUCHI[2]

From the [1]Department of Pediatrics, Kurume University School of Medicine, Kurume and the [2]Research Center for Medical Mycology, Teikyo University, Tokyo Japan

During August and September, 1992, we experienced 4 cases of Hansenula anomala (H. anomala, synonym Pichia anomala) fungemia in immunocompromised patients. Two patients had been suffering from a malignant disease, 3 of them had received broad-spectrum antibiotics and a central venous catheter (CVC) had been inserted in all of them. H. anomala was isolated as the sole pathogen from all 4 patients. Three of them responded favorably to fluconazole after withdrawal of the catheter, but one failed. H. anomala should be considered as a possible cause of catheter-related infections.

Sh. Yamada, MD, Department of Pediatrics, Kurume University School of Medicine, 67 Asahi-machi, Kurume 830, Japan

INTRODUCTION

Infections caused by H. anomala, particularly in children, have rarely been reported previously. H. anomala, the perfect state of Candida pelliculosa, is an ascosporogenous yeast belonging to the class Hemiascomycetes, division Ascomycetes. To identify H. anomala, it is necessary to confirm the formation of hat-shaped ascospores which are characteristics of this yeast.

H. anomala is thought to dwell as a member of normal or transient microbial flora in the human throat and/or the alimentary tract, and is ubiquitous plants, soil, and fruit. It can cause various types of infectious diseases, such as interstitial lung disease (1), fungemia (2–8), endocarditis (9) and urinary tract infection (10) in immunocompromised patients, although it appears to be only mildly virulent.

We report 4 cases of catheter-related H. anomala fungemia and review all cases previously reported in the English-language literature.

CASE REPORTS

Case 1

A 27-month-old boy with a diagnosis of non-Hodgkin lymphoma (T-cell, stage IV) developed a fever with no other symptoms during chemotherapy through a CVC. The WBC count was 1,500/μl with 85% neutrophils, the hemoglobin concentration 89 g/l, the platelet count 24,000/μl and CRP 71 mg/l. Five serial sets of blood cultures proved positive for Candida albicans. Therefore, the cathether was removed, anti-neoplastic chemotherapy interrupted and i.v. administration of fluconazole (5 mg/kg) was started. The patient's fever subsided after 5 days and the follow-up cultures were negative. A new CVC was inserted 2 weeks later to restart the course of chemotherapy. However, the fever recurred in a few days. Although there was no specific finding by a physical examination, nor definitive change in any of the laboratory tests performed, 3 serial sets of blood cultures yielded H. anomala. The catheter was removed again and fluconazole was administered in an increased dose (10 mg/kg). Fever subsided in 48 h and blood cultures were negative.

Case 2

An 8-year-old male with acute myelocytic leukemia developed a fever with general fatigue, oral and abdominal pain 2 weeks after commencing chemotherapy through a CVC. The WBC count was 300/μl (agranulocytosis), the hematocrit level 25.7%, the hemoglobin concentration 101 g/l, the platelet count 7,000/μl and CRP 142 mg/l. There was no palpable lymphadenopathy and no significant finding from pulmonary, abdominal and oral examinations. The fever persisted and a combined regimen of parenteral cefzonam and tobramycin did not afford any clinical improvement. These antibiotics were replaced by imipenem/cilastatin and fluconazole (10 mg/kg). Six serial sets of initial blood cultures proved positive for H. anomala. The catheter was removed and H. anomala was isolated in pure culture from the catheter tip. The fever subsided 24 h after removal of the catheter and follow-up blood cultures were all negative.

Case 3

A female infant born after normal pregnancy and delivery had been well until the age of 4 months when she was referred to our hospital for afebrile convulsions with severe watery diarrhea subsequently. She appeared lethargic, and laboratory examinations showed: WBC 8,200/μl (84% neutrophils), hematocrit level 36.8%, hemoglobin concentration 136 g/l. Hypocalcemia (41 mg/l) causing convulsions and hypoproteinemia (44 g/l) with hypogammaglobulinemia were also found. Primary intestinal lymphangiectasia was suspected from her clinical history and laboratory data, and was confirmed later by intestinal biopsy. Following administration of parenteral nutrition through a CVC line, the patient suddenly developed a fever with no specific symptoms. The WBC count fell to 1,800/μl and CRP was 50 mg/l. The fever persisted for 72 h without any significant clinical change despite treatment with intravenous cefotiam. H. anomala was isolated from 2 sets of blood cultures. The catheter was removed and fluconazole therapy (9.5 mg/kg) was started. A culture from the tip of the catheter yielded H. anomala. The patient's fever subsided after 24 h, and follow-up cultures were negative.

Case 4

A 12-day-old female infant born after a normal pregnancy and delivery was referred to the hospital to investigate poor weight gain and a heart murmur. A cardiac catheterization disclosed

 ISSN 0036-5548

transposition of the great arteries, a ventricular septal defect, patent ductus arteriosus (PDA) and coarctation of the aorta. Open heart surgery involving coarctectomy using a subclavian flap and ligation of PDA was performed at 35 days of age. A CVC was inserted postoperatively for prophylactic administration of intravenous ampicillin. Her temperature increased on the tenth day after the antibiotic therapy was started. The WBC count was 9,600/μl and CRP 140 mg/l. The fever continued after ampicillin was replaced by amikacin and flomoxef, and H. anomala was isolated from peripheral blood specimens. Then the catheter was removed and treatment with fluconazole (10 mg/kg) was started. The fever did not subside and 18 days after starting fluconazole treatment the WBC count was 18,600/μl and CRP 112 mg/l. Since the patient did not respond to fluconazole, it was replaced by miconazole (10 mg/kg) and flucytosine (120 mg/kg). The patient then gradually defervesced over 4 days and improved clinically. However, she later died of the underlying congenital heart disease.

MYCOLOGICAL STUDIES

In all cases, cultures of blood samples obtained through both CVCs and peripheral vessels grew yeasts, later identified as H. anomala.

The yeasts grew well on 5% horse blood agar and Candida GE agar (Nissui Pharm. Co., Tokyo, Japan) at 35°C, producing visible white, opaque, smooth glistening colonies within 48 h. Identification of the yeasts was achieved by biochemical characterization using the automated testing VITEK identification system (bioMérieux Vitek Inc., Hazelwood, U.S.A.) which showed positive reactions for the assimilation of glucose, maltose, sucrose, raffinose, trehalose, melezitose, palatinose, glycerin and erythritol and negative reactions for the assimilation of lactose and urease production. Hat-shaped ascospores were demontrated by Nomarski differential interference contrast microscopy (Olympus BH2-NIC, ×1,000) after incubation for 2 weeks at 20°C on 5% malt extract agar.

Susceptibilities of H. anomala isolates to amphotericin B, flucytosine, miconazole, and fluconazole were studied by a micro broth dilution method in synthetic aminoacid medium, fungal (SAAMF) (pH 7.4) using the viable count technique (11). Microtiter plates (Nippon Becton Dickinson Co., Tokyo, Japan) were used for the preparation of dilutions. Yeast suspensions were prepared from 2-day-old cultures grown on Candida GE agar (Nissui Pharm. Co., Tokyo, Japan) at room temperature. Inocula were prepared in sterile saline to give 95% transmission at 540 nm, yielding a concentration of 10^5 CFU/ml as determined by plate counts. A 10 μl volume was used for the inoculation into each well of microtitre plates (Nippon Becton Dickinson Co.), and the plates were incubated for 24 ~ 48 h at 30°C before the MIC was determined. The MIC was defined as the lowest concentration of antibiotic showing no growth by naked eye inspection. One well was kept drug free and was used as a control. As regards fluconazole, MICs of 3 isolates from cases 1 to 3 were 1.56–3.13 μg/ml and an isolate from case 4 showed an MIC of 12.5 μg/ml. All isolates were susceptible to amphotericin B, flucytosine and miconazole with MICs of 0.78–1.56 μg/ml, 0.20–0.78 μg/ml and 0.39–0.78 μg/ml, respectively. Sandven et al. (12) tested 224 strains of C. albicans for susceptibility to fluconazole and stated that the strains for which the MIC was ≤1.56 μg/ml were susceptible, while ≥12.5 μg/ml were resistant. Therefore, the strain of case 4 was resistant to fluconazole and the other strains were susceptible or showed decreased sensitivity.

DISCUSSION

Diagnosis of invasive mycosis is made by either isolation of fungi from pathogenic specimens, or demonstration of a significant increase in antibodies to etiologic fungi with consideration of the patient's underlying disease. It is not always easy to identify any etiologic fungus as the causative agent of the disease with a single isolation. Moreover, in immunocompromised patients, increasing antibody or other immunological response to invasive microorganism usually decreased.

The first description of H. anomala infection in the clinical literature was made by Csillag & Brandstein in 1953 (13), including a case of a $2\frac{1}{2}$-month-old male infant who died of interstitial pneumonia, and from whom yeasts were isolated. However, this isolate was later identified as Pneumocystis carinii (1).

Infections caused by H. anomala in children have been reported in only 13 cases in the English-language literature (Table I) (3, 6, 8, 14).

We initially suspected that all our 4 patients cases were nosocomial infections, because H. anomala was serially isolated from them within a period as short as 1 month and all the patients had used a CVC. The breach in the defence mechanism of the skin caused by inserting a CVC was regarded as a direct route for invasion by microorganisms into the blood. Dickensheets (6) suggested that the catheter-related sepsis due to H. anomala was secondary and amphotericin B therapy for a short period after removing the catheter would probably succeed in controlling the infection. Any patient having a CVC inserted should therefore be carefully monitored.

Two of our 4 patients had been suffering from malignant disease and 3 had previously received broad-spectrum antibiotics. Murphy et al. (3) described an outbreak of infection due to H. anomala in a neonatal intensive care unit in England. All of those affected had had an umbilical arterial and a peripheral venous cannula inserted in situ and had previously been treated with broad-spectrum antibiotics. Previous studies have shown several risk factors for fungemia: the duration of CVC insertion, neutropenia, lymphopenia, hypoproteinemia, administration of chemotherapy, radiation therapy, use of antibiotics or steroids, and surgical operation (15, 16). Numerous risk factors were also observed in our cases.

The optimal therapy for infection by H. anomala is not yet clearly established. H. anomala was the sole pathogen isolated in all previously reported cases and almost all of them had been treated with a combination of amphotericin B and flucytosine or amphotericin B alone. We chose a new azole antifungal agent, fluconazole, for the treatment of all our cases, because of its low toxicity after withdrawal of the catheter.

In 1994, Sherman & Jane (14) described the case of a 4-year-old boy with H. anomala fungemia during fluconazole therapy for C. albicans. Fluconazole was then replaced by amphotericin B. The MICs of amphotericin B and fluconazole for the isolates were 0.8 and 25 μg/ml, respectively. In case 1 in this report, H. anomala emerged while

Table I. *Cases of Hansenula anomala infection in children*

Patient No.	Reference	Age	Site(s) of infection	Underlying disease	Treatment	Central venous catheterization	Outcome
1	Murphy et al. 1986	74 d	Blood	LBW	AmB, 5-FC	+	Recovered
2		9 d	Blood	LBW	AmB, 5-FC	+	Died
3		16 d	Blood	LBW	AmB, 5-FC	+	Recovered
4		44 d	Blood	LBW	AmB, 5-FC	+	Recovered
5		17 d	Blood	LBW	AmB, 5-FC	+	Recovered
6		19 d	CSF	LBW	None	+	Died
		28 d	Blood				
7		36 d	CSF	LBW	AmB, 5-FC	+	Recovered
8		21 d	Blood	LBW	AmB, 5-FC	+	Recovered
			CSF				
9	Dickensheets, 1989	10 y	Blood	NEC	AmB	+	Recovered
10	Mozes et al. 1991	5 m	Blood, urine	NEC	AmB ~ KCZ	−	Recovered
			Peritoneal fluid				
11		17 m	Peritoneal fluid	HUS	None	−	Recovered
12		15 y	Peritoneal fluid	Renal failure	None	−	Recovered
13	Sherman et al. 1994	4 y	Blood	Traumatic injuries	FLCZ ~ AmB	+	Recovered

* LBW = low birth weight; NEC = necrotizing enterocolitis; HUS = hemolytic-uremic syndrome; AmB = amphotericin B; 5-FC = flucytosine; KCZ = ketoconazole; FLCZ = fluconazole; MCZ = miconazole.

the patient was receiving fluconazole therapy for C. albicans. Failure of the fluconazole treatment in case 4 was thought to be caused by an insufficient dosage to an isolate with low susceptibility.

Clinicians should be aware of appropriate choice and doses of antifungal agents, and the potential for emergence of fluconazole-insusceptible or -resistant opportunistic fungi in immunocompromised patients, particularly those given fluconazole therapy.

REFERENCES

1. Wang CJK, Schwarz J. The etiology of interstitial pneumonia: Identification as Hansenula anomala of a yeast isolated from lungs of infants. Mycopathologia 9: 299–306, 1958.
2. Milstoc M, Siddiqui NA. Fungemia due to Hansenula anomala. N Y State J Med 86: 541–542, 1986.
3. Murphy N, Damjanovic V, Hart CA, Buchanan CR, Whitaker R, Cooke RWI. Infection and colonisation of neonates by Hansenula anomala. Lancet 1: 291–293, 1986.
4. Haron E, Anaissie E, Dumphy F, McCredie K, Fainstein V. Hansenula anomala fungemia. Rev Infect Dis 10: 1182–1186, 1988.
5. Klein AS, Tortora GT, Malowitz R, Greene WH. Hansenula anomala: a new fungal pathogen. Two case reports and a review of the literature. Arch Intern Med 148: 1210–1213, 1988.
6. Dickensheets DL. Hansenula anomala infection. Rev Infect Dis 11: 507–508, 1989.
7. Munoz P, Leoni MEG, Berenguer J, Quiros JCLB, Bouza E. Catheter-related fungemia by Hansenula anomala. Arch Intern Med 149: 709–710, 1989.
8. Moses A, Maayan S, Shvil Y, Dudin A, Ariel I, Thalji A, Polacheck I. Hansenula anomala infections in children: from asymptomatic colonization to tissue invasion. Pediatr Infect Dis J 10: 400–402, 1991.
9. Nohinek B, Zee-Cheng CS, Barnes WG, Dall L, Gibbs HR. Infective endocarditis of a bicuspid aortic valve caused by Hansenula anomala. Am J Med 82: 165–168, 1987.
10. Qadri SMH, Dayel FA, Strampfer MJ, Cunha BA. Urinary tract infection caused by Hansenula anomala. Mycopathologia 104: 99–101, 1988.
11. Yamaguchi H, Uchida K, Kawasaki K, Matsunaga T. In vitro activity of fluconazole, a novel bistriazole antifungal agent. Jpn J Antibiot 42: 1–16, 1989.
12. Sandven P, Bjørneklett A, Maeland A, The Norwegian Yeast Study Group. Susceptibilities of Norwegian Canadian albicans strains to fluconazole: Emergence of resistance. Antimicrob Agents Chemother 37: 2443–2448, 1993.
13. Cssillag A, Brandstein L. The role of a Blastomyces species in the genesis of interstitial pneumonia of the premature infant: a preliminary report. Acta Microbiol Hung 9: 299–306, 1954.
14. Sherman JA, Jane F. Development of Hansenula anomala infection in a child receiving Fluconazole therapy. Pediatr Infect Dis J 13: 158–159, 1994.
15. Maksymiuk AW, Thongprasert S, Hopfer R, Luna M, Fainstein V, Bodey GP. Systemic candidiasis in cancer patients. Am J Med 77 (suppl 4D): 20–27, 1984.
16. Bodey GP. Candidiasis in cancer patients. Am J Med 77 (suppl 4D): 13–19, 1984.

Submitted September 26, 1994; accepted November 20, 1994

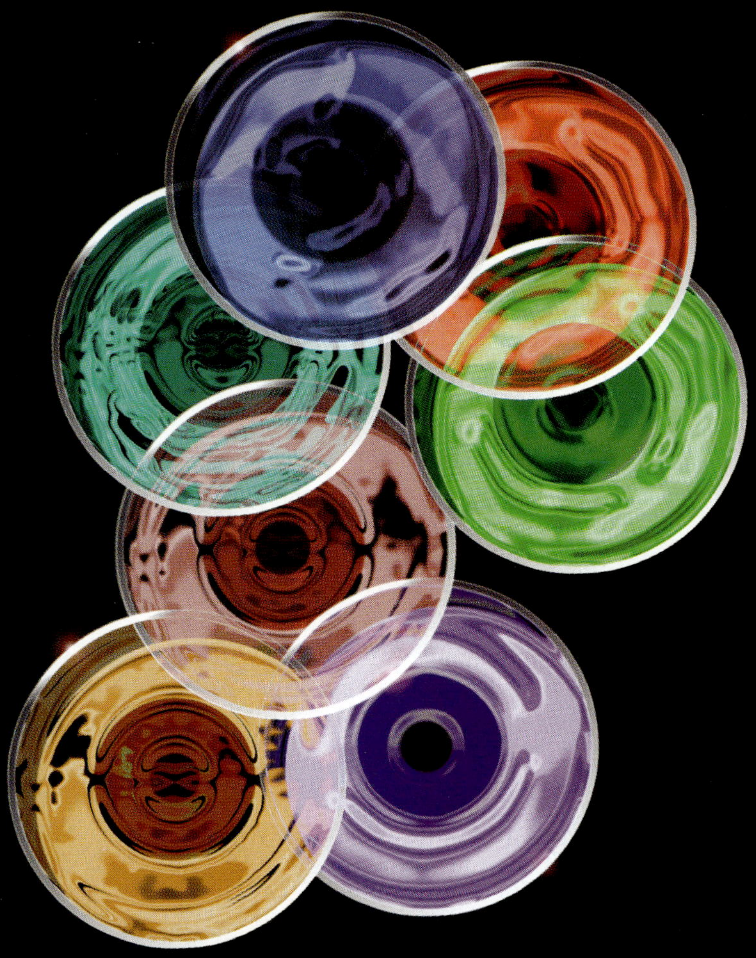

REFERENSER

Pizzo PA, Hathorn JW, Miemenz J et al. N Engl J Med 1986; 315: 552-8.
De Pauw BE, Feld R, Deresinski S et al. 6th International Symposium on infections in the immunocompromised Host. Peebles, Scotland June 3-6, 1990.
Novakova I, Donnelly P, de Pauw B. Scand J Infect Dis 22: 705-71 (1990)
Parr MD, Hansen LA, Rapp RP. Drug Intell Clin Pharm 1988; 22:628-31.
Mondorf AW, Mondorf W, Banzer S. 5th Mediterranean Congress of Chemotherapy, Cairo 1986: Abst. 0196.
Sanders JW, Powe NR, Moore RD. J Infect Dis 1991; 164:907:16.

Scand J Infect Dis 27: 89–91, 1995

CASE REPORT

Histoplasma Capsulatum Infection in Three AIDS Patients Living in Africa

ROBERT COLEBUNDERS[1,2], KOEN VAN DEN ABBEELE[1,2], ESTHER HAUBEN[2], TOM VERSTRAETEN[1,2], TOM HEREMANS[2], JOZEF VAN DEN ENDE[1,2] and ERIC VAN MARCK[2]

From the [1]Institute of Tropical Medicine, and [2]University Hospital Antwerp, Edegem, Antwerp, Belgium

Three AIDS patients are reported, 2 European and 1 African. All 3 developed Histoplasma capsulatum infection while living in Africa. Two developed a pulmonary infiltrate, and 2 had skin lesions. One patient was successfully treated with itraconazole, 400 mg daily; in a second patient, itraconazole was partially successful; the third patient was lost to follow-up before adequate treatment could be started. Histoplasma infection is probably an often undiagnosed complication in African AIDS patients.

R. Colebunders, MD, Institute of Tropical Medicine, Nationalestraat 155, B-2000 Antwerpen, Belgium

INTRODUCTION

Cases of disseminated histoplasmosis in AIDS patients have been reported mainly from the United States (1–3) but by now also from all continents (4–13). So far histoplasma infection has been observed in only a few AIDS patients living in Africa (4–10). In most cases the diagnosis of histoplasma infection was made at autopsy. Both Histoplasma duboisii and Histoplasma capsulatum infections have been reported (4–10).

We describe 3 cases of Histoplasma capsulatum infection in AIDS patients living in Africa.

METHODS

The diagnosis of Histoplasma capsulatum infection was made by histology in all 3 cases, using the following staining methods: Periodic acid-schiff (PAS) staining, PAS staining after diastase, and silver methenamine staining. Histoplasma capsulatum organisms were identified by standard morphological criteria.

CASE REPORTS

Case 1

This patient, a 41-year-old Belgian teacher, a heterosexual, was living in Zaire. In 1981 he was treated for liver amebiasis. In 1985, during a routine check-up he was found to be HIV seropositive. In August 1990, when seen at the Institute of Tropical Medicine, Antwerp, for an annual medical check-up, he had no complaints. Physical examination was normal. His CD4 lymphocyte count was 0 cells/mm^2. A chest X-ray revealed a pulmonary infiltrate in the lower right lobe. Bronchoscopy did not reveal any abnormalities. Histological examination of a transbronchial biopsy specimen confirmed Histoplasma capsulatum infection. The patient was treated with itraconazole 400 mg daily, zidovudine 250 mg twice daily, cotrimoxazole 960 mg daily and isoniazid 300 mg daily. The pulmonary infiltrate regressed slowly. Itraconazole 400 mg daily was continued for 1 year, followed by 100 mg daily.

In April 1991 the patient developed Kaposi's sarcoma lesions of the conjunctivae, gingiva and skin. In October 1991 a brônchoscopy revealed Kaposi's sarcoma lesions in the bronchi. Histoplasma could not be cultured from the broncho-alveolar lavage (BAL) fluid. Chemotherapy for the Kaposi's sarcoma was started. In March 1992 he presented with bilateral hemorrhagic pleuritis. Culture of the pleural fluid revealed a Mycobacterium avium complex infection. He was treated with rifabutin and ciprofloxacin but finally died, in September 1992. Post-mortem examination revealed disseminated Kaposi's sarcoma lesions and pulmonary embolism, but no evidence of histoplasma infection.

Case 2

A 41-year-old Polish priest living in Zaire. In February 1991 he developed fever, cough and weight loss (>10% of his body weight). On physical examination, oral candidiasis was observed. He was found to be HIV seropositive and to have a Plasmodium ovale infection. His CD4 lymphocyte count was 40 cells/mm^3. He received anti-malaria treatment, zidovudine 250 mg b.i.d. and cotrimoxazole 960 mg daily. In August 1993 he was admitted to the hospital because of fever lasting more than 2 months, severe weight loss, and cough with episodes of hemoptysis. Physical examination revealed severe anemia, a large ulcerative skin lesion on his right shoulder, and hemorrhoids. A chest X-ray revealed an infiltrate with a central cavity in the upper right lobe. The following laboratory abnormalities were noted: hemoglobin 72 g/l, CD4 lymphocyte count 40×10^6/l. On blood culture and culture of BAL fluid, Rhodococcus equi was grown. Histological examination of the skin lesion showed Histoplasma capsulatum infection (Fig. 1).

The patient was treated with a blood transfusion, itraconazole 400 mg daily, cotrimoxazole 960 mg t.i.d. minocycline 100 mg daily, amikacin 1.5 g i.v. daily. Hemorrhoidectomy was performed. The ulcerative skin lesion gradually regressed, the fever abated and his general condition improved. There was a slow regression of the pulmonary infiltrate but the cavitary lesion did not decrease in size. In November 1993, he was readmitted because of a perianal tumour. Histological examination of this tumour showed a non-Hodgkin lymphoma. In December 1993 he died. At postmortem examination a non-Hodgkin lymphoma was observed involving the bone marrow, liver, lymph nodes and anus. Histoplasma yeasts were observed in the histiocytes surrounding a pulmonary cavity in the right lung. Postmortem cultures did not reveal persistent Rhodococcus infection.

Case 3

A 44-year-old Zairian physician, a heterosexual, who lived in Zaire, Rwanda and Cameroon. He also had travelled to Europe on several occasions. In December 1992, he was admitted to the hospital because of chronic fever and diarrhoea, nocturnal sweating, cough, anorexia, and weight loss (>10% of his body weight). Physical examination revealed severe anemia, small non-pruritic

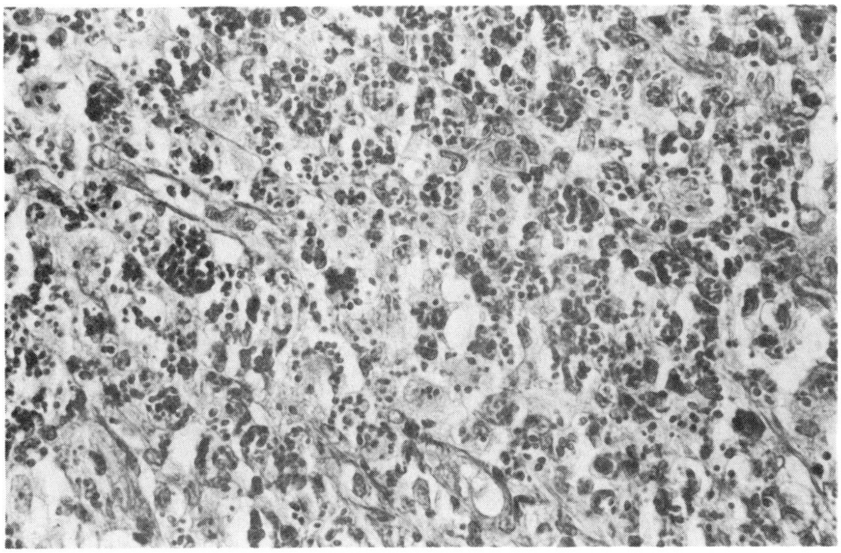

Fig. 1. A skin biopsy in Case 2, showing a microphotograph of a dermal inflammatory infiltrate, with numerous histiocytic cells with intracytoplasmic yeast forms (small black dots), morphologically compatible with Histoplasma capsulatum (PAS stain, ×360).

papules on his forehead, slight splenomegaly and malleolar edema. He was found to be HIV seropositive. Moreover the following laboratory adnormalities were noted: hemoglobin 59 g/l, CD4 lymphocyte count 4×10^6/l. Culture of blood and bone marrow revealed Mycobacterium avium complex infection. Histological examination of a biopsy sample from a papule on the forehead showed Histoplasma capsulatum infection. He was treated with a blood transfusion, fluconazole 100 mg daily, and cotrimoxazole 960 mg daily. When results of blood and bone marrow cultures became available, antituberculous treatment was added, initially with rifampicin 600 mg daily, isoniazid 300 mg daily and pyrazinamide 1500 mg daily and later clarithromycin 500 mg twice daily and lamprene 100 mg daily. The fever and diarrhoea disappeared and his general condition improved. During follow-up he developed a genital herpes simplex infection which was successfully treated with acyclovir 200 mg five times daily. In April 1993 he returned to Africa and died in December that year.

DISCUSSION

Histoplasmosis, in contrast to cryptococcosis, has not been reported as a frequent complication in African AIDS patients (8–10). It may be, however, that histoplasmosis often remains undiagnosed in the absence of histological examination of tissue or culture. In a postmortem study of 360 patients with HIV infection in Abidjan Cryptococcus neoformans infection was found in 10 (3%) and a Histoplasma capsulation infection in 6 (2%) (10). At the Institute of Tropical Medicine in Antwerp, among 100 AIDS patients who had lived at least 1 year in Africa, a diagnosis of Histoplasma capsulatum infection was made in 3.

To increase histoplasma case detection rates, a cheap histoplasma antigen test which is easy to perform would be most useful. Histoplasma antigen tests with fairly good sensitivity and specificity (also in HIV-infected individuals) have been developed but are not yet commercially available (14). Such an antigen test would also be useful in evaluating the response to treatment.

Disseminated histoplasma infection in persons with HIV infection is now considered to be an AIDS-defining disease (3). The 3 patients described in this report were all in an advanced stage of HIV infection and had CD4 lymphocyte counts $<40 \times 10^6$/l. In case 1 the histoplasma infection was his first opportunistic infection. In the 2 other patients, other AIDS-defining illnesses were present when the histoplasma infection was diagnosed.

Until recently amphotericin was the preferred treatment for disseminated histoplasmosis (1). Approximately 85% of AIDS patients with disseminated histoplasmosis respond to primary amphotericin B treatment (1, 3). However, such treatment has several disadvantages: it requires an intravenous infusion, it is associated with several side effects (fever, chills, headache, and myalgia), and has significant nephro- and hematotoxicity (15). Moreover, relapses occur in as many as 20% of the patients who receive 50 to 100 mg of amphotericin weekly or bi-weekly as maintenance therapy (16). More recently it was shown that itraconazole is effective as initial treatment for disseminated histoplasmosis (17, 18). Itraconazole is probably also the best drug for maintenance therapy (18). In a study performed in the U.S.A., 95% of patients receiving itraconazole as histoplasmosis maintenance therapy remained free of histoplasmosis during 97 patient-years of follow-up (19). In that study, itraconazole was well tolerated, only 1 patient being withdrawn from the study because of itraconazole toxicity (hypopotassemia) (19). Itraconazole was also effective in at least 1/2 patients who received such treatment.

A histoplasma infection should be included in the differential diagnosis of AIDS patients with unexplained fever, pulmonary infiltrates and skin or mucosal lesions. Other opportunistic infections that may cause such symptoms are Mycobacterium tuberculosis infection, Mycobacterium avium complex infection and other fungal infections, e.g. disseminated cryptococcal infection. If a diagnosis of histoplasma infection is made sufficiently early, itraconazole will probably be able to cure the patient.

ACKNOWLEDGEMENTS

We thank Prof. Dr. K. P. Schaal for the identification of the Rhodococcus equi infection and Annemie Van der Meer for preparing the manuscript.

REFERENCES

1. Wheat JL. Histoplasmosis in Indianapolis. Clin Infect Dis 14: S91–99, 1992.
2. Cohen PR, Grossman ME, Silvers DN. Disseminated histoplasmosis and human innumodeficiency virus infection. Int J Dermatol 9: 614–622, 1991.
3. Sarosi GA, Johnson PC. Disseminated histoplasmosis in patients infected with human immunodeficiency virus. Clin Infect Dis 14: S60–67, 1992.
4. Arendt V, Coremans-Pelseneer J, Gottlob R, Bril T, Bujan-Boza W, Fondu P. African histoplasmosis in a Belgian AIDS patient. Mycoses 34: 59–61, 1991.
5. Carme B, Ngaporo AI, Ngolet A, Ibara JR, Ebikili B. Disseminated African histoplasmosis in a Congolese patient with AIDS. J Med Vet Mycol 30: 245–248, 1992.
6. Smith E, Franzmann M, Mathiesen LR. Disseminated histoplasmosis in a Danish patient with AIDS. Scand J Infect Dis 21: 573–577, 1989.
7. Macher AM, Nelson AM, De Vinatea M. Disseminated infection by Histoplasma duboisii in an African patient with AIDS. US and Canadian Academy of Pathology, Annual Meeting, Washington, DC, 1988 (abstract).
8. Nelson AM, Kalengayi MR. The pathology of AIDS in Africa. In: AIDS in Africa (ed. M. Essex, S. Mboup, P. Kauki, M. Kalengayi). New York: Raven Press, 283–323, 1994.
9. Lucas SB, Honnou A, Peacock C, Beaumel A, Djomand G, N'Gbichi JM, Yeboue K, Hondé M, Diomande M, Giordano C, Doorly R, Brattegaard K, Kestens L, Smithwick R, Kadio A, Ezani N, Yapi A, De Cock KM. The mortality and pathology of HIV infection in a West African city. AIDS 7: 1569–1579, 1993.
10. Kakou A, Kra O, Bissagnene E, Coulibaly M, Aoussi E, Koffi K, Eholie S, Honde M, Lucas S, De Cock K, Odenhouri K, Kadio A. Etude rétrospective de 24 cas de mycoses profondes associées à l'infection à VIH à Abidjan. VIIIth International Conference on AIDS in Africa & VIIIth African Conference on STDS, Marrakech, Abstract ThB 047, p. 255, December 12–16. 12. 1993.
11. Dietrich PY, Bille J, Fontolliet C, Regamey C. Disseminated histoplasmosis due to Histoplasma capsulatum in a patient with acquired immunodeficiency syndrome (AIDS). Schweiz Med Wochenschr 117: 1289–1296, 1987.
12. Alados JC, Miranda C, Ortiz F, Cano R. Disseminated histoplasmosis in an AIDS patient in Spain. AIDS 12: 793, 1993.
13. Heyligenberg R, Kuijper EJ, Danner SA. Gegeneraliseerde histoplasmose bij 3 patiënten met een HIV-infectie. Ned Tijdschr Geneeskd 37: 1793–1796, 1990.
14. Wheat J. Diagnosis of histoplasmosis – Review of current methods. In: Dimorphic Fungy in Biology and Medicine (ed. H. Vanden Bossche et al.). New York: Plenum Press, 333–340, 1993.
15. Utz JP, Bennet JE, Brandriss MW. Amphotericin B toxicity. Ann Intern Med 61: 334, 1964.
16. McKinsey DS, Gupta MR, Driks MR, Smith DL, O'Connor M. Histoplasmosis in patients with AIDS: efficacy of maintenance amphotericin B therapy. Am J Med 92: 225–227, 1992.
17. Sharkey-Mathis PK, Velez J, Fetchick R, Graybill JR. Histoplasmosis in the Acquired Immunodeficiency Syndrome (AIDS): Treatment with itraconazole and fluconazole. J Acquir Immune Defic Syndr 6: 809–819, 1993.
18. Kell PD, Smith DE, Barton SE, Midgley J, Samarasinghe PL, Gazzard BG. Disseminated histoplasmosis in an AIDS patient treated with itraconazole. Genitourin Med 67: 342–344, 1991.
19. Wheat J, Hafner R, Wulfsohn M, Spencer P, Squires K, Powderly W, Wong B, Rinaldi M, Saag M, Hamill R, Murphy R, Connolly-Stringfield P, Briggs N, Owens S, and the National Institute of Allergy and Infectious Diseases Clinical Trials and Mycoses Study Group Collaborators. Prevention of relapse of histoplasmosis with itraconazole in patients with the acquired immunodeficiency syndrome. Ann Intern Med 118: 610–616, 1993.

Submitted June 27, 1994; accepted November 20, 1994

Scand J Infect Dis 27: 93–94, 1995

CASE REPORT

Hypersensitivity Hepatitis due to Pyrazinamide

XAVIER CORBELLA, MIQUEL VADILLO, CARMEN CABELLOS, PEDRO FERNANDEZ-VILADRICH and GABRIEL RUFI

From the Department of Infectious Diseases, Hospital de Bellvitge, University of Barcelona, Barcelona, Spain

Pyrazinamide hepatotoxicity is considered secondary to a direct and dose-related toxic effect. At currently used doses, pyrazinamide provides effective short-term treatment and is free from serious side effects. We report a case of pyrazinamide-induced hepatitis for which the rechallenge data strongly suggest a hypersensitivity mechanism.

X. Corbella, MD, Infectious Disease Service, Hospital de Bellvitge, Feixa Llarga s/n, L'Hospitalet de Llobregat, E-08907 Barcelona, Spain

INTRODUCTION

At a time when the occurrence of tuberculosis is on the increase all over the world, pyrazinamide at currently used dosages constitutes effective short-term treatment, free from serious adverse effects.

Pyrazinamide is a synthetic analog of nicotinamide which is bactericidally active against intracellular mycobacteria. Toxic hepatitis is regarded as the major side effect of pyrazinamide. The use of current dosage of pyrazinamide (25–30 mg/kg daily) has reduced hepatotoxicity, but not completely suppressed it (1).

In a large series of cases, the addition of pyrazinamide at doses of 25–40 mg/kg daily to regimens containing rifampicin and isoniazid did not increase the incidence of hepatitis (2). However, even at standard dosages, sporadic cases of fulminant hepatitis due to pyrazinamide have been reported (1, 3). Pyrazinamide hepatotoxicity is considered secondary to a direct, dose-related toxic effect (3, 4). To our knowledge, our report is the first concerning a case of pyrazinamide-induced hepatitis in which the rechallenge data strongly suggest a hypersensitivity mechanism.

CASE REPORT

A 59-year-old white woman was first admitted to the hospital because of fever and a non-ketotic hyperosmolar syndrome. The investigations revealed diabetes mellitus type II and pulmonary tuberculosis. At this first admission, the aminotransferase levels and eosinophil counts were normal. In relation to her weight (42 kg) therapy was initiated with a once daily dose of isoniazid (225 mg), rifampicin (450 mg), ethambutol (1000 mg), and pyrazinamide (1,250 mg). One month later, she presented with abdominal pain, vomiting, and fever. Blood pressure was 135/70 mmHg, temperature 38.2°C, respiratory rate 20 min, and pulse 92 per min. Physical examination revealed both scleral and cutaneous jaundice. The liver edge was felt 3 cm below the right costal margin. No splenomegaly, enlarged lymph nodes, arthritis, or skin lesions were present.

Laboratory data were as follows: alanine aminotransferase (ALT) 1,260 U/l (normal <40 U/l); asparate aminotransferase (AST) 1,680 U/l (normal <40 U/l); total bilirubin 136 μmol/l; glucose 6.3 mmol/l; red-cell count 4.2×10^{12}/l; hematocrit 0.37; hemoglobin 120 g/l; white-cell count 11.4×10^{9}/l, with 28% lymphocytes, 54% neutrophils, and 14% eosinophils (1596×10^{6}/l eosinophils); platelet count was 190×10^{9}/l. Prothrombin time was 15 s (control, 14 s), and partial thromboplastin time, 41 s (control, 35 s).

There was no previous background of alcohol abuse, hypersensitivity reactions, liver disease, or medications other than antituberculous treatment and NPH insulin. Serological markers of hepatitis B and C virus, Epstein-Barr virus, cytomegalovirus, and human immunodeficiency virus were negative. Drug-induced hepatitis was suspected.

On day 1 of admission her tuberculostatic treatment was withdrawn, while therapy was NPH insulin was continued. The patient improved, and 9 days after discontinuation of the antituberculous treatment she was afebrile and laboratory values were: ALT 204 U/l, AST 78 U/l and eosinophil count 320×10^{6}/l. At that time, her weight was 46 kg. Treatment with ethambutol (1,200 mg/d) was resumed on day 10, and with rifampicin (450 mg/d), on day 14. On day 28, the patient was asymptomatic, and the hepatic biochemical values and blood eosinophil count were normal. At that time, pyrazinamide (1,500 mg/d) was reintroduced. Two hours after the first dose of pyrazinamide, the patient presented acute malaise, fever of 40°C, generalized pruritus, arthralgia, perioral paresthesia, and vomiting. 12 hours later the aminotransferase values were: ALT 3,240 U/l; AST 4,140 U/l; and the white-cell count 6.6×10^{9}/l, with 13% eosinophils (858×10^{6}/l eosinophils) (Fig. 1). Tuberculostatic treatment was again withdrawn and the clinical symptoms improved dramatically within 48 h. Six days after the withdrawal, the aminotransferase values were: ALT 720 U/l and AST 120 U/l, and eosinophil count 280×10^{6}/l. On day 39, oral rifampicin (450 mg/d), oral ethambutol (1,200 mg/d), and intramuscular streptomycin (750 mg/d) were readministered and tolerated. To date, the patients remains healthy, with normal laboratory data, after one year of follow-up.

DISCUSSION

Acute hepatitis associated with pyrazinamide has been described as secondary to a direct toxic mechanism, and, being dose-related, it is usually predictable (3, 4). In this case, since the first episode of hepatitis was associated with fever and blood hypereosinophilia, and since it rapidly recurred with clear hypersensitivity symptoms a few hours following a second exposure to pyrazinamide, we believe that the liver injury was secondary to a hypersensitivity mechanism.

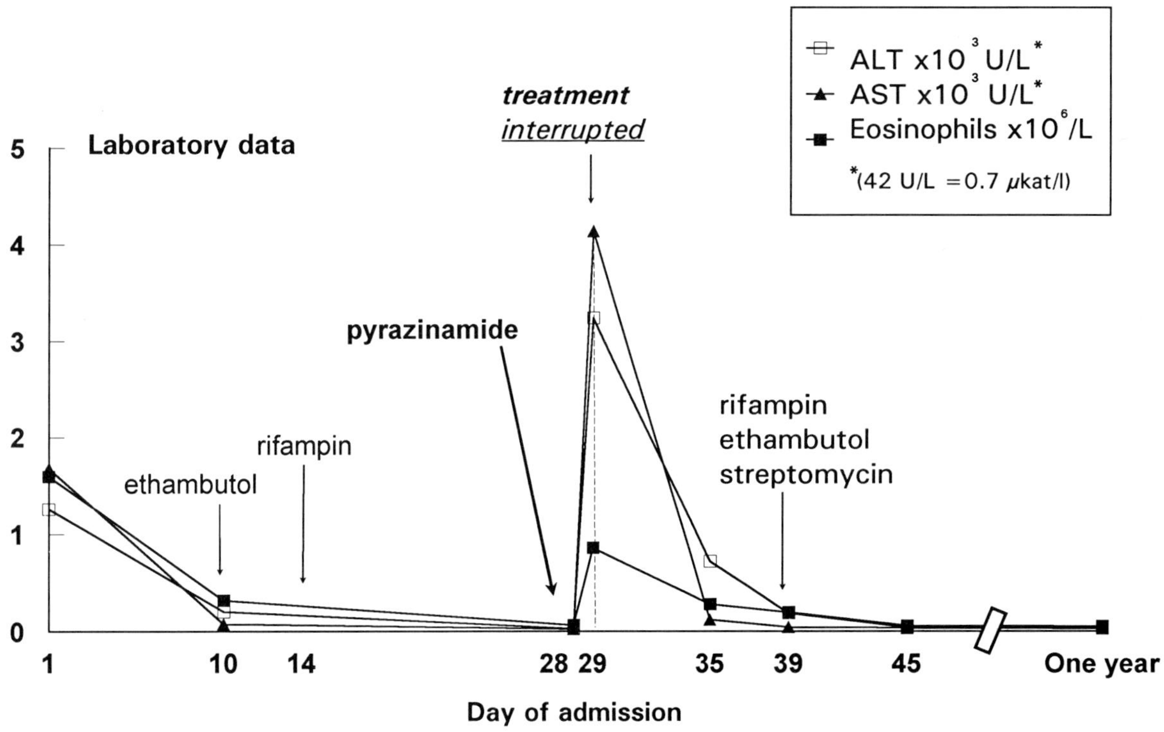

Fig. 1. Evolution of laboratory data in a 59-year-old woman with pyrazinamide-induced hepatitis.

In general, hypersensitivity hepatitis is not dose-related and is therefore unpredictable and commonly associated with hypersensitivity manifestations (5). Halothane, methyl dopa, and clomethacin are examples of this type of hepatitis (5, 6). In such cases, antibodies and cytotoxic T-lymphocytes directed against proteins of the hepatocyte modified by the reactive metabolites of the drug are hypothetically responsible for the hepatotoxicity (5, 6). In conclusion, we believe that hypersensitivity hepatitis should be included among the causes of pyrazinamide-induced hepatitis.

REFERENCES

1. Danan G, Pessayre D, Larrey D, Benhamou JP. Pyrazinamide fulminant hepatitis: an old hepatotoxin strikes again. Lancet 7: 1056–1057, 1981.
2. British Thoracic Association. A controlled trial of six months chemotherapy in pulmonary tuberculosis. First report: results during chemotherapy. Br J Dis Chest 75: 141–153, 1981.
3. Roden S, Lagneau M, Homasson JP. Hépatite fulminante au pyrazinamide. Rev Pneumol Clin 46: 43, 1990.
4. Girling DJ. The hepatic toxicity of antituberculosis regimens containing isoniazid, rifampicin and pyrazinamide. Tubercle 59:13–32, 1978.
5. Pessayre D. Physiopathologie des hépatopathies médicamenteuses. Gastroenterol Clin Biol 17 (suppl 5): H3–H17, 1993.
6. Kenna JG, Satoh H, Christ DD, Pohl LR. Metabolic basis for a drug hypersensitivity: antibodies in sera from patients with halothane hepatitis recognize liver neoantigens that contain the trifluoacetyl group derived from halothane. J Pharmacol Exp Ther 245: 1103–1109, 1988.

Submitted June 27, 1994; accepted November 11, 1994

Scand J Infect Dis 27: 95, 1995

Moraxella catarrhalis Bacteræmia in an Immunocompetent Adult

PERE DOMINGO, MIREIA PUIG, ROSER PERICAS, BEATRIZ MIRELIS and GUILLEM PRATS

From the Department of Infectious Diseases and Microbiology, Hospital de la Santa Creu i Sant Pau, Universitat Autonoma de Barcelona, Barcelona, Spain

P. Domingo, MD, Department of Internal Medicine, Hospital de la Santa Creu i Sant Pau, Avgda. Sant Antoni Mª Claret, 167, E-08025 Barcelona, Spain

SIR – Moraxella catarrhalis (formerly Branhamella catarrhalis) has long been considered a harmless oral commensal rarely implicated in human infection. When associated with human disease it has usually been restricted to acute, self-limiting infections of the upper respiratory tract in children, such as otitis and maxillary sinusitis (1). However, since the mid-seventies, bronchopulmonary infection with M. catarrhalis has been recognized as a significant cause of exacerbation of chronic pulmonary diseases (2). In addition, isolated cases of invasive disease such as endocarditis, septicæmia, and meningitis caused by this organism have been reported since the beginning of the twentieth century (3).

We have recently treated an immunocompetent patient with chronic obstructive pulmonary disease (COPD) who presented an episode of M. catarrhalis bacteræmia in the setting of acute exacerbation of his COPD.

A 76-year-old man was admitted to the hospital because of an 8 day history of fever, cough producing small amounts of mucopurulent sputum, and progressive dyspnea. The patient had been a heavy smoker and his past medical history was only remarkable for COPD. He had never been treated with corticosteroids nor had he received immunosuppressive therapy. His temperature was 38.4°C, respiratory rate 56/min, pulse 128, and blood pressure 150/100 mmHg. Physical examination on admission disclosed use of accessory respiratory muscles, cyanosis, and flapping tremor. Inspiratory and expiratory wheezing was audible over both lungs and scattered rales over the left. The physical examination was otherwise unremarkable. An X-ray film of the chest revealed chronic changes consistent with COPD but no infiltrate. Arterial blood gases when breathing room air were: PO_2 46 mmHg, PCO_2 41, and pH 7.42. The hæmoglobin was 149 g/l and white blood cell count 13.6×10^9/l, with 9% band forms and 76% neutrophils. Blood cultures taken on admission grew M. catarrhalis. The MICs of penicillin and cefotaxime were ≤ 0.03 μg/ml and ≤ 0.06 μg/ml, respectively. The strain did not produce β-lactamase (nitrocephin test), and was also susceptible to ciprofloxacin, ofloxacin, chloramphenicol, rifampicin, and cotrimoxazole. Complement and immunoglobulin levels were within the normal range. The patient was initially treated with oxygen, aerosolized bronchondilators and corticosteroids, and cefotaxime 4 g a day. 24 h after admission, fever was no longer detected. The patient rapidly improved and he was discharged 3 days later in good health.

Well over 50 cases of M. catarrhalis bacteræmia have been reported to date, and most cases share at least 1 of the 2 following conditions: a well-identified source, e.g. pneumonia, endocarditis, meningitis, upper respiratory tract infection, or underlying immunosuppression (3). To our knowledge, among the primary foci of M. catarrhalis bacteræmia, bronchitis has not been described yet. This may be explained by the fact that bronchitis in otherwise healthy adults is generally treated on an outpatient basis with oral antibiotics, and blood cultures are not routinely done (4).

There is a clear-cut association between immunosuppressive conditions and M. catarrhalis bacteræmia (3). However, in more than 40% of the patients with bacteræmia due to this organism, no identifiable immunosuppression can be found (3), as in our patient. Thus, M. catarrhalis remains a microorganism capable of striking healthy subjects, sometimes with a fatal outcome despite aggressive care (5, 6).

Our report provides further evidence of the ability of M. catarrhalis to cause invasive disease even in immunocompetent patients with a 'superficial' source, such as bronchitis, that may frequently be overlooked.

REFERENCES

1. Kovatch AL, Wald ER, Michaels RH. β-lactamase-producing Branhamella catarrhalis causing otitis media in children. J Pediatr 102: 261–264, 1983.
2. Hager H, Verghese A, Alvarez S, Berk SL. Branhamella catarrhalis respiratory tract infections. Rev Infect Dis 9: 1140–1149, 1987.
3. Wallace MR, Oldfield III EC. Moraxella (Branhamella) catarrhalis bacteremia. A case report and literature review. Arch Intern Med 150: 1332–1334, 1990.
4. Eng C, Aronson MD. Pneumococcal bacteræmia in two immunocompetent adults with otitis media and bronchitis. Lancet 2: 1266, 1990.
5. Barber PV, Stanbridge TN. Bacterial septicæmia with multiple organisms complicating influenzal pneumonia. BMJ 1: 1511–1512, 1977.
6. Bannatyne RM, Kolodej V. Branhamella catarrhalis bacteremia and immunosuppression-part of a larger problem? Diagn Microbiol Infect Dis 3: 65–67, 1985.

Submitted September 14, 1994; accepted October 11, 1994

Dapsone as Prophylaxis for Disseminated Mycobacterium avium Complex Infection

ANDRÉ CABIÉ, SOPHIE MATHERON, MARIE-AUDE KHUONG, OLIVIER BOUCHAUD, ADRIEN GÉRARD SAIMOT and JEAN-PIERRE COULAUD.

From the Infectious and Tropical Diseases Service, Service des Maladies Infectieuses et Tropicales, Hôpital Bichat – Claude Bernard, Paris, France

A. Cabié, Service des Maladies Infectieuses et Tropicales, Hôpital Bichat – Claude Bernard, 46 rue Henri Huchard F-75018 Paris, France

Disseminated infection due to the Mycobacterium avium complex (MAC) is the most common systemic bacterial infection among patients with AIDS in developed countries. Usually, the median CD4 cell count in patients with disseminated MAC infection is in the range 10–50/mm^3 (1). Rifabutine is the only recommended drug, at the present time, for prophylaxis of disseminated MAC infection (1). Dapsone, a dihydropteroate synthase inhibitor, has been shown to be active in vitro against M. tuberculosis and MAC (2, 3). In addition, dapsone is recommended for prophylaxis of Pneumocystis carinii pneumonia and neurotoxoplasmosis in association with pyrimethamine (4). Thus, dapsone is a potential agent against "multiple opportunistic pathogen prophylaxis".

The purpose of this study was to assess the prophylactic effectivity of dapsone against disseminated MAC infection. We evaluated, retrospectively, the frequency of disseminated MAC infection among patients receiving different types of PCP prophylaxis regimen: cotrimoxazole (480 or 960 mg, daily), dapsone (50 mg, daily), or aerosolized pentamidine (300 mg, monthly). We included the patients receiving one and the same prophylactic regimen for at least 4 weeks. Differences in MAC infection rate between different types of prophylaxis were analysed by χ^2-test.

From July 1992 to December 1993, 665 patients receiving PCP prophylaxis were followed at our Department. 22 (3.3%) developed disseminated MAC infection. The distribution of these patients according to the different types of prophylaxis regimen is presented in Table I. Disseminated MAC infection was observed with the same frequency in the dapsone group as in the cotrimoxazole group. The low frequency of disseminated MAC infection observed in the aerosolized pentamidine (AP) group probably stands in proportion to the highest CD4 cell count observed among these patients: dapsone = 112 ± 102/mm^3; cotrimoxazole = 123 ± 109/mm^3; AP = 282 ± 168/mm^3 ($p = 0.001$ for dapsone vs AP). To confirm this hypothesis, we analysed the data of the patients with < 100 CD4 cells/mm^3. The distribution of these patients according to the different types of prophylaxis regimen is presented in Table I. In this subgroup of patients, there was no difference between the 3 prophylactic regimens.

Although this study was retrospective, we conclude that dapsone is ineffective in preventing disseminated MAC infection.

Table I. *Distribution of patients with disseminated MAC infection according to the different types of prophylaxis regimen*

Prophylaxis	MAC infection: No. (%)	p^a
Dapsone (n = 155)	9 (6)	–
Cotrimoxazole (n = 276)	11 (4)	0.3
Aerosolized pentamidine (n = 234)	2 (1)	0.01
Patients with CD4 cells < 100/mm^3		
Dapsone (n = 45)	9 (20)	
Cotrimoxazole (n = 78)	11 (14)	> 0.1
Aerosolized pentamidine (n = 9)	2 (22)	> 0.1

[a] Comparison between dapsone and the other prophylactic treatment.

REFERENCES

1. Masur H. Recommendations on prophylaxis and therapy for disseminated Mycobacterium avium complex disease in patients infected with the human immunodeficiency virus. N Engl J Med 329: 898–904, 1993.
2. Rastogi N, Goh K, Labrousse V. Activity of subinhibitory concentrations of dapsone alone and in combination with cell-wall inhibitors against Mycobacterium avium complex organisms. Eur J Clin Microbiol Infect Dis 329: 1922–1926, 1993.
3. Gonzalez A, Berlin O, Bruckner D. In vivo activity of dapsone and two potentiators against Mycobacterium avium complex. J Antimicrob Chemother 24: 19–22, 1989.
4. Decker C, Masur H. Current status of prophylaxis for opportunistic infections in HIV-infected patients. AIDS 8: 11–20, 1994.

Submitted August 29, 1994; accepted September 13, 1994

Scandinavian Journal of

INFECTIOUS DISEASES

Vol. 27, no. 2, 1995
pp. 97–188

SCANDINAVIAN
UNIVERSITY PRESS

Oslo - Copenhagen -
Stockholm - Boston

Scand J Infect Dis 27: 99–104, 1995 ORIGINAL ARTICLE

Risk Factor Exposure Among Hepatitis C Virus RNA Positive Swedish Blood Donors – The Role of Parenteral and Sexual Transmission

STEVEN SHEV[1,5], SVANTE HERMODSSON[2], ANNIKA LINDHOLM[3], EWA MALM[1], ANDERS WIDELL[4] and GUNNAR NORKRANS[1]

From the Departments of [1]Infectious Diseases, East Hospital, [2]Virology, Sahlgrenska Sjukhuset, Göteborg, [4]Virology, Malmö General Hospital, Malmö, [5]Internal Medicine, Varberg Hospital, Varberg, and the [3]Blood Bank, East Hospital, Göteborg, Sweden

The potential modes of transmission for hepatitis C virus (HCV) infections were studied using a multivariate analysis of risk factor exposure among 51 2nd generation anti-HCV and HCV-RNA positive and matched anti-HCV negative blood donors. The following variables were found to be independently associated with anti-HCV and HCV-RNA positivity: intravenous drug use (IVDU) ($p < 0.001$), blood transfusion ($p < 0.01$), tattoos ($p < 0.001$), previous hospitalization ($p < 0.05$), history of sexually transmitted disease (STD) ($p < 0.001$) and lack of travels outside of Europe ($p < 0.05$). Among the 23 HCV-RNA positive donors without a history of IVDU or blood transfusion, an increased frequency of hospitalization ($p = 0.017$) and history of STD ($p = 0.023$) were found. Five of 22 sexual partners of the 51 index blood donors were HCV-RNA positive and in one of these couples sexual transmission was suspected. Anti-HCV and HCV-RNA positive donors were more often seropositive for herpes simplex virus type 2 (HSV-2) antibodies than were HCV-negative controls ($p = 0.015$). Sexual transmission of HCV may occur, but the possible role of HSV-2 requires further investigation.

S. Shev, MD, Department of Infectious Diseases, Östra Sjukhuset, S-416 85 Göteborg, Sweden

INTRODUCTION

Intravenous drug use (IVDU) and blood transfusion are important risk factors in the transmission of the hepatitis C virus (1, 2). Hepatitis C transmission following minor blood exposure such as needle-stick injuries and tattooing has also been reported (3, 4). Even in the absence of blood transfusion, major surgery (5) and nosocomial transmission at hemodialysis units (6, 7) have been discussed as potential risk factors for the transmission of hepatitis C. On the other hand, staff members at a dialysis unit and health-care workers (8) have not experienced an increased prevalence of hepatitis C antibodies (anti-HCV) despite occupational risks.

The mode of transmission in about half of all hepatitis C infections is still far from being completely understood. In some studies conducted with 1st generation anti-HCV assays among heterosexual partners of patients with acute (9) or chronic (9–11) NANB/C hepatitis, anti-HCV has either not been found at all or found at a very low frequency. Using 2nd generation anti-HCV assays, evidence for (12) and against (13) the heterosexual transmission of HCV has been presented. Prostitutes (14) and homosexual men (15) have been found to have a higher frequency of anti-HCV than has been reported in studies on blood donors, but, at least among male homosexuals, hepatitis B and HIV antibodies are more prevalent. Mother to child transmission of hepatitis C does occur, but probably not to any great extent (16). Conflicting findings regarding intrafamilial (but not necessarily sexual) transmission of hepatitis C infections have been reported (10, 17).

The aim of this study was to investigate the potential modes of transmission for hepatitis C infections in 2nd generation anti-HCV ELISA and HCV-RNA-positive blood donors.

MATERIALS AND METHODS

Blood donor screening for anti-HCV in Göteborg

Between February 1990 and January 1992, 47 of approximately 20,000 (0.23%) regular and 36 of 7,422 (0.48%) first-time blood donors were tested positive with either the 1st or 2nd generation anti-HCV ELISA (Orthos HCV test systems, Ortho Diagnostic Systems, Raritan, NJ, USA) and confirmed by a recombinant immunoblot assay (RIBA; Chiron Emeryville, CA, USA).

Blood donors

Blood donors identified as anti-HCV positive between February 1990 and January 1992 were included in the study. All 1st generation anti-HCV ELISA-positive donors were retested with the 2nd generation anti-HCV ELISA when it became available (May 1991). The first 100 consecutive 2nd generation anti-HCV ELISA-positive blood donors (originally screened with either 1st or 2nd generation anti-HCV ELISA), irrespective of RIBA results, were tested for HCV-RNA and 51 donors were found to be viremic, i.e. had chronic hepatitis C infections, thereby eliminating not only donors with resolved HCV infections but also those with false-positive anti-HCV results. These 51 (18 first-time) HCV-RNA-positive donors (44 men and 7 women) with a median age of 32 years (range 25–53) and 51 age- and sex-matched anti-HCV-negative donors found at the same blood banks were included in the study. Matching was done without any consideration of the socioeconomic status of the donors. All blood donors had, when enrolling as donors, signed a questionnaire denying present or past i.v. drug abuse. No male donor was bi- or homosexual. Each donor, after inclusion in the study, was interviewed by the same interviewer using a questionnaire dealing with potential risk factors for hepati-

 ISSN 0036-5548

tis C transmission. Both the interviewer and the interviewed blood donors were aware of the donor's HCV status.

This study was approved by the local Ethics Committee and all blood donors and relatives gave informed consent.

Household contacts and relatives

62 relatives (22 regular monogamous sexual partners, 19 children, 13 parents, and 8 siblings) to anti-HCV and HCV-RNA positive donors were tested with the 2nd generation anti-HCV ELISA. None of the 22 couples reported regular use of barrier contraceptives.

Laboratory procedures

Hepatitis B surface antigen (HBsAg), antibodies to hepatitis B core antigen (anti-HBc IgG) and anti-HIV were determined by commercial immunoassays. Serum alanine aminotranferase (s-ALAT) levels were also determined (reference <0.7 μkat/l). Herpes simplex type 2 IgG-antibodies were determined by ELISA as described elsewhere (18, 19) and titres greater than or equal to 1:200 were considered positive. The specificity of the anti-HSV-2 test versus antibodies to HSV type 1 has been shown to be good (19–21).

Hepatitis C virus RNA detection

HCV RNA was determined by the polymerase chain reaction (PCR) using primers from the 5′ non-coding region as described previously (22). PCR was performed on sera from all sexual partners to index blood donors.

Genotyping of hepatitis C virus

Genotyping was performed on sera from blood donors and their sexual partners who were PCR-positive.

Genotyping by PCR was done with type-specific primers directed against the HCV core gene, based on the principal of Okamoto et al. (23) but with several modifications (24). The typing terminology suggested by Chan et al. (25) was used. Our assay also identified the important type 3a by Chan, which was never identified by the original Okamoto assay. Briefly, typing was started with a consensus amplification of bp 467–751 with primers 5′-TAGATTGGGTGTGCGCGCGA (sense, s), 5′-ATGTACCC-CATGAGGTCGGC (antisense, as); thereafter typing for each isolate was done in 2 different reactions under stringent conditions (annealing temperature of 63°C, 25 cycles). Typing primer for type 1a was 5′-TGGGGATAGGCTGACGTCTACCT (as), for 1b 5′-CCATCCTGCCCACCCCA (as), for 2a 5′-CCAAGAGG-GACGGGAACCTC (as) and for 2b 5′-GCAACCCTCGTTTCC-(GA)TACAGAG (as); these primers were run against an upstream primer 5′-AGGAAGACTTCCGAGCGGTC (s). Type 3a was identified with a primer 5′-GTGTGCGCGACGCGTAAA (s) and a consensus primer 5′-GCA(TC)GT(AG)AGGGTA-TCGATGAC(TC)T (as), in this reaction type 1b was also confirmed with primer 5′-AACCTCGTGGAAGGCGACAA (s). Bases within parentheses denote a redundant base at this position.

Statistical analysis

Statistical analysis was performed using Fisher's Exact Test with 2-sided p-values for univariate analysis and Mantel's Test for multivariate analysis (26). Wilcoxon's Signed Rank Test for paired data (2-tailed test) was also used when appropriate. In all tests 2-tailed p-values <0.05 were considered statistically significant.

RESULTS

The results of a univariate analysis of risk factor exposure among 51 anti-HCV, PCR-positive and 51 anti-HCV-negative matched blood donors are shown in Table I. Using a multivariate procedure, the following variables were found to be independently associated with anti-HCV and PCR positivity: IVDU, blood transfusion, tattoos, previous hospitalization, history of STD and no travels outside Europe.

18 anti-HCV ELISA, PCR-positive donors had a history of IVDU, 7 others had received blood transfusions and 3 donors had a history of both IVDU and blood transfusion. When focusing on risk factor exposure (including tattooing) in the remaining 23 PCR-positive blood donors and 23 matched anti-HCV-negative control donors, a statistically significant difference was found in only 2 categories: previ-

Table I. *Univariate and multivariate analyses of risk factor exposure among 51 anti-HCV and polymerase chain reaction (PCR) positive and 51 age- and sex-matched anti-HCV-negative blood donors*

Risk factor	Anti-HCV, PCR pos blood donors ($n = 51$)	Anti-HCV neg blood donors ($n = 51$)
IVDU	21	0***
Blood transfusion	10	0**
Tattoos	19	3***
Acupuncture	5	4
Intravenous drips	22	9 [**]
I.m. gammaglobulin	20	31 [*]
Surgery	34	25
Hospitalization	43	32*
Health-care worker	4	4
Exposure to human blood	3	8
Exposure to hepatitis	15	9
Sex partner of IVDU	4	0
History of STD	20	5***
Alcohol abuse	6	0 [*]
Travels outside Europe	16	28*

I.m. = Intramuscular.
IVDU = Intravenous drug user, STD = Sexually transmitted disease.
* $p < 0.05$, ** $p < 0.01$, *** $p < 0.001$; significant differences by both uni- and multivariate analyses are expressed as *, **, ***, whereas differences only significant by univariate analysis are written within brackets; [*] and [**].

Table II. *Risk factor exposure, HCV-RNA as determined by polymerase chain reaction (PCR) results and hepatitis C virus (HCV) genotypes in 5 anti-HCV-positive blood donors and their anti-HCV-positive sex partners*

BLOOD DONOR/SEX PARTNER			
Risk factor	Sex	HCV-RNA	HCV genotype
IVDU/IVDU	f/m	+/+	3a/3a
Tattoos/Tattoos	m/f	+/+	3a/2b
SEX CONTACT			
with IVDU/IVDU	f/m	+/+	2b/2b
with IVDU/IVDU	m/f	+/+	1b/3a
with IVDU/IVDU	f/m	+/neg	la/neg

IVDU = intravenous drug user; m = male; f = female; neg = negative.

Table III. *Herpes simplex virus type 2 (HSV-2) enzyme-linked immunosorbent assay (ELISA) results in 41 anti-HCV ELISA, polymerase chain reaction (PCR) positive and 41 age- and sex-matched anti-HCV ELISA negative blood donors*

	HSV-2 pos			
Donors	No	(%)	p-value	Odds ratio (95% confidence interval)
anti-HCV + PCR pos ($n = 41$)	18	(43.9)	0.015	3.8 (1.4–10.2)
anti-HCV neg ($n = 41$)	7	(17)		
anti-HCV + PCR pos IVDU ($n = 19$)	10	(53)	n.s.	4.2 (1.0–16.7)
anti-HCV neg ($n = 19$)	4	(21)		
anti-HCV + PCR pos (excluding IVDU and blood transfused) ($n = 16$)	8	(50)	n.s.	4.3 (0.9–20.3)
anti-HCV neg ($n = 16$)	3	(19)		

n.s. = not significant; pos = positive; neg = negative; IVDU = intravenous drug user.

ous hospitalization ($p = 0.017$) and a history of sexually transmitted diseases ($p = 0.023$). A multivariate analysis found these 2 risk factors to be independently associated with HCV viremia as detected by PCR.

None of the children, parents or siblings to the anti-HCV-positive donors were anti-HCV positive. Five monogamous heterosexual partners were found to be anti-HCV positive (Table II) and parenteral risk factor exposure could not be established for at least one of the partners in 3 of these couples. In one of these 3 couples an identical set-up of genotypes was found. None of the anti-HCV-negative sexual partners to PCR-positive blood donors ($n = 17$) was PCR-positive. None of these sexual partners had a history of IVDU.

The number of estimated 'lifetime' sexual partners for 15 of the 23 anti-HCV, PCR-positive donors (no accurate estimates available for 8 donors) who did not have a history of IVDU or blood transfusion (median 10; range 0–200) was significantly increased ($p = 0.017$) vis-à-vis matched anti-HCV-negative ($n = 15$) control donors (median 6; range 0–15).

Anti-HCV, PCR-positive blood donors ($n = 41$) were more often seropositive for herpes simplex type 2 virus (HSV-2) antibodies ($p = 0.015$) than were 41 matched anti-HCV-negative donors (no sera available for HSV-2 determination in 10 anti-HCV-negative controls) (Table III). The prevalence of HSV-2 seropositivity was not increased among anti-HCV, PCR-positive IVDU vis-á-vis anti-HCV, PCR-positive donors without a history of IVDU or blood transfusion.

10 anti-HCV-positive donors (but none of the anti-HCV-negative control donors) were anti-HBc IgG positive (7/10 with a history of IVDU). No donor was anti-HIV or HBsAg positive. 13 of 51 (25%) PCR-positive blood donors had a normal s-ALAT level when enrolled in the study.

DISCUSSION

In this study, blood transfusion, tattooing and IVDU were independently associated with anti-HCV and PCR positivity, findings which correlate well with previous studies on the modes of transmission for hepatitis C (1, 2, 27). Previous IVDU and/or blood transfusion represented 28 of 51 (55%) PCR-positive blood donors. This is in agreement with Esteban et al. (28) and Serfaty et al. (5) who found that 43% and 49%, respectively, of 2nd generation recombinant immunoblot assay (RIBA 2)-confirmed 1st generation anti-HCV ELISA positive blood donors had a history of IVDU or blood transfusion. The lack of travels outside of Europe was also a factor associated with PCR positivity but this may merely reflect our donors' socioeconomic status.

The greater incidence of hospitalization among PCR-positive donors (and even when excluding IVDU and blood transfused) as compared with seronegative controls raises the question of HCV as a nosocomial infection. Hepatitis C infections among nontransfused dialysis patients has been reported (6, 7). Previous surgery was not a risk factor for PCR positivity in our study, which is in agreement with a study on non-transfused patients undergoing open-heart surgery (29). However, major surgery has been suggested to be a risk factor for HCV infection (5) and even for non-A, non-B hepatitis (30).

Although occupational exposure may be a risk factor in certain circumstances, i.e. after needle-stick injuries (3), we did not find a greater proportion of healthcare workers among anti-HCV and PCR positive blood donors than among matched controls. This compares well with findings from southern Sweden where staff at a dialysis unit and infectious diseases clinic did not have a greater anti-HCV positivity than healthy blood donors (8).

We found no parents, children or siblings who were anti-HCV positive. In Spain, Riestra and co-workers found that hepatitis C transmission to household contacts was correlated to the duration of contact with family members and the severity of liver disease in the index patient (31). We do not know when our seropositive donors contracted hepatitis C, so the duration of exposure is also unknown and may have been too short to cause transmission to household contacts. Infectiousness of hepatitis C may of course also depend on other factors such as the serum level of HCV. HCV transmission from mother to child has been suggested to be dependent on the level of viremia (32). Other, hitherto unrecognized factors, may also contribute to hepatitis C transmission. In Japan, where intrafamilial transmission has been suggested (33), percutaneous exposure to infected blood during medical treatments could have been directly involved in the spread of hepatitis C (34).

Five regular monogamous sexual partners were anti-HCV positive. In one couple with only 9 months of cohabitation and where the female blood donor had no history of parenteral risk factor exposure, both partners had the same HCV genotype. In this case, sexual transmission of the HCV virus is highly probable. In another pair where different HCV genotypes (1b/3a) were found, the male index blood donor had a history of alcohol abuse. Viremia could not be detected by PCR in anti-HCV-negative partners of HCV-RNA-positive donors.

A history of STD and the estimated number of lifetime sex partners was greater in the anti-HCV, PCR positive blood donors with community-acquired hepatitis C as compared with matched controls. Multiple heterosexual partners have been reported to be a risk factor in the transmission of non-A, non-B hepatitis (35). A history of prostitution exceeding 6 months has also been shown to be a significant risk factor for HCV infection (14).

In one study among 1st generation anti-HCV ELISA screened, RIBA 2 confirmed blood donors, multiple sex partners and a history of STD were found not to be significant risk factors as compared with negative controls (5). Other studies also based on the 1st generation anti-HCV ELISA, confirmed by RIBA 2 or a neutralization ELISA, have produced similar results (36, 37). The 2nd generation anti-HCV ELISA, with newer HCV antigens, has an increased sensitivity (38–40) and this may explain the different findings in our study.

In 2 previous investigations, HCV-RNA was not found in bodily secretions from patients with chronic hepatitis C infections (41, 42), while in other studies HCV RNA was found in saliva (43–45) and urine (45) of some patients with hepatitis C. HCV-related antigen has been found in semen from patients with non-A, non-B hepatitis (46). Sexual transmission of hepatitis C is probably uncommon but when it does occur it may be dependent on the existence of a co-factor. HIV has been suspected of being such a co-factor (47). However, none of the blood donors or anti-HCV-positive sexual partners in our study were HIV-positive. The herpes simplex type 2 virus has been suspected of being a co-factor in the transmission of HIV (48–50). In our study, PCR-positive blood donors were more often seropositive for antibodies to HSV-2 virus than were matched controls. Co-infection with HSV-2 may facilitate the sexual transmission of HCV but on the other hand may only represent an indication of increased risk of STD. Only one of our blood donors reported clinical symptoms of genital HSV-2 infection. Each donor was asked if he or she had a history of STD but not specifically questioned as to previous HSV-2 infections. This may explain the discrepancy between serological findings and donor responses to the questionnaire.

21 of 51 anti-HCV and PCR-positive voluntary blood donors admitted to previous IVDU in spite of written denials made at the blood bank before blood donation. Many of these donors had not used narcotics for many years or only had a history of sporadic IVDU. Donors may be unaware of the fact that hepatitis C infections are often chronic but asymptomatic. Even routine check-ups of s-ALAT levels may show normal values. 25% of PCR-positive blood donors in our study had a normal s-ALAT level. This has also been observed in other studies (40, 51).

To sum up, sexual transmission of hepatitis C, though it does occur, seems to be uncommon. The role of HSV-2 infections in facilitating the sexual transmission of HCV needs further study. Nosocomial hepatitis C infections cannot be excluded, but here again, more studies are required to elucidate these findings. Despite signed denials, previous IVDU was found among blood donors. More vigorous checks at blood banks are needed to avoid this problem in the future.

ACKNOWLEDGEMENTS

The authors thank Dr Lars Bohlin, Nancy Nehonen, Clementina Garcia and the staff of the hepatitis and serology laboratories at the Department of Virology, Sahlgrenska Sjukhuset, Göteborg and Lena Widerström and Ann Paterson, Department of Infectious Diseases, Östra Sjukhuset, Göteborg, for technical assistance. Siv Månsson of Malmö Allmänna Sjukhus performed the genotyping of HCV. Special thanks go to Dr Sven-Olof Jansson, Department of Internal Medicine, Varberg Sjukhus, Sweden, for technical and computer assistance. Dr Anders Odén helped with statistical analysis. This study received grants from University of Göteborg, University of Lund, and the Medical Society of Göteborg.

REFERENCES

1. Widell A, Hansson BG, Berntorp E, Moestrup T, Johansson HP, Hansson H, Nordenfelt E. Antibody to a hepatitis C virus related protein among patients at high risk for hepatitis B. Scand J Infect Dis 23: 19–24, 1991.
2. Alter HJ, Purcell RH, Shih JW, Melpolder JC, Houghton M, Choo Q-L, Kuo G. Detection of antibody to hepatitis C virus in prospectively followed transfusion recipients with acute and chronic non-A, non-B hepatitis. N Engl J Med 321: 1494–1500, 1989.

3. Marranconi F, Mecenero V, Pellizzer GP, Bettini MC, Conforto M, Vaglia A, Stecca C, Cardone E, de Lalla F. HCV infection after accidental needlestick injury in health-care workers. Infection 20: 111, 1992.
4. Abildgaard N, Peterslund NA. Hepatitis C virus transmitted by tattooing needle. Lancet 338: 460, 1991.
5. Serfaty L, Giral P, Elghouzzi MH, Jullien AM, Poupon R. Risk factors for hepatitis C virus infection in hepatitis C virus antibody ELISA-positive blood donors according to RIBA-2 status: A case-control survey. Hepatology 17: 183–187, 1993.
6. Nordenfelt E, Löfgren B, Widell A, Hansson B-G, Zhang YY, Hagstam K-E, Kurkus J. Hepatitis C virus infection in hemodialysis patients in southern Sweden: Epidemiological, clinical and diagnostic aspects. J Med Virol 40: 266–270, 1993.
7. Allander T, Medin C, Jacobson SH, Grillner L, Persson MAA. Hepatitis C transmission in a Hemodialysis Unit: Molecular evidence for spread of virus among patients not sharing equipment. J Med Virol 43: 415–419, 1994.
8. Norrgren H, Flodman-Norrlund I-G, Lindholm T, Hansson BG, Nordenfelt E. Prevalence of antibodies against hepatitis B and C viruses among different groups of medical staff. Scand J Infect Dis 24: 553–554, 1992.
9. Shev S, Wejstål R, Wahl M, Hermodsson S, Norkrans G. The lack of transmission of NANB/C hepatitis between acute and chronically infected patients and their heterosexual partners. Scand J Infect Dis 23: 407–411, 1991.
10. Everhart JE, Di Bisceglie AM, Murray LM, Alter HJ, Melpolder JJ, Kuo G, Hoofnagle JH. Risk for non-A, non-B (type C) hepatitis through sexual or household contact with chronic carriers. Ann Intern Med 112: 544–545, 1990.
11. Gordon SC, Patel AH, Kulesza GW, Barnes RE, Silverman AL. Lack of evidence for the heterosexual transmission of hepatitis C. Am J Gastroenterol 87: 1849–1851, 1992.
12. Kao J-H, Chen P-J, Yang P-M, Lai M-Y, Sheu J-C, Wang T-H, Chen D-S. Intrafamilial transmission of hepatitis C virus: The important role of infections between spouses. J Infect Dis 166: 900–903, 1992.
13. Bresters D, Mauser-Bunschoten EP, Reesink HW, Roosendaal G, van der Poel CL, Chamuleau RAFM, Jansen PLM, Weegink CJ, Cuypers HTM, Lelie PN, van den Berg HM. Sexual transmission of hepatitis C virus. Lancet 342: 210–211, 1993.
14. Wu J-C, Lin H-C, Jeng F-S, Ma G-Y, Lee S-D, Sheng W-Y. Prevalence, infectivity and risk factor analysis of hepatitis C virus infection in prostitutes. J Med Virol 39: 312–317, 1993.
15. Westh H, Worm A-M, Jensen BL, Kroon S, Kvinesdal B, Nielsen CM, Wantzin P. Hepatitis C virus antibodies in homosexual men and intravenous drug users in Denmark. Infection 21: 115–117, 1993.
16. Wejstål R, Widell A, Månsson A-S, Hermodsson S, Norkrans G. Mother-to-infant transmission of hepatitis C virus. Ann Intern Med 117: 887–890, 1992.
17. Honda M, Kaneko S, Unoura M, Kobayashi K, Murakami S. Risk of hepatitis C virus infections through household contact with chronic carriers: Analysis of nucleotide sequences. Hepatology 17: 971–976, 1993.
18. Jeansson S, Forsgren M, Svennerholm B. Evaluation of solubilized herpes simplex virus membrane antigen by enzyme-linked immunosorbent assay. J Clin Microbiol 18: 1160–1166, 1983.
19. Svennerholm B, Olofsson S, Jeansson S, Vahlne A, Lycke E. Herpes simplex virus type-selective enzyme-linked immunosorbent assay with Helix pomatia lecitin-purified antigens. J Clin Microbiol 19: 235–239, 1984.
20. Olofsson S, Lundström M, Marsden H, Jeansson S, Vahlne A. Characterization of a herpes simplex virus type 2-specified glycoprotein with affinity for N-acetylgalactosamine-specific lectins and its identification as g92K or gG. J Gen Virol 67: 737–744, 1986.
21. Ho DWT, Field PR, Sjögren-Jansson E, Jeansson S, Cunningham AL. Indirect ELISA for the detection of HSV-2 specific IgG and IgM antibodies with glycoprotein G (gG-2). J Virol Methods 36: 249–264, 1992.
22. Widell A, Månsson A-S, Sundström G, Hansson BG, Nordenfelt E. Hepatitis C virus RNA in blood donor sera detected by the polymerase chain reaction: Comparison with supplementary hepatitis C antibody assays. J Med Virol 35: 253–258, 1991.
23. Okamoto H, Sugiyama Y, Okada S, Kurai K, Akahane Y, Sugal Y, Tanaka T, Sato K, Tsuda F, Miyakawa Y, Mayumi M. Typing hepatitis C virus by polymerase chain reaction with type-specific primers: application to clinical surveys and tracing infectious sources. J Gen Virol 73: 673–679, 1992.
24. Widell A, Shev S, Månsson S, Zhang YY, Foberg U, Norkrans G, Frydén A, Weiland O, Kurkus J, Nordenfelt E. Genotyping of hepatitis C virus isolates by a modified PCR assay using type specific primers: Epidemiological applications. J Med Virol 44: 272–279, 1994.
25. Chan SW, McOmish F, Holmes EC, Dow B, Peutherer JF, Follett E, Yap PL, Simmonds P. Analysis of a new hepatitis C virus type and its phylogenetic relationship to existing variants. J Gen Virol 73: 1131–1141, 1992.
26. Mantel N. Chi-square tests with one degree of freedom; Extensions of the Mantel-Haenszel procedure. J Am Statistical Assoc 58: 690–700, 1963.
27. Ko Y-C, Ho M-S, Chiang T-A, Chang S-J, Chang P-Y. Tattooing as a risk of hepatitis C virus infection. J Med Virol 38: 288–291, 1992.
28. Esteban JI, López-Talavera JC, Genescà J, Madoz P, Viladomiu L, Muñiz E, Martin-Vega C, Rosell M, Allende H, Vidal X, González A, Hernández JM, Esteban R, Guardia J. High rate of infectivity and liver disease in blood donors with antibodies to hepatitis C virus. Ann Intern Med 115: 443–449, 1991.
29. Mattsson L, Åberg B, von Sydow M, Weiland O. Incidence of hepatitis and seroconversion to hepatitis C virus after open-heart surgery in transfused and non-transfused patients in Sweden. Scand J Infect Dis 23: 25–29, 1991.
30. Hollinger B, Mosley J, Szmuness W, Aach R, Melnick J, Abdelmomen A, Stevens C, Kahn R. Non-A, non-B hepatitis following blood transfusion: Risk factors associated with donor characteristics. In: Szmuness W, Alter HJ, Maynard JE, eds. Viral Hepatitis 1981 International Symposium. Philadelphia: The Franklin Institute Press, 361–376, 1981.
31. Riestra Menéndez S, Rodriguez Garcia M, Sánchez San Román F, Menéndez Tévar F, Suárez González A, Alvarez Navascués C, Pérez Alvarez R, Rodrigo Sáez L. Intrafamilial spread of hepatitis C virus. Infection 19: 431–433, 1991.
32. Ohto H, Terazawa S, Sasaki N, Sasaki N, Hino K, Ishiwata C, Kako M, Ujiie N, Endo C, Matsui A, Okamoto H, Mishiro S. The Vertical Transmission of Hepatitis C Virus Collaborative Study Group. Transmission of hepatitis C virus from mothers to infants. N Engl J Med 330: 744–750, 1994.
33. Kiyosawa K, Sodeyama T, Tanaka E, Shimizu S, Furuta S, Miyazaki Y, Akahane Y, Suzuki H. Intrafamilial transmission of hepatitis C virus in Japan. J Med Virol 33: 114–116, 1991.
34. Kiyosawa K, Furuta S. Transmission and prevention of hepatitis C infection. Abstract. Fourth International Symposium on HCV. Tokyo, Japan, 7–9 May, 1993.
35. Alter MJ, Coleman P, Alexander J, Kramer E, Miller JK, Mandel E, Hadler SC, Margolis HS. Importance of heterosex-

ual activity in the transmission of hepatitis B and non-A, non-B hepatitis. JAMA 262: 1201–1205, 1989.
36. Weinstock HS, Bolan G, Reingold AL, Polish LB. Hepatitis C virus infection among patients attending a clinic for sexually transmitted diseases. JAMA 269: 392–394, 1993.
37. Osmond DH, Padian NS, Sheppard HW, Glass S, Shiboski SC, Reingold A. Risk factors for hepatitis C virus seropositivity in heterosexual couples. JAMA 269: 361–365, 1993.
38. Aach RD, Stevens CE, Hollinger FB, Mosley JW, Peterson DA, Taylor PE, Johnson RG, Barbosa LH, Nemo GJ. Hepatitis C virus infection in post-transfusion hepatitis. N Engl J Med 325: 1325–1329, 1991.
39. Chemello L, Cavalletto D, Pontisso P, Bortolotti F, Donada C, Donadon V, Frezza M, Casarin P, Alberti A. Patterns of antibodies to hepatitis C virus in patients with chronic non-A, non-B hepatitis and their relationship to viral replication and liver disease. Hepatology 17: 179–182, 1993.
40. Shev S, Foberg U, Frydén A, Hermodsson S, Lindh G, Lindholm A, Månsson A-S, von Sydow M, Weiland O, Widell A, Norkrans G. Second generation hepatitis C ELISA antibody tests confirmed by the four-antigen recombinant immunoblot assay correlate well with hepatitis C viremia and chronic liver disease in Swedish blood donors. Vox Sanguinis 65: 32–37, 1993.
41. Fried MW, Shindo M, Fong T-L, Fox PC, Hoofnagle JH, Di Bisceglie AM. Absence of hepatitis C viral RNA from saliva and semen of patients with chronic hepatitis C. Gastroenterology 102: 1306–1308, 1992.
42. Hsu H, Wright T, Luba D, Martin M, Feinstone S, Garcia G, Greenberg H. Failure to detect hepatitis C virus genome in human secretions with the polymerase chain reaction. Hepatology 14: 763–767, 1991.
43. Wang J-T, Wang T-H, Sheu J-C, Lin J-T, Chen D-S. Hepatitis C virus RNA in saliva of patients with posttransfusion hepatitis and low efficiency of transmission among spouses. J Med Virol 36: 28–31, 1992.
44. Young K-C, Chang T-T, Liou T-C, Wu H-L. Detection of hepatitis C virus RNA in peripheral blood mononuclear cells and in saliva. J Med Virol 41: 55–60, 1993.
45. Numata N, Ohori H, Hayakawa Y, Saitoh Y, Tsunoda A, Kanno A. Demonstration of hepatitis C virus genome in saliva and urine of patients with type C hepatitis: Usefulness of the single round polymerase chain reaction method for detection of the HCV genome. J Med Virol 41: 120–128, 1993.
46. Kotwal GJ. Routine laboratory diagnosis of hepatitis C virus infection. J Hepatol 17 (suppl 3): S83–S89, 1993.
47. Eyster ME, Alter HJ, Aledort LM, Quan S, Hatzakis A, Goedert JJ. Heterosexual co-transmission of hepatitis C virus (HCV) and human immunodeficiency virus (HIV). Ann Intern Med 115: 764–768, 1991.
48. Holmberg SD, Stewart JA, Gerber AR, Byers RH, Lee FK, O'Malley PM, Nahmias AJ. Prior herpes simplex virus type 2 infection as a risk factor for HIV-infection. JAMA 259: 1048–1050, 1988.
49. Stamm WE, Handsfield HH, Rompalo AM, Ashley RL, Roberts PL, Corey L. The association between genital ulcer disease and acquisition of HIV-infection in homosexual men. JAMA 260: 1429–1433, 1988.
50. Hook EW III, Canno RO, Nahmias AJ, Lee FF, Campbell CH Jr, Glasser D, Quinn TC. Herpes simplex virus infection as a risk factor for human immunodeficiency virus infection in heterosexuals. J Infect Dis 165: 251–255, 1992.
51. Alberti A, Morsica B, Chemello L, Cavalletto D, Noventa F, Pontisso P, Ruol A. Hepatitis C viraemia and liver disease in symptom-free individuals with anti-HCV. Lancet 340: 697–698, 1992.

Submitted October 5, 1994; accepted January 10, 1995

Scand J Infect Dis 27: 105–108, 1995 ORIGINAL ARTICLE

Prevalence of HTLV-I/II Antibodies in HIV Seropositive and HIV Seronegative STD Patients in Vellore Region in Southern India

PALLA-GEORGE BABU[1], TAKAFUMI ISHIDA[2], JOYCE NESADOSS[1] and T. JACOB JOHN[1]

From the [1]Retrovirus Laboratory, Department of Virology and Microbiology, Christian Medical College Hospital, Vellore, India, and the [2]Department of Anthropology, Faculty of Science, University of Tokyo, Tokyo, Japan

This retrospective study was designed to determine the relationship between human T-lymphotropic virus (HTLV) type-I/II infection and human immunodeficiency virus (HIV) infection among sexually promiscuous persons in southern India. Stored sera collected between 1986 and 1993 from 822 male and 488 female patients attending clinics for sexually transmitted diseases (STD), for the purpose of HIV serosurveillance, were used. They comprised 376 HIV-positive sera and 934 HIV-negative sera. They were screened for HTLV-I/II antibody by a particle agglutination test and repeatedly reactive sera were confirmed by an immunofluorescence test and a western blot test. Five (2.4%) of 212 HIV-seropositive men were confirmed positive for HTLV-I/II antibody, while none of the 610 HIV-seronegative men were positive; the difference in prevalence between HIV-seropositive and seronegative men was statistically significant ($p < 0.001$). Nine (5.5%) of 164 HIV-seropositive women and 3 (0.9%) of 324 HIV-seronegative women were positive for HLTV-I/II antibody ($p < 0.005$). All HIV-seropositives taken together, had a significantly higher prevalence of HTLV-I/II (3.7%; 14/376) compared with HIV seronegatives (0.3%; 3/934; $p < 0.001$). Thus, in southern India, HTLV infection, like HIV infection, is sexually transmitted, though less effectively.

P.-G. Babu, MD, Retrovirus Laboratory, Christian Medical College Hospital, Vellore-632004, Tamilnadu, India

INTRODUCTION

Human T-lymphotropic virus type-I (HTLV-I) has been epidemiologically linked to adult T cell leukemia/lymphoma (ATLL) and to tropical spastic paraparesis, also known as HTLV-I associated myelopathy (TSP/HAM) (1). More recently, it has been associated with several other diseases and with immunosuppression (2). HTLV-I is found in clusters in endemic areas such as Southern Japan, the Caribbean basin, South America, Sub-Saharan Africa and the South Pacific Islands (3). HTLV-II, which is closely related to HTLV-I and serologically indistinguishable from HTLV-I, is not known to have a clear epidemiological association with any specific disease (1, 2). HTLV-I and II have several modes of transmission; the main modes are mother to child via breast milk, sexual intercourse, blood transfusion and re-use of contaminated needles (4).

In India, the epidemiological features of HTLV-I have not yet been elucidated, though clinical conditions resembling TSP which are known to have HTLV-I aetiology in other parts of the world, have long been described (5–7). Only recently, studies done at Vellore (5, 6) and Bombay (7) have shown that HTLV-I may play an aetiological role, at least in a few cases of ATLL and TSP. In addition, in southern India, HTLV-I/II infection was detected among persons who are known to be at high risk for HIV infection, namely female commercial sex workers and patients attending clinics for sexually transmitted diseases (STD) (8), but not among the non-professional blood donors who are known to be at low risk for HIV infection (8). Interestingly, the prevalence of HIV antibody among HTLV-I/II seropositives was found to be very high (86%; 6/7), indicating that HIV infection itself may have some influence on the transmission of HTLV-I/II among the sexually promiscuous. To examine this possibility, we estimated the prevalence of HTLV-I/II antibodies in HIV-seropositive and HIV-seronegative STD patients as reported in this paper.

MATERIALS AND METHODS

Between 1986 and 1993, serum samples collected from male and female patients with STD for the purpose of HIV serosurveillance at Vellore were used for this study after obtaining clearance from the research and ethical committees of our institutions. A large proportion of these sera (85%) were collected from the STD clinics in Vellore itself, while the remainder were collected from neighbouring towns and cities in the southern states of Tamilnadu, Andhra Pradesh and Kerala. They were initially screened for HIV-1 or 2 antibody by a commercial ELISA kit (Electronucleonics, HIV-1, USA; Wellcozyme, HIV-1, Wellcome Laboratories, GB; Vironostika Uniform, HIV-1 or Vironostika MixT, HIV-1/2, Organon Teknika, The Netherlands; Genelavia MixT, HIV-1/2, Diagnostic Pasteur, France; Detect HIV, HIV-1/2, International Biochemical Corporation, Montreal, Canada or Abbott 3rd Generation, HIV-1/2, Abbott Laboratories, USA) within 24 h of collection. The sera which were reactive in screening ELISA were retested in duplicate by the same ELISA test; repeatedly reactive sera were aliquoted and stored at -20°C until tested further with Western Blot test (WBT) (HIV-1 IgG, Dupont Laboratories, USA or HIV-1/2 IgG, Diagnostic Biotechnology, Singapore) for confirmation of HIV antibody. Sera which had at least 1 antibody against each of the 3 structural gene products of HIV (*env, gag & pol*) were defined as positive and those with no antibody at all were classified as negative (9). After WBT, one aliquot of each sample irrespective of WBT result, was saved separately at −70°C for future use.

From among our collection of WB tested samples from male and female STD patients, 1,800 sera were selected randomly. Of these, 490 were rejected because they either had equivocal patterns in WBT or were highly haemolysed, icteric or turbid. The remaining 1,310 samples were coded and screened for the presence of HTLV-I/II antibody by a particle agglutination test (Serodia HTLV-I, Fujirebio Inc, Tokyo, Japan). Reactive sera were retested in duplicate and repeatedly reactive sera were subjected to an indirect immunofluorescence test (IFT) and a WBT. For IFT, acetone-fixed smears of MT-1 cells which are known to express HTLV-I antigens were used; the presence of HTLV antibody was identified by FITC-labelled anti-human IgG goat serum (Cappel Laboratories, USA) under a fluorescent microscope (Leitz, Germany). Sera showing reactivity at a dilution of 1:10 were considered IFT-positive (10). For WBT, native HTLV-I antigens were electrophoresed and blotted onto nitrocellulose paper and goat anti-human IgG conjugated to horseradish peroxidase was used to capture the bound antibody. Occasionally, a commercial WBT kit was used (Problot, Fujirebio Inc, Tokyo, Japan). Sera with antibody to *gag* and *env* gene products of HTLV were classified as positive (11). Student's *t*-test or χ^2-test was used to test for statistical significance.

RESULTS

The mean age of the 212 HIV seropositive male STD patients was 27 years (range: 18–54 years), of the 610 seronegatives, 38 years (range: 13–60 years). The mean age of the 164 HIV seropositive female STD patients was 31 years (range: 16–46 years), of the 324 seronegatives, 33 years (range: 16–44 years). By statistical analysis, no significant difference was found between the mean ages of the seropositive and seronegative groups of either male or female STD patients.

The prevalences of HTLV-I/II antibody among HIV-seropositive and seronegative STD patients are summarized in Table I. The HIV-seropositive patients, irrespective of sex, had a significantly higher prevalence of HTLV antibodies (3.7%; 14/376) compared with the HIV-seronegative patients (0.3%; 3/934) ($p < 0.0001$). Male STD patients who were HIV-positive had a prevalence of 2.3% (5/212), while none of the 610 seronegative controls had antibodies ($p < 0.001$). Similarly, the female HIV seropositives had a significantly higher prevalence of HTLV antibodies (5.5%; 9/164) than the HIV seronegatives (0.9%; 3/324) ($p < 0.005$). All female STD patients taken together, had a higher prevalence (2.5%) than their male counterparts (0.6%) ($p < 0.025$). In contrast, the female STD patients who were HIV-seropositive had a higher prevalence (5.5%) than their male counterparts (2.4%) but the difference was statistically insignificant.

DISCUSSION

Among the modes of transmission for HTLV-I/II, sexual contact was postulated to be important (4, 12). If this is so, then factors affecting it must be characterized. Based upon the results of our previous study (8), we suspected that HIV infection may be one of the factors influencing the transmission of HTLV among the sexually promiscuous. If HIV seropositivity is indeed an influencing factor, then the prevalence of HTLV antibodies among the HIV-seropositive individuals is expected to be higher than among the HIV seronegatives.

To test such possibility, this retrospective serological study was made. Sera from HIV antibody positive and negative STD patients were examined for the presence of HTLV antibodies. Since there is extensive antigenic cross-reactivity between HTLV-I and HTLV-II and since genomic analysis was not attempted in this study to distinguish between the two types, the HLTV prevalence documented herein represents the presence of HTLV-I or II antibody. No attempt was made to trace the patients from whom sera had previously been collected. Attending an

Table I. *Prevalence of HTLV-I antibodies in male and female STD patients attending STD clinics in southern India*

Sex	HIV status	Number tested in PAT	Number reactive in PAT	Number positive by IFT & WBT	Per cent positive for HTLV	*P*-value
Male	Positive	212	6	5	2.4	<0.001
	Negative	610	3	0		
	Total	822	9	5	0.6	
Female	Positive	164	10	9	5.5	<0.005
	Negative	324	4	3	0.9	
	Total	488	14	12	2.5	
Both	Positive	376	16	14	3.7	<0.0001
	Negative	934	7	3	0.3	
Grand total		1310	23	17	1.3	

PAT = particle agglutination test for HTLV-I/II; WBT = Western blot test for HTLV-I/II.

STD clinic itself was assumed to be a marker of sexual promiscuity.

Our results show a significantly higher prevalence of HTLV antibodies in HIV-seropositive patients, irrespective of sex. The reasons for this difference are not clear. One explanation could be that HIV infection *per se*, or immunological alterations mediated by HIV, may be conducive to the successful seeding of HTLV in the genital tract. On the other hand, it is also conceivable that HIV infection may play no part whatsoever in influencing the transmission of HTLV infection. Some individuals simply get dually infected by sexual contact with persons who are carriers of both viruses; particularly so if the dually infected person is male and had ulcerative genital lesion(s) at the time of sexual intercourse. This view is supported by the finding of the Jamaican study which ascribed a critical role to ulcerative genital disease in the transmission of HTLV among male STD patients (12).

Compared with males, the female STD patients were found to have a higher prevalence of HTLV antibodies, irrespective of their HIV status. This was not unexpected, as previous studies have reported a higher prevalence of HTLV in women attending STD clinics than in men (12). Also, transmission of HTLV from man to woman was estimated to be at least 100-fold greater than from woman to man (4, 12, 13), suggesting that female partners act as reservoirs of infection. Since the major risk factor for HTLV among the female STD patients was the number of sexual partners (14) it is possible that at least some of the HTLV seropositive women in our study were not spouses/single-partners of HTLV infected men but were commercial sex workers with numerous sexual partners.

Detection of dual infection among our patients is not unusual. Previous studies had shown the presence of concomitant infection of HTLV with HIV among groups of individuals who were at high risk of contracting HIV infection (14, 15). In one study (14) in which the prevalence of HTLV in HIV seropositives (but not seronegatives) had been estimated, persons who were intravenous drug abusers (IVDA) were found to have the highest prevalance (12.4%; 26/209) while the homosexual/bisexual men had low prevalence (1.8%; 3/168). In contrast, none of the 27 transfusion recipients were positive for HTLV antibody. Only 2.4% (2/85) of the spouses of HIV-positive individuals were positive; interestingly, these positives were women and were sexual partners of IVDAs but were otherwise risk-free (14). In other words, if the male sexual partner is an IVDA, then the risk of transmitting HTLV to the female partner is high whether it is a high HTLV prevalence region (14) or low prevalence region (16). In our study, we examined the heterosexual route only because it is the main mode of transmission in southern India; IVDAs are common in northeastern India but are rare in southern India. The magnitude of HIV infection in homo/bisexual individuals is believed to be extremely low (9, 17).

Our results show that in India, as in other regions of the world, HTLV infections are not limited to rare disorders or to endemic areas. HTLV, like HIV, is sexually transmitted in southern India, but less efficiently than HIV. However, our data are inadequate to support the contention that HIV seropositivity plays a role in accelerating the transmission of HTLV infection. Carefully designed prospective studies may resolve its role. Other important factors such as the number, duration and type of sexual contacts, the STD profile, the duration and the serotype of HIV infection, the type of HIV variant existing at the time of sexual contact, immunological status and other host factors may also influence HTLV transmission.

ACKNOWLEDGEMENTS

We thank Fujirebio Co Ltd, Japan, for their generous donation of Serodia PA kits and HTLV-1 Western Blot kits. This study was supported in part by the Fleming Memorial Research Laboratory Fund of the Christian Medical College Hospital, Vellore, and in part by the Indian Council of Medical Research, New Delhi and the Ministry of Education, Science and Culture, Japan.

REFERENCES

1. Manns A, Blattner WA. The epidemiology of the human T-cell lymphotropic virus type I and type II: etiologic role in human disease. Transfusion 31: 67–75, 1991.
2. Debakan GA, Oger JJF, Foti D, King EE, Waters DJ, Picard FJ, Arp J, Werker D, Rice GPA. HTLV-1 infection associated with disease in aboriginal Indians from British Columbia: a serological and PCR analysis. Clin Diagn Virol 2: 67–78, 1994.
3. Blattner WA. Epidemiology of HTLV-1 and associated diseases. In: Blattner WA, ed. Human Retrovirology. New York: Raven Press, 251–265, 1990.
4. Murphy EL. The epidemiology of HTLV-1: Modes of transmission and their relation to patterns of seroprevalence. In: Blattner WA, ed. Human Retrovirology: HTLV. New York: Raven Press, 295–305, 1990.
5. Chandy M, Babu P-G, Saraswathi NK, Ishida T, John TJ. HTLV-1 infection in patients with leukemia in Southern India. Lancet 338: 380, 1991.
6. Babu P-G, Gnanamuthu C, Saraswathi NK, Nerurkar VR, Yanagihara R, John TJ. HTLV-1 associated myelopathy in south India. AIDS Res Hum Retroviruses 6: 499–500, 1993.
7. Hashimoto K, Lalkaka J, Fujisawa JI, Singhal BS, Machigashira K, Kubota R, Suehara M, Osame M, Yoshida M. Limited sequence divergence of HTLV-1 from a prototype Japanese isolate. AIDS Res Human Retroviruses, 9: 495–498, 1993.
8. Babu P-G, Saraswathi NK, John TJ, Ishida T, Imai J, Murphy E, Varney K. Sexual transmission of HTLV infections in southern India. J Acquir Immune Defic Syndr 5: 317, 1992.
9. Kaur A, Babu P-G, Jacob M, Narasimhan C, Ganesh A, Saraswathi NK, Mathai D, Pulimood BM, John TJ. Clinical and laboratory profile of AIDS in India. J Acquir Immune Defic Syndr 5: 883–889, 1992.
10. Ishida T, Yamamoto K, Kanek R, Tokita E, Hinuma Y. Seroepidemiological study of antibodies to adult T cell leukemia virus-associated antigen (ATLA) in free-ranging Japanese Monkeys (Macaca fuscata). Microbiol Immunol 27: 297–301, 1983.

11. Centres for Disease Control. Licensure of screening tests for antibody to human T-lymphotropic virus type I. MMWR 37: 736–747, 1988.
12. Murphy EL, Fuguera JP, Gibbs WN, Braithwaite A, Holding-Cobham M, Waters D, Crauston B, Howchar B, Blattner WA. Sexual transmission of HTLV-1. Ann Intern Med 111: 555–560, 1989.
13. Yamaguchi K, Nishimura Y, Kiyokawa T, Yoshihara N, Takatsuki K. Sexual transmission of Human T-lymphotropic virus type I (HTLV-1) and serologic diagnosis of HTLV-1 infection. In: Takatsuki K, Hinuma Y, Yoshida M, eds. Advances in Adult T-cell leukemia and HTLV-1 research. Tokyo: Japan Scientific Societies Press, Gann Monograph on Cancer Research 39: 185–194, 1992.
14. Hall WW, Kaplan MH, Salahuddin SZ, Oyaizu N, Gurgo C, Coronesi M, Nagashima K, Gallo RC. Concomitant infections with human T-cell leukemia viruses (HTLVs) and human immunodeficiency virus (HIV): identification of HTLV-II infection in intravenous drug abusers (IVDAs). In: Blattner WA, ed. Human Retrovirology: HTLV. New York: Raven press, 115–128, 1990.
15. Krook A, Blomberg J. HTLV-II among injecting drug users in Stockholm. Scand J Infect Dis 26: 129–132, 1994.
16. Blomberg J, Moestrup T, Frimand J, Hansson BG, Krogsgaard K, Grillner L, Nordenfelt E. HTLV-I and -II in intravenous drug users from Sweden and Denmark. Scand J Infect Dis 26: 23–26, 1994.
17. John TJ, Babu P-G, Saraswathi NK, Jayakumari H, Selvaraj R, Kaur A, Chacko S, Jacob M, Ramachandran P, Tripathy SP. The epidemiology of AIDS in Vellore region in southern India. AIDS 7: 421–424, 1993.

Submitted August 29, 1994; accepted December 10, 1994

Scand J Infect Dis 27: 111–117, 1995
ORIGINAL ARTICLE

Complement Analysis in Adult Patients with a History of Bacteremic Pneumococcal Infections or Recurrent Pneumonia

KARL EKDAHL[1], LENNART TRUEDSSON[2], ANDERS G. SJÖHOLM[2], and JEAN HENRIK BRACONIER[1]

From the Departments of [1]Infectious Diseases, and [2]Medical Microbiology, Lund University Hospital, Lund, Sweden

Complement deficiencies are known to be associated with increased susceptibility to bacterial infections. In the present study we investigated 80 patients with either a history of pneumococcal bacteremic infection, or recurrent pneumonia, or both. Hemolytic screening tests for complement deficiency were performed and serum concentrations of C1q, C1s, C2, C3, C4, C4 isotypes, factor B, factor D, and properdin were determined. Complete deficiencies of single complement proteins were not found. 10 patients (12%) had a C4 isotype deficiency, but the frequency of homozygous C4A and C4B deficiency was not significantly increased. Seven patients (9%) had hypocomplementemia with low concentrations of at least 2 complement proteins. One of these patients had profound depletion of classical pathway components and findings suggesting acquired C1 esterase inhibitor deficiency. 16 patients (20%) had minor complement aberrations. A majority of the patients with hypocomplementemia suffered from other conditions associated with pneumococcal infections. However, impaired complement function could be a significant predisposing factor in some patients with invasive pneumococcal infections or recurrent pneumonia.

K. Ekdahl, MD, Department of Infectious Diseases, Lund University Hospital, S-221 85 Lund, Sweden

INTRODUCTION

Inherited deficiencies of the classical complement activation pathway (C1, C4, C2) and of C3 are associated with increased susceptibility to invasive pneumococcal infections, which probably reflects the critical role of this pathway in opsonization (1–3). During activation of the classical pathway, C4 binds to target surfaces (4). C4 exists as 2 isotypes, both coded for within the major histocompatibility complex (5). The C4B isotype binds preferably to hydroxyl groups, which could be important for reactions involving bacterial polysaccharides (6). Association between C4B deficiency and susceptibility to infections with encapsulated bacteria has been suggested, but this issue is controversial (7–9).

Streptococcus pneumoniae is the most common cause of pneumonia and bacterial meningitis in adults (10, 11). In patients with bacteremic pneumococcal infections (BPI) pneumonia is the most common clinical manifestation (12). Some patients suffer from recurrent pneumonia (RP), and in a large, retrospective study we recently described patients with a history of at least 3 episodes of pneumonia (13). As for pneumonia in general, pneumococcal etiology dominates in RP (14).

Only a few defined groups of patients have been systematically examined for the presence of complement deficiency. Reports of complement deficiencies in groups of patients with pneumococcal infections are sparse (15), and to our knowledge no group of adult patients with a history of recurrent pneumonia has been investigated. In the present study, complement analysis was performed in adult patients treated earlier for BPI (i.e. severe pneumococcal disease) and RP (i.e. recurrent pneumococcal disease could be suspected).

MATERIAL AND METHODS

Patients

From the records of the Department of Infectious Diseases, Lund University Hospital, 119 adults with a history BPI and 54 adults with a history of RP were identified. 51 patients (16–83 years of age, median age 57) with BPI, and 39 patients (27–82 years of age, median age 62) with RP agreed to participate in the study. 10 patients had a history of both BPI and RP. Thus 80 patients were investigated. 48 of the bacteremic episodes were associated with concomitant pneumonia, 3 with meningitis, 2 with sinusitis, and 1 each with pharyngitis, peritonitis, and acute otitis media. In 1 patient, no focus of infection was found. The patients with RP had a history of 3–18 (mean 5) X-ray verified pneumonic episodes. Of a total of 211 episodes 184 (87%) were community-acquired. Serum and EDTA plasma for investigation of complement and immunoglobulins were obtained when the patients were free from infection. The blood sample was taken 6 weeks to 6 years (median 2 years) after the last infection (BPI or pneumonia). The study was approved by the Ethics Committee, Lund University.

Complement analysis

All samples were stored in aliquots at −70°C pending analysis. Screening for defects of the classical and alternative pathways was performed with hemolytic gel assays, using sensitized sheep erythrocytes and guinea pig erythrocytes, respectively (16). Complement proteins were determined by electroimmunoassay (17–19). C3, C4, C1q, and C1s were quantified in serum from all the patients. C2 was determined in 4 patients with impaired hemolysis of sensitized sheep erythrocytes. Properdin, factors B and D, and alternative pathway-mediated hemolysis of rabbit erythrocytes (20) were studied in patients with impaired hemolysis of guinea pig erythrocytes. Complement protein concentrations were given in mg/l, assuming that the pooled reference serums used contained each protein at the normal concentration reported by Cooper (21). Reference areas were based on those reported by Johnson et al. (22): C1q 53–95 mg/l, C1s 22–45 mg/l, C2 20–41 mg/l, C3 910–1846 mg/l, C4 360–996 mg/l, factor B 118–308 mg/l, factor D 0.75–1.41 mg/l, and properdin 14–38 mg/l. In the rabbit erythrocyte hemolysis assay (20) the observed range in 20 healthy adults was 65–161%. Phenotyping of C4 was performed as described earlier (23). We also quantified the C4A and C4B isotypes in the patients with BPI and RP, using an ELISA (24) based on the use of monoclonal antibodies to C4A and C4B (Biotest AG, Dreieich, Germany) essentially as described by Chrispeels et al. (25). The prevalence of C4A deficiency as determined in a reference population of 121 healthy blood donors was 5.8% (23). The prevalence of C4B deficiency in the same material was 3.3%.

Immunoglobulin analysis

Immunoglobulins (IgG, IgA and IgM) were determined at the Department of Clinical Chemistry, Lund University Hospital, using immunoturbidimetry. IgG subclasses were kindly determined by Dr Vivi-Anne Oxelius, Department of Pediatrics, Lund University Hospital, using polyclonal rabbit antisera (26). The following reference areas were used: IgA 0.5–3.0 g/l, IgM 0.4–2.0 g/l, IgG 7.0–15.0 g/l, IgG1 4.01–9.25 g/l, IgG2 1.3–6.13 g/l, IgG3 0.12–1.27 g/l, and IgG4 < 0.01–1.12 g/l.

Pneumococcal serotyping

Serotyping of the pneumococcal strains from the acute bacteremic infections were performed at the Clinical Microbiology Laboratory, Lund University Hospital, using the quellung reaction (27) with antisera from Statens Seruminstitut, Copenhagen, Denmark. Further typing within serogroups was not performed.

Statistics

Student's t-test for paired observations was used to examine differences of complement protein levels (C1q, C1s, C3, and C4) between the 2 patient groups and 100 healthy blood donors (22). The Pearson correlation test was used to measure the relationship between serum levels of C1q and IgG. The χ^2-test was used to test differences in the frequency of homozygous C4A and C4B deficiency between the patients and healthy blood donors. Quotients between C4B and C4A were determined, and the Wilcoxon signed rank test was used to measure any differences in the C4B/C4A quotients between the groups.

RESULTS

Concentrations of the complement proteins C1q, C1s, C3, and C4 in the patients are shown in Fig. 1. The concentrations of C1q, C1s, C3, and C4 in serum varied widely in the patient groups, but the mean values were similar to those of healthy controls (no statistically significant difference). The relationship between C1q and IgG is shown in Fig. 2.

Low concentrations of at least two complement proteins were seen in 7 patients, 6/51 (12%) with a history of BPI and in 2/39 (5%) with a history of RP (Table I). The patient H.G. was profoundly hypocomplementemic with depletion of classical pathway components, and findings consistent with acquired C1 esterase inhibitor deficiency (28). The patient I.N. showed markedly impaired alternative pathway activity with reduced hemolysis of rabbit erythrocytes. The other 5 patients showed more or less pronounced abnormalities of the classical pathway.

The distribution of C4 allotypes in the patients did not deviate from that in the control population. C4 isotype deficiency was seen in 10 patients (Table II). Homozygous C4B deficiency (phenotype B0) was observed in 1 patient, who had both a history of BPI (1/51; 2%) and RP (1/39; 3%). Homozygous C4A deficiency (phenotype A0) was seen in 6/51 (12%) patients with BPI, and in 4/39 (10%) patients with RP. In 2 patients from the BPI group (Patients H.G. and K.L.), C4 phenotyping was not possible due to low concentrations of C4. The mean C4B/C4A quotients were

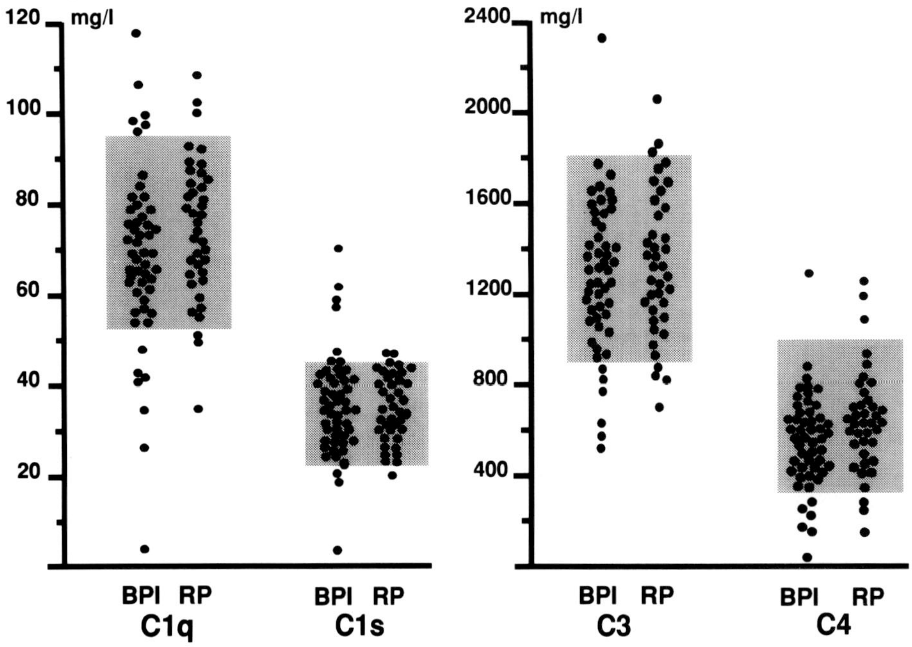

Fig. 1. Complement protein concentrations in patients with a history of bacteremic pneumococcal infection (BPI) and patients with a history of recurrent pneumonia (RP). The reference areas for each protein are indicated with shadowed areas.

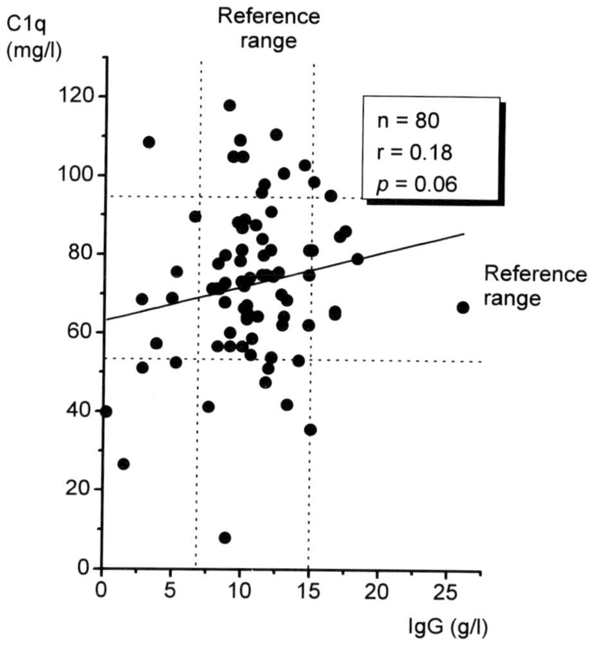

Fig. 2. Relationship between serum levels of C1q, and IgG. The correlation (Pearson correlation test) between concentrations of C1q and IgG is not significant ($p = 0.06$).

1.29, 1.47, and 1.35 for the BPI patients, the RP patients and the control subjects, respectively. Differences between the patient groups and healthy controls were not statistically significant.

Minor complement aberrations, with moderately low levels of individual complement proteins or impaired alternative pathway function as detected by the hemolytic gel assay with guinea pig erythrocytes, were seen in 9/51 (18%) BPI patients and in 8/39 (21%) RP patients (Table III). One of these patients had both a history of BPI and RP. Among these minor aberrations, moderately low concentrations of complement proteins were found in 7/51 (14%) BPI patients and in 7/39 (18%) RP patients. Nine of the 16 patients with minor complement aberrations had unrelated conditions that could predispose to infection. Six patients (Table I, III) showed impaired activity in hemolytic gel assay with guinea pig erythrocytes. Except for the patient I.N., only minor complement aberrations were observed in these patients with normal or only slightly reduced function in the rabbit erythrocyte hemolysis assay (Table III).

Pneumococcal serotypes/groups causing bacteremic disease are listed for the BPI patients with low concentrations of at least two complement proteins (Table I) and partial C4 deficiency (Table II).

DISCUSSION

Opsonization with type-specific antibodies and complement proteins is necessary for efficient phagocytosis, which is the principal host defence mechanism against infections caused by S. pneumoniae (29, 30). The effects of IgG and IgM are believed to be mediated through their ability to activate the classical pathway of the complement system (31).

Inherited complement deficiencies are known to be associated with susceptibility to invasive infections caused by encapsulated bacteria, i.e. S. pneumoniae, Haemophilus influenzae, and Neisseria meningitidis (1–3). Several studies have dealt with the prevalence of complement deficiencies among patients with meningococcal disease (1, 2), but little information is available concerning other types of infections. In a study of 101 patients with pneumococcal meningitis Densen et al. found 1 complement deficient

Table I. *Low concentrations of ≥2 complement proteins in patients with a history of bacteremic pneumococcal infection (BPI) or recurrent pneumonia (RP)*

The pneumococcal serotypes/groups are given in the patients with a history of BPI.

Patient	Patient group (serotypes in parentheses)	Hemolytic gel assay	Low level of C1q, C1s, C2, C3, C4, factor B, factor D, or properdin (values in % of normal)	Other conditions predisposing to pneumococcal infection
H.G.	BPI (6, 6)	CP[a]	C1q (<10), C1s (<10), C2 (74), C3 (44), C4 (<10)	Non-Hodgkin lymphoma, splenectomy, IgGs deficiency, IgM M-component (15 g/l)
U.H.	BPI (8)	CP[a]	C1q (38), C4 (45)	Common variable immunodeficiency
K.L.	BPI (9)	CP[a]	C3 (49), C4 (27)	Hyper IgG
K.H.	BPI (22)		C1q (57), C1s (51)	Common variable immunodeficiency
I.N.	BPI (14)	AP (18%)[b]	C1q (68), C1s (62), C3 (39), factor B (46)	Splenectomy
K.K.	BPI (6, 14) + RP	CP[a]	C1q (51), C1s (68), C3 (21), C4 (26)	Splenectomy, IgG2-IgA deficiency
L.B.	RP		C3 (66), C4 (46)	Hyper IgM

[a] Hemolysis of sensitized sheep erythrocytes (impaired function of the classical activation pathway).

[b] Hemolysis of guinea pig erythrocytes (impaired function of the alternative activation pathway). Result from rabbit erythrocyte hemolysis assay in parenthesis.

Table II. *Partial C4 deficiency in patients with a history of bacteremic pneumococcal infection (BPI) or recurrent pneumonia (RP)*

The pneumococcal serotypes/groups are given in the patients with a history of BPI. In 2 patients from the BPI group (patients H.G. and K.L., Table I) analysis of C4 variants was not possible due to low C4 levels.

Patient	Patient group (serotypes in parentheses)	C4 phenotype	Hemolytic gel assay	Low level of C1q, C1s, C2, C3, C4, factor B, factor D, or properdin (values in % of normal)	Other conditions predisposing to pneumococcal infection
G.D.	BPI (9)	A0; B1	AP (43%)[a]	C3 (67)	Splenectomy, alcohol abuse
C.K.	BPI (22)	A0; B1, 2			
H.A.	BPI (14)	A0; B1, 2			Polycythemia vera
A.N.	BPI (23)	A0; B1			
G.S.	BPI (7)	A0; B1			
K.K.	BPI (6, 14) + RP	A0; B2	CP[b]	C1q (51), C1s (68), C3 (21), C4 (26)	Splenectomy, IgG2-IgA deficiency
S.T.	BPI (9) + RP	A3; B0			
J.L.	RP	A0; B1	AP (45%)[a]	Properdin (50)	Chronic lymphocytic leukemia, IgG1-IgG2 deficiency
M.O.	RP	A0; B1, 2		C3 (56)	Chronic lymphocytic leukemia, IgG1-IgG2 deficiency
H.P.	RP	A0; B1		C1q (73)	Common variable immunodeficiency

[a] Hemolysis of guinea pig erythrocytes (impaired function of the alternative activation pathway). Result from rabbit erythrocyte hemolysis assay in parentheses.
[b] Hemolysis of sensitized sheep erythrocytes (impaired function of the classical activation pathway).

Table III. *Minor complement aberrations in patients with a history of bacteremic pneumococcal infection (BPI) or recurrent pneumonia (RP)*

Patient	Patient group	Hemolytic gel assay	Low level of C1q, C1s, C2, C3, C4, factor B, factor D, or properdin (values in % of normal)	Other conditions predisposing to pneumococcal infection
L.J.	BPI	AP (70%)[a]		
M.A.O.	BPI	AP (114%)[a]		Malignant lymphoma, IgG1 deficiency
G.D.	BPI	AP (43%)[a]	C3 (67)	Splenectomy, alcohol abuse
A.H.	BPI		C1q (59)	
M.B.	BPI		C1q (60)	
I.G.	BPI		C1q (73)	
G.G.	BPI		C4 (42)	
E.D.	BPI		C3 (60)	Rheumatoid arthritis (systemic steroids)
K.N.	BPI + RP		C4 (44)	Systemic lupus erythematosus, hyper IgG
J.L.	RP	AP (45%)[a]	Properdin (50)	Chronic lymphocytic leukemia, IgG1-IgG2 deficiency
A.M.	RP	AP (131%)[a]		Sarcoidosis
K.D.	RP		C1q (75)	IgG deficiency
H.P.	RP		C1q (73)	Common variable immunodeficiency
M.O.	RP		C3 (56)	Chronic lymphocytic leukemia, IgG1-IgG2 deficiency
E.S.	RP		C3 (66)	

[a] Alternative activation pathway. Result from rabbit erythrocyte hemolysis assay in parentheses.

patient (15). Apart from the 10 patients with C4 isotype deficiency, we did not identify any patient with inherited complement deficiency in the present study.

It has been suggested that homozygous C4B deficiency is a risk factor for invasive disease with encapsulated bacteria (7, 8). This view has been disputed by Cates et al., whose large study found no correlation between C4B deficiency and meningitis or bacteremia caused by such organisms (9). The results from our study did not support such a relationship, since the prevalence of C4A and C4B deficiency was not significantly increased in the patient groups. The possibility that a low concentration of C4B – and not only its complete absence – could be of importance was ruled out from the results of specific C4 isotype measurements.

Various forms of acquired hypocomplementemia were found, and might be considered in relation to the immune status of the patients. The patient K.K., who has been described earlier (32), had hypocomplementemia and a pronounced IgG2-IgA deficiency. Findings in the patient H.G. were consistent with acquired C1 esterase inhibitor deficiency. This condition has been observed in patients with lymphoproliferative disease and M-components. Previously this deficiency has been associated with angio-edema (28), but not with increased susceptibility to infection (2).

Another 5 patients with low concentrations of 2 or more complement proteins had abnormalities involving the classical pathway. The classical pathway works in concert with type-specific immunoglobulins, and deficiencies of this part of the complement system are well known to predispose to pneumococcal infection (1, 2, 30). It is therefore possible that the hypocomplementemia in these patients contributed to the infections.

The role of the alternative pathway in defence against pneumococci is less certain. Pneumococci recruit the alternative as well as the classical pathway in vitro (30, 33), but pneumococcal infections appear to be rare in patients with inherited deficiencies of alternative pathway proteins (1, 2). Patient I.N. had a pronounced, but unexplained, impairment of alternative pathway function and, prior to the development of BPI, had been splenectomized during surgery for a carcinoma of the ventricle. It is possible that the splenectomy was more important than the defect in complement function as a predisposing factor to the invasive pneumococcal infection.

We believe the results to be largely representative of the groups investigated, despite the fact that less than half of the patients with a history of BPI and/or RP participated in the study. On the other hand, the retrospective design precluded assessment of complement function in patients with fatal infections. Another limitation derives from the time lapse between infection and sampling, which implies that complement function at the time of infection was not documented. This could be of relevance in patients with acquired hypocomplementemia and should be borne in mind, even if the findings in most of the hypocomplementemic patients might be expected to be persistent.

Screening with hemolytic gel assays has long been used as a reliable and simple means to exclude or detect hereditary complement deficiencies and other forms of profound hypocomplementemia (16). Moderate complement aberrations are known not to reduce hemolysis in assays of this kind, but a variety of factors may occasionally interfere with hemolysis, which implies that findings of impaired hemolysis should be further investigated with other assays, as was also done in the study. With the design used, moderately low concentrations of C2, properdin and the factors B and D might well have escaped detection. However, such aberrations are not likely to be clinically significant, since heterozygosity for complement deficiency has not been shown to be associated with disease (1–3).

Several patients had unrelated chronic diseases that could interfere with the functioning of the immune system. Conditions such as splenectomy, immunoglobulin deficiencies and impaired complement function could act in synergism with regard to decreased immunity. Splenectomy itself is probably not a cause of hypocomplementemia (34). However, synergistic interaction between splenectomy and cobra venom factor induced depletion of complement has been reported in an experimental rat model, where the animals subjected to total splenectomy and complement depletion had a more severe pneumococcemia and higher mortality than was attributable to either factor alone (35).

In a previous study of immunoglobulins in 68 patients with bacteremic pneumococcal disease we found that 18% had depressed values of total IgG or of IgG subclasses (36). In the present study, immunoglobulin deficiency was the most common associated condition, both in the patients with more pronounced complement deficiencies (Table I) and in those with minor complement aberrations (Table III). Six of 10 patients with low C1q had low levels of IgG or any of the IgG subclasses. However, we did not find a statistically significant correlation between C1q and IgG (Fig. 2). Kohler et al. have earlier found a significant correlation between decreased concentrations of C1q and deficient synthesis of IgG (37), and Atkinson et al. have shown that such low C1q concentrations in patients with hypogammaglobulinemia could be corrected by gammaglobulin infusion (38).

In patients with properdin deficiency and other defects of the complement system, meningococcal infections with uncommon serogroups (W-135 and Y) predominate (3). Various pneumococcal capsular polysaccharide types have differing abilities to activate the complement system (39, 40). In our study no single serotype/group dominated in the BPI patients with partial C4 deficiency or decreases of 2 or more complement proteins. All serotypes in these patients were among the 10 most common observed in 253 pneumococcal bacteremic infections in southern Sweden (unpublished data).

In conclusion, severe inherited and acquired complement deficiencies are rate in patients with a history of BPI or RP, but should not be disregarded as possible predisposing factors for the development of invasive pneumococcal disease. Minor aberrations of complement were common in the patients, but the clinical significance of this is questionable. The relative role of complement aberrations compared with other risk factors for pneumococcal infection is still uncertain.

ACKNOWLEDGEMENTS

This study was supported by grants from the Faculty of Medicine, University of Lund, the Swedish Medical Research Council (projects no. 10381 and no. 7921), the Royal Physiographic Society, Lund, the King Gustaf V 80th Birthday Foundation, Greta and Johan Kock's Foundation, the Professor Nanna Swartz trust, and the Alfred Österlund Foundation.

REFERENCES

1. Ross SC, Densen P. Complement deficiency states and infection: epidemiology, pathogenesis and consequences of neisserial and other infections in an immune deficiency. Medicine (Baltimore) 63: 243–272, 1984.
2. Figueroa JE, Densen P. Infectious diseases associated with complement deficiencies. Clin Microbiol Rev 4: 359–395, 1991.
3. Sjöholm AG. Inherited complement deficiency states: implications for immunity and immunologic disease. APMIS 98: 861–874, 1990.
4. Porter RR, Reid KBM. The biochemistry of complement. Nature 275: 699–704, 1978.
5. O'Neill GJ, Yang SY, Dupont B. Two HLA-linked loci controlling the fourth component of human complement. Proc Natl Acad Sci USA 75: 5165–5169, 1978.
6. Isenman DE, Young JR. Covalent binding properties of C4A and C4B isotypes of the fourth component of human complement on several C1-bearing cell surfaces. J Immunol 136: 2542–2550, 1986.
7. Rowe PC, McLean RH, Wood RA, Leggiadro RJ, Winkelstein JA. Association of homozygous C4B deficiency with bacterial meningitis. J Infect Dis 160: 448–451, 1989.
8. Bishof NA, Welch TR, Beischel LS. C4B deficiency: A risk factor for bacteremia with encapsulated organisms. J Infect Dis 162: 248–250, 1990.
9. Cates KL, Densen P, Lockman JC, Levine RP. C4B deficiency is not associated with meningitis or bacteremia with encapsulated bacteria. J Infect Dis 165: 942–944, 1992.
10. Burman LÅ, Trollfors B, Andersson B, Henrichsen J, Juto P, Kallings I, Lagergård T, Môllby R, Norrby R. Diagnosis of pneumonia by cultures, bacterial and viral antigen detection tests, and serology with special reference to antibodies against pneumococcal antigens. J Infect Dis 163: 1087–1093, 1991.
11. Durand ML, Calderwood SB, Weber DJ, Miller SI, Southwick FS, Caviness VS Jr, Swartz MN. Acute bacterial meningitis in adults. A review of 493 episodes. N Engl J Med 328: 21–28, 1993.
12. Burman LÅ, Norrby R, Trollfors B. Invasive pneumococcal infections: incidence, predisposing factors and prognosis. Rev Infect Dis 7: 133–142, 1985.
13. Ekdahl K, Braconier JH, Rollof J. Recurrent pneumonia: a review of 90 adult patients. Scand J Infect Dis 24: 71–76, 1992.
14. Winterbauer RH, Bedon GA, Ball WC Jr. Recurrent pneumonia: predisposing illness and clinical patterns in 158 patients. Ann Intern Med 70: 689–700, 1969.
15. Densen P, Sanford M, Burke T, Densen E, Wintermeyer L. Prospective study of the prevalance of complement deficiency in meningitis. In: Program and abstracts, 30th Interscience Conference on Antimicrobial Agents and Chemotherapy (ICAAC), Atlanta, Georgia. Abstr. 320, 140, 1990.
16. Truedsson L, Sjöholm AG, Laurell AB. Screening for deficiencies in the classical and alternative pathways of complement by hemolysis in gel. Acta Pathol Microbiol Scand [C] 89: 161–166, 1981.
17. Sjöholm AG. Complement components in normal serum and plasma quantitated by electroimmunoassay. Scand J Immunol 4: 25–30, 1975.
18. Laurell A-B, Mårtensson U, Sjöholm A. The development of simple tests for C1q, C1r, C1s, C2 and properdin. In: Opferkuch W, Rother K, eds. Clinical aspects of the complement system. Stuttgart: Georg Thieme Publishers, 12–14, 1978.
19. Sturfelt G, Truedsson L. Complement factor D concentrations in normal sera: comparison of immunochemical and functional determinations. Acta Pathol Microbiol Immunol Scand [C] 93: 383–389, 1983.
20. Nilsson UR, Nilsson B. Simplified assays of hemolytic activity of the classical and alternative complement pathways. J Immunol Methods 72: 49–59, 1984.
21. Cooper NR. Laboratory investigation of complement proteins and complement receptors. Baillière's Clin Immunol Allergy 2: 263–293, 1988.
22. Johnson U, Truedsson L, Gustavii B. Complement components in 100 newborns and their mothers determined by electroimmunoassay. Acta Pathol Microbiol Immunol Scand [C] 91: 147–150, 1983.
23. Bucin D, Truedsson L, Hammarström L, Smith CIE, Sjöholm AG. C4 polymorphism and major histocompatibility complex haplotypes in IgA deficiency: association with C4 null haplotypes. Exp Clin Immunogenet 8: 233–241, 1991.
24. Truedsson L, Gullstrand B, Jönsson T, Klint C. Serum concentrations of C4 isotypes and factor B in type I C2 deficiency suggest haplotype dependent quantitative expression of MHC class III complement genes. Exp Clin Immunogenet. [in press]
25. Chrispeels J, Bank S, Rittner C, Bitter-Suermann D. Sandwich enzyme-linked immunosorbent assays for the quantification of the C4 isotypes (C4A and C4B) in human plasma. J Immunol Methods 125: 5–12, 1989.
26. Oxelius V-A. Crossed immunoelectrophoresis and electroimmunoassay of human IgG subclasses. Acta Pathol Microbiol Scand [C] 86: 109–116, 1978.
27. Lund E, Henrichsen J. Laboratory diagnosis, serology and epidemiology of Streptococcus pneumoniae. In: Bergan T, Norris JR, eds. Methods in microbiology. London: Academic Press, 12: 241–262, 1978.
28. Gelfand JA, Boss GR, Conley CL, Reinhart R, Frank MM. Acquired C1 esterase inhibitor deficiency and angioedema: a review. Medicine (Baltimore) 58: 321–328, 1979.
29. Guckian JC, Christensen GD, Fine DP. The role of opsonins in recovery from experimental pneumococcal pneumonia. J Infect Dis 142: 175–190, 1980.
30. Winkelstein JA. The role of complement in the host's defense against Streptococcus pneumoniae. Rev Infect Dis 3: 289–298, 1981.
31. Bruyn GAW, Zegers BJM, van Furth R. Mechanisms of host defense against infections with Streptococcus pneumoniae. Clin Infect Dis 14: 251–262, 1992.
32. Prellner K, Braconier JH, Sjöholm AG. Combined IgG2, IgG4 and IgA deficiency: low C1q concentrations and the presence of excess C1r and C1s in an adult patient with recurrent pneumococcal infections. Acta Pathol Microbiol Immunol Scand [C] 93: 257–263, 1985.
33. Braconier JH, Odeberg H, Sjöholm AG. Granulocyte phagocytosis of Streptococcus pneumoniae in properdin deficient serum. Infect Immun 40: 219–224, 1983.
34. Truedsson L, Sturfelt G, Offenbartl K, Sjöholm AG. The spleen is not a major synthetic site of alternative pathway components. Complement and Inflammation 7: 52–56, 1990.
35. Van Wyck DB, Witte MH, Witte CL. Synergism between the spleen and serum complement in experimental pneumococcemia. J Infect Dis 145: 514–519, 1982.
36. Ekdahl K, Rollof J, Oxelius VA, Engellau J, Braconier JH. Analysis of immunoglobulin isotype levels in acute pneumococcal bacteremia and in convalescence. Eur J Clin Microbiol Infect Dis 13: 374–378, 1994.
37. Kohler PF, Müller-Eberhard HJ. Complement-immunoglobulin relation: Deficiency of C'1q associated with impaired immunoglobulin synthesis. Science 163: 474–475, 1969.
38. Atkinson JP, Fisher RI, Reinhard R, Frank MM. Reduced concentrations of the first component of complement in hypogammaglobulinemia: correction by infusion with γ-globulin. Clin Immunol Immunopathol 9: 350, 1978.

39. Winkelstein JA, Bocchini JA Jr, Schiffman G. The role of the capsular polysaccharide in the activation of the alternative pathway by the pneumococcus. J Immunol 116: 367–370, 1976.

40. Giebink GS, Verhoef J, Peterson PK, Quie PG. Opsonic requirements for phagocytosis of Streptococcus pneumoniae types VI, XVIII, XXIII, and XXV. Infect Immun 18: 291–297, 1977.

Submitted August 4, 1994; accepted December 8, 1994

Scand J Infect Dis 27: 119–121, 1995 ORIGINAL ARTICLE

DNA Fingerprinting of Streptococcus pyogenes from Patients with Recurrent Pharyngotonsillitis by Means of Random Amplified Polymorphic DNA Analysis

ANDERS ÖSTERLUND and LARS ENGSTRAND

From the Department of Clinical Microbiology, University Hospital, Uppsala, Sweden

In recent years, several DNA fingerprinting methods have been tried for the epidemiological investigation of Streptococcus pyogenes isolates. We chose the Random Amplified Polymorphic DNA (RAPD) method for the typing of pre- and post-antibiotic treatment S. pyogenes isolates obtained from 14 patients with pharyngotonsillitis. Isolates from 4 patients had been collected 10 years earlier than from the others. Hence epidemiological connections between the strains were unlikely. Both pre- and post-antibiotic treatment isolates showed identical RAPD patterns, indicating that recurrences in these patients had been caused by homologous strains of S. pyogenes. It was possible by means of RAPD to differentiate between 12 different T-types and occasionally between clones of the same serotype of S. pyogenes. The RAPD method is an easier alternative to traditional DNA-typing techniques and provides quick results with minimal technical complexity.

A. Österlund, MD, Department of Clinical Microbiology, University Hospital, S-751 85 Uppsala, Sweden

INTRODUCTION

Recurrence of pharyngotonsillitis caused by Streptococcus pyogenes after seemingly adequate antibiotic treatment has puzzled scientists for over 40 years (1). Serotyping of T and M antigens is the standard method for epidemiological typing of S. pyogenes (2). Until recently this has been the most sensitive tool with which to distinguish between recurrences caused by a new strain of S. pyogenes and by persistence of the original strain. In recent years, genomic typing methods, such as restriction endonuclease analysis (REA) of genomic DNA (2 – 5), typing of ribosomal DNA (ribotyping) (2, 5) and pulsed field gel electrophoresis (6, 7) have been successfully used to obtain information for epidemiological studies on S. pyogenes. All of these methods are time-consuming, technically demanding and expensive (4).

A faster, technically easier and more economical method for detecting DNA polymorphisms is random amplified polymorphic DNA (RAPD) (8). This method has been used successfully for epidemiological typing of different microorganisms (9–12). RAPD has proved superior to REA by virtue of its ability to differentiate between isolates of different strains of S. pyogenes (4). Furthermore, RAPD has been shown to provide valuable information for serotyping when distinguishing between original strains and new strains in recurrent pharyngotonsillitis (5). The aim of this study was to apply the RAPD method as an epidemiological tool for comparison of pre- and post-treatment strains of S. pyogenes.

MATERIALS AND METHODS

Bacterial strains

Clinical isolates of S. pyogenes from 14 patients with recurrent pharyngotonsillitis were obtained from the Department of Clinical Microbiology, Uppsala University, Sweden. Bacterial strains, obtained before antibiotic treatment and 2–4 weeks afterwards were isolated in 1984 from 4 patients and in 1994 from 10 patients. In addition, isolates from 6 patients with differing T-types were obtained. By choosing strains isolated 10 years apart, epidemiological connections were excluded. The strains are listed in Table I.

Extraction of bacterial DNA

All bacteria were grown in Todd-Hewitt broth. S. pyogenes DNA for RAPD was prepared as follows: bacterial cells were harvested by centrifugation, washed twice in phosphate-buffered saline (PBS), resuspended in 200 μ/ml GTEL buffer (50 mM glucose, 50 mM Tris-HCl, pH 8.0, 50 mM EDTA, 10 mg/ml lysozyme) and incubated at 37°C for one hour. 500 μl of lysis buffer (50 mM Tris-HCl, pH 8.0, 50 mM EDTA, 1% SDS, 50 mg/ml proteinase K) was then added, followed by 2 h of incubation at 55°C. RNAse (final concentration 20 μg/ml) was added and the mixtures were incubated for 10 min at 55°C. Phenol extraction and ethanol precipitation were performed by standard procedures. DNA was dissolved in 100 μl of distilled water and the amount of DNA obtained was measured.

RAPD analysis

PCR was accomplished in a volume of 50 μl, containing 40 ng of S. pyogenes DNA, 200 ng of each primer, 1 U of Ampli Taq DNA polymerase (Perkin-Elmer Cetus), 200 μM each of dCTP. dGTP, dATP, and dTTP (Boehringer Mannheim) in 10 × buffer. A Perkin-Elmer 9600 thermocycler was used for amplification. The cycling program run was for 10 cycles of (95°C, 5 min, 36°C, 5 min, 72°C, 2 min), 30 cycles of (94°C, 30 s, 55°C, 30 s, 72°C,

 ISSN 0036-5548

Table I. *Strains of S. pyogenes used in the study*

Strain	Isolated (year)	T-type
A1[a]	1994	1
A2[b]	1994	1
A3[a]	1994	1
A4[b]	1994	1
A5[a]	1994	3
A6[b]	1994	3
A7[b]	1994	2
A8[b]	1994	13
A9[b]	1994	14
A10[a]	1984	4
A11[b]	1984	4
A12[a]	1994	4
A13[b]	1994	4
A14[a]	1994	4
A15[b]	1994	4
A16[a]	1994	11
A17[b]	1994	11
B1[a]	1984	6
B2[b]	1984	6
B3[a]	1984	6
B4[b]	1984	6
B5[b]	1994	6
B6[b]	1994	25
B7[b]	1994	B3264
B8[a]	1984	12
B9[b]	1984	12
B10[a]	1994	12
B11[b]	1994	12
B12[a]	1994	12
B13[b]	1994	12
B14[a]	1994	28
B15[b]	1994	28
B16[a]	1994	28
B17[b]	1994	28

[a] Before antibiotic treatment.
[b] After antibiotic treatment.

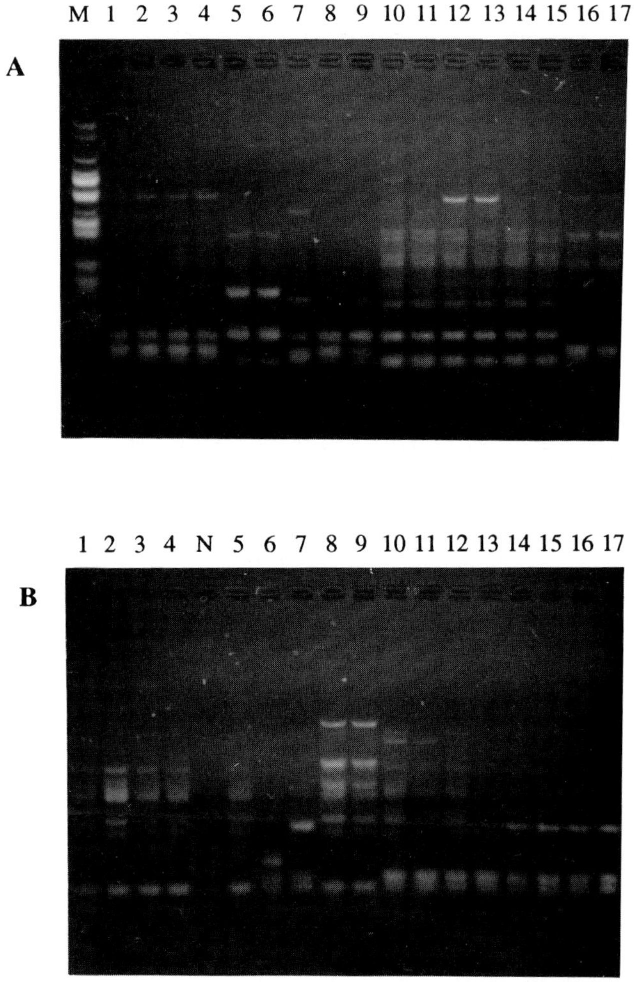

Fig. 1. Comparison of random amplified polymorphic DNA (RAPD) patterns from 34 clinical isolates of S. pyogenes belonging to 12 serotypes. DNA-fragments were electrophoresed in 1.5% agarose gels along with DNA molecular weight marker VI from Boehringer-Mannheim (M) and stained with ethidiumbromide. A, from left to right: M (marker), T1, T1, T1, T1, T3, T3, T2, T13, T14, T4, T4, T4, T4, T11 and T11. The patterns in B, from left to right: T6, T6, T6, T6, N (negative control), T6, T25, TB3264, T12, T12, T12, T12, T12, T12, T28, T28, T28 and T28. A10–11, B1–4 and B8–9 were isolates from 1984, the others from 1994. A1, A3, A5, A10, A12, A14, A16, B1, B3, B8, B10, B12, B14 and B16 were pre-treatment isolates, the other strains were isolated after antibiotic treatment. Identical pre-treatment and post-treatment patterns are seen. Different T-types show distinctly differing RAPD patterns. The patterns from lane A12–13 clearly differ from the patterns in A9–19 and A13–14, and the patterns in B8–9, B10–11 and B12–13 are all different, whereas the other isolates show similar RAPD patterns within the same T-type.

2 min), followed by a 10 min incubation at 72°C. 15 µl of PCR-products were electrophoresed in 1.5% agarose gels along with a DNA molecular weight marker VI from Boehringer-Mannheim. Gels were stained with ethidiumbromide and photographed under UV light. The primers used, pMav 17B (5′ CACTCGTCGGG-AATGCCCT; G + C content, 60% and HSVP1 (5′ CGACTTT-GCCAGCCTGTACC; G + C content, 60%, were designed for other purposes and arbitrarily chosen for this experiment. It has been found that these primers can be used in various typing assays with DNA prepared from such unrelated bacteria as Helicobacter pylori, Legionella pneumophila, Proteus sp., Klebsiella sp. and Listeria sp. (unpublished data).

RESULTS

Identical RAPD patterns were found in all pre- and post-treatment isolates (Fig. 1). Isolates with twelve different T-types also demonstrated distinctly differing RAPD patterns. One patient with S. pyogenes T-type 4 (A12–13 in Fig. 1) generated clearly different RAPD patterns from those of identical T-types isolated 10 years earlier (A10–11 in Fig. 1). In addition 3 patients with S. pyogenes T-type 12 (B8–9, B10–11 and B12–13 in Fig. 1) were found to generate different RAPD patterns. No obvious differences were seen among the remaining strains with identical T-types (Fig. 1).

DISCUSSION

In the evaluation of recurrent S. pyogenes pharyngotonsillitis, it is of interest to distinguish between infections caused by the original strain and by new strains. Different DNA 'fingerprinting' methods, such as REA, ribotyping, pulsed field gel electrophoresis, and RAPD have been shown to provide information additional to serotyping for the analysis of epidemiologically related strains of S. pyogenes (3–7). Bingen et al., using REA, differentiated between relapses and recurrences when treating failures of S. pyogenes pharyngitis (6). When using a single primer, Seppälä et al. (5) found RAPD to be more sensitive than REA for the differentiation of isolates of both identical and differing serotypes of S. pyogenes. The discriminatory power of RAPD has been shown to increase by using 2 primers (14, 15). We used RAPD with two primers, designed for other purposes, to compare pre- vs. post-antibiotic treatment strains of S. pyogenes. Although a limited number of strains were studied in our experiments, the results showed: that RAPD differentiated well between the serotypes, that in some cases RAPD could distinguish between 2 clones of the same serotype, and that the pre- and post-treatment isolates studied gave identical RAPD patterns. These findings tally with earlier results, indicating that recurrent pharyngotonsillitis is usually caused by the recurrence of homologous strains of S. pyogenes rather than by the acquisition of new, unrelated strains (5, 13).

RAPD is a practical alternative method for detecting DNA polymorphisms. It adds information to serological typing systems in studies on S. pyogenes epidemiology. It could prove to be of particular value in the study of serologically non-typable strains (3, 17), and further studies of such strains using RAPD should be undertaken.

ACKNOWLEDGEMENTS

We thank Helena Berglund for skilful technical assistance. This study was supported by The Swedish Medical Research Council (grants 10 617 and 10 848).

REFERENCES

1. Markowitz M, Gerber MA, Kaplan EL. Treatment of streptococcal pharyngotonsillitis: reports of penicillin's demise are premature. J Pediatr 123: 679–685, 1993.
2. Lancefield RC. A serological differentiation of human and other groups of hemolytic streptococci. J Exp Med 57: 571–595, 1933.
3. Seppälä H, Vuopio-Varkila J, Österblad M, Jahkola M, Rammukainen M, Holm SE, Huovinen P. Evaluation of methods for epidemiologic typing of group A streptococci. J Infect Dis 169: 519–525, 1994.
4. Mylvaganam H, Bjorvatn B, Hofstad T, Hjetland R, Hoiby EA, Holm SE. Small-fragment restriction endonuclease analysis in epidemiological mapping of group A streptococci. J Med Microbiol 40: 256–260, 1994.
5. Seppäla H, He Q, Österblad M, Houvinen P. Typing of group A streptococci by random amplified polymorphic DNA analysis. J Clin Microbiol 32: 1945–1948, 1994.
6. Bingen E, Denamur E, Lambert-Zechovsky N, Braimi N, el Lakany M, Elion J. DNA restriction fragment length polymorphism differentiates recurrence from relapse in treatment failures of Streptococcus pyogenes pharyngitis. J Med Microbiol 37: 162–164, 1992.
7. Single LA, Martin DR. Clonal differences with M-types of the group A Streptococcus revealed by pulsed field gel electrophoresis. FEMS Microbiol Lett 70: 85–89, 1992.
8. Lefevre JC, Faucon G, Sicard AM, Gase AM. DNA fingerprinting of Streptococcus pneumoniae strains by pulsed-field gel electrophoresis. J Clin Microbiol 31: 2724–2728, 1993.
9. Welsh J, McClelland M. Fingerprinting genomes using PCR with arbitrary primers. Nucleic Acids Res 18: 7213–7218, 1990.
10. Barbut F, Mario N, Frottier J, Petit JC. Use of the arbitrary primer polymerase chain reaction for investigating an outbreak of Clostridium difficile-associated diarrhea in AIDS patients [letter]. Eur J Clin Microbiol Infect Dis 12: 794–795, 1993.
11. Woods JP, Kersulyte D, Tolan RW Jr, Berg CM, Berg DE. Use of arbitrarily primed polymerase chain reaction analysis to type disease and carrier strains of Neisseria meningitidis isolated during a university outbreak. J Infect Dis 169: 1384–1389, 1994.
12. van Belkum A, Struelens M, Quint W. Typing of Legionella pneumophila strains by polymerase chain reaction-mediated DNA fingerprinting. J Clin Microbiol 31: 2198–2200, 1993.
13. van Belkum A. DNA fingerprinting of medically important microorganisms by use of PCR. Clin Microbiol Rev 7: 174–184, 1994.
14. Welsh J, McClelland M. Fingerprinting genomes using arbitrarily primed PCR and a matrix of pairwise combinations of primers. Nucleic Acids Res 19: 5275–5279, 1991.
15. Micheli MR, Bova P, Calissano P, D'Ambrosio E. Randomly amplified polymorphic DNA fingerprinting using combinations of oligonucleotide primers. BioTechniques 15: 388–390, 1993.
16. Musser J, Gray BM, Schlievert PM, Pichichero ME. Streptococcus pyogenes pharyngitis: characterization of strains by multilocus enzyme genotype, M and T protein serotype, and pyrogenic exotoxin gene probing [published erratum appears in J Clin Microbiol 1992 Jul; 30(7): 1905]. J Clin Microbiol 30: 600–603, 1992.
17. Tran PO, Johnson DR, Kaplan EL. The presence of M protein in nontypeable group A streptococcal upper respiratory tract isolates from Southeast Asia. J Infect Dis 169: 658–661, 1994.

Submitted December 6, 1994; accepted December 22, 1994

Scand J Infect Dis 27: 125–130, 1995 ORIGINAL ARTICLE

Correlation between Serum TNFα and IL6 levels and Severity of Group A Streptococcal Infections

ANNA NORRBY-TEGLUND[1], KARLIS PAUKSENS[2], MARI NORGREN[1] and STIG E. HOLM[1]

From the Departments of [1]Clinical Bacteriology, Umeå University, Umeå, and of [2]Infectious Diseases, Akademiska sjukhuset, Uppsala, Sweden

The multiorgan failure syndrome caused by group A streptococci (GAS) designated streptococcal toxic shock syndrome (STSS) is believed to be mediated by cytokines induced by superantigens. In order to study the relationship between superantigen production, cytokine levels in patient sera, and clinical GAS manifestation we examined acute-phase sera and strains from 25 patients with GAS bacteremia. The patients had various disease manifestations, including STSS (44%), erysipelas (28%), septicemia (24%), wound infections (16%), and pneumonia (12%). Serotype T1M1 dominated, representing 56% of the isolates, but also strains of other serotypes were identified. The strains were found to produce the streptococcal pyrogenic exotoxins (Spe) A, B, and F, as determined by immuno-blot analyses. There was no difference in amounts of toxin produced between strains isolated from patients with different manifestations of disease. Levels of TNFα, IL1α, IL6, IL8, and IFNγ in acute-phase sera were determined by use of ELISA and RIA assays. The analyses showed higher levels of IL6 in sera from patients with STSS than in sera from patients with bacteremia without shock. TNFα was elevated in sera from patients with STSS, as compared to sera from patients with uncomplicated pharyngotonsillitis. No increase in the levels of IL1α, IL8, and IFNγ could be found in the patient sera and there was no difference in the level of those cytokines between the various patient categories.

S. Holm, MD, Department of Clinical Bacteriology, Umeå University, S-901 85 Umeå, Sweden

INTRODUCTION

Toxic shock syndrome (TSS) is an acute clinical manifestation with a high mortality. The disease is characterized by high fever, general malaise, and multiorgan failure in an early stage of infection. TSS caused by Staphylococcus aureus is rather well studied and it has been shown to be caused by the toxic shock syndrome toxin-1 (TSST-1) (1, 2). Less is known about the streptococcal toxic shock syndrome (STSS), a multiorgan failure defined as late as 1987 by Cone et al. (3). However, recent studies of clinical group A streptococcal (GAS) isolates and patients' humoral response against streptococcal virulence factors have indicated that the streptococcal pyrogenic exotoxins (Spe) are involved in the development of STSS (3–8).

TSST-1 and the streptococcal pyrogenic exotoxins (Spe) A, B, C and F have been shown to belong to the superantigen family, which include a group of proteins with high immunomodulatory potential (9–14). Streptococcal superantigens also include SSa (15), and M-proteins (16). Superantigens differ from conventional antigens in their interaction with T cells and antigen presenting cells (APCs). They bind outside the antigen-binding groove of the MHC class II molecule on APCs and to the Vβ-chain of the T cell receptor (TcR) (13, 17–21). Superantigens can therefore activate a large proportion of T cells to massive proliferation and subsequent high production of cytokines (9, 13, 22).

Cytokines are necessary for the regulation and activation of the human immune system, but can at elevated levels be harmful. SpeA, SpeB, and SpeF have been shown to induce massive production of cytokines in human mononuclear cells (23–27) and it has also been reported that sera collected from patients with GAS bacteremia contain elevated cytokine levels, as compared to sera from patients with uncomplicated GAS infections (28). In an attempt to examine the relation between severity of GAS infection, characteristics of the infecting strains, and the levels of secreted cytokines we analyzed acute-phase sera and GAS strains isolated from patients with GAS bacteremia.

MATERIAL AND METHODS

Patient material

25 patients admitted to the Department of Infectious Diseases at the Akademiska sjukhuset in Uppsala, Sweden, during 1988–92, with GAS bacteremia were included in this study. Only individuals with a blood culture positive for GAS from whom an acute-phase serum was obtained were included. Sera were drawn within 7 days of the initial symptoms before initiation of antibiotic treatment. They were collected in vacutainer tubes (Becton Dickinson, Sweden) and stored at −80°C until further processed. The clinical data of the patients are presented in Table I. Patient number 1–5 were admitted during 1988, no. 6–15 during 1989, no. 16–20 during 1990, no. 21–24 during 1991, and no. 25 during 1992. Isolates from all patients were serotyped and 22 strains were saved for analyses of toxin production.

The material included STSS cases, which were defined by high fever, hypotension, and multiorgan failure at an early stage of the infection.

Acute-phase sera collected from patients with uncomplicated pharyngotonsillitis in Sweden during 1988/89 were included as controls. Sera were collected and stored as described above.

 ISSN 0036-5548

Table I. *Clinical data of patients with GAS bacteremia*

Patient no.	Sex	Age	Serotype of bacterial isolate	Clinical background	Clinical condition
1	M	31	T22	Healthy	Wound infection
2	F	44	T1M1	Healthy	Pneumonia, STSS
3	F	82	T1M1	Diabetes Mellitus Myeloma	STSS
4	F	62	T22	R.A.	Pneumonia, Empyema, STSS
5	M	60	T12	Etylismus	Erysipelas
6	M	77	T1M1	Myocardial infarct	STSS
7	M	61	T1M1	Cancer of the urinary bladder	Pneumonia, STSS
8	M	76	T1M1	Chronic myeloic leukemia	Masteoditis, Meningitis
9	M	72	T1M1	Uremia, dialysis	Infected AV-fistula, Sepsis
10	M	76	T1M1	Uremia, dialysis	STSS[a]
11	F	55	T1M1	Healthy	Erysipelas, Sepsis
12	F	67	T1M1	R.A., immunosuppressed	Pansinuitis, STSS
13	F	38	T1M1	Brain tumor	Erysipelas, STSS
14	F	80	T1M1	Healthy	Wound infection, STSS[a]
15	F	79	T28	Healthy	Wound infection
16	F	25	T1M1	Diabetes mellitus	Epiglottis
17	F	71	T28	M.S.	Erysipelas, STSS
18	M	67	T11	Healthy	Erysipelas
19	M	53	T1M1	Heart transplant	Otitis media, Wound infection
20	M	79	T28	Healthy	Erysipelas
21	F	5	T1M1	Leukemia, Mb Down	Sepsis, Varicella
22	F	42	T12	Healthy	Tonsillitis, STSS
23	M	69	T8	Healthy	Sepsis, Erysipelas
24	M	14	T4	Healthy	Sepsis, Sinusitis
25	M	83	T14	Cancer prostate	Sepsis, UTI

[a] Fatal outcome.
M = male; F = female; STSS = streptococcal toxic shock syndrome; R.A. = rheumatoid arthritis; M.S. = multiple sclerosis; UTI = urinary tract infection.

Typing of group A streptococci

T-typing was performed according to Griffith (29) by agglutination using anti-T sera (Sevac) from the Institute of Sera and Vaccines, Prague, the Czech Republic. The serum opacity reaction was performed for further discrimination of serotypes, as described by Maxted and Widdowson (30).

Determination of TNFα, IL6, IFNγ, IL1α and IL8

The levels of various cytokines in patient sera were determined by use of ELISA and RIA assays. TNFα and IL6 were detected by Genzymes ELISA assays (Novakemi, Sweden), the detection limits are 15 pg/ml for both assays. The levels of IFNγ was determined by using a Medgenix IFN-gamma kit (Novakemi, Sweden), with a detection limit of 100 pg/ml. The level of IL1α was measured by a RIA assay with a detection limit of 79 pg/ml (Novakemi, Sweden). IL8 was measured using a modified Pharmacia sandwich-fluorescent ELISA (FEIA) assay (31). The catching antibody used in the FEIA was a murine monoclonal antibody specific for IL8 and as tracer a goat anti-IL8-antibody conjugated to β-galactosidase were used. The detection limit of this assay was 20 pg/ml.

Extracellular antigen (EC) preparation

Supernatants from overnight cultures were precipitated by ethanol for 16 hours. The sediments were dialyzed against dH_2O, lyophilized, and dissolved in 1 ml of dH_2O, which corresponded to a 10-fold concentration of the culture filtrate. The method has been described previously in detail and is especially designed for isolation of the Spes, but may also contain other streptococcal antigens (5).

Semiquantitative determination of SpeA, SpeB, and SpeF

The ECs were analyzed for the presence of SpeA, SpeB, and SpeF, by immuno-blot analyses. The toxins were semiquantitatively determined by transfer of dilution series of ECs to nitrocellulose filters by a dot-blot technique. The toxins were detected by an enzyme immunoassay using polyclonal mono-specific rabbit antibodies against each toxin, as described previously in detail (5).

Statistical analysis

Willcoxon rank's test and Willcoxon Gehan's test with sensored data was used to evaluate significant differences between groups.

RESULTS

Serotype of infecting strain

25 patients with GAS bacteremia were included in this study. The clinical background, age, and clinical condition of the patients, as well as the results obtained from serotype analysis of the strains are presented in Table I. 56% of the patients had underlying conditions, such as diabetes, rheumatoid arthritis, and cancer, which might have contributed to the development of severe manifestations (Table I). Serotype T1M1 dominated in the material and was isolated from 56% of the patients, but also strains of serotype T22, T12, T28, T11, T8, T4, and T14 could be identified (Table I). 44% of the patients included in this study developed STSS and 73% of the strains isolated from

Table II. *Serotype and exotoxin production of clinical GAS isolates*

Clinical isolate of patient no.	SOR	Serotype	Exotoxin production[b]		
			SpeA	SpeB	SpeF
1	–	T22	5	10	2
2[a]	–	T1M1	8	9	4
3[a]	–	T1M1	8	5	7
4[a]	–	T22	5	9	4
5	–	T12	5	5	7
6[a]	–	T1M1	7	9	2
7[a]	–	T1M1	ND	ND	ND
8	–	T1M1	ND	ND	ND
9	–	T1M1	6	9	3
10[a]	–	T1M1	8	9	7
11	–	T1M1	9	9	5
12[a]	–	T1M1	ND	ND	ND
13[a]	–	T1M1	8	10	7
14[a]	–	T1M1	7	9	4
15	+	T28	5	9	9
16	–	T1M1	5	9	9
17[a]	+	T28	7	9	5
18	–	T11	9	9	5
19	–	T1M1	7	9	2
20	+	T28	9	9	5
21	–	T1M1	9	8	4
22[a]	ND	T12	8	9	4
23	ND	T8	5	9	4
24	ND	T4	5	5	9
25	ND	T14	5	9	5

[a] STSS patients.
[b] Median values of exotoxin after $\log_2$ dilution. Value of 6 is equal to 64 times higher amount of toxin.
SOR = serum opacity reaction; ND = not determined.

those patients were of T1M1 serotype. Two of the STSS cases had fatal outcome and both patients were infected with strains of T1M1 serotype. Other manifestations commonly noted among the patients were erysipelas (28%), septicemia (24%), wound infections (16%), and pneumonia (12%).

Determination of exotoxin production

The production and secretion of SpeA, SpeB, and SpeF were tested by immuno-blot technique (Table II). All 3 exotoxins could be detected in the supernatants of all 22 strains. The highest production was noted for SpeB, followed by SpeA, and last SpeF. No difference in amounts of toxin produced could be noted between isolates from patients with STSS and the non-shock patients.

Determination of cytokine levels in serum

Levels of TNFα, IL6, IL1α, and IL8 sera were determined in sera taken from the patients during the acute phase of infection and the results are presented in Tables III and IV. Table III shows the levels of TNFα and IL6 in each individual sera. Sera isolated from STSS patients had significantly higher IL6 values, than sera from non-shock patients ($p < 0.01$). Sera from the STSS cases also contained elevated levels of TNFα ($p < 0.05$), as compared to sera from patients with uncomplicated GAS infections (Table IV). No difference could be noted in the levels of IL1α or IL8 between sera obtained from patients with uncomplicated pharyngotonsillitis or patients with bacteremia (Table IV). The levels of IFNγ was also measured, but only very low amounts could be detected (data not shown).

DISCUSSION

Gram-negative bacteria, and its endotoxin, LPS, have long been in focus for the discussion of the pathogenesis of septicemia, but due to an increase in septicemia cases caused by gram-positive bacteria more attention has lately been given to gram-positive septicemia and shock. It has been shown that superantigens are responsible for development of TSS caused by S. aureus and research in the streptococcal field has indicated a similar role for superantigens in STSS (1, 7, 13, 22, 32, 33). A recent study by

Table III. *Cytokine levels in acute phase sera isolated from patients with GAS bacteremia*

Patient no.	Days of serum sampling[b]	Cytokine levels (pg/ml)	
		TNFα[c]	IL6[d]
1	5	550	78
2[a]	5	700	>1800
3[a]	2	80	992
4[a]	7	1500	>1800
5	5	470	505
6[a]	2	900	>1800
7[a]	2	450	ND
8	1	830	32
9	1	300	116
10[a]	3	190	>1800
11	2	400	974
12[a]	2	980	>1800
13[a]	1	640	>1800
14[a]	4	560	750
15	3	260	>1800
16	2	620	740
17[a]	1	330	443
18	2	290	87
19	4	1030	386
20	5	200	>1800
21	3	1140	<15
22[a]	1	860	>1800
23	1	200	1064
24	1	640	>1800
25	1	290	221

[a] STSS patients.
[b] Also days after first symptoms. All sera were drawn before initiation of antibiotic treatment.
[c] TNFα was higher in STSS patients than in patients with uncomplicated infections.
[d] Levels of IL6 in sera from STSS patients were significantly higher than in sera from other patients ($p < 0.01$) as evaluated in Willcoxon-Gehan's test with sensored data.
ND = not determined.

Table IV. *Levels of TNFα, IL6, IL1α, and IL8 in acute-phase sera collected from patients with GAS bacteremia of uncomplicated GAS infections*

Patient category	TNFα[a] (pg/ml)		IL6[b] (pg/ml)		IL1α[c] (pg/ml)		IL8[d] (pg/ml)	
	No. of sera	Mean ± SD	No. of sera	Mean ± SD	No. of sera	Mean ± SD	No. of sera	Mean ± SD
Bacteremia[e]	25	576 ± 350*	25	1016 ± 735	18	255 ± 191	24	78 ± 189
Uncomplicated pharyngotonsillitis	12	358 ± 90	ND	ND	12	310 ± 42	15	265 ± 561

[a] Determined by use of Genzyme ELISA kit from Novakemi.
[b] Determined by use of Medgenix ELISA kit from Novakemi. The levels of IL6 in healthy individuals are <16 pg/ml.
[c] Determined by use of RIA kit from Novakemi.
[d] Determined by use of a modified Pharmacia FEIA (31).
[e] Includes all patients with a blood culture positive for GAS.
* Significantly higher levels of TNFα in sera from bacteremia patients than in sera from patients with uncomplicated infections ($p < 0.05$).
ND = not determined.

Watanabe-Ohnishi et al. revealed that certain T cells were depleted during the acute phase of STSS. Since T cell depletion is a common phenomenon induced by superantigens those results provided in vivo data that supported the involvement of superantigens in STSS (34). In vitro studies have shown that superantigens produced by gram-positive bacteria can induce massive cytokine production, which are central mediators of septicemia and toxic shock (23–27, 35, 36). Determination of the cytokine induction profiles of the streptococcal SpeA, SpeB, SpeF, the staphylococcal enterotoxin A, and the gram-negative endotoxin LPS revealed that gram-positive toxins induced a different cytokine production profile than LPS did (23, 27). Thus, if immunotherapy is to be used as a possible treatment of toxic shock it might have to be directed against different cytokines or effector molecules based on the infecting organism.

In this study we have tried to determine the relationship between exotoxin production, the cytokine levels in acute phase sera, and clinical manifestation. Strains were isolated from 25 patients with GAS bacteremia and characterized with respect to serotype and exotoxin production. Serotyping of the strains showed a dominance of T1M1, which was the serotype that caused an outbreak of serious GAS infections in Sweden 1988/89 (5). In the present study serotype T1M1 was especially prevalent among strains isolated from STSS cases. T1M1 is believed to be somewhat more virulent and invasive than other serotypes, but as can be seen in this study also other serotypes are capable of causing STSS.

The strains were analyzed for the production of SpeA, SpeB, and SpeF and all 3 superantigens were found to be produced by the isolates. There were no differences in exotoxin production between isolates from shock and non-shock patients. This is in accordance with a previous study, which showed that Swedish GAS strains isolated from patients with different clinical manifestation during 1988–89 all had a similar toxin production profile (5). However, the strains included in that study produced high amounts of SpeB and SpeF, while only low amounts of SpeA. This is different from the results obtained in the present study where SpeA and SpeB were produced in higher amounts than SpeF; however, the data are consistent with our previous suggestion that there is not one single toxin responsible for the development of STSS, but rather, the repertoire of toxins produced and the reactivity/sensitivity of the patient are important (7, 27).

The acute-phase sera of the patients in the present study were included in a previous study where the ELISA antibody titers against SpeA, SpeB, and SpeF, as well as the ability of the sera to inhibit the toxins mitogenicity were tested (7). The study showed that the majority (58%) of sera collected from the patients in the present study lacked toxin-neutralizing capacity against at least 2 of the toxins. There was no difference in toxin-neutralizing capacity between sera from patients with STSS and patients with bacteremia without shock (7). Thus, the majority of patients lacked protection against the toxins in the acute-phase of infection.

Analyses of the presence of cytokines in the acute phase sera showed that TNFα was significantly higher in sera from STSS patients than in sera from patients with uncomplicated pharyngotonsillitis. This is in accordance with the suggestion that TNF has a central role as mediator of shock. Other studies have also reported elevated levels in sera from septic patients (37, 38). Another cytokine commonly associated with sepsis is IL6, which in this study was found to be markedly higher in patients with shock than in patients with non-shock septicemia ($p < 0.01$). Since the patients did not differ in toxin-neutralizing capacity it is conceivable that the elevated levels of IL6 in sera from STSS patients results from a stronger immune response due to highly reactive lymphocytes of the patients. In contrast, no difference could be noted in serum levels of IL1α, IL8 between different patient categories. The absence of IL1α in serum contradicts the findings by Müller-Alouf et al. (39) who reported induction as well as release of IL1α after in vitro T-cell stimulation with Spes'. Furthermore, elevated levels of IL8 have previously been reported to correlate to shock in both gram-positive and gram-negative septicemia (40). Since cytokines have very short half-life times and appear at different stages of infection it is possible that we have missed the peak of production of IL1α and IL8 in the patients included in this study. Thus, although not proven the significance of these cytokines for the septic shock in STSS can not be excluded.

We have previously proposed that the manifestation of disease is dependent on the humoral response of the host, the reactivity of the hosts immune cells, with respect to the T cell Vβ repertoire and the HLA class II molecules, as well as the toxin production of the infecting bacteria (7, 27). In this study we have shown that the infecting bacteria had ability to produce at least 3 superantigens and that the sera of the patients contained elevated levels of cytokines. Furthermore, the level of IL6 correlated to the development of STSS. Since we in a previous study showed that the patients in the present study had low toxin-neutralizing capacity we find it highly likely that the noted elevated levels of cytokines reflects the action of superantigens produced by the infecting strains and that they contribute to the pathogenesis of STSS.

ACKNOWLEDGEMENT

The technical assistance of Lena Elfman at Pharmacia Diagnostic Uppsala, is gratefuly acknowledged. This study was supported by grants from the Swedish Medical Research Council to SEH (10844) and to MN (8876). SEH was also supported by a grant from Claes Groshinskys Foundation and MN by a grant from the Medical Faculty, Umeå University. AN was supported by the Kempe Foundation, Lennanders Foundation, and the Swedish Society for Medical Research.

REFERENCES

1. Choi Y, Lafferty JA, Clements JR, Todd JK, Gelfand E, Kappler J, Marrack P, Kotzin B. Selective expansion of T cells expressing Vβ2 in toxic shock syndrome. J Exp Med 172: 981–984, 1990.
2. Todd JK. Toxic shock syndrome. Clin Microbiol Rev 1: 432–436, 1988.
3. Cone LA, Woodard DR, Schlievert PM, Tomory GS. Clinical and bacteriological observations of a toxic-shock-like syndrome due to Streptococcus pyogenes. N Engl J Med 317: 146–149, 1987.
4. Hauser AR, Stevens DL, Kaplan EL, Schlievert PM. Molecular analysis of pyrogenic exotoxins from Streptococcus pyogenes isolates associated with toxic shock-like syndrome. J Clin Microbiol 29: 1562–1567, 1991.
5. Holm SE, Norrby A, Bergholm A-M, Norgren M. Aspects of the pathogenesis of serious group A streptococcal infections in Sweden, 1988–1989. J Infect Dis 166: 31–37, 1992.
6. Musser JM, Hauser AR, Kim MH, Schlievert PM, Nelson K, Selander RK. Streptococcus pyogenes causing toxic-shock-like syndrome and other invasive diseases: clonal diversity and pyrogenic exotoxin expression. Proc Natl Acad Sci USA 88: 2668–2672, 1991.
7. Norrby-Teglund A, Pauksens K, Holm SE, Norgren M. Relation between low capacity of human sera to inhibit streptococcal mitogens and serious manifestation of disease. J Infect Dis 170: 585–591, 1994.
8. Stevens DL, Tanner MH, Winship J, Swartz R, Ries KM, Schlievert PM, Kaplan E. Severe group A streptococcal infections associated with a toxic shock-like syndrome and scarlet fever toxin A. N Engl Med 321: 1–7, 1989.
9. Alouf JE, Knöll, H, Köhler W. The family of mitogenic, shock-inducing and superantigenic toxins from staphylococci and streptococci. In: Alouf JE, Freer JH, eds. Sourcebook of bacterial protein toxins. San Diego: Academic Press, 367–414, 1991.
10. Fleisher B, Gerardy-Schahn R, Metzroth B, Carrel S, Gerlach D, Köhler W. An evolutionary conserved mechanism of T cell activation by microbial toxins. Evidence for different affinities of T cell receptor-toxin interaction. J Immunol 146: 11–17, 1991.
11. Janeway CA, Yagi J Jr, Conradt PJ, Katz ME, Jones B, Vroegop S, Buxser S. T-cell responses to Mls and to bacterial proteins that mimics its behaviour. Immunol Rev 107: 61–88, 1989.
12. Tomai M, Schlievert PM, Kotb M. Distinct T cell receptor Vβ gene usage by human T lymphocytes stimulated with the streptococcal pyrogenic exotoxins and M protein. Infect Immun 60: 701–705, 1992.
13. Marrack P, Kappler J. The staphylococcal enterotoxins and their relatives. Science 248: 705–711, 1990.
14. Norrby-Teglund A, Newton D, Kotb M, Holm SE, Norgren M. Superantigenic properties of the group A streptococcal exotoxin SpeF (MF). Infect Immun 62: 5227–5233, 1994.
15. Mollick JA, Miller GG, Musser JM, Cook RG, Grossman D, Rich RR. A novel superantigen isolated from pathogenic strains of Streptococcus pyogenes with amino terminal homology to staphylococcal enterotoxins B and C. J Clin Invest 92: 710–719, 1993.
16. Tomai M, Kotb M, Majumdar G, Beachey EH. Superantigenicity of streptococcal M protein. J Exp Med 172: 359–362, 1990.
17. Fleisher B, Schrezenmeizer H, Conradt PJ. T lymphocyte activation by staphylococcal enterotoxins: role of class II molecules and T cell surface structures. Cell 120: 92–101, 1989.
18. Fraser JD. High affinity binding of staphylococcal enterotoxins A and B to HLA-DR. Nature 339: 221–223, 1989.
19. Mollick JA, Cook RG, Rich RR. Class II MHC molecules are specific receptors for staphylococcus enterotoxin A. Science 244: 817–820, 1989.
20. Scholl P, Diez A, Mourad W, Parsonnet J, Geha RS, Chatila T. Toxic schock syndrome toxin 1 binds to major histocompatibility complex class II molecules. Proc Natl Acad Sci USA 86: 4210–4214, 1989.
21. Uchiyama T, Imanishi K, Saito S, Araake M, Yan X-J, Fujikawa H, Igarashi H, Kato H, Obata F, Kashiwagi, Inoko H. Activation of human T cells by toxic shock syndrome toxin-1: the toxin binding structures expressed on human lymphoid cells acting as accessory cells are HLA class II molecules. Eur J Immunol 19: 1803–1809, 1989.
22. Kotb M. Role of superantigens in the pathogenesis of infectious diseases and their sequelae. Curr Opin Infect Dis 5: 364–374, 1992.
23. Andersson J, Nagy S, Björk L, Abrams J, Holm S, Andersson U. Bacterial toxin-induced cytokine production studied at the single-cell level. Immunol Rev 127: 69–96, 1992.
24. Fast DJ, Schlievert PM, Nelson RD. Toxic shock syndrome-associated staphylococcal and streptococcal pyrogenic toxins are potent inducers of tumor necrosis factor production. Infect Immun 59: 291–294, 1989.

25. Hacket SP, Stevens DL. Streptococcal toxic shock syndrome: synthesis of tumor necrosis factor and interleukin-1 by monocytes stimulated with pyrogenic exotoxin A and streptolysin O. J Infect Dis 165: 879–885, 1992.
26. Hackett SP, Stevens DL. Superantigens associated with staphylococcal and streptococcal toxic shock syndrome are potent inducers of tumor necrosis factor-β synthesis. J Infect Dis 168: 232–235, 1993.
27. Norrby-Teglund A, Norgren M, Holm SE, Andersson U, Andersson J. Similar cytokine induction profiles of a novel streptococcal exotoxin, MF, and the pyrogenic exotoxins A and B. Infect Immun 62: 3731–3738, 1994.
28. Norrby A, Norgren M, Holm SE. Elevated levels of interleukin 6 in serum from patients with serious group A streptococcal infections. Infection 20: 369–370, 1992.
29. Griffith G. The serological classification of Streptococcus pyogenes. J Hygien 34: 542–584, 1934.
30. Maxted WR, Widdowson JP. The protein antigens of group A streptococci. In: Wannamaker JW, Matsen JM, eds. Streptococci and streptococcal diseases. New York: Academic Press, 256–261, 1972.
31. Peichl P, Ceska M, Effenberger F, Haberhauer G, Broell H, Lindley IJD. Presence of NAP-1/IL-8 in synovial fluids indicates a possible pathogenic role in rheumatoid arthritis. Scand J Immunol 34: 333–339, 1991.
32. Stevens D, Bryant AE, Hackett SP. Sepsis syndromes and toxic shock syndromes: concepts in pathogensis and a perspective of future treatment strategies. Curr Opin Infect Dis 6: 374–383, 1993.
33. Schlievert PM. Role of superantigens in human disease. J Infect Dis 167: 997–1002, 1993.
34. Watanabe-Ohnishi R, Low DE, Mcgeer A, Stevens DL, Schlievert PM, Newton D, Schwartz B, Kreiswirth B, Ontario streptococcal study project, and Kotb M. Selective depletion of Vβ-bearing T cells in patients with severe invasive group A streptococcal infections and streptococcal toxic shock syndrome. J Infect Dis 171: 74–84, 1995.
35. Jupin C, Andersson S, Damais C, Alouf JE, Parant M. Toxic shock syndrome toxin 1 as an inducer of human tumor necrosis factors and γ interferon. J Exp Med 167: 752–761, 1988.
36. Uchiyama T, Kamagata Y, Yan X-J, Kohno M, Yoshioko M, Fujikawa M, Igarashi H, Okubo M, Awano F, Saito-Taki T, Nakano M. Study on the biological activities of toxic shock syndrome toxin-1. II. Induction of the proliferative response and the interleukin-2 production by T cells from human peripheral blood mononuclear cells stimulated with the toxin. Clin Exp Immunol 68: 638–647, 1987.
37. Cannon JG, Tompkines RG, Gelfand JA, Michie HR, Stanford GG, Van de Meer JWM, Endres S, Lonneman G, Corsetti J, Chernow B, Wilmore DW, Wolff SM, Burke JF, Dinarello CA. Circulating interleukin-1 and tumor necrosis factor in septic shock and experimental endotoxin fever. J Infect Dis 161: 79–84, 1990.
38. Waage A, Brandtzaeg P, Halstensen A, Kierulf P, Espevik T. The complex pattern of cytokines in serum from patients with meningococcal septic shock. J Exp Med 169: 333–338, 1989.
39. Müller-Alouf H, Alouf JE, Gerlach D, Ozegowski J-H, Fitting C, Cavaillon J-M. Comparative study of cytokine release by human peripherial blood mono nuclear cells stimulate with Streptococcal pyogenes superantigenic erythrogenic toxins, heat-killed streptococci, and lipopolysaccharide. Infect Immun 62: 4915–4921, 1994.
40. Hack SE, Hart M, Strack van Schijndel RJM, Eerenberg AJM, Nuijens JH, Thijs LG, Aarden LA. Interleukin-8 in sepsis: relation to shock and inflammatory mediators. Infect Immun 60: 2835–2842, 1992.

Submitted October 25, 1994; accepted February 9, 1995

Scand J Infect Dis 27: 131–134, 1995 ORIGINAL ARTICLE

Are Penicillin Treatment Failures in Arcanobacterium haemolyticum Pharyngotonsillitis Caused by Intracellularly Residing Bacteria?

ANDERS ÖSTERLUND

From the Department of Clinical Microbiology, University Hospital, Uppsala, Sweden

Arcanobacterium haemolyticum is an infrequent agent of pharnygotonsillitis in children and young adults. Despite the fact that A. haemolyticum is fully sensitive to penicillin in vitro, penicillin treatment failures are frequent. The ability of A. haemolyticum to invade HEp-2 cells and survive intracellularly was investigated. All 12 strains tested, of which 10 were isolated from patients with pharyngotonsillitis, and 2 were reference strains, were internalized by the HEp-2 cells. Four strains tested further, one of the reference strains and 3 of the clinical isolates, proved able to survive intracellularly for 4 days, thus creating intracellular reservoirs of bacteria. It was also shown that erythromycin, an antibiotic known to penetrate well intracellularly, efficiently killed these bacteria.

A. Österlund, MD, Department of Clinical Microbiology, University Hospital, S-571 85 Uppsala, Sweden

INTRODUCTION

Arcanobacterium haemolyticum [formerly Corynebacterium haemolyticum (5, 7)] is known primarily as a causative agent of pharyngitis in children and young adults (3–7), but is also seen as an infrequent cause of other infectious diseases (8–11). A. haemolyticum is known to be sensitive in vitro to phenoxymethylpenicillin, oral cephalosporins, erythromycin and clindamycin (6, 12). In spite of this, many clinical and microbiological failures have been described after penicillin therapy (3, 11, 13). Nyman et al. have reported penicillin tolerance in A. haemolyticum (14) and suggested penicillin tolerance as an explanation for the treatment failures.

It is known that Haemophilus influenzae (15), β-hemolytic group G streptococci (16) and Streptococcus agalactiae (17), are capable of invading respiratory epithelial cells. The aim of this study was twofold: to ascertain (i) whether A. haemolyticum could invade respiratory epithelial cells and survive there, thus creating an intracellular reservoir of bacteria, and (ii) whether these intracellular bacteria could be killed by erythromycin, an antibiotic known to penetrate intracellularly (18).

MATERIALS AND METHODS

Bacterial strains

Two reference strains were used, Arcanobacterium haemolyticum, NCTC 9697, isolated in 1946 and probably of human origin and Arcanobacterium haemolyticum, NCTC 10514, isolated from a patient with tonsillitis and exanthema in 1967. In addition, 10 clinical isolates of A. haemolyticum, obtained from the Department of Clinical Microbiology, Malmö General Hospital, Sweden, were used as test strains. The clinical isolates were collected from patients with pharyngotonsillitis.

Antibiotics

Phenoxymethylpenicillin and erythromycin were kindly supplied by Pharmacia Therapeutics, Sweden, and Abbot Scandinavia AB, Sweden, respectively. Solutions were prepared according to Anhalt and Washington (19). Gentamicin, 10 mg/ml, was purchased from the Schering Corporation, USA. Phenoxymethylpenicillin and erythromycin were tested at concentrations of 10 and 4 mg/l, respectively, in the tissue culture medium. These are the approximate maximum peak serum concentrations of antibiotic attained after oral administration of 1 g phenoxymmethylpenicillin (20, 21) and 500 mg erythromycin (22, 23).

Minimal inhibitory concentrations (MICs)

MICs were determined using the E test (AB Biodisk, Solna, Sweden) on Iso-Sensitest agar (Oxoid) supplemented with 5% horse blood. The MICs were measured after 18 h of incubation at 35°C in 5% CO_2, by direct reading of the intercept of the antibiotic gradient strip and the zone of inhibition.

Epithelial cell invasion assay

Bacteria were grown overnight in Todd-Hewitt broth supplemented with 10% fetal calf serum (FCS), washed twice in phosphate-buffered saline (PBS, pH 7.2), and resuspended in RPMI-1640 tissue culture medium containing 10% FCS. Each strain of A. haemolyticum was inoculated onto HEp-2 cell monolayers in 24-well tissue culture plates (each well with an area of 1.9 cm^2) at approximately 10^6 CFU/ml. Four strains, one reference strain, Arcanobacterium haemolyticum, NCTC 9697, and 3 clinical isolates were inoculated onto 3 tissue culture plates. Plates were centrifuged at 2500*g* for 5 min and incubated at 35°C in 5% CO_2 for 6 h. Extracellular non-adherent bacteria were removed by washing 3 times with tissue culture medium containing gentamicin (100 mg/l), and infected monolayers were then incubated overnight at 35°C in tissue culture medium containing gentamicin (100 mg/l) to remove all extracellular bacteria (24). This was followed by viable counts as described below.

Four strains, 1 reference strain, Arcanobacterium haemolyticum, NCTC 9697, and 3 clinical isolates, were tested further as follows.

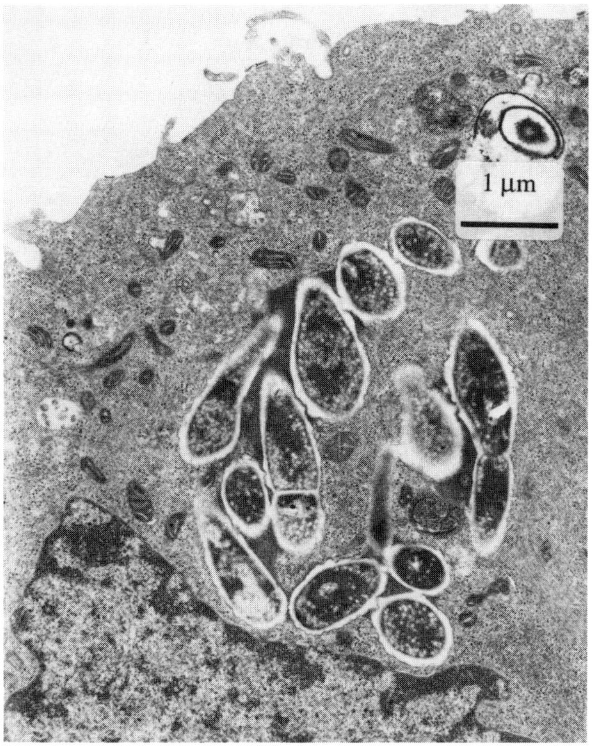

Fig. 1. Transmission electron micrograph showing HEp-2 cells invaded by A. haemolyticum.

Tissue culture media were removed from 2 of the 3 tissue culture plates, and the HEp-2 cell monolayers were washed 3 times with tissue culture medium containing phenoxymethylpenicillin (10 mg/l) or erythromycin (4 mg/l) respectively, to remove the gentamicin. Finally, the infected monolayers were incubated at 35°C in 5% CO_2 with tissue culture medium containing either gentamicin (100 mg/l), phenoxymethylpenicillin (10 mg/l) or erythromycin (4 mg/l) in the corresponding tissue culture plate. Culture media were changed once daily.

A. haemolyticum cultures were also incubated overnight in RPMI-1640 tissue culture medium containing 10% FCS and gentamicin (100 mg/l), to ensure that all bacteria in the extracellular fluid were nonviable.

Viable counts were performed as follows: tissue culture medium was removed, HEp-2 cell monolayers were washed 4 times with PBS to remove antibiotics, then lysed by osmotic chock for 10 min in sterile, distilled water. The lysate was transferred to sterile plastic tubes and vortexed vigorously for 30 s to separate the bacterial cells. 100-μl aliquots from serial dilutions of the lysate were inoculated on blood-agar plates to determine the number of viable intracellular bacteria. Experiments were performed in triplicate and reproduced 3 times.

Electron microscopy

A. haemolyticum in HEp-2 monolayers was prepared as described above. Infected HEp-2 cells in 24-well tissue culture plates were harvested from the wells after 24 h, washed twice in PBS and fixed with 3% glutaraldehyde in cacodylate buffer, pH 7.2. Preparations were postfixed with 1% osmium tetroxide for 1 h. After a wash in PBS and dehydration in ethanol, cells were embedded in Epon. Ultrathin sections of the embedded cells were stained with uranyl acetate and lead citrate, then examined with a Philips EM 420 transmission electron microscope.

RESULTS

The cell invasion assay relies on poor penetration of gentamicin into mammalian cells, thus enabling selective killing of extracellular bacteria (24). After overnight incubation with gentamicin in the tissue culture medium, viable counts revealed approximately 10^4 CFU/well for all 12 strains tested. No viable bacteria could be found in the extracellular medium of the controls after 24 h. Transmission electron microscopy confirmed the intracellular presence of A. haemolyticum in the cytoplasm of HEp-2 cells (Fig. 1).

The 4 strains when tested further survived for 4 days in HEp-2 cells (Fig. 2). MICs for phenoxymethylpenicillin and erythromycin were 0.016 mg/l and for gentamicin 0.75–1.5 mg/l (Table I). The antibiotic concentrations in the culture media exceeded the MIC approximately 100-fold for gentamicin, 250 times for erythromycin, and 600 times for phenoxymethylpenicillin. After 3 days of incubation, viable counts revealed approximately 10 times more intracellular A. haemolyticum in the cell layers incubated with phenoxymethylpenicillin or gentamicin in the cell culture medium than in those incubated with erythromycin (Fig. 2). At any time when antibiotics were excluded from the tissue culture medium, bacteria were released from the HEp-2 cells and extracellular growth was established within a day. This was easy to observe, as the tissue culture medium turned acid and turbid, and the HEp-2 cell monolayers were destroyed.

DISCUSSION

Treatment of patients suffering from A. haemolyticum pharyngitis with penicillin may fail despite the fact that the bacteria are usually fully sensitive to penicillin in vitro (11, 12). Nyman et al. suggested that such failures are a result of penicillin tolerance (14), but this hypothesis has not been confirmed.

It is shown here that A. haemolyticum can invade HEp-2 cells and survive there for 4 days, thus creating an intracellular reservoir of bacteria. The HEp-2 cells, which are immortalized upper respiratory epithelial cells, were chosen in order to produce an experimental situation as close as possible to the in vivo situation. It was also shown that erythromycin, an antibiotic known to have good intracellular penetration (18), kills the intracellularly residing bacteria more efficiently than does phenoxymethylpenicillin. Failures after erythromycin treatment of patients with A. haemolyticum pharyngitis are fewer than after penicillin treatment (11, 13), possibly due to intracellular invasion bacteria.

ACKNOWLEDGEMENTS

I thank Lillemor Fredriksson, Department of Clinical Microbiology, Malmö General Hospital, Sweden, for kindly supplying clinical isolates of A. haemolyticum and Tapio Niketa for technical assistance with TEM.

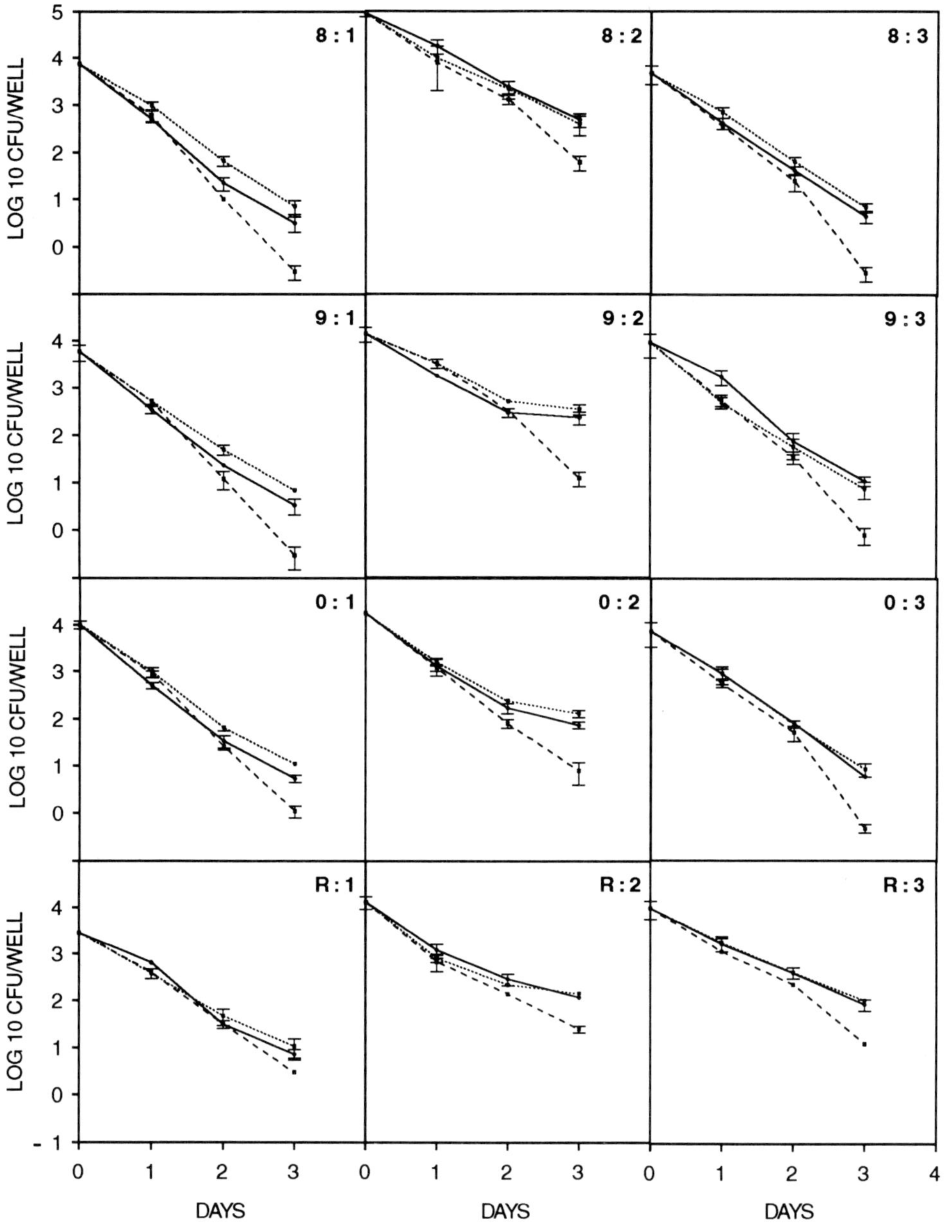

Fig. 2. Intracellular survival of 4 different strains of A. haemolyticum in HEp-2 cells on 3 different occasions. The strains used were A. haemolyticum NCTC 9697 (R), and 3 clinical isolates of A. haemolyticum (8, 9 and 0). Antibiotics used in the assay were gentamicin 100 mg/l (continuous line), phenoxymethylpenicillin 10 mg/l (dotted line) and erythromycin 4 mg/l (dashed line). Data are expressed as $\log_{10}$ cfu/well ± SD.

Table I. *Minimal inhibitory concentrations (MICs) of gentamicin, phenoxymethylpenicillin and erythromycin for the 4 strains of A. haemolyticum used in the experiments*

	Minimal inhibitory concentration (MIC) of		
A. haemolyticum strain	Gentamicin (mg/l)	Phenoxymethylpenicillin (mg/l)	Erythromycin (mg/l)
Clinical isolate (8)	0.75	0.016	0.016
Clinical isolate (9)	1.0	< 0.016	0.016
Clinical isolate (0)	1.5	0.016	0.016
NCTC 9697 (R)	1.0	< 0.016	< 0.016

REFERENCES

1. MacLean PD, Liebow AA, Rosenberg AA. A hemolytic corynebacterium resembling Corynebacterium ovis and Corynebacterium pyogenes in man. J Infect Dis 79: 69–90, 1946.
2. Collins MD, Jones D. Reclassification of Corynebacterium pyogenes (Glage) in the genus Actinomyces, as Actinomyces pyogenes comb. nov. J Gen Microbiol 128: 901–903, 1982.
3. Miller RA, Brancato F, Holmes KK. Corynebacterium hemolyticum as a cause of pharyngitis and scarlatiniform rash in young adults. Ann Intern Med 105: 867–872, 1986.
4. Selander B, Ljungh A. Corynebacterium haemolyticum as a cause of nonstrepotocccal pharyngitis [letter]. J Infect Dis 154: 1041, 1986.
5. Wickremsinghe RS, Weeratne WM. Corynebacterium haemolyticum. An uncommon cause of throat infection. Ceylon Med J 23: 61–63, 1978.
6. Carlson P, Renkonen O-V, Kontiainen S. Arcanobacterium haemol-yticum and streptococcal pharyngitis. Scand J Infect Dis 26: 283–287, 1994.
7. Cambier M, Janssens M, Wauters G. Isolation of Arcanobacterium haemolyticum from patients with pharyngitis in Belgium. Acta Clin Belg 47: 303–307, 1992.
8. Kain KC, Noble MA, Barteluk RL, Tubbesing RH. Arcanobacterium haemolyticum infection: confused with scarlet fever and diphtheria. J Emerg Med 9: 33–35, 1991.
9. Ben-Yaacob D, Waron M, Boldur I, Gil I, Sompolinsky D. Septicemia due to Corynebacterium haemolyticum. Isr J Med Sci 20: 431–433, 1984.
10. Chhang WH, Ayyagari A, Sharma BS, Kak VK. Arcanobacterium haemolyticum brain abscess in a child. Indian J Pathol Microbiol 34: 145–148, 1991.
11. Waagner DC. Arcanobacterium haemolyticum: biology of the organism and diseases in man. Pediatr Infect Dis J 10: 933–939, 1991.
12. Carlson P, Kontiainen S, Renkonen O-V. Antimicrobial susceptibility of Arcanobacterium haemolyticum. Antimicrob Agents Chemo-ther 38: 142–143, 1994.
13. Banck G, Nyman M. Tonsillitis and rash associated with Corynebacterium haemolyticum. J Infect Dis 154: 1037–1040, 1986.
14. Nyman M, Banck G, Thore M. Penicillin tolerance in Arcanobacterium haemolyticum. J Infect Dis 161: 261–265, 1990.
15. Forsgren J, Samuelsson A, Ahlin A, Jonasson J, Rynnel-Dagöö B, Lindberg A. Haemophilus influenzae resides and multiplies intracellularly in human adenoid tissue as demonstrated by in situ hybridization and bacterial viability assay. Infect Immun 62: 673–679, 1994.
16. Nath SK. Invasion of HeLa cells by beta-hemolytic group G streptococci. Can J Microbiol 35: 515–517, 1989.
17. Rubens CE, Smith S, Hulse M, Chi EY, van Belle G. Respiratory epithelial cell invasion by group B streptococci. Infect Immun 60: 5157–5163, 1992.
18. Williams JD, Sefton AM. Comparison of macrolide antibiotics. J Antimicrob Chemother 31: 11–26, 1993.
19. Anhalt JP, Washington JA. Preparation and storage of antimicrobial solutions. In: Balows A, Hausler WJ, Herrmann KL, Isenberg HD, Shadomy HJ, eds. Manual of Clinical Microbiology, 5th edn. Washington, D.C.: American Society for Microbiology, 1199–1200, 1991.
20. Josefsson K, Bergan T. Pharmacokinetics of phenoxymethylpenicillin in volunteers. Chemother 28: 241–246, 1982.
21. Josefsson K, Magni L. Absorption of phenoxymethylpenicillin from mixtures and tablets in healthy volunteers. J Int Med Res 11: 380–384, 1983.
22. Walstad RA, Hellum KB. Penetration of erythromycin in respiratory tract infections. Acta Otolaryngol (Stockh) Suppl 407: 50–54, 1984.
23. Sundberg L, Edèn T, Ernstson S. Penetration of erythromycin in Waldeyer's ring-tonsil tissue. Acta Otolaryngol (Stockh) Suppl 384: 10–17, 1981.
24. Holmes B, Quie PG, Windhorst DB, Pollara B, Good R. Protection of phagocytized bacteria from the killing action of antibiotics. Nature 210: 1131–1132, 1966.

Submitted November 14, 1994; accepted January 18, 1995

Scand J Infect Dis 27: 135–138, 1995 ORIGINAL ARTICLE

Treatment of Tuberculous Meningitis in Turkey*

MEHMET DOĞANAY[1], SEMRA ÇALANGU[2], HÜSEYIN TURGUT[3], MEHMET BAKIR[4] and BILGEHAN AYGEN[1]

From the Department of Infectious Diseases, [1]Erciyes University, Kayseri, [2]İstanbul University, İstanbul, [3]Dicle University, Diyarbakır, and the [4]Cumhuriyet University, Sivas, Turkey

A prospective study was performed on 72 cases of tuberculous meningitis studying various treatments. 37 patients were treated with a combination of isoniazid, rifampicin, pyrazinamide and streptomycin for 2 months, followed by a combination of isoniazid and rifampicin for 6 months. 35 patients were treated with various combinations of antituberculous drugs for 12–16 months. Disappearance of symptoms took (mean) 17 days. Mean duration of therapy for the hospitalized patients was 36 ± 4 days. Seven (9.7%) patients died, 5 in the short-course therapy group and 2 in the long-course therapy group. Sequelae persisted in 18 (31%) cases, 8 of which cases were in the short-course therapy group and 10 in the long-course therapy group. No relapse was observed in either of the groups.

M. Doğanay, MD, Erciyes Üniversitesi, Tıp Fakültesi, İnfeksiyon Hastalıkarı Kliniği, 38039 Kayseri, Turkey

INTRODUCTION

Tuberculous meningitis is a disease that still often results in residual sequelae, and has a fatality rate ranging between 15 and 51% (1–4). In contrast to rapid advances in the management of pulmonary tuberculosis, there have been few clinical studies for the treatment of tuberculous meningitis (4, 5). There is currently no general consensus regarding chemotherapy or the optimal duration of treatment. Some studies suggest that a 6–9-month regimen as appropriate (6, 7). Conversely, a recent study noted that short-course chemotherapy was inadequate (8). The aim of our study was to evaluate the results of therapy in cases of tuberculous meningitis at four centres in Turkey.

MATERIALS AND METHODS

This study was carried out between January 1989 and April 1993 at 4 university clinics (Kayseri, Sivas, Diyarbakır and İstanbul). Three clinics (Kayseri, Sivas, Diyarbakır) studied short-course chemotherapy, while the centre in İstanbul used long-course therapy. The study was approved by the Ethics Committee of the Faculty of Medicine at Erciyes University.

Patients over 15 years old with diagnosed tuberculous meningitis were enrolled in the study. The diagnosis of tuberculous meningitis was based on the following: 1) clinical findings of subacute and chronic meningitis (meningeal symptoms lasting for >4 days); 2) cerebrospinal fluid findings – clear or xanthochromic, elevated cell count with predominance of lymphocytes, glucose level <400 mg/l, protein level >1 g/l; 3) demonstration of acid-fast bacilli in CSF by microscopic examination and/or culture; 4) evidence of any associated extrameningeal tuberculous lesion. Liver function tests and routine examination of peripheral blood and urine were carried out. Roentgenography was performed routinely. CT scans were also performed as indicated.

The clinical condition of the patients upon admission was classified into stages (4). Stage I: No definite neurological symptoms. Stage II: Signs of meningeal irritation with no clouding of consciousness and no neurologic deficit. Stage III: Severe clouding of consciousness, stupor or coma, gross paresis and involuntary movements.

Patients dying within 5 days of admission were not evaluated. Additionally, patients were excluded from short-course therapy if they were given a different antituberculous regimen for >1 week or if therapy lapsed for 10 days during the treatment period, or if the patients had been treated for tuberculosis within the last 2 years.

Short-course chemotherapy included a combination of isoniazid (300 mg/day) and rifampicin (600 mg/day) for 8 months and pyrazinamide (1500 mg/day for 2 months) and streptomycin (1 g daily for 1 month, thereafter on alternate days, to a total of 45 g). Long-course chemotherapy included 4 antituberculous drugs initially for 4 or 6 months followed by a combination of 2 or 3 antituberculous drugs. The course of therapy was completed in 12–16 months. 19 patients were given a combination of isoniazid, rifampicin, pyrazinamide and ethambutol, 6 received isoniazid, rifampicin, ethambutol and streptomycin, 6 isoniazid, rifampicin, pyrazinamide and streptomycin, 3 isoniazid, rifampicin, pyrazinamide, ethambutol and streptomycin and 1 patient isoniazid, rifampicin and ethambutol. Protainamide was also given to 3 patients.

Prednisolone was initially given for 4 or 6 weeks to patients in stage III of the short-course therapy group. In the long-course therapy group, a steroid such as prednisolone or dexamethasone was given in the presence of papilloedema, cranial nerve palsies, clouding of consciousness and/or coma. Pyridoxine (100 mg/day) was added to all regimens.

Clinical recovery, side effects of drugs, the rate of residual sequelae and death were assessed. After the completion of therapy, the relapse rate was also followed.

RESULTS

72 patients were evaluated. Characteristics of the patients with tuberculous meningitis are summarized in Table I. Their ages ranged between 16 and 65 years (mean 30.4 years). There were 32 patients and 40 males. 38 had only meningitis. Meningitis and extrameningeal tuberculous lesions were found in 34 cases. Seven patients were in clinical stage I, 34 in stage II and 31 in stage III. Steroid therapy was given in 48 cases.

* Presented at the 6th International Congress on Infectious Diseases, April 26–30, 1994, in Prague, Czech Republic.

 ISSN 0036-5548

Table I. *Characteristics of cases of tuberculous meningitis*

Number of patients	72
Age (mean ± SD)	30.4 ± 2.1
Sex	
Female	32
Male	40
Meningitis only	38
Meningitis + extrameningeal lesion	34
Miliary tuberculosis	5
Pulmonary tuberculosis	22
Spondylitis	4
Intracerebral tuberculoma	1
Tuberculous lymphadenitis	1
Previous history of tuberculosis	3
Clinical stage	
I	7
II	34
III	31
Steroid therapy	48

Table II. *Results of therapy in cases of tuberculous meningitis*

Number of patients	72
No. completing therapy	55
No. lost to follow-up	10
No. of deaths	7 (9.7%)
No. with side effects	14 (19.4%)
Median days to disappearance of symptoms (range)	17 (5–210)
Duration of hospital stay, in days (mean ± SD)	36 ± 4
No. recovered	
With sequelae	18 (31%)
Without sequelae	40
No. unevaluated	7
No. of cases followed after therapy	48
Median duration of follow-up, in months (range)	
Short-course therapy group	10 (6–24)
Long-course therapy group	13 (4–36)
Relapse	
Short-course therapy group	0
Long-course therapy group	0

37 cases received short-course and 35 long-course therapy. The results of therapy in 72 cases of tuberculous meningitis are summarized in Table II. 55 of 72 patients completed their therapy plans. 10 patients were lost to follow-up after their symptoms had disappeared. Seven patients (9.7%) died. 25/37 patients who were given short-course therapy completed their therapy protocols. The duration of therapy was prolonged in 2 of 25 (8%) patients in one for 9 months, in the other 10 months. Treatment regimen was modified in 1 patient (2.7%) because of inadequate clinical response. Five (13.5%) patients died in the short-course group. The characteristics of patients who died are reported in Table III.

In the long-course therapy group, 25 patients were treated for 12 months, 2 for 15 months and 3 for 16 months. Two patients interrupted treatment after 3 and 5 months and relapsed. Treatment was reinstituted and continued for an additional 12 months. Two (5.7%) patients died, the first one after 10 days of treatment, due to cardiac arrest and the second after 5 months of therapy, due to therapeutic failure. Both patients were in stage III. Time of disappearance of symptoms varied between 5 and 210 days, mean 17 days. Mean duration of hospital treatment was 36 ± 4 days.

Side effects were observed in 14/72 (19.4%) patients of whom 6 (16.2%) were in the short-course therapy group and 8 (22.8%) in the long-course therapy group. Toxic hepatitis was observed in 10 cases, nausea and vomiting in 2 and hearing loss in 2.

Residual sequelae developed in 18/58 (31%) patients who survived and were evaluated; of those, 8 (30.7%) were in the short-course therapy group and 10 (31.2%) in the long-course group. Hemiparesis/monoparesis persisted in 8 cases, visual impairment in 4, imbalance in 3, and hydrocephalus in 3. Other sequelae were less frequently observed (Table IV). Ventriculoperitoneal shunt operations were performed in the 3 patients who developed hydrocephalus.

48 cases were followed up after completion of the therapy. The mean duration of following-up was 10 months (range 6–24) in the short-course therapy group and 13

Table III. *Characteristics of patients dying in the short-course therapy group*

	Patient no.				
Characteristic	1	2	3	4	5
Age/sex	28/M	23/M	46/M	45/F	18/M
Clinical stage	II	II	III	III	III
Underlying disease	pulmonary TB	–	–	–	pulmonary TB
Day of death	5	24	16	60	7
Cause of death	Respiratory failure	Hydrocephalus	Meningo-encephalitis	Sepsis arachnoidit	Respiratory failure

Table IV. *Residual sequelae*

Sequelae	Short-course ($n = 8$)	Long-course ($n = 10$)	Total ($n = 18$)
Hemiparesis/ monoparesis	3	5	8
Visual impairment	2	2	4
Imbalance	3	0	3
Hydrocephalus	0	3	3
Sense loss	1	1	2
Cerebral atrophy	1	0	1
Hearing loss	0	1	1

months (range 4–36) in the long-course group. No relapse was observed in either group.

DISCUSSION

Before the introduction of modern chemotherapy, tuberculous meningitis was invariably fatal. The introduction of isoniazid reduced mortality to between 23 and 36% (4, 5, 9). The addition of rifampicin to isoniazid-containing regimens further reduced mortality, to <20% (9). In our previous study (2), we showed that the regimen including rifampicin for tuberculous meningitis was no better than a combination of isoniazid, ethambutol and streptomycin, given for 12 months. Total mortality was 21% in that study. In the present study, both regimens also included rifampicin and total mortality was 9.7%. The patients dying in the first 5 days of treatment were excluded from both studies. The results of various treatment regimens available for adult tuberculous meningitis are summarized in Table V.

Mortality is known to be higher in clinical stage III (4, 9). Ogawa et al. (9) presented a mortality of 78% for patients in stage III. In the present study, 5 of the 7 patients who died were in stage III. Two patients in stage II progressed to clinical stage III and ultimately died.

Treatment for tuberculous meningitis should be initiated as soon as the disease is suspected. Three drugs readily penetrating into CSF must be given initially for sterilization and to prevent the development of resistant microorganisms. Isoniazid and rifampicin are accepted as a mainstay of such regimens. Pyrazinamide is added for 2 months to the regimen of short-course therapy for tuberculous meningitis. If resistance is suspected in the endemic area for tuberculosis, 1 of 2 drugs – streptomycin or ethambutol – is recommended in addition to the combination of isoniazid, rifampicin and pyrazinamide for 2 months at the beginning of therapy (5). Tuberculosis is still an endemic disease in Turkey (10). Primary resistance of M. tuberculosis to isoniazid is 11.7% and the sum of primary and secondary resistance to isoniazid is about 47.6% (11). For this reason, in Turkey short-course therapy must include streptomycin or ethambutol to the combination of isoniazid, rifampicin and pyrazinamide. The combination of pyrazinamide with isoniazid and rifampicin increases the hepatotoxicity, though rarely to an unacceptable level (6, 7, 12). In our study, during treatment, 10 patients showed a moderate increase in hepatic enzyme levels. Isoniazid and rifampicin were discontinued in these cases for a short time (3–5 days) and, after recovery, reinstituted. The rate of hepatotoxicity was acceptable. Streptomycin was stopped in 2 patients cases who developed hearing loss due to ototoxicity.

After clinical improvement and bacteriological cure, the major therapeutic goal in tuberculous meningitis is to avoid permanent neurological damage and relapse. 18 (31%) of the surviving patients were left with one or more neurolog-

Table V. *Treatment regimens available for adult tuberculous meningitis and results*

Literature ref.	No. of patients	Regimen of therapy	Duration of treatment (months)	Death rate (%)	Sequelae (%)	Toxicity (%)
Phuapradit-Vejjajiva 1987	24	2IRPS;7IR	9	2 (8.3)	3 (12.5)	1 (4.2)
Ogawa et al. 1987	45	IERS	NS	14 (31)	7/22 (32)	14 (31)
Doğanay et al. 1989	29	2IRS;10IR 2IES;10IR	12	6 (21)	9 (31)	8 (27.5)
Alarcon et al. 1990	22	2IRP;4IR	6	9 (40.9)	3 (23)	6 (27.2)
Girgis et al. 1991	166 144	24IE;(6wks)S	24	151 (54)	41 (14.6)	NS
Chotmongkol 1991	29	4IRPS;2IR	6	4/25 (16)	3/21 (14.2)	1/25 (4)
Present study	37	2IRPS;6IR	8	5 (13.5)	8 (30.7)	6 (16.2)
	35	see text	12–16	2 (5.7)	10 (31.2)	8 (22.8)

I: isoniazid, R: rifampicin, E: ethambutol, P: pyrazinamide, S: streptomycin, NS: not stated.

ical deficits (Table IV). A short-course regimen did not increase the number of neurological sequelae in our study. A neurological deficit was present in 12–24% of the patients with tuberculous meningitis treated for a period of 6–9 months in various studies (6, 12, 13), and in 14–32% of those treated <1 year (2–4).

In our study, no relapse was observed after completion of treatment. The results were not compared in the 2 therapy groups because the cases could not be randomized. This study did provide us with a fund of information about the results of short-course therapy in tuberculous meningitis in Turkey. To our knowledge, this is the first study on treatment of tuberculous meningitis with a short-course regime in our country.

Short-course therapy has shortened the duration of the therapy in tuberculous meningitis and is less expensive. It does not entail unacceptable toxic risks (6, 7, 12). However, there are opinions to the contrary. One study (8) from India presented 35 cases of recurrent central nervous system tuberculosis treated with chemotherapy for <2 years. 20/35 patients received chemotherapy for <6 months, which is known to be insufficient to eradicate tuberculous meningitis. The authors of that study therefore concluded that a treatment period of <2 years is inadequate. Girgis et al. (3) and Parsons (14) also advocate a period of therapy >18 months for tuberculous meningitis. Additionally, socio-economic circumstances are very important in the treatment of tuberculosis. When short-course therapy is contemplated, physicians should consider those conditions.

ACKNOWLEDGEMENTS

The authors would like to thank Prof. Dr. Osman Günay for useful criticism and assistance in the statistical analyses and Patrichia Shapiro for assistance in editing the text.

REFERENCES

1. Kennedy DH, Fallon RJ. Tuberculous meningitis. JAMA 241: 264–268, 1979.
2. Doğanay M, Bakır M, Dökmetaş İ. Treatment of tuberculous meningitis in adults with a combination of isoniazid, rifampicin and streptomycin: a prospective study. Scand J Infect Dis 21: 81–85, 1989.
3. Girgis NI, Farid Z, Kilpatrick ME, Sultan Y, Mikail IA. Dexamethasone adjunctive treatment for tuberculous meningitis. Pediatr Infec Dis J 10: 179–183, 1991.
4. Molavi A, LeFrock JL. Tuberculous meningitis. Med Clin North Am 69: 315–331, 1985.
5. Holdiness MR. Management of tuberculosis meningitis. Drugs 39: 224–233, 1990.
6. Alarcon F, Escalante L, Perez Y, Banda H, Chacon G, Duenas G. Tuberculous meningitis: short course chemotherapy. Arch Neurol 47: 1313–1317, 1990.
7. Jacobs RF, Sunakorn P, Chotpitayasunonah T, Pope S, Kelleher K. Intensive short course chemotherapy for tuberculous meningitis. Pediatr Infect Dis J 11: 194–198, 1992.
8. Goel A, Pandya SK, Satoskar AR. Whither short-course chemotherapy for tuberculous meningitis? Neurosurgery 27: 418–421, 1990.
9. Ogawa SK, Smith MA, Brennessel DJ, Lowy FD. Tuberculous meningitis in an urban medical center. Medicine 66: 317–326, 1987.
10. Bahar B, Demir R, Özesmi M. An analysis of the cases hospitalized in Kayseri NNY Chest Diseases Hospital in the last eight years. Tüberküloz ve Toraks 37: 59–63, 1989.
11. Özesmi M. The treatment of multi-resistant tuberculous cases. Solunum 18: 24–28, 1993.
12. Phuapradit P, Vejjajiva A. Treatment of tuberculous meningitis: role of short-course chemotherapy. Q J Med 62: 249–258, 1987.
13. Chotmonkol V. Treatment of tuberculous meningitis with 6 month course of chemotherapy. Southeast Asian J Trop Med Public Health 22: 372–374, 1991.
14. Parsons M. The treatment of tuberculous meningitis. Tubercle 70: 79–82, 1989.

Submitted September 16, 1994; accepted February 2, 1995

Scand J Infect Dis 27: 139–144, 1995 ORIGINAL ARTICLE

Epidemiological, Clinical and Microbiological Features of Shigellosis among Hospitalized Children in Northern Israel

OSNAT ADMONI[1], PABLO YAGUPSKY[2], AVIVIT GOLAN[1], YORAM KENES[3], GALIA SCHIFRONI[4] and IOSEF HOROWITZ[1]

From the [1]Pediatric Department A, and [3]Clinical Microbiology Laboratory, Haemek Medical Center, Afula, [2]Clinical Microbiology Laboratories, Soroka Medical Center, Ben-Gurion University of the Negev, Beer Sheva, and [4]Department of Medicine, Health and Epidemiology, Carmel Hospital, Haifa, Israel

The epidemiological, clinical, and bacteriological aspects of shigellosis were studied in a population of hospitalized children in northern Israel. During the 6-year period 1987–92, 262 children were hospitalized due to shigella infection. Shigellosis represented 10% of pediatric admissions for diarrhea. Admissions for the disease peaked during the summer and autumn. The median age of the patients was 3 years. Shigella sonnei was isolated in 74% of patients and S. flexneri in 21%, compared with relative frequencies of 87% and 10%, respectively, in the non-hospitalized population of the area, detected during the same period ($p < 0.001$). Shigella sonnei represented 82% of isolates of hospitalized Jewish patients but only 60% of hospitalized Arab children, many of whom live in poverty and overcrowding ($p < 0.001$). Shigella flexneri was particularly frequent among hospitalized infants, and was associated with Arab origin, large families and residence in agricultural settlements. Duration of hospitalization was 4.7 ± 2.3 days for S. sonnei infections and 5.8 ± 3.6 days for S. flexneri ($p < 0.005$). No cases of shigella sepsis, hemolytic uremic syndrome, or fatalities were observed. Overall, 37% of all shigella isolates from hospitalized children were resistant to ampicillin, 71% to cotrimoxazole, 28% to both and 13% were resistant to ≥ 3 different drugs. It is concluded that shigellosis is an important cause of hositalization in northern Israel. Resistance to antimicrobial drugs is widespread among all Shigella spp. Although S. sonnei is the most common species, S. flexneri is particularly frequent in infants.

P. Yagupsky, MD, Clinical Microbiology Laboratory, Soroka Medical Center, Ben-Gurion University of the Negev, Beer Sheva 84101, Israel

INTRODUCTION

Enteric infections caused by Shigella species continue to be a major universal cause of diarrheal diseases, including the Middle East countries (1, 2). Despite the continuous improvement of sanitary conditions and in the socioeconomic level of the population over the last 4 decades, shigellosis remains a serious public health problem in Israel. Recently published data even suggest that the incidence of the disease is increasing and current Israeli figures are 20-fold higher than those in the USA (3, 4).

We conducted a retrospective review of the medical charts of all pediatric patients hospitalized on account of shigellosis at a single hospital located in northern Israel during a 6-year period and collected data of non-hospitalized patients with positive stool cultures for Shigella spp. identified during the same period. The aims of the study were 1) to assess the impact of shigellosis as a cause of children's hospitalization; 2) to define the population at risk of serious morbidity; 3) to describe the clinical presentation of the disease among hospitalized children; 4) to define the Shigella species causing shigellosis in the area and those responsible for hospitalization of children; 5) to investigate the prevalence of antimicrobial resistance of shigellae in the area.

MATERIALS AND METHODS

Background

The Emek region of northern Israel has a population of 312,000, of whom 155,000 are Jews and 157,000 are of Arab origin. About 20% of the inhabitants live in agricultural settlements. In general terms, the majority of the Jewish population is urban, enjoying lower middle class socioeconomic standards, whereas a large proportion of the Arab population is rural, living in poverty with suboptimal sanitary facilities.

Outpatient medical services are provided at numerous health clinics distributed all over the region. With the exception of part of the Arab population, all patients in the area are referred for hospitalization to the Emek Central Hospital, located in the City of Afula, and all diagnostic bacteriology services are provided by the Clinical Microbiology Laboratory of this hospital.

Bacteriological methods

Stool samples from patients with diarrhea, collected from all the outpatient clinics and in-patients' hospial wards are sent to the hospital laboratory, either fresh or in modified stewart transport medium, 6 days-a-week. Samples are plated onto SS-agar, MacConkey agar and Campylobacter medium within 4 h. In addition a thetrahionate tube is also inoculated to enhance the detection of salmonellae. Identification of Shigella organisms is performed according to accepted bacteriological procedures and completed by agglutination with specific antisera (Wellcome Labs, Poole, Dorset, England) (5). Determination of antimicrobial susceptibility to ampicillin, cotrimoxazole, tetracycline, chloramphenicol, nalidixic

 ISSN 0036-5548

acid, neomycin and colistin is performed by the disc diffusion method of Bauer et al. (6).

Collection of data

Records of the Clinical Microbiology Laboratory were reviewed to identify patients who were hospitalized on the pediatric wards from January 1st, 1987 to December 31st, 1992 and from whom Shigella organisms were isolated from stool cultures. The medical records of these patients were reviewed and demographic, clinical, and bacteriological data were extracted. Demographic data included: age, sex, ethnic origin (Jew or Arab), place of residence (urban or rural), family size and date of specimen collection. Clinical data comprised: duration of hospital stay, occurrence of fever, vomiting, diarrhea, presence of blood in the stool, abdominal pain, convulsions, encephalopathy (defined as confusional state, stupor or coma), seizures, sepsis, hemolytic-uremic syndrome, or death. Laboratory data included: blood hemoglobin, leukocyte and differential counts, thrombocyte count, and serum urea and electrolyte concentration. Bacteriological data collected included Shigella species isolated and results of antimicrobial susceptibility testing.

To assess the impact of Shigella infections upon hospitalized pediatric patients, the total number of children hospitalized during the study period as well as the number of children admitted with gastroenteritis and the duration of the hospital stay were obtained from the hospital records.

In addition, records of the Clinical Microbiology Laboratory were reviewed to identify cultures of non-hospitalized patients resident in the area, from whom Shigellae were isolated during the same period, and the following data were collected: sex, ethnic origin, date of specimen collection, Shigella species isolated and results of the antibiotic susceptibility testing. Although the vast majority of these patients were probably children, age was inconsistently recorded and this information was therefore not considered in the data analysis.

Statistical analysis

Statistical analysis was performed by using the Statistical Package for Social Sciences (SPSS, Chicago, IL, 1990). Means of continuous variables were compared with a 2-tailed t-test. A χ^2-test was used to compare distributions of variables between groups. Logistic regression was used to adjust for potential confounding effects. A backward elimination procedure with $p \leq 0.10$ was used to screen variables for inclusion in the final analysis. A p-value of 0.05 or less was considered statistically significant.

RESULTS

Patients

During the 6-year period, 262 children with culture-confirmed shigellosis were hospitalized, representing 1% of all pediatric hospitalizations and 10.2% of all children's admissions for diarrheal diseases during the study period. 141 (54%) of all hospitalized patients were males and 121 (46%) females. 164 (64%) were Jews and 94 (36%) were Arabs. The median age of the patients was 3 years (range 1 month–13 years). Arab children were overrepresented in the youngest age group. Below the age of 12 months, 35.8% of the patients were Jews and 64.2% Arab children, whereas between 12 and 24 months of age, 53.7% were Jewish and 46.3% of Arab origin ($p < 0.001$). With the exception of 1 child admitted with diarrhea and failure to thrive, all other children showed a normal nutritional status.

Seasonal distribution

As expected, a seasonal distribution of hospitalizations was observed: 48 children (18.3%) were admitted during the coldest months of the year (December–February), 44 (16.8%) in the spring (March–May), 89 (33.6%) during the summer (June–August) and 81 (30.9%) in the autumn (September–November).

Clinical features

At the time of hospital admission, patients had been sick for a mean of 3.8 ± 2.6 days (median 3 days, range 1–14 days). Chief complaints on admission were fever in 162 children (62.6%), watery diarrhea in 144 (55.0%), vomiting in 111 (42.4%), convulsions in 37 (14.1%) and bloody diarrhea in 13 (5.0%). In 9 of the 37 (14.1%) children admitted with convulsions, no history of diarrhea prior to the onset of seizures was elicited.

Children were hospitalized for a mean of 5.0 ± 2.7 days (median 4.0 days, range 1–24 days). In the course of the hospital stay, fever (temperature > 38.3°C) was recorded in 95% of the patients, vomiting in 76%, watery diarrhea was observed in 76%, bloody diarrhea in 42%, dehydration in 22.5%, febrile convulsions in 17% and encephalopathy in 7%. Dehydration was significantly more frequent among infants younger than 12 months but vomiting was significantly less common than in other age groups (data not shown). No cases of Shigella sepsis, hemolytic-uremic syndrome or fatalities attributable to the enteric infection were observed during the study period, but 1 child developed Streptococcus pneumoniae bacteremia in the course of the disease.

Bacterial isolates

Shigella sonnei was isolated in 193 of 262 hospitalized children (74%), S. flexneri in 54 (21%), S. boydii in 10 (3.8%) and S. dysenteriae in 5 (1.9%), compared with relative frequencies of 87.1%, 9.6%, 2.8% and 0.6%, respectively among 2,038 non-hospitalized patients ($p < 0.001$). The proportions of the different species changed significantly over the 6-year period. Whereas the proportion of patients infected with S. sonnei increased among both hospitalized children and non-hospitalized patients, that of S. flexneri diminished in both populations (Table I). In 9 children, other enteric pathogens such as salmonellae, Campylobacter species and Giardia lamblia were found.

To assess the relative virulence of the 2 most common Shigella species, the proportions of S. sonnei and S. flexneri among hospitalized and non-hospitalized patients were compared. However, because these organisms were unequally distributed among the 2 ethnic groups [S. sonnei represented 137/168 (81.5%) of isolates of hospitalized Jewish children but only 56/94 (59.6%) of hospitalized Arab children ($p < 0.001$)], the proportion of the 2 species was calculated in the two populations, separately (Table II). In both groups S. flexneri was significantly more common

Table I. *Proportions of infections caused by S. sonnei and S. flexneri among hospitalized children and non-hospitalized patients in 1987–89 and 1990–92*

		Population					
		Hospitalized			Non-hospitalized		
Organism	Period	children	(%)	*P*	patients	(%)	*P*
S. sonnei	1987–89	96/156	(61.5)	< 0.001	784/958	(81.8)	< 0.001
	1990–92	97/106	(91.5)		989/1,080	(91.5)	
S. flexneri	1987–89	47/156	(30.1)	< 0.001	138/958	(14.4)	< 0.001
	1990–92	7/106	(6.6)		58/1,080	(5.4)	

Table II. *Frequencies of S. sonnei and S. flexneri among hospitalized children and non-hospitalized patients, according to ethnic grouping*

Population		Hospitalized		Non-hospitalized		
n	Organism	children	(%)	patients	(%)	*P*
Jews	S. sonnei	137/168	(81.5)	1,633/1,859	(87.8)	0.026
(2,027)	S. flexneri	24/168	(14.3)	163/1,859	(8.8)	0.027
Arabs	S. sonnei	56/94	(59.6)	140/179	(78.2)	0.002
(273)	S. flexneri	30/94	(31.9)	32/179	(17.9)	0.013

among hospitalized children than in non-hospitalized patients.

Demographic and clinical features of patients with infections caused by the 2 most common species are compared in Table III. The ages of hospitalized patients did not vary according to Shigella species, but the proportion of Shigella species varied significantly in the different age groups: S. flexneri represented 45.8% of isolates in infants younger than 12 months, 17.2% in the 1–5 year-old group and 28.6% in children older than 5 years ($p < 0.03$). Below the age of 12 months and among children older 3 years, the proportions of S. sonnei and S. flexneri were equal in the ethnic groups. Among children between the ages of 12 and 24 months, S. flexneri constituted 32% of organisms isolated from Arab children but only 5.6% of those recovered from Jewish children ($p < 0.006$); in the >24–36 month age group this species represented 38.9% of all isolates from Arab children and 9.3% of those from Jewish children ($p < 0.006$).

Because the occurrence of different Shigella species was found to vary with age and ethnic origin, a multivariate analysis of data was performed to investigate risk factors for infection with S. flexneri and to control for confounding factors (Table IV). Results of the analysis demonstrated that whereas Arab origin was a risk factor for infection with this species among both hospitalized and non-hospitalized patients, living in an agricultural settlement and belonging to a large family were significantly associated with S. flexneri in Jewish children.

Overall, high fever, watery diarrhea and predominance of polymorphonuclear cells in the peripheral blood count were more frequent among children with S. sonnei infection, whereas bloody diarrhea and lower serum sodium concentration characterized infection with S. flexneri. Frequency of vomiting, dehydration or neurological signs did not differ significantly between the 2 species.

Antibiotic susceptibility

Overall, 36.6% of all Shigella isolates of hospitalized children were resistant to ampicillin, 70.6% to cotrimoxazole, 28.2% to both and 13.4% were multiresistant (resistant to ≥3 different drugs). Only 1.9% were resistant to nalidixic acid. Antimicrobial resistance differed between Shigella species: 9.5% of all S. sonnei isolates were susceptible to all antimicrobial drugs tested, 73.5% were resistant to 1 or 2 drugs and 16.9% were multiresistant; among S. flexneri isolates, 24.4% were susceptible to all antimicrobials, 57.4% were resistant to 1 or 2 drugs and 18.5% were multiresistant ($p < 0.02$).

Of the isolates from non-hospitalized patients, 41.3% were resistant to ampicillin and 83.1% to cotrimoxazole, while 35.6% were resistant to both drugs. Resistance of individual species to the antimicrobial drugs tested was not statistically different from that observed among isolates from hospitalized children (data not shown).

Therapy

84 (32%) patients were given oral fluid therapy and 178 (68%) required intravenous fluid replacement for 1–17 days (median 3 days). 177 (68%) children did not receive antibiotic therapy. Of those treated with antibiotics, 45 received ampicillin or amoxicillin, 14 cephalosporins, 8 trimetho-

Table III. *Demographic, clinical and laboratory features in hospitalized children with S. sonnei and S. flexneri infections*

	S. sonnei ($N = 193$)	S. flexneri ($N = 54$)	P
Demographic features			
Age (months)	3.3 ± 2.1	3.5 ± 2.6	NS
Jewish origin (%)	71.0	44.4	<0.001
No. of siblings	2.7 ± 1.3	3.6 ± 2.4	<0.001
Clinical and laboratory features			
Days of illness prior to admission	4.2 ± 3.1	3.3 ± 2.1	NS
Hospital stay (in days)	4.7 ± 2.3	5.8 ± 3.6	<0.005
Fever ≥39.0°C on admission (%)	54.5	42.6	<0.05
Bloody diarrhea on admission (%)	38.7	53.7	<0.05
Dehydration on admission (%)	20.9	29.6	NS
Neurological signs (%)	23.8	25.9	NS
Na concentration (mEq/l)	136.3 ± 3.6	133.8 ± 3.3	<0.005
Percentage of PMNs in blood count	60.6	52.3	<0.05

Table IV. *Risk factors for S. flexneri infections (by multivariate analysis)*

	Odds ratio	95% Confidence intervals	P
Hospitalized children			
Arab origin	2.5	1.8–3.3	<0.02
Large family	1.6	1.4–1.8	<0.001
Bloody diarrhea	2.9	2.2–3.6	<0.004
Jews only			
Large family	1.7	1.4–2.1	<0.002
Bloody diarrhea	5.1	4.0–6.2	<0.004
Arabs only			
Susceptible strain	12.9	11.3–14.6	<0.003
Non-hospitalized patients			
Residence in an agricultural settlement	3.1	2.7–3.5	<0.0001
Arab origin	2.6	2.1–3.1	0.001
Susceptible strain	3.3	2.8–3.7	<0.0001

prim-sulphamethoxazole, 6 nalidixic acid and the remaining 12 a wide array of other antimicrobial drugs.

DISCUSSION

The present data demonstrate that shigellosis is widespread in northern Israel and is an important cause of hospitalization for diarrhea among children. Although the number of culture-proven cases of shigellosis detected in the community tended to increase during the study period, the number of hospital admissions decreased during the last years of the study. This tendency probably reflects both a decline in the frequency of the more virulent S. flexneri during the study period and a better primary care of children with shigellosis.

Our results show that 2 species, S. sonnei and S. flexneri, together caused over 90% of infections among both the hospitalized and non-hospitalized populations and that the relative frequency of S. sonnei increased during the study period. Data collected by the Israeli Health Ministry over the years indicate that countrywide the most common species of Shigella in Israel has shifted in the late 1970s from S. flexneri to S. sonnei (4, 7). This shift has been attributed to an improvement in standards of living and hygiene in Israel over the last 4 decades, which tend to select for less virulent organisms (1, 11). It appears that in Israel, the shift to S. sonnei has occurred later than in other developed countries. The reasons for this delay are not altogether clear. It should be pointed out, however, that a relatively large proportion of the Israeli population serves in the army, in which S. flexneri is hyperendemic because of suboptimal sanitary conditions, and that pockets of poverty persist among the Arab population and among Jews living in rural areas in which the organism is especially prevalent, as shown by the results of the present study (4). In a recent report, S. flexneri was found to be the most common species also among the indigent semi-nomadic Bedouins of southern Israel, whereas the Jewish population of the area suffered mainly from infections caused by S. sonnei (12). These findings demonstrate that even in a small country such as Israel, the shift from S. flexneri to S. sonnei does not occur simultaneously in the entire population. Replacement of the virulent species by S. sonnei is probably attributable to improvements in living conditions, and S. flexneri may persist for long periods of time within populations living in poverty.

Analysis of the clinical data shows that the clinical features differed between the two Shigella species. Whereas high temperatures were significantly more common among patients with S. sonnei infections, bloody diarrhea, lower sodium levels and a trend towards more frequent signs of dehydration characterized S. flexneri. Similar findings were reported by Keusch in the USA and by Stoll in Bangladesh who found that S sonnei infections frequently caused watery diarrhea only, whereas the most virulent species, i.e. S. dysenteriae and S. flexneri, presented as a dysenteric syndrome with typical bloody stools (1, 8). In the individual patient, however, there is no accurate way to distinguish between infections caused by the different species on the basis of clinical features. It should be pointed out that despite the overall greater severity of the enteric disease caused by S. flexneri, the frequency of neurological signs was similar to that observed with S. sonnei, indicating that these two aspects of the disease are caused by different mechanisms (9).

Although our population comprised a large group of hospitalized infants and young children, no cases of Shigella sepsis, hemolytic-uremic syndrome or fatalities were observed over the 6-year period. Failure to detect life-threatening conditions in our study population demonstrates that when the less virulent S. sonnei infections prevail, the incidence of such complications is low (1). Occurence of pneumococcal bacteremia in 1 child admitted with culture-proven shigellosis, however, should remind us that invasive disease caused by unrelated organisms may complicate the course of diarrheal diseases in the very young (10).

The presented results show that antimicrobial resistance is widespread among Shigella species in northern Israel and, as observed in other countries, is especially frequent in S. sonnei isolates, making the choice of adequate empiric therapy of clinical dysentery particularly difficult (13). Antimicrobial resistance patterns frequently included ampicilln and cotrimoxazole, alone or in combination, but only a small proportion of isolates were resistant to nalidixic acid. Although emergence of resistance to nalidixic acid has been reported in populations exposed to the drug, this drug appears for the time being to be an attractive choice for the oral treatment of children with shigellosis. It should be noted that the distribution of antimicrobial resistance was similar among isolates obtained from Arab and Jewish patients. This finding suggests that the antimicrobial drug prescription pattern is similar in both communities, resulting in comparable antibiotic pressures on the microbial flora, or that Jews and Arabs share a common pool of Shigella organisms. There is no obvious explanation for the unexpected finding that infection with strains of S. flexneri susceptible to antimicrobials increases the need for hospitalization among Arab children. It is speculated that the lack of resistance to antimicrobials exhibited by these isolates implies the recent introduction of these strains in a community and the unexpected hospitalization rate resulted from absence of immunity to these organisms.

Control of shigellosis has traditionally been based on the improvement of sanitary conditions (supply of potable water, foodhandling regulations and proper disposal of human waste), personal hygiene and administration of antimicrobial drugs to interrupt the chain of person-to-person transmission of the disease (1). These measures are frequently insufficient, however, because of the extremely low infecting dose of Shigella species and the high prevalence of antibiotic resistance among members of the genus.

The global impact of shigellosis and the difficulties faced in gaining control over it have aroused interest in the development of a vaccine as a means to a more efficacious prevention, and recent advances in this area have heralded the possible advent of such a vaccine in the near future (14). To implement a correct vaccination program it will be necessary to ascertain the need for such a vaccine, and to define the target population and shigella antigens to be included in the preparation in every country. The present results indicate that to prevent serious shigella infections necessitating hospital admission in northern Israel, any future vaccine formulation will have to be administered at an early age and protect against both S. sonnei and S. flexneri.

REFERENCES

1. Keusch GT. Shigella infections. Clin Gastroenterol 8: 645–662, 1979.
2. Al-Eissa Y, Al-Zamil F, Al-Kharashi M, Kambal A, Chowdhury M, Al-Ayed I. The relative importance of Shigella in the aetiology of childhood gastroenteritis in Saudi Arabia. Scand J Infect Dis 24: 347–351, 1992.
3. Lee LA, Shapiro CN, Hargrett-Bean N, Tauxe RV. Hyperendemic shigellosis in the United States: a review of surveillance data for 1967–1988. J Infect Dis 164: 894–900, 1991.
4. Green MS, Block C, Cohen D, Slater P. Four decades of shigellosis in Israel: epidemiology of a growing problem. Rev Infect Dis 13: 248–253, 1991.
5. Kelly MT, Brenner DJ, Farmer JJ III. Enterobacteriaceae. In: Lennette EH, Balows A, Hausler WJ Jr, Shadomy HJ, eds. Manual of Clinical Microbiology, 4th edn. Washington, DC: American Society for Microbiology, 263–277, 1985.
6. Bauer AM, Kirby WMM, Sherris JC, Turck M. Antibiotic susceptibility testing by standardized single disk method. Am J Clin Pathol 45: 493–496, 1966.
7. Ashkenazi S, May-Zahav M, Dinari G, Gabbay U, Zilberberg R, Samra Z. Recent trends in the epidemiology of Shigella species in Israel. Clin Infect Dis 17: 897–899, 1993.
8. Stoll BJ, Glass RI, Huq MI, Khan MU, Banu H, Holt J.

Epidemiologic and clinical features of patients infected with Shigella who attended a diarrheal disease hospital in Bangladesh. J Infect Dis 146: 177–183, 1982.
9. Ashkenazi S, Cleary KR, Pickering LK, Murray BE, Cleary TG. The association of Shiga toxins and other cytotoxins with the neurologic manifestations of shigellosis. J Infect Dis 161: 961–965, 1990.
10. Mitra AK, Albert J, Alam AN. Bacteraemia and meningitis among hospital patients with diarrhoea. Trans Roy Soc Trop Med Hyg 87: 560–563, 1993.
11. Ewald PW. Waterborne transmission and the evolution of virulence among gastrointestinal bacteria. Epidemiol Infect 106: 83–119, 1991.
12. Finkelman Y, Yagupsky P, Fraser D, Dagan, R. Epidemiology of Shigella infections in two ethnic groups in a geographic region in southern Israel. Eur J Clin Microbiol Infect Dis 13: 367–373, 1994.
13. Tauxe RV, Puhr ND, Wells JG, Hargrett-Bean N, Blake PA. Antimicrobial resistance of Shigella isolates in the USA: the importance of international travelers. J Infect Dis 162: 1107–1111, 1990.
14. Li A, Cam PD, Islam D, Binh Minh N, Huan PT, Rong ZC, Karlsson K, Lindberg G, Lindberg AA. Immune responses in Vietnamese children after a single dose of the auxotrophic, live Shigella flexneri Y vaccine strain SFL_{124}. J Infect 28: 11–23, 1994.

Submitted August 10, 1994; accepted December 18, 1994

Scand J Infect Dis 27: 145–148, 1995

ORIGINAL ARTICLE

A Survey of Campylobacter Bacteremia in Three Danish Counties, 1989 to 1994

HENRIK C. SCHØNHEYDER[1,2], PER SØGAARD[2] and WILHELM FREDERIKSEN[3]

From the Departments of [1]Clinical Microbiology, Aalborg Hospital, Aalborg, [2]Clinical Microbiology, Århus University Hospital, Århus, and [3]Clinical Microbiology, Statens Seruminstitut, København S, Denmark

Over a 5-year period (April 1989 to March 1994) bacteremia caused by Campylobacter species was diagnosed in 15 patients in a population of 1.3 million in three counties in Jutland province, Denmark. The incidence was 0.2/100,000/year and the ratio of blood to fecal isolates, was 0.008. Campylobacter coli and Campylobacter jejuni accounted for 6 cases each, Campylobacter fetus for 2, and in 1 case the species diagnosis was uncertain. Seven patients were males and 8 females; median age was 42 (range 15–90) years. 11 patients had underlying disorders, including immunological, neoplastic and vascular disease. In a 67-year-old man a Starr-Edwards prosthesis of the aortic valve was probably infected by C. fetus, as recurrent bacteremia resolved following valve replacement. Eight patients had pyrexia and diarrhea, whereas 7 had pyrexia with only slight intestinal discomfort or none at all. In 4 patients the bacteremia was associated with cutaneous cellulitis or vasculitis. 14 of 15 patients survived. Campylobacter bacteremia seems to be more common in Denmark than hitherto thought.

H. C. Schønheyder, MD, Department of Clinical Microbiology, Aalborg Hospital, Box 365, DK-9100 Aalborg, Denmark

INTRODUCTION

The role of Campylobacter jejuni and Campylobacter coli in foodborne gastroenteritis is well known and poultry is the leading source of infection (1). Consumption of Danish poultry has been recognized as an important risk factor in Norway (2). The registered rate of fecal isolations in Denmark was 1,458 in 1985 and 1,776 in 1993 (3, 4), but bacteremic infections with C. jejuni and C. coli are considered to be rare. We are aware of only a single Danish report of Campylobacter jejuni bacteremia (5), and as information is sparse, regarding epidemiological and clinical aspects of bacteremic campylobacteriosis in Scandinavian countries, we undertook a retrospective 5-year survey, identifying a total of 15 cases in three Danish counties. We now present these 15 cases of Campylobacter bacteremia as this entity may be more frequent than hitherto thought.

MATERIALS AND METHODS

The 3 counties of Århus, Viborg and Northern Jutland had a combined population of 1.32 million (1991 census). All blood cultures were processed by the Department of Clinical Microbiology at either Århus University Hospital or Aalborg Hospital. The last 6 months of the survey period did not include the County of Viborg (population 230,000) as a local Department of Clinical Microbiology had then been established. Patients were identified by manual review of laboratory records covering the period April 1, 1989 to March 31, 1994. For patients with Campylobacter species detected by blood culture the hospital record was reviewed with emphasis on coexisting disease, exposure, clinical picture, therapy, and outcome. The study was approved by the regional scientific ethics committee.

Blood cultures

Counties of Århus and Viborg: A traditional blood culture system with multiple tubes of bacteriological media (6) was replaced in 1990 by the BACTEC 460/660 blood culture system (Becton-Dickinson, USA) which in turn was replaced in 1993 by the BacT/Alert blood culture system (Organon Teknika, Holland). For the whole survey period, 1 blood culture set included 1 aerobic and 1 anaerobic blood culture bottle for adult patients. *County of Northern Jutland:* In 1992 the traditional blood culture system was replaced by Colorbact (Statens Seruminstitut, København) (7). One blood culture set included 2 aerobic and 1 anaerobic blood culture bottle for adult patients.

Bacteriology

Micro-aerophilic Gram-negative curved, 'gull-wing' or spiral-shaped rods were tentatively identified as Campylobacter species and submitted to the Department of Clinical Microbiology at Statens Seruminstitut, Copenhagen for confirmation and species identification.

Isolates that grew at 22°C were identified as Campylobacter fetus; C. jejuni proved positive and C. coli negative for hippurate hydrolysis. Susceptibility testing by disc diffusion was performed in a micro-aerophilic atmosphere on Danish horse blood agar either by Thomsen's method (8) using locally prepared discs, or by the commercially available NeoSensitabs system (9).

Fecal culture

Bacteriological examination of fecal specimens was done by Statens Seruminstitut, Copenhagen. Isolates of C. jejuni and C. coli were not routinely differentiated. Annual numbers of isolates of Campylobacter species were available for each county for the years 1991–93 (4, 10, 11).

RESULTS

A total of 15 patients with Campylobacter bacteremia were identified (Table I). The incidence was approximately 0.2/100,000/year in the 3 counties. The numbers of fecal isolates were 345, 277 and 368 for the years 1991, 1992 and 1993, respectively, being equivalent to a rate of approximately 25/100,000/year. The ratio between blood and fecal isolates could thus be estimated to 0.008.

The patients had a median age of 42 (range 15–90) years. Seven were males, 8 females. In 2 cases, poultry was

 ISSN 0036-5548

Table I. *Clinical and microbiological characteristics of 15 patients with Campylobacter bacteremia in 3 Danish counties 1989–1994*

Patient no.	Sex[a]	Age (years)	Blood isolate	Detection time[b] (days)	Fecal culture	Underlying disease	Clinical picture
1	M	15	C. coli	3	Positive	None	Febrile gastroenteritis
2	F	21	C. jejuni	3	Positive	None	Febrile gastroenteritis
3	M	33	C. coli	5	Positive	X-linked hypogammaglobulinemia	Protracted fever, weight loss
4	M	38	Campylobacter sp.	4	Negative	HIV-infection	Fever, erythema nodosum, cellulitis
5	M	38	C. coli	3	Not done[c]	Chronic alcoholism	Febrile gastroenteritis, cellulitis
6	F	40	C. jejuni	3	Positive	None	Febrile gastroenteritis
7	F	41	C. coli	3	Positive	Panhypopituitarism, diabetes mellitus	Febrile gastroenteritis
8	F	42	C. coli	4	Not done	Malignant lymphoma, systemic lupus erythematosus, leukopenia, steroid therapy	Fever, hypoglycemia
9	F	57	C. jejuni	2	Not done	Myelomatosis, leukopenia, steroid therapy	Fever, erythema multiforme
10	F	58	C. coli	3	Negative	Renal allotransplantation, splenectomy, liver cirrhosis, carcinoma of urinary bladder	Coma, fever
11	M	67	C. fetus	4	Not done	Aortic valve prosthesis abdominal aortic aneurism, chronic obstructive pulmonary disease	Fever, erysipelas
12	F	69	C. jejuni	5	Positive	None	Febrile gastroenteritis
13	M	76	C. fetus	7	Not done	Choledocholithiasis, abdominal aortic aneurism	Cholangitis
14	M	76	C. jejuni	3	Positive	Chronic obstructive pulmonary disease, steroid therapy	Febrile gastroenteritis
15	M	90	C. jejuni	7	Positive	Diabetes mellitus	Febrile gastroenteritis

[a] M = Male; F = Female.
[b] Number of days from sampling of blood until notification of positive blood culture.
[c] Fecal specimen negative after start of antibiotic therapy.

a suspected source of infection, and 1 patient kept 9 budgerigars. One patient had recently been on holiday in Spain and another in Portugal.

Eight patients were admitted to hospital with pyrexia and acute gastroenteritis, but none had signs of hemorrhagic colitis. The remaining 7 patients had pyrexia as the predominant finding, any enteric symptoms beng mild. One of the 7 patients (no. 13) presented with cholangitis, whereas 2 had relapsing pyrexia of 4 weeks and 22 months duration, respectively (nos. 3 and 11).

On admission, 4 of the 15 patients had a rectal temperature below 38.5°C, whereas 11 were febrile with a temperature between 38.9 and 39.8°C. Four patients had acute cutaneous manifestations described as erythema multiforme, erythema nodosum, erysipelas and an extensive cellulitis, respectively. It is noteworthy that in none of the 4 cases was the cutaneous disorder suspected to be a manifestation of a systemic infection, nor was an association with Campylobacter bacteremia indicated.

Patient no. 3 with hypogammaglobulinemia had 2 febrile episodes with positive blood cultures 4 weeks apart. On the first occasion the patient was discharged before the blood culture report was obtained, as defervescence had occurred soon after commencement of penicillin treatment. After the clinical and bacteriological relapse, a 10-day intravenous course of netilmicin was administered together with intravenous gammaglobulin, and this was followed by complete recovery. Patient no. 11 had several bacteremic episodes during a period of 22 months despite courses of antibiotic therapy including betalactams, gentamicin and clindamycin. A Starr-Edwards aortic valve prosthesis was the probable focus of infection as the patient was clinically and bacteriologically cured after replacement of the valve; however, bacteriological culture of the valve was negative.

Of the remaining 13 patients, 9 received antibiotic therapy, and in 6 the regimen included penicillin or ampicillin in combination with an aminoglycoside. A betalactam was given as monotherapy in 3 (penicillin in 2 and ceftriaxone in 1). One patient with advanced hepatic cirrhosis (no. 10) died from hepatic coma, but the fatal outcome seemed not to be directly related to the Campylobacter bacteremia.

With the exception of patients 3 and 11, in whom the infection ran a protracted course, no clinical or bacteriological recurrences were observed. This also pertained to 4 patients who did not receive antibiotic therapy.

Bacteriology

The median time until detection of positive blood culture was 3 days, range 2–7 days. One isolate was obtained with the traditional blood culture system with multiple tubes of bacteriological media. The remaining 14 isolates were recovered from bottle culture systems, 11 of these with the BACTEC 440/460 system, 2 with BacT/Alert and 1 with Colorbact.

The bacteriological diagnoses were C. coli and C. jejuni in 6 patients each. C. fetus was isolated in 2 patients (nos. 11 and 13), and 1 isolate was lost before speciation could be done. Fecal specimens were submitted from 10 patients prior to antibiotic therapy and C. coli/C. jejuni were reported in 8.

All isolates were susceptible to gentamicin, netilmicin, ciprofloxacin, tetracycline and chloramphenicol. However, of 14 isolates tested 43% were resistant to ampicillin, 57% to cefotaxime, and 14% to erythromycin.

DISCUSSION

Members of the genus Campylobacter are micro-aerophilic and fastidious, and it is probable that the type of blood culture system affects the isolation rate (12, 13). It is noteworthy that although Campylobacter isolates were obtained with all 4 types of blood culture system used, 11 were found with the BACTEC 460/660 system. This corroborates a recent report from Spain (14) and experience with a similar microorganism, Helicobacter cinaedi in the USA (15).

An invasive role is well established for C. fetus (16), but studies in Britain, Australia and Bangladesh have confirmed that C. jejuni and C. coli do play the same role (17–19). An enteral route of infection was likely in our series, as C. jejuni/C. coli was isolated from feces in 8 out of 10 cases sampled properly. With the exception of 2 patients the infection was acquired in Denmark, but the specific source of infection remained unknown except in 2 cases where poultry was incriminated.

The ratio between blood and fecal isolates was in the order of 0.01, and this figure may both reflect the invasiveness of the pathogen and the extent to which bacteriological culture is performed in cases of diarrhea. Skirrow et al. (17) found a figure of 0.001 in England for the 10-year period 1981–91. Comparable statistics are not available for salmonellosis in our region, but we consider that Campylobacter bacteremia deserves as much concern as the upsurge of salmonellosis. Patients with compromised immunity seem to be especially affected, and X-linked hypogammaglobulinemia (patient no. 3) has repeatedly been recognized as a risk factor (18, 20, 21). Patient no. 11 had a likely diagnosis of prosthetic valve endocarditis, and a role in foreign body infections has previously been documented (22, 23). This emphasizes the need to be able to culture fastidious and micro-aerophilic bacteria when investigating foreign body infections.

The clinical pattern of Campylobacter bacteremia described here is very similar to that of Skirrow et al. (17). One of our patients had cholangitis, and this entity seems to be rare (23). Four patients had prominent acute, though differing cutaneous manifestations, and the triad of pyrexia, diarrhea and cutaneous cellulitis should alert clinicians to the possibility of invasive campylobacteriosis (20, 21).

Due to the prolonged detection time, several patients had already been discharged, and no serious complications of withholding antibiotic therapy were on record. Only 1 of the 15 patients died, and the death was apparently not directly related to Campylobacter bacteremia. Skirrow et al. (17) reported a mortality of 2.5% among 3,954 patients with Campylobacter bacteremia. Although the prognosis is favourable, antibiotic therapy is indicated in patients at increased risk and patients with serious focal infections such as endocarditis. McNulty (24) has made a valuation of different therapeutic regimens, recommending aminoglycosides, macrolides and fluoroquinolones. We found all isolates sensitive to gentamicin/netilmicin and ciprofloxacin, but 14% of our isolates were resistant to erythromycin. Fluoroquinolone resistance is well documented in Scandinavia (25, 26), and we therefore consider aminoglycosides to be first choice.

To conclude, modern blood culture systems seem to be effective for the diagnosis of Campylobacter bacteremia, an invasive form of a common zoonosis. It affects mostly patients with underlying disorders, and may present with pyrexia without diarrhea and sometimes with cutaneous cellulitis. The course is generally benign, but serious complications and death may occur.

REFERENCES

1. Skirrow MB. Campylobacter. Lancet 336: 921–923, 1990.
2. Kapperud G, Skjerve E, Bean NH, Ostroff SM, Lassen J. Risk factors for sporadic Campylobacter infections: Results of a case-control study in southeastern Norway. J Clin Mirobiol 30: 3117–3121, 1992.
3. Andreasen JJ. In vitro susceptibility of Campylobacter jejuni and Campylobacter coli isolated in Denmark to fourteen an-

timicrobial agents. Acta Pathol Microbiol Immunol Scand Sect B 95: 189–192, 1987.

4. Tarmbakteriologisk laboratorium. Bakterielle tarminfektioner i Denmark: fordeling af bakterietyper på amt og indsenderkategori i perioden fra 1.1.93 til 31.12.93. København: Statens Seruminstitut, 1994. [in Danish]
5. Kelbæk H, Sørensen TS. Campylobacter jejuni infektioner. Ugeskr Læger 144: 556–557, 1982.
6. Bruun B, Sloth K, Weis Bentzon M, Frederiksen W. A study of bacteremias in Denmark from 1977–1978. Acta Pathol Microbiol Immunol Scand Sect B 90: 309–317, 1982.
7. Prag J, Jensen J, Lebech K. Colorbact, a visually read blood culture system using darkening of haemoglobin in aerobic blood cultures as an early growth indicator, compared with Bactec 6A and 7A. APMIS 99: 1089–1095, 1991.
8. Thomsen VF. Om teknikken ved resistensbestemmelse med særligt henblik på anvendelse af prædiffusion. Thesis, Nyt Nordisk Forlag, Arnold Busck, København, 1967. [in Danish]
9. Casals JB, Pringler N. Antibacterial and antifungal sensitivity testing using NeoSensitabs, 9th edn. Taastrup, Denmark: Rosco Diagnostica, 1991.
10. Tarmbakteriologisk laboratorium. Bakterielle tarminfektioner i Danmark: fordeling af bakterietyper på amt og indsenderkategori i perioden fra 1.1.91 til 31.12.91. København: Statens Seruminstitut, 1992. [in Danish]
11. Tarmbakteriologisk laboratorium. Bakterielle tarminfektioner i Danmark: fordeling af bakterietyper på amt og indsenderkategori i perioden fra 1.1.92 til 31.12.92. København: Statens Seruminstitut, 1993. [in Danish]
12. Pasternak J, Bolivar R, Hopter RL, Fainstein V, Mills K, Rios A, Bodey GP, Fennell CL, Totten PA, Stamm WE. Bacteraemia caused by Campylobacter-like organisms in two male homosexuals. Ann Intern Med 101: 339–341, 1984.
13. Wang W-LL, Blaser MJ. Detection of pathogenic Campylobacter species in blood culture systems. J Clin Microbiol 23: 709–714, 1986.
14. de Guevara CL, Gonzalez J, Pena P. Bacteraemia caused by Campylobacter spp. J Clin Pathol 47: 174–175, 1994.
15. Kiehlbauch JA, Tauxe RV, Baker CN, Wachsmuth IK. Helicobacter cinaedi-associated bacteremia and cellulitis in immunocompromised patients. Ann Intern Med 121: 90–93, 1994.
16. Guerrant RL, Lahita RG, Winn WC, Roberts RB. Campylobacteriosis in man: pathogenic mechanisms and review of 91 bloodstream infections. Am J Med 65: 584–592, 1978.
17. Skirrow MB, Jones DM, Sutcliffe E, Benjamin J. Campylobacter bacteraemia in England and Wales, 1981–1991. Epidemiol Infect 110: 567–573, 1993.
18. Spelman DW, Davidson N, Buckmaster ND, Spicer WI, Ryan P. Campylobacter bacteraemia, a report of 10 cases. Med J Aust 145: 503–505, 1986.
19. Hossain MA, Kabir I, Albert MJ, Kibriya AKMG, Alam K, Alam AN. Campylobacter jejuni bacteraemia in children with diarrhoea in Bangladesh: report of six cases. J Diarrhoeal Dis Res 10: 101–104, 1992.
20. LeBar WD, Menard RR, Check FE. Hypogammaglobulinemia and recurrent Campylobacter jejuni infection. J Infect Dis 152: 1099–1100, 1985.
21. Kerstens PJSM, Endtz HP, Meis JFGM, Oyen WJG, Koopman RJI, van den Broek PJ, van der Meer JWM. Erysipelas-like skin lesions associated with Campylobacter jejuni septicemia in patients with hypogammaglobulinemia. Eur J Clin Microbiol Infect Dis 11: 842–847, 1992.
22. Peterson MC, Farr RW, Castiglia M. Prosthetic hip infection and bacteremia due to Campylobacter jejuni in a patient with AIDS. Clin Infect Dis 16: 439–440, 1993.
23. Blaser MJ, Perez GP, Smith PF, Patton C, Tenover FC, Lastovica AJ, Wang W-LL. Extraintestinal Campylobacter jejuni and Campylobacter coli infections: host factors and strain characteristics. J Infect Dis 153: 552–559, 1986.
24. McNulty CAM. The treatment of campylobacter infections in man. J Antimicrob Chemother 19: 281–284, 1987.
25. Sjögren E, Kaijser B, Werner M. Antimicrobial susceptibilities of Campylobacter jejuni and Campylobacter coli isolated in Sweden: a 10-year follow-up report. Antimicrob Agents Chemother 36: 2847–2849, 1992.
26. Rautelin H, Renkonen O-V, Kosunen TU. Emergence of fluoroquinolone resistance in Campylobacter jejuni and Campylobacter coli in subjects from Finland. Antimicrob Agents Chemother 35: 2065–2069, 1991.

Submitted November 7, 1994; accepted January 18, 1995

Scand J Infect Dis 27: 149–151, 1995 ORIGINAL ARTICLE

Helicobacter pylori Infection in Dentists – a Case-control Study

NICHOLAS BANATVALA[1], YASIN ABDI[2], LOUISA CLEMENTS[1], ANN-MARIE HERBERT[3], JUNE DAVIES[3], JEREMY BAGG[4], JONATHAN P. SHEPHERD[3], ROGER A. FELDMAN[1] and JEREMY M. HARDIE[2]

From the Departments of [1]Epidemiology and Medical Statistics and [2]Oral Microbiology, London Hospital Medical College, London, [3]Oral Surgery, Medicine & Pathology, University of Wales College of Medicine Dental School, Cardiff, [4]Oral Sciences, Glasgow Dental Hospital and School, Glasgow, UK

To test the null hypothesis that frequent and multiple salivary exposure is not a risk factor for developing H. pylori infection, serum anti-H. pylori IgG from 179 dentists and dental students and 179 age-, sex- and socioeconomic-matched controls were assayed using an ELISA. Seroprevalence in dentists was 16% (11/70); clinical dental students 6% (3/47); and pre-clinical dental students 10% (6/62). There were no differences in H. pylori seropositivity between cases and controls. There was an increase in H. pylori seropositivity with age (χ^2_{trend} 9.04, $p = 0.003$). These data provide evidence that adults are not at high risk of developing H. pylori infection as a result of exposures to saliva from multiple sources.

N. Banatvala, MD, Department of Epidemiology and Medical Statistics, London Hospital Medical College at QMW, Mile End Road, London E1 4NS, UK

INTRODUCTION

Helicobacter pylori frequently colonises the stomach in UK adults (1) and is a cause of type B gastritis and duodenal ulceration (2). In addition, H. pylori is associated with gastric ulcer disease and gastric cancer (3–5).

Transmission of H. pylori remains poorly understood. There is evidence to suggest that H. pylori is spread orally from person-to-person (6, 7) and H. pylori has been detected in saliva and dental plaque both by primary culture and PCR (8–10). It might therefore be expected that frequent and multiple salivary exposure is a risk factor for developing H. pylori infection. We tested the null hypothesis that frequent and multiple salivary exposure is not a risk factor for developing H. pylori infection by examining serum anti-H. pylori IgG from dentists and individually matched controls.

Although 2 other studies have suggested a lack of association between H. pylori seroprevalence and dentists (11, 12), neither study individually matched cases to controls and more importantly, as dentists are from high socio-economic class, neither included socio-economic status as a matched variable. Increasing age and low socio-economic status are 2 important risk factors for developing H. pylori infection.

MATERIALS AND METHODS

H. pylori seropositivity was compared in dentists, dental students and controls using sera collected for a previous study (13).

Case selection

Dentists. A mailed invitation to participate in the original study (13) was sent to 150 Dental Practitioners from Cardiff, Wales. Dentists from Cardiff were selected randomly from the General Dental Council Register. The response rate to participate in this study was 69% (103/150). Of the 103 sera initially collected, there was sufficient remaining sera from 70 (68%) of the dentists to test for H. pylori antibody in this study.

Clinical dental students. Clinical dental students from The University of Wales College of Medicine Dental School, Cardiff were invited prior to a lecture to enrol in the study. Of 60 invitations, 88% (53/60) agreed to participate (13). Of these 53 sera, 47 sera (89%) remained and were available for this study.

Pre-clinical dental students. Pre-clinical dental students from The University of Wales College of Medicine Dental School, Cardiff were invited prior to a lecture to enrol in the original study (13). Of 90 invitations, 90% (81/90) agreed to participate. Of these 81 sera, 62 sera (77%) remained and were available for this study.

Control selection.

The same age-, sex- and socio-economic-matched controls were used both in the original and this study. Socioeconomic status was determined using the England & Wales Registrar-General's occupation-based socio-economic measure. This social class classification has 6 categories from I and II (professional occupations) to V (unskilled occupations). Class III is divided into 2 categories. Controls had no significant past medical history.

Dentists and clinical dental student controls. Controls matched for age, sex and socio-economic status were obtained from 3 sources. First volunteers were recruited from staff working at the Welsh National Blood Transfusion Service, Rhydlafa, Cardiff, South Wales; second, from police officers attending a police training college in South Wales and third from patients attending clinics for routine dental treatment at The University of Wales College of Medicine Dental School, Cardiff.

Pre-clinical dental student controls. Controls matched for age, sex and socio-economic status were obtained from pharmacy and arts students attending Cardiff University.

Demographic details

All cases and controls were asked to complete a questionnaire that included demographic and occupational details.

Table I. *H. pylori seropositivity by age in dentists, clinical students, preclinical students and their controls*

	Dental practitioners		Clinical students		Pre-clinical students	
Age group	case	control	case	control	case	control
10–19[a]					4/43	1/43
20–29	4/31	6/31	3/47	3/47	2/19	5/19
30–39	4/18	5/18				
40–49	1/14	3/14				
50–59	2/5	0/5				
60+	0/2	2/2				
Total	11/70	18/70	3/47	3/47	6/62	6/62
Odds Ratio	0.6 (95% CI = 0.2–1.5)		1.0 (95% CI = 0.3–3.7)		1.0 (95% CI = 0.2–5.4)	
p value	0.2		1.0		1.0	

[a] No subjects below age 18 in this group.

H. pylori serology

H. pylori IgG status was determined using the ELISA with an H. pylori acid-glycine extract as antigen (14). All sera were run in duplicate, with negative and postive controls.

Statistical analyses

Initial power calculations, matched pair analyses, odds ratios, confidence intervals, multiple logistic regression and tests of statistical significance were calculated using Stata (Computing Resource Center, 1640 Fifth Street, Santa Monica, CA 90401, USA) and Epi-Info (CDC, Atlanta, GA 30333, USA).

RESULTS

Seroprevalence in dentists was 16% (11/70); clinical dental students 6% (3/47); and pre-clinical dental students 10% (6/62). There were no differences in H. pylori seropositivity between dentists and controls, clinical dental students and controls or pre-clinical dental students and their controls (Table I). There was no difference in the rates of seropositivity in cases and controls when the data for dentists and clinical students were combined. There was no significant difference in rates of H. pylori seropositivity between clinical and pre-clinical dental students.

Combining H. pylori seropositivity in cases and controls demonstrated an increase in H. pylori seropositivity with age (χ^2_{trend} 9.04, $p = 0.003$). There was no consistent gender difference in H. pylori seropositivity. There was no relationship between length of practice and H. pylori seropositivity, independent of age.

DISCUSSION

In this, the largest study assessing H. pylori seropositivity in dentists and dental students, members of the dental profession were not found to be at higher risk of H. pylori infection than age-, sex- and socio-economically-matched controls.

A total of 300 individuals were invited to participate in the original study (13). Of these individuals, 69% of dentists and 90% of dental students participated in that study (13). It is unlikely that the consenting individuals were different to non-consenting individuals with regards to H. pylori seropositivity. Selection would not have been influenced by either the presence or the absence of risk factors or symptoms associated with H. pylori infection.

The sera used in this study were a subset of the original study (13); 70 (68%) of 103 sera from dental practitioners were available for H. pylori antibody determination. The 70 sera were not unrepresentative of the sera from the 103 dentists initially bled. Data from the 70 available and the 33 unavailable sera were compared: there were no statistically significant age or gender differences between available and unavailable sera. In addition, there were no statistical differences in seropositivity between available and unavailable sera with respect to the following antibodies assayed previously (13, 15); herpes simplex virus 1 (HSV1), human herpes virus 6 (HHV6), influenza A, influenza B, adenovirus and respiratory syncytial virus (RSV).

Although this is the largest study assessing H. pylori seropositivity in dentists and dental students, the size of the serum bank was limited. As a result it is possible that the study failed to detect an increased risk of H. pylori seropositivity in dentists if such a difference really existed. Calculations based on an unmatched design and analysis prior to the study, suggested that if age-adjusted seroprevalence in the dental and clinical student controls was 49.2%, the same as a study based on Welsh individuals from Social Classes I and II (1), the study would detect a seroprevalence in dentists and clinical students of 68% (an odds ratio of 2.19) with 80% power at the 0.05% significant level. The effect of the matched design and analysis on the study was not undertaken as the degree of confounding removed by the match was unknown.

Although it was initially planned to select controls from one source, it became necessary to select controls from a variety of sources to ensure that close age- and socio-economic-matching with cases occurred. The control groups used in this study enable the higher prevalance of H. pylori infection seen in dentists compared with students to be explained as an age effect rather than as a result of increased exposure to H. pylori. These data suggest that adults are not at high risk of developing H. pylori infection as a result of exposure to saliva from multiple sources.

The sera from the dental practitioners and their controls were previously tested for IgG antibody to common viral agents. Unlike HSV1, CMV, EBV and HHV6, antobodies to influenza A, influenza B, adenovirus and RSV were significantly higher in dentists compared with controls (13, 15). Cytomegalovirus and herpes simplex virus type 1 are both agents transmitted by saliva but only transiently present in saliva; no difference in the seroprevalence of these 2 viruses was seen in dentists compared with controls. Interpretation of these data suggest that either H. pylori is not spread by saliva, or if it is then adults are at low risk of infection from saliva.

The 2 major determinants of H. pylori seropositivity are age and socio-economic status (1). H. pylori seropositivity in this series is lower than that in other UK studies (1, 16) and is probably a reflection of the high socio-economic status of dentists and dental students and that Sitas's study combined H. pylori seroprevalence from socio-economic groups I and II (1).

ACKNOWLEDGEMENTS

We thank all those participating subjects in the study. We thank Dr Gillian Urwin for her critical review of this manuscript.

REFERENCES

1. Sitas F, Forman D, Yarnell JW, Burr ML, Elwood PC, Pedley S, Marks KJ. Helicobacter pylori infection rates in relation to age and social class in a population of Welsh men. Gut 32: 25–28, 1991.
2. Warren JR, Marshall B. Unidentified curved bacilli on gastric epithelium in active chronic gastritis. Lancet 1: 1273–1275, 1983.
3. Taylor DN, Blaser MJ. The epidemiology of Helicobacter pylori infection. Epidemiol Rev 13: 42–59, 1991.
4. Forman D, Newell DG, Fullerton F, Yarnell JW, Stacey AR, Wald N, Sitas F. Association between infection with Helicobacter pylori and risk of gastric cancer: evidence from a prospective investigation. BMJ 302: 1302–1305, 1991.
5. Parsonnet J, Friedman GD, Vandersteen DP, Chang Y, Vogelman JH, Orentreich N, Sibley RK. Helicobacter pylori infection and the risk of gastric carcinoma. N Engl J Med 325: 1127–1131, 1991.
6. Banatvala N, Feldman R. The epidemiology of Helicobacter pylori: missing pieces in a jigsaw. CDR Review 3: R56–R59, 1993.
7. Drumm B, Perez Perez GI, Blaser MJ, Sherman PM. Intrafamilial clustering of Helicobacter pylori infection. N Engl J Med 322: 359–363, 1990.
8. Ferguson DA Jr, Li C, Patel NR, Mayberry WR, Chi DS, Thomas E. Isolation of Helicobacter pylori from saliva. J Clin Microbiol 31: 2802–2804, 1993.
9. Shames B, Krajden S, Fuksa M, Babida C, Penner JL. Evidence for the occurrence of the same strain of Campylobacter pylori in the stomach and dental plaque. J Clin Microbiol 27: 2849–2850, 1989.
10. Banatvala N, Lopez CR, Owen R, Abdi Y, Davies G, Hardie J, Feldman R. Helicobacter pylori in dental plaque. Lancet 341: 380, 1993.
11. Reiff A, Jacobs E, Kist M. Seroepidemiological study of the immune response to Campylobacter pylori in potential risk groups. Eur J Clin Microbiol Infect Dis 8: 592–596, 1989.
12. Malaty HM, Evans DJ Jr, Abramovitch K, Evans DG, Graham DY. Helicobacter pylori infection in dental workers: a seroepidemiology study. Am J Gastroenterol 87: 1728–1731, 1992.
13. Herbert AM, Davies KJ, Westmoreland D, Bagg J, Walker DM. The seroepidemiology of herpes virus infections among dental personnel. J Dent. [in press]
14. Newell DG, Johnston BJ, Ali MH, Reed PI. An enzyme-linked immunosorbent assay for the serodiagnosis of Campylobacter pylori-assisted gastritis. Scand J Gastroenterol Suppl 142: 53–57, 1988.
15. Davies KJ, Herbert AM, Westmoreland D, Bagg J. Seroepidemiological study of respiratory virus infections among dental surgeons. Br Dent J 176: 262–265, 1994.
16. Banatvala N, Mayo K, Megraud F, Jennings R, Deeks JJ, Feldman R. The cohort effect and Helicobacter pylori. J Infect Dis 168: 219–221, 1993.

Submitted November 22, 1994; accepted January 29, 1995

Scand J Infect Dis 27: 153–155, 1995 ORIGINAL ARTICLE

Capnocytophaga (Capnocytophaga ochracea group) Bacteremia in Hematological Patients with Profound Granulocytopenia

BRIAN KRISTENSEN[1], HENRIK C. SCHØNHEYDER[1,2], NIELS A. PETERSLUND[3], STEEN ROSTHØJ[4], NIELS CLAUSEN[5] and WILHELM FREDERIKSEN[6]

From the Departments of [1]Clinical Microbiology and [4]Pediatrics, Aalborg Hospital, Aalborg, and the Departments of [2]Clinical Microbiology, [3]Hematology and [5]Pediatrics, Aarhus University Hospital, Århus and the Department of [6]Clinical Microbiology, Statens Seruminstitut, Copenhagen, Denmark

The clinical and microbiological features of 7 cases of bacteremia due to Capnocytophaga (Capnocytophaga ochracea group) are reported. They were diagnosed during 1991–93 at three hospital clinics. Five patients were <10 years old and all had hematological disorders, 4 acute lymphoblastic leukemia and 1 each had aplastic anemia, non-Hodgkin lymphoma, and myelodysplastic syndrome. All were profoundly granulocytopenic with an absolute granulocyte count $<0.13 \times 10^9$/l, and all but 1 had oral lesions as a possible portal of entry. A favourable response to antibiotic therapy was recorded in all patients but one who, being profoundly granulocytopenic, rapidly succumbed to Pseudomonas aeruginosa septicemia. None of the isolates were beta-lactamase producers. In addition to penicillin the isolates were susceptible to broad-spectrum cephalosporins and ciprofloxacin, but resistant to aminoglycosides.

B. Kristensen, MD, National Center of Hygiene, Statens Seruminstitut, DK-2300 Copenhagen S, Denmark

INTRODUCTION

Capnocytophaga is a genus of fastidious Gram-negative rods occurring in the oral cavity (1). Species of the Capnocytophaga ochracea group (formerly CDC biogroup DF-1) have been reported to cause post-partum endometritis (2), septic arthritis (3), endocardititis (4) pericardial abscess (5), pleural empyema (6) and bacteremia (6–8). We present 7 cases of bacteremia with isolates belonging to the C. ochracea group diagnosed in granulocytopenic patients during a 3-year period at three Danish hospitals. Our purpose is to draw attention to pertinent clinical and microbiological aspects of Capnocytophaga bacteremia.

MATERIALS AND METHODS

Prompted by 2 cases of bacteremia at Aalborg Hospital in 1993, we identified 5 additional cases with similar bacterial isolates during the 3-year period 1991–93 by reviewing the laboratory files of the Departments of Clinical Microbiology at Aarhus University Hospital and Aalborg Hospital. The hospital records of the 7 patients were reviewed, particularly regarding underlying disease, length of hospital stay, leukocyte count, antibiotic treatment before and after the report of positive blood culture, oral pathology, and outcome. The blood isolates were obtained with 2 different blood culture systems, either Colorbact (Statens Seruminstitut, Copenhagen) (2 isolates) or Bactec NR 660® (Becton Dickinson Diagnostic Instrument Systems, Sparks, MD, USA) (5 isolates). Bacteriological diagnosis of C. ochracea was established according to the following test results: Gram-negative rods requiring CO_2 for growth, yellowish pigmentation on blood agar, gliding motility on blood agar, and production of neither oxidase, catalase nor indole. All strains fermented sucrose, raffinose and maltose, whereas their ability to ferment glucose, galactose, lactose and fructose varied. Most strains hydrolysed esculin and all exhibited β-galactosidase activity. Susceptibility testing was peformed on enriched chocolate agar with disc diffusion employing NeoSensitabs (Rosco Diagnostica, Taastrup, Denmark) (9, 10). Apart from one isolate lost on subculturing, all isolates were found to be fully susceptible to penicillin, ampicillin, cefuroxime, cefotaxime, imipenem and ciprofloxacin, but resistant to gentamicin and trimethoprim. No strains exhibited β-lactamase production when tested by a chromogenic assay (Nitrocefin, BBL, Microbiology Systems, Cockeysville, MD, USA).

RESULTS

The clinical characteristics of the 7 patients appear in Table I. Four were females and 3 males (age range from 2 to 70 years), 5 patients were <10 years old. All patients suffered from hematological disorders (for hematological diagnoses, see Table I) and were profoundly granulocytopenic at the time of positive blood culture with an absolute granulocyte count $<0.13 \times 10^9$/l. A body temperature >38.9°C was noted in 6 patients and an elevation of C-reactive protein (normal <10 mg/l) was seen in 6 patients (range: 90–162 mg/l) at the time of positive blood culture. In 2 patients, blood cultures were obtained on the day of admission and in 5 between day 13 and day 48. All but 1 had oral lesions; 4 with ulceration and 1 each with periodontitis and periodontal abscess, respectively. Six patients had received antibiotics before positive blood culture (range: 3–14 days) (Table I). In 5 cases, Capnocytophaga was isolated from blood culture bottles after 3 days of incubation and in 2 cases after 1 and 2 days, respectively. In all cases Capnocytophaga was isolated in pure culture, but in 3 cases other microorganisms (Pseudomonas aeruginosa,

 ISSN 0036-5548

Table I. *Clinical characteristics of patients with Capnocytophaga (Capnocytophaga ochracea group) bacteremia*

Case number	1	2	3	4	5	6	7
Sex	Female	Female	Female	Male	Male	Female	Male
Age (years)	9	5	2	17	70	2	8
Underlying disease	ALL[a]	ALL	Aplastic anemia	Non-Hodgkin lymphoma	Myelodys-plastic syndrome	ALL	ALL/AML[b]
Leukocyte-count ($\times 10^9$/l)	0.4	0.5	1.1	0.3	0.6	0.1	0.2
Absolute granulocyte-count ($\times 10^9$/l)	0	0	0	0.03	0.13	0	0
Oral lesion	Ulceration	Ulceration	Ulceration	Periodontitis	Periodontal abscess	Ulceration	None
Prior antibiotic therapy[c]	Fluconazole	Ampicillin Gentamicin Fluconazole	Ampicillin Ceftriaxone Vancomycin Fluconazole	Piperacillin Netilmicin Metronidazole Fluconazole	None	Ampicillin Gentamicin Fluconazole	Co-trimoxazole
Therapy[d]	Ceftazidime Methicillin	Ampicillin Gentamicin →[e] Ceftriaxone Vancomycin	Ceftriaxone Vancomycin → Ceftriaxone Gentamicin	Piperacillin Netilmicin → Ciproflocaxin	Penicillin G Netilmicin, Imipenem + cilastatin	Methicillin Metronidazole → Cefotaxime	Ampicillin Gentamicin Fluconazole Acyclovir
Outcome	Recovered	Recovered	Recovered	Recovered	Recovered	Died	Recovered

[a] Acute lymphoblastic leukemia.
[b] Acute myeloblastic leukemia.
[c] Antibiotics given within 14 days before cultivation of Capnocytophaga.
[d] Therapy given empirically and later changed according to cultivation of Capnocytophaga.
[e] Treatment changed to.

Candida species and Acinetobacter calcoaceticus) were isolated within 7 days of the Capnocytophaga isolation. All patients but 1 recovered from the septicemia with Capnocytophaga. The patient who did not recover was a 2-year-old girl with a granulocyte count $<0.1 \times 10^9$/l who had a fatal P. aeruginosa bacteremia 6 days after Capnocytophaga had been found.

DISCUSSION

Capnocytophaga are capnophilic microorganisms, and although C. ochracea is the commonly listed clinical isolate in humans, the bacteriological diagnosis may be valid only to the genus level due to problems in species differentiation (11, 12). Therefore the name C. ochracea group may be more appropriate. The CDC biogroup DF-2 has also been included into the genus as Capnocytophaga canimorsus, but this member of the canine oral flora are not a subject of this report.

In immunocompetent hosts, Capnocytophaga has mainly associated been with periodontitis (13) and localized infections of the respiratory tract (6). Systemic infections such as septicemia have been reported mostly in the immunocompromised host (6–8). Most of the listed cases were pediatric patients who were profoundly granulocytopenic, which agrees with our findings. Oral mucosal lesions and oral infections are frequently seen in hematological patients (14). We found oral lesions in the majority of our cases, but attempts to isolate Capnocytophaga from these lesions were not successful. This may be due to inappropriate culture methods and the slow growth of Capnocytophaga. Still, we consider the oral cavity the most likely portal of entry. The entry of Capnocytophaga into systemic circulation may be facilitated by a factor that impedes the active locomotion of granulocytes (15), as well as IgAl- and IgG-proteases that inactivate local humoral immune defence mechanisms (16).

A mortality of 43% (3/7) for patients with Capnocytophaga bacteremia has been noted (8), but as in a previous study (7) we found that the prognosis seemed to be more favourable. Just 1 of our 7 patients died and that was directly related to a subsequent P. aeruginosa bacteremia. This patient (case no. 6) had the most pronounced granulocytopenia.

Six patients were given appropriate antibiotics as part of empirical antibiotic treatment and this reflects the susceptibility to penicillin, broad-spectrum cephalosporins as well as fluoroquinolones. This profile of susceptibility is in agreement with other reports (10, 17, 18), whereas Capnocytophaga was resistant to aminoglycosides (10, 19).

Recently, a case of multidrug-resistant Capnocytophaga sputigena has been reported in a bacteremic granulocytopenic patient (20) and 6/19 Capnocytophaga isolates from clinical sources were β-lactamase producers (19). Our isolates remained susceptible, but the aforementioned reports underline the importance of being aware of emergence of antimicrobial resistance in new bacterial groups.

REFERENCES

1. Leadbetter ER, Holt SC, Socransky SS. Capnocytophaga: New genus of gram-negative gliding bacteria. I. General characteristics, taxonomic considerations and significance. Arch Microbiol 122: 9–16, 1979.
2. Paerregaard A, Gutschik E. Capnocytophaga bacteremia complicating premature delivery by cesarean section. Eur J Clin Microbiol 6: 580–581, 1987.
3. Winn RE, Chase WF, Lauderdale PW, McCleskey FK. Septic arthritis involving Capnocytophaga ochracea. J Clin Microbiol 19: 538–540, 1984.
4. Buu-Hoi AY, Joundy S, Acar JF. Endocarditis caused by Capnocytophaga ochracea. J Clin Microbiol 26: 1061–1062, 1988.
5. Matlow A, Vellend H. Capnocytophaga: A pathogen in immunocompetent hosts. J Infect Dis 152: 233–234, 1985.
6. Parenti DM, Snydman DR. Capnocytophaga species: Infections in nonimmunocompromised and imunocompromised hosts. J Infect Dis 151: 140–147, 1985.
7. Forlenza SW, Newman MG, Lipsey AI, Siegel SE, Blachman U. Capnocytophaga sepsis: A newly recognised clinical entity in granulocytopenic patients. Lancet i: 567–568, 1980.
8. Warren JS, Allen SD. Clinical, pathogenetic, and laboratory features of Capnocytophaga infections. Am J Clin Pathol 86: 513–518, 1986.
9. Casals JB, Pringler N. Antibacterial sensitivity testing using Neo-sensitabs. 9th edn. Taastrup, Denmark: Rosco 1991.
10. Bremmelgaard A, Pers C, Kristiansen JE, Korner B, Heltberg O, Frederiksen W. Susceptibility testing of Danish isolates of Capnocytophaga and CDC group DF-2 bacteria. APMIS 97: 43–48, 1989.
11. Kristiansen JE, Bremmelgaard A, Busk HE, Heltberg O, Frederiksen W, Justesen T. Rapid identification of Capnocytophaga isolated from septicemic patients. Eur J Clin Microbiol 3: 236–240, 1984.
12. Collins MD, Shah HN, McKee AS, Kroppenstedt RM. Chemotaxonomy of the genus Capnocytophaga (Leadbetter, Holt & Socransky). J Appl Bacteriol 52: 409–415, 1982.
13. Newman MG, Socransky SS, Savitt ED, Propas DA, Crawford A. Studies of the microbiology of periodontosis. J Periodontol 47: 373–379, 1976.
14. Bergman OJ. Oral infections and septicemia in immunocompromised patients with hematologic malignancies. J Clin Microbiol 26: 2105–2109, 1988.
15. Shurin SB, Socransky SS, Sweeny E, Stossel TP. A neutrophil disorder induced by Capnocytophaga, a dental micro-organism. N Engl J Med 301: 849–854, 1979.
16. Kilian M. Degradation of immunoglobulins A1, A2, and G by suspected principal periodontal pathogens. Infect Immun 34: 757–765, 1981.
17. Arlet G, Sanson-Le Pors MJ, Casin IM, Ortenberg M, Perol Y. In vitro susceptibility of 96 Capnocytophaga strains, including a beta-lactamase producer, to new beta-lactam antibiotics and six quinolones. Antimicrob Agents Chemother 31: 1283–1284, 1987.
18. Hawkey PM, Smith SD, Haynes J, Malnick H, Forlenza SW. In vitro susceptibility of Capnocytophaga species to antimicrobial agents. Antimicrob Agents Chemother 31: 331–332, 1987.
19. Roscoe DL, Zemcov SJV, Thornber D, Wise R, Clarke AM. Antimicrobial susceptibilities and beta-lactamase characterization of Capnocytophaga species. Antimicrob Agents Chemother 36: 2197–2200, 1992.
20. Gomez-Garces J-L, Alos J-I, Sanchez J, Cogollos R. Bacteremia by multidrug-resistant Capnocytophaga sputigena. J Clin Microbiol 32: 1067–1069, 1994.

Submitted October 17, 1994; accepted January 19, 1995

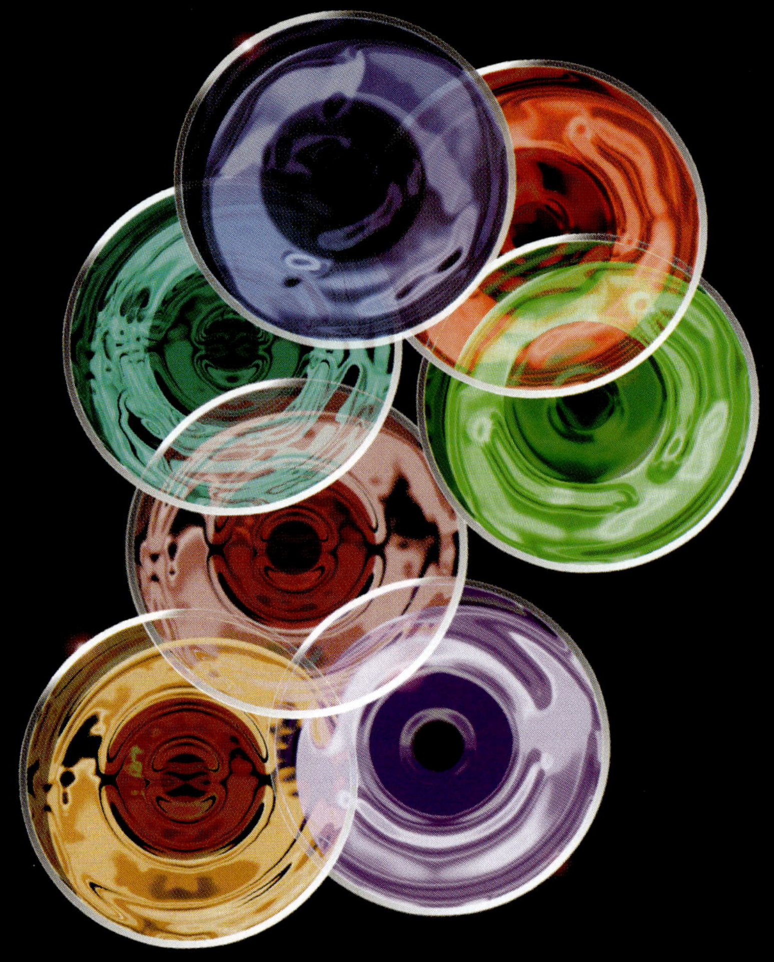

REFERENSER

Pizzo PA, Hathorn JW, Miemenz J et al. N Engl J Med 1986; 315: 552-8.
De Pauw BE, Feld R, Deresinski S et al. 6th International Symposium on infections in the immunocompromised Host. Peebles, Scotland June 3-6, 1990.
Novakova I, Donnelly P, de Pauw B. Scand J Infect Dis 22: 705-71 (1990)
Parr MD, Hansen LA, Rapp RP. Drug Intell Clin Pharm 1988; 22:628-31.
Mondorf AW, Mondorf W, Banzer S. 5th Mediterranean Congress of Chemotherapy, Cairo 1986: Abst. 0196.
Sanders JW, Powe NR, Moore RD. J Infect Dis 1991; 164:907:16.

Open Lung Biopsy Provides a Higher and More Specific Diagnostic Yield Compared to Broncho-Alveolar Lavage in Immunocompromised Patients

MICHAEL E. ELLIS[1], DAVID SPENCE[2], ABDERREZAK BOUCHAMA[1], JOHN ANTONIUS[3], MAHER BAZARBASHI[1], FAREED KHOUGEER[4], EDWARD B. DE VOL[5] and the FUNGAL STUDY GROUP*

From the Departments of [1]Medicine, [2]Oncology, [3]Pathology and Laboratory Services, [4]Cardiovascular Diseases, [5]Biomedical Statistics and Scientific Computing Department and [6]Radiology, King Faisal Specialist Hospital and Research Centre, Riyadh, Kingdom of Saudi Arabia

In order to examine the feasibility and safety of undertaking a larger prospective study to compare the diagnostic yield from concurrent open lung biopsy (OLB) and bronchoalveolar lavage (BAL) in febrile neutropenic patients with pulmonary infiltrates and the impact of such knowledge on clinical outcome, a pilot exploratory study was performed. 13 immunocompromised patients (mainly with haematological malignancy or bone marrow transplantation recipients) were investigated. At least one diagnostic finding in 12 of 13 patients was provided by OLB compared to 4 of 13 patients by BAL. BAL provided 7 specific diagnoses (pneumocystis 1, fungal infection 3, bacterial pneumonia 1, pulmonary haemorrhage 2) whilst OLB provided 12 specific diagnosis (CMV 2, pneumocystis 3, fungal infection 1, bacterial pneumonia 1, pulmonary haemorrhage 4, pulmonary embolism 1). Five patients with nonspecific interstitial/alveolar inflammation were diagnosed only by OLB. The concordance that the exact same specific diagnoses present in the OLB were found in the BAL was zero. There were 2 minor complications (1 wound infection by OLB, 1 moderate haemorrhage by BAL). Mortality at 28 days was 8 of 13 patients which in no case was related to either procedure. We suggest that OLB is a safe procedure in such patients, provides superior and more complete diagnostic information compared to BAL and a larger controlled study to investigate the impact of early OLB on the outcome of these patients appears to be justified.

M. Ellis, MD, Department of Medicine, King Faisal Specialist Hospital and Research Centre, Box 3354, Riyadh 11211, Kingdom of Saudi Arabia

INTRODUCTION

Pulmonary disease is a leading cause of death in immunocompromised patients and its management controversial. Empirical antimicrobial therapy is one approach but is unsatisfactory since pathogens or non-infectious processes responsible for the pulmonary infiltrates may not be appropriately treated, polymicrobial regimens are toxic, expensive and associated with emergence of resistant organisms. Attempting a specific diagnosis by an invasive technique most often fibreoptic bronchoscopy with bronchoalveolar lavage (BAL), and then directing specific treatment is another approach (1–3). However, variability in specificity and sensitivity of the findings have been reported (1, 3, 4–7). Although open lung biopsy (OLB) is generally accepted as the diagnostic gold standard, patients usually do not routinely undergo this procedure at an early stage in their illness because of concerns over technique-associated mortality and morbidity, but are often submitted to the procedure when other investigations have proved negative and they have advanced hypoxaemia and/or systemic toxicity. It is not known whether the high mortality rate in such immunocompromised patients is due to failure to make a specific diagnosis (and hence offer specific treatment) early enough in the course of the patient's illness and conversely, whether it can be improved by obtaining such information. However, before this issue can be addressed a catch-all diagnostic technique with the highest sensitivity and specificity together with an acceptable degree of technique-related moribidity and mortality needs to be established. Although information from retrospective studies has suggested that OLB will provide this there are no properly controlled prospective studies (1, 8–15). This pilot exploratory study was designed to gather preliminary information relating to safety and diagnostic yield of OLB and BAL performed concurrently, in order to assess the feasibility of embarking on such a larger study.

METHODS

Immunocompromised patients with suspected acute pulmonary opportunistic infection were sequentially recruited. The objective was to recruit the first 20 patients who fulfilled the admission criteria (see below) but an interim analysis would be performed if the investigators observed trends either related to safety or diagnostic issues. The study was approved by the Hospital's Clinical Protocol Committee.

* [2]Hugh Clink, [2]Peter Ernst, [1]Magid A. Halim, [6]Walther von Sinner

 ISSN 0036-5548

Patients were eligible if the following criteria were fulfilled: (a) age 14–65 years; (b) immunocompromised as a result of bone marrow or solid organ transplantation or leukaemia; (c) presumptive evidence of pulmonary infection (that is the presence of fever $\geq 38°C$, tachypnoea ≥ 20 breaths/min, cough $\pm$ sputum, auscultatory physical signs, crepitations, rhonchi, wheeze) and diffuse radiological infiltrates (presence of bilateral pulmonary infiltrates involving at least 4 zones); (d) non-response (that is continuing fever, non-improvement of clinical, radiological and ventilatory parameters of the pulmonary process) to broad spectrum antimicrobials. All patients received an amnioglycoside and a 3rd generation cephalosporin for 72 h, if no defervescence they then received in addition vancomycin for 72 h; if no defervescence then amphotericin B for at least 48 h.

The following patients were excluded from the study: those with (a) incorrectible coagulopathy; (b) ventilated with PEEP requirement of at least 20 cm; (c) those not giving their full informed consent.

After correction of coagulopathies with platelet transfusions and other appropriate blood products, the patient proceeded to general anaesthesia. Following induction, an appropriate sized bronchoscope was introduced without suction through the endotracheal tube into an appropriate segmental bronchus (corresponding to the area of maximal pulmonary infiltrate). A protected specimen brush (PSB) catheter was inserted through the bronchoscope, positioned in the appropriate terminal bronchiole, unsheathed, and brushing was performed. The brush was covered and withdrawn, and processed for culture. 50 mls of non-bacteriostatic normal saline at 37°C was then instilled into the same anatomical area, allowed to dwell for 15 s and aspirated into a sterile container. This was repeated until 200 mls had been infused. Immediately following these 2 procedures, the patient proceeded to open lung biopsy of the same segment via a small thoracotomy.

Specimen processing and analysis

The lung biopsy tissue (fresh), BAL and PSB specimen were sent to the laboratory. A piece of the tissue was removed under sterile technique and forwarded to the microbiology laboratory, as well as an aliquot of the BAL together with the PBB specimen.

Bacteriology

A Gram stain for bacteria and fungal hyphae and a Kinyoun stain for acid fast bacilli were performed on the BAL and OLB specimens. The PSB specimen, BAL and portions of the OLB were submitted for bacteriological, fungal and viral culture by standard techniques. The number of colony forming units/ml of bacteria in the specimen was measured. Semiquantitative bacteriological analysis of the brush was performed by aseptically removing the brush from the tubing. The brush was cut off and suspended in 1.0 ml sterile saline and agitated on a Vortex mixture for 2.0 min. Volumes of 0.1, 0.01 and 0.001 ml were plated on chocolate agar and incubated in a CO_2 incubator for 24–48 h. The number of colonies were counted and multiplied by the dilution factor. The isolates were identified by standard techniques. Biopsy tissues (1 g) for semiquantitative analysis were ground in 5 ml sterile saline and plated in 0.1, 0.01 and 0.001 ml quantities as stated above. Volumes of 0.1, 0.01 and 0.001 ml of BAL were used for semiquantitative bacteriological counts. Details of the methodology were the same as stated above for the brush specimen.

Cytological/histological evaluation of the BAL

The remainder of the BAL specimen was centrifuged at 1500 rpm × 10 min, and the sediment distributed between 10 slides, 6 of which were air dried and 4 fixed in methanol. The 6 air dried slides were stained for pneumocystis, fungal organisms, acid-fast bacilli, bacteria and iron. Of the 4 methanol fixed slides, 1 was stained by the Gruenwald-Giemsa method (Diff-Quick) and 3 post fixed in papanicolau stain. Evaluation of this material included the cell differential on the papanicolau smear (also studied for malignant cells and viral inclusions). The iron and papanicolaou stains were used to quantitate the number of macrophages and the intensity of the iron pigment.

Histological evaluation of OLB tissue

The tissue was fixed in formalin, paraffin embedded and sectioned the following day. The acid-fast, pneumocystis, Gomori-fungal, Gram's and hemosiderin (Prussian Blue) stains were performed. The intensity of color was graded 1 to 4 on the hemosiderin stain and this was subjectively assessed along with the number of alveolar histiocytes. When a few positively stained histiocytes were found, the appearance was graded 1 and not considered relevant. Any grading greater or equal to 2 through 4 was considered as indicating significant pulmonary haemorrhage (PH). Hematoxylin-eosin stains were screened for evidence of viral changes such as multi-nucleation and active nucleoli. CMV changes were identified by large nucleoli, nuclear halos and cytoplasmic granules. Other herpes changes were identified by ground glass glass nuclei. When suspicious, the tissue was stained with specific antibody by means of the immunoperoxidase technique. The presence of polymorphs, lymphocytes and plasma cells was noted and a search for malignant cells was made. The biopsy diagnosis was either specific, indicating the presence of an infectious agent, or non-specific. In the latter case, the presence of changes of non-specific lymphoid interstitial infiltration or swollen alveolar lining cells detached from the alveolar wall containing fluid/fibrin exudate of diffuse interstitial fibrosis in the absence of a diagnosis were classified as non-specific interstitial/alveolar inflammation (NSIAI: non-specific changes).

Statistical analysis

The analysis consisted of comparing the OLB findings with those from the BAL and assumed that OLB provided 100% sensitivity and specificity for any pulmonary diagnosis present or absent. It was performed in the following ways:

Analysis of patients

It was examined which patients were found to have the exact same specific diagnosis (or diagnoses, in the case of patients with multiple specific diagnoses) from the OLB and the BAL. This could be considered as a stringent measure of BAL sensitivity among patients.

Analysis of diagnostic occurrences

First, a comparison was made for which the unit of analysis was occurrence of some specific diagnosis (for which there were 11 such occurrences – see results section), and examined was the number of those in which both the OLB and the BAL yielded some specific diagnosis. This would be a gross measure of BAL sensitivity for whenever some specific diagnosis existed. Second, a comparison was made for which the unit of analysis was investigation for pneumocystis. The motivation behind this comparison is as follows. For each patient, both OLB and BAL were employed to detect whether pneumocystis was present or not. To the extent that BAL detected pneumocystis for a patient in which OLB also detected it, then BAL would be sensitive for pneumocystis. This same comparison was also carried out for the other specific diagnoses.

In each of the 3 instances above (the analysis of patients and the 2 types of analyses of diagnostic occurrences) the findings from the BAL were compared to those of the OLB by using a 2 × 2 contingency table in which 1 margin of the table recorded the findings from the OLB and the other recorded that from the BAl. (Note, in the statistical analyses, comparisons were made between patients with, or occurrences of, only those opportunistic infections or pathological processes which have the potential of being diagnosed by BAL. Therefore, NSIAI was excluded from this.)

RESULTS

It was decided to perform an interim analysis once the 13th patient had been recruited, since it was perceived that the OLB appeared to be yielding more information than the BAL. 11 of the 13 patients were immunocompromised as a result of haematological malignancy/bone marrow transplantation/aplastic anaemia and 2 had solid organ transplants (1 liver, 1 renal). Demographic patient data are given in Table I.

Our patients had been febrile for at least (since some patients were admitted from another institution already febrile) 9.5 ± 4.5 days (range 1–21 days) prior to the surgical procedure. 10 patients had a platelet count below the normal range immediately prior to the surgery the mean platelet count being 68.6 ± 68.2 × 10^9/L (range 8–207, normal = 150–430). In 8 patients who received platelet infusions, the mean platelet count at operation was 72.1 ± 31.6 (range 43–132) × 10^9/L. The prothrombin time was prolonged in 8 patients – the mean for the group as a whole was 15.68 ± 3.64 seconds (normal = 11–14.4).

The recovery volume of fluid from the BAL was between 60 to 80% of that instilled. Results of the analysis of cell type were available from 12 of the 13 patients (Table II) (1 specimen was damaged during processing). The cell count was raised in all 12 patients, showing predominance of lymphocytes (1 patient), polymorphs (5 patients) and macrophages (6 patients). There was no obvious relationship between the cell type and the findings on open lung biopsy.

OLB provided at least 1 definite diagnosis in 12 of these 13 patients (92%) compared to BAL which provided a definite diagnosis in 4 of 13 patients (31%) (Table II). Among these 12 patients there were 17 different diagnoses (12 specific, 5 non-specific). Eight of these 12 patients had at least 1 specific finding – compared to 7 specific findings from BAL in 4 of the 13 patients. Infections were diagnosed by OLB in 6 patients (7 instances, 1 patient had 2 different pathogens), pulmonary haemorrhage in 4 patients, pulmonary embolism in 1 patient and non-specific interstitial/alveolar inflammation (NSIAI) in 5 patients. Infections were diagnosed by BAL in 4 patients (5 instances, 1 patient had 2 different pathogens), and pulmonary haemorrhage confidently in 2 patients. The sensitivity of BAL for yielding the exact same specific diagnosis/diagnoses as provided by OLB was 0/8 (0%) (95% Cl 0.0% to 36.9%) i.e. in no patient did the BAL identify all the specific diagnoses that were detected by OLB. At best, BAL detected the same 2 specific diagnoses in 1 patient (patient no 6) that were present at OLB, but falsely diagnosed fungal infection.

Table I. *Demographic data on the 13 patients included*

No	Sex	Age (yr)	Underlying disease
1	M	32	Aplastic Anaemia
2	M	39	Hodgkins
3	M	25	BMT(CGL)
4	M	36	Liver Tx
5	M	27	AML/Lymphoma
6	M	15	BMT (AML)
7	M	30	BMT (AML)
8	M	46	Renal Tx
9	M	25	ALL
10	F	38	BMT(Aplastic anaemia)
11	F	21	AML/Lymphoma
12	F	48	BMT (NHL)
13	F	18	Aplastic Anaemia

Tx = transplant, BMT = bone marrow transplant, CGL = chronic granulocytic leukemia, AML = acute myeloid leukemia, ALL = acute lymphocytic leukemia, NHL = non-hodgkin's lymphoma.

BAL was not able to diagnose any of the patients with NSIAI seen on OLB – however, these 5 patients had either uncertain findings ("pulmonary haemorrhage" – 4 patients) or false fungal diagnosis (2 patients) on the BAL.

If the results are analysed in terms of detecting each of the individual specific diagnoses (diagnostic occurrences) proven by OLB, (a total of 12), BAL sensitivity was 5/12 (42%) (95% Cl, 15.1% to 72.3%). The individual sensitivity figures for pneumocystis, cytomegalovirus, pulmonary haemorrhage, fungus, bacterial pneumonia and pulmonary embolism were 33%, 0%, 50%, 100%, 100% and 0% respectively.

There were 2 patients with complications – 1 with a thoracotomy site infection which resolved and 1 with moderate bleeding following bronchoscopy which resolved following infusions of platelets and coagulation factors.

Eight of the 13 patients died (6 from sepsis) within 28 days of the procedures but the cause of death was not related to either procedure in any patient.

Eight of 13 patients received modification of their antimicrobial regime as a result of the OLB. Patient 1 was receiving empirical antibiotic treatment for antibiotic resistant neutropenic fever – neither the BAL nor the OLB confirmed fungal elements and amphotericin B was discontinued on the basis of these findings. The patient, however, died of biopsy confirmed fungal brain abscess 18 days later. Patient 11 died from CMV pneumonia (confirmed by follow-up BAL) 21 days following the BAL/OLB findings which were originally negative for cytomegalovirus.

The protected specimen brush (PSB) revealed 2,000 cfu/ml of Pseudomonas spp in 1 patient (pneumonia confirmed by OLB). In 5 other patients, organisms were found by PSB, but the quantitative culture count was < 10^3 cfu/ml and in none of these patients was bacterial pneumonia confirmed at OLB.

Table II. *Results of BAL and OLB performed concurrently in the 13 patients*

No	BAL Cytology	BAL Diagnosis	OLB Diagnosis	ALT Mx	Survival (days)	Notes
1	M	?-PH	NSIAI	+	18	Fungal brain abscess
2	P	Neg	PCP	+	28	Staph sepsis
3	P	?-PH	NSIAI	+	19	Intracran haem
4	M	Neg	CMV; PCP	+	>100	0
5	ND	?-PH	NSIAI	0	10	Gram negative sepsis
6	M	PCP; Fungi; PH	PCP; PH	+	>220	Relapse of AML
7a	M	PH	Aspergillus; PH	+	>200	0
8	P	Bacterial* pneumonia	PH; Bacterial pneumonia	0	14	Idiopathic PH
9	M	?-PH	PE	0	>21	0
10	P	Neg	CMV	+	14	Multiorgan failure
11	P	Fungal	PH; NSIAI	+	21	CMV pneumonia
12b	M	Neg	Neg	0	3	Sepsis MOF
13	L	?PH	NSIAI	0	5	Sepsis MOF

PH = pulmonary haemorrhage, PCP = pneumocystis carinii pneumonia, NSIAI = non-specific interstitial/alveolar inflammation, ALT Mx = management altered by findings of OLB, MOF = multi-organ failure, * = diagnosed by PSB, PE = pulmonary embolism, a = thoracotomy infection, b = brush bleeding, M = macrophage, P = polymorph, L = lymphocyte, ND = not done.

DISCUSSION

The diagnostic yield and technique-related morbidity and mortality of both BAL and OLB may be dependent upon the clinical operator's technical skills, specimen processing and the pathologist's methodology and expertise. Such factors may account for the variability in published results. In addition, data from OLB/BAL procedures cannot be precisely compared in the situations where they have been performed at different stages of the patient's illness, by different operators or where the results have been compared from different centers (1, 8, 9, 16). By concurrently performing the 2 techniques in a standardised fashion by the same operator and processing the specimens by standard protocols in the same laboratory and reading the histopathology by 1 person (JA) it was hoped to minimize the influence of such variables. Our results suggest that OLB may be performed safely with minimum technique-related morbidity and mortality despite the adverse immunocompromisation and coagulation status in the majority of our patients. This is in accord with other published data, which suggest safety of OLB is at least on a par with transbronchial biopsy or fine needle aspiration, although some series had reported a higher incidence of complications (1, 9, 11, 17–19). Direct control of bleeding, control of pneumothorax and adequate sampling of tissue are major advantages of OLB over blind transbronchial biopsy (hence transbronchial biopsy was not done in any of our patients). However, in patients with uncontrolled coagulopathy or other contraindications to OLB then BAL may be preferred. The common reluctance to perform OLB through fear of substantial mortality and morbidity is not substantiated by our findings.

The PSB gave a diagnosis of pseudomonas pneumonia (confirmed by open lung biopsy) in 1 patient. There were no false positive/negative findings from this technique in any patient, confirming its usefulness for the diagnosis of bacterial pneumonia.

This study has supported previous findings that OLB provides a high diagnostic yield; in only 1 patient was no information forthcoming. Two thirds of these diagnoses were specific for pathogenic or non-infectious processes. The study further demonstrates that both the yield of specific diagnoses and the concordance of the diagnoses provided by BAL compared to concurrent open lung biopsy is much less. Only 1 previously published study prospectively examined the diagnostic utility of OLB compared to BAL performed synchronously (13). In that study of 15 bone marrow transplant recipients, BAL gave a 33% yield (all CMV) compared to 60% (CMV mainly, a few patients with fungal disease and pulmonary haemorrhage) for OLB. Our study supports these findings that OLB is a more useful diagnostic tool.

If antimicrobial management had been based on BAL findings alone, failure to treat 2 patients with pneumocystis carinii pneumonia and 2 patients with cytomegalovirus pneumonia would have resulted.

The diagnostic information provided by OLB led to discontinuation of or adding antimicrobial therapy in 8 patients. Patient 9 (pulmonary embolism) is of some interest since the presentation mimicked an infectious process and may have been overlooked, if OLB had not been performed. In patient 1, neither the BAL nor the OLB revealed the presence of a fungal organism, and, on the basis of this finding, amphotericin B was discontinued. The patient died 18 days later with biopsy proven fungal brain abscess. A likely source was the lower respiratory tract and if this indeed was the case, then it highlights the fear that even OLB can fail to diagnose some opportunistic infections (6, 9, 12). Discontinuation of the amphotericin B in this patient cannot be excluded as a factor leading to his death. Patient 11 died of proven CMV pneumonia 3 weeks after BAL and OLB was negative for this pathogen. In this case, however, CMV infection may have supervened after the OLB had bee performed.

The high mortality rate in this series raises the question as to whether the acquisition of optimal diagnostic data and subsequent alteration in management has any impact on outcome. Although alteration in management often occurs as a result of the information provided by the OLB (9, 20) conflicting evidence exists regarding the impact on the patient's outcome (12, 14, 21). However, many such studies were published 10–15 years ago when some important antimicrobial agents including ganciclovir, liposomal amphotericin B and colony stimulating factors were not available. Recent studies have suggested that clinically significant benefit accrues from OLB one-third of patients (9, 11). Delay in performing invasive diagnostic procedures may contribute to the adverse outcome of these patients (12). Patients with diffuse pulmonary infiltrates may deteriorate more rapidly than those with local disease, and if OLB has any chance of influencing survival, it should be done early (20). However, in some patients e.g., bone marrow transplant recipients, diagnostic yield may be significantly lower if investigations are performed too early (22). We chose, however, to investigate our patients after an initial therapeutic trial of broad spectrum antibiotics and antifungals since some patients may have had bacterial bronchopneumonia or very early fungal infection and might be expected to respond to such an empirical approach. Clearly the optional timing of diagnostic intervention remains conjectural.

This initial exploratory study suggests that OLB may be safely performed in most immunocompromised patients with febrile pulmonary infiltrates, and the diagnostic yield from OLB is higher than BAL. The result should provide a basis for a larger prospective study in which further information related to technique-related morbidity and mortality can be obtained, as well as assessing of the impact the knowledge of specific diagnosis on patient outcome.

ACKNOWLEDGEMENTS

We are grateful to our colleagues for reporting on their patients; and to Ms Bernadette Martinez for her secretarial assistance.

REFERENCES

1. Wilson WR, Cockerill FR, Rosenow III EC. Pulmonary disease in the immuncompromised host. Mayo Clin Proc 60: 610–631, 1985.
2. Blic de J, Mckelvie P, Bourgeois le M, Blanche S, Benoist MR, Scheinmann. Value of bronchoalveolar lavage in the management of severe acute pneumonia and interstitial pneumonitis in the immunocompromised child. Thorax 42: 759–765, 1987.
3. Stover DE, Zaman MB, Hajdu Sl, Lange M, Gold J, Armstrong D. Bronchoalveolar lavage in the diagnosis of diffuse pulmonary infiltrates in the immunosuppressed host. Ann Intern Med 101: 1–7, 1984.
4. Cordonnier C, Bernaudin J-F, Fleury J, Feuilhade M, Haoiun C, Payen D, Huet Y, Atassi K, Vernant J-P. Diagnostic yield of bronchoalveolar lavage in pneumonitis occurring after allogeneic bone marrow transplantation. Am Rev Respir Dis 132: 1118–1123, 1985.
5. Milburn HJ, Prentice HG, Bois du RM. Role of bronchoalveolar lavage in the evaluation of interstitial pneumonitis in recipients of bone marrow transplants. Thorax 42: 766–772, 1987.
6. Crawford SW, Bowden RA, Hackman RC, Gleaves CA, Meyers JD, Clark JG. Rapid detection of cytomegalovirus pulmonary infection by bronchoalveolar lavage and centrifugation culture. Ann Intern Med 108: 180–85, 1988.
7. Ruutu P, Ruutu T, Volin L, Tukiainen P, Ukkonen P, Hovi T. Cytomegalovirus is frequently isolated in bronchoalveolar lavage fluid of bone marrow transplant recipients without pneumonia. Ann Intern Med 112: 913–16, 1990.
8. Cockerill III FR, Wilson WR, Carpenter HA, Smith TF, Rosenow III EC. Open lung biopsy in immunocompromised patients. Arch Intern Med 145: 1398–1404, 1985.
9. Snyder CL, Ramsay NK, McGlave PB, Ferrell KL, Leonard AS. Diagnostic open-lung biopsy after bone marrow transplantation. J Ped Surg 25: 871–877, 1990.
10. Venn GE, Kay PH, Midwood CJ, Goldstraw P. Open lung biopsy in patients with diffuse pulmonary shadowing. Thorax 40: 931–935, 1985.
11. Gururangan S, Lawson RAM, Morris Jones PH, Stevens RF, Campbell RHA. Evaluation of the usefulness of open lung biopsies. Pediatr Hematol Oncol 9: 107–113, 1992.
12. Rossiter SJ, Miller C, Churg AM, Carrington CB, Mark JBD. Open lung biopsy in the immunosuppressed patient. Is it really beneficial? J Thorac Cardiovasc Surg 77: 338–345, 1979.
13. Springmeyer SC, Hackman RC, Holle R, Greenberg GM, Weems CE, Myerson D, Meyers JD, Thomas ED. Use of bronchoalveolar lavage to diagnose acute diffuse pneumonia in the immunocompromised host. J Infect Dis 154: 604–610, 1986.
14. Haverkos HW, Dowling JN, Pasculle AW, Myerowitz RL, Lerberg DB, Hakala T. Diagnosis of pneumonitis in immunocompromised patients by open lung biopsy. Cancer 52: 1093–1097, 1983.
15. Burt ME, Flye W, Webber BL, Wesley RA. Prospective evaluation of aspiration needle, cutting needle, transbronchial, and open lung biopsy in patients with pulmonary infiltrates. Ann Thorac Surg 32: 146–153, 1981.
16. Toledo-Pereyra LH, DeMeester TR, Kincaley I, MacMahon H, Churg A, Colomb H. The benefits of open lung biopsy in patients with previous non-diagnostic transbronchial lung biopsy. A guide to appropriate therapy. Chest 77: 647–650, 1980.
17. Prober CG, Whyte H, Smith CR. Open lung biopsy in immunocompromised children with pulmonary infiltrates. Am J Dis Child 138: 60–63, 1984.
18. Graeve AH, Saul VA, Akl BF. Role of different methods of lung biopsy in the diagnosis of lung lesions. Am J Surg 140: 742–746, 1980.
19. Gaensler EA, Carrington CB. Open biopsy for chronic diffuse

infiltrative lung disease: clinical, roentgenographic, and physiological correlations in 502 patients. Ann Thorac Surg 30: 411–426, 1980.
20. Mason WH, Siegel SE, Tucker BL. Diagnostic open lung biopsy for diffuse pulmonary disease in immunocompromised pediatric patients. Am J Pediatr Hematol Oncol 4: 355–359, 1982.
21. Puksa S, Hutcheon MA, Hyland RH. Usefulness of transbronchial biopsy in immunosuppressed patients with pulmonary infiltrates. Thorax 38: 146–150, 1983.
22. Crawford SW, Hackman RC, Clark JG. Open lung biopsy diagnosis of diffuse pulmonary infiltrates after marrow transplantation. Chest 94: 949–953, 1988.

Submitted August 22, 1994; accepted December 8, 1994

Scand J Infect Dis 27: 163–164, 1995

Serological Screening for Toxoplasmosis in Pregnancy in Slovenia

JERNEJ LOGAR[1], ŽIVA NOVAK-ANTOLIČ[2] and ANDREJ ZORE[2]

From the [1]Institute of Microbiology, Department of Parasitology, Medical Faculty, University of Ljubljana and the [2]Department of Gynaecology and Obstetrics, Medical Centre, Ljubljana, Slovenia

In the period from 1981 to 1994, serological screening for toxoplasmosis was carried out in 20,953 pregnant women in Slovenia. Seropositivity among pregnant women was found to have decreased from 52% in the 1980s to 37% in the recent period, 1991–94, while during the same period the incidence of suspected primary infections acquired in pregnancy rose from 0.33% to 0.75%. These latest figures ought to promote an informed debate on the possible need for obligatory serological screening of pregnant women in Slovenia for toxoplasmosis.

J. Logar, MD, Institute of Microbiology, Medical Faculty, Zaloška* 4, 61105 *Ljubljana, Slovenia

INTRODUCTION

Toxoplasmosis, especially its congenital form caused by the parasite Toxoplasma gondii, is a universal health problem. Primary infection acquired in pregnancy may result in severe fetal morbidity and even death. Congenital toxoplasmosis can only be prevented by informing women on how to avoid infection during pregnancy (primary prevention), or by routine serological screening of pregnant women (secondary prevention) for a recent Toxoplasma infection, which renders prenatal diagnosis and timely treatment possible. In keeping with these observations and in view of the estimated prevalence and incidence of Toxoplasma infection in pregnant women and congenital toxoplasmosis in Slovenia, primary prevention and serological screening was proposed in the early 1980s (1).

MATERIAL AND METHODS

Non-obligatory serological screening of pregnant women for toxoplasmosis, similar to the screening program in Austria, has been practised in Slovenia since 1981 (2–5). From May 1981 to end-September 1994, 20,953 pregnant women attending antenatal clinics from all parts of Slovenia, were tested for Toxoplasma infection. Serological tests were performed at the Institute of Microbiology, Medical Faculty of Ljubljana.

Three years ago, the basic screening dye test (SFT) was replaced by the indirect fluorescent antibody test (IFAT). Our current policy is to test pregnant women as soon as possible, at the latest by 10–12 weeks of gestation. Those who are seronegative on the first visit, are re-tested at 20–24 weeks and in the 3rd trimester of pregnancy in order to detect possible acute infection acquired in pregnancy. Women with a positive low-titre antibody test (1:16, 1:64 and 1:256) are re-tested 2 to 3 weeks later for definitive confirmation or ruling out of a probable previous infection. In women with titres $\geqslant 1024$, or seroconversion, suspected of having acquired recent infection during pregnancy, repeat testing is done on the first serum sample, as well on another sample obtained as soon as possible. In addition, primary infection is evaluated by testing for detection of specific IgM antibodies (Sanofi Diagnostics Pasteur). Recently, tests were introduced for detection of IgA antibodies (Sanofi Diagnostic Pasteur) and for determination of circulating antigens (Novum Diagnostica). Women primarily infected with Toxoplasma are treated with pyrimethamine and sulphadiazine with addition of folinic acid. Spiramycin is used before the 20th gestational week. All primarily infected women are followed up at the Department of Gynaecology and Obstetrics, University Medical Centre, Ljubljana (6).

RESULTS

Over a period of 14 years, 20,953 pregnant women were tested for toxoplasmosis in Slovenia, 55% of whom were found to be seronegative, while 0.60% were suspected of having acquired primary infection during pregnancy. Interestingly, infection rates have considerably decreased during the past 14 years, i.e. from 52% at the early 1980s (1981–85) to 37% in the recent period 1991–94, while seronegativity among pregnant women of all age groups has increased, from 48% to 63%. In the same period, the proportion of pregnant women with suspected primary infection increased from 0.33% to 0.75% (Table I).

DISCUSSION

It is well known that the incidence rate of Toxoplasma gondii infection depends on the prevailing climatic conditions and consequently varies from one geographic area to another. Factors related to the life style of the population seem to be of epidemiological significance in this infection.

Table I. *Results of screening for toxoplasmosis in pregnancy in Slovenia*

Study period	Screened *n*	Seronegative *n* (%)	Primary infections *n* (%)
1981–85	5,108	2,460 (48)	8 (0.33)
1986–90	7,591	3,859 (51)	22 (0.57)
1991–94	8,254	5,204 (63)	39 (0.75)
Total	20,953	11,523 (55)	69 (0.60)

 ISSN 0036-5548

A study carried out in Israel in 1993 showed a 21% prevalence rate for Toxoplasma antibodies in women of childbearing age. The seropositivity rate detected was lower than was found 20 years earlier. The incidence rate for infection acquired in pregnancy, which had previously not been determined in Israel, was 1.4% (7). A decrease in Toxoplasma seropositivity in pregnant women was also reported by several European investigators. In Switzerland, the incidence of antibody positivity fell from 52.7% in 1982 to 42.6% in 1992. Toxoplasma seropositivity in pregnant women in Belgium decreased from 70% in 1966 to 47% in 1987, but there was also a decrease in the rate of seroconversions, from 6.4% to 1.2% (8, 9). Aspöck and Pollak found that seropositivity among pregnant women in Austria had decreased, from nearly 50% in the late 1970s to 36.7% in recent years (1989–91). In the same period, however, the incidence of suspected primary infections acquired in pregnancy rose from less than 0.4% to 0.83% (10).

The incidence and prevalence of Toxoplasma antibodies in pregnant women in Slovenia and Austria were found to be nearly identical, most probably because of similarities in climatic conditions and life styles of the 2 populations. In Slovenia, seropositivity among pregnant women fell from 52% in 1981 to 37% in the period 1991–94, while in the same period, the incidence rate of suspected primary infections in pregnancy increased from 0.33% to 0.75%. The observed decline in the seropositive prevalence rate may be due to a general improvement in personal hygiene in the intervening period. In Slovenia the incidence rate of 0.75% for infections acquired during pregnancy might be expected to increase in the future if there is a continuing decrease in the prevalence of seropositivity in women of reproductive age, leading to a larger proportion of high-risk population in that group.

The results of screening of pregnant women for toxoplasmosis in Slovenia should defray the cost of obligatory preventive screening for this infection in pregnancy.

REFERENCES

1. Logar J. Prevention of congenital toxoplasmosis. Zdrav Vestn 50: 295–97, 1981.
2. Logar J. Congenital toxoplasmosis in Slovenia. Zdrav Vestn 54: 369–73, 1985.
3. Thalhammer O, Heller-Szöllösy E. Erfahrungen mit routinemässigem Toxoplasma-Screening bei Schwangeren zwecks Verhütung angeborener Toxoplasmose. Eine prospektive Untersuchung. Wien Klin Wochenschr 91: 20–25, 1979.
4. Aspöck H, Flamm H. Die Toxoplasmose-Überwachung während der Schwangerschaft. apibio Merieux-Monographien I: 10–26, 1984.
5. Aspöck H. Toxoplasmosis. In: WHO, ed. Prenatal and perinatal infections. Report on a WHO meeting, Graz, 24–26 May, 1982. EURO Reports and Studies 93: 43–51, 1985.
6. Logar J, Novak-Antolič Ž, Zore A, Cerar V, Likar M. Incidence of congenital toxoplasmosis in the republic of Slovenia. Scand J Infect Dis 24: 105–108, 1992.
7. Franklin DM, Dror Z, Nishri Z. The prevalence and incidence of Toxoplasma antibodies in pregnant women. Isr J Med Sci 29: 285–86, 1993.
8. Berger R, Stürchler D, Rudin C. Cord blood screening for congenital toxoplasmosis: detection and treatment of asymptomatic newborns in Basel, Switzerland. Scand J Infect Dis Suppl 84: 46–50, 1992.
9. Thoumsin H, Senterre J, Lambotte R. Twenty-two years screening for toxoplasmosis in pregnancy: Liège-Belgium. Scand J Infect Dis Suppl 84: 84–85, 1992.
10. Aspöck H, Pollak A. Prevention of prenatal toxoplasmosis by serological screening of pregnant women in Austria. Scand J Infect Dis Suppl 84: 32–38, 1992.

Submitted November 11, 1994; accepted December 18, 1994

Scand J Infect Dis 27: 165–169, 1995

CASE REPORT

Cytomegalovirus Ventriculoencephalitis in AIDS Patients

ALBERT SALAZAR[1], DANIEL PODZAMCZER[1], RAMON REÑE[2], MIGUEL SANTIN[1], JOSE LUIS PEREZ[3], ISIDRE FERRER[4], PEDRO FERNANDEZ-VILADRICH[1] and FRANCESC GUDIOL[1]

From the [1]Infectious Disease, [2]Neurology, [3]Microbiology Services, and the [4]Neuropathology Unit, Ciutat Sanitaria de Bellvitge, University of Barcelona, Barcelona, Spain

We report 4 autopsy-proven cases of cytomegalovirus ventriculoencephalitis (CMV-VE) and a further case with dramatic clinical and radiological response to ganciclovir therapy. The diagnoses were based upon clinical features, cerebrospinal fluid (CSF) examination and either brain computerized tomography (CT) or magnetic resonance imaging (MRI), and confirmed by autopsy findings in 4 cases. All patients had previously had an AIDS-defining condition. CMV retinitis was diagnosed in 3 patients, 2 of them before the onset of encephalitis. CMV viremia was present in 4 patients. Examination of CSF demonstrated elevated protein and hypoglycorachia in all cases. CSF culture was negative for CMV in 3 of 3 patients. Periventricular enhancement was detected by MRI in 2 of 3 patients, but in only 1 of 5 patients by CT. Three patients received ganciclovir and 2 patients foscarnet therapy. All 4 patients died. Pathologic examination revealed periventriculitis with ependymal necrosis and CMV intranuclear inclusion bodies all 4 patients. One showed a marked neurological improvement and radiological resolution by MRI after 4 weeks of ganciclovir therapy. We conclude that CMV-VE should be suspected in HIV-infected patients who present with altered neurological status, CMV viremia or retinitis, hypoglycorachia and ventriculitis as demonstrated by MRI. Although more effective therapy is needed, ganciclovir may be beneficial, as shown in one of our patients.

D. Podzamczer, MD, Infectious Diseases Service, Ciutat Sanitaria de Bellvitge, Feizxa Llarga s/n, 08907 L'Hospitalet de Llobregat, Barcelona, Spain

INTRODUCTION

Autopsy series have shown evidence of central nervous system (CNS) infection by CMV in about 30% of AIDS patients (1), whereas antemortem diagnosis of CMV infection of the CNS is uncommon. Thus, most cases of autopsy-diagnosed CMV encephalitis are not suspected in vivo. Known CMV neurological manifestations in AIDS patients include ascending lumbosacral polyradiculopathy (2–4) and meningoencephalitis (5–8).

We report 4 autopsy-proven cases of CMV-VE and a presumed case with a dramatic clinical and radiological response to ganiclovir therapy. The charts of these 5 patients have been reviewed, concentrating on their clinical features, CSF findings, and brain imaging studies.

CASE REPORTS

Case 1

A 40-year-old homosexual (HS) man with AIDS presented in April 1992 with headache and fever of 1 month's duration. Pneumocystis carinii pneumonia (PCP) and cutaneous Kaposi sarcoma (KS) had developed 17 and 15 months earlier, respectively. CMV retinitis had been diagnosed 8 months earlier, and he received ganciclovir therapy, followed by a maintenance dose of 10 mg/kg 3 days a week. A CD4 cell count was $7 \times 10^6/l$.

On admission, body temperature was 37.2°C. He was lethargic, and mildly confused. Sensory and motor examination were normal. A CT scan of the head showed cerebral atrophy. CSF Data are given in Table I. Cryptococcal antigen detection in CSF was negative, as were bacterial, mycobacterial, viral, and fungal cultures. Active CMV retinitis was observed in the right eye and a blood culture grew CMV.

The ganciclovir dose was increased to 10 mg/kg per day. On therapy, the patient developed generalized seizures, right-sided hemiparesis, disconjugate gaze and upward gaze-directed nystagmus. On the 31st day of ganciclovir treatment, he developed bacterial pneumonia and died.

Case 2

A 32-year-old (HS) male with AIDS was admitted for evaluation of fever and cholestasis. Cutaneous KS had developed 11 months earlier and CMV retinitis was diagnosed 3 months earlier, for which he received a 3-week induction course of ganciclovir, followed by a maintenance dose of 10 mg/kg 3 days a week.

On presentation, body temperature was 38°C and physical examination showed generalized cutaneous KS, oral candidiasis, and hepatomegaly. Neurologic examination was normal. An endoscopic retrogade cholangiography was performed and culture of the papilla proved positive for CMV. Ganciclovir was replaced by foscarnet, 180 mg/kg per day. His subsequent course was notable for the development of candida esophagitis, tracheobronchitis due to Pseudomonas aeruginosa, and increasing lethargy. A CT scan of the head disclosed cerebral atrophy. Table I shows his CSF data. CSF cryptococcal antigen detection, bacterial, mycobacterial, and fungal cultures all proved negative. A gadolinium-enhanced MRI study of the head demonstrated increased signal intensity in the periventricular region characteristic of ventriculitis.

Despite foscarnet therapy, he was febrile every day, confusion and lethargy progressed, and the patient died from aspiration pneumonia 2 months later.

Case 3

A 31-year-old male intravenous drug abuser with AIDS presented in August 1992 with headache and fever. PCP was diagnosed in May 1991. Gastritis, duodenitis, and pancreatitis due to CMV were diagnosed in November 1991, for which he was receiving foscarnet, 120 mg/kg for 3 days per week. Blood cultures at that time also

 ISSN 0036-5548

Table 1. *Demographic data in 5 AIDS patients with CMV ventriculoencephalitis*

Case no.	Age	Sex	HIV risk factor	Prior AIDS defining condition	CD4 cells/μ/l	CMV disease (therapy)	Viremia	Symptoms on admission	CT/MRI	CSF Profile: WBC cells × 10^6/l	CSF Profile: Glucose mmol/l (serum)	CSF Profile: Protein g/l	CSF Profile: Viral culture	Treatment	Outcome
1	40	M	HS	PCP/KS	7	Retinitis (Ganciclovir)	+	Headache Fever Lethargy	Atrophy/ND	0	1.8 (4.1)	1.33	—	Ganciclovir (10 mg/kg/day)	Generalized seizures, hemiparesis, nystagmus and death
2	32	M	HS	KS	ND	Retinitis (Ganciclovir)	ND	Fever Cholestasis (ERCP-CMV+)	Atrophy/ Periventriculitis	0	1.4 (7.1)	1.29	ND	Foscarnet (180 mg/kg/day)	Persistent fever, confusion, lethargy and death
3	31	M	IVDU	PCP/MAI	ND	Pancreatitis Gastritis Duodenitis (Foscarnet)	+	Headache Fever Diminished concentration	Atrophy, ventriculomegaly periventricular enhancement/ ND	5	3.3 (8.1)	1.57	—	Ganciclovir (10 mg/kg/day)	Generalized seizures, confusion and death
4	33	M	HS	PCP	8	Retinitis	+	Aphasia Disorientation Loss of vision	Atrophy/ Atrophy	2	1.5 (5.1)	1.60	ND	Foscarnet (180 mg/kg/day)	Death
5	44	M	HS	WS	3	No	+	Fever Confusion Disorientation Lethargy	Atrophy/ Periventriculitis	3	2.1 (6.1)	1.90	—	Ganciclovir (10 mg/kg/day)	Afebrile, clinical improvement. MRI: resolution of lesions

CMV = Cytomegalovirus; VE = Ventriculoencephalitis; M = Male; HS = Homosexual; IVDU = Intravenous Drug User; PCP = Pneumocystis carinii Pneumonia; KS = Kaposi Sarcoma; MAI = Mycobacterium avium intracellulare; WS = Wasting Syndrome; ERCP = Endoscopic Retrograde Cholangiopancreatography; CT = Computerized Tomography; MRI = Magnetic Resonance Imaging; CSF = Cerebrospinal Fluid; WBC = White Blood Cells Count; ND: Not Done grew Mycobacterium avium complex. In June 1992 he was readmitted with a recurrence of PCP.

On admission his temperature was 38°C, he was alert, oriented, but had diminished concentration. Neurologic examination was negative and there was no retinitis. A CT scan of the head demonstrated mild cerebral atrophy, ventriculomegaly, and periventricular enhancement. His CSF data are given in Table I. Cryptococcal antigen detection, bacterial, mycobacterial, viral, and fungal cultures of the CSF proved negative, but a blood culture for CMV was positive.

Ganciclovir therapy was initiated. By the 2nd hospital day the patient had developed generalized seizures and confusion. He became comatose and died on the 28th hospital day.

Case 4

A 33-year-old HS male with AIDS was admitted in September 1993 for evaluation of desorientation, and loss of vision of the right eye of approximately 2 weeks' duration. PCP had been diagnosed 5 years earlier with a relapse in March 1992. The CD4 cell count was 8×10^6/1.

On examination the patient was disoriented, and his temperature was 38°C. Neurologic examination revealed no abnormalities. Retinitis due to CMV was recognized in the right eye, and a blood culture for CMV proved positive. A CT scan and a gadolinium-enhanced MRI of the head demonstrated diffuse cerebral atrophy. CSF data are given in Table I. Cryptococcal antigen detection was negative and CSF cultures proved negative for bacteria, mycobacteria, and fungi.

Therapy with foscarnet was begun, but the patient's condition deteriorated until his death 1 month later.

Case 5

A 44-year-old HS man with AIDS presented in August 1993 with a 3-week history of fever, confusion and disorientation. Wasting syndrome had been diagnosed 11 months earlier. A CD4 cell count was 3×10^6/1.

His temperature was 37.8°C. He was lethargic, disoriented, and confused. Neurologic examination showed no evidence of cranial neuropathy, meningism, or sensory and motor abnormalities. Oph-

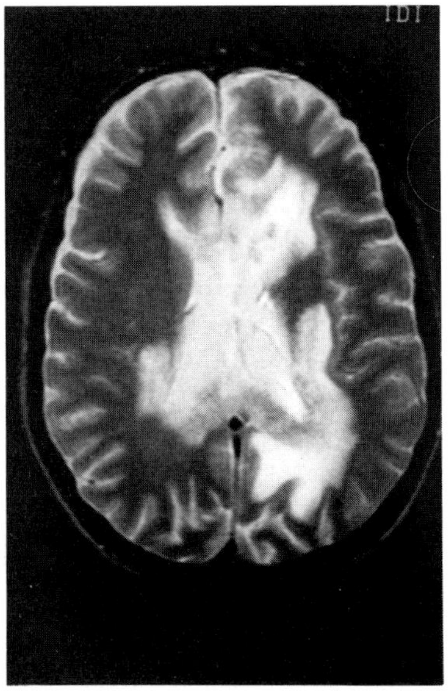

Fig. 1. Axial T2-weighted magnetic resonance images of the head in case no. 5 demonstrating increased signal intensity in the periventricular white matter.

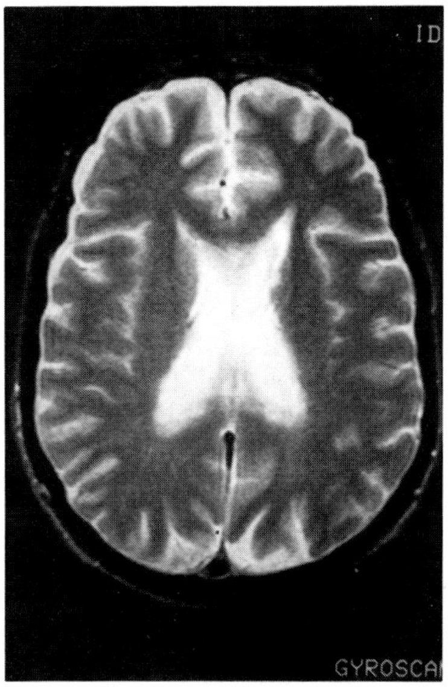

Fig. 2. Axial T2-weighted image in case no. 5 obtained after 4 weeks of ganciclovir treatment, showing resolution of the previously noted lesions.

thalmologic examination revealed no evidence of CMV retinitis. Cultures of blood yielded CMV. A CT scan of the head was unremarkable except for diffuse cerebral atrophy. CSF data are shown in Table I. Results of CSF cryptococcal antigen detection, bacterial, mycobacterial, viral, and fungal cultures were negative. An MRI of the head demonstrated increased signal intensity in the periventricular white matter visualized on T2-weighted images (Fig. 1).

The patient was given ganciclovir (5 mg/kg every 12 h) for 6 weeks, followed by a maintenance dosage of 10 mg/kg/day 3 days a week. On therapy, he became afebrile and showed a marked improvement with a complete recovery of his mental status. After 4 weeks of ganciclovir therapy a repeated lumbar puncture revealed no cells, glucose 2.6 mmol, and protein 0.56 g/l. At this time, another MRI revealed resorption of the previously visualized lesions (Fig. 2).

Neuropathology findings

Neuropathologic examination in each case (patients 1–4) disclosed necrotizing CMV-VE. Inclusion bodies were observed in hematoxylin–eosin stained sections (Fig. 3). Diagnosis was confirmed by immunohistochemistry, using well characterized anti-CMV bodies (clones E13 + 2A2; Clonatec, Paris) used at a dilution of 1:40 g following the avidin–biotin peroxidase (ABC, Vectastain, Vector Labs, Burlingame, Calif.) method. There was no histologic evidence of other co-existent CNS processes in any of the brains autopsied.

DISCUSSION

CMV may produce encephalopathy with ventriculitis in patients with HIV infection. Autopsy series have shown that about 30% of AIDS patients have evidence of CMV inclusions in CNS (1). However, symptomatic disease is uncommon. Petito et al. (1) found CMV encephalitis in the

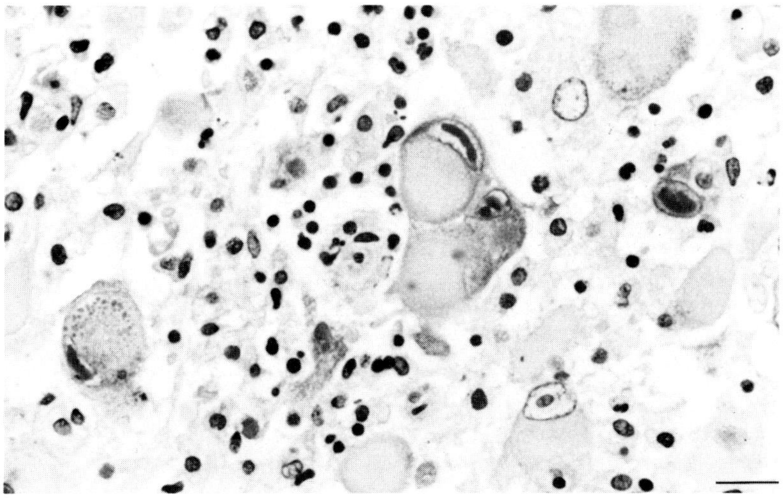

Fig. 3. Necrotizing ventriculitis with giant cells showing typical CMV intranuclear inclusions (case no. 3). (Hematoxilin and eosin bar = 20 μ.)

brain in 40 (26%) of 153 adult patients dying with AIDS. The CMV encephalitis was characterized by multiple microglial nodules. Ventriculitis with subependymal necrosis and CMV inclusions were present in 5 of the 40 patients. Morgello et al. (6) found necrotizing ventriculo-encephalitis in 3 of 30 patients with AIDS and CMV encephalitis. Microglial nodules were found in all of the 30 patients.

CMV infection of the CNS in AIDS occurs most often in profoundly immunocompromised hosts who have evidence of widespread CMV infection, such as viremia, retinitis, or colitis (5). CMV-VE has no consistent clinical picture, since patients may be completely asymptomatic or may present with dementia (6). Kalayjian et al. (9) observed a distinct clinical presentation with encephalitis often associated with cranial nerve deficits and gaze-directed nystagmus.

In the present AIDS patients, CMV-VE developed 23 months (median) (range, 11–60 months) after the onset of their first AIDS-defining condition. CMV retinitis had been diagnosed in 3 patients, 2 of them 6 months (median) before the onset of encephalitis. Encephalitis developed in 3 patients while receiving maintenance treatment with ganciclovir or foscarnet. This agrees with the findings of Berman and Kim (10), who reported development of fatal CMV-VE in 5 patients receiving ganciclovir for CMV retinitis. CMV was isolated from the blood in 4 patients. In contrast to the high frequency of neuro-ophthalmologic impairment reported by Kalayjian et al. (9), only 1 of our patients (case no. 1) presented with an ocular motor palsy. According to these authors (9), examination of CSF in our patients demonstrated elevated protein, hypoglycorachia and negative viral cultures in all cases. CMV polymerase chain reaction (PCR) analysis of CSF samples could not be undertaken in our patients. Recent reports have suggested that PCR is a sensitive marker for active CMV infection of the CNS (11–13). However, Achim et al. (14), using specimens from patients with neuropathology confirmed at autopsy, found that PCR assay of CSF was not a very specific marker of CNS disease. Further studies are needed to determine the precise role and interpretation of PCR in the diagnosis of CMV CNS infection. Brain imaging studies, particularly MRI, have become a helpful tool for the diagnosis (15, 16). In our experience, MRI was more sensitive than a CT scan for detecting periventricular abnormalities. MRI exhibited increased periventricular signal intensities on T2-weighted images, which strongly support the diagnosis of CMV-VE, though it is not a specific finding, as this may be observed in patients with CNS lymphoma, toxoplasmosis, and pyogenic brain abscesses (17). Three patients received ganciclovir and 2 patients foscarnet therapy. Though viral sensitivity testing would be helpful in proving drug resistance, this was not done. No patient was given combined ganciclovir and foscarnet therapy. Encouraging results with combination therapy for CMV infection in AIDS patients has been reported (18).

In our investigation, death occurred in 4 patients a median of 5 weeks after the onset of neurologic symptoms. Pathologic examination revealed periventriculitis with ependymal necrosis associated with intranuclear inclusion bodies characteristic of CMV in 4 of our patients. One patient (case 5) showed neurological improvement, with reduction of CSF protein, and radiological resolution of the ventriculitis by MRI after 4 weeks of ganciclovir treatment.

Foscarnet, which penetrates the blood–brain barrier, has been suggested to be the best choice for treatment of CMV infection in the CNS (19, 20). Patient no. 5 in the present series of CMV-VE demonstrated a marked clinical improvement on ganciclovir therapy. In a retrospective study of 14 autopsy-confirmed cases of CMV-VE recently published (21), 9 patients had received either ganciclovir or foscarnet; none of the patients had improved. Two further reports on CMV encephalitis in HIV-infected individuals treated with ganciclovir failed to show clinical improvement despite radiological improvement of the lesions (22, 23).

We conclude that CMV-VE should be suspected in HIV-infected patients at an advanced stage of disease who present with altered neurological status, concomitant CMV viremia or retinitis, hypoglycorachia and ventriculitis demonstrated by MRI. Although more effective therapy is needed for this fatal disease, one of our patients responded to prompt initiation of ganciclovir therapy.

REFERENCES

1. Petito CK, Cho ES, Lemann W, Navia BA, Price RW. Neuropathology of acquired immunodeficiency syndrome (AIDS): an autopsy review. J Neuropathol Exp Neurol 45: 635–646, 1986.
2. Behar R, Wiley C, McCutchan JA. Cytomegalovirus polyradiculopathy in acquired immune deficiency syndrome. Neurology 37: 557–561, 1987.
3. Miller RG, Storey JR, Greco CM. Ganciclovir in the treatment of progressive AIDS-related polyradiculopathy. Neurology 40: 569–574, 1990.
4. So YT, Olney RK. Acute lumbosacral polyradiculopathy in acquired immunodeficiency syndrome: experience in 23 patients. Ann Neurol 35: 53–58, 1994.
5. Vinters HV, Kwok MK, Ho HW, Anders KH, Tomiyasu U, Wolfson WL, Robert F. Cytomegalovirus in the nervous system of patients with the acquired immune deficiency syndrome. Brain 112: 245–268, 1989.
6. Morgello S, Cho ES, Nielsen S, Devinsky O, Petito CK. Cytomegalovirus encephalitis in patients with acquired immunodeficiency syndrome. Hum Pathol 18: 289–297, 1987.
7. Gray F, Gherardi R, Scaravilli F. The neuropathology of the acquired immune deficiency syndrome (AIDS). A review. Brain 111: 245–266, 1988.
8. Schmidbauer M, Budka H, Ulrich W, Ambros P. Cytomegalovirus (CMV) disease of the brain in AIDS and connatal infection: a comparative study by histology, immunocytochemistry and in situ DNA hybridization. Acta Neuropathol 79: 286–293, 1989.
9. Kalayjian RC, Cohen ML, Bonomo RA, Flanigan TP. Cytomegalovirus ventriculoencephalitis in AIDS. A syndrome with distinct clinical and pathologic features. Medicine 72: 67–77, 1993.
10. Berman SM, Kim RC. The development of cytomegalovirus encephalitis in AIDS patients receiving ganciclovir. Am J Med 96: 415–419, 1994.
11. Cinque P, Vago L, Brytting M, Castagna A, Accordini A, Sundqvist V-A, Zanchetta N, d'Arminio Monforte A, Wahren B, Lazzarin A, Linde A. Cytomegalovirus infection of the central nervous system in patients with AIDS: Diagnosis by DNA amplification from cerebrospinal fluid. J Infect Dis 166: 1408–1411, 1992.
12. Wolf DG, Spector SA. Diagnosis of human cytomegalovirus central nervous system disease in AIDS patients by DNA amplification from cerebrospinal fluid. J Infect Dis 166: 1412–1415, 1992.
13. Gozlan J, Salord JM, Rullet E, Baudrimont M, Caburet F, Picard O, Meyohas M-C, Duvivier C, Jacomet Ch, Petit J-C. Rapid detection of cytomegalovirus DNA in cerebrospinal fluid of AIDS patients with neurologic disorders. J Infect Dis 166: 1416–1421, 1992.
14. Achim CL, Nagra RM, Wang R, Nelson JA, Wiley CA. Detection of cytomegalovirus in cerebrospinal fluid autopsy specimens from AIDS patients. J Infect Dis 169: 623–627, 1994.
15. Barloon TJ, Yuh WTC, Knepper LE, Biller J, Ryals TJ, Sato Y. Cerebral ventriculitis: MR findings. J Comput Assist Tomogr 14: 272–275, 1990.
16. Grafe MR, Press GA, Berthoty DP, Hesselink JR, Wiley CA. Abnormalities of the brain in AIDS patients: correlation of postmortem MR findings with neuropathology. AJNR 11: 905–911, 1990.
17. Whelan MA, Kricheff II, Handler M, Ho V, Crystal K, Gopinathan G, Laubenstein L. Acquired immunodeficiency syndrome: cerebral computed tomographic manifestations. Radiology 149: 477–484, 1983.
18. Dieterich DT, Poles MA, Lew EA, Mendez PE, Murphy R, Addesi A, Holbrook JT, Naughton K, Friedberg DN. Concurrent use of ganciclovir and foscarnet to treat cytomegalovirus infection in AIDS patients. J Infect Dis 167: 1184–1188, 1993.
19. Hengge UR, Brockmeyer NH, Malessa R, Ravens U, Goos M. Foscarnet penetrates the blood–brain barrier: rationale for therapy of cytomegalovirus encephalitis. Antimicrob Agents Chemother 37: 1010–1014, 1993.
20. Raffi F, Taburet AM, Ghaleh B, Huart A, Singlas E. Penetration of foscarnet into cerebrospinal fluid of AIDS patients. Antimicrob Agents Chemother 37: 1777–1780, 1993.
21. Holland NR, Power C, Mathews VP, Glass JD, Forman M, McArthur JC. Cytomegalovirus encephalitis in acquired immunodeficiency syndrome (AIDS). Neurology 44: 507–514, 1994.
22. Masdeu JC, Small CB, Weiss L, Elkin CM, LLena J, Mesa-Tejada R. Multifocal cytomegalovirus encephalitis in AIDS. Ann Neurol 23: 97–99, 1988.
23. Price TA, Digioia RA, Simon GL. Ganciclovir treatment of cytomegalovirus ventriculitis in a patient infected with human immunodeficiency virus. Clin Infect Dis 15: 606–608, 1992.

Submitted September 21, 1994; accepted December 10, 1994

Scand J Infect Dis 27: 171–172, 1995

Primary Group A Streptococcal Peritonitis

J. CLIVE GRAHAM, PETER J. MOSS and MICHAEL W. MCKENDRICK

From the Department of Infectious Diseases and Medicine, Royal Hallamshire Hospital, Sheffield, England

Primary peritonitis caused by Group A β-haemolytic streptococci (GAS) is extremely rare and is usually only seen in the presence of underlying disease. This report describes the case of a previously fit young woman who developed primary GAS peritonitis. She had a laparotomy performed at which large amounts of intra-peritoneal pus was identified but no focus of infection was found. Broad spectrum antibiotics were initially used, these were changed to intravenous benzylpenicillin when GAS was isolated. She made a good recovery and was discharged 2 weeks after admission on oral amoxycillin. The organism was serotyped as T3/M3/R3 (opacity factor negative) and it is interesting that the same serotype was isolated from a throat swab taken from her daughter. We also discuss the possible routes of infection and the epidemiology of invasive GAS disease.

J. C. Graham, MD, Department of Infectious Diseases and Medicine, Royal Hallamshire Hospital, Glossop Road, Sheffield, S10 2JF, England

INTRODUCTION

There has recently been a resurgence of interest in disease caused by group A streptococci (GAS). Epidemics of particular serotypes of GAS have been described in Scandinavia and Britain (1, 2) associated with an increased incidence of serious illness and invasive disease. Despite this, primary peritonitis caused by GAS remains an extremely rare condition, and in adults is usually related to an underlying medical problem. We report a case of primary group A streptococcal peritonitis in a previously healthy adult, caused by a strain of GAS known to be associated with invasive disease.

CASE REPORT

A 39-year old lady presented with a 3 day history of diarrhoea, abdominal pain and distension. She had been unwell for a week before admission with fever, rigors and severe myalgia. She also described a generalised rash and headaches. Apart from treated depression and menorrhagia she was healthy, and there was no history of illness in her family at the time of admission.

On examination she was unwell, with a temperature of 40°C. Her abdomen was exquisitely tender and silent with rebound and guarding, but she was not shocked and there were no signs of infection elsewhere. Initial investigations showed a neutrophilia of 30.6×10^9/l and reduced haemoglobin at 97 g/l. Biochemical profile including amylase was normal, erect chest X-ray was unremarkable with no pneumoperitoneum and abdominal X-ray revealed only slightly distended loops of small bowel.

A clinical diagnosis of acute peritonitis was made and a laparotomy was performed after starting treatment with intravenous cefotaxime and metronidazole. At operation a large amount of intraperitoneal pus was found, but no focus of infection could be identified. The pus was drained, and she made a good recovery post-operatively.

Samples taken from the peritoneum grew a group A β-haemolytic Streptococcus, subsequently identified as serotype T3/M3/R3, (opacity factor negative). Swabs taken from the throat and cervix grew only commensals and blood cultures (taken before the first dose of antibiotics) were negative. In view of the microbiological findings her therapy was changed to intravenous benzylpenicillin and subsequently to oral amoxycillin as she continued to improve. She was discharged home 2 weeks after admission, and although she developed erythema nodosum she eventually made a complete recovery.

In view of the unusual nature of her illness an extensive search was made for an underlying cause, but subsequent investigations (including assays of immunoglobulins and IgG subclasses, serum complement levels and a blood film to look for hyposplenism) did not reveal any evidence of immunodeficiency.

Although the patient had no clinical or microbiological evidence of pharyngitis her 10-year-old daughter developed tonsillitis while her mother was in hospital, and a group A streptococcus was grown from her throat swab which was the same serotype as her mothers.

DISCUSSION

Primary peritonitis is a relatively uncommon condition, usually seen in patients with hepatic ascites, nephrotic syndrome, immunosuppression and in otherwise healthy children (3). The most commonly identified causes are pneumococci and Gram-negative enteric bacilli (3). It is very rarely seen as part of the spectrum of invasive group A streptococcal disease: in a review of the recent literature we found only 8 cases of primary GAS peritonitis in adults without the predisposing conditions described above (4–10). Of these, 1 was diabetic (5), 1 had abnormal liver enzymes secondary to alcohol consumption (4), 1 had a history of non-A non-B hepatitis (7), 1 had anorexia nervosa (9) and 1 was 87 years old (5). Our patient, by contrast, was a completely healthy young woman with no evidence of any underlying medical problems.

Various mechanisms have been proposed for the pathogenesis of primary GAS peritonitis. Simultaneous isolation of the organism from the trachea, blood and peritoneum indicates haematogenous spread from the pharynx (7), as does a history of preceding tonsillitis (11). Group A streptococci are occasionally found in the vagina, both as pathogenic organisms and as asymptomatic commensals (10, 12). This, along with the preponderance of women among the reported cases of primary GAS peritonitis, suggests that ascending infection from the genital tract may sometimes

 ISSN 0036-5548

be responsible. Direct transluminal spread from intact bowel has also been suggested as a route of infection (13). In the case reported here throat swabs, high vaginal swabs and blood cultures did not grow GAS, and the mode of infection remains uncertain.

It has been suggested that there has been an overall increase in invasive GAS disease on both sides of the Atlantic in the past 15 years (1, 14, 15). At the Royal Hallamshire Hospital (A Teaching Hospital of 730 beds located in central Sheffield) the number of cases of GAS bacteraemia has risen from 8 cases over a 10-year period up to 1980 (16) to 10 cases in the last 2 years. In this country, however, although there are annual fluctuations in the prevalence of more invasive strains of GAS a recent review did not show any sustained increase in the incidence of invasive disease (2). Instead there appears to be a pattern of epidemics, sometimes lasting for years, superimposed on a stable endemic disease.

In situations where there is an increased incidence of invasive GAS infection a higher incidence of M1 and M3 strains of GAS has been found, and these are the strains most commonly isolated from patients with invasive disease (1, 5, 17). However, the occurrence of epidemics of invasive GAS M1 disease has not always been associated with changes in the incidence of the isolation of this serotype from patients with uncomplicated pharyngitis, suggesting that virulence may be strain or toxin-associated rather than broadly related to serotype (18, 19). Such outbreaks may be the result of the appearance of a unique clone of particularly invasive bacteria (20). Along with localised epidemics there also appears to be considerable fluctuation in the numbers of sporadic cases in previously healthy adults, implying that host susceptibility may also play a part in determining the course of illness (15). This was certainly true in this case where the same serotype caused invasive disease in the mother but not the daughter.

REFERENCES

1. Martin PR, Hoiby EA. Streptococcal serogroup A epidemic in Norway 1987–1988. Scand J Infect Dis 22: 421–429, 1990.
2. Colman G, Tanna A, Efstratiou A, Gawozewska ET. The serotypes of Streptococcus Pyogenes in Britain during 1980–1990 and their association with disease. J Med Microbiol 39: 165–178, 1993.
3. Mandell GL, Douglas RG, Bennet JE. Principles and Practice of Infectious Diseases, 3rd ed.
4. Gribbin JC, Cox CJ. Spontaneous bacterial peritonitis in a healthy adult male. Aust NZJ Surg 60: 723–725, 1990.
5. Casadevall A, Pirofski LA, Catalano MT. Primary group A peritonitis in adults (review). Am J Med 88: 63–64, 1990.
6. Christen RD, Moser R, Schlup P, Neftel KA. Fulminant group A streptococcal infections. Report of 2 cases. Klinische Wochenscroft 68: 427–430, 1990.
7. Brase R, Kuckelt W, Manhold C, Bohmert F. Spontaneous bacterial peritonitis without ascites. Anasthesiol Intensivmed Notfallmed Schmerzther 27: 325–327, 1992.
8. Golden GT, Stevenson TR, Ritchie WP. Primary peritonitis in adults. South Med J 68: 413–414, 1975.
9. Khoury GA, Wall RA. Streptococcal peritonitis associated with the cathartic colon. Br J Surg 69: 327, 1982.
10. Bibler MR, Rouan GW. Cryptogenic group A streptococcal bacteremia: Experience at an urban general hospital and review of the literature. Rev Infect Dis 8: 941–951, 1986.
11. Golden GT, Shaw A. Primary peritonitis. Surg Gynecol Obstet 135: 513–516, 1972.
12. Monif GR, Williams BT, Dase DF. Group A streptococcus as a cause of endometritis/salpingitis/peritonitis in a nongravid female. Obstet Gynecol 50: 509–510, 1977.
13. Schweinburg FB, Seligman AM, Fine J. Transmural migration of intestinal bacteria: A study based on the use of radioactive Escherichia coli. N Engl J Med 242: 747–751, 1950.
14. Begovac J, Gmajnic B, Kuzmanovic N. Invasive streptococci (letter). Lancet 335: 109, 1990.
15. Stevens DL. Invasive group A streptococcus infections. Clin Infect Dis 14: 2–13, 1992.
16. Goepel JR, Richards DG, Harris DM, Henry L. Fulminant streptococcus pyogenes infection. BMJ 281: 1412, 1980.
17. Demers B, Simor AE, Vellend H, Schlievert PM, Byrne S, Jamieson F, Walmsey S, Low DE. Sever invasive group A streptococcal infections in Ontario, Canada: 1987–1991. Clin Infect Dis 16: 792–800, 1993.
18. Johnson DR, Stevens DL, Kaplan EL. Epidemiologic analysis of group A streptococcal serotypes associated with severe systemic infections, rheumatic fever, or uncomplicated pharyngitis. J Infect Dis 166: 374–382, 1992.
19. Krause RM. Dynamics of emergence. J Infect Dis 170: 265–271, 1994.
20. Cleary PP, Kaplan EL, Handley JP, Wlazlo A, Kim MH, Hauser AR, Schlievert PM. Clonal basis for the resurgance of serious Streptococcus pyogenes disease in the 1980s. Lancet 339: 518–521, 1992.

Submitted October 17, 1994; accepted December 7, 1994

Scand J Infect Dis 27: 173–174, 1995

CASE REPORT

Non-typhoid Salmonella Subdural Empyema in a Patient with AIDS

CRISTINA MUSSINI, FEDERICA TRENTI, GIOVANNA MANICARDI, NICOLA MONGIARDO, MAURO CODELUPPI, LEONARDO D'ANDREA, GIOVANNI GUARALDI, FRANCO SQUADRINI and BRUNO DE RIENZO

From the Department of Infectious Diseases, University of Modena School of Medicine, Modena, Italy

In AIDS patients, non-typhoid salmonella metastatic abscesses in lung and brain due to bacteremia have ben described previously. Here we present a case in which a group B Salmonella, serotype Copenhagen, caused right parietal subdural empyema. The etiologic diagnosis was based on culture of pus obtained from the lesion. The patient was treated for bacterial meningitis and made a good recovery. He is at present reasonably well and is taking ciprofloxacin as prophylaxis against salmonella relapse.

C. Mussini, MD, Department of Infectious Diseases, Policlinico Universitario, via del Pozzo, 71, 41100 Modena, Italy

INTRODUCTION

Non-typhoid (NT) salmonella can produce a clinical syndrome characterized by protracted episodes of intermittent fever, anorexia and persistent bacteremia. Intestinal complaints and concomitant positive stool cultures are uncommon in these cases (1). Recurrent salmonella bacteremia is an AIDS-defining diagnosis in HIV-infected patients (2), and NT salmonella metastatic abscesses in different localizations (lung and brain) have previously been described in AIDS patients (3–5). We report here a patient with AIDS who had an abscess in the right parietal subdural space. As far as we know, this is the first description of a NT salmonella subdural empyema.

CASE-REPORT

Our patient was a 29-year-old male intravenous drug user with AIDS, in whom cerebral toxoplasmosis was diagnosed in October, 1992, after taking zidovudine since November, 1991. He was also taking aerosolized penthamidine as PCP prophylaxis. In early October, 1992, he was admitted to our Clinic because of fever and persistent headache. A brain CT scan showed a contrast enhancing focal cerebral lesion affecting the basal nuclei. On the basis of the clinical and radiological findings and of his response to the therapy (pyrimethamine 75 mg/day and sulphadiazine 4 g/day), a new diagnosis of cerebral toxoplasmosis was made. A new CT scan, made at the conclusion of the treatment for acute encephalitis, showed almost complete resolution of the lesion, whereafter the patient was discharged, with a prescription of pyrimethamine 50 mg/day and sulphadiazine 2 mg/day as secondary prophylaxis against toxoplasmosis. Two months later, in January, 1993, he was readmitted with fever (38.5°C), headache and left hemianopsia. There was no neck rigidity. Left hemianopsia was the only neurological finding. When hospitalized, his WBC count was 4.51×10^9/l; neutrophil count, 3.07×10^9/l; total lymphocyte count, 0.95×10^9/l and CD4 cell count, 18×10^6/l. Blood and urine cultures were negative for bacteria, mycobacteria and fungi.

A lumbar puncture showed pleocytosis (18×10^6/l) and elevated total protein content (0.89 g/l). A cryptococcal antigen test on CSF and blood proved negative. The CT scan showed presence of an encapsulated extracerebral subdural mass measuring 1.5 cm × 3 cm. The mass was located to the right parietal side. No lesions compatible with the toxoplasma relapse were found in the brain. The radiological findings were consistent with subdural empyema.

The patient was transferred to the Department of Neurosurgery where he underwent trepanation. He received chloramphenicol 2 g/day and cefotaxime 12 g/day for *ex adjuvantibus* treatment of bacterial meningitis. The pus obtained from the lesion contained mainly PMNs; a polymerase chain reaction for toxoplasma was negative and no fungi were found. From the evaluated pus, group B, non-typhoid salmonella, serotype Copenhagen, was grown. The salmonella strain was sensitive to amikacin, cefoxitin, chloramphenicol, ciprofloxacin and trimethoprim/sulphamethoxazole. The patient was discharged 2 weeks after drainage ciprofloxacin 500 mg b.i.d. was begun as prophylaxis against NT salmonella relapse. A CT scan 2 month later showed complete resolution of the subdural empyema. During hospitalization the patient continued his prophylaxis for toxoplasmosis and his zidovudine treatment. At present he is alive in good health and no relapse of salmonella has occurred.

DISCUSSION

NT salmonella metastatic abscesses have been found in many organs, in both immunocompetent and immmunosuppressed hosts (6). This shows that immune alterations, and in particular those caused by HIV infection, increase susceptibility to septic salmonella infections (7, 8). Thus, Celum et al. (9) reported an incidence of NT salmonella bacteremia of 45%, vs. only 9% in HIV-patients with salmonellosis. In general, involvement of the central nervous system is not rare and includes meningitis, brain abscesses, infected subdural hematoma and epidural abscesses (3, 6). The patient reported here had an unusual localization of a NT salmonella, which has not previously been reported in AIDS cases.

Salmonella can affect tissues which have been previously diseased. Other authors have reported the presence of intracranial salmonella infections in areas of pre-existing hematomas, metastatic tumours, and primary brain tumours (10). Our patient had no history of traumatic events, but had had a previous cerebral toxoplasmosis, diagnosed

 ISSN 0036-5548

on the basis of radiological findings and response to treatment. A brain CT scan performed during the second hospitalization showed no evidence of toxoplasma lesions in the right parietal area or in other locations and the response to the antibiotic treatment for salmonella was complete.

In our patient salmonella could not be isolated from the blood, urine or faeces. The subdural empyema was, however, probably caused by hematogenous spread of the organism.

Zidovudine has been described to be effective in vitro against Gram-negative bacteria such as Salmonella (11). Accordingly, Salmon et al. (12) noted the efficacy of zidovudine at dosage ≥400 mg/day in preventing relapses of salmonella bacteremia in AIDS patients. The patient we studied has been taking zidovudine 400 mg per day since 1991 which, however, failed to have any primary prophylactic effect. It is noteworthy that the patient developed a subdural abscess caused by NT salmonella eventhough he was taking sulphadiazine as secondary prophylaxis for toxoplasmosis and although the Salmonella strain isolated was sensitive to sulphamethoxazole. Possibly the dose of sulphadiazine was sufficient to prevent recurrence of toxoplasmosis but not the onset of a salmonella infection. A further explanation for the development of the abscess was that the isolated Salmonella strain was sensitive to sulphadiazine but not to sulphamethoxazole.

Considering that, without maintenance therapy, the frequency of recurrences is approximately 45% (13), we decided to give secondary proplylaxis with ciprofloxacin. This drug has previously been recommended for secondary prophylaxis against salmonella infections in AIDS patients who have had salmonella septicemia and in whom ciprofloxacin had not been used for primary treatment (4). Thus, in agreement with Nelson et al. (4), we propose that maintenance treatment for salmonella bacteremia in AIDS patients should be continued on a life-long basis. This patient could also take advantage of a Pneumocystis carinii prophylaxis with co-trimoxazole instead of aerosolized penthamidine. Thus since this drug is effective not only against P. carinii and toxoplasma, but also against salmonella.

The presence of the unusual NT salmonella serotype has previously been described as more prevalent in AIDS patients than in immunocompetent hosts (9). The salmonella serotype (group B, Copenhagen) in our patient is quite common in this part of Italy, and may be related to exposure to natural food products. Taking into account that, in an immunocompromised host, the development may result after ingestion of a small inoculum of Salmonella (14), the importance of giving adequate advice to AIDS patients about cooking and food preparation has to be stressed.

ACKNOWLEDGEMENTS

This study was supported in part by grants from M.U.R.S.T. and from Istituto Superiore di Sanità (VI Progetto di Ricerche AIDS) to B.D.R. The authors wish to thank Dr Andrea Cossarizza, Univ. of Modena, for helpful suggestions.

REFERENCES

1. Fischl MA, Dickinson GM, Sinave C, Pitchenik AE, Cleary TJ. Salmonella bacteremia as manifestation of acquired immunodeficiency syndrome. Arch Intern Med 146: 113–115, 1986.
2. Centers for Disease Control. Revision of the CDC surveillance case definition for acquired immunodeficiency syndrome. MMWR Morb Mortal Wkly Rep 36: 15, 1987.
3. Fraimow SH, Wormser PG, Coburn DK, Small Butkus C. Salmonella meningitis and infection with HIV. AIDS 4: 1271–1273, 1990.
4. Nelson MR, Shanson DC, Hawkins DA, Gazzard BG. Salmonella, Campylobacter and Shigella in HIV-seropositive patients. AIDS 6: 1495–1498, 1992.
5. Ankobiah WA, Salehi F. Salmonella lung abscess in a patient with acquired immunodeficiency syndrome. Chest 100: 591, 1991.
6. Cohen IJ, Bartlett AJ, Corey R. Extra-intestinal manifestations of Salmonella infections. Medicine 66: 349–388, 1987.
7. Polsky B, Gold JWM, Whimbey E, Dryjansky J, Brown AE, Schiffman G, Armstrong D. Bacterial pneumonia in patients with the Acquired Immunodeficiency Syndrome. Ann Intern Med 104: 38–41, 1986.
8. Whimbey E, Gold JWM, Polsky B, Dryjansky J, Hawkins C, Blevins A, Brannon P, Kiehn TE, Brown AE, Armstrong D. Bacteremia and fungemia in patients with acquired immunodeficiency syndrome. Ann Intern Med 104: 511–514, 1986.
9. Celum CL, Chaisson RE, Rutherford GW, Barnhart JL, Echenberg DF. Incidence of salmonellosis in patients with AIDS. J Infect Dis 6: 998–1002, 1987.
10. Rodriguez RE, Valerno V, Watanakunakorn C. Salmonella focal intracranial infections: review of the world literature and report of an unusual case. Rev Infect Dis 8: 31–41, 1986.
11. Elwell LP, Ferone R, Freeman A. Antibacterial activity and mechanism of action of 3′-azido-3′ desoxythymidine. Antimicrob Agents Chemother 31: 274–280, 1987.
12. Salmon D, Detruchis P, Leport C, Bouvet E, Karam D, Meyohas MC, Coulaud JP, Vildé JL. Efficacy of zidovudine in preventing relapses of salmonella bacteremia in AIDS. J Infect Dis 163: 415–416, 1991.
13. Sperber SJ, Schleupner CJ. Salmonellosis during infection with Human Immunodeficiency Virus. Rev Infect Dis 9: 925–934, 1987.
14. Lipson A, Meikle H. Porcine pancreatin as a source of salmonella infection in children with cystic fibrosis. Arch Dis Child 52: 569–572, 1977.

Submitted November 23, 1994; accepted January 18, 1995

Scand J Infect Dis 27: 177–178, 1995 CASE REPORT

Recurrent Salmonella enteritidis Meningitis in a Patient with AIDS

ALFONSO GUTIÉRREZ[1], RAMÓN TEIRA[2], MERCEDES VARONA[1],
SANTIAGO GONZÁLEZ DE ETXABARRI[2] and JUAN MIGUEL SANTAMARÍA[2]

From the Departments of [1]Emergency Medicine and [2]Infectious Diseases, Hospital de Basurto, Bilbao, Spain

The profound impairment of cellular immunity associated with HIV infection predisposes to salmonella infections with recurrent bacteremia as a well recognized opportunistic infection in patients with AIDS. However, salmonella meningitis is extremely rare in this group of patients and only 4 cases have been reported so far. We present 1 case of recurrent Salmonella enteritidis meningitis in an AIDS patient. The infection recurred despite prolonged antimicrobial therapy. Treatment of salmonella infections in AIDS patients may be very difficult and, in some cases, lifelong maintenance therapy may be required.

A. Gutiérrez Macías, MD, Servicio de Urgencias, Hospital de Basurto, Avenida de Montevideo, 18, 48013 Bilbao (Vizcaya), Spain

INTRODUCTION

Non-typhoidal salmonella infections are manifestations of immunosuppression in patients with HIV infection (1); recurrent salmonella bacteremia was identified early in the AIDS epidemic (2–5) and included in the AIDS surveillance definition in 1987 (6). While recurrent bacteremia is the most common manifestation, focal infections have rarely been reported (7, 8) and only 4 cases of meningitis have been reported in patients with HIV infection so far (9, 10). We present a HIV-seropositive patient with recurrent meningitis caused by Salmonella enterica serotype enteritidis (Salmonella enteritidis).

CASE REPORT

A 35-year old man, HIV seropositive, with oral candidiasis and CD4+ cell count 4×10^6/l, treated with zidovudine and prophylaxis for Pneumocystis carinii pneumonia with pyrimethamine-sulfadoxine was admitted because of worsening headache, fever and vomiting in the preceding week. He had been treated with amoxicillin-clavulanate, but without improvement. Physical examination was negative except for neck stiffness and oral thrush. Computerized tomography (CT) of the cranium was normal. A lumbar puncture was performed, obtaining a turbid cerebrospinal fluid (CSF) with glucose 1.16 mmol/l (21 mg/dl), total protein 2.28 g/l and leukocytes 1200×10^6/l with 850×10^6/l neutrophils. Gram stain allowed the identification of Gram-negative bacilli and culture showed growth of Salmonella enteritidis susceptible to ampicillin, sulfonamides, chloramphenicol, third generation cephalosporins and ciprofloxacin. CSF fungal and mycobacterial cultures, blood and stool cultures proved negative. The white blood cell count was 1.4×10^9/l with 0.6×10^9/l neutrophils and platelet count was 54×10^9/l. Blood chemical and hematological values were otherwise within normal limits. Therapy commenced with intravenous cefotaxime 2 g every 4 h and 48 h later the fever and neck stiffness had disappeared. CSF obtained after 1 week of antimicrobial therapy disclosed 5×10^6/l white cells, total protein 0.31 g/l and glucose 2.83 mmol/l (51 mg/l). Gram stain and culture now proved negative. Cefotaxime was continued for 21 days and meanwhile the patient remained asymptomatic and was discharged. Three days after, headache and fever recurred and altered consciousness and agitation appeared. On physical examination, there was no neck stiffness, nor clinical data of elevated intracraneal pressure or neurological signs. A new spinal tap was performed and CSF showed 10×10^6/l white cells, total protein 0.36 g/l and glucose 1.77 mmol/l (32 mg/dl). Blood and CSF cultures yielded Salmonella enteritidis with the same susceptibility to antimicrobial agents. CT scan of the cranium, bone scan and X-ray of paranasal sinuses were all normal. Cefotaxime at the same dose as earlier was resumed, with good clinical response. On the 20th day of therapy, CSF was sterile and cefotaxime was continued to complete 30 days of treatment. He was discharged with ciprofloxacin at a daily dose of 1,500 mg and completed 6 additional weeks of therapy. Four days after ciprofloxacin was withdrawn, symptoms recurred, neutrophilic pleocytosis was observed in a spinal tap and Salmonella enteritidis was again recovered from CSF, with identical antibiotic susceptibility. Parenteral cefotaxime was administered for 2 additional weeks and the patient was discharged with ciprofloxacin at the same dose in order to maintain a life-long suppressive therapy.

DISCUSSION

Salmonella meningitis has been extensively described in neonates and children, but reports in adults are scanty and predominate in patients with impaired cellular immunity or following neurosurgery (11). In spite of the severe immunosuppression related to advanced HIV infection, Salmonella meningitis is extremely rare in this groups of patients and only 4 cases have been reported so far (9, 10); although it has been suggested that its incidence appears to be much higher than reported in non-AIDS patients (9).

It has been noticed that AIDS not only renders patients susceptible to serious salmonella infections with bacteremia and relapse despite standard antibiotic treatment, but also compromises their capacity to eradicate these bacteria (3, 5). The ability of salmonella to cause recurrent infections rests in the fact that it is an intracellular facultative organism, able to survive and even multiply into macrophages. Thus, therapeutic failures are usually associated with persistence and incomplete clearance of the infection, rather than with the emergence of antibiotic-resistant strains (12).

Our case underscores the fact that management of salmonella infections in AIDS patients poses a significant clinical problem; we believe that recurrent infections probably require at least 4 weeks of parenteral antibiotics with bactericidal activity, followed by oral therapy for 2 or 3 months (4); but in some cases, as in the one presented here, a life-long maintenance therapy may be required. The choice of the antimicrobial agent deserves consideration. The use of aminopenicillins and third generation cephalosporins may be hampered by their inadequate penetration in phagocytic cells, while trimethoprim-sulfamethoxazole is a bacteriostatic agent that frequently produces serious side effects in this category of patients (12). Fluoroquinolones with high bactericidal activity and good intracellular penetration probably are the best antimicrobials for suppressive therapy. The optimal dose for ciprofloxacin is not established, but 500 or 750 mg twice a day seems a reasonable alternative (12).

REFERENCES

1. Celum CL, Chaisson RE, Rutherford GW, Barnhart JL, Echenberg DF. Incidence of salmonellosis in patients with AIDS. J Infect Dis 156: 998–1002, 1987.
2. Glaser JB, Morton-Kute L, Berger SR, Weber J, Siegal FP, López C, Robbins W, Landesman SH. Recurrent salmonella typhimurium bacteremia associated with the acquired immunodeficiency syndrome. Ann Intern Med 102: 189–193, 1985.
3. Nadelman RB, Malthur-Wagh U, Yancovitz SR, Mildvan D. Salmonella bacteremia associated with the acquired immunodeficiency syndrome. Arch Intern Med 145: 1968–1971, 1985.
4. Jacobs JL, Gold JWM, Murray HW, Roberts RB, Armstrong D. Salmonella infections in patients with the acquired immunodeficiency syndrome. Ann Intern Med 102: 186–188, 1985.
5. Fischl MA, Dickinson GM, Sinave C, Pitchenik AE, Cleary TJ. Salmonella bacteremia as manifestation of acquired immunodeficiency syndrome. Arch Intern Med 146: 113–115, 1986.
6. Centers for Disease Control. Division of the CDC surveillance case definition for acquired immunodeficiency syndrome. MMWR 36 (suppl 1): 1S–15S, 1987.
7. Spreber SJ, Schleupner CJ. Salmonellosis during infection with human immunodeficiency virus. Rev Infect Dis 9: 925–934, 1987.
8. Mastroianni CM, Vullo V, Delia S. Cranial salmonella abscess with parietal bone osteomyelitis in an HIV-infected patient. AIDS 6: 749–750, 1992.
8. Fraimow HS, Wormser GP, Coburn KD, Small CB. Salmonella meningitis and infection with HIV. AIDS 4: 1271–1273, 1990.
10. Jimémez-Mejías ME, Castillo MJ, García-Luaces M, Pachón Díaz J. Meningitis por Salmonella no typhi, hemofilia e infección por virus de la inmunodeficiencia humana. Med Clin (Barc) 94: 156–157, 1990.
11. Cohen JI, Bartlett JA, Corey GR. Extra-intestinal manifestations of Salmonella infections. Medicine (Baltimore) 66: 349–388, 1987.
12. Jacobson MA, Hahn SM, Gerberding JL, Lee B, Sande MA. Ciprofloxacin for Salmonella bacteremia in the acquired immunodeficiency syndrome. Ann Intern Med 110: 1027–1029, 1989.

Submitted November 23, 1994; accepted January 18, 1995

Scand J Infect Dis 27: 179–182, 1995 CASE REPORT

Chlamydia pneumoniae and Chronic Pharyngitis

GÖRAN FALCK[1], LENA HEYMAN[2], JUDY GNARPE[3] and HÅKAN GNARPE[3]

From the Departments of [1]Family Medicine, Uppsala University, Uppsala; [3]Clinical Microbiology, Gävle Central Hospital, Gävle and [2]Community Health Centre, Solsidan, Ludvika, Sweden

Chlamydia pneumoniae has been implicated as an etiological agent for both upper and lower respiratory tract infections. We describe 4 cases of chronic pharyngitis where Chlamydia pneumoniae appears to be the etiological agent. All the patients were non-smokers, and had symptoms of more than 6 months' duration. Disease symptoms seemed to resolve following appropriate antibiotic treatment.

G. Falck, MD, Apoteksgårdens Vårdcentrum, S-714 22, Kopparberg, Sweden

INTRODUCTION

Chlamydia pneumoniae has been implicated as an etiological agent in various types of respiratory tract infection (1–5). On the basis of serological findings, it has earlier been suggested that C. trachomatis could be a common cause of pharyngitis (6), though this proposal has later been withdrawn and judged to be the result of misinterpretation of serological findings (7, 8). Thus Greber et al. in a prospective study, found no evidence of C. trachomatis infection (9). In 1989, Huovinen et al. (10) presented evidence that C. pneumoniae could be an etiological agent causing pharyngitis. C. pneumoniae has since been found by different authors to cause acute pharyngitis in 0.7 to 20% of such cases (3, 8, 10, 11).

Acute pharyngitis often accompanies a generalized infection of the mucous membranes of the upper respiratory tract. Chronic pharyngitis is usually considered to be due not to infectious agents, but rather to irritants of various kinds, e.g. smoking or alcohol. The potential importance of bacterial pathogens has not yet been assessed.

During an earlier investigation (12) we found that several patients with serologic evidence of C. pneumoniae infection had granulations in the pharynx. During the spring of 1994 we detected C. pneumoniae in throat specimens taken from patients with granulations on mucous membranes. These observations prompted us to include diagnostic procedures for the detection of C. pneumoniae in the investigation of patients with chronic pharyngitis. In this report, 4 cases of chronic pharyngitis with findings positive for C. pneumoniae are described.

MATERIAL AND METHODS

Patients

Four patients seeking medical advice for persistent symptoms of pharyngitis were investigated repeatedly with serology, culture, and polymerase chain reaction (PCR) for the presence of Chlamydia pneumoniae. None of the individuals studied were smokers.

Specimens

Specimens were taken for culture and PCR detection of Chlamydia pneumoniae by means of a CTA (Chlamydia trachomatis alginate) swab (13), normally used for sampling C. trachomatis specimens. The retropharyngeal wall was swabbed vigorously whereafter the swab was immersed in chlamydia transport medium (2SP) and sent by mail to the laboratory (distance 200 km). Specimens were transported at ambient temperatures, and frozen at −70°C on arrival at the laboratory. The time for transportation varied between 18 and 28 h. On several occasions, blood was sampled by venipuncture in each patient for serological purposes.

Polymerase chain reaction

Specimens from the pharyngeal mucosa, frozen at −70°C, were thawed, and after a rigorous vortexing, transferred to a 0.5 ml Eppendorf reaction tube. These specimens were then centrifuged at 10,000 rpm for 10 min at +4°C using an IEC MicroMax bench centrifuge. Supernatants were removed, and 50 µl of proteinase K (10 mg/ml) (Boehringer-Mannheim, GmbH, Mannheim, Germany) dissolved in 0.01 M Tris-HCl buffer with an added 1% Triton-X 100 was added to each cell pellet. All tubes were incubated at 55°C for 60 min, followed by incubation at 90°C for 10 min. Specimens thus processed were tested using a PCR method according to Campbell (14). Amplified products were electrophoresed in 1.5% agarose (International Biotechnologies Inc., New Haven, Conn., USA) and visualized by staining with ethidium bromide under UV-transillumination. Positive specimens were rerun using the same PCR procedure.

Culture

Throat specimens were cultured for C. pneumoniae in Human Lung (HL) cells as described previously (12), except that specimens were passaged 4–8 times before staining. All culture-positive specimens were recultured from the original specimen to rule out possible contamination. Cultures were stained using a genus-specific fluorescein isothiocyanate conjugated monoclonal antibody (Pathfinder, Kallestad, Chaska, Minn. USA), and, when positive inclusions were identified, these were reconfirmed using a specific C. pneumoniae monoclonal (Chlamydia-Cel TWAR I.F. Test, Cellabs Diagnostics Pty Ltd., Brookvale 2100, Australia).

Serology

Serum specimens were analysed for IgG, IgA and IgM antibodies by microimmunofluorescence (MIF) to C. pneumoniae strain IOL-

207 according to a method described elsewhere (12). Sera positive for IgA antibodies were absorbed using Protein-A sepharose (CL-4B) (Pharmacia, Uppsala) to remove possible interference from IgG antibodies, and then retested. All serum specimens from the same patient were retested in parallel.

CASE REPORTS

Case 1

A 52-year-old previously healthy man who after a respiratory tract infection in May 1993 had persisting difficulty in swallowing, a sense of swollen throat necessitating frequent clearing of the throat, periodic purulent nasal discharge, plugged ears and head congestion.

The patient had consulted several general practitioners as well as an ear, nose and throat specialist on numerous occasions. The symptoms were interpreted as being caused by yeasts, by Hemophilus influenzae, but also as globus syndrome. On the basis of suspected Hemophilus influenzae infection, he was given lymecycline 300 mg bid for 2 weeks late in 1993. He improved during treatment, but returned in January 1994 with complaints of unchanged throat symptoms, and was constantly clearing his throat during the examination. The tonsils were slightly swollen, the pharyngeal mucous membrane was red and swollen, with hyperplastic lymph noduli. Specimens were taken which proved positive for C. pneumoniae by PCR and culture. Serology showed an IgG titre of 128, and an IgA titre of 16 for C. pneumoniae, but no specific IgM antibodies.

On January 24th he noted deterioration, with symptoms from the ears and head congestion so severe that he remained in bed. Treatment was initiated with azithromycin for 4 days, followed by 250 mg biw for 5 weeks. The symptoms abated after 1 week of treatment, and were almost gone after 1 month. A certain irritation in the throat remained, although the mucous membranes were not visibly reddened and the lymph noduli had disappeared.

On March 25th, 3 weeks after the end of treatment throat symptoms reappeared, and hyperplastic lymph noduli were again noted on examination. PCR tests for C. pneumoniae were negative; serological analysis showed the same titres as in January. Azithromycin was given for 4 weeks, whereupon the symptoms disappeared during treatment. At a visit on June 3rd the patient reported throat irritation when speaking. Both tonsils were slightly swollen but pharyngeal wall was normal on inspection. PCR and culture were positive for C. pneumoniae. Antibody titres remained unchanged. Four weeks later, symptoms persisted and occasional lymph noduli could be seen in the throat. As the symptoms were rather mild, no treatment was given.

Cases 2 and 3

A 35-year-old, previously healthy, active orienteer fell ill in late 1992 with persistent common cold, sore throat, and headache. In December 1992 the pharyngeal mucosa appeared to be covered by granulations. A culture for C. pneumoniae from the tonsils proved negative. The patient had an IgG antibody titre to C. pneumoniae of 1024, and an IgA titre of 32. No IgM could be demonstrated, and no treatment was given.

Two months later, the patient was healthy, but a specimen taken for C. pneumoniae culture from the back of the throat proved positive. Antibody titres were unchanged. Shortly thereafter he became ill with acute bronchitis and was given doxycycline, 100 mg bid for 2 weeks. Virus serology taken at this time indicated an Influenza B infection. His IgG antibody titre to C. pneumoniae was 512 and his IgA titre 32. After this episode, he was healthy until April 1994, when he became ill with a sore throat, cough and mucus aggregation in the throat. As the symptoms persisted, he visited a general practitioner and was found to have a positive culture for C. pneumoniae. No record was made of the appearance of the back of the throat. Serology demonstrated an IgG titre of 256, and an IgA titre of 32 to C. pneumoniae.

Case no. 3 a 30-year-old woman, the wife of case 2, had had problems with sore throat, and mucus aggregation necessitating frequent clearing of the throat since 1990. The symptoms worsened every time she had an upper respiratory tract infection, and an allergy to moulds was suspected. Her respiratory infections persisted throughout the autumn of 1993, with fatigue, plugged nose, and purulent sputum in the mornings. She sought medical advice in December 1993, when a granulated mucus membrane in the retropharynx was observed. Culture for C. pneumoniae proved negative. IgG antibody titres to C. pneumoniae were 64 and for IgA and IgM, <16. She was treated with erythromycin, 250 mg bid for 10 days whereafter the symptoms disappeared for several months. Pharyngeal symptoms eventually returned, necessitating a visit to her physician in August 1994. No record was made of the macroscopic appearance of the throat at that time. Culture of samples taken from the retropharyngeal mucosa proved negative, but PCR was positive for Chlamydia. IgG antibodies remained at a titre of 64 and the IgA titre was still 16.

The couple were given azithromycin, 250 mg $\times$ 2 initially, then 250 mg daily for 4 days. The husband recovered, but his wife's symptoms returned 20 days post-treatment. She received an additional course of azithromycin, 250 $\times$ 2 initially, then 250 mg daily for 4 days, followed by 250 mg biw for 5 weeks.

Case 4

A 68-year-old man who since 1984 suffered from congestion and plugged nose, particularly during the night, mucus aggregation in the throat, periodic hoarseness and cough. He was basically healthy, besides being treated with atenolol for hypertension. In 1988 he was treated with doxycycline for bronchopneumonia. He had repeatedly complained of nasopharyngeal symptoms each time he had visited his general practitioner to check his blood pressure.

On examination, August 2nd 1994, a granulated retropharyngeal mucous membrane was noted. ESR was 30 mm, and PCR was positive for C. pneumoniae. IgG antibody titres to C. pneumoniae were 128, and for IgA, 16. Treatment was initiated with azithromycin 250 mg $\times$ 2, followed by 250 mg once daily for 4 days, and then 250 mg biw for another 5 weeks.

The patient reported marked improvement after 2–3 days of treatment, and for the first time in many years he was able to sleep through the entire night without having to get up and clear his passages. The irritation and mucous aggregation disappeared. At examination on Sept 1st no hyperplastic lymph noduli were found. His antibody titres have not decreased since treatment.

DISCUSSION

All 4 patients presented had a variety of symptoms in the upper respiratory tract, but those from the throat predominated, especially the aggregation of viscous mucous in the throat. We have earlier reported similar findings from the upper respiratory tract in patients with serologically verified C. pneumoniae infection (15). Our cases indicate that C. pneumoniae may be the causative agent of pharyngeal infections persisting for more than one year. Our findings are in agreement with those of Hammerschlag and coworkers (17), who presented 5 cases of persistent infections: one started as bronchitis, while the other 4 began with influenza-like symptoms and pharyngitis.

With the exception of Case 2, our patients did not fulfill the serological criteria of Grayston et al. (3) for acute C. pneumoniae infection. All 5 had had symptoms for a lengthy period of time before seeking medical attention, and it is possible that they may have had specific IgM antibodies initially which had disappeared. The relatively low IgG titres (1/128) are also in agreement with the findings of Kleemola et al. (16) and Hammerschlag et al. (17), who speculated whether treatment with antibiotics may have modified the antibody response. Our 4 patients had specific IgA antibody titres which have been interpreted as a sign of persistent or chronic infection (18).

Specimens were taken from retropharyngeal wall. We have earlier failed to verify the presence of C. pneumoniae by culture (12). At that time specimens were taken from the tonsils, and particularly from the crypts. Only one earlier patient had positive findings by this sampling technique. When the specimens were taken from the retropharynx for the convalescent work-ups, 4 patients were found positive by culture. This is in agreement with our experience and that of other research workers (19). Tonsillitis, however, is not a part of C. pneumoniae infection. Our present technique is to take specimens from the back of the throat by rather vigorous rubbing with a swab. The possibilities offered by the PCR technique have contributed to the improved quality of diagnostic procedures, since even non-viable C. pneumoniae may be detected, which most likely compensated for the suboptimal transportation conditions.

A granular mucous membrane in the throat is a common finding, and has been regarded as being non-specific. However, we have made this clinical observation in patients with verified C. pneumoniae infection. In the cases described above, the granulation paralleled the clinical picture and disappeared following azithromycin treatment. It is known that lymph follicles may appear in Chlamydia trachomatis infections. Lymph follicles under the upper eyelid are one of the classical signs of trachoma (20). Similar findings have been observed in the genital area (21).

Like Hammerschlag et al. (17) we found that persistent C. pneumoniae infections can be very difficult to treat successfully. Extended periods of treatment may be necessary. Azithromycin has a pharmacokinetic profile suitable for treatment of intracellular organisms with a high degree of intracellular penetration (22), long halflife and good in vitro effect on C. pneumoniae (23, 24). The extended treatment period was chosen in order to sustain a high intracellular concentration. The period of treatment was determined empirically.

C. pneumoniae may be one etiological agent causing chronic pharyngitis, at least in some patients. Further studies on the clinical significance of throat granulation in C. pneumoniae infections are necessary.

REFERENCES

1. Saikku P, Wang SP, Kleemola M, Brander R, Rusanen E, Grayston JT. An epidemic of mild pneumonia due to an unusual strain of Chlamydia psittaci. J Infect Dis 151: 832–839, 1985.
2. Marrie TJ, Grayston JT, Wang SP, Kuo CC. Pneumonia associated with the TWAR strain of Chlamydia. Ann Intern Med 106: 507–511, 1987.
3. Grayston JT, Campbell LA, Kuo CC, Mordhurst CH, Saikku P, Thom DH, Wang SP. A new respiratory tract pathogen: Chlamydia pneumoniae strain TWAR. J Infect Dis 161: 618–625, 1990.
4. Ogawa H, Hashiguchi K, Kazuyama Y. Recovery of Chlamydia pneumoniae in six patients with effusion. J Laryngol Otol 106: 490–492, 1992.
5. Hashiguchi K, Ogawa H, Suzuki T, Kazuyama Y. Isolation of Chlamydia pneumoniae from the maxillary sinus of a patient with purulent sinusitis. Clin Infect Dis 15: 570–571, 1992.
6. Komaroff AL, Aronsson MD, Pass TM, Ervin CT, Branch WI, Schachter J. Serologic evidence of chlamydial and mycoplasmal pharyngitis in adults. Science 222: 927–929, 1983.
7. Schachter J. Human Chlamydia psittaci infection. In: Oriel JD, Ridgway G, Schachter J, Taylor-Robingson J, eds. Chlamydial infections. Cambridge: Cambridge University Press, 311–320, 1986.
8. Komaroff AL, Branch WI, Aronson MD, Schachter J. Chlamydial pharyngitis. Ann Intern Med 111: 537–538, 1989.
9. Greber MA, Ryan RW, Tilton RC, Watson JE. Role of Chlamydia trachomatis in acute pharyngitis in young adults. J Clin Microbiol 20: 993–994, 1984.
10. Huovinen P, Lahtonen R, Ziegler T, Meurman O, Hakkarianen K, Miettinen A, Arstila P, Eskola J, Saikku P. Pharyngitis in adults: The presence and coexistence of viruses and bacterial organisms. Ann Intern Med 110: 612–616, 1989.
11. Hargreaves JE, Zajac RA, Kuo CC, Wang SP, Grayston JT. Chlamydia pneumoniae strain TWAR pharyngitis in US Air Force basic trainees. JOAO 94: 51–54, 1994.
12. Falck G, Heyman L, Gnarpe J, Gnarpe H. Chlamydia pneumoniae (TWAR): a common agent in acute bronchitis. Scand J Infect Dis 26: 179–187, 1994.
13. Gnarpe H, Andersson G, Svensson L, Belsheim J. Comparison of Chlamydia trachomatis alginate (CTA) and ear, nose and throat (ENT) swabs for isolation of C. trachomatis. Genitourin Med 61: 139, 1985.
14. Campbell LA, Perez Melgosa M, Hamilton DJ, Kuo CC, Grayston JT. Detection of Chlamydia pneumoniae by Polymerase Chain Reaction. J Clin Micro 30: 434–439, 1992.
15. Falck G, Engstrand I, Persson K. TWAR-infektion vanlig diagnos vid öppenvårdsmottagning. Läkartidningen 89: 1473–1476, 1992. [in Swedish]
16. Kleemola M, Saikku P, Visakorpi R, Wang SP, Grayston JT. Epidemics of pneumonia caused by TWAR, a new Chlamydia organism, in military trainees in Finland. J Infect Dis 157: 230–236, 1988.
17. Hammerschlag MR, Chirgwin K, Roblin PM, Dumornay W, Mandel L, Smith P, Schachter J. Persistent infection with Chlamydia pneumoniae following acute respiratory illness. Clin Infect Dis 14: 178–182, 1992.
18. Saikku P, Leinonen M, Tenkanen L, Linnanmäki E, Ekman MR, Manninen V, Mänttäri M, Frick MF, Huttunen JK. Chronic Chlamydia pneumoniae infection as a risk factor for coronary heart disease in the Helsinki Heart Study. Ann Intern Med 116: 273–278, 1992.
19. Hone SW, Moore J, Fenton J, Gormley PK, Hone R. The role of Chlamydia pneumoniae in acute tonsillitis. J Laryngol Otol 108: 135–137, 1994.

20. Schachter J. The pathogenesis of Chlamydial infection. In: Mårdh P-A, La Placa M, Ward M, eds. Proceedings of the European Society for Chlamydia Research. Uppsala, 67–72, 1992.
21. Hare MJ, Toone E, Taylor-Robinson D, Evans RT, Furr PM, Cooper P, Oates JK. Follicular cervicitis-colposcopic appearances and association with Chlamydia trachomatis. Br J Obstet Gynaecol 1981; 88: 174–180.
22. Foulds G, Shepard RM, Johnson RB. The pharmacokinetics of azithromycin in human serum and tissues. J Antimicrob Chemother, Suppl A, 25: 73–82, 1990.
23. Agacfidan A, Moncada J, Schachter J. In vitro activity of azithromycin (CP-62,993) against Chlamydia trachomatis and Chlamydia pneumoniae. Antimicrob Agents Chemother 37: 1746–1748, 1993.
24. Hammerschlag MR, Qumei KK, Roblin PM. In vitro activities of azithromycin, clarithromycin, L-ofloxacin, and other antibiotics against Chlamydia pneumoniae. Antimicrob Agents Chemother 36: 1573, 1992.

Submitted October 25, 1994; accepted December 11, 1994

Scand J Infect Dis 27: 183–185, 1995 CASE REPORT

Fulminant Disseminated Toxoplasmosis in an HIV Patient

ABDULSALAM K. AL-KASSAB[1], EYASSU HABTE-GABR[1], WILLYS F. MUELLER[2], and QAZI AZHER[2]

From the Department of [1]Internal Medicine Education and [2]Pathology, Hurley Medical Center/Michigan State University College of Human Medicine, Flint, Michigan, USA

Disseminated toxoplasmosis in AIDS is a rare condition. We present an unusual case of a fulminant form of disseminated toxoplasmosis in a young male homosexual. He was a 30-year-old HIV-positive (diagnosed 4 months earlier), admitted with a 5-day history of diarrhea, vomiting, fever, and cough. He had been generally healthy except for an 8-week history of weight loss and malaise. On admission, except for a temperature of 37.6°C, the physical examination was normal. He was treated symptomatically. Four days after admission he suddenly became short of breath. Despite intensive management, he continued to deteriorate and expired 6 h later. Postmortem examination revealed disseminated toxoplasmosis involving the heart, lungs, brain, stomach, small intestine, and colon. This is an unusual presentation of disseminated toxoplasmosis because of its rapid course with no prior indication of infection. To our knowledge, such an atypical and rapid downhill course of toxoplasmosis (with minimal clinical and laboratory features) has not been reported previously. Increased awareness of this infection in all HIV patients and its possibly rapid course is needed.

E. Habte-Gabr, MD, Hurley Medical Center, Two Hurley Plaza, Suite 212, Flint, MI 48503, USA

INTRODUCTION

Toxoplasma gondii is an important protozoan which causes opportunistic infections in patients with AIDS, involving particularly the central nervous system. We report here an unusual case of severe fulminant disseminated toxoplasmosis in a young homosexual male.

CASE REPORT

A 30-year-old homosexual male, found HIV-positive 4 weeks earlier, was referred to the Infectious Diseases Clinic by his family physician. The patient reported a history of fever, night sweats, and weight loss over the past 6 months prior to admission. He had no thrush.

Anamnesis included 1 episode of sudden diarrhea and dehydration 1 year before the present condition, which had been treated symptomatically. At that time his HIV serology was negative. He also had a history of Bell's palsy 2 years earlier, which had resolved completely. It was believed that the patient seroconverted for HIV sometime during the past 12 months.

The patient has been working in the sales department of a major company. He did not keep pet animals and had never been in contact with cats or other pets, nor had he handled pet litter.

Initial laboratory evaluation at the clinic revealed a hemoglobin concentration of 138 g/l, and a platelet count of 258×10^9/l. His white cell count was 2×10^9/l (30% lymphocytes). His absolute CD4+ cell count was 19×10^6/l, CD8+ count was 270×10^6/l resulting in CD4/CD8 ratio of 0.07. He had a negative stool examination for ova and parasites. Serological tests (IgM Ab) for CMV, herpes virus types I and II, were all negative. Toxoplasma IgM antibody was negative, while the IgG antibody level was 1.12. Hepatitis and VDRL serology were negative.

The patient was started on Zidovudine (AZT) (200 mg orally t.i.d.), but he developed severe nausea, vomiting, and diarrhea. He was noncompliant with his follow-up, which prevented further management and chemoprophylaxis consideration for opportunistic infections.

He was admitted to the hospital 3 months after his initial presentation, because of a 5-day history of severe watery diarrhea and vomiting. Physical examination on admission revealed a slight fever of 37.6°C, but was otherwise entirely normal. Initial laboratory work-up was normal, including negative cultures for blood, urine, stool, and sputum. Examination of his stool for ova, parasites, etc. was negative. His chest X-ray was normal. The patient was treated symptomatically, but on the fourth day he suddenly became breathless and tachypneic. He was transferred to the intensive care unit. His chest X-ray at that time revealed extensive bilateral infiltrates with bilateral pleural effusion. Despite intensive management, he continued to deteriorate and developed ventricular fibrillation from which he could not be resuscitated and he expired within 6 hours of this deterioration.

An autopsy was performed and showed the body of a fairly well-developed, well-nourished male, 178 cm in length and weighing 77.3 kg. There was no evidence of wasting or significant weight loss. Externally, there were no significant findings.

Internally, there was minimal fluid within the chest cavities. The lungs filled in both cavities and were consolidated and quite firm in consistency. The heart weighed 400 g, but the myocardium and endocardium were unremarkable. The liver and spleen were not enlarged and were unremarkable. The pancreas had numerous small (3 mm in diameter) nodules. The stomach had numerous small nodules throughout its mucosal surface, measuring 5 to 10 mm in diameter, but the mucosal lining of the small and large intestines appeared unremarkable. The brain weighed 1,420 g; no significant gross abnormalities noted.

Microscopically, Toxoplasmosis gondii cysts and free tachyzoites (trophozoites) were visualized in the tissues by H&E stain and silver stain. They were found in the heart (Fig. 1a), lungs (Fig. 1b), stomach (Fig. 1c), appendix, pancreas (Fig. 1d), brain (Fig. 1e), and colon (Fig. 1f). The severe respiratory distress was readily explained by the extensive involvement by Toxoplasma and the pneumonitic response. In addition to inflammation, hyaline membranes lined many of the alveoli. No other infectious agent was identified.

 ISSN 0036-5548

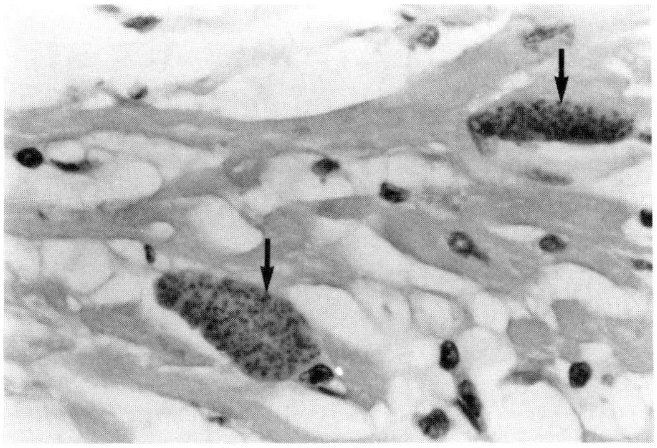

Fig. 1a

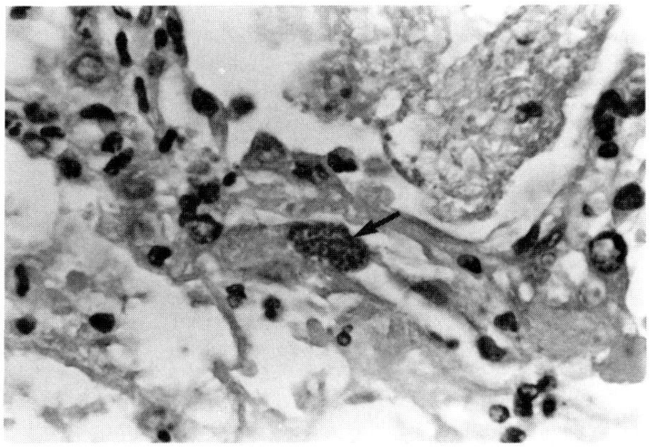

Fig. 1b

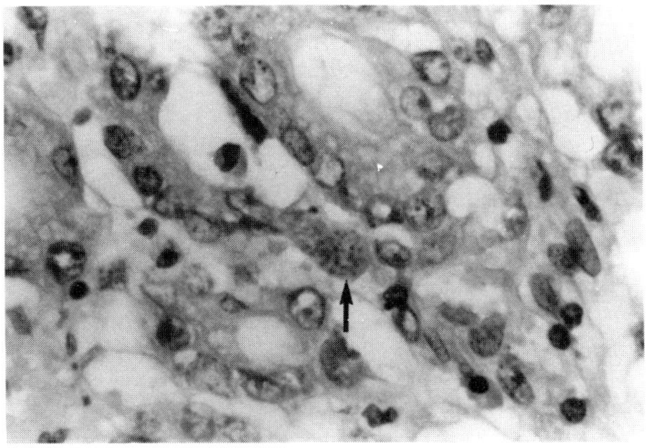

Fig. 1c

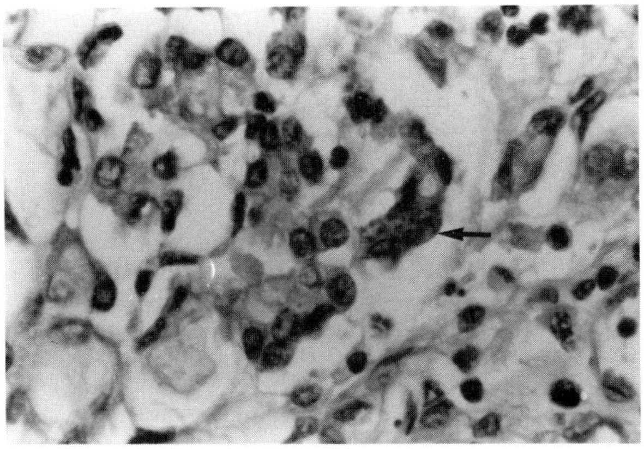

Fig. 1d

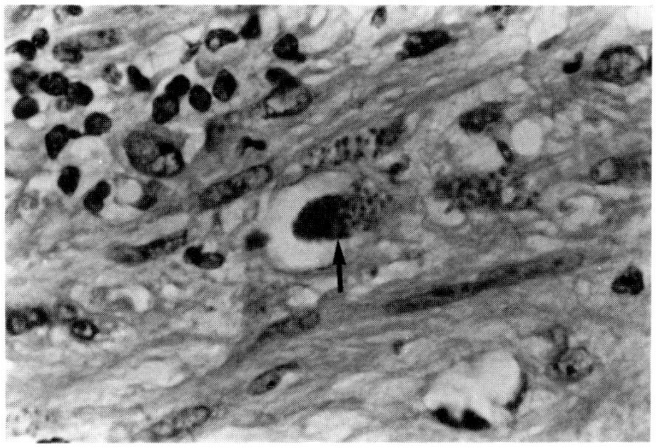

Fig. 1e

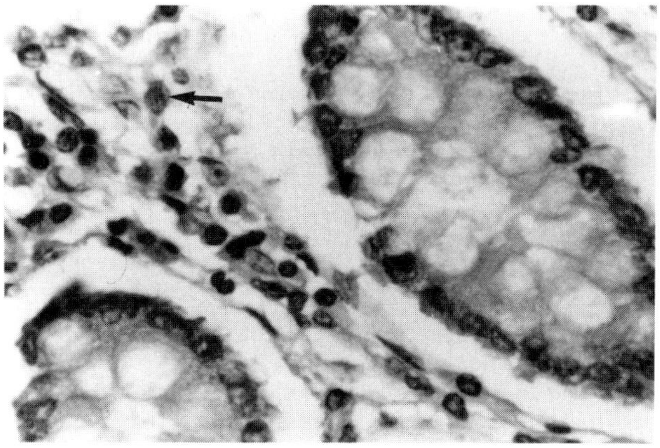

Fig. 1f

Fig. 1. Toxoplasma cysts and trophozoites (*arrows*) in sections of myocardium (*a*), lungs (*b*), gastric mucosa (*c*), pancreas (*d*), brain (*e*), and colon (*f*). All sections, ×200, and stained with H&E.

DISCUSSION

Toxoplasmosis in the immunocompromised host is a well known but relatively uncommon infection (1). In HIV-infected patients, it commonly invades the central nervous system and other organs can also be involved (2). Furthermore, it can also be disseminated especially if the immune deficiency is severe (3), but a fulminant rapid downhill course has not been described previously. Our case had several unusual features. There was severe immunodeficiency (judging by the extremely low CD4+ cell count), yet the patient did not show any clinical or laboratory evidence of an opportunistic infection.

The diarrhea episode that occurred during the terminal illness was short (5 days). No parasites were recovered from the stools. An autopsy examination confirmed the extensive invasion of the gastrointestinal tract by Toxoplasma gondii. This was similar to a previous report (4) describing a case of symptomatic toxoplasmosis involving both the gastrointestinal tract and the lungs, which was diagnosed at autopsy.

Pulmonary toxoplasmosis is being encountered with increasing frequency in patients with AIDS (5). Very often it is associated with fever and bilateral pulmonary infiltrates

(5, 6). The vast majority of patients (>92%) show positive serology. The clinical picture resembles that of Pneumocystis carinii pneumonia (5, 7). Our patient, by contrast, had a normal clinical examination and a normal chest X-ray at presentation but succumbed quickly to an acute respiratory distress within 5 days. Toxoplasma titers were negative. This picture of adult respiratory distress syndrome (ARDS) has been described recently (8). Septic shock secondary to toxoplasmosis has also been described recently (9). Clinical clues to this syndrome include fever and recent onset of dyspnea, and markedly elevated LDH (all of which were present in our patient). Other clues are thrombocytopenia, and initially abnormal chest radiographs, neither of which was present in our patient (who had a normal platelet count, and a normal chest X-ray at the onset of his terminal illness).

Fatal disseminated toxoplasmosis has been attributed mostly to central nervous system infection (10). In one large series evaluating the immediate cause of death in AIDS patients, Moskowitz et al. (11) found that 60% of the patients died of respiratory failure, none of which was due to Toxoplasma infection. In our case, respiratory failure developed suddenly and was most likely related to extensive toxoplasma infection and hyaline membrane formation, as found at autopsy. It is also possible that the patient developed acute pulmonary edema secondary to heart failure as a consequence of the extensive invasion of his myocardium by Toxoplasma.

Disseminated toxoplasmosis is often encountered with the more severe forms of immunodeficiency. The disease is potentially treatable, but the diagnosis is difficult and requires a high index of suspicion on the part of the treating clinician. Our case illustrates the difficulty of making the diagnosis, since all laboratory tests were negative. In addition, it demonstrates the precipitate course that this infection may have. Recently, it became possible to use polymerase chain reaction (PCR) to amplify Toxoplasma gondii DNA in biological samples from AIDS patients with Toxoplasmosis. This facilitates more sensitive detection of Toxoplasma gondii presence in the samples. However, this technique is not yet widely available and was not used in our case. A rapid confirmatory test for Toxoplasmosis would have helped to institute therapy at an earlier stage in this case.

Presently, there are no guidelines for chemoprophylaxis against Toxoplasma infection in severely immunocompromised patients, based on prospective studies. But a recent review (12) has recommended the use of trimethoprim-sulfamethoxazole in HIV patients with CD4 counts $<10 \times 10^6$/l and who have anti-toxoplasma IgG antibodies. It is also not certain which chemotherapeutic agent should be used for this purpose. The fact that an increasing number of disseminated toxoplasmosis cases are being encountered requires the development of guidelines and the establishment of appropriate chemoprophylaxis against it in the severely immunodeficient patients, in the same way that guidelines exist for Pneumocystis carinii pneumonia and Mycobacterium avium intracellulare infections.

REFERENCES

1. Trotter JA, Haglund LA, Greenfield RA, Slater CN, Harris SL, Huchmore HG, Fine DP. Clinical experience with HIV infected patients at the University of Oklahoma Health Science Center. J Ok State Med Assoc 82: 257–261, 1989.
2. Pauwels A, Meyohas MC, Eliaszewicz M, Legendrec C, Momgeot G, Frottier J. Toxoplasma colitis in the acquired immunodeficiency syndrome. Am J Gastroenterol 87: 518–519, 1992.
3. Oksenhandler E, Matheron S. Toxoplasmosis: new aspects, diagnosis and treatment (review). Revue du Praticien 42: 155–159, 1992.
4. Garcia LW, Hemphill RB, Marasco WA, Ciano PS. Acquired immunodeficiency syndrome with disseminated toxoplasmosis presenting as an acute pulmonary and gastrointestinal illness. Arch Pathol Lab Med 115: 459–463, 1991.
5. Pomeroy C, Filice GA. Pulmonary toxoplasmosis: A review. Clin Infect Dis 14: 863–870, 1992.
6. Oksenhandler E, Cadranel J, Sarfati C, Katlama C, Datry A, Marche C, Wolf M, Roux P, Derouin F, Clauvel JP. Toxoplasma gondii pneumonia in patients with the acquired immunodeficiency syndrome. Am J Med 88: 184–214, 1990.
7. Bergin C, Murphy M, Lyons D, Gaffney E, Mulcahy FM. Toxoplasma pneumonitis: fatal presentation of disseminated toxoplasmosis in patients with AIDS. Eur Respir J 5: 1018–1020, 1992.
8. Gandhi S, Lyubsky S, Jimenez-Lucho V. Adult respiratory distress syndrome associated with disseminated toxoplasmosis. Clin Infect Dis 19: 169–171, 1994.
9. Lucet JC, Bailly MP, Bedos JP, Wolff M, Gachot B, Vachon F. Septic shock due to toxoplasmosis in patients infected with human immunodeficiency virus. Chest 104: 1054–1058, 1993.
10. Tschirhart D, Klatt EC. Disseminated toxoplasmosis in the acquired immunodeficiency syndrome. Arch Pathol Lab Med 112: 1237–1241, 1988.
11. Moskowitz L, Hensley GT, Chan JC, Adams K. Immediate cause of death in acquired immunodeficiency syndrome. Arch Pathol Lab Med 109: 735–738, 1985.
12. Gallant JE, Moore RD, Chaisson RE. Prophylaxis for opportunistic infections in patients with HIV infection. Ann Intern Med 120: 932–944, 1994.

Submitted September 6, 1994; accepted January 9, 1995

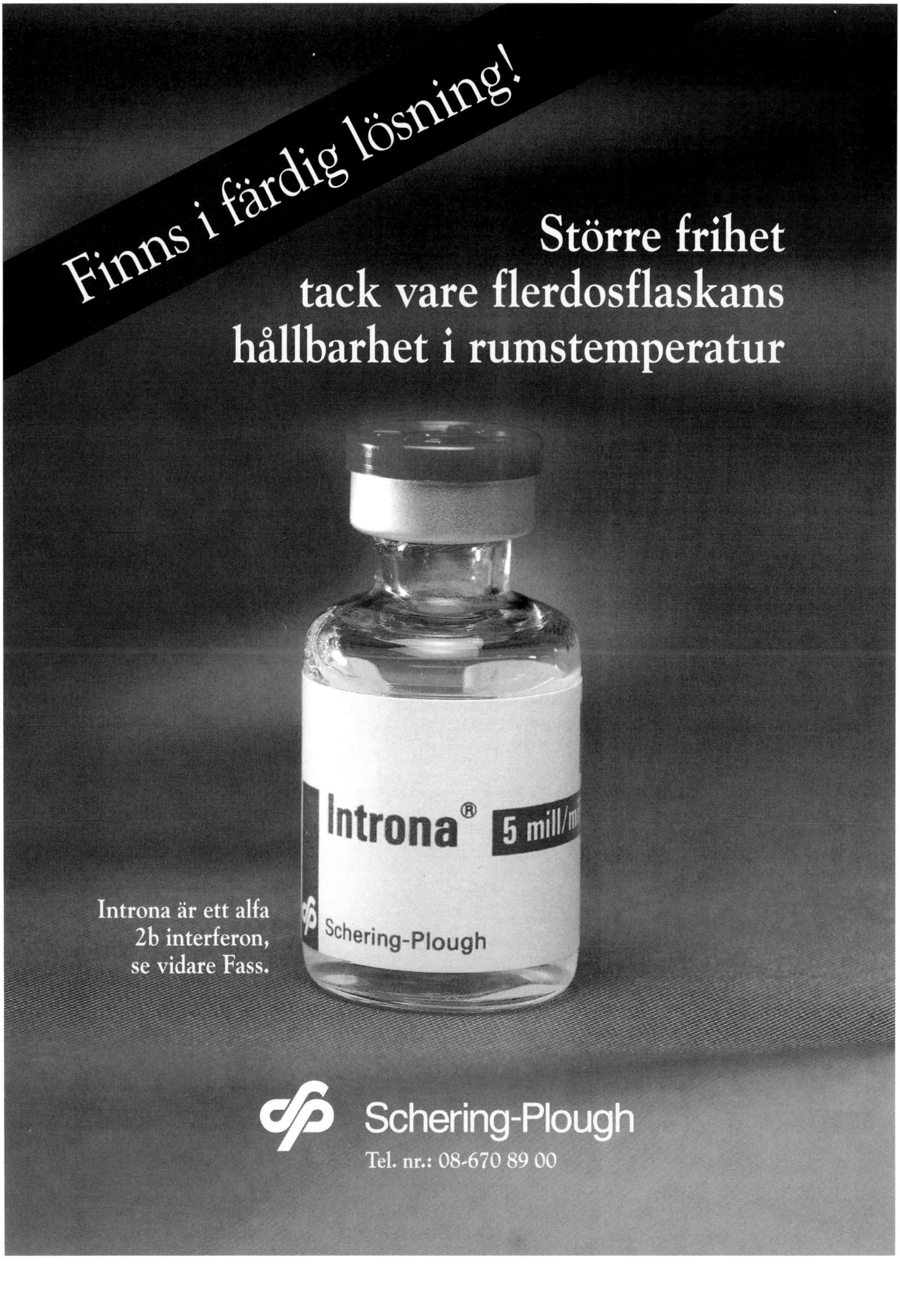
Finns i färdig lösning!
Större frihet
tack vare flerdosflaskans
hållbarhet i rumstemperatur
Introna®
5 mill/m
Schering-Plough
Introna är ett alfa
2b interferon,
se vidare Fass.
Schering-Plough
Tel. nr.: 08-670 89 00

Scand J Infect Dis 27: 187–188, 1995

Campylobacter upsaliensis, C. sputorum sputorum and C. concisus as Common Causes of Diarrhoea in Swedish Children

GUN-BRITT LINDBLOM, EVA SJÖGREN, JANE HANSSON-WESTERBERG and BERTIL KAIJSER

From the Department of Clinical Bacteriology, Göteborg University, Göteborg, Sweden

It has recently been reported that Campylobacter sp. other than Campylobacter jejuni/coli are likely to be the cause of gastroenteritis in humans. Examples are C. upsaliensis, C. jejuni doylei, C. concisus, C. lari and C. mucosalis (1–4).

The routine method today in many clinical microbiological laboratories for isolation of Campylobacter from stool specimens is cultivation on blood-free selective (BFS) agar (5) and incubation for 48 h in 42°C in a micro-aerophilic atmosphere. This procedure generally does not permit the growth of Campylobacter species other than C. jejuni/coli.

In order to investigate the prevalence of Campylobacter species other than C. jejuni/coli in human faeces, we have added a filter technique (0.65 μm) plus a blood agar plate (FTB) which was incubated for 5 days at 37°C in a micro-aerophilic atmosphere (5). For species identification, suspected colonies were subcultivated at 25°, 37° and 42°C for 2–5 days. Besides Gram-staining, the following biochemical tests were used: oxidase, catalase, hippurate, indoxyl-acetate and H_2S/TSI. Sensitivity to nalidixic acid and cephalotin was also tested (6).

During 1993, 2 different Campylobacter studies were carried out on stool specimens sent for routine testing of enteropathogens with standard methods. The first study (study A) included 864 specimens, from as many adults, with diarrhoea, two-thirds of whom were infected abroad. The second study (study B) included 1,077 specimens from as many children <10 years of age, 90% with diarrhoea. Half the children with diarrhoea had been infected abroad. In study A, 85% of the Campylobacter isolates were C. jejuni/coli and in study B, 53% (Table).

In both studies, C. upsaliensis was the most common species next to C. jejuni (Table). C. upsaliensis was twice as common among children (study B) as among adults (study A). Of 16 C. upsaliensis isolates, only 3 were also isolated with the standard method. Among the children, next to C. upsaliensis (18%), C. sputorum sputorum and C. concisus were common, 14 and 6% respectively. These 2 species were isolated only by using the FTB processing of samples and not at all with BFS agar.

Of 16 patients (3 adults and 13 children) positive for C. upsaliensis, 11 had diarrhoea, in some cases severe and with abdominal cramps. Five children, newly adopted or immigrants, had no symptoms. All 10 children positive for C. sputorum sputorum had diarrhoea, in 1 case bloody, and in some cases also with vomiting and fever. C. concisus was isolated from 4 children, all with diarrhoea, and 2 cases also had fever.

In only 3 cases were mixed bacterial infections present, 1 patient with C. upsaliensis and Shigella flexneri, 1 with C. sputorum sputorum and Yersinia enterocolitica and 1 with Salmonella enteritidis together with a non-typable Campylobacter.

We conclude that in some patient groups, e.g. children and immunocompromised persons, Campylobacter infections caused by species other than C. jejuni/coli are likely to occur. We found that certain Campylobacter species that are not routinely searched for, are capable of inducing diarrhoea, especially in children. In 47% of

Table I. *Isolation of Campylobacter species from human stool specimens by 2 different methods*

1) Blood-free selective (BFS) agar; 2) filter technique (0.65 μm) plus blood (FTB) agar. Study A ($n = 864$) adults. Study B ($n = 1,077$) children <10 years.

	Study A (adults) specimens proved positive by					Study B (children) specimens proved positive by					Study A + B specimens positive	
	BFS only	FTB only	BFS & FTB	Total		BFS only	FTB only	BFS & FTB	Total		Total	
Species	*n*	*n*	*n*	*N*	(%)	*n*	*n*	*n*	*N*	(%)	*N*	(%)
C. jejuni	13	1	16	30	(77)	2	2	25	29	(40)	59	(53)
C. coli	2	0	1	3	(8)	2	3	4	9	(3)	12	(11)
C. upsaliensis	0	3	0	3	(8)	0	10	3	13	(18)	16	(15)
C. sput. sputorum	0	0	0	0		0	10	0	10	(14)	10	(9)
C. concisus	0	0	0	0		0	4	0	4	(6)	4	(4)
C. jejuni doylei	0	0	0	0		0	1	1	2	(3)	2	(2)
C. lari	0	0	1	1	(3)	0	1	0	1	(1)	2	(1)
C. non-typable	0	2	0	2	(5)	0	4	0	4	(6)	6	(5)
Total *N*	15	6[a]	18	39		4	35[a]	33	72		111	
(%)	(39)	(15)	(46)		(100)		(49)	(46)		(100)		(100)

[a] $p < 0.01$

 ISSN 0036-5548

the children with Campylobacter an 'uncommon' Campylobacter species was isolated, among whom the frequent occurrence of C. sputorum sputorum (14%) was the most remarkable finding. Until now, this species has only rarely been identified as a pathogen for humans and its clinical significance has to be further clarified (7). In addition to C. sputorum sputorum, C. upsaliensis and C. concisus were common isolates in children. We recommend that laboratories use isolation methods such as the present filter technique that permit detection of these Campylobacter species.

REFERENCES

1. Lastovica AJ, Le Roux E. Prevalence and distribution of Campylobacter species in paediatric patients. Microb Ecol Health Dis Suppl 4: 86, 1991.
2. Lauwers S, Devreker T, Van Etterijck R, Breynaert J, Van Zeebroek A, Smekens L, Kersters K, Vandamme P. Isolation of Campylobacter concisus from human faeces. Microb Ecol Health Dis Suppl 4: 91, 1991.
3. Figura N, Zanchi A, Partini N, Bugnoli M, Guglielmetti P, Signori R, Rossolini A. Campylobacters of unusual species in Siena, Italy. Acta Gastroenterol Belg Suppl 56: 15, 1993.
4. Lastovica AJ, Le Roux E, Warren R, Klump H. Clinical isolates of Campylobacter mucosalis. J Clin Microbiol 31: 2835–2836, 1993.
5. Bolton FJ, Hutchinson DN, Parker G. Reassessment of selective agars and filtration techniques for isolation of Campylobacter species from faeces. Eur J Clin Microbiol Infect Dis 7: 155–160, 1988.
6. Penner JL. The genus Campylobacter: A decade of progress. Clin Microbiol Rev 1: 157–172, 1988.
7. Borczyk A, Lior H, McKeown A, Svendsen H. Isolations of Campylobacter sputorum associated with human infections. In: B. Kaijser, E. Falsen, eds. Campylobacter IV. University of Göteborg, Göteborg, Sweden, 1987 (abstract 211).

Submitted October 26, 1994; accepted December 5, 1994

Scandinavian Journal of

INFECTIOUS DISEASES

Vol. 27, no. 3, 1995
pp. 189–300

SCANDINAVIAN
UNIVERSITY PRESS

Oslo - Copenhagen -
Stockholm - Boston

Scand J Infect Dis 27: 191–194, 1995 ORIGINAL ARTICLE

Antibodies against Hepatitis Viruses in Merchant Seamen

HENRIK L. HANSEN[1], PAUL L. ANDERSEN[2], LARS BRANDT[1] and OLE BROLØS[3]

From the [1]Institute of Maritime Medicine, South Jutland University Centre, Esbjerg, the [2]Department of Infectious Diseases, Marselisborg Hospital, Aarhus, and the [3]Medical Office, Danish Shipowners Association, Copenhagen, Denmark

Seamen constitute a special group of international travellers who may run an increased risk of contracting hepatitis, because of visits to foreign ports and the particular environment on board ship. The purpose of the survey was to assess the prevalence of serological markers for hepatitis A, B and C virus infection among seamen and to identify present and previous risk factors for infection. 515 seamen were studied. The prevalence of antibodies against hepatitis A was 0.3% in subjects below 40 years of age, increasing with age above 40 years, and highest among those who had sailed in international trade. The prevalence of antibodies against hepatitis B was 2.7% in subjects below 40 years of age, increasing to 35.7% in the group above 60 years of age. Hepatitis C antibodies occurred in 1.2%. Vaccination of sailors against hepatitis A should follow the same recommendations as to other travellers. The prevalence of hepatitis B was higher than in reference groups of non-seamen but, because hepatitis B is only one of many blood-borne diseases, prevention should be directed towards changes in behaviour rather than vaccination, except for special groups. Young seamen in international trade were found to be most at risk of contracting sexually transmitted diseases.

H. Hansen, MD, Institute of Maritime Medicine, South Jutland University Centre, Niels Bohrs Vej 9, DK-6700 Esbjerg, Denmark

INTRODUCTION

Seamen are a special group of travellers who may run an increased risk of acquiring hepatitis by exposure to risk factors on board the ships and in foreign ports. Consumption of contaminated water and food on board and ashore can lead to hepatitis A virus (HAV) infection (1, 2). Faecal contamination of ships water supplies has occurred, especially on cruise ships (3). Sexual contacts with persons in high-endemic areas, tattoos, unsatisfactory medical treatment and crowded living conditions are all factors carrying a potential risk for hepatitis B virus (HBV) infection (2, 4, 5).

The maritime trade is important in all Scandinavian countries, and Denmark alone has a merchant navy employing more than 15,000 persons. Most of the vessels, are engaged in foreign trade all over the world.

The purposes of this study were: to assess the prevalence of serological markers for hepatitis A, B, and C virus infection in seamen on board Danish ships and to identify risk factors and risk groups. The intention was to assess preventive measures, including vaccination of sailors seamen against hepatitis A and B. As serological results describe the past, we also wanted to identify the present level of risk behaviour in order to estimate the future risk of transmission of blood-borne diseases among seamen.

MATERIAL AND METHODS

A cross-sectional survey was undertaken at 5 different clinics in various parts of Denmark performing mandatory health examinations of seamen. After written and oral explanation of the purpose of the study, 639 consecutive persons attending any of the five clinics between April and December 1993 for a health examination were invited to participate. Of the 639 subjects, 551 (86.2%) answered a questionnaire providing details of age, sex, country of birth, citizenship, seniority at sea, types of ships, and service in different regions of the world. Furthermore, questions were put regarding tattoos, medical treatment abroad, sexual contacts abroad, previous vaccination against hepatitis A and B, recent injections with immunoglobulin and previous episodes of icterus. Of the 551, 515 (80.6% of all) also agreed to give a blood sample.

The 515 serum samples were screened with ELISA for the presence of total anti-HAV, anti-HBc and anti-HCV using commercially available ELISA kits (HAVAB®, CORE™, ABBOT HCV EIA 2nd Generation, Abbott Lab. USA), and for HBsAg by an ELISA kit (AUSZYME® monoclonal Abbott, USA). Additional retesting of samples positive for anti-HCV in screening was done with a 2nd generation RIBA (Chiron Corporation, USA).

All data were analysed with Epi Info Version 5, (CDC, Atlanta, GA, USA). Logistic regression was performed with Statistix® Version 4.0 (Analytical Software, Tallahassee, FL, USA).

The study was approved by the local Medical Ethics Committee and all participants gave informed consent.

RESULTS

Serology

Seropositivity for HAV was related to age and origin (Tables I and II). Of the seamen below 40 years of age of Scandinavian origin, 248 (75.4%) had been to sea previously and 173 (49.6%) had sailed to ports outside Europe and North America where HAV is endemic. None in this group except one vaccinated seaman was anti-HAV positive. Among the 154 Scandinavians over 40 years old, seroprevalence increased with age (Table II). In a Mantel-Haenszel analysis stratifying for age (10-year age groups), the odds ratio between the group who had sailed to endemic areas and the unexposed group was 2.1 (95% CI 0.4–11.5).

Table I. *Prevalence of antibodies against HAV, HBV and HCV and history of jaundice in seamen attending a fit-for-duty health examination*

		Anti-HAV pos	Anti-HBc pos	Anti-HCV pos	History of jaundice
Group	No. tested	No. (%)	No. (%)	No. (%)	No. (%)
Total	515	79 (15.3)	47 (9.1)	6 (1.2)	11 (2.1)
Male	441	78 (17.7)	45 (10.2)	6 (1.4)	10 (2.3)
Female	74	1 (1.4)	2 (2.7)	0	1 (1.6)
Scandinavian origin	483	62 (12.8)	38 (7.9)	5 (1.0)	8 (1.7)
Non-scandinavian origin	21	11 (52.4)	6 (28.5)	1 (4.8)	2 (4.8)
Uncertain origin	11	6 (54.5)	3 (27.3)	0	1 (9.1)

Table II. *Prevalence of antibodies against HAV, HBV and HCV in seamen of Scandinavian origin attending a fit-for-duty health examination according to age and years in occupation (percentages in parentheses); both sexes included*

		Anti-HAV positive (%)			
		Total	Vaccinated excluded[a]	Anti-HBc pos	Anti HCV pos
	No. tested	No. (%)	No. (%)	No. (%)	No. (%)
Age-group					
<20	11	0 (0.0)	0 (0.0)	0 (0.0)	0
20–29	177	1 (0.6)	1 (0.6)	2 (1.1)	0
30–39	141	1 (0.7)	0 (0.0)	7 (5.0)	3 (2.1)
40–49	71	10 (14.1)	10 (14.1)	14 (19.7)	2 (2.8)
50–59	69	39 (56.5)	38 (55.1)	10 (14.5)	0
60–69	14	11 (78.6)	10 (71.4)	5 (35.7)	0
Years in occupation					
No experience	87	2 (2.3)	2 (2.3)	2 (2.3)	0
0–9 years	144	2 (1.4)	1 (0.7)	4 (2.8)	0
10–19 years	93	2 (2.2)	2 (2.2)	3 (3.2)	3 (3.2)
20–29 years	62	7 (11.3)	7 (11.3)	10 (16.1)	2 (3.2)
30 or more years	84	47 (56.0)	45 (53.6)	17 (20.2)	0
Unknown	13	2 (15.4)	2 (15.4)	2 (15.4)	0

[a] Subjects with positive hepatitis A serology and a history of vaccination or immunoglobulin injection within one year subtracted.

Table III. *Prevalence odds ratios (POR) for variables independently associated with hepatitis B seropositivity calculated by use of multible logistic regression*

Males only and only subjects of Scandinavian origin; CI = confidence interval.

Variable	Adjusted POR (95% CI)	
Age (10-year groups)	1.86	(1.35–2.55)
Sex abroad	1.68	(0.55–5.13)
Tattooing	1.76	(0.85–3.64)
Operation and/or blood transfusion abroad	3.01	(0.88–10.23)

47 seamen were anti-HBc-positive (9.1%). One of these, a 54-year-old master of Danish origin was both HBsAg-positive and HBeAg-positive. The importance of individual risk factors was also evaluated using logistic regression (Table III). In a Mantel-Haenzel analysis stratifying for age (10-year age groups), the odds ratio between Scandinavian non-officer seamen and officers was 1.49 (95% CI 0.66–3.29).

Six subjects were anti-HCV-positive, all confirmed by RIBA. Five were Danes and 1 non-Scandinavian. The prevalence among subjects from Scandinavia was 1.0% and for males 1.2% (95% CI 0.4–2.8%). Three of the 5 positive Scandinavians were also positive for anti-HBc. All 5 had tattoos and had had sex abroad. One had also been operated in hospital abroad.

Jaundice

Among persons of Scandinavian origin, 11 recalled an episode of jaundice in the past. Of these, 3 were anti-HAV-positive, 3 anti HBc-positive and one had antibodies against HAV, HBV, and HCV. We know of the interval between the first employment at sea until the time of the survey in 379 of 396 subjects. This group had been seamen for an average of 17.6 years and for a total of 6,668 years. One anti-HAV-positive person possibly had icterus while at sea. From this the risk of clinical hepatitis A can roughly be estimated to be below 0.15 cases per 1,000 seamen per year. The risk of clinical hepatitis B can correspondingly be estimated to be below 0.45 cases per 1,000 seamen per year (90% exact binomial confidence interval 0.12–1.16).

Table IV. *Frequency of having had sexual contacts abroad and having had a sexually-transmitted disease (STD) within the last 4 years in different age groups in relation to geographic area of sailing*

Only males of Scandinavian origin[a].

Age group	Sexual contact abroad within the last 4 years Area of sailing: World wide No/total no	(%)	North European only No/total no.	(%)	Sexual transmitted disease within the last 4 years Area of sailing: World wide No/total no.	(%)	North European only No/total no.	(%)
<20	3/3	(100.0)	0/3	(0.0)	2/3	(66.7)	0/3	(0.0)
20–29	30/70	(42.9)	7/29	(24.1)	7/70	(10.0)	0/29	(0.0)
30–39	32/75	(42.7)	3/39	(7.7)	6/75	(8.0)	2/39	(5.1)
40–49	17/48	(35.4)	2/17	(11.8)	0/48	(0.0)	0/17	(0.0)
50–59	6/51	(11.8)	0/16	(0.0)	1/51	(2.0)	0/16	(0.0)
60–69	3/10	(30.0)	0/3	(0.0)	0/10	(0.0)	0/3	(0.0)
Total	91/257	(35.4%)	12/107	(11.2%)	16/257	(6.2%)	2/107	(1.9%)

[a] 4 subjects with incomplete information excluded from the table.

Present risk behaviour

The frequency of sexual contacts abroad and the occurrence of sexually transmitted diseases (STD) was investigated in all males of Scandinavian origin who answered the questionnaire, irrespective of whether a blood sample was taken or not (Table IV). The difference between the group who had been in world-wide trade (35.4%) and those who had sailed in North European waters only (11.2%) was statistically significant ($p < 0.001$). STD also occurred more frequently in sailors in world-wide trade (6.2%) than in those who had sailed in North European waters (1.9%, (n.s.)).

A total of 143 (32.9%) Scandinavian males had tattoos, and 113 stated the year they had their first tattoos performed. The mean age at time of first tattoo was calculated for each 10-year age group and was found to be between 17.6 and 20.1 years. In all age groups, more than 90% had their first tattoo before 28 years of age. 61% reported that they had their first tattoo within the first 4 years of going to sea.

DISCUSSION

Vaccination against HAV was introduced in Denmark a few months before the conclusion of this study and Ig had not been recommended routinely to seamen. The results therefore reflect the seroprevalence in a population who have had a limited exposure to HAV and who were generally unprotected. The risk of contracting hepatitis A in the surveyed group was limited. This is in agreement with 1 study from 2 U.S. Navy ships deployed to South America, West Africa and the Mediterranean where none seroconverted during a 6-month follow-up period (6). In another study from the U.S. Navy, 1.3% seroconverted during a 6-month deployment in the Western Pacific and the Indian Ocean (2). The same trend was found in a Norwegian study from 1985–86 (7). On the basis of the results of our and other studies (2, 6, 7) we conclude that merchant seamen should be vaccinated against HAV according to general recommendations (8). Life on board a modern merchant ship does not appear to be a serious risk factor for acquiring hepatitis A.

Scandinavia has one of the lowest prevalence rates of hepatitis B markers in the world (9). Nevertheless, Scandinavian seamen had a higher age-adjusted seroprevalence than other Scandinavians generally. In the most recent Danish study, from 1984, in non-risk persons, no 10-year age group had a prevalence above 5% (10). In a survey from 1977 of 960 Danish blood donors, the prevalence reached a maximum of 7% in subjects aged 55 years and older (11). In a 20-year old survey of 1,000 hospital patients, the prevalence was below 5% for patients born after 1930, but increased to 17% in those born between 1920 and 1930 (12). The estimated incidence of clinical hepatitis B is above the incidence in Denmark for the period 1986–90 (13). Similar results have been found in a survey among Norwegian seamen (7).

In a study from the U.S. Navy, the annual seroconversion rate was 4.1/100 person-years among sailors deployed in the Western Pacific and the Indian Ocean (2). The high rate could not be explained by heterosexual transmission and it was concluded that transmission probably occurred in a variety of ways, including living in the crowded environment on board in combination with a large proportion of HBsAg carriers among the crew (1%). However, in another study of American sailors, only 2/1744 seroconverted during a 6-month deployment to South America, West Africa, and the Mediterranean (6). Only 0.2% of the sailors were HBsAg-carriers. Shipboard transmission cannot be excluded on the basis of the results of our survey. But life on board merchant ships is no longer crowded and implies no more physical contact than at workplaces ashore.

One of the 38 Scandinavians (2.6%) in this study had persistent hepatitis B infection as in other studies (14). The risk of contracting chronic hepatitis B virus infection among Danish seamen is limited. HBV is only one of several blood-borne and sexually transmitted diseases of importance for seamen; i.e. HIV is another (15). Prophylaxis should therefore be directed primarily against blood-borne and sexually transmitted diseases in general, and HBV vaccination should be reserved for special categories, such as ships officers whose duties include repeated medical interventions (16). This group should be informed about the risks of blood-borne diseases associated with medical treatment.

The prevalence of anti-HCV was much higher among seamen than among blood donors in Northern Europe where only 0.04% are positive (17). Those positive for anti-HCV all had had sex and tattooing abroad, both risk factors which may transmit HCV (18, 19). Former or present intravenous drug abuse may possibly be of importance. Anti-HCV positivity is very common among Danish drug addicts (20). The results of this survey cannot explain the mode of transmission but may indicate that hepatitis C is considerably more common in Scandinavia than estimated from the prevalence figures among blood donors (17).

The present risk behaviour and the prevalence of sexually transmitted diseases show that the target group for preventitive measures should be the young seamen, in world-wide trade. The extent to which safe sex is practised in different age groups is not known but almost all cases of sexually transmitted diseases occurred among the young. Information about the risks of having tattoos performed should be given to very young seamen, since it is then that the majority get their first tattoos.

ACKNOWLEDGEMENTS

This study was supported by grants from the J. Lauritzen Foundation, Sygekassernes Helsefond, Novo Nordisk Foundation and The Foundation for Public Health Research (Ribe/Ringkøbing, Denmark). We gratefully acknowledge the assistance from Dr J. Brix, Dr B. Bertelsen, Dr Schouesboe, Dr Rørth, Dr N. Stiggård, Dr O. Gamst, Dr L. Kruse, Dr Witmeur and their staff for assistance in recruiting participants for the study. We also want to thank the staff at the Blood Bank, Esbjerg Central Hospital, Denmark, for technical assistance.

REFERENCES

1. Goethe WHG. Hepatitis on board of seagoing vessels and trawlers. Bull Inst Marit Trop Med Gdynia 19: 31–38, 1968.
2. Hooper R, Cunion S, Conwill D, Merrel B, Wallace J, Batchelor R. Hepatitis A and B in a naval population. Mil Med 153: 350–355, 1988.
3. Addiss DG, Yashuk JC, Clappe DE, Blake PA. Outbreaks of diarrheal illness on passenger cruise ships, 1975–85. Epidemiol Infect 103: 63–72, 1989.
4. Struve J. Hepatitis B virus infection among Swedish adults: Aspects on seroepidemiology, transmission and vaccine response. Scand J Infect Dis Suppl 82: 1–57, 1992.
5. Limentani AE, Elliott LM, Lamborn JK. An outbreak of hepatitis B from tattooing. Lancet 2: 86–88, 1979.
6. Hawkins RE, Malone JD, Cloninger LA, Rozmajzl PJ, Lewis D, Butler J, Cross E, Gray S, Hyams KC. Risk of viral hepatitis among military personnel assigned to US Navy ships. J Infect Dis 165: 716–719, 1992.
7. Siebke JC, Wessel N, Kvandal P, Lie T. The prevalence of hepatitis A and B in Norwegian merchant seamen – a serological study. Infection 17: 77–80, 1989.
8. WHO. International Travel and Health. Vaccination Requirements and Health Advice. Geneva: World Health Organisation, 1994.
9. Sobêslavsky O. Prevalence of markers of hepatitis B virus infection in various countries: a WHO Collaborative Study. Bull World Health Organ 58: 621–628, 1980.
10. Rothgardt NP, Schouenborg PO, Foldspang A. Hepatitis B among physicians in the county of Vejle. Ugeskr Læger 149: 2282–2284, 1987. [in Danish]
11. Hardt F, Aldershvile J, Dietrichson O, Juhl E, Nielsen JO, Schlichting P, Skinhøj P, Tage Jensen U. Hepatitis B virus infection among Danish surgeons. J Infect Dis 140: 972–974, 1979.
12. Skinhøj P. Epidemiology of hepatitis B antigen and antibody in hospital patients in Copenhagen. Scand J Infect Dis 7: 85–89, 1975.
13. Gade, K. Hepatitis B 1991–92. Weekly Report, The State Serum Institute (Epi Nyt) 46: 1, 1993.
14. Shah N, Ostow D, Altman N, Baker AL. Evolution of acute hepatitis B in homosexual men to chronic hepatitis B. Arch Intern Med 145: 881–882, 1985.
15. Hansen HL, Brandt L, Jensen J, Balslev U, Skarphendinsson S, Jørgensen AF, David K, Black FT. HIV Infection among seafarers in Denmark. Scand J Infect Dis 26: 27–31, 1994.
16. Nelsing S, Nielsen TL, Nielsen JO. Occupational blood exposure among health care workers: I Frequency and reporting. Scand J Infect Dis 1993; 25: 193–198.
17. Krarup HB, Krogsgaard K. Hepatitis C. Ugeskr Læger 156: 4129–4134, 1994.
18. Shev S, Wejstål R, Wahl M, Hermodsson S, Norkrans G. The lack of transmission of NANB/C Hepatitis between acute and chronically infected patients and their heterosexual partners. Scand J Infect Dis 23: 407–411, 1991.
19. Ollero M, Marino D, Pujol E, Marquez P, Gimeno A, Angulo C. Tattoos and hepatitis C virus infection (Abstract). VIII International Converence on AIDS: PuC 8163, 1992.
20. Westh H, Worm AM, Jensen BL, Kroon S, Kvinesdal B, Nielsen CM, Wantzin P. Hepatitis C virus antibodies in homosexual men and intravenous drug users in Denmark. Infection 21: 115–117, 1993.

Submitted November 24, 1994; accepted February 6, 1995

Scand J Infect Dis 27: 195–199, 1995 ORIGINAL ARTICLE

Decline of Herpes Simplex Virus Type 2 and Chlamydia trachomatis Infections from 1970 to 1993 Indicated by a Similar Change in Antibody Pattern

KENNETH PERSSON, ANNSOFIE MÅNSSON, EVA JÖNSSON and ERIK NORDENFELT

From the Department of Clinical Virology, Malmö General Hospital, Malmö, Sweden

Antibodies to herpes simplex virus type 2 (HSV-2) and Chlamydia trachomatis (Ct) were determined in sera from pregnant women from 1970 and at intervals up to 1993. The trends for HSV-2 and Ct infections were deduced from the observed antibody rates in different age groups during the observation period. Total antibody rates for HSV-2 tended to decline toward the end of the period when age-matched groups were compared, while the Ct antibody rates peaked in 1979 and then declined gradually. Age-specific antibody rates showed declining frequencies in women younger than 20 years for both HSV-2 and Ct over the study period. Women 35 years of age and older in the early 1990s had significantly higher antibody rates than younger women at that time or than women of similar age in the early 1970s. This group of slightly older women with high antibody rates in the 1990s were 15–20 years of age in 1970 when a high antibody frequency was noted in this age group. High antibody rates against both HSV-2 and Ct in older pregnant women in the early 1990s may thus reflect a high incidence of these infections around 1970. The declining rates of antibodies in the youngest women would suggest a declining incidence of primary infections in this group.

K. Persson, MD, Department of Clinical Virology, Malmö General Hospital, S-214 01 Malmö, Sweden

INTRODUCTION

The prevalences of different sexually transmitted diseases (STD) change over time. Social and individual factors translating into a life style will determine the risk of acquiring STDs ciculating in the population. Effective control programs would tend to reduce the prevalence of such infections. Epidemiological trends can be deduced from the statistics of notifiable diseases. In Sweden, public statistics for gonorrhea are available from the beginning of the century. The reported number of cases soared during the 2 World Wars. During the 1960s the prevalence of gonococcal infections increased and peaked in 1970 with about 40,000 cases reported, since when the continuing decline has led to its virtual eradication. Effective treatment and control measures have contributed to this development.

The diagnostic facilities for Chlamydia trachomatis (Ct) became more generally available during the 1980s. The number of cases detected during the first half of the decade most probably reflected the extent of testing rather than the real prevalence of infection (1). After 1987 when 38,000 cases were reported a genuine decline seems to have occured and the number of cases has decreased by 10–15% each year. Country-wide screening programs are now in operation and must be assumed to have influenced the prevalence of C. trachomatis infections during the last 5–10 years.

Herpes simplex virus type 2 (HSV-2) is associated with genital infections and is primarily sexually transmitted. After the primary infection, the virus remains in a latent state but may be activated at intervals with bouts of clinical disease. Treatment to prevent recurrences has been available for some years but has not been widely used in our population. Limited information is available on the prevalence of genital HSV-2 infection but 4 studies from Sweden have noted increased antibody rates during the 1970s and 1980s (2–5).

The prevalence of antibodies to different human pathogens ought to reflect the frequency of current and previous infections in the population. In order to elucidate the epidemiological trends since 1970 for Ct and HSV-2 infections, a serological study was performed. Pregnant women were used in the study to represent a large segment of the average female population, but non-childbearing women were not included. Changes in the incidences of chlamydial and especially HSV-2 infections may reflect changes in sexual behaviour which are of importance for the prevalence of other STDs, including HIV.

MATERIALS AND METHODS

Sera from 3,244 pregnant women were tested for antibodies to HSV-2 and Chlamydia trachomatis. Women who gave birth during the months March to May, inclusive, at Malmö General Hospital were included. The hospital is the only hospital serving the population of Malmö and most women give birth at the hospital. Only women with Swedish-sounding names were included in the study in order to exclude immigrants who may have experienced a different epidemiological situation. Post-partum sera from consecutive women who gave birth in 1970, 1973, 1979, 1987, 1989, 1991 and

 ISSN 0036-5548

1993 were tested. 300 women were selected from each year, but subsequently the number of sera were doubled from the early and the late parts of the study period in order to obtain large enough groups for statistical analysis. In a few cases, sera could not be located.

HSV-2 antibodies were determined by an enzyme immuno assay (ELISA) using a HSV-2-specific antigen of glycoprotein G (gG2) as described (5) and validated elsewhere (6). Only IgG antibodies were measured. For control purposes, appropriate positive and negative sera were included in the test. In order to confirm the specificity of the test, sera from 15 patients with labial herpes and with a titre rise against a common herpes antigen were tested for HSV-2 antibodies; no such antibodies were detected. Sera from one patient with clinical genital herpes infection and with a positive isolation of HSV-2 showed a titre rise of HIV-2 antibodies. To check for cross-reactive antibodies between HSV-2 and Ct, paired sera from 6 patients with salpingitis and a titre rise against Ct were tested for HSV-2 antibodies. No indication of cross-reactive antibodies between HSV-2 and Ct was found.

Chlamydial IgG antibodies were detected by the micro immunofluorescence method (7). Antigens from representative strains of Ct, C. psittaci and C. pneumoniae (TWAR) were prepared from yolk sacs of infected embryonated hens' eggs. Formalin-treated antigen dots of the different species were placed in clusters of three on microscopic slides. Sera were screened for antibody reactivity in dilution 1/16 and titrated to end point if positive. Reactivity to the different species of chlamydia could be differentiated. Cross-reactive antibodies between HSV-2 and Ct were tested for, using paired sera with titre rise in the HSV-2 test from 5 patients and an additional two individual sera with high titres of HSV-2 antibodies. No antibodies to Ct were detected.

Statistical comparisons between groups were performed by χ^2-tests including Yates' correction. No provision was made for multiple comparisons. Weighted frequecies were calculated for the different years of observation, using the age distribution of 1970 as reference.

RESULTS

HSV-2 antibodies

The total annual rates of HSV-2 antibody in pregnant women from 1970 to 1993 varied between different years from 21% up to 25% (see Table I). Mean age rose from 25 years in 1970 to 29 years in 1993. When weighted antibody frequencies were calculated from the age distribution of women in 1970, a decline in total antibody rates was evident at the end of the period. Increasing mean age inflated observed total antibody frequencies during the 1980s and 1990s.

The age-specific results shown in Table I disclosed a changing antibody pattern during the period. The youngest age-group, consisting of women up to 20 years of age, showed HSV-2 antibodies in 23% in 1970 + 1973. The antibody rates then declined in this age-group during the period to a mean rate of 4% during 1990, 1991 and 1993. In the early 1990s the antibody rates gradually increased with age. The highest rate of 37% was seen in women older than 35 years. These women had been 15 to 20 years of age in 1970 when the antibody rate was high in this age category. The high rate of HSV-2 antibodies in the early 1990s in older women therefore to a large extent reflected infections contracted around 1970. The age-related increase in HSV-2 antibodies seen at the end of the period was probably a cohort effect of a declining incidence of HSV-2 infections since 1970 in women younger than 20 years.

Comparisons of antibody frequencies in different age groups between 1970 + 1973 and 1990 + 1991 + 1993 demonstrated a statistically significant decrease in antibody rate in women younger than 25 years and a significant increase in women over 35 years of age from the beginning to the end of the period. The total antibody rate was 21% in both groups. Again, when weighted frequencies were calculated, there was a significantly lower antibody rate at the end of the period than at the beginning. Differences in mean age tend to obscure this decline in antibody rate.

Different STD agents may share epidemiological features and will thus show a mutual association. Therefore the presence of antibodies to one agent may increase the likelihood of finding antibodies to another sexually transmitted agent. When HSV-2 antibodies were analyzed in those with vs. without antibodies to Chlamydia trachomatis, a clear association between these two agents was observed (Table II).

Chlamydia trachomatis antibodies

Antibodies to Chlamydia trachomatis showed a distribution similar to that of HSV-2 (Table III). In 1970 + 1973 the youngest women had a relatively high rate of antibodies, which declined markedly toward the end of the study

Table I. *Antibodies to herpes simplex virus type 2 in pregnant women 1970–93*

Age group	1970 + 1973	(%)	1979	(%)	1987 + 1989	(%)	1990 + 1991 + 1993	(%)	*p*-values[a]
– 20	28/121	(23)	4/22	(18)	2/43	(5)	2/45	(4)	0.002
21 – 25	107/479	(22)	16/102	(16)	32/174	(18)	35/283	(12)	<0.001
26 – 30	73/401	(18)	26/104	(25)	45/176	(31)	67/436	(15)	
31 – 35	35/139	(25)	12/50	(24)	42/118	(36)	89/284	(31)	
36 –	8/58	(14)	3/16	(19)	15/51	(33)	53/142	(37)	<0.01
Total	255/1,198	(21)	61/294	(21)	138/562	(25)	246/1,190	(21)	
Weighted frequency	21%		20%		23%		16%		<0.001

[a] *p*-values of comparisons between 1970 + 1973 and 1990 + 1991 + 1993.

Table II. *Correlation between HSV-2 and Chlamydia trachomatis antibodies in pregnant Swedish women*

Year	HSV-2 + /Chlamydia + (%)		HSV-2 + /Chlamydia − (%)		*p*-values
1970	67/199	(34)	94/430	(22)	<0.01
1973	47/184	(26)	47/385	(12)	<0.001
1979	40/138	(29)	21/156	(13)	<0.01
1987	35/117	(30)	33/150	(22)	NS
1989	34/111	(31)	36/162	(22)	NS
1990	40/111	(36)	29/186	(16)	<0.001
1991	37/113	(33)	18/180	(10)	<0.001
1993	77/227	(34)	45/373	(12)	<0.001

NS = statistically not significant.

Table III. *Antibodies to Chlamydia trachomatis in pregnant women, 1970–93*

Age group	1970 + 1973 (%)		1979 (%)		1987 + 1989 (%)		1990 + 1991 + 1993 (%)		*p*-values[a]
– 20	48/121	(40)	11/22	(50)	17/43	(40)	6/45	(13)	<0.001
21 – 25	154/479	(32)	48/102	(47)	71/174	(41)	86/283	(30)	
26 – 30	117/401	(29)	50/104	(48)	67/176	(38)	167/436	(38)	<0.01
31 – 35	43/139	(31)	18/50	(36)	52/118	(44)	124/284	(44)	<0.002
36 –	21/58	(36)	11/16	(69)	21/51	(41)	64/142	(45)	
Total	383/1,198	(32)	138/294	(47)	228/562	(41)	447/1,190	(38)	<0.01
Weighted frequency	32%		47%		40%		33%		

[a] *p*-values of comparisons between 1970 + 1973 and 1990 + 1991 + 1993.

period. An age-related increase in antibody frequency was noted during the 1990s, parallel to that observed for HSV-2 antibodies, although the peak rates in older women were not as marked for Ct antibodies. High antibody rates in the youngest age group during the 1970s may be reflected in the increasing antibody rates in older women at the end of the period in a way similar to that of HSV-2 antibodies. The antibody rates for the different years between 1970 and 1993 showed higher total rates at the middle of the period for Ct and then a decline which was clearly evident when weighted frequencies were compared. The decline in Ct antibodies may therefore have been lagging somewhat behind that of HSV-2 antibodies, although the groups for the individual years may not all be large enough to give reliable information.

When comparing aggregate figures for 1970 + 1973 and 1990 + 1991 + 1993, the decline in Ct antibodies between the beginning and the end of the study period among the youngest women was statistically highly significant (Table III). The increase in antibody rates in women 26 to 35 years of age is also statistically significant. The difference of 9% in women older than 36 years was not statistically significant, however.

The MIF test utilizes whole elementary bodies as antigen. Both species-specific and genus-reactive antibodies can be detected. When prototype strains for both C. psittaci, C. pneumoniae and Ct are included in the test, cross-reactive antibodies can be distinguished from the species-specific reactivity. In order to verify that specific antibodies to Ct were measured, the frequency of Ct antibodies was compared in women with and without concurrent antibodies to C. pneumoniae. It was found that the rate of Ct antibodies did not differ in women with vs. without such antibodies (Table IV). Cross-reactive antibodies therefore did not seem to flaw the results.

DISCUSSION

Total antibody rates for 1970 + 1973 and 1990 + 1991 + 1993 demonstrated an increase of chlamydial anti-

Table IV. *Correlation between antibodies to Chlamydia trachomatis and Chlamydia pneumoniae in pregnant Swedish women*

Year	C. trachomatis + /C. pneumoniae + (%)		C. trachomatis + /C. pneumoniae − (%)		*p*-value
1973	58/173	(34)	36/128	(28)	NS
1991	65/170	(38)	47/126	(37)	NS
1993	133/321	(41)	94/279	(34)	NS

NS = statistically not significant.

bodies but showed similar HSV-2 antibody frequencies during the early 1970s compared with the early 1990s. This development of antibody rates was partly explained by a change in mean age of the groups of women of the different years. An increasing mean age towards the end of the period tended to inflate antibody rates. When weighted antibody rates were calculated, a marked decline in the 1990s was obvious for HSV-2, while the prevalence of Ct antibodies was the same at the beginning as at the end of the period. Peak antibody rates were observed at the middle of the period for Ct and to a lesser extent for HSV-2. There were also marked changes in age-specific antibody rates between the individual years. The prevalence of both HSV-2 and Ct antibodies declined at the end of the period in the youngest age groups, suggesting a lower infection rate at that time. The highest prevalence of Ct infections is known to occur around 20 years of age in women and might be expected to be similar for primary HSV-2 infections, which is the time when antibodies first appear. At the beginning of the period, similar levels of antibodies were detected in the different age groups. At the end of the period this pattern had altered and a gradual increase with age was found for both HSV-2 and Ct antibodies. Women older than 36 years in the 1990s and with high antibody rates at that time had been 15 to 20 years of age in 1970 when relatively high antibody frequencies occurred in women younger than 20 years. Therefore the high antibody rate in older women in the early 1990s probably reflected infections contracted around 1970. The peak at the end of the period is not so marked for Ct as for HSV-2 antibodies but the persistence of antibody is also likely to be different. HSV-2 is a lifelong infection, although latent most of the time, while Ct infection is of limited duration and will clear after a time. Older women are more likely to have lost earlier C. trachomatis antibodies than HSV-2 antibodies. The observed frequencies of C. trachomatis antibodies in older women in the early 1990s are thus probably unduly low.

The peak in the middle of the period, which was prominent for C. trachomatis antibodies and indicated for HSV-2 antibodies, ought to be predicted by a high incidence of infections around 1970 in young women. The mean age of childbearing women is close to 30 years, which is some 10 years after the incidence peak of C. trachomatis infection (and presumably of HSV-2 infections). The full impact of such infections occurring around 1970 would therefore be evident in pregnant women around 1980. The observed weighted frequencies seem to vindicate that prediction.

Neonatal herpes simplex virus infection is usually a complication of primary herpes infection. In the population studied, we have diagnosed 5 cases with this condition between 1981 and 1984. This is in contrast to the period before 1981 when no case had been detected for several years. Again, neonatal herpes simplex infections virtually disappear in the late 1980s and early 1990s. This pattern could be compatible with the epidemiological situation described above. An increased awareness and a change in the management of genital herpes simplex virus infection during pregnancy may have influenced the situation at the end of the period. It is of interest that a peak of neonatal herpes simplex virus infections was also observed in Seattle at the same time (8).

A clinical indicator of Ct infection in women would be non-gonococcal salpingitis, especially in women younger than 25 years where at least a third may be expected to be associated with Ct infection. In our population there was a peak in the number of annual cases of non-goncoccal salpingitis around 1970, since when a parallel decline has been observed in the prevalence of both gonococcal and non-gonococcal salpingitis. The decline of gonococcal salpingitis faithfully reflects the decrease in the total number of detected gonococcal infections in women in Malmö and in Sweden as a whole.

Between 1989 and 1993, isolates of herpes simplex virus from the genital tract of pregnant women were type 2 in 59–67% of the cases and type 1 in the remainder of 70 to 100 isolates a year. A larger proportion of type 2 strains may have been present earlier in the study period, but no direct information is available. An increase in the proportion of HSV-1 isolates in Edinburgh from 1978 to 1991, when some 40% were type 1, has recently been reported (10). The effect of such a change – if it occurred – would be only marginal on the observed antibody rates in this study and could not account for the detected trends in the HSV-2 antibody pattern.

The specificity of the antibody testing is of prime concern. The HSV-2 antibody test using a gG2 preparation as antigen has been thoroughly described elsewhere (6, 7). In this study a small panel of sera from patients with HSV-1 and HSV-2 infections were included as controls of the test performance. An association between HSV-2 and Ct antibodies was demonstrated. No cross-reactive antibodies were observed in a number of paired sera with titre rises against one antigen when tested for antibodies against the other antigen. Antibody reactivity against both Ct and C. pneumoniae is often found together, as two-thirds of adults are expected to have C. pneumoniae antibodies. Inclusion of a C. psittaci antigen as well in the test will make cross-reactive antibodies easy to detect. The results obtained in this study show that Ct antibodies are equally common in patients with concurrent C. pneumoniae antibodies as in those without such antibodies. Antibodies to C. pneumoniae therefore did not flaw the results of Ct antibody rates.

The association between HSV-2 and Ct antibodies is likely to be an indirect one. The number of lifetime sex partners will influence the risk of contracting any STD agent. The association of antibodies reflects lifetime exposure rather than an increased risk of concurrent transmission. The observed antibody patterns for HSV-2 and Ct from 1970 to 1993 suggest a relatively high incidence of infections around 1970 in young women, leaving a trace of antibodies to be detected in increasingly older segments of the pregnant women over the observation period. The decreasing antibody rates in the youngest women suggest declining incidences of both Ct and HSV-2 infections during the period. The decline in the incidence of HSV-2 infections would suggest a change in sexual behaviour with decreasing risk of acquiring infection. The incidence of Ct infections is expected to have declined as a result of an extensive control programme implemented during the second half of the 1980s. Whether a decline in incidence had started earlier during the period cannot be concluded from the serological results. Antibody rates in women older than 36 years in the coming few years may clarify the situation.

Reported numbers of gonococcal infections evidence a gradual decrease in the prevalence of this infection since 1970. The serological results in this study would suggest a similar decline for herpes simplex virus type 2 infections. The antibody pattern for C. trachomatis also indicates a declining incidence of this infection. Serological surveys may be helpful in detecting long-term changes in the prevalence of some STD agents where other means of information may be lacking. Changes in antibody frequencies may reflect changes in sexual behaviour either in terms of the number of sex partners or in the adoption of safe sex practices such as condom use. Such changes would influence the prevalence of different STD agents, including HIV.

REFERENCES

1. Ripa T. Epidemiological control of genital Chlamydia trachomatis infections. Scand J Infect Dis Suppl 69: 157–167, 1990.
2. Nahmias AJ, Lee FK, Beckman-Nahmias S. Sero-epidemiological and -sociological patterns of herpes simplex virus infection in the world. Scand J Infect Dis Suppl 69: 19–36, 1990.
3. Forsgren M. Genital herpes simplex virus infection and incidence of neonatal disease in Sweden. Scand J Infect Dis Suppl 69: 37–41, 1990.
4. Löwhagen GB, Jansen E, Nordenfelt E, Lycke E. Epidemiology of genital herpes infections in Sweden. Acta Derm Venereol 70: 330–334, 1990.
5. Forsgren M, Skoog E, Jeansson S, Olofsson S, Giesecke J. Prevalence of antibodies to herpes simplex virus in pregnant women in Stockholm in 1969, 1983 and 1989: implications for STD epidemiology. Int J STD AIDS 5: 113–116, 1994.
6. Olofsson S, Lundström M, Marsden H, Jeansson S, Vahlne A. Characterization of a herpes simplex type 2-specific glycoprotein and affinity for N-acetylgalactosamine-specific lectins and its identification as 92 K or gG. J Gen Virol 67: 737–744, 1986.
7. Ho DWT, Field PR, Sjögren-Jansson E, Jeansson S, Cunningham L. Indirect ELISA for the detection of HSV-2 specific IgG and IgM antibodies with glycoprotein G (gG-2). J Virol Methods 36: 249–264, 1992.
8. Wang SP, Grayston JT. Immunologic relationship between genital TRIC, lymphogranuloma venereum, and related organisms in a new microtiter indirect immunofluroescence test. Am J Ophthalmol 70: 367–374, 1970.
9. Corey L. Herpes simplex virus infections during the decade since the licensure of acyclovir. J Med Virol Suppl 1: 7–12, 1993.
10. Ross DC, Smith IW, Elton RA. The epidemiology of herpes simplex types 1 and 2 infection of the genital tract in Edinburgh. Genitourin Med 69: 381–383, 1993.

Submitted October 12, 1994; accepted February 21, 1995

Scand J Infect Dis 27: 201–206, 1995

ORIGINAL ARTICLE

Severe Community-acquired Pneumococcal Pneumonia

PIERRE MOINE[1], JEAN BAPTISTE VERCKEN[1], SYLVIE CHEVRET[2], PHILIPPE GAJDOS[1] and THE FRENCH STUDY GROUP OF COMMUNITY-ACQUIRED PNEUMONIA IN ICU[3]

From the [1]Service de Réanimation Médicale, Hôpital Raymond Poincaré, Garches, and the [2]Département de Biostatistique et Informatique Médicale, Hôpital Saint-Louis, Paris, France

Streptococcus pneumoniae is the most frequent pathogen of severe community-acquired pneumonia (CAP) necessitating hospitalization. The main objective of this multicentre prospective study was to determine the value of clinical, biological, and radiological features for predicting pneumococcal etiology and to define prognostic factors. Streptococcus pneumoniae was isolated in 43/132 patients (33%) with CAP requiring ICU treatment. The mean age of the patients with pneumococcal pneumonia was 55 ± 17 (SD) yrs and 34 were male. On admission, 14 patients with pneumococcal pneumonia were in shock, 24 were mentally confused, and 27 required mechanical ventilation during their hospitalization. Among the clinical, biological, and radiological features, fever >39°C, pleuritic chest pain, lobar distribution or alveolar consolidation, and an increase in immature granulocytes ≥5% of WBC were more frequent in pneumococcal pneumonia than in other etiologies. Mortality was 35%. Fatal outcome was significantly related to the presence of impaired alertness, septic shock, mechanical ventilation, acute renal failure, and bacteremic pneumonia.

P. Moine, MD, Service de Réanimation Médicale, Hôpital Raymond Poincaré, 92380-Garches, France

INTRODUCTION

Severe community-acquired pneumonia (CAP) requiring intensive care treatment is frequent, and represents some 18–36% of CAP patients requiring hospitalization (1, 2). Mortality rates of 47–76% have been reported (3, 4). Streptococcus pneumoniae remains the predominant pathogen of CAP in adults requiring hospitalization, often accounting for 35% or more of the identified agents (1, 2, 5–11). Despite the availability of penicillin to which most pneumococcal strains are fully sensitive, pneumococcal pneumonia continues to pose considerable problems in the 1990's in terms of morbidity and mortality. Moreover, the emergence of penicillin-resistant S. pneumoniae strains will become a major concern in the future. Many authors (12–16) have pointed out the difficulty of determining pneumococcal etiology during the first 48 h after admission. The lack of discriminant clinical, biological and radiological criteria may explain this difficulty. Although a recent report has partially addressed this issue (17), little is still known regarding the incidence, prognostic factors, and outcome of patients with severe community-acquired pneumococcal pneumonia.

The main aim of this study was to describe the clinical, radiological and biological features of patients with severe pneumococcal pneumonia admitted to an intensive care unit (ICU), as well as to clarify features that could predict this etiology. A secondary goal involved a prognostic study which attempted to define a subset of patients with a high risk of death.

METHODS AND PATIENTS

From June 1987 to December 1989, 132 consecutive patients with severe CAP requiring ICU treatment were prospectively included in this study. There were 15 French participating centres. Pneumonia was defined as any acute septic episode with respiratory symptoms and radiological pulmonary shadowing which was neither pre-existing nor of other known cause. The presence of at least one of the following conditions justified defining the pneumonia as severe: respiratory frequency >30 breaths/min, the need of mechanical ventilation, chest X-ray showing bilateral involvement or involvement of multiple lobes, or shock (systolic blood pressure <80 mmHg). All non-immunocompromised adults (≥15 years) with a simplified acute physiologic score (SAPS) (18) ≥8 were eligible [patients with chronic bronchitis or emphysema who developed pneumonia (acute septic illness with evidence of a new infiltrate) were also included]. Patients with pulmonary edema or pulmonary tuberculosis were excluded, as were patients with lymphoma, cancer, organ transplantation, and treatment with corticosteroids or immunosuppressants. HIV-positive patients and those suffering from agranulocytosis and hypogammaglobulinemia were also excluded.

For each case, a questionnaire was filled out reporting medical symptoms and signs on admission, in addition to radiological and laboratory findings. Clinical parameters during the first 24 h were also noted. Each type of bronchopulmonary sampling [expectorated sputum (ES), transtracheal aspiration (TTA), distal aspiration (Matthew's method) (19) (DA), or plugged telescoping catheter (PTC) brush (Wimberley's method) (20, 21)], as well as blood cultures, cultures of pleural effusions of CSF, direct IF for Legionella, soluble antigen detection for pneumococcal antigen by latex agglutination, and serological tests for Mycoplasma pneumoniae, Chlamydia, Legionella species, Rickettsia, or virus (Influenza

[3] B. Schlemmer, M-T. Garrouste (Paris), J-F. Muir, C. Defouilloy (Amiens), F. Thaler (Suresnes), A. Tenaillon (Evry), J. Carlet, J-F. Timsit (Paris), J-B. Vercken, Ph. Gajdos, P. de Rohan-Chabot (Garches), J-M. Boles (Brest), H. Outin (Poissy), J-D. Tempe, F. Schneider (Strasbourg), L. Holzapfel (Bourg en Bresse), J-P. Sollet (Argenteuil), P. Petitpretz (Clamart), F. Fraisse (Saint Denis), G. Gbikpi-Benissian, J-P. Cardinaud (Bordeaux) and C. Brun-Buisson (Creteil).

 ISSN 0036-5548

Virus type A and B, Parainfluenza Virus, Adenovirus, Respiratory Syncytial Virus) were not required but recommended. The ES, TTA, and DA samples were submitted to the local microbiological laboratory where cultures (quatitative culture for TTA or DA) and Gram stains were performed. Each centre carried out its own serologic tests. The choice of antibiotics was left to the discretion of each centre.

Etiological diagnosis

All blood culture isolates were considered to be etiologic agents of the pneumonia, except for Staphylococcus aureus and aerobic Gram-negative bacteria (Enterobacteriaceae and Pseudomonadaceae), which in addition were required to be isolated from the bronchopulmonary sample. All pleural fluid culture isolates were considered as causal agents of the pneumonia.

S. pneumoniae was considered to be the etiological agent if it was isolated in pure culture from ES or TTA, irrespective of the Gram stain result. Purulence was evaluated by microscopy, and only purulent samples (>5 leukocytes/epithelial cell) were cultured. Staph. aureus, Haemophilus influenzae, Moratecca catarrhalis, or enterobacteria were regarded as the etiological agent if isolated in pure culture from ES or TTA, and if the morphological correlates of the bacterium predominated on Gram stain. S. pneumoniae, Staph. aureus, H. influenzae, M. catarrhalis, or Gram-negative bacilli were considered to be the cause of the pneumonia only if the micro-organism was isolated in a quantitative culture with $\geq 10^3$ cfu/ml from DA or PTC brush specimens.

Pneumococcal infection was considered definite when pneumococcal antigen was detected in serum or pleural fluid.

A 4-fold or greater rise in virus serological test titre was regarded as evidence of viral infection. A 4-fold rise in titre $\geq$1:128, or a single titre $\geq$1:256 in Legionella immunofluorescent antibody tests, was regarded as evidence of Legionella infection. A 4-fold rise in titre $\geq$1:64, or a single titre $\geq$1:256 in the Mycoplasma specific IgG immunofluorescent antibody test, was considered evidence of Mycoplasma infection. A 4-fold rise in titre $\geq$1:16, or a single titre $\geq$1:128 in complement fixing tests, was considered evidence of Chlamydia psittaci infection.

The DFA examination of respiratory tract secretion established a diagnosis of Legionella infection.

Dual aerobic or anaerobic bacteria were considered to be the etiological agents if they were isolated simultaneously in the same culture.

Statistical methods

Statistical analysis was performed using the S.A.S. software package. Comparisons between pneumococcal pneumonia and the other etiologies were based on χ^2-tests for categorical variables, and on the non-parametric Wilcoxon test for the continuous variables. Such predictive analysis used 2-tailed tests of significance, and a type I-error of 5%. For patients with pneumococcal pneumonia, overall survival was estimated by the Kaplan-Meier method. The prognostic value of the baseline parameters assessed at admission and during hospitalization was evaluated using the logrank test.

RESULTS

S. pneumoniae was isolated in 43/132 patients (33%) with CAP requiring ICU treatment. The organisms in the entire group and their relative frequencies are listed in Table I. The mean age of the 43 patients was 55 ± 17 (SD) years, and 34 were males. 28 (65%) had pre-existing disease. 15 had COPD, 19 had chronic alcoholism, there were 4 cases of diabetes mellitus and 3 patients presented neurological diseases. Seven patients had received antibiotics before admission; beta-lactams in 4 cases, macrolides in 2 cases and tetracyclines in 1 case.

Table I. *Microbiological Diagnosis*[a] *and Mortality*[b] *of 132 patients with severe pneumonia which required ICU treatment*

	Organism n (%)	Death n (%)
Streptococcus pneumoniae[c]	43 (33)	15 (33)
Streptococcus species	9 (7)	2 (22)
Staphylococcus aureus	5 (4)	3 (60)
Haemophilus influenzae	14 (11)	4 (29)
Escherichia coli	7 (5)	3 (43)
Klebsiella pneumoniae	6 (5)	2 (33)
Pasteurella multocida	1 (1)	1
Legionella pneumophila	4 (3)	1 (25)
Mycoplasma pneumoniae	1 (1)	
Chlamydiae psittaci	1 (1)	
Moraxella catarrhalis	2 (2)	
Moraxella lacunata	1 (1)	
Coxiella Burnetii	2 (2)	1
Viruses[d]	7 (5)	
Anaerobes	1 (1)	
Etiology determined	95 (72)	29 (31)
Undetermined etiology	37 (28)	3 (8)

[a] Included 9 patients with dual etiologies (S. pneumoniae + H. influenzae, 2; S. pneumoniae + K. pneumoniae, 1; Staph. pneumoniae + S. aureus, 1; Streptococcus species + Staph. aureus, 1; Streptococcus species + H. influenzae, 1; H. influenzae + anaerobes, 1; K. pneumoniae + L. pneumophila, 1; E. coli + Enterococcus, 1).

[b] Included 3 patients with dual etiologies (S. pneumoniae + Staph. aureus; H. influenzae + Streptococcus species; S. pneumoniae + H. influenzae).

[c] Included 4 patients with dual etiologies (S. pneumoniae + H. influenzae, $n = 2$; S. pneumoniae + K. pneumoniae, $n = 1$; S. pneumoniae + Staph. aureus, $n = 1$).

[d] Varicella-Zoster Virus, $n = 2$; Influenza A or B Virus, $n = 2$; Parainfluenza Virus, $n = 3$.

had COPD, 19 had chronic alcoholism, there were 4 cases

Clinical findings and investigation results: In patients with pneumococcal pneumonia, the mean duration of illness prior to admission was 3.7 ± 2.7 days (SD) with a range of <1 up to 10 days. 12 patients presented symptoms for <24 h prior to admission. On admission to the ICU, 14 patients were in shock, 24 were mentally confused, 29 had a respiratory frequency >30 breaths/min, 7 were already reveiving mechanical ventilation, 30 had a PaO_2/FiO_2 ratio <250 mmHg, and 16 had renal failure (BUN > 10 mmol/l). During the first 24 h in the ICU, 18 additional patients required intubation and mechanical ventilation. The mean value for the simplified acute physiologic score (SAPS) was 14 ± 5 (range 8–29). The clinical, biological, and radiological data on ICU admission are summarized in Table II. Chest X-rays showed bilateral involvement in 18 cases and involvement of multiple lobes in 27 cases. During

Table II. *Clinical features and investigation results on admission*

	Streptococcus pneumoniae ($n = 43$) Number of cases (%)	Other etiologies ($n = 89$) Number of cases (%)	p
Age (years, mean-SD)	55 ± 17	60 ± 18	
Mean duration of symptoms before admission to ICU (days, mean-SD)	3.7 ± 2.7	4.9 ± 4.2	0.057
Symptoms on admission			
Temperature (°C, mean-SD)	39.4 ± 1	38.5 ± 3.2	0.06
High fever (≥39°C)	29 (67)	42 (47)	0.05
Chills	10 (23)	19 (21)	
Cough	25 (58)	60 (67)	
Purulent expectoration	27 (63)	53 (60)	
Rusty-brown expectoration	4 (9)	4 (4)	
Chest pain	11 (26)	8 (9)	0.01
Wheezing	2 (5)	17 (19)	
Upper respiratory symptoms	3 (7)	7 (8)	
Confusion, stupor, coma	24 (56)	47 (53)	
Abdominal pain	7 (16)	9 (10)	
Hepatomegaly	17 (40)	22 (25)	0.06
Jaundice	8 (19)	9 (10)	
Laboratory tests on admission			
Leukocytosis WBC ≥ 8,000 cells/mm3	32 (74)	65 (73)	
WBC ≥ 15,000 cells/mm3	12 (28)	20 (22)	
Leukopenia WBC ≤ 3,000 cells/mm3	4 (9)	5 (6)	
Increased percentage of immature granulocytes (≥5% of WBC)	11 (26)	8 (9)	0.046
Chest x-ray on admission			
Lobar distribution	28 (65)	40 (45)	0.027
Homogeneous infiltrates	29 (67)	43 (48)	0.030
Reticular or reticulonodular infiltrates	0	5	
Mixed infiltrates	13 (30)	40 (45)	
Pleural effusion	13 (30)	18 (20)	

hospitalization, 27 patients (63%) required mechanical ventilation.

The results from this prospective study showed that a temperature >39°C, chest pain, increase in immature granulocytes ≥5% of WBC, lobar distribution, and alveolar consolidation were more frequently associated with severe pneumococcal pneumonia when compared with the other etiologies (Table II). However, the positive/negative predictive values of the symptoms that were more common in patients with pneumococcal pneumonia than in those with other etiologies were respectively 0.38/0.71, 0.58/0.72, 0.58/0.72, 0.42/0.77 and 0.40/0.77. The association of 4 of these symptoms was found in only 21% of the 43 pneumococcal infections and 3 of them in 49% of the pneumococcal infections.

Bacteriologic procedures: 52 bronchopulmonary samples were obtained from 38 patients (88%) with pneumococcal pneumonia during the first 24 h. Gram staining was performed on 42 samples (ES, TTA, and DA) in 34 patients. Gram staining could not be done in 4 cases in which PTC brush only was performed. Gram-positive cocci on a Gram stain were found in 26 samples. For the 132 patients, Gram-positive cocci on Gram stain had a positive predictive value of 0.67 and a negative predictive value of 0.79. In 6 patients, the diagnosis was based solely on non-protected cultures (sputum or TTA) and compatible Gram stain findings.

Blood cultures were performed in 41 patients with pneumococcal pneumonia. 22 patients (54%) had positive results of blood cultures. In 25 patients, both blood-soluble antigen detection for pneumococcal antigen and blood cultures were performed; soluble antigen detection was positive in only 5/13 cases of bacteremic pneumococcal pneumonia, and in 1/12 cases of non-bacteremic pneumonia. The diagnostic yield of the various tests is shown in Table III.

The influence of antibiotics before admission on microbiological diagnosis: Taking all patients into account, antibiotic treatment before admission had a significant effect on mi-

Table III. *Yield of various diagnostic tests used in investigations in 43 patients with severe pneumococcal pneumonia*

Test	No. performed	Gram-positive cocci on Gram's stain	No. of positive pneumococci cultures
ES	15	11	14
TTA	5	2	5
DA	22	13	17
PTC brush	10		7
Blood cultures	41		22
Pleural fluid cultures	7		1

crobiological diagnosis ($p = 0.001$). Microbiological diagnosis could be made in 79% of the 86 patients who had not received antibiotics before admission, and in 59% of the 46 patients who had. Only 16% of the 43 patients with a confirmed pneumococcal infection had received antibiotics before admission. Pneumococcal infection was diagnosed in 42% of the 86 patients who had not received antibiotics, compared with 15% of the 46 who had.

Treatment course: All patients received antibiotic treatment at the time of admission. Single therapy was prescribed in 27 cases, dual therapy in 14 cases, and triple therapy in 2 cases. Penicillin was the most frequently prescribed antibiotic (22 patients, 51%), and was used either alone or in combination with other antimicrobial agents. Amoxicillin-clavulanic acid was prescribed for 15 patients, and ampicillin, macrolides and third-generation cephalosporins for 2 patients respectively. The most frequently prescribed antibiotic combination was amoxicillin-clavulanic acid plus a macrolide agent (8 patients). The initial treatment was changed later in 21 patients. These changes were due to allergy to the treatment in 3 patients and to nosocomial infections in 6 patients. In 12 patients, the therapy was changed in favour of a simpler and equally effective treatment even when the initial response had been good.

Of the 43 patients with a pneumococcal pneumonia, 15 (35%) died. 12 of these 15 patients were males, and their mean age was 64 ± 11 years (range 44–84). The mean SAPS of the 15 patients who died was 18.1 ± 5.3 compared with 11.7 ± 2.9 for the patients who survived ($p = 0.0001$). Two patients died within 24 h and another one within 48 h of admission to ICU. Eight patients died after >2 weeks' treatment in ICU. Nosocomial infection was related to 2 late deaths. 10 of the 22 patients with bacteremic pneumococcal pneumonia died.

Septic shock at the onset of the disease ($p = 0.001$), presence of impaired alertness ($p = 0.026$), mechanical ventilation requirement on admission ($p = 0.0009$) and during hospitalization ($p = 0.003$), acute renal failure ($p = 0.01$), and bacteremic pneumonia ($p \leq 0.05$) were individually predictive of death. On the other hand, absence of antibiotics before admission, presence of debilitating diseases, hypoxemia, leukocyte count, initial radiological pattern, and age ≥ 65 year old were not significantly related to the outcome.

DISCUSSION

S. pneumoniae was found to be the most causative agent of severe CAP requiring ICU treatment, accounting for 33% of the patients in this study. This result is not substantially different from the 32%, 33%, and 27% incidence of pneumococcal pneumonia in patients with severe CAP admitted to the ICU reported in previous studies (2, 5, 22). However, it differs from the low 18% and 20% incidence of pneumococcal pneumonia in patients with severe CAP reported in 2 Spanish studies (23, 17). Nevertheless, pneumococcal pneumonia was probably underdiagnosed in our study. The large number of patients (35%) in the entire group who received antibiotics before admission could explain this underestimation. Indeed we found that prior antibiotic therapy significantly changed the rate of etiologic diagnosis. Our results indicated that the use of antibiotic therapy regularly active against S. pneumoniae before admission reduced the rate of culture of pneumococci. This has already been underlined in previous studies (6, 7).

The attribution of specific clinical features to an etiologic agent is a common clinical practice. However, previous studies have suggested that it is difficult to predict microbial aetiology during the first 48 h after admission on the basis of clinical and radiological features because of the lack of discriminant clinical and radiological criteria (12–16, 24). In our study, temperature over 39°C, thoracic pain, lobar consolidation, homogeneous infiltrate, and immature white blood cells $\geq 5\%$ were the features most frequently associated with severe pneumococcal pneumonia. However, the positive/negative predictive values of such symptoms remained low. These results provide a quantitative assessment to the difficulty encountered in the differential diagnosis of the infecting organism at the time of admission to the ICU of patients who have community-acquired pneumonia. Therefore the idea that pneumococcal pneumonia may be clinically difficult to distinguish from other bacterial causes of pneumonia is reinforced. These findings point out the importance of obtaining a rapid and specific microbiologic diagnosis in order to correctly manage the initial antibiotic therapy in these critically ill patients.

In our study, the type of bronchopulmonary sample was not specified in the protocol because no data in the literature had definitely proved the superiority of one procedure over another for CAP. Moreover, it was not the primary goal of the study. A pure culture of sputum or bronchial secretion was accepted as evidence of pneumococcal pneumonia. In 6 patients, the diagnosis was based solely on non-protected cultures (sputum or TTA) and compatible Gram stain findings. the value of Gram stain and sputum and TTA cultures in the diagnosis of pneumonia is still controversial (25–29). Even when a microorganism is isolated from sputum, one cannot be sure that it is the etiologic agent rather than an upper-airway contaminant. Some investigators do not consider the results of a sputum culture as sufficient to determine the etiology of pneumonia. A compromise would be to use the guidelines that Fang et al. (30) proposed for categorizing the etiology of CAP as definite or probable. Presumably, DA and PTC brush would give better and more definite results. In the present study, cultures of DA and PTC brush gave a pneumococcal diagnosis in 17/22 (77%) and 7/10 (70%) cases, respectively. Moreover, the diagnostic threshold we retained ($\geq 10^3$ cfu/ml) was probably unnecessarily strict in patients with CAP. This quantitative threshold of 10^3 cfu/ml remains to be evaluated in CAP. Nevertheless, we consider bronchoscopy using protected brush analysis to be of value for the management of patients by establishing an etiologic diagnosis, thus preventing severe bacterial pneumonia from being inadequately treated.

The overall mortality of 35% was in the same range as in some studies (2), but higher than in others (17, 22) relating to severe pneumococcal pneumonia. The mortality rate we found was associated with the high incidence of bacteremia (51%), which may very well reflect the severity of illness in these patients. In the present study, the great impact of septic shock and pneumococcal bacteremia on mortality at the time of admission is in complete agreement with other reports (4, 7, 17, 23, 31). We also found that confusion or impairment of alertness on admission, mechanical ventilation requirement, and acute renal failure were strongly related to mortality. Other groups have shown identical results in previous studies (1, 7, 17, 31, 32). The simplified acute physiological score (SAPS) was closely correlated with death. Interestingly, age was not related to mortality. However, 7/15 patients who died were ≥ 65 years old, compared with 6/28 surviving patients who were ≥ 65 years old. These results do not agree with other reports concerning bacteremic pneumococcal pneumonia (4, 33, 34), possibly because of the small size of our population. Nevertheless, Örtqvist et al., in a retrospective study, showed that the fatality rate in elderly patients was no higher than in other age groups (35). Regarding other factors already found to correlate with high risk of death, we were unable to confirm the importance of underlying clinical conditions of the patients, alcoholism, antibiotic administration prior to admission, leukocyte count, or radiographic spread of pneumonia (1, 4, 7, 17, 31, 32).

Taking into account our results, the choice of antibiotherapy for severe CAP should always be guided by its effectiveness against S. pneumoniae, – as the latter is by far the most common causative agent in severe CAP. Antibiotic treatment of severe pneumococcal pneumonia may be a problem, since pneumococci with reduced penicillin sensitivity as well as multiple antibiotic resistant pneumococci have been described. In 1991 in France (36), 7% of bacteremic pneumococcal pneumonia cases were due to strains with diminished penicillin sensitivity ($0.125 \leq \mathrm{MIC} \leq 4$ mg/l). Given the current situation concerning the penicillin sensitivity of S. pneumoniae in France, it is conceivable that high-dose penicillin [or high-dose amoxicillin] continues to be the drug of first choice for the treatment of patients with severe community-acquired pneumococcal pneumonia.

REFERENCES

1. Marrie TJ, Durant H, Yates L. Community-acquired pneumonia requiring hospitalization: 5-year prospective study. Rev Infect Dis 11: 586–599, 1989.
2. Sörensen J, Forsberg P, Håkanson E, Maller R, Sederholm C, Sören L, Carlsson C. A new diagnostic approach to the patient with severe pneumonia. Scand J Infect Dis 21: 33–41, 1989.
3. Van Eeden SF, Coetzee AR, Joubert JR. Community-acquired pneumonia. Factors influencing intensive care admission. S Afr Med J 73: 77–81, 1988.
4. Hook EW, Horton CA, Schaberg DR. Failure of intensive care unit support to influence mortality from pneumococcal bacteremia. JAMA 249: 1055–1057, 1983.
5. Woodhead MA, Macfarlane JT, Rodgers FG, Laverick A, Pilkington R, Macrae AD. Aetiology and outcome of severe community-acquired pneumonia. J Infection 10: 204–210, 1985.
6. Lim I, Shaw DR, Stanley D, Lumb R, McLennan G. A prospective hospital study of the aetiology of community-acquired pneumonia. Med J Aust 151: 87–91, 1989.
7. Research Committee of the British Thoracic Society and the Public Health Laboratory Service. Community-acquired Pneumonia in adults in British hospitals in 1982–1983: a survey of aetiology, mortality, prognostic factors outcome. Q J Med 62, 239: 195–200, 1987.
8. Berntsson E, Blomberg J, Lagergard T, Trollfors B. Etiology of community-acquired pneumonia in patients requiring hospitalization. Eur J Clin Microbiol 4: 268–272, 1985.
9. Macfarlane JT, Ward MJ, Finch RG, Macrae AD. Hospital study of adult community-acquired pneumonia. Lancet 31: 255–258, 1982.
10. Örtqvist A, Hedlund J, Grillner J, Jalonen E, Kallings I, Leinonem M, Kalin M. Aetiology, outcome and prognostic factors in community-acquired pneumonia requiring hosptialization. Eur Resp J 3: 1105–1113, 1990.
11. Holmberg H. Aetiology of community-acquired pneumonia in hospital treated patients. Scand J Infect Dis 19: 491–501, 1987.
12. Helms CM, Viner JP, Sturm RH, Reneer ED, Johnson W. Comparative features of pneumococcal, mycoplasmal, and Legionnaires' disease pneumonias. Ann Intern Med 90: 543–547, 1979.
13. Gajdos Ph, Vercken JB, Charpak Y, Andremont A, Brun Buisson C, Carlet J, Raphaël JC, Schlemmer B, Tenaillon A, Thaler F. Concordance study of empiric antibiotic therapy in patients with acute community acquired pneumonia admitted in intensive care units. Réan Soins Intens Méd Urg 4: 67–72, 1988.
14. Macfarlane JT, Miller AC, Roderick Smith WH, Morris AH, Rose DH. Comparative radiographic features of community acquired legionnaires' disease, pneumococcal pneumonia, mycoplasma pneumonia, and psittacosis. Thorax 39: 28–33, 1984.
15. Tew J, Calenoff, Berlin BS. Bacterial or nonbacterial pneumonia: accuracy of radiographic diagnosis. Radiology 124: 607–612, 1977.

16. Woodhead MA, Macfarlane JT. Comparative clinical and laboratory features of Legionella with pneumococcal and mycoplasma pneumonias. Br J Dis Chest 81: 133–139, 1987.
17. Torres A, Serra-Batlles J, Ferrer A, Jimenez P, Celis R, Cobo E, Rodriguez-Roisin R. Severe community-acquired pneumonia epidemiology and prognostic factors. Am Rev Respir Dis 144: 312–318, 1991.
18. Le Gall JR, Loirat Ph, Alperovitch A. Simplified acute physiological score for intensive care patients. Lancet 2: 741, 1983.
19. Matthew AB, Holstrom FMG, Kaspar RL. A simple method for diagnosing pneumonia in intubated or tracheostomized patients. Crit Care Med 5: 76–81, 1977.
20. Wimberley N, Faling LJ, Bartlett JG. A fiberoptic bronchoscopy technique to obtain uncontaminated lower airway secretions for bacterial culture. Am Rev Respir Dis 119: 337–343, 1979.
21. Wimberley NW, Bass JB, Boyd BW, Kirkpatrick MB, Serio RA, Pollock HM. Use of a bronchoscopic protected catheter brush for the diagnosis of pulmonary infections. Chest 81: 556–561, 1982.
22. Örtqvist A. Prognosis in community-acquired pneumonia requiring treatment in hospital. Importance of predisposing and complicating factors and of diagnostic procedures. Scand J Infect Dis Suppl 65, 1990.
23. Pachon J, Prados MD, Capote F, Cuello JA, Garnacho J, Verano A. Severe community-acquired pneumonia. Am Rev Respir Dis 142: 369–373, 1990.
24. Farr BM, Kaiser DL, Harrison BDW, Conolly CK. Prediction of microbial etiology at admission to hospital for pneumonia from the presenting clinical features. Thorax 44: 1031–1035, 1989.
25. Tobin MJ. Diagnosis of pneumonia: techniques and problems. Clin Chest Med 8: 513–527, 1987.
26. Bartlett RC. Diagnosis of bacterial infections of the lung. Clin Chest Med 8: 119–134, 1987.
27. Bartlett RC, Melmick A. Usefulness of Gram stain and routine and quantitative culture of sputum in patients with and without acute respiratory infection. Conn Med 34: 347–351, 1970.
28. Rein MF, Gwaltney JM, O'Brien W, Jennings RH, Mandell GL. Accuracy of Gram's strain in identifying pneumococci in sputum. JAMA 239: 2671–2673, 1978.
29. Bartlett JG. Diagnostic accuracy of transtracheal aspiration bacteriologic studies. Am Rev Respir Dis 115: 777–782, 1977.
30. Fang GD, Fine M, Orloff J, Arisumi D, Yu VL, Kapoor W, Grayston JT, Wang SP, Kohler R, Muder RR. New and emerging etiologies for community-acquired pneumonia with implications for therapy. Medicine 69: 307–316, 1990.
31. Petit JY, Philit F, Thomas X, Gaussorgues PH, Blanchin M, Gérard M, Robert D. Pronostic des insuffisances respiratoires aiguës d'origine pneumococcique nécessitant la ventilation mécanique. Press Méd 19: 362–366, 1990.
32. Farr BM, Sloman AJ, Fisch MJ. Predicting death in patients hospitalized for community-acquired pneumonia. Ann Intern Med 115: 428–436, 1991.
33. Austrian R, Gold J. Pneumococcal bacteremia with special reference to bacteremic pneumococcal pneumonia. Ann Intern Med 60: 759–776, 1964.
34. Mufson MA, Kruss DM, Wasil RE, Metzger WI. Capsular types and outcome of bacteremic pneumococcal disease in the antibiotic era. Arch Intern Med 134: 505–510, 1974.
35. Örtqvist A, Kalin M, Julander I, Mufson MA. Deaths in bacteremic pneumococcal pneumonia. A comparison of two populations – Huntington, WVa, and Stockholm, Sweden. Chest 103: 710–716, 1993.
36. Geslin P, Fremaux A, Sissia G. Evolution de la résistance des pneumocoques responsables des infections des voies respiratoires en France. Méd Mal Infect 22S: 74–86, 1992.

Submitted May 2, 1994; accepted February 13, 1995

Scand J Infect Dis 27: 207–210, 1995 ORIGINAL ARTICLE

Role of Aeromonas Isolated from Feces of Finnish Patients

HILPI RAUTELIN[1], AULIKKI SIVONEN[1], ARJA KUIKKA[1], OLLI-VEIKKO RENKONEN[1], VILLE VALTONEN[2], HEIKKI LEHTI[3], ASKO KAHANPÄÄ[4] and TIMO U. KOSUNEN[1]

From the [1]Department of Bacteriology and Immunology, and [2]Second Department of Medicine, University of Helsinki, the [3]Garrison Hospital of the Air Defence Regiment of Helsinki, and the [4]Municipal Nursing Home Kustaankartano, Helsinki, Finland

Aeromonas species were isolated from 249/13,027 (1.9%) stool samples submitted to the Dept. of Bacteriology and Immunology, University of Helsinki, during 1 year, to be cultured for bacterial enteropathogens. Aeromonas was the third most common enteropathogen isolated, after campylobacter (3.6%) and salmonella (3.3%). Isolates and clinical information from 234 Aeromonas patients were available for further study. A. caviae (41%), A. hydrophila (27%), and A. veronii biovar sobria (22%) were the most frequent isolates. In 15% of the patients, other enteropathogens were found along with aeromonas. Only 2% of all aeromonas-positive patients were found to be asymptomatic, whereas no aeromonas isolates were detected in the stools of 343 asymptomatic individuals. Almost all (96%) patients with aeromonas in their feces had gastroenteritis. Patients infected with A. veronii biovar sobria had a shorter illness course and had more often travelled abroad. In conclusion, Aeromonas spp. were found to be a potential cause of diarrhea in Finnish patients.

H. Rautelin, MD, Department of Bacteriology and Immunology, P.O. 21 FIN-00014, University of Helsinki, Finland

INTRODUCTION

Aeromonads are Gram-negative, oxidase-positive rods commonly found in water and soil. Aeromonas species have been isolated in various human extra-intestinal infections, as in wounds and in septicaemia, especially in immunocompromised individuals (1). Reports have also suggested that Aeromonas species could be important pathogens in human gastroenteritis (2, 3). The most common clinical isolates of aeromonas include A. hydrophila, A. caviae and A. veronii biovar sobria (3). These 3 species also predominate in aeromonas-associated gastroenteritis (4). Altwegg et al. have reported that a strain of aeromonas identical to the one isolated from a patient with diarrhea was detected in food ingested prior to the illness (5). Otherwise, the role of aeromonads as enteropathogens remains controversial, however, as animal models and documented outbreaks are still awaited. Furthermore, aeromonas isolates used in challenge trials have mostly failed to induce diarrhea in volunteers (6).

The present prospective study was undertaken to determine the role of Aeromonas species isolated from feces of Finnish patients and the prevalence of aeromonas in asymptomatic individuals.

MATERIALS AND METHODS

Patients and controls

Stool samples (13,027) submitted in 1990 to the Dept. of Bacteriology and Immunology, University of Helsinki, to be cultured for Salmonella, Shigella, Yersinia, Campylobacter, Aeromonas and Plesiomonas spp. were studied. In positive cases of aeromonas the physicians who had submitted the stool specimens were contacted and questionnaires regarding the details of the illness, possible underlying disorders, antibiotic treatment within 1 month and travel abroad within 3 months prior to the illness were sent to the corresponding patients. The isolates and clinical information were available for further study for 234/249 (94%) aeromonas-positive patients. Two repeat stool cultures for enteropathogens with an interval of about 2 weeks were performed in most cases to study the clearance of aeromonas from feces.

To determine the prevalence of Aeromonas spp. in the stools of asymptomatic individuals, fecal sampels from a total of 343 persons were studied. These persons included 131 medical and medical-technological students (females 94, age range 20–40, mean 23; males 37, age range 21–31, mean 23), 26 members of laboratory staff (females 22, age range 20–58, mean 28; males 4, age range 26–52, mean 36), 57 persons at a municipal nursing home (females 42, age range 61–96, mean 82; males 15, age range 58–97, mean 76) and 129 conscript soldiers at a garrison (all males, age range 18–26, mean 20). Their stool specimens were cultured for all the above-mentioned enteric pathogens.

Isolation of enteric pathogens

Stool samples submitted in Stuart tubes to the Dept. of Bacteriology and Immunology were cultured within 48 h of sampling. For the isolation of thermotolerant Campylobacter spp., stool samples were inoculated on campylobacter blood-free selective agar (Oxoid Ltd., Basingstoke, Hants., England) and incubated at 43°C in an atmosphere of 5% O_2, 10% CO_2, and 85% N_2 for 48 h. For the other bacteria, stool specimens were routinely cultured by inoculating them on cystine lactose electrolyte-deficient (CLED) agar (Oxoid), xylose lysine deoxycholate (XLD) medium (BBL, Cockeysville, MD, USA), yersinia selective agar (Oxoid), and 5% horse blood agar containing 20 µg of ampicillin/ml (7); agar plates were incubated at 35°C for 18 h. For the enrichment of Salmonella species, a sample of feces was inoculated into selenite broth (Oxoid), which was subcultured on XLD after 24 h of incubation. For the identification of the pathogens, routine methods were applied.

Identification of Aeromonas species

For the identification of Aeromonas spp., colonies resembling aeromonas from any plate used were screened for the production of oxidase. Presumed Aeromonas spp. were tested for resistance to vibriostatic agent O/129 and were further characterized by the API 20 E test (Bio Merieux, Marcy-l'Etoile, France). For the identification of aeromonas isolates to the species level, additional tests were used: hemolytic activity on sheep blood agar, production of gas from glucose, susceptibility to cephalothin, hydrolysis of esculin, and fermentation of salicin (1).

Statistical methods

For statistical analysis the patients were divided into subgroups in two ways: 1) polymicrobial infections versus Aeromonas sp. as the only positive finding, and 2) grouping by Aeromonas species. The statistical methods used were the Pearson's χ^2-test and Fisher's two-tailed exact test for categorized variables and the Mann-Whitney rank sum test and the Kruskal-Wallis test for continuous variables. A p-value ≤ 0.05 was considered significant. Computations were made with BMDP programs.

RESULTS

Aeromonas species were isolated from 249/13,027 stool samples, an isolation rate of 1.9% (repeat stool cultures of aeromonas-positive patients excluded). Other enteropathogens isolated included Campylobacter jejuni/coli (3.6%), Salmonella sp. (3.3%), Yersinia enterocolitica (1.7%), Shigella sp. (0.4%), and Plesiomonas shigelloides (0.2%). Aeromonas isolates were found throughout the year but were least common in May and most frequent in July–October. No aeromonas isolates were found in the feces of a total of 343 asymptomatic persons, 2 of whom had Salmonella sp. isolated from their feces. Furthermore, 186 of these stool samples were stored at +4°C and cultured daily on agar plates for 4 days, but no aeromonads were isolated.

Isolates from 234 aeromonas patients were available for further study. On the basis of the biochemical characteristics of these isolates, 96 (41%) patients were shown to be infected with A. caviae, 64 (27%) with A. hydrophila, 52 (22%) with A. veronii biovar sobria, 9 (4%) with Aeromonas sp. (could not be identified to the species level) and 13 (6%) patients had two aeromonads with different biochemical characteristics obtained from the same stool sample. A total of 35 (15%) aeromonas-positive patients also had other enteropathogens isolated: 12 patients had Campylobacter jejuni/coli, 11 had Salmonella sp., 6 had Yersinia enterocolitica, and 4 Plesiomonas shigelloides. Two patients were infected with Campylobacter jejuni, Yersinia enterocolitica and aeromonas. Polymicrobial infections were not associated with any particular aeromonas species.

Of the 234 aeromonas patients, only 4 patients (2%) were found to be asymptomatic: 1 of them was positive for A. hydrophila and 3 had A. caviae in their feces. In these 4 cases, stool cultures had been taken merely as a part of health examinations. All the other patients reported various symptoms and the majority of them had gastroenteritis with watery diarrhea (Table I). Five patients (3% of pure aeromonas infections) reported reactive arthritis (synovitis only or with arthralgia) following aeromonas enteritis.

At least one stool sample for follow-up was available for 182 patients and 150 patients had two such samples taken with an interval of about 2 weeks. Two weeks after the primary culture, repeat stool cultures proved negative for aeromonas in 39% of the patients, and after 4 weeks in 80%. There were no significant differences in the clearance times between the different species of aeromonas.

To define the clinical significance of aeromonas isolates, the characteristics of the infections with aeromonas as the sole enteropathogen and those of polymicrobial infections with well-established enteric pathogens were compared (Tables I, II). There was no significant difference between the

Table I. *Results of questionnaires from patients with Aeromonas sp. isolated from their feces*

Patient characteristic	No. of patients[a] with: Aeromonas only ($n = 199$)	Mixed infection ($n = 35$)
Mean age	38.4 (SD 23.8)	34.2 (SD 19.7)
Females	108 (54%)	16 (46%)
Outpatients	146 (73%)	30 (86%)
Asymptomatic	4 (2%)	0 (0%)
Gastroenteritis	151 (96%)	30 (100%)
Diarrhea		
watery	124 (80%)	23 (77%)
bloody	22 (15%)	2 (7%)
mucous	52 (35%)	8 (27%)
Frequency of diarrhea (per day)		
3–4 stools	51 (41%)	11 (40%)
5–9	50 (40%)	8 (30%)
≥10	23 (19%)	8 (30%)
Duration of illness[b]		
≤7 d	37 (26%)	14 (48%)
8–14 d	33 (23%)	7 (24%)
≥15 d	72 (51%)	8 (28%)
First symptom[c]		
pain	47 (34%)	17 (57%)
diarrhea	46 (33%)	5 (17%)
fever	8 (6%)	6 (20%)
Worst symptom		
pain	61 (46%)	15 (52%)
diarrhea	49 (37%)	11 (38%)
fever	4 (3%)	2 (7%)
Fever (≥37.5°C)[d]	65 (42%)	23 (77%)
Hospitalized because of diarrhea	29 (17%)	4 (14%)
Antimicrobials because of diarrhea	27 (19%)	10 (33%)

[a] Percentages in parentheses have been calculated from those cases whose questionnaires gave adequate information.
Significant differences (Pearson's χ^2-test or Fisher's two-tailed exact test if needed): [b] $p = 0.03$, [c] $p = 0.006$, [d] $p < 0.001$.

Table II. *Predisposing factors according to questionnaires answered by patients with Aeromonas sp. isolated from their feces*

Predisposing factors	No. of patients[a] with Aeromonas only	Mixed infection
Disease/prior medication	100 (69%)	10 (44%)
Underlying disease[b]	77 (48%)	8 (27%)
Diabetes	12 (8%)	0 (0%)
Malignancy	5 (3%)	0 (0%)
Cardiovascular	28 (18%)	3 (10%)
Gastrointestinal	23 (14%)	1 (3%)
Medication prior to illness	58 (38%)	8 (29%)
Antimicrobials[c]	33 (28%)	0 (0%)
NSAIDs	9 (6%)	1 (4%)
Gastrointestinal	7 (5%)	1 (4%)
Corticosteroids	3 (2%)	2 (7%)
Foreign travel[d]	74 (45%)	26 (84%)

[a] Percentages in parentheses have been calculated from those cases whose questionnaires gave adequate information.
Significant differences (Pearson's χ^2-test or Fisher's two-tailed exact test if needed): [b] $p < 0.05$, [c] $p < 0.01$, [d] $p < 0.001$.

groups regarding the occurrence of diarrhea, or the duration of fever, of pain or of diarrhea. The close contacts of the patients with mixed infections did not have diarrhea more often than those of other patients. However, some differences could be discerned (Tables I, II). Patients with mixed infections more often had fever than had patients with aeromonas as the only finding (Table I). Furthermore, most patients with mixed infections (82%) had high temperatures (>38.5°C) whereas the corresponding figure for infections with aeromonas as the sole pathogen was 40% ($p = 0.0011$). Mixed infections were over within 2 weeks in 72% of the cases, whereas in pure aeromonas infections it was only in 49% of cases ($p = 0.0256$). Furthermore, there was a longer delay from the onset of the symptoms to the submission of the stool samples for culture in pure aeromonas infections (mean 23.2 days, SD 6.5), than in polymicrobial infections (mean 7.8 days, SD 44.5). Thus, mixed infections seemed to be more acute in nature.

A larger proportion of patients with polymicrobial infections had travelled abroad within 3 months prior to their illness than among patients infected with aeromonas only (Table II). The most common travel destinations were Southern Europe, the Soviet Union, the Far East and the Middle East. In 19 (10%) cases of aeromonas infection (polymicrobial infections excluded) the criteria for a hospital infection were fulfilled.

When the characteristics of the infections with different Aeromonas species were compared, A. veronii biovar sobria infections differed from others in several respects. The differences were significant even when polymicrobial infections were excluded. A greater proportion of patients with A. sobria infection had travelled abroad than of others (82% vs. 42%, $p = 0.0003$, polymicrobials excluded), and their disease had also often begun abroad (51%). Furthermore, the duration of their illness was shorter than in patients infected with other Aeromonas species. In 72% of cases of A. sobria infection the disease was over within 2 weeks, whereas in patients infected with other species it was so in 43% of cases ($p = 0.0066$). The duration of illness was longer for A. hydrophila patients than for others, as 66% of patients infected with A. hydrophila still had symptoms 2 weeks after the onset of the illness ($p = 0.0372$). The proportion of patients infected with A. veronii biovar sobria who had been swimming outdoors in untreated water ($p = 0.003$) was greater and their close contacts (family members, travelling companions) more often had diarrhea ($p = 0.007$).

DISCUSSION

Aeromonas sp. was isolated from 1.9% of stool samples, which is comparable to the figures (ranging from 0.61% to 1.8%) reported by others (4, 8–10). In the present study, aeromonas was the third most common enteropathogen after campylobacter and salmonella which have previously been the most frequent fecal isolates in Finnish patients (11). In the USA (8) and in India (10) aeromonas could not be isolated from the stools of controls, whereas an Italian study reported similar isolation rates in children with and without gastroenteritis (12). The prevalence of aeromonas in the feces of asymptomatic Finnish persons was very low. Only 2% of the patients with aeromonas in their feces were found retrospectively not to have diarrhea. Furthermore, none of the 343 asymptomatic control subjects had aeromonas-positive stool cultures.

Seasonal variations in the isolation rate of aeromonas have been reported (8, 13). In our study, aeromonas isolates were most frequent in late summer and in the autumn, which might reflect the increase of aeromonas in the environment as well as domestic and foreign travel during summer holidays. Furthermore, contact with untreated water was found to be a risk factor, especially for A. veronii biovar sobria infections.

In 15% of cases, aeromonas was isolated concomitantly with other enteropathogens. Our results do not differ significantly from those of others (4, 13), and for instance for campylobacters, rates of mixed infections as high as 16% have been reported (14). Infections with aeromonas as the only positive finding were more frequent than mixed infections of a subacute or chronic nature. Moyer (13) has reported that A. caviae was more often associated with an illness of longer duration. In the present study this was true of A. hydrophila, whereas A. veronii biovar sobria was significantly more often isolated in infections with a shorter duration.

Antimicrobial therapy and underlying diseases are known risk factors for aeromonas infections (15). In the present study, however, 31% of infections with aeromonas as the only positive finding occurred in patients without these two predisposing factors. This supports the idea that aeromonas could cause enteritis also in previously healthy people.

In summary, Aeromonas sp. was the third most common enteropathogen isolated at our Department but it could not be isolated from any of the asymptomatic individuals. The majority of aeromonas patients reported varying symptoms of gastroenteritis. In comparison with polymicrobial infections, infections with aeromonas as the only positive finding were more chronic in nature and were more often domestic in origin, except for A. veronii biovar sobria infections which were associated with acute disease usually after foreign travel. Our study suggests that aeromonas is an important enteropathogen also in previously healthy persons.

REFERENCES

1. Janda JM, Duffey PS. Mesophilic aeromonads in human disease: Current taxonomy, laboratory identification, and infectious disease spectrum. Rev Infect Dis 10: 980–977, 1988.
2. Altwegg M, Geiss HK. Aeromonas as a human pathogen. CRC Crit Rev Microbiol 16: 253–286, 1989.
3. Janda JM. Recent advances in the study of the taxonomy, pathogenicity, and infectious syndromes associated with the genus Aeromonas. Clin Microbiol Rev 4: 397–410, 1991.
4. Kuijper EJ, Bol P, Peeters MF, Steigerwalt AG, Zanen HC, Brenner DJ. Clinical and epidemiological aspects of members of Aeromonas DNA hybridization groups isolated from human feces. J Clin Microbiol 27: 1531–1537, 1989.
5. Altwegg M, Martinetti Lucchini G, Lüthy-Hottenstein J, Rohrbach M. Aeromonas-associated gastroenteritis after consumption of contaminated shrimp. Eur J Clin Microbiol Infect Dis 10: 44–45, 1991.
6. Morgan DR, Johnson PC, DuPont HL, Satterwhite TK, Wood LV. Lack of correlation between known virulence properties of Aeromonas hydrophilia and enteropathogenicity for humans. Infect Immun 50: 62–65, 1987.
7. Kelly MT, Stroh EMD, Jessop J. Comparison of blood agar, ampicillin blood agar, MacConkey-ampicillin-tween agar, and modified cefsulodin-irgasan-novobiocin agar for isolation of Aeromonas spp. from stool specimens. J Clin Microbiol 26: 1738–1740, 1988.
8. Agger WA, McCormick JD, Gurwith MJ. Clinical and microbiological features of Aeromonas hydrophila-associated diarrhea. J Clin Microbiol 21: 909–913, 1985.
9. Altwegg M, Jöhl M. Isolation frequency of Aeromonas species in relation to patient age. Eur J Clin Microbiol Infect Dis 6: 55–56, 1987.
10. Deodhar LP, Saraswathi K, Varudkar A. Aeromonas spp. and their association with human diarrheal disease. J Clin Microbiol 29: 853–856, 1991.
11. Rautelin HI, Renkonen OV, von Bonsdorff CH, Lähdevirta J, Pitkänen T, Järvinen A, Reinikainen P, Kosunen TU. Prospective study of the etiology of diarrhea in adult outpatients and inpatients. Scand J Gastroenterol 24: 329–333, 1989.
12. Figura N, Marri L, Verdiani S, Ceccherini C, Barberi A. Prevalence, species differentiation, and toxigenicity of Aeromonas strains in cases of childhood gastroenteritis and in controls. J Clin Microbiol 23: 595–599, 1986.
13. Moyer NP. Clinical significance of aeromonas species isolated from patients with diarrhea. J Clin Microbiol 25: 2044–2048, 1987.
14. Lassen J, Kappererud G. Epidemiological aspects of enteritis due to Campylobacter spp. in Norway. J Clin Microbiol 19: 153–156, 1984.
15. King GE, Werner SB, Kizer KW. Epidemiology of aeromonas infections in California. Clin Infect Dis 15: 449–452, 1992.

Submitted November 7, 1994; accepted March 16, 1995

Scand J Infect Dis 27: 211–215, 1995

Association of Bacteroides fragilis with Childhood Diarrhea

VENUSTO H. SAN JOAQUIN,[1] JUDY C. GRIFFIS,[1] CHRISTOPHER LEE[2] and CYNTHIA L. SEARS[2]

From the [1]Section of Infectious Diseases, Department of Pediatrics, University of Oklahoma Health Sciences Center, Oklahoma City, Oklahoma and the [2]Divisions of Infectious Diseases and Gastroenterology, Department of Medicine, The Johns Hopkins University School of Medicine, Baltimore, Maryland, USA

Enterotoxigenic strains of Bacteriodes fragilis (ETBF) have recently been found to be associated with diarrheal illness in Apache and Bangladeshi children. This study was conducted to define the role of ETBF in diarrhea of children in an urban setting. Fecal specimens from 991 children with diarrhea and 581 asymptomatic age-matched controls were cultured for B. fragilis (BF). The isolates were tested for enterotoxin production using a human colonic epithelial cell line. BF was isolated from 318 (32.1%) of the patients and 123 (21.2%) of the controls ($p < 0.001$). In children < 1 year old which comprised about 50% of both patients and controls, the BF isolation rates were comparable (26.5% vs 25.7%; $p = 0.812$), contrasting with the significant difference in isolation rates for children ≥ 1 year (37.6% vs 16.5%; $p = < 0.001$). Overall, ETBF were identified in 4.4% of patients and 3.1% of controls ($p = 0.2$). However, ETBF were significantly associated with diarrheal disease in children 1–5 years (5.4% vs 1.8%; $p = 0.033$) and 1–10 years (4.8% vs 1.5%; $p = 0.021$) in age. ETBF were isolated the year round and comprised 14.4% and 15% of the BF isolated from the patients and controls, respectively, suggesting that part of the indigenous BF are inherently enterotoxin producers. In this study, BF and ETBF were associated with diarrheal illness in children 1–10 years old.

V. H. San Joaquin, MD, The University of Oklahoma Health Science Center, Department of Pediatrics, Box 26901, Oklahoma City, OK 73190-3030, U.S.A.

INTRODUCTION

Acute diarrheal disease remains a scourge of children worldwide. In developing countries, it is one of the 2 main causes of childhood mortality, accounting for some 4–4.5 million deaths every year (1, 2). In the USA, it is estimated that 16.5 million children < 5 years old develop at least one episode of diarrhea every year. Of these, 220,000 are hospitalized, and 325–425 die (3). In the past 2 decades, tremendous advances have been achieved in the identification of various enteropathogens and in our understanding of their pathogenic mechanisms. Still, the etiologies of up to 50% of acute diarrheal illness in American children remain unknown (4, 5). Identifying as yet unrecognized enteropathogens will contribute immensely to our knowledge of childhood diarrhea.

In 1984, Myers et al. (6) described the association between a severe diarrheal illness in lambs and enterotoxin-producing strains of Bacteroides fragilis (ETBF). This novel veterinary enteropathogen was characterized by the ability to induce a secretory response in ligated ileal loops of lambs and calves. Subsequently, ETBF was also associated with diarrheal disease in other young domestic animals (7–12) and was shown to induce diarrhea in gnotobiotic pigs (13). Until recently, the ability of ETBF to produce the enterotoxin was demonstrable only with the use of animal models. Weikel et al. have since developed a tissue culture assay for ETBF using a cloned human colonic epithelial cell line, HT29/C1 (14).

The isolation of ETBF from feces of humans with diarrhea was first described in 1987 (15). Of the 8 patients whose stools were positive for ETBF, 6 were children 3 years old or younger. Recognized enteropathogens were not detected in the stools of 7/8 patients. Following this report, Sack and his associates studied Apache children with and without diarrhea who were attending an outpatient facility in Whitewater, Arizona. They found a significant association between ETBF and acute diarrhea in these Native American children (16). A more recent study involving Bangladeshi children also demonstrated an association between ETBF and diarrhea (17).

We hypothesized that ETBF is a common cause of childhood diarrhea in an urban setting, and that ETBF-associated gastroenteritis accounts for a proportion of childhood diarrhea which at present does not have an identifiable etiology. Our study was conducted to test this hypothesis.

SUBJECTS AND METHODS

Study population

Children who were seen for diarrhea at the Children's Hospital of Oklahoma were enrolled consecutively into the study if a stool culture was requested by their physician. Patients were enrolled from July 1, 1990 through June 30, 1991. A cohort of asymptomatic children, who were comparable to the patients regarding age, and month of enrollment, were designated as controls. The patients' feces or rectal swabs were cultured for the usual bacterial enteropathogens, i.e. Salmonella, Shigella, Campylo-

 ISSN 0036-5548

bacter, Aeromonas, and Yersinia. In addition, they were cultured for Bacteriodes fragilis. Assays for rotavirus and enteric adenoviruses and examination for enteric parasites were not made routinely. Rectal swabs from controls were cultured solely for B. fragilis.

Isolation of B. fragilis

The fecal specimens were inoculated onto a selective solid medium consisting of tryptose blood agar, polymyxin B, irgasan (triclosan), novobiocin, and nalidixic acid (PINN agar) (17). Plates were incubated anaerobically at 35°C for 48 h. Colonies on the PINN agar were viewed under a stereoscope and those with the characteristic internal mottling were presumptively identified as B. fragilis. A colony with the mottled internal structure was subcultured, then tested for catalase and indole reactions and ability to ferment trehalose, rhamnose, and mannitol. The isolate was identified as B. fragilis if it was catalase positive, indole negative, and did not ferment trehalose, rhamnose, and mannitol. The isolates of B. fragilis were inoculated into chopped-meat broth and stored in a CO_2 incubator at 35°C until assayed for enterotoxin production 1–6 months after isolation. Seven strains of B. fragilis known to be enterotoxigenic and 2 non-enterotoxigenic strains (courtesy of Dr. Lyle L. Myers) were stored and assayed in identical manner.

Preparation of B. fragilis supernatants for enterotoxin assay

A swab of 24- to 48-h-old blood plate culture of B. fragilis was inoculated in 45 ml of Difco brain heart infusion broth and incubated anaerobically at 35°C for 48 h. The broth culture was centrifuged at 12,000 *g* (10.000 rmp) for 45 min at 4°C. The supernatant was separated from the bacterial pellet and concentrated 20-fold using an Amicon Centriprep-10 concentrator (14). The concentrated supernatant was filter-sterilized through a 45 μm Amicon filter, then stored in a polypropylene tube at −75°C until assayed for the presence of enterotoxin within 1 month.

Enterotoxin assay

$HT29/C_1$ cells were grown in Dulbecco's modified Eagle's medium, with 10% fetal bovine serum, 1 mM pyruvate, 44 mM $NaHCO_3$, 10 μm of human transferrin (Boehringer Mannheim)/ml and penicillin (3 μm/ml)—streptomycin (50 μm/ml) in 10% CO_2; medium was replenished 6 days/week. Cells were suspended 1 : 15 at 80 to 90% confluency by using 0.005% trypsin—0.053 mM EDTA, plated into 8-well LabTek slides, and allowed to grow for 2 to 3 days. B. fragilis supernatants were diluted 1/4 directly into tissue culture media on the cells (final volume, 400 μl well). Following a 3-h incubation time, the medium was aspirated from the cells, and the cells fixed with 90% methanol and strained with Giemsa. Slides were read at ×100 magnification with standard bright-field light microscopy. Rounding and separation of cells in the monolayer from their neighbouring cells indicated the presence of the B. fragilis enterotoxin. This tissue culture assay has previously been demonstrated to be 89% sensitive and 100% specific in detecting ETBF strains as defined by the lamb ligated intestinal loop assay (14).

Statistical analysis

Using SAS/STAT version 6 (Cary, NC), patients and controls were compared by χ^2 analysis supplemented by Fisher's Exact test when necessary due to sample size. A p value ≤ 0.05 was considered statistically significant.

RESULTS

991 children with diarrhea and 581 asymptomatic controls were enrolled in the study during the 12-month period. 46% of the patients and 53% of the controls were females. The age distributions of the children in both groups are depicted in Table I. Infants < 1 year comprised 50.3% and 52.2% of patients and controls respectively. More than two-thirds of the patients (76.5%) and controls (77.3%) were < 3 years. The number of symptomatic children and of asymptomatic controls studied during each quarter, approximating seasonal distribution, is shown in Fig. 1. The numbers of children enrolled each month ranged between 55 and 110 for patients, and 33–72 for controls.

As shown in Table I, B. fragilis was isolated in fecal specimens from 318 (32.1%) of the 991 patients and 123 (21.2%) of the 581 controls. The overall isolation rate of B. fragilis in patients was significantly different ($p < 0.001$) from the overall isolation rate in controls. When stratified by age, the differences in rates attained statistical significance in children who were ≥1 year old, and were particularly marked in children 1–3 years old. However, in children < 1 year, the difference was not significant even

Table I. *Isolation rates of Bacteroides fragilis (BF) distributed by age groups*

Age (yrs)	Patients			Controls			Odds Ratio (95% Confidence Limits)	p-value
	No.	BF+	Rate (%)	No.	BF+	Rate (%)		
<1	498	132	26.5	303	78	25.7	1.04 (0.75–1.44)	0.812
1–5	340	136	40.0	221	40	18.1	3.02 (2.01–4.52)	<0.001*
1	175	74	42.3	91	16	17.6	3.43 (1.85–6.37)	<0.001*
2	85	39	45.9	55	13	23.6	2.74 (1.29–5.82)	0.008*
3	40	13	32.5	32	2	6.3	7.22 (1.49–34.95)	0.006*
4	21	6	28.6	25	6	24.0	1.27 (0.34–4.74)	0.725
5	19	4	21.1	18	3	16.7	1.33 (0.25–7.01)	0.734
6–10	69	18	26.1	51	5	9.8	3.25 (1.12–9.45)	0.025*
1–10	409	154	37.6	272	45	16.5	3.05 (2.09–4.44)	<0.001*
>10	84	32	38.1	6	0	—	—	
Total	991	318	32.1	581	123	21.2	1.76 (1.38–2.24)	<0.001*

* Statistically significant difference.

Table II. *Isolation rates of Enterotoxigenic Bacteroides fragilis (ETBF) distributed by age groups*

Age (yrs)	Patients No.	Patients ETBF+	Patients Rate (%)	Controls No.	Controls ETBF+	Controls Rate (%)	Odds Ratio (95% Confidence Limits)	p-value
<1	490	20	4.1	300	14	4.7	0.87 (0.43–1.75)	0.694
1–5	331	18	5.4	221	4	1.8	3.12 (1.04–9.35)	0.033*
1	172	10	5.8	91	2	2.2	2.75 (0.59–12.81)	0.181
2	80	4	5.0	55	2	3.6	1.40 (0.25–7.90)	0.706
3	40	1	2.5	32	0	0.0	2.47 (0.10–62.65)	0.368
4	20	2	10.0	25	0	0.0	6.89 (0.31–152.19)	0.106
5	19	1	5.3	18	0	0.0	3.00 (0.11–78.53)	0.324
6–10	67	1	1.5	51	0	0.0	2.32 (0.09–58.22)	0.381
1–10	398	19	4.8	272	4	1.5	3.36 (1.13–9.99)	0.021*
>10	84	4	4.8	6	0	0.0	—	—
Total	972	43	4.4	578	18	3.1	1.44 (0.82–2.51)	0.200

* Statistically significant difference.

though these children accounted for 50.3% and 52.2% of patients and controls, respectively.

The isolates of B. fragilis from 19 patients and 3 controls were not viable on subculture, and were therefore not tested for enterotoxin production. Of the isolates tested, B. fragilis from 43 (4.4%) of 972 patients and 18 (3.1%) of 578 controls produced the enterotoxin ($p = 0.25$). ETBF was isolated in all age groups among patients, but among controls only in children < 3 years. However, the zero isolation rates in controls ≥ 3 years were not significantly different from the isolation rates observed in patients in the corresponding age groups (Table II). Three patients harbored ETBF concomitantly with a recognized bacterial enteropathogen; one was also positive for Clostridium difficile, the other 2 were also positive for Campylobacter jejuni.

The difference between the isolation rates of ETBF (Table II) in patients and controls was not significant when compared overall or when compared according to age in individual years, i.e. 1-year-old patients vs 1-year-old controls, 2-year-old patients vs 2-year-old controls, etc. However, when patients 1–5 years old were compared as a group vs. controls 1–5 years old, ETBF were significantly associated with diarrheal disease ($p = 0.033$; Odds Ratio 3.12, 95% confidence interval 1.041–9.346). The significant association holds when 1–10 year old patients and controls were compared $p = 0.021$: Odds Ratio 3.35, 95% confidence interval 1.13–9.985). The pattern of significant association between ETBF and diarrheal illness in children 1–10 years old is similar to that observed with B. fragilis. Children > 10 years in age were not analysed separately as a group because there were only 6 controls.

ETBF was isolated in the feces of patients and controls all the year round. The respective numbers of isolates by season, spring through winter, were 13, 12, 9, and 9 in patients, and 6, 4, 4, and 4 in controls. The seasonal

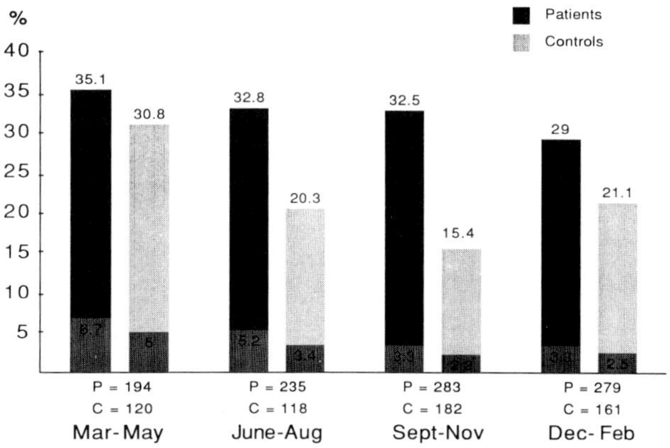

Fig. 1. Seasonal isolation rates of B. fragilis and ETBF. In each season, the first bar represents patients and the second represents controls. The base of each bar denotes ETBF. The numbers of patients (P) and controls (C) studied during each season are listed below the bars.

variations in the isolation rate of B. fragilis and ETBF are depicted in Fig. 1.

Enterotoxigenic strains comprised 14.4% (43 of 299) of the B. fragilis isolated from patients and 15% (18 of 120) of those isolated from controls ($p > 0.5$). The ratio of ETBF to the total isolates of B. fragilis was not affected significantly by the age of the children, by the season of the year, or by the presence or absence of diarrhea in the hosts.

Review of the presenting clinical manifestations of the children with ETBF-associated diarrhea did not reveal any characteristic features. Four had recurrent diarrhea for more than 2 weeks, the others had acute diarrheal disease. The stools were most often described as watery and loose, with 8 reporting the presence of blood. Approximately one-fourth of the children had fever and a third had vomiting.

DISCUSSION

A fascinating association between both B. fragilis and ETBF and diarrheal illness in children in an urban setting is demonstrated in our study. The association with ETBF is confined to children ≥1 year old. The difference in isolation rates of ETBF between patients and controls attains statistical significance when the study subjects are cohorted into and compared as groups of children 1–5 years or 1–10 years old. Inclusion of infants <1 old into the groupings or comparison of patients and controls as stratified by age in individual years result in ETBF isolation rates that are not significantly different. These observations conform with findings of other investigators. In 1992, Sack et al. (16) reported isolation of ETBF to be significantly associated with diarrheal disease in Apache children between the ages 13–36 months but not in children <1 year. In the former age group, the ETBF isolation rates of 20–24% observed among patients were significantly different from the 8–9% observed among controls. As in our study, the difference in rates between cases and controls lost its significance when the age category was separated into 13–24 months and 25–36 months. In a study involving Bangladeshi children, ETBF was also found to be significantly associated with diarrhea in patients between the ages of 1 and 5 years but not in children <1 year of age; older children were not studied (17).

The intriguing and unexpected finding in this study is the significant association between B. fragilis and diarrhea. As observed with ETBF, the association is not demonstrable in children <1 old, despite the predominance (>50%) of patients and controls in this age group. But the power of the relationship between B. fragilis and diarrheal illness in older infants and children is such that statistical significance persists when overall isolation rates for patients and controls are compared. The latter observation is not true for ETBF.

Our data show that approximately 15% of the B. fragilis isolated from fecal specimens were enterotoxin producers regardless of whether they were isolated in diarrheal stools of patients or in feces of controls, and regardless of the age of the children and the season of collection of the specimens. These appear to accord with the findings that 9.3% of the isolates of B. fragilis in municipal sewage were enterotoxigenic (18). These observations suggest that ETBF comprise a considerable fraction of the B. fragilis flora of the intestinal tract and, possibly, the apparent association between ETBF and childhood diarrhea observed in this study may be a 'piggy back effect' of the highly significant association between B. fragilis and diarrhea. Alternatively and potentially akin to the diversity of diarrheagenic E. coli (19), B. fragilis may have additional virulence factors important in the pathogenesis of diarrheal disease that remain to be identified.

The meaning of the association between B. fragilis and ETBF with diarrhea is not clear from our data. The higher rate of shedding of both organisms may have been related to the purging effect of diarrhea on these indigenous bacteria. If this be the case, the association of B. fragilis and ETBF with diarrhea may stem from mechanical factors rather than from causal relationship. The patients were not routinely tested for parasites, rotavirus, or other enteropathogenic viruses which may have been responsible for the diarrhea. On the other hand, the apparent age-related susceptibility of children to B. fragilis-ETBF-associated diarrhea suggests that certain age-dependent host factor(s) determines the child's response to the disruption, by whatever mechanism, of the symbiotic relationship between the host and B. fragilis. These findings are reminiscent of the epidemiology of Clostridium difficile-associated diarrhea in childhood (20–22). C. difficile and its toxin are prevalent in feces of young infants but are not commonly associated with diarrheal disease until later in childhood. Analogous to C. difficile enteritis, B. fragilis-ETBF-associated diarrhea may have been precipitated by antibiotic therapy; this possibility is not addressed in the present study and needs to be investigated. Recently, a significant association between diffusely adherent E. coli with diarrhea was observed in children ≥18 months in age (23), an age-related pattern similar to that observed in our study. The significant association between B. fragilis and diarrheal disease found in our study differs from the findings of Sack and his associates in Apache children (16). In that study the isolation rates of B. fragilis did not differ significantly between patients and controls. Moreover, the overall B. fragilis isolation rates of 32.1% in patients and 21.1% in controls in the present study were less that one-half of the corresponding rates observed by Sack et al. The frequency of isolation of B. fragilis in the feces may vary with the population being studied. 45% of specimens from 20 normal adults had B. fragilis in one study (24); in another, B. fragilis was isolated in only 4% of feces from 10 patients with colonic cancer (25). The higher rate of shedding of B. fragilis observed in our patients with diarrhea could be related to methodological differences in the processing of the specimens for culture or to geographic factors. The Bangladeshi study (17) did not provide information on the isolation rates of B. fragilis in patients and controls. In the present study, only one colony with the characteristic appearance of B. fragilis on the PINN agar was processed for confirmatory identification from the stool of each child. Conceivably, some ETBF may have been missed by the initial testing although the proportion of missed ETBF in patients should be comparable to that in controls. However, this is probably not a major concern because Sack et al. (16) found that in persons harbouring ETBF, this strain constituted the predominant B. fragilis flora, and that approximately 84% of multiple isolates of B. fragilis from these persons proved enterotoxigenic when tested.

In our study population of urban children, B. fragilis, including ETBF, is significantly associated with acute diarrheal illness in children > 1 year old. Enterotoxin production may be an inherent characteristic of some strains of the B. fragilis flora of the intestinal tract. Whether enterotoxin production alone as a virulence trait is sufficient to lead to B. fragilis-associated diarrhea in children is not yet known. The findings of our study suggest that in favorable biologic surroundings B. fragilis and ETBF may act as enteropathogens in children. Further studies are evidently indicated to delineate the role of B. fragilis and ETBF in diarrheal disease.

ACKNOWLEDGEMENTS

The advice and invaluable help by Lyle L. Myers, Ph.D. are truly appreciated (VSJ). We thank A. Abdelhamid, M.D.; Jason Sigmon; P. Sarvepalli, M.D.; Joseph Covington; and Pirtham Raj for technical assistance.

This study was supported by the Oklahoma Center for Advancement of Science and Technology (VSJ), and by an Institutional Grant Award (to CLS) from the NIH Biomedical Research Support Grant (no. S07 RR05378) awarded to the Johns Hopkins University School of Medicine.

REFERENCES

1. Claeson M, Merson MPH, Merson M. Global progress in the control of diarrheal diseases. J Pediatr Infect Dis 9: 345–355, 1990.
2. Snyder JD, Merson MH. The magnitude of the global problem of acute diarrheal disease: A review of active surveillance data. Bull World Health Organ 60: 605, 1982.
3. Glass RI, Lew JF, Gangarosa RE, LeBaron CW, Ho MS. Estimates of morbidity and mortality rates for diarrheal diseases in American children. J Pediatr 118: S27–33, 1991.
4. Cohen MB. Etiology and mechanisms of acute infectious diarrhea in infants in the United States. J Pediatr 118: S34–39, 1991.
5. Kotloff KL, Wasserman SS, Steciak JY. Acute diarrhea in Baltimore children attending an outpatient clinic. J Pediatr Infect Dis 7: 753–759, 1988.
6. Myers LL, Firehammer BD, Shoop DS, Border MM. Bacteroides fragilis: a possible cause of acute diarrheal disease in newborn lambs. Infect Immum 44: 241–244, 1984.
7. Border M, Firehammer BD, Shoop DS, Myers LL. Isolation of Bacteroides fragilis from the feces of diarrheic calves and lambs. J Clin Microbiol 21: 472–473, 1985.
8. Myers LL, Shoop DS. Association of enterotoxigenic Bacteriodes fragilis with diarrheal disease in young pigs. Am J Vet Res 48: 774–775, 1987.
9. Myers LL, Shoop DS, Byars TD. Diarrhea associated with enterotoxigenic Bacteroides fragilis in foals. Am J Vet Res 48: 1565–1567, 1987.
10. Myers LL, Shoop DS, Collins JE, Bradbury WC. Diarrheal disease caused by enterotoxigenic Bacteroides fragilis in infant rabbits. J Clin Microbiol 27: 2025–2030, 1989.
11. Collins JE, Bergeland ME, Myers LL, Shoop DS. Exfoliating colitis associated with enterotoxigenic Bacteroides fragilis in a piglet. J Vet Diagn Invest 1: 349–351, 1989.
12. Myers LL, Collins JE, Shoop DS. Ultrastructural lesions of enterotoxigenic Bacteroides fragilis in rabbits. Vet Pathol 28: 336–338, 1991.
13. Duimstra JR, Myers LL, Collins JE, Benfield DA, Shoop DS, Bradbury WC. Enterovirulence of enterotoxigenic Bacteroides fragilis in gnotobiotic pigs. Vet Pathol 28: 514–518, 1991.
14. Weikel CS, Grieco FD, Reuben J, Myers LL, Sack RB. Human colonic epithelial cells, $HT29/C_1$, treated with crude Bacteroides fragilis enterotoxin dramatically alter their morphology. Infect Immun 60: 321–327, 1992.
15. Myers LL, Shoop DS, Stackhouse LL, Newman FS, Flaherty RJ, Letson GW, Sack RB. Isolation of enterotoxigenic Bacteroides from humans with diarrhea. J Clin Microbiol 25: 2330–2333, 1987.
16. Sack RB, Myers LL, Almeido-Hill J, Shoop DS, Bradbury WC, Reid R, Santosham M. Enterotoxigenic Bacteroides fragilis: epidemiologic studies of its role as a human diarrhoeal pathogen. J Diarrhoeal Dis Res 10: 04–09, 1992.
17. Sack RB, Albert MJ, Alam K, Neogi PKB, Akbar MS. Isolation of enterotoxigenic Bacteroides fragilis from Bangladeshi children with diarrhea: a controlled study. J Clin Microbiol 32: 960–963, 1994.
18. Shoop DS, Myers LL, LeFever JB. Enumeration of enterotoxigenic Bacteroides fragilis in municipal sewage. Appl Envi Microbiol 56: 2243–2244, 1990.
19. Levine MM. Escherichia coli that cause diarrhea: enterotoxigenic, enteropathogenic, enteroinvasive, enterohemorrhagic, and enteroadherent. J Infect Dis 3: 377–389, 1987.
20. Jarvis WR, Feldman RA. Clostridium difficile and gastroenteritis: how strong is the association in children? Pediatr Infect Dis 3: 4–6, 1984.
21. Donta ST, Myers MG. Clostridium difficile toxin in asymptomatic neonates. J Pediatr 100: 431–434, 1982.
22. Mårdh PA, Helin I, Colleen I, Öberg M, Holst E. Clostridium difficile toxin in faecal specimens of healthy children with diarrhoea. Acta Paediatr Scand 71: 275–278, 1982.
23. Gunzberg ST, Chang B, Simon E, Burke V, Gracey M. Diffuse and enteroaggregative patterns of adherence of enteric Escherichia coli isolated from aboriginal children from the Kimberley region of Western Australia. J Infect Dis 167, 1993.
24. Duerden BI. The isolation and identification of Bacteroides spp. from the normal human faecal flora. J Med Microbiol 13: 69–78, 1980.
25. Namavar F, Theunissen EB, Verweij-Van Vught AM, Peerbooms PG, Bal M, Hoitsma HF, MacLaren DM. Epidemiology of the Bacteroides fragilis group in the colonic flora in 10 patients with colonic cancer. J Med Microbiol 29: 171–6, 1989.

Submitted December 27, 1994; accepted March 20, 1995

Scand J Infect Dis 27: 217–220, 1995 ORIGINAL ARTICLE

Randomized Study of Sulfamethoxazole-trimethoprim versus Aerosolized Pentamidine for Secondary Prophylaxis of Pneumocystis carinii Pneumonia in Patients with AIDS

THYGE L. NIELSEN[1], BIRGITTE N. JENSEN[2], SUZANNE NELSING,[2] LARS R. MATHIESEN[1], PETER SKINHØJ[2] and JENS O. NIELSEN[1]

From the Departments of Infectious Diseases at [1]University Hospital Hvidovre, and at the [2]State University Hospital, Copenhagen, Denmark

In a prospective, randomized open-label trial, the efficacy of sulfamethoxazole-trimethoprim (SMX-TMP) 400/80 mg b.i.d. was compared with the efficacy of aerosolized pentamidine (AP) 60 mg every 2nd week as secondary prophylaxis (SP) against recurrence of Pneumocystis carinii pneumonia (PCP) in AIDS patients. 94 patients participated in the study, 47 in each group. The patients were observed for a mean period of 17.2 months. PCP recurred in the AP group in 8 cases, while 1 relapse occurred in the SMX-TMP group. The one-year cumulative relapse rate was 9.0% (95% CI 0–19%) in the AP group compared with 2.4% (95% CI 0–8%) in the SMX-TMP group ($p < 0.05$). The odds ratio was 4.2 (95% CI 0.5–39.8) in favour of SMX-TMP. Furthermore, we found a tendency towards a protective effect against toxoplasmosis in the SMX-TMP group, though there was no difference in survival between the two groups. There was no statistical difference in frequency of crossover from one therapy form to the other. Based on these data we recommend SMX-TMP for secondary PCP prophylaxis.

T. Lynghøj Nielsen, MD, Department of Internal Medicine B, Hillerød Sygehus, Helsevej 2, Dk-3400 Hillerød, Denmark

INTRODUCTION

Pneumocystis carinii pneumonia (PCP) is one of the most common opportunistic infections (OI) that establishes the diagnosis of AIDS (1). In Denmark, PCP occurred as the AIDS-defining diagnosis in about half of the patients before primary PCP prophylaxis was introduced as standard treatment (2). Relapses are frequent when no prophylaxis is given (>60% by 1 year), and although the prognosis has improved during recent years, PCP is still a major cause of morbidity and mortality in AIDS patients (3–4). Prophylaxis against PCP has therefore become an important part of the management of HIV disease. Several drugs have proved effective in both primary and secondary prophylaxis against PCP (SMX-TMP, AP, parenteral pentamidine, dapsone ± pyrimethamine, pyrimethamine with sulfadoxine, clindamycin with primaquine). Of these, AP and SMX-TMP are most often used. We compared the efficacy and safety of AP 60 mg every 2nd week vs. SMX-TMP 400/80 mg b.i.d. as secondary PCP prophylaxis in a prospective randomized trial.

PATIENTS AND METHODS

Patients

The patients were recruited from the 2 Departments of Infectious Diseases in Copenhagen (Hvidovre Hospital and Rigshospitalet). All patients who had suffered a previous episode of histologically verified PCP were invited to enroll in the study. Patients were enrolled from November 1988 to December 1991. The patients were followed either to termination of the study on 1st January, 1993, or to their decease.

Exclusion criteria were: age <18 years, lactating women, drug abusers, patients who were unlikely to keep appointments, patients who used sulfonamides or clindamycin for other purposes. All the patients had been treated with high-dose SMX-TMP during the primary episode of PCP. 41 patients (44%) (95% CI 33–54%) experienced adverse effects during this therapy, mainly rashes (34 patients). These adverse effects were treated with either dose reduction, temporary discontinuation of therapy, or antihistamines. None of patients were switched to pentamidine on suspicion of intolerance of SMX-TMP. The study was approved by the local Ethics Committee.

Study design

The trial was prospective, randomized and non-blinded, comparing AP versus SMX-TMP as secondary PCP prophylaxis. After giving their informed consent, the patients were allocated by block randomization to either group. AP was given with a loading dose of 300 mg, followed by 60 mg every 2nd week. The pentamidine isothionate was dissolved in 5 ml of sterile water and nebulized with System 22 Mizer linked to compressed air with a flow rate of 8 litres/min. The AP treatment was given under the supervision of specially trained staff, and patients were sitting in an upright position inhaling at tidal volume. If needed, bronchodilator was administered before each inhalation. SMX-TMP were administered as two tablets of 400/80 mg daily.

At entry, after 6 week and then every 3 months, each patient was evaluated by a physician.

End-points

The primary end-point was recurrence of histologically verified PCP. The secondary end-points were death, or the occurrence of

 ISSN 0036-5548

toxoplasmosis. Side effects due to 1 or 2 regimens that required a shift to another regimen were registered, but did not lead to discontinuation of the study. Survival data for all patients were evaluated on termination of study January 1993.

Statistical analysis

Data were analysed according to the intention-to-treat principle.

Numerical data are expressed as mean (range) values. Baseline data were compared using the Mann-Whitney test for unpaired data. Relapse rates, survival data and the cumulative incidence of adverse events were estimated using Kaplan-Meier Plots and compared using the Log-Rank test. Frequencies of events are expressed at 95% confidence intervals (CI). A p-value of 0.05 or less was considered to indicate a statistical significant difference. P-values above 0.05 are expressed as non-significant (NS).

Relative risk with 95% (CI) was used to monitor the variation in the primary end-point.

RESULTS

94 participants (47 patients in each group) were randomly assigned to either AP or SMX-TMP. The study period lasted 17 months (2.6–40.6) in the AP group and 17.5 months (1.9–48.9) in the SMX-TMP group. Four patients were lost to follow-up. The two groups matched well with respect to age, primary AIDS diagnosis, CD4-cell count at entry, and the number of patients receiving antiviral therapy (zidovudine) during the study (Table I). 84 patients (89%) were homosexual men.

Efficacy

Nine patients had a recurrence of PCP, 8 in the AP group and 1 in the SMX-TMP group. All the episodes were histologically verified after bronchoalveolar lavage. The one-year relapse rate was 9.0% (95% CI 0–19%) in the AP group and 2.4% (95% CI 0–8%) in the SMX-TMP group; the 18-month relapse rates were 16.5% (95% CI 8–32%) and 2.4% (95% CI 0–8%) respectively, $p < 0.05$ (Fig. 1). The relative risk of recurrent PCP after 1 year of prophylaxis was 4.2 (95% CI 0.5–39.8) times as high in the AP group as in the SMX-TMP group.

Table I. *Baseline data of the 2 groups on entering the study*

Characteristics	AP	SMX-TMP
No. of patients	47	47
Age, years	40	40
range	(25–63)	(24–65)
Sex		
Female	5	0
Male	42	47
Primary AIDS diagnosis		
PCP	45	43
Other	2	4
CD4 cell count at study entry	74	0.059[a]
($\times 10^6$/l)	(0–612)	(0–500)
Patients on antiviral therapy	44	45
Days on antiviral therapy	641	646[a]
(range)	(30–1745)	(27–1825)

[a] Not significant; AP = aerosolized pentamidine; SMX-TMP = sulfamethoxazole-trimethoprim.

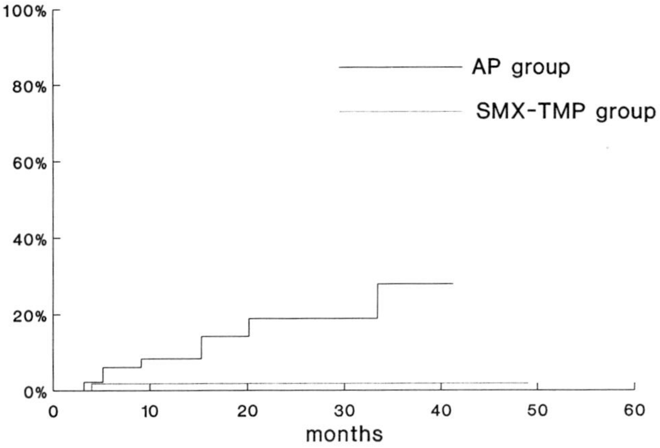

Fig. 1. The cumulative incidence of PCP relapse, according to the initial PCP prophylaxis, showed as Kaplan Meier curves.

Mortality

Two patients died during a repeat episode of PCP; one patient was randomized to AP, the other to SMX-TMP. Altogether 66 patients died during the study period. The mean survival time in the AP group was 25 months (4.5–66.1) and in the SMX-TMP group, 21.1 months (3.0–62.0) calculated from the time of the AIDS diagnosis, (NS).

Toxoplasmosis

Six cases of toxoplasmosis were diagnosed during the study period, 5 cases in the AP group and 1 in the SMX-TMP group, (NS). The latter patient was shifted to AP due to severe rash 3.8 months before he had toxoplasmosis diagnosed.

Crossovers between treatment

19 Patients crossed over to the reverse therapy: 11 patients in the AP group switched to SMX-TMP after 9.7 months (0.1–29.7), whereas 8 SMX-TMP patients switched to AP after 8.0 months (0.1–20.9), (NS). All the patients on SMX-TMP changed therapy due to rash. In the AP group, 4 patients shifted therapy of their own volition, whereas 3 patients had a severe cough and one had several episodes of bacterial pneumonia. The last 3 patients were preterminal in their AIDS disease and were unable to cooperate in the inhalation therapy. Patients who shifted from AP received SMX-TMP for 13.2 months (2.0–26.0) and patients who switched from SMX-TMP received AP for 13.5 months (3.8–23.5), (NS). None of the patients who changed therapy had relapse of PCP.

DISCUSSION

In this prospective, randomized, unblinded study we demonstrated that SMX-TMP is superior to AP as secondary PCP prophylaxis. We found that the use of SMX-TMP is approximately 4 times as effective as AP after one year of prophylaxis. These data agree closely with a recently published prospective study by Hardy et al. who found the difference in efficacy between the two treatments to be 3.25 times in favour of SMX-TMP (5). Three other studies dealing with primary PCP prophylaxis have found comparable results in favour of SMX-TMP (6–8). We found no difference in the survival data between the 2 groups, calculated from the time when AIDS was diagnosed. Similar data have been reported from other studies (5).

A tendency towards a protective effect against toxoplasmosis was demonstrated in the SMX-TMP group. All the 6 patients who had toxoplasmosis received AP as PCP prophylaxis at the time of the diagnosis. One patient was initially randomized to SMX-TMP but switched to AP approximately 4 months before the diagnosis of toxoplasmosis. This effect has been noticed in a few other prospective studies (5, 8–9).

Adverse reactions to SMX-TMP therapy and prophylaxis are well known. Although 44% of our patients experienced adverse effects during the initial high-dose SMX-TMP treatment of PCP, only 17% of all patients had to discontinue SMX-TMP as secondary PCP prophylaxis. These data suggest that intolerance might be a dose-related phenomenon (10–11). An equal number of patients crossed over from one prophylactic therapy to the other. All the patients in the SMX-TMP group changed treatment due to rashes. In the AP group, 11 patients switched to SMX-TMP. This is notably more than reported from other studies (5–8). In our study this might be due to the fact that 4 patients wished to change and a further 3 patients were transferred to the other therapy because of advanced AIDS disease that precluded inhalation therapy. Only 3 patients were shifted because of severe cough.

The optimal medical regime for PCP prophylaxis is debated. The Center for Disease Control (USA) recommended in 1989 either SMX-TMP 800/160 mg b.i.d. or AP delivered via a Respirgard II nebulizer 300 mg a month. This recommendation was amended in favour of SMX-TMP in 1992 (12, 13).

Though the SMX-TMP dose has been reduced in many studies, mainly because of adverse effects, the lower limit for an effective dose is still not known. SMX-TMP doses of 400/80 mg/day or maybe even less seems to be effective (5, 14–17). AP in doses of 300 mg delivered by Respirgard seems to be the golden rule (18–19). With a breakthrough rate of approximately 10% a year for both primary and secondary PCP prophylaxis, we have demonstrated in previous studies, that the regimen of 60 mg every 2nd week delivered by System 22 Mizer is at least as effective as 300 mg every 4th week delivered with a Respirgard (20).

In conclusion, these data demonstrate that SMX-TMP in a dose 400/80 mg b.i.d. is superior to AP in dose of 60 mg every 2nd week as secondary PCP prophylaxis. Furthermore there seems to be an additional prophylactic effect against cerebral toxoplasmosis. We therefore recommend SMX-TMP as the primary choice for secondary PCP prophylaxis.

REFERENCES

1. Kovacs JA, Masur H. Pneumocystis carinii pneumonia: Therapy and prophylaxis. J Infect Dis 158: 254–259, 1988.
2. Smith E, Orholm M. Trends and patterns of opportunistic diseases in Danish Aids patients, 1980–1990. Scand J Infect Dis 22: 665–672, 1990.
3. Kovacs JA, Masur H. Prophylaxis for pneumocystis carinii pneumonia in patients infected with human immunodeficiency virus. Clin Infect Dis 14: 1005–1009, 1992.
4. Nielsen TL, Schattenkerk JKME, Jensen BN, Lundgren JD, Gerstoft J, Steenwijk RP, Bentsen K, Frissen PHJ, Gaub J, Orholm M, Hansen JE, Mathiesen L, Skinhøj P, Danner SA, Nielsen JO. Adjunctive corticosteroid therapy for pneumocystis carinii pneumonia in AIDS. A randomized European multicenter open label study. J Acquir Immune Defic Syndr 5: 726–731, 1992.
5. Hardy D, Feinberg J, Finkelstein D, Power M, He W, Kaczka C, Frame P, Holmes M, Waskin H, Fass R, Powderly W, Steigbigel R, Zuger A, Holtzman R. A Controlled trial of trimethoprim-sulfamethoxazole or aerosolized pentamidine for secondary prophylaxis of pneumocystis carinii pneumonia in patients with the acquired immunodeficiency syndrome. N Engl J Med 327: 1842–1848, 1992.
6. Schneider MME, Hoepelman AIH, Schattenkerk JKME, Nielsen TL, Graff Y, Frissen J, Ende IME, Kolsters A, Borleffs JCC and the Dutch AIDS Treatment Group. A controlled trial of aerosolized pentamidine or trimethoprim-sulfamethoxazole as primary prophylaxis against pneumocystis carinii pneumonia in patients with human immunodeficiency virus infection. N Engl J Med 327: 1836–1841, 1992.
7. Mallolas J, Zamora L, Gatell JM, Miró JM, Vernet E, Valls ME, Soriano E, San Miguel JG. Primary prophylaxis for pneumocystis carinii pneumonia: a randomized trial comparing cotrimoxazole, aerosolized pentamidine and dapsone plus pyrimethamine. AIDS 7: 59–64, 1993.
8. May T, Beuscart J, Reynes B, Marchou B, Leclercq P, Lebas B, Saba J, Micoud M, Mouton M, Canton Ph. Trimethoprim-sulfamethoxazole versus aerosolized pentamidine for primary prophylaxis of pneumocystis carinii pneumonia: A prospective, randomized, controlled trial. J Acquir Immune Defic Syndr 7: 457–462, 1994.
9. Jakobson MA, Besch CL, Child C, Hafner R, Matts JP, Muth K, Wentworth DN, Neaton JD, Abrams D, Rimland D, Perez G, Grant IH, Saravoaltz LD, Brown LS, Deyton L. Primary prophylaxis with pyrimethamine for toxoplasmic encaphalitis in patients with advanced human immunodeficiency virus disease: Results of a randomized trial. J Infect Dis 169: 384–394, 1994.
10. Schneider MME, Nielsen TL, Hoepelman AIM, Nelsing S, Graaf Y, Kolsters AFP, Borleffs JCC. Two doses of trimethoprim-sulfamethoxazole as primary prophylaxis against pneumocystis carinii pneumonia in HIV-infected patients. 33nd ICAAC New Orleans M097, 1993.
11. Shafer RW, Seitzman PA, Tapper ML. Successful prophylaxis of Pneumocystis carinii pneumonia with trimethoprim-sulfamethoxazole in AIDS patients with previous allergic reactions. J Acquir Immune Defic Syndr 2: 389–393, 1989.
12. Center for Disease Control. Guidelines for prophylaxis against Pneumocystis carinii pneumonia for persons infected with human immunodeficiency virus. MMWR 38: 1–9, 1989.
13. Center for Disease Control. Recommendations for prophylaxis against Pneumocystis carinii pneumonia for adults and adolescents infected with human immunodeficiency virus. MMWR 41: 1–11, 1992.

14. Nielsen TL, Jensen BN, Nelsing S, Pedersen C, Mathiesen LR, Skinhøj P, Nielsen JO. Prevention of pneumocystis carinii pneumonia relapse in AIDS patients. Dan Med Bull 40: 503–505, 1993.
15. Carr A, Tindall B, Penny R, Cooper DA. Trimethoprim-sulfamethoxazole appears more effective than aerosolized pentamidine as secondary prophylaxis against pneumocystis carinii pneumonia in patients with AIDS. AIDS 6: 165–171, 1992.
16. Raviglione MC, Nash EN, Cortes H, Mariuz P, Sanjana Veeraf. Intermittent co-trimoxazole prophylaxis against Pneumocystis carinii pneumonia. Lancet 336: 180, 1990.
17. Ruskin J, Laviriere M. Low-dose cotrimoxazole for prevention of Pneumocystis carinii pneumonia in human immunodeficiency virus disease. Lancet 468–471, 1991.
18. Hirschel B, Lazzaran A, Chopard P, Opravil M, Furrer HJ, Ruttimann S, Vernazza P, Chave JP, Acarani F, Gabriel V, Heald A, Nicod L, Loredana S, Vivirito MC, Zerboni R, and the Swiss group for clinical studies on AIDS. A controlled study of inhaled pentamidine for primary prevention of Pneumocystis carinii pneumonia. N Engl J Med 324: 1079–1083, 1991.
19. Leoung GS, Feigal DW, Montgomery B, Corkery K, Wardlaw L, Adams M, Busch D, Gordon S, Jacobseon MA, Volberding P, Abrams D. Aerosolized pentamidine for prophylaxis against Pneumocystis carinii pneumonia. N Engl J Med 323: 769–775, 1990.
20. Jensen BN, Nielsen TL, Backer V, Nelsing S, Simonsen L, Flaschs H, Gaub J, Højlyng N, Nielsen JO, Mathiesen L, Skinhøj P. Aerosolized pentamidine for primary prophylaxis of Pneumocystis carinii pneumonia: A controlled, randomized trial. J Acquir Immune Defic Syndr 6: 472–477, 1993.

Submitted October 27, 1994; acccepted January 22, 1995

Scand J Infect Dis 27: 221–228, 1995 ORIGINAL ARTICLE

Is Penicillin the Appropriate Treatment for Recurrent Tonsillopharyngitis? Results from a Comparative Randomized Blind Study of Cefuroxime Axetil and Phenoxymethylpenicillin in Children

STIG HOLM[1], CLAES HENNING[2], EVA GRAHN[1], HELENA LOMBERG[3] and HEATHER STALEY[4] on behalf of the Swedish study group*

From the [1]Department of Clinical Microbiology, University of Umeå, the [2]Clinical Bacteriological Laboratory, Söder Hospital, Stockholm, [3]Glaxo Sweden AB, Mölndal, Sweden, and [4]Glaxo Research and Development Limited, Uxbridge, Middlesex, England

The efficacy of cefuroxime axetil compared with phenoxymethylpenicillin (PcV) was studied in group A β-haemolytic streptococci (GAS) culture-proven tonsillitis in children aged 3–12 years with a history of at least 1 episode of tonsillopharyngitis requiring antibiotic therapy during the previous 3 months. This was a comparative, randomized, investigator-blind, multicentre study. A total of 236 children received either cefuroxime axetil suspension or PcV syrup. Inclusion criteria were a positive, rapid, group A strep test verified by bacteriological culture and clinical signs and symptoms of tonsillopharyngitis. Cefuroxime axetil treatment gave a significantly higher bacteriological eradication rate and clinical cure rate than PcV. At day 2–5 post treatment the eradication rates were 99/114 (87%) for cefuroxime axetil vs 61/109 (56%) for PcV ($p < 0.001$). The clinical cure rates were 98/114 (86%) and 73/109 (67%) respectively ($p < 0.01$). Up to 21–28 days post-treatment, 9/114 (8%) cefuroxime axetil patients and 37/109 (34%) PcV patients were treatment failures or had recurrence/reinfection of GAS tonsillopharyngitis ($p < 0.001$). More than 90% of the patients who experienced bacteriological treatment failure at either the first or second follow-up had the same serotype isolated pre- and post-treatment. During the study period, 21/114 (18%) patients in the cefuroxime axetil group and 50/109 (46%) patients in the PcV group received additional antibiotics ($p < 0.001$). No serious adverse events were noted and the mild adverse events were equally distributed among the patients in the 2 study groups: 15% for cefuroxime axetil and 14% for PcV.

S. Holm, MD, Department of Clinical Microbiology, University of Umeå, S-901 85 Umeå, Sweden

INTRODUCTION

Penicillin has been the preferred treatment for Group A β-haemolytic streptococcal (GAS) tonsillopharyngitis for several decades and is the standard against which other antibiotics are compared. Penicillin efficacy was originally demonstrated in the 1950s when prevention of rheumatic fever was a key objective. Denny et al. (1) showed that use of injectable long-acting procaine benzylpenicillin formulations provided consistently good efficacy and contributed significantly to reduction in rheumatic fever as a sequel to streptococcal tonsillopharyngitis.

Penicillin treatment failure has been documented and the failure rates are usually 10–30% (2–4). Recent comparative studies have questioned whether Phenoxymethylpenicillin (PcV) is still the most appropriate treatment for GAS, especially in patients suffering recurrent infections or who fail on PcV therapy (5, 6). Cephalosporins offer an alternative treatment and have been shown in meta-analyses to have an equivalent or superior activity to PcV (7). Reasons for penicillin failure are multifaceted and include poor patient compliance, re-infection from nearest family and friends, low antibiotic levels at the site of infection, treatment duration, penicillin tolerance of streptococci, disturbed ecological balance of the tonsillopharyngeal flora and presence of β-lactamase-producing bacteria in the throat (8). An antibiotic with good activity against GAS, β-lactamase stability and causing minimal disturbance to the normal flora of the mouth, would offer a useful alternative for the treatment of GAS tonsillopharyngitis. Cefuroxime axetil fulfils these criteria. It is an oral pro-drug of the active compound cefuroxime, a β-lactamase-stable cephalosporin. Cefuroxime axetil (CA) is inactive during intake and is de-esterified to cefuroxime during absorption through the gut. The aim of the study was to compare the efficacy of CA with PcV for treatment of recurrent tonsillopharyngitis.

* Members of the Swedish study group at health care centres in Sweden: K. Nordmark, Björknäs, Boden, H. Ingvarsson, Björkskatan, Luleå, S. Salmonsson, Blåsippan, Härnösand, C. Brändström, Gammelstad, T. Sturesson, Hörnefors, G. Eriksson, Ljustadalen, Sundsbruk, E. Johansson, Nacksta, Sundsvall, G. Johansson, Matfors, N. Ernstdotter, Mjölkudden, Luleå, Y. Johansson, Skönsberg, Sundsvall, A.-M. Georén, Sävar, L. Lönneborg, Söråker, C. Carlsten, Hammarkullen, Angered, I. MacDowall, Krokslätt, Mölndal, C. Gundevall, Kungsbacka, S.-E. Åhlander, Hisings Kärra, G. Hedelin, Lerum, S. Mårild, Mölndal, B. Danielsson, Mölnlycke, B. Hedelin, Onsala, C. Hegen, Torpa, Vänersborg and P. Bandrup, Angered.

 ISSN 0036-5548

PATIENTS AND METHODS

This study was designed as a multicentre, investigator blind, randomized study, to compare cefuroxime axetil (CA) suspension with PcV syrup for the treatment of children with recurrent tonsillopharyngitis. It was conducted at 23 health centres in Sweden between January 1990 and May 1992. Parental informed consent was obtained for all patients and the co-operation of the child was confirmed. The study protocol was approved by the Ethics Committees concerned and by the Swedish Medical Products Agency.

Patients. A total of 236 children with recurrent tonsillopharyngitis, fulfilling the criteria listed below, were entered into the study and received treatment.

Inclusion criteria were: 1) children aged 3–12 years, 2) clinical signs/symptoms of tonsillopharyngitis, including presence of tonsillar and/or oropharyngeal erythema and ≥1 of the following: sore throat, tonsillar exudate, fever (>37.5°C) and tender cervical lymphadenitis, 3) evidence of the presence of GAS by a rapid antigen detection test, 4) a history of ≥1 episode of tonsillopharyngitis (GAS not culture proven) requiring antibiotic treatment during the previous 3 months documented by a physician.

Exclusion criteria were: 1) known hypersensitivity to penicillins or cephalosporins, 2) antimicrobial therapy in the preceding 3 days, 3) diagnosis of epiglottitis or other life threatening infection, 4) clinical evidence of viral infection (rhinorrhea, cough), 5) previous entry to the study.

Treatment. Patients were randomly assigned by a study nurse to receive either CA suspension or PcV syrup. Patients randomized to cefuroxime axetil (Zinnat, Glaxo, England) ($n = 119$) received 250 mg twice daily. Patients randomized to PcV (Kåvepenin syrup, Astra, Sweden) ($n = 117$) received 250 mg or 500 mg twice daily, depending on their weight (≤20 kg or >20 kg respectively, the standard recommended dose in Sweden). Treatment duration was 10 days. The investigator was not informed as to which treatment the patient had been assigned.

Procedures. Following the initial clinical examination, a throat swab was taken to determine the presence of GAS by rapid antigen test (Testpack Strep A, Abbott Diagnostics). If positive, a second throat swab was obtained for bacteriological culture and saliva was collected for determination of β-lactamase activity. If growth of GAS was not confirmed by bacteriological culture, patients were withdrawn from the evaluation of efficacy.

Each patient was scheduled for 2 follow-up visits: 1) 2–5 days post-treatment, and 2) 21–28 days post-treatment. At each visit, throat swabs were obtained for bacteriological culture and saliva was collected for determination of β-lactamase activity. A clinical examination was performed and symptoms of tonsillopharyngitis (tonsillar and/or oropharyngeal erythema, sore throat, tonsillar exudate, fever, cervical lymphadenitis) were recorded. A standard question was asked to determine whether any adverse event had occurred. Compliance was checked by the study nurse who collected any unused study medication and asked the parents if any doses of medication had been missed. Unused medication was documented.

If a patient returned to the clinic between scheduled visits due to clinical symptoms, a throat swab was taken before any further antibiotic treatment was given. Patients discontinued the study if new antibiotic treatment was given for any reason.

Bacteriological methods. Throat swabs were placed in a semisolid Stuarts' transport medium and promptly sent to 1 of the 2 reference microbiology laboratories where they were cultured immediately. For the pre-treatment throat swabs, 10 or more colonies of GAS were required for the sample to be regarded as positive for

Table I. *Patient demography*

Patients	Cefuroxime axetil	Penicillin V
Male/Female	66/53	62/55
Age (years) mean, range	6.8 (3–12)	6.4 (3–12)
Weight (kg) mean, range	27.3 (13.7–66)	25.4 (13–55)
Total randomized	119	117
Total treated	119	116

inclusion in the study according to the European Society of Clinical Microbiology and Infectious Disease guidelines for the clinical evaluation of anti-infective drugs. GAS were identified serologically. The GAS strains were frozen at −70°C. Patients who had a positive GAS culture during follow-up had all their isolates subsequently typed by T agglutination (using sera from Seravac Prague, Czech Republic) and by testing for opacity factor as described by Maxted and Widdowson (9).

M-typing was performed by immunodiffusion-in-gel analysis using an HCl extract of the streptococcal cells and specific M-typing sera kindly provided by Dr Maxted, Reference at The Colindale Laboratory; UK. All isolates were tested for susceptibility to PcV and cefuroxime, using the antibiotic paper disc method of Ericsson and Sherris (10). The non-stimulated sample of saliva was frozen at −20°C and subsequently tested for the presence of β-lactamase activity with chromogenic cephalosporin according to the method of O'Callaghan (11) using both the salivary pellet after centrifugation and the supernatant (12).

Patient evaluation. The efficacy of the therapy was assessed, both clinically and bacteriologically at each follow-up assessment (2–5 days post-treatment and 21–28 days post-treatment). However, a patient could be assessed outside the scheduled visits if they returned spontaneously due to clinical symptoms. Any patient re-treated with antibiotic discontinued the study, with no further follow-up (for details, see Table I).

The clinical response was assessed as: 1) cured: signs and symptoms subsided, 2) improved: incomplete resolution of signs and symptoms, 3) failure: persistence of symptoms, 4) recurrence: subsequent deterioration after initial cure or improvement.

The bacteriological response was assessed as: 1) cleared: original GAS serotype eradicated, 2) failure: original pathogen persisted, 3) relapse: same pathogen serotype isolated after initial clearance, 4) reinfection: new GAS serotype was isolated.

Outcome assessment. A retrospective assessment of the outcome of patients during the entire study period taking account of non GAS upper respiratory tract symptoms and adverse events in addition to GAS tonsillopharyngitis. The endpoints were: 1) successful – able to tolerate study medication, no further symptoms of upper respiratory tract infection or no further antibiotic prescribed up to 21–28 days post-treatment; 2) Unsuccessful – unable to tolerate study medication, persistence or recurrence of symptoms of upper respiratory tract infection with or without a new antibiotic prescribed up to 21–28 days post-treatment. Asymptomatic patients treated with a new antibiotic due to presence of GAS were not defined as either successful or unsuccessful, but listed separately.

Statistical analysis. The study was designed to detect at least a 15% difference in the bacteriological clearance rate. This was based on an expected bacteriological clearance rate of 75% in the PcV treatment group, a type I error rate of 5% and a type II error rate

Table II. *Patient tonsillopharyngitis history*

Patient history	Number of patients	
	Cefuroxime axetil	Penicillin V
Physician-documented previous episode(s) of tonsillopharyngitis	119	117
Treatment of previous episode		
Penicillin V	106	103
Other antibiotic[a]	13	14
Days since last episode[b]		
3–7	46	40
8–21	41	39
22– <90	31	37
Current episode		
Rapid antigen test positive	119	117
Confirmed by culture	114	109
Patients excluded because GAS was not confirmed by culture	5	8

[a] Cefaclor, cefadroxil, amoxicillin, erythromycin, clindamycin, or unknown.
[b] Two patients have missing data.

of 20%. Thus 95 evaluable patients were required per treatment group.

Demographics and other relevant characteristics were compared between the treatment groups, using Student's *t*-test for quantitative data and the log-likelihood ratio test for multinomial data. Bacteriological and clinical efficacy results and incidence of adverse events were compared between groups, using Fisher's exact test (2-sided) ($p < 0.05$), and 95% confidence limits on difference between groups were estimated. The data presented were analysed on an intention-to-treat basis.

RESULTS

Study population: There were no significant differences between the treatment groups with regard to age, sex, and weight (Table I). Of the 236 randomized patients, 119 received cefuroxime axetil and 116 received PcV, one patient randomized to penicillin did not take any medication. All of the patients had a history of tonsillopharyngitis documented by a physician (Table II) and most, 209/236 (89%) had received PcV treatment for an earlier episode of tonsillopharyngitis. The mean interval since the previous episode of tonsillopharyngitis was also similar for the 2 groups, with 166/236 (70%) of patients having had an episode within 3 weeks of entry to the present study.

In the current episode of tonsillopharyngitis, signs/symptoms and severity of infection were not significantly different in the 2 treatment groups. The rapid antigen test was positive in a very high proportion of cases 231/236 (97.9%) and was also confirmed by culture (Table II). Only 13 patients were excluded from the analysis because GAS was not cultured. 223 patients had a bacteriologically-confirmed positive, pre-treatment throat culture and these constituted the intent-to-treat population used in the analysis. 208 patients received treatment for 10–11 days according to the protocol; compliance was similar in both treatment groups. Four patients in each group took antibiotic for <3 days.

Patients withdrawn during treatment: Three patients receiving CA and 5 in the PcV treatment group were withdrawn during treatment. In the CA group, 2 patients refused to take the study medication and 1 experienced moderately severe diarrhea which was probably related to the antibiotic. In the PcV group, 2 patients refused to take the antibiotic and 3 others experienced an adverse event: otitis media, nausea and vomiting and urticaria, respectively. All events were moderately severe but urticaria was considered the only event related to the study drug. All 8 patients were treated with alternative antibiotics.

Eradication of GAS: Cefuroxime axetil was significantly more effective than PcV in eradicating GAS ($p < 0.001$) (Table III). At the first assessment, 2–5 days after a standard 10-day treatment, GAS was still detected in 42 patients who had received PcV (39%) compared with only 3% in the CA group. This was a significantly different result ($p < 0.001$) suggesting that PcV may be less effective in the treatment of recurrent tonsillopharyngitis if GAS eradication is used as the endpoint. GAS was eradicated, but other non-Group A haemolytic streptococci were isolated from 2 patients receiving CA and 1 patient in the PcV group. 15 patients were either unable to attend for assessment or did not have a throat swab taken (Table III). In addition to the 8 patients withdrawn during treatment (see above), 6 patients in the CA group and 21 patients in the PcV group ended the study after a first assessment and were given alternative antibiotics – see clinical responses. At the second assessment 21–28 days post-treatment, 80/105 (76%)

Table III. *A comparison of the efficacy of Cefuroxime axetil and Penicillin V in eradicating GAS in children with recurrent tonsillopharyngitis*

Assessment	Number of patients (%) Cefuroxime axetil	Penicillin V	p-value (95% CI)
2–5 days post-treatment	$n = 114$	$n = 109$	
GAS eradicated	99 (87%)	61 (56%)	<0.001 (20–42%)
GAS present	6 (3%)	42 (39%)	<0.001 (26–46%)
Outcome unknown – either patient or throat swab not available	9	6	
21–28 days post-treatment	$n = 105$	$n = 83$	
GAS eradicated	80 (76%)	46 (55%)	<0.01 (8–34%)
GAS present	18 (17%)	31 (37%)	<0.01 (8–32%)
Outcome unknown – either patient or throat swab not available	7	6	

of patients in the CA group remained bacteriologically free from GAS ($p < 0.01$); in contrast, 37% of patients in the PcV group still harboured the organism (Table III). Non-group A β-haemolytic streptococci were isolated from 1 PcV-treated patient and four CA treatment patients.

GAS serotyping: At the first assessment, all but 2 GAS strains, 1 in each treatment group, were of the same M and T types as the corresponding pre-treatment isolate. Nine different M and T types were identified at this time, of which T_{12}, M_{12} was the most common, occurring in 14 patients. At the second assessment, of patients from whom GAS had apparently been eradicated, the organism was cultured from an additional 26 people. Of these, only 2 patients in the CA group and 3 in the PcV group were re-infected and the remainder were judged to be relapses. Five strains were not typed: 2 from CA group and 2 from the PcV group.

Clinical responses: At the first assessment, the clinical cure rates, regardless of positive GAS throat culture, were 98/114 (86%) in the CA group compared with 73/109 (67%) in

Table IV. *Cefuroxime axetil vs Penicillin V in the treatment of recurrent tonsillopharyngitis in children: patient outcome 21–28 days post-treatment*

Patient outcome	Number of patients (%) Cefuroxime axetil	Penicillin V	p-value (95% CI)
Successful[a] No further experience of upper respiratory tract infections and no re-treatment with antibiotic	89 (78%)	55 (50%)	< 0.001 (16–40%)
Unsuccessful	18 (16%)	50 (46%)	< 0.001 (19–42%)
Intolerance to study medication	3	5	
Clinical symptoms of upper respiratory tract infection	15	45	
– GAS tonsillopharyngitis	9	37	
– Tonsillopharyngitis not culture proven	2	3	
– Non GAS URTI	4	5	
New antibiotic treatment due to GAS present despite lack of symptoms	5 (4%)	3 (3%)	
No final assessment performed	2 (2%)	1 (1%)	
Total	114	109	

[a] Includes 18 patients with GAS present without symptoms: 8 patients in the cefuroxime axetil group and 10 in the PcV group.

the PcV group ($p < 0.01$). Six patients in the CA group and 21 in the PcV group discontinued the study at or before the first assessment because GAS was still detected and/or clinical symptoms persisted. These patients were retreated with an alternative antibiotic.

Detailed reasons for re-treatment were: among the CA treated patients, 3 had GAS-positive culture with persistent clinical symptoms, 1 had a positive culture but was judged clinically to have been sucessfully treated, and 2 patients were GAS-negative but still had clinical symptoms. In the PcV group, 17 patients still had a GAS-positive culture with persistent clinical symptoms, 2 were culture-positive but judged to be clinically cured, 1 was culture-negative but still had clinical symptoms, and 1 patient still had clinical symptoms but a swab was not cultured. 105 patients in the CA group and 83 in the PcV group remained in the study. At the second assessment, 91/105 (87%) in the CA group and 56/83 (67%) for the PcV group remained clinically cured ($p < 0.01$). Thus at the end of the study period, 21–28 days after completion of the treatment, the overall clinical success rates were 91/114 (80%) for the CA group and 56/109 (51%) for the PcV group ($p < 0.001$, Confidence Interval 17–40%).

An overview of treatment outcome, incorporating both bacteriological and clinical findings is shown in Table IV. 78% of patients (89/114) in the CA group had a successful outcome compared with 50% (55/109) of patients given PcV ($p < 0.001$). 'Successful' meant that patients were able to tolerate study medication, had no further symptoms of GAS tonsillopharyngitis, had no other upper respiratory tract infection and no re-treatment with antibiotic up to 21–28 days after the initial 10-day treatment course. Patients with GAS, but not treated with a new antibiotic and without clinical symptoms were classified as having a successful outcome (8 patients in the CA group and 10 patients in the PcV group).

Treatment failures: At the first assessment, 3% of the 114 patients in the CA group had treatment failure, both clinically and bacteriologically. The corresponding rate for the PcV group was 23% (25/109; $p < 0.001$); 14 patients in this arm of the study were judged to be clinically improved, of whom 8 were left untreated and were scheduled for a second assessment. All other patients with GAS-positive culture and clinical symptoms were re-treated with antibiotic and left the study (Tables IV and V). Three patients in the CA group and 17 in the PcV group had GAS present but were deemed clinically cured.

At the second assessment, 6/105 (6%) of the CA group and 20/83 (24%) of the PcV group had recurrence of clinical GAS tonsillopharyngitis, $p < 0.001$. Altogether, during the study period, 9/114 (8%) CA patients were either treatment failures or had a recurrence/reinfection of clinically diagnosed and culture-confirmed GAS tonsillopharyngitis (3 diagnosed at first assessment and 6 at the second assessment). The corresponding results for PcV-treated patients were 37/109 (34%), 17 diagnosed at first assessment and 20 at the second ($p < 0.001$). Four patients with culture-confirmed GAS tonsillopharyngitis at the second assessment were not retreated with an alternative antibiotic, 1 in the CA group and 3 in the PcV group. Most patients who had GAS present after 2–5 days, but were left untreated because they were asymptomatic or had improved, clinically relapsed within the subsequent follow-up period: 1/2 in the CA group and 14/23 in the PcV group. Three patients, 1 in the CA group and 2 in the PcV group cleared spontaneously and 7 patients in the PcV group still had GAS at the second assessment but remained asymptomatic. Including patients intolerant to study medication and those with non-GAS upper respiratory tract infections, the total unsuccessful outcome for the study period was 16% for the CA group and 46% for the PcV group ($p < 0.001$) (Table IV). All patients judged to have been unsuccessfully treated

Table V. *Reasons for re-treatment with new antibiotic; study period up to 21–28 days post-treatment*

Reasons	Number of patients (%) Cefuroxime axetil ($n = 114$)	Penicillin V ($n = 109$)	p-value (95% CI)
Study drug terminated			
– adverse event	1	3	
– patient's refusal to take medication	2	2	
GAS + /symptoms of tonsillopharyngitis[a]	8	34	
Not cultured/symptoms of tonsillopharyngitis	2	3	
GAS + /no symptoms of tonsillopharyngitis	5	3	
Upper respiratory tract infection unrelated to GAS	3	5	
Total	21 (18%)	50 (46%)	< 0.001 (16–40%)

[a] Additional four patients, one in the CAE group and 3 in the PcV group, had recurrence of GAS tonsillopharyngitis at second follow-up. They were not retreated with a new antibiotic during the study period.

or who were withdrawn from the study had a new treatment prescribed within the study period. The reasons for re-treatment are listed in Table V.

Beta-lactamase activity: The incidence of β-lactamase activity detected in patients' saliva was low in both pre- and post-treatment samples. Initially, β-lactamase was detected in 28/104 (27%) of saliva samples from patients randomized to receive CA and in 19/102 (19%) samples from patients destined to have PcV. Saliva samples were not analysed for 10 patients in the CA group or for 7 in the PcV group. Post-treatment, there was no significant change in the incidence of β-lactamase activity in either of the study groups, neither was there a correlation between presence of the enzyme in saliva and bacteriological failure. In the CA group, 2/25 (8%) of patients who had detectable β-lactamase pre-treatment, failed bacteriologically, compared with 4/73 (6%) patients for whom no β-lactamase was detected. The corresponding correlation rates for the PcV group were 6/18 (33%) and 34/80 (43%), respectively.

Safety: Most reported adverse events were classified as being of mild or moderate severity. 18/119 (15%) patients in the CA group experienced at least 1 adverse event, compared with 16/116 (14%) patients in the PcV group, which was not significant. The events considered to be drug related by the investigator were, for CA and PcV: gastrointestinal (6 and 2), urticaria requiring withdrawal from the study (0 and 1) and myalgia (1 and 0).

DISCUSSION

The study shows that CA is statistically significantly superior to PcV for the treatment of recurrent antibiotic-treated tonsillopharyngitis in children. Higher cure rates with cephalosporins vis-à-vis PcV have also been observed in studies on primary infections (13–18). The greatest differences in treatment outcome were found among patients experiencing bacterial treatment failure or those with recurrent tonsillopharyngitis. When earlier PcV treatment had been given, failure rates as high as 70% have been reported (5, 6, 19). In this study all patients had experienced an episode of tonsillopharyngitis requiring antibiotic treatment (89% PcV) in the preceding 3 months and most of these (63%) had occurred within 2 weeks of enrolment in the study.

Recent papers have debated whether PcV should remain the preferred drug for treatment of streptococcal tonsillopharyngitis (20–22). Although 2 authors recommend PcV (21, 22) their conclusions are based on studies of primary tonsillopharyngitis rather than recurrent episodes. Our results, together with earlier studies (5, 6, 19), suggest that PcV treatment is not appropriate for patients with recurrent tonsillopharyngitis, particularly if PcV treatment has already been given. Of the PcV-treated patients, 46% had an unsuccessful treatment outcome during the 21–28 day follow-up period, as compared with 16% in the CA group. Unsuccessful treatment was defined as intolerance to study medication, treatment failure, recurrence of tonsillopharyngeal infection or other upper respiratory infection, which required retreatment with a new antibiotic within the study period.

The reasons for the superior efficacy of the cephalosporins may be attributed to factors such as stability to β-lactamase produced by micro-organisms in the throat (12, 16, 23), lack of tolerance by GAS to cephalosporins (24, 25), favourable pharmacokinetics (26), minimal disturbance to the normal flora of the mouth (27) and patient compliance. The presence of β-lactamase-producing bacteria in the throat is considered a major contributory factor to PcV treatment failure and these organisms have been termed co-pathogens by some authors (16, 28).

Tunér and Nord (23) and Brook (28) have demonstrated emergence of β-lactamase-producing bacteria, both aerobes and anaerobes, in the oropharynx during PcV therapy; the latter noted that this occurred in about a third of patients after 1 course of PcV treatment and that co-pathogens could be transferred to household contacts.

The observation that a study with erythromycin, which is unaffected by β-lactamase did not demonstrate better efficacy than PcV, suggests that other factors are also involved (15). In this study there seemed to be no correlation between recurrence after PcV therapy and high rates of β-lactamase activity in saliva samples, a correlation that has been demonstrated by others (23, 25). The most likely explanation is that the method of sampling was not sufficiently sensitive to detect β-lactamase activity at the site of infection and in the tonsillar crypts, where many co-pathogens, especially anaerobes, reside.

Ecological disturbance of the oropharyngeal flora is a common finding after PcV treatment and is reflected in the increase in β-lactamase-producing bacteria and concomitant decrease in the α-streptococci (27). If antibiotic is given as a syrup or a suspension, the extremely high concentration in the oropharynx could influence throat flora, whereas use of a microbiologically inactive pro-drug should theoretically diminish the risk of ecological disturbances of the normal throat flora. The important role played by the normal throat flora in protecting against recurrent streptococcal tonsillopharyngitis has recently been demonstrated in re-implantation experiments in man (29).

In this study there were no differences in compliance rates between children given oral PcV and CA, but the importance of patient compliance should not be overlooked as treatment needs to be continued after the patient's clinical symptoms have resolved. Shorter, 5-day courses of penicillin have been shown to be less effective than 10 days (14); in contrast, 5 days of treatment with a cephalosporin has been shown to be as effective as 10 days of PcV treatment in terms of GAS eradication (15).

It has been suggested that GAS carriers might influence study results (30). The carrier status of the patients enrolled in the present study was not known, but the carrier rate among children in Sweden has been reported to be between 5.9 and 11.3% with no obvious season-dependent variation and the highest rate amongst the 4-year-olds (31). Since the present study was large and randomized, any GAS carriers would have been equally distributed among the treatment groups.

In addition, to reduce the risk of enrolling GAS carriers with concurrent viral pharyngitis, we excluded patients with symptoms such as rhinorrhea or cough. It is therefore conceivable that inclusion of potential GAS carriers is unlikely to affect the comparison between the 2 treatment groups. It should be emphasized that most patients from whom GAS was isolated at the first assessment despite being asymptomatic and who were left untreated, experienced symptoms of tonsillopharyngitis during the study period and needed further treatment (14 patients in the PcV group and one patient in the CA group).

The role of cephalosporins in preventing rheumatic fever is unproven and may remain so because of the very large studies which would be needed to demonstrate prophylactic efficacy. Nevertheless, more effective bacteriological eradication can be demonstrated for cephalosporins (13, 15, 17). In the USA, outbreaks of rheumatic fever have led to a debate about current therapeutic regimens, although outbreaks appear to have been associated with specific serotypes rather than being attributable to antibiotic failure. Nevertheless, with increasing numbers of children in day-care centres in industrially developed countries and with overcrowding in the developing world, it would seem prudent to use therapeutic regimens which offer a high likelihood of GAS eradication from the oropharynx in culture-positive patients, in order to limit the spread. The 46% failure rate of PcV in this study endorses the view that, at least for recurrent tonsillopharyngitis, PcV no longer offers an appropriate likelihood of GAS eradication.

PcV has been shown to be less efficacious in eradicating GAS and of eliminating clinical symptoms, than were cephalosporins in more than 30 studies (7). The present study further underlines the superior efficacy of cephalosporins and focuses on cefuroxime axetil as a valuable alternative for the treatment of recurrent GAS tonsillopharyngitis in children.

It is conceivable that patients with an unsuccessful outcome after antibiotic therapy would need an additional visit to a health centre for further treatment and microbiological assessment, with inconvenience for both patient and parent. When the total costs of management of treatment failures are considered, it is likely that cefuroxime axetil suspension represents a cost-effective treatment alternative to PcV for patients with recurrent infection. Now is the time to review the place of PcV in the treatment of recurrent GAS tonsillopharyngitis.

ACKNOWLEDGEMENT

This study received financial support from Glaxo Research and Development Ltd., Greenford, Middlesex, England.

REFERENCES

1. Denny FW, Wannamaker LW, Brink WR, et al. Prevention of rheumatic fever: treatment of the preceding streptococcal infections. JAMA 143: 151–153, 1950.
2. Gastanaduy AS, Kaplan EL, Huwe BB, et al. Failure of penicillin to eradicate Group A streptococci during an outbreak of pharyngitis. Lancet 2: 498–501, 1980.
3. Stillerman M. Comparison of oral cephalosporins with penicillin therapy for Group A streptococcal pharyngitis. Pediatr Infect Dis J 5: 649–654, 1986.
4. Pichichero ME. The rising incidence of penicillin treatment failures in Group A streptococcal tonsillopharyngitis: an emerging role for the cephalosporins? Pediatr Infect Dis J 10: 50–55, 1991.
5. Brook I. Treatment of patients with acute recurrent tonsillitis due to Group A β-haemolytic streptococci: a prospective randomized study comparing penicillin and amoxycillin/clavulanate potassium. J Antimicrob Chemother 24: 227–233, 1989.
6. Kaplan EL, Johnsson DR. Clinical and laboratory observations: Eradication of Group A streptococci from the upper respiratory tract by amoxicillin with clavulanate after oral penicillin V treatment failure. J Pediatr 113: 400–403, 1988.
7. Pichichero ME, Margolis PA. A comparison of cephalosporins and penicillin in the treatment of Group A beta-hemolytic streptococcal pharyngitis: a meta-analysis supporting the concept of microbial copathogenicity. Pediatr Infect Dis J 10: 275–281, 1991.
8. Holm SE. Reasons for failures in penicillin treatment of streptococcal tonsillitis and possible alternatives. Pediatr Infect Dis J 13: 66–69, 1994.
9. Maxted WR, Widdowson JP. The protein antigens of Group A streptococci. In: Wannamaker LW, Matsen JM, eds. Streptococci and Streptococcal Diseases. New York: Academic Press, 251–264, 1972.
10. Ericsson HM, Sherris JS. Antibiotic sensitivity testing: Report of an international collaborative study. Acta Pathol Microbiol Scand [B] Suppl 217, 1971.
11. O'Callaghan CH, Morris A, Kirkby SM, Shingler A. Novel method for detection of beta-lactamase by using a chromogenic cephalosporin substrate. Antimicrob Agents Chemother 1: 283–288, 1972.
12. Roos K, Grahn E, Holm SE. Evaluation of beta-lactamase activity and microbial interference in treatment failures of acute streptococcal tonsillitis. Scand J Infect Dis 18: 313–319, 1986.
13. Holm SE, Roos K, Strömberg A. A randomised study of treatment of streptococcal tonsillopharyngitis with cefadroxil or phenoxy-methylpenicillin (penicillin V). Pediatr Infect Dis J 10: 68–71, 1991.
14. Strömberg A, Schwan A, Cars O. Five versus 10 days treatment of group A streptococcal tonsillopharyngitis: a randomized controlled clinical trial with phenoxymethylpenicillin and cefadroxil. Scand J Infect Dis 20: 37–46, 1988.
15. Milatovic D. Evaluation of cefadroxil, penicillin and erythromycin in the treatment of streptococcal tonsillo-pharyngitis. Pediatr Infect Dis J 10: 61–63, 1991.
16. Milatovic D, Knauer J. Cefadroxil versus penicillin in the treatment of pharyngitis. Eur J Clin Microbiol Infect Dis 8: 282–288, 1989.

17. Pichichero ME, Disney EA, Aronowitz GH, et al. Randomised, single-blind evaluation of cefadroxil and phenoxymethyl penicillin in the treatment of streptococcal pharyngitis. Antimicrob Agents Chemother 31: 903–906, 1987.
18. Pichichero ME, McLinn SE, Gooch MW, et al. Ceftibuten vs penicillin V in Group A beta-hemolytic streptococcal pharyngitis. Pediatr Infect Dis J 12: 64–69, 1993.
19. Stjernquist-Desatnik A, Orrling A, Kamme C, Schalén C. Eradication of group A streptococci from the throat after oral penicillin V treatment failure: A comparison between clindamycin and penicillin V. Proceedings of XII Lancefield symposium on streptococci and streptococcal diseases, St Petersburg, Sept 1993. [in press]
20. Pichichero M. Cephalosporins are superior to penicillin for treatment of streptococcal tonsillopharyngitis: is the difference worth it? Pediatr Infect Dis J 12: 268–274, 1993.
21. Shulman ST, Gerber MA, Tanz RR, Markowitz M. Streptococcal pharyngitis: the case for penicillin therapy. Pediatr Infect Dis J 13: 1–7, 1993.
22. Markowitz M, Gerber MA, Kaplan EL. Treatment of streptococcal tonsillopharyngitis: Reports of penicillin's demise are premature. J Pediatr 123: 679–685, 1993.
23. Tunér K, Nord CE. Emergence of beta-lactamase producing bacteria in the tonsils during penicillin treatment. Eur J Clin Microbiol 5: 399–404, 1986.
24. Grahn E, Holm SE, Roos K. Penicillin tolerance in beta-streptococci isolated from patients with tonsillitis. Scand J Infect Dis 19: 421–426, 1987.
25 Kim KS, Kaplan EL. Association of penicillin tolerance with failure to eradicate Group A streptococci from patients with pharyngitis. J Pediatr 107: 681–684, 1985.
26. Wise R, Bercnet SA, Dent J. The pharmacokinetics of orally absorbed cefuroxime compared with amoxycillin-clavulanic acid. J Antimicrob Chemother 13: 603–610, 1984.
27. Grahn E, Holm SE. Bacterial interference in the throat flora during a streptococcal tonsillitis outbreak in an apartment house area. Zbl Bakt Hyg A 256: 72–79, 1983.
28. Brook I. The role of β-lactamase-producing bacteria in the persistence of streptococcal tonsillar infection. Rev Infect Dis 6: 601–607, 1984.
29. Roos K, Holm SE, Grahn E, Lind L. Alpha-streptococci as supplementary treatment of recurrent streptococcal tonsillitis: a randomized placebo controlled study. Scand J Infect Dis 25: 31–35, 1993.
30. Kaplan EL, Gastanaduy AS, Huwe BB. The role of the carrier in treatment failures after antibiotic treatment for group A streptococci in the upper respiratory tract. J Lab Clin Med 98: 326–335, 1981.
31. Strömberg A, Schwan A, Cars O. Throat carrier rates of beta-haemolytic Streptococci among healthy adults and children. Scand J Infect Dis 20: 411–417, 1988.

Submitted November 12, 1994; accepted March 14, 1995

Scand J Infect Dis 27: 229–234, 1995 ORIGINAL ARTICLE

Treatment of Acute Maxillary Sinusitis – Comparing Cefpodoxime Proxetil with Amoxicillin

CARL VON SYDOW[1], SEPPO SAVOLAINEN[2] and ANITA SÖDERQVIST[3]

*From the E.N.T. Departments of [1]Lundby Hospital, Göteborg, Sweden and [2]Central Military Hospital, Helsinki, Finland, and [3]Roussel Nordiska AB, Stockholm, Sweden**

In order to evaluate the clinical efficacy and tolerance of cefpodoxime proxetil, compared with that of amoxicillin in the treatment of acute bacterial maxillary sinusitis, a randomized, double-blind, parallel group comparative study was performed. A total of 286 adults patients were included at 12 centres, each treatment group consisting of 143 patients. Each patient was treated for 10 days and observed before and after treatment. The observations included clinical, roentgenological, bacteriological and laboratory examinations. At inclusion, the most common pathogens were Haemophilus influenzae (24%) and Streptococcus pneumoniae (17%). In the per protocol analysis, 117 patients in the cefpodoxime group and 113 in the amoxicillin group were evaluable for clinical efficacy. The clinical response rates were 96% and 91%, respectively. The corresponding figures in the intent-to-treat analysis were 130 and 128 patients, with clinical response rates of 93% and 88%, respectively. Cefpodoxime proxetil proved clinically as effective as amoxicillin in the treatment of acute bacterial maxillary sinusitis. It was more effective in eradicating H. influenzae and was more efficient in improving the radiological score. Adverse events were reported in 20% of cefpodoxime cases and in 16% of amoxicillin cases. There was no statistically significant difference between the groups.

C. von Sydow, MD, ENT Department, Lundby Hospital, S-417 17 Göteborg, Sweden

INTRODUCTION

Acute maxillary sinusitis is a bacterial complication of rhinitis or the common cold. Penicillins, tetracyclines, cephalosporins and macrolides are the antibiotics most commonly used, and the therapeutic outcome seems to differ very little among the drugs used (1). Drainage is recommended as the most important way to combat purulent maxillary sinusitis (2). However, general practitioners, who see most of these patients, are as a rule not skilled in antral puncture technique.

Although we regard sinusitis as a common disease, it is not easily diagnosed clinically (3, 4). Its symptoms are often indistinct from those of uncomplicated rhinitis, needing a different kind of therapy. To ensure a correct diagnosis of purulent maxillary sinusitis, the clinical symptoms must be supplemented with a combination of radiological (or ultrasonic) examination and sinus puncture (5, 6).

The bacterial panorama of acute maxillary sinusitis has changed over the last decades and is now dominated by Haemophilus influenzae and Streptococcus pneumoniae (1, 6–10), while the β-hemolytic streptococci, more common in the 1950s (8), are now rarely encountered (5–10%) (7, 11). Other bacteria, usually found in small numbers (today, as well as 20 years ago) are Moraxella catarrhalis and anaerobic bacteria (1, 11). Large numbers of anaerobic bacteria (or a mixture of anaerobic and aerobic bacteria) are mostly seen in chronic sinusitis or sinusitis of dental or other origin (12). Staphylococcus aureus is a known pathogen in chronic sinusitis, but in acute maxillary sinusitis cases it is probably found merely as a result of contamination (13).

An increasing occurrence of β-lactamase-producing strains of M. catarrhalis and H. influenzae has been reported, the current prevalence figures for Sweden estimated to 80% and 8(−15)%, respectively (8).

Cefpodoxime proxetil (CP) is the inactive prodrug of cefpodoxime, a new oral cephalosporin (Orelox®, Roussel). CP is characterized by its stability to bacterially produced β-lactamases, and by its broad-spectrum activity against Gram-positive and Gram-negative bacteria, including the common pathogens associated with acute sinusitis (14–16). A previous sinusitis study has indicated that CP is more effective than cefaclor (17). Significant advantages in clinical efficacy were also evident with twice daily CP, compared with thrice daily amoxicillin/clavulanic acid in the treatment of acute otitis media in children (18).

In order to further evaluate the usefulness of CP in the treatment of acute bacterial maxillary sinusitis, the current study was conducted to compare its clinical and bacteriological efficacy with that of amoxicillin. Amoxicillin, with its well-documented efficacy against acute maxillary sinusitis (6, 8, 9, 19), was chosen as the comparative drug because of its similarity of bacteriological spectrum, though CP has an extended spectrum regarding

---

* Study group. H. Kiukaanniemi (Oulu), E. Lappalainen (Helsinki), K. Roos (Göteborg), B. Synnerstad (Västervik), C. Sjölin, C. Björklund (Kristianstad), L. Sundberg, P. Jansson (Karlskrona), R. Berglund (Oskarshamn), O. Spandow, Å. Dahlqvist, D. Berggren (Umeå), P. Persson, H. Harder (Linköping), O. Olsson, H-E. Persson (Sundsvall), M. Tvinnereim (Bergen), A. Orrling (Eslöv).

 ISSN 0036-5548

β-lactamase-producing strains of M. catarrhalis and H. influenzae.

MATERIAL AND METHODS

Study design

This multicentre study was performed at 12 centres in 3 Nordic countries: Sweden (9 centres), Finland (2 centres) and Norway (1 centre), engaging 20 ENT specialists. It was designed as a comparative, randomized, double-blind, double-dummy, parallel group study. Out-patients, >18 years old, with a history of sinus pain or pressure sensation, purulent nasal discharge and/or nasal obstruction for <30 days were enrolled. Patients with symptomatic frontal and ethmoidal sinusitis, allergic sinusitis, acute attacks of chronic sinusitis or maxillary sinusitis of dental origin were excluded. The clinical diagnosis was confirmed radiologically, followed by an antral puncture for the demonstration and bacteriological examination of pus.

Patients were also excluded for the following reasons: pregnancy or nursing, localized treatment or surgery within 2 weeks, impaired renal or liver function, history of hypersensitivity to β-lactam antibiotics, concomitant treatment with probenecid and other antibiotics, antibiotic treatment within 4 days of enrolment, or concomitant treatment with nasal preparations containing steroids.

Ethical considerations

This study was reviewed by the local ethics committees and was conducted according to the Declaration of Helsinki. All patients were informed, orally and in writing, of the aim, nature and duration of the study and of possible adverse events. All patients' oral consent had to be obtained prior to entering the study.

Study drugs

To obtain a total of 224 clinically evaluable patients, a number of at least 270 outpatients with acute maxillary sinusitis were to be enrolled and treated for 10 days. They were to be allocated at random to either

cefpodoxime 200 mg BID or
amoxicillin 750 mg BID

All patients also received a nasal decongestant (xylometazoline) for not more than 7 days – any other concomitant treatment was specified in the case record form.

Bacteriology

A microbiological sample was obtained by antral aspiration before inclusion and – if the clinical and radiological recovery was considered unsatisfactory by the clinician – again, at the end of treatment. Aspirated material was transported in a carefully plugged syringe or in Stuart medium to the laboratory for bacteriological examination.

The samples were incubated at 37°C aerobically and under 5% CO_2 and examined after 24 and 48 h. For anaerobic screening, Brucella agar was used at 37°C anaerobically and examination after 48–72 h. The samples were also enriched in BHI broth or PYG broth at 37°C for 48–72 h. The microorganisms were identified by Gram stain and according to standardized methods. The anaerobic bacteria were identified by Gram stain, biochemical tests and gas-liquid chromatography according to Holdeman et al. (20). Susceptibility tests of cefpodoxime and amoxicillin were performed at the different laboratories using Oxoid or Biodisc disks loaded with 30 and 10 µg of antibiotics, respectively, and β-lactamase tests were performed using chromogenic tests. The isolated resistant microorganisms were sent to the National Bacteriological Laboratory in Stockholm for MIC determinations.

Radiological signs

The pre- and post-treatment radiological examinations were made according to the routine of each centre, but an occipito-mental projection, with an additional occipito-mental side view, was recommended for the best demonstration of small amounts of sinus secretion (21).

In order to be enrolled in the study, sinus secretion had to be demonstrated. Completely opaque sinuses were always punctured to verify pus, thus excluding sinuses where the radiological opacity was caused by polyps or cysts, or by mucous or serous fluid. The roentgenological state of each sinus was classified according to a 6-point scale (22):

Mucous membrane thickening ≤6 mm	1 point
Mucous membrane thickening >6 mm	2 points
Secretion	2 points
Mucous membrane thickening ≤6 mm + secretion	3 points
Mucous membrane thickening >6 mm + secretion	4 points
Complete opacity	6 points

Follow-up

The patients were to be observed on 3 occasions: the pretreatment visit (day 0), the post-treatment visit (days 11–20) and the follow-up visit (days 28–35). The follow-up visit could be replaced by a telephone interview, if the results at the second visit had been satisfactory or improved, and if there were no clinical symptoms related to maxillary sinusitis.

Cinical efficacy

The clinical efficacy was to be based on 2 examinations of each patient: before and after treatment. At the post-treatment visit, the clinical response was to be judged as *satisfactory* (i.e., absence of all clinical signs – with the exception of partial nasal obstruction – plus absence or improvement of radiological signs/points), *improved* (i.e., clinical signs improved, plus improved or unchanged radiological signs/points), *unsatisfactory* (i.e., clinical and sinus X-ray points unchanged or worsened) or *unevaluable* (i.e., due to a protocol violation, or if a prohibited treatment had been administered). In the criteria of clinical efficacy evaluation, patients were not considered evaluable if microorganisms isolated from the pretreatment aspirates were resistant to either CP or amoxicillin.

Bacteriological response

Bacteriological response was deemed *satisfactory* if the causative agent (isolated from the sinus aspirate at enrolment) was eradicated by the end of the treatment period or, if no post-treatment maxillary aspiration had been performed, due to clinical recovery. *Unsatisfactory* response was due either to *failure* (i.e., the causative agent still present, or – in the case of multiple pathogens – partial eradication of one or more microorganisms) or to *superinfection* (i.e., the causative agent had been eradicated at the end of treatment, but a new pathogen was detected with clinical signs of infection). The bacteriological response was *unevaluable* when the pretreatment culture was sterile, lost, or not performed, when the organism isolated was a commensal or not causative, or if it was not tested for antibiotic susceptibility.

Follow-up evaluation

Based on the clinical and bacteriological evaluations, each patient was classified at the follow-up visit as *cured* (i.e., had no clinical signs of persisting sinusitis or of a new infection), *relapse* (i.e., clinical signs of sinusitis, with or without the continuous presence of the causative agent/s), *reinfection* (i.e., clinical signs of sinusitis and new pathogen/s found), or *unevaluable* (i.e., failure at the end of treatment, concomitant treatment with antibiotics, or no follow-up visit).

In the protocol it was stated that a per protocol analysis of the study was to be performed. Discussions about the relevance of bacteriological analysis in phase III studies (23) resulted in the addition of a modified intent-to-treat analysis. In this, all randomized patients, including those with resistant strains of bacteria at inclusion, were accepted.

Safety and tolerance

The safety evaluation was based on adverse events and on laboratory tests. Adverse events recorded from the spontaneous report by the patient or from the active questioning by the examiner were specified with regard to onset, severity and duration. The laboratory tests were made before and after treatment. Blood tests included hemoglobin, leukocytes and a differential count. Bilirubin and C-reactive Protein (CRP), as well as creatinine and liver tests (ASAT, ALAT and ALP) were compulsory. Urine analysis included glucose and protein.

Statistical methods

A total of 112 patients per group were needed to satisfy the condition that the 95% confidence limit for a difference in efficacy should not exceed $\partial = 0.10$ (with 80% probability) in favour of amoxicillin, while a true success rate of 90% was assumed.

Demographic data, baseline recordings and adverse events for the two treatment groups were compared, using the Student's *t*-test, χ^2-test or Mann-Whitney U-test as appropriate. A 5% significance level in two-tailed tests was used throughout the study.

Differences between pre- and post-treatment laboratory values (related to normals) were tested with the McNemar test of symmetry, and between groups with a test for homogeneity.

Wherever possible, success rates were calculated, and *success* was defined as "Satisfactory" and "Improved" (or the corresponding categories). For efficacy variables, two-sided 95% confidence intervals were used for the difference between success rates and means. When such an interval includes zero, equivalence between the groups *can* be assumed with 95% confidence – and when it lies entirely on one side (positive or negative), equivalence *cannot* be assumed (cf. notes No. 3 and 4, respectively, in Table III).

RESULTS

Patients

A total of 286 patients were enrolled. Their ages ranged from 18 to 78, with a mean of 33 years. There was an even sex distribution (149 males and 137 females) and a good balance between the groups regarding age, sex, weight and height.

The two groups were well balanced regarding the incidence of clinical signs on admission. Other baseline assessments of demographic and background characteristics, basic illness, previous therapy and bacteriological status, showed no significant differences between the groups.

The radiological status of all patients at admission was comparable in the two treatment groups (4.4 and 4.3, respectively).

In all, 282 patients were treated and were therefore evaluated for tolerance (1 patient in each group failed to return for the second visit, and 2 patients in the CP group did not take the study drugs as planned).

According to the per protocol analysis, 230 patients (117 in the CP and 113 in the amoxicillin group) were evaluable for clinical efficacy. Bacteria resistant to amoxicillin (in samples from 4 patients in the CP group and from 10 patients in the amoxicillin group), protocol violation at enrolment (6 and 10 patients, respectively) or during the trial (11 and 4 patients, respectively), interruption due to intercurrent illness (2 patients in the amoxicillin group) or withdrawal, due to adverse events (2 and 3 patients, respectively) were reasons for exclusion.

The radiological status at enrolment was here 4.4 in both groups, and the mean radiological recovery values (i.e., reduction of the 6-point scale) at follow-up were 3.4 and 2.9 points, respectively. With 95% confidence, a true difference in favour of CP can be assumed (confidence interval for difference between means: -1.06 to -0.07).

No major differences were noted at the post-treatment visit, regarding the elimination of *clinical baseline symptoms*.

The post-treatment *clinical response* was rated as successful (i.e., satisfactory or improved clinical response) or unsuccessful (i.e., with sinusitis symptoms still present at post-treatment visits). The success rate for overall clinical efficacy was 112/117 (95.7%) in the CP group and 103/113 (91.2%) in the amoxicillin group. Equivalence between the groups could be assumed with 95% confidence (confidence interval for difference in success rate -1.6 to 10.8).

In 125 cases (44%), aspirates were negative for bacteriological culture, or the patient could not be included in further bacteriological follow-up. Of 161 patients with identified pathogens, altogether 122 (65 and 57, respectively) were evaluable for both clinical and *bacteriological efficacy*. The most common pathogens were H. influenzae (24%) and S. pneumoniae (17%) (Table I). In the CP group, 63/65 patients (96.9%) had a satisfactory bacteriological response. In the amoxicillin group the corresponding figure was 51/57 (89.5%). Equivalence between the groups could be assumed with 95% confidence (confidence interval for difference in success rate -1.3 to 16.2).

The proportion of the patients with eradication of H. influenzae were 100% (30/30 patients) in the CP group and 83.9% (26/31 patients) in the amoxicillin group. Thus, a difference in favour of CP with 95% confidence could be assumed (confidence interval for difference in success rate, 3.3 to 29.0). All evaluable patients in both groups with S. pneumoniae (26 and 20 patients, respectively) had a satisfactory bacteriological result.

Altogether 38 patients (19 in each group) had received antimicrobial treatment within 30 days before enrolment in the study. Most common drugs were phenoxymethyl penicillin (8 patients in the CP group and 10 in the amoxicillin group), doxycycline (5 patients in each group) and amoxicillin (4 and 5 patients, respectively). Only 26 of these 38 patients (15 and 11, respectively) were evaluated for clinical efficacy: no failures were reported in the CP group, while in the amoxicillin group 3 failures were noted (for patients having been treated with narrow-spectrum penicillin, tetracycline and broad-spectrum penicillin, respectively).

Table I. *Initial bacteriological findings*

Findings	Treatment group: Cefpodoxime proxetil n (%)	Treatment group: Amoxicillin n (%)	Total n (%)
Aerobic pathogens			
Haemophilus influenzae	35 (25)	40 (28)	75 (26)
Streptococcus pneumoniae	29 (20)	23 (16)	52 (18)
Streptococcus species (other)	7 (5)	7 (5)	14 (5)
Staphylococcus aureus	6 (4)	4 (3)	10 (4)
Moraxella catarrhalis	3 (2)	3 (2)	6 (2)
Other aerobes	7 (5)	4 (3)	11 (4)
Anaerobic pathogens			
Bacteroides species	1		1
Eikonella corrodens	1		1
Fusobacterium necrophorum	1		1
Prevotella melaninogenica	1		1
Peptostreptococcus micros	1		1
Veillonella parvula	1		1
Anaerobic Gram negative rod		1	1
Anaerobic mixed flora		1	1
Total number of pathogens	93	83	176
Number of patients with			
Identified pathogens	82 (57.3)	79 (55.2)	161 (56.3)
Negative culture or non-pathogenic flora	61 (42.7)	64 (44.8)	125 (43.7)
Total number of patients	143 (100.0)	143 (100.0)	286 (100.0)

Table II. *Results of treatment*

Clinical efficacy	Per protocol: Cefpodoxime proxetil	Per protocol: Amoxicillin	Intent to treat: Cefpodoxime proxetil	Intent to treat: Amoxicillin
No. of evaluable patients	117	113 (230)	130	128 (258)
Satisfactory	74%	66%[a]	70%	64%[c]
Improved	22%	25%	23%	24%
Unsatisfactory	4%	9%	7%	12%
Bacteriological efficacy				
No of evaluable patients	65	57 (122)	78	72 (150)
Satisfactory	97%	89%[b]	87%	79%[d]
Unsatisfactory	3%	11%	3%	11%
Unevaluable		10%	10%	10%

95% confidence intervals for difference in success rate:
[a] −1.6 to +10.8 percent units.
[b] −1.3 to +16.2 percent units.
[c] −2.2 to +11.9 percent units.
[d] +0.9 to +18.0 percent units.

Intent-to-treat analysis

In addition to the per protocol analysis, results were analysed using an intent-to-treat analysis. For these patients ($n = 258$), the clinical success rate was 93% for the CP group and 88.2% for the amoxicillin group. Equivalence between the groups could be assumed with 95% confidence. The overall *bacteriological response*, on the other hand (97.1% and 87.7% satisfactory response, respectively), showed with 95% confidence a true difference in response (95% confidence interval for difference in success rate 0.9 to 18.0; $n = 150$) (Table II).

Table III. *Adverse drug events*

	Treatment group							
	Cefpodoxime proxetil ($n = 140$)				Amoxicillin ($n = 142$)			
	Total	Mild	Moderate	Severe	Total	Mild	Moderate	Severe
Patients	28 (20%)	17	8	3	23 (16.2%)	10	11	2
Symptoms	36				24			
Gastro-intestinal	29				12			
Diarrhea		17	7			6	2	
Abdominal pain				1		2	1	
Nausea		1	1					
Gastroenteritis			1					
Vomiting			1					
Dry mouth						1		
Skin & appendages	5				9			
Urticaria		1					3	1[a]
Rash, erythematous		1					3	
Pruritus, genital			2	1			1	
Skin disorder							1	
Platelets, bleeding & clotting	1				1			
Epistaxis				1[a]				1[a]
Hearing & vestibular	0				1			
Deafness (reversible)						1		
Musculo-skeletal	1				0			
Joint stiffness			1					
General	0				1			
Allergic reaction							1	

[a] Serious adverse events.

Adverse events

The number of patients included in the analysis of safety was 282: 140 in the CP group and 142 in the amoxicillin group.

Altogether 28 patients (20%) in the CP group reported 36 adverse events, while 23 patients (16.2%) in the amoxicillin group reported 24 events. There was no statistically significant difference between the two groups ($p > 0.05$).

The most common adverse events were gastro-intestinal disorders – 26 patients (19%) in the CP group, and 12 patients (9%) in the amoxicillin group ($p = 0.013$). Of these, diarrhea was most common (24 and 8, respectively) (Table III). The total of gastro-intestinal adverse events was higher in the CP group, whereas the amoxicillin group had a significantly higher incidence of moderate to severe skin reactions considered to be related to drug treatment ($p = 0.033$). Most adverse events were mild or moderate – only 3 patients in the CP group and 2 in the amoxicillin group had severe adverse events. Eleven patients (4 in the CP group and 7 in the amoxicillin group) did not complete their treatment due to adverse events. Three of these events were considered as serious according to the FDA definition: 1 patient in each group with nose-bleeding requiring hospitalization, and a third patient (in the amoxicillin group) needing hospital treatment due to urticaria and dyspnea. All patients recovered from these events.

Laboratory examinations

No abnormal results were noted in the haematology or biochemistry tests. During the treatment, a normalization of high leukocyte counts (elevated WBC at enrolment in 38 and 43 patients, respectively) was seen in 79% of the patients in the CP group and in 81% of the patients in the amoxicillin group. Also, high CRP values (in 54 and 68 of cases, respectively) returned to normal in 85% of the patients in both groups, reflecting the abatement of inflammation.

For urinary glucose and for urinary protein findings, there was no clinically significant change in either group.

DISCUSSION

In the present study, no significant difference was found in the per protocol analysis, regarding either clinical or bacteriological efficacy. In the intent-to-treat analysis, patients with bacteria resistant to amoxicillin were also included.

Here, a significant difference in bacteriological efficacy was found in favour of CP. This result suggests that CP is a better choice than amoxicillin in complicated or recurrent sinusitis cases, where a higher incidence of resistant bacterial strains can be expected. In uncomplicated sinusitis cases, on the other hand, CP should have no expected advantage, compared with amoxicillin.

A special sinusitis study, selectively including patients with recurrence or treatment failure after phenorymethyl penicillin or amoxicillin, would be of interest. In these cases we can expect a higher frequency of β-lactamase-producing bacteria (and especially H. influenzae), and the results of the present study seem to indicate an increased CP efficacy in sinusitis cases with a high percentage of H. influenzae.

Patients in the CP group also showed a significantly better radiological recovery, comparing the X-ray results at visits one and two. This result must be considered to be of special interest, as the radiological score is an objective diagnostic parameter, proved to be more reliable than the clinician's subjective evaluation of the clinical effect (4).

In our study, bacteriological findings from aspirates at inclusion were positive in 58% of all clinically evaluable patients (133/230). This low percentage may seem untoward, but similar results are commonly seen, as were recently reported from another multi-centre sinusitis treatment study (24).

In conclusion, cefpodoxime proved as clinically effective as amoxicillin in the treatment of acute bacterial maxillary sinusitis. It was more effective in eradicating H. influenzae, and was more efficient in improving the radiological score. Cefpodoxime occasioned a somewhat higher frequency of gastro-intestinal troubles, which is the most common adverse event for both of these drugs. However, most of the gastrointestinal disorders in the cefpodoxime groups were mild.

ACKNOWLEDGEMENT

The investigation was financially supported by Roussel Nordiska AB.

REFERENCES

1. von Sydow C, Axelsson A, Jensen C. Acute maxillary sinusitis. A comparison between 27 different treatment modes. Rhinology 20: 223–229, 1982.
2. Engquist S, Lundberg C, Venge P. Effects of drainage in the treatment of acute maxillary sinusitis. Acta Otolaryngol (Stockh) 95: 153–159, 1983.
3. Berg O, Carenfelt C. Analysis of Symptoms and Clinical Signs in the Maxillary Sinus Empyema. Acta Otolaryngol (Stockh) 105: 343–349, 1988.
4. Axelsson A, Runze U. Symptoms and signs of maxillary sinusitis. ORL J Borderl 38: 298–308, 1976.
5. Berg O, Bergstedt H, Carenfelt C, Lind MG, Perols O. Discrimination of purulent from nonpurulent maxillary sinusitis. Clinical and radiographic diagnosis. Ann Otol Rhinol Laryngol 90: 272–275, 1981.
6. Nord CE. Efficacy of penicillin treatment in purulent maxillary sinusitis. A European multicenter trial. Infection 16: 209–214, 1988.
7. Carenfeldt C, Melén I. Ödkvist l, Olsson O, Prellner K, Rudblad S, Savolainen S, Skaftason S, Sorri M, Synnerstad B. Treatment of Sinus Empyema in Adults. Acta Otolaryngol (Stockh) 110: 128–135, 1990.
8. Berg O, Carenfeldt C, Kronvall G. Bacteriology of maxillary sinusitis in relation to character of inflammation and to prior treatment. Scand J Infect Dis. 20: 511–516, 1988.
9. Camacho AE, Cobo R, Otte J. Spector SL, Lerner CJ, Garrison NA, Miniti A, Mydlow PK, Ciguere GC, Collins JJ. Clinical comparison of cefuroxime axetil and amoxicillin/clavulanate in the treatment of patients with acute bacterial maxillary sinusitis. Am J Med 93: 271–276, 1993.
10. Sydnor TA, Scheld WM, Gwaltney JJ, Nielsen RW, Huch W, Therasse DG. Loracarbef (LY 163892) vs amoxicillin/clavulanate in bacterial maxillary sinusitis. Ear Nose Throat J 71: 225–232, 192.
11. Ylikoski J, Savolainen S, Jousimies-Somer H. The bacteriology of acute maxillary sinusitis. J Otolaryngol Relat Spec 51: 175–181, 1989.
12. Frederick J, Braude AI. Anaerobic infection of the paranasal sinuses. N Engl J Med 290: 135–137, 1974.
13. Jousimies-Somer H, Savolainen S, Ylikoski J. Bacteriological findings of acute maxillary sinusitis in young adults. J Clin Microbiol 26: 1919–1925, 1988.
14. Jones RN, Barry AL. In vitro evaluations of U-76252 (CS 807): antimicrobial spectrum, β-lacatamase stability and enzyme inhibition. Diagn Microbiol Infect Dis 8: 245–249, 1987.
15. Fass RJ, Helsel VL. In vitro activity of U-76252 (CS 807) a new oral cephalosporin. Antimicrob Agents Chemother 32: 1082–1085, 1988.
16. Wise R, Andrews JM, Ashby JP, Thornber D. The in-vitro activity of cefpodoxime: a comparison with other cephalosporins. J Antimicrob Chemother 25: 541–550, 1990.
17. Gehanno P, Depondt J, Barry B, Simonet M, Denever H. Comparison of cefpodoxime proxetil with cefaclor in the treatment of sinusitis. J Antimicrob Chemother 26 Suppl E: 87–91, 1990.
18. Gehanno P, Barry B, Bobin S, Safran C. Twice daily cefpodoxime proxetil compared with thrice daily amoxicillin/clavulanic acid for treatment of acute otitis media in children. Scand J Infect Dis 26: 577, 1994.
19. Karma P, Pukander J, Penttilä M, Ylikoski J, Savolainen S, Olén L, Melén I, Löth S. The comparative efficacy and safety of clarithromycin and amoxicillin in the treatment of outpatients with acute maxillary sinusitis. J Antimicrob Chemother 27 Suppl A: 83–90, 1991.
20. Holdeman LV, Cato EC, Moore WEC. Anaerobe Laboratory Manual, 4th edn. Virginia Polytechnic Institute and State University, Blacksburg, Virginia, 1977.
21. Axelsson A, Grebelius N, Chidekel N, Jensen C. The correlation between the radiological examination and the irrigation findings in maxillary sinusitis. Acta Otolaryngol (Stockh) 69: 302–306, 1970.
22. Axelsson A, Jensen C. The roentgenological demonstration of sinusitis. Am J Roentgenol Radium Ther Nucl Med 122: 621–627, 1974.
23. European Guidelines for the Clinical Evaluation of Anti-Infective Drug Products 1992. European Society of Clinical Microbiology and Infectious Diseases.
24. Scandinavian Study Group. Loracarbef versus doxycycline in the treatment of acute bacterial maxillary sinusitis. J Antimicrob Chemother 31: 949–961, 1993.

Submitted November 3, 1994; accepted February 13, 1995

Scand J Infect Dis 27: 235–237, 1995 ORIGINAL ARTICLE

Fluconazole for Primary Prophylaxis of AIDS-associated Cryptococcosis: A Case-control Study

ADRIANA AMMASSARI, ANGELA LINZALONE, RITA MURRI, GIUSEPPE MARASCA, GIULIA MORACE,* and ANDREA ANTINORI

*From the Department of Infectious Diseases and *Institute of Microbiology, Catholic University, Rome, Italy*

In order to verify whether fluconazole has a prophylactive effect against the occurrence of cryptococcosis in HIV-infected patients and to identify other factors capable of increasing or reducing the risk of this infection, we arranged a case-control study of 17 patients with cryptococcal infection. 34 controls were selected, matched by presence of an AIDS-defining event, CD4 cell count, and date of T-cell phenotyping. No significant difference in exposure to fluconazole, in total days of treatment, or in total dose administered was observed between cases and controls. However, control patients took a significantly higher average daily dosage of fluconazole and a linear tendency in risk reduction ($p = 0.04$) in relation to increasing dosage was observed. Antiretroviral therapy and an average daily fluconazole dose exceeding 150 mg both each reduced the risk of a cryptococcal infection.

A. Antinori, MD, Department of Infectious Diseases, Catholic University, L. go A. Germelli, 8, 00168 Rome, Italy

INTRODUCTION

Systemic mycotic infections are an important cause of morbidity and mortality in patients with HIV infection (1). Cryptococcosis has been reported in some 6–10% of American and in 29% of African AIDS patients (2). At our Department, cryptococcosis has been diagnosed in 5% of patients with AIDS. Some authors observed that patients with a CD4 cell count below 50×10^6/l are more likely to develop cryptococcal meningitis (3). Therefore, the identification of a safe and efficacious drug for use in a primary prophylaxis regimen for the prevention of cryptococcal infection, especially in these high-risk patients, seems to be of crucial importance (4).

Maintenance therapy with fluconazole against cryptococcal menigitis has proved highly effective in preventing relapses (5–6). Moreover, a non-randomized study showed a significantly lower 1-year incidence of systemic fungal infections in patients treated daily with 100 mg fluconazole, when compared with historical controls (7). We conducted this case-control study in order to ascertain the conceivably protective role of fluconazole on the occurrence of cryptococcosis among HIV-infected patients and to identify other factors which increase or reduce the risk of this infection.

PATIENTS AND METHODS

Cases and controls were designated in a study population formed of all HIV-infected patients observed at the Department of Infectious Diseases from January 1986 to December 1992. The inclusion criteria for cases and controls were: documented HIV infection and a follow-up at our Department of 12 months before matching. Infection due to Cryptococcus neoformans was established by a positive blood or cerebrospinal fluid (CSF) culture, associated (or not) with a serum or CSF cryptococcal-antigen titre. Moreover, the presence of a serum cryptococcal-antigen titre of >32 with or without confirmatory blood or CSF culture, has been considered as diagnostic. Of the 54 observed patients showing cryptococcal infection, 17 met these criteria and were included in the study as cases. The remaining 37 patients were excluded because the preceding follow-up spanned less than one year. Files of T-cell phenotyping and clinical records were used to identify control subjects, matched with cases according to the following criteria determined at the time of cryptococcal infection: 1) presence or absence of a previous AIDS-defining event; 2) CD4 cell count ($\pm 50 \times 10^6$/l); 3) date of T-cell phenotyping (± 90 days). The first 2 criteria were chosen in order to match cases with their controls having the same stage of HIV disease. The third variable was used to minimize the influence of changes in medical approach over the years. Two controls were selected for each case. In all, 34 controls were designated as the comparison group.

Exposure of cases and controls to fluconazole during the previous 12 months was established on the basis of prescriptions indicated in the patients' clinical records. In presence of exposure, the total number of treatment days, total dose administered, and average daily dosage were registered. Fluconazole was administered exclusively for the treatment of oral or esophageal candidiasis. Data regarding demographical and epidemiological characteristics, history of a previous AIDS-defining event, interval since AIDS diagnosis, CD4 cell count, and main haematologic parameters were collected at diagnosis of cryptococcosis for cases and for matching controls. Moreover, any history of antiretroviral therapy with zidovudine and number of medical visits during the previous 12 months were also recorded.

Statistical analyses were performed using exact 2×2 tables, χ^2-test, and Fisher's exact test for categorical variables. The relative risk of developing cryptococcosis for each variable was estimated as an odds ratio and presented with a 95% confidence interval. Continuous variables were analysed using Student's t-test and Wilcoxon's rank sum test. An unstratified exact trend test was performed on rank-ordered continuous variables. In order to check for confounding factors and to assess the independent value of variables, a conditional logistic regression analysis was performed. The p-value for variables to be entered in the stepwise regression model was 0.1.

Table I. *Demographical, epidemiological, immunological and haematological characteristics at the time of diagnosis of cryptococcosis for 17 cases and 34 matching controls*

	Cases ($n = 17$)	Controls ($n = 34$)	p-value
Age (y)	34 ± 5	36 ± 6	NS
Sex (M/F)	16/1	30/4	NS
HIV transmission mode			
IVDUs	10	17	NS
Homosexual	4	11	NS
Heterosexual	–	4	NS
IVDUs/Homosexual	3	1	NS
Not determined	–	1	NS
No. of patients with previous AIDS diagnosis	13	26	NS
Median time from AIDS diagnosis (days)	359 ± 421	293 ± 262	NS
Mean CD4 cell count ($\times 10^6$/l)	18 ± 15	20 ± 24	NS
Haematological parameters			
Hb (g/l)	107 ± 17	111 ± 17	NS
WBC ($\times 10^9$/l)	2.45 ± 0.93	2.82 ± 1.16	NS
Neutrophils ($\times 10^9$/l)	1.59 ± 0.85	1.77 ± 0.96	NS

Table II. *Comparison of exposure to fluconazole and other considered variables among cases and controls*

	Cases ($n = 17$)	Controls ($n = 34$)	Univariate analysis O.R. (95% C.I.)	p-value
No. of patients exposed to fluconazole	9	23	0.54 (0.14–2.11)	0.47
Total days of treatment[a]	89 ± 75	76 ± 60	n.c.[b]	0.61
Total dose administered (g)[a]	9.9 ± 7.9	11.9 ± 10.4	n.c.[b]	0.63
Average daily dosage (mg)[a]	112 ± 27	146 ± 39	n.c.[b]	0.02
Never exposed	8	11	1.00	
1–100 mg	5	6	1.14 (0.20–6.48)	1.00
101–150 mg	4	4	1.36 (0.19–9.87)	1.00[c]
≥ 151 mg	–	13	0.00 (0.00–0.65)	0.01
History of antiretroviral therapy	11	31	0.18 (0.03–1.04)	0.06
No. of patients on PCP prophylaxis	12	28	0.52 (0.11–2.61)	0.53
No. of medical visits (mean)	8.7 ± 7.3	13.4 ± 9.7	n.c.[b]	0.08

[a] Only for exposed patients.
[b] n.c. = not calculable.
[c] Unstratified exact trend test $p = 0.04$.

RESULTS

Of the 17 cases included in the study, 8 had cryptococcal meningitis and 9 extraneural infection. In 7 of the 8 patients with cryptococcal meningitis the diagnosis was based on a positive CSF culture and in 1 at autopsy. Eight of 9 patients with extraneural cryptococcosis had a serum cryptococcal-antigen titre >1,024. Cryptococcus neoformans was isolated simultaneously from blood in 4 of these cases. The remaining patient had cutaneous and pulmonary cryptococcis and a serum cryptococcal antigen titre >256.

Demographical, epidemiological, immunological characteristics, and the principal haematological parameters did not differ significantly between cases and controls (Table I).

Table II shows that no significant difference in previous use of fluconazole, in total days of treatment or in total dose administered was recorded between cases and controls. However, because of the shorter duration of treatment and the higher total dose administered, a significantly higher average daily dosage of fluconazole ($p = 0.02$) was recorded for controls. Furthermore, none of the patients who developed cryptococcal infection took an average daily dosage above 150 mg. A linear trend in risk reduction ($p = 0.04$) in relation to increasing daily dosage was identified. Cases and controls did not differ regarding antiretroviral therapy, previous PCP prophylaxis or medical follow-up during the preceding 12 months.

Antiretroviral therapy (O.R. 0.05; 95% C.I. 0.004–0.7; $p = 0.03$) and an average daily dosage of more than 150 mg of fluconazole (O.R. 0.1; 95% C.I. 0.01–1.0; $p = 0.05$) were found to have an independent effect on the occurrence of cryptococcosis in the logistic regression analysis.

DISCUSSION

Our study shows that fluconazole at a daily dosage above 150 mg clearly reduces the risk of AIDS-related cryptococcosis. Our data would therefore appear to confirm a previous suggestion that the use of systemic antifungal therapy in early stages of HIV disease has a protective effect against cryptococcosis (8). Moreover, as earlier reported (9), we found that the presence of antiretroviral treatment decreases the frequency of opportunistic infections, such as that caused by Cryptococcus neoformans. Since all our patients who developed cryptococcal infection had a CD4 cell count below 50×10^6/l, it seems as if these patients may form a high-risk group which might benefit from primary prophylaxis, although a danger of selecting drug-resistent yeasts and moulds might exist. Since fluconazole administered regularly at a high dosage might have a protective effect against the development of cryptococcal infections, randomized, placebo-controlled trials are needed to further evaluate its efficacy and to find the most adequate dose for primary prophylaxis against AIDS-associated cryptococcosis.

REFERENCES

1. Saag M, Powderly W, Cloud G, Robinson P, Grieco M, Sharkey P, Thompson S, Sugar A, Tuazon C, Fisher J, Hyslop N, Jacobson J, Hafner R, Dismukes W, the NIAID Mycoses Study Group, the AIDS Clinical Trials Group. Comparison of Amphotericin B with fluconazole in the treatment of acute AIDS-associated cryptococcal meningitis. N Engl J Med 326: 83–89, 1992.
2. Holmberg K, Meyer R. Fungal Infections in patients with AIDS and AIDS-related complex. Scand J Infect Dis 18: 179–192, 1986.
3. Douglas W, Pietroski N, Buckley M, Braffman M, Stern J. Incidence of cryptococcal meningitis in HIV positive patients with low CD4 cells. VII International Conference on AIDS, Florence 16–21 June, (M.C. 3111), 1991.
4. Perfect RJ. Antifungal prophylaxis: to prevent or not. Am J Med 94: 233–234, 1993.
5. Bozzette S, Larsen R, Chiu J, Leal M, Jacobsen J, Rothman P, Robinson P, Gilbert G, McCutchan J, Tilles J, Leedom J, Richman D, the Californian Collaborative Treatment Group. A placebo-controlled trial of maintenance therapy with fluconazole after treatment of cryptococcal meningitis in the acquired immunodeficiency syndrome. N Engl J Med 324: 580–584, 1991.
6. Powderly W, Saag M, Cloud G, Robinson P, Meyer R, Jacobson J, Graybill J, Sugar A, McAuliffe V, Follansbee S, Tuazon C, Stern J, Feinberg J, Hafner R, Dismukes W, the NIAID AIDS Clinical Trials Group, the NIAID Mycoses Study Group. A controlled trial of fluconazole or amphotericin B to prevent relapse of cryptococcal meningitis in patients with the acquired immunodeficiency syndrome. N Engl J Med 326: 793–798, 1992.
7. Nightingale S, Cal S, Peterson D, Loss S, Gamble B, Watson D, Manzone C, Baker J, Jockusch J. Primary prophylaxis with fluconazole against systemic fungal infections in HIV-positive patients. AIDS 6: 191–194, 1992.
8. Pradier C, Bernard E, Lubick C, Toussaint-Gari M, Pinier Y, Durant J, Mondain V, Le Fichoux Y, Dellamonica P. Does fluconazole prevent cryptococcal meningitis in human immunodeficiency virus-infected patients? J Infect Dis 165: 787, 1992.
9. Fischl M, Richman D, Grieco M, Gottlieb M, Volberding P, Laskin O, Leedom J, Groopman J, Mildvan D, Schooley R, Jackson G, Durack D, King D, the AZT Collaborative Working Group. The efficacy of azidothymidine (Azt) in the treatment of patients with AIDS and AIDS-related complex: A double-blind, placebo-controlled trial. N Engl J Med 317: 185–197, 1987.

Submitted October 25, 1994; accepted January 22, 1995

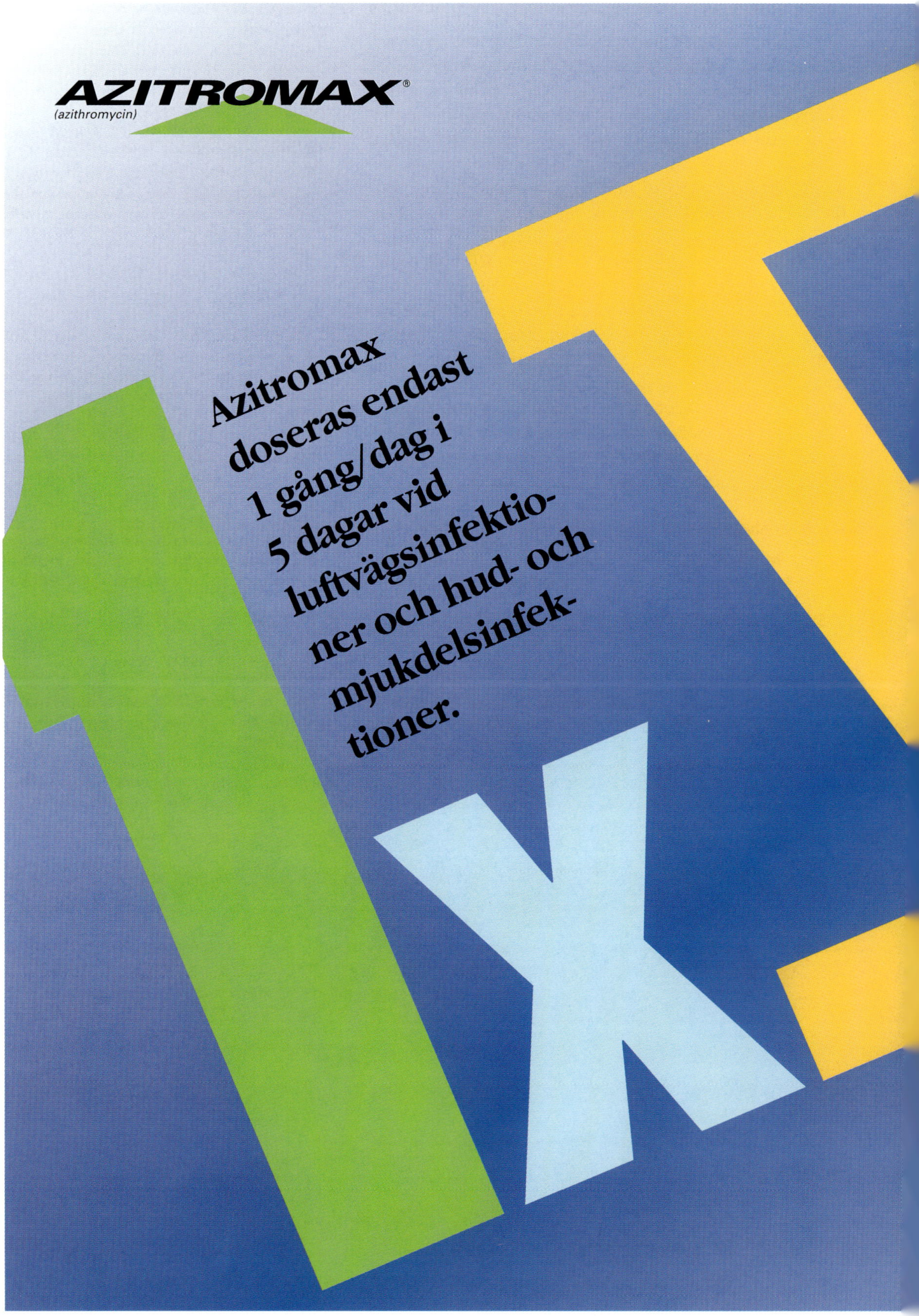
AZITROMAX®
(azithromycin)
Azitromax doseras endast 1 gång/dag i 5 dagar vid luftvägsinfektioner och hud- och mjukdelsinfektioner.
1X.

Scand J Infect Dis 27: 241–243, 1995 ORIGINAL ARTICLE

Intravenous Immunoglobulin Treatment in Children with Guillain-Barre Syndrome

NURAN GÜRSES, SERAP UYSAL, FEYZULLAH ÇETINKAYA, İSMAIL İŞLEK, and AYHAN GAZI KALAYCI

From the Department of Pediatrics, Ondokuz Mayıs University School of Medicine, Samsun, Turkey

Guillain-Barre syndrome is an acquired demyelinating polyneuropathy that is presumed to be immune-mediated. On the basis of this assumption, intravenous immunoglobulin (IVIG) has been used in the treatment of Guillain-Barre syndrome in recent years and found to be effective. To test this we performed a randomized study in patients with Guillain-Barre syndrome by giving IVIG (1 g/kg body weight per day over 2 consecutive days) in 9 children who were compared with 9 patients who were observed but not given specific therapy. We concluded that intravenous immunoglobulin is a safe and effective treatment for childhood Guillain-Barre syndrome which shortens the time to recovery.

N. Gürses, MD, Department of Pediatrics, Ondokuz Mayıs University School of Medicine, 55139 Samsun, Turkey

INTRODUCTION

Guillain-Barre syndrome (GBS) is an acute inflammatory demyelinating neuropathy characterized by progressive symmetric loss of motor strength, reflexes, and variable sensory loss (1). Although the precise mechanism is unknown, it is believed to be autoimmune. There is strong evidence that demyelination in the peripheral nerves and consequent neurologic deficit in GBS are the result of an immunologic attack on the peripheral nervous system myelin or possibly Schwann cells (2). High-dose intravenous immunoglobulin (IVIG) has been reported to be effective in numerous potentially immune-mediated diseases, such as GBS (3–5). Only a few studies concerning IVIG therapy in childhood GBS have been reported (6). We present our experience regarding the effect of IVIG on the clinical course of childhood GBS.

MATERIAL AND METHODS

Between January 1991 and March 1993, 18 children who fulfilled the criteria for acute GBS (Table I) were enrolled in the study (1, 7). After verbal explanation of its purpose, subjects and parents agreed to participate in the study. Approval of the study was given by the local Ethics Committee. The children with GBS were randomly chosen for either IVIG or no therapy, according to the hospital admission sequence. The IVIG group received intravenous immunoglobulin (Sandoglobulin) 1 g/kg body weight/day in continuous infusions lasting 4–6 hours over 2 days. The patients were monitored for side effects, including alterations in heart rate, respiratory rate, blood pressure, and temperature.

In addition to the clinical examination, cerebrospinal fluid cell count and protein level and electrodiagnostic studies the following data were also evaluated in all patients; time interval from onset of symptoms to hospitalization; interval from onset of symptoms to maximum weakness (days); interval from maximum weakness to improvement; duration of mechanical ventilation; duration of hospitalization.

Statistical analysis was done with the Mann-Whitney U-test. The patients were followed for $1-2\frac{1}{2}$ years after the acute disease.

RESULTS

Altogether 18 (12 male and 6 female) children were included in the study. The mean age of the patients given IVIG was 10.4 (7–14) years compared with 9.5 (6–11) years in the non-IVIG (control) group and mean weight 28.4 (18.5–41) and 27.2 (17–36.5) kg respectively. Two patients from each group required mechanical ventilation, and one from the non-IVIG (control) group died during treatment. Comparisons between groups are seen in Table II. The interval from onset to maximum symptoms, from maximum weakness to improvement and duration of hospitalization was significantly shorter in the IVIG group than in the controls ($p < 0.05$). The duration of mechanical ventilation was also shorter in the IVIG group. No relapse or any other complication occurred in any of the patients in the following period ($1-2\frac{1}{2}$ years) after the acute disease.

DISCUSSION

Guillain-Barre syndrome is the most common cause of acute neuro-muscular paralysis in both adults and children, with an incidence of 0.38–1.7 cases per 100,000 (8, 9). The underlying pathology in GBS is a variable, with a multifocal pattern of inflammation and demyelination in the spinal roots and the spinal and cranial nerves (10). It has been suggested that GBS has a different natural history and a better prognosis in children than in adults (11, 12). Thus 8 of our patients in the control group recovered spontaneously. Since serious and sometimes life threatening conditions occur and long periods of hospitalization and rehabilitation are often necessary, specific therapy and supportive care is important for GBS patients. Supportive measures are still the mainstay of therapy, but in addition, plasmapheresis and intravenous immunoglobulin are promising therapeutic modalities (13, 14). Firm evidence

 ISSN 0036-5548

Table I. *Criteria used for diagnosis of patients with Guillain-Barre syndrome according to treatment group.* IVIG = intravenous immunoglobulin

	IVIG group	Controls
Features required for diagnosis		
Progressive motor weakness in more than one limb	9	9
Areflexia or appreciable hyporeflexia	9	9
CSF cell count not exceeding $10/mm^3$ mononuclear leukocytes	9	9
Features strongly supportive of the diagnosis		
Progression over some days to a few weeks	9	9
Relative symmetry		
Mild sensory symptoms	7	6
Autonomic dysfunction		
Cranial nerve involvement	4	5
Incipient recovery 2–4 weeks after progression stops	9	8

Table II. *Comparison of the outcome of IVIG-treated and untreated control children with Guillain-Barre syndrome*

	IVIG group ($n = 9$) Mean (range)	Controls ($n = 9$) Mean (range)
Interval from symptoms to hospitalization (days)	4.6 (2–6)	4.2 (1–6)
Interval from onset to maximum symptoms (days)	9.3 (7–11)*	12.5 (9–17)*
Interval from maximum weakness to improvement (days)	7.5 (5–11)*	11.8 (8–16)*
Duration of mechanical ventilation (days)	3 (2.5–3.5)	4.5 (4–5)
Duration of hospitalization (days)	16.5 (11–20)	23.8 (13–23)*

*$p < 0.05$

from several studies has indicated that plasma exchange shortens the duration of the paralysis (14–16). A serious drawback with plasma exchange is that it can be performed only in major hospitals with appropriate equipment and trained personnel. On the other hand, a few studies have demonstrated improvement in patients with GBS after intravenous immune globulin treatment (17, 18). In a randomized study, Van der Meche & Schimitz (18) demonstrated the efficacy of IVIG when given during 2 weeks of disease. Shahar et al. (6) reported a rapid improvement of muscle strength in 3 children with GBS following IVIG treatment. Obvious and quick improvement was seen in all of our patients treated with IVIG. Apart from the patients who required mechanical ventilation, almost all the IVIG-treated patients were able to sit and walk within 7 days, whereas this took at least 12 days for untreated control patients.

Four patients (2 from each group) required mechanical ventilation, but the ventilation period was significantly shorter in children treated with IVIG. Unlike in adults, mechanical ventilation has not been considered to be a poor prognostic factor in children (12).

Different relapse rates have been reported after IVIG therapy (19–21). Although Irani et al. (20) reported a high rate of relapse after IVIG therapy in adult patients with GBS, we did not see any relapse during follow-up.

We conclude that IVIG treatment seems to be safe, practical, and effective for GBS in children. Larger and more comprehensive studies are needed, however, to confirm the benefit of IVIG for routine use in the treatment of GBS in children.

REFERENCES

1. Asbury AK, Cornblath DR. Assessment of current diagnostic criteria for Guillain-Barre syndrome. Ann Neurol 27 (Suppl): S21–24, 1990.
2. Rostami AM. Pathogenesis of immune-mediated neuropathies. Pediatr Res 33 (Suppl): S90–94, 1993.
3. Dwyer JM. Manipulating the immune system with immune globulin. N Engl J Med 326: 107–116, 1992.
4. NIH Consensus Conference. Intravenous immunoglobulin: Prevention and treatment of diseases. JAMA 264: 3189–3193, 1990.
5. Kaveri SV, Dietrich G, Hurez V, Kazatchkine D. Intravenous immunoglobulin (IVIG) in the treatment of autoimmunc diseases. Clin Exp Immunol 86: 192–198, 1991.
6. Shahar E, Murphy EG, Roifman CM. Benefit of intravenously administered immune serum globulin in patients with Guillain-Barre syndrome. J Pediatr 116: 141–144, 1990.
7. The Guillain-Barre Study Group. Plasmapheresis and acute Guillain-Barre syndrome. Neurology 35: 1096–1104, 1985.
8. Briscoe DM, McMenamin JB, O'Donohoe NV. Prognosis in Guillain-Barre syndrome. Arch Dis Child 62: 733–735, 1987.

9. Rantala H, Uhari M, Niemala M. Occurrence, clinical manifestations, and prognosis of Guillain-Barre syndrome. Arch Dis Child 66: 706–709, 1991.
10. Ropper AH. The Guillain-Barre syndrome. N Engl J Med 326: 1130–1136, 1992.
11. Winer JB, Hughes RAC, Greenwood RJ, Perkin GD, Healy MJR. Prognosis in Guillain-Barre syndrome. Lancet i: 1202–1203, 1985.
12. Cole GF, Matthew DJ. Prognosis in severe Guillain-Barre syndrome. Arch Dis Child 62: 288–291, 1987.
13. Hughes RAC. The management of Guillain-Barre syndrome. Hosp Pract 30: 107–125, 1992.
14. Thorton CA, Griggs RC. Plasma exchange and intravenous immunoglobulin treatment of neuromuscular diseases. Ann Neurol 35: 260–268, 1994.
15. Jansen PW, Perkin RM, Ashwal S. Guillain-Barre syndrome in childhood: Natural course and efficacy of plasmapheresis. Pediatr Neurol 9: 16–20, 1993.
16. Epstein MA, Sladky JT. The role of plasmapheresis in childhood Guillain-Barre syndrome. Ann Neurol 28: 65–69, 1990.
17. Sharar, Gordon, Kleyweg RP, van der Meche FGA, Meulstee J. Treatment of Guillain-Barre syndrome with high-dose gammaglobulin. Neurology 38: 1639–1641, 1988.
18. Van der Meche FGA, Schimitz PIM, Dutch Guillain-Barre Syndrome Study Group. A randomized trial comparing intravenous immune globulin and plasma exchange in Guillain-Barre syndrome. New Engl J Med 326: 1123–1129, 1992.
19. Bleck TP. IVIG for GBS: Potential problems in the alphabet soup. Neurology 43: 857–858, 1993.
20. Irani DN, Cornblath DR, Chaudhry V, Borel C, Hanley DF. Relapse in Guillain-Barre syndrome after treatment with human immune globulin. Neurology 43: 872–875, 1993.
21. Castro LH, Ropper AH. Human immune globulin infusion in Guillain-Barre syndrome: worsening during and after treatment. Neurology 43: 1034–1036, 1993.

Submitted October 31, 1994; accepted January 26, 1995

Scand J Infect Dis 27: 245–251, 1995

ORIGINAL ARTICLE

Bacteremia at a Danish University Hospital during a Twenty-five-year Period (1968–1992)

MAGNUS ARPI[1], JAN RENNEBERG[1], HANS-KRISTIAN ANDERSEN[1], BENNY NIELSEN[1] and SEVERIN OLESEN LARSEN[2]

From the [1]Department of Clinical Microbiology, Frederiksberg Hospital and the [2]Department of Biostatistics, Statens Seruminstitut, Copenhagen, Denmark

In the 25-year period 1968–92, 3,317 out of 477,420 patients admitted to Frederiksberg Hospital experienced 3,491 episodes of bacteremia. Enterobacteriaceae dominated as causative agents (57%), following by Gram-positive cocci (31%) and anaerobes (7%). Polymicrobial bacteremia was found in 8% of the episodes. The incidence of Enterobacteriaceae bacteremia culminated in the middle (1978–82) of the period (4.7/1,000 admissions) and decreased during the last decade. Gram-positive bacteremia increased throughout the period (from 1.8 to 2.9; $p < 0.001$), due mainly to increasing incidences of bacteremia caused by non-hemolytic streptococci, Streptococcus pneumoniae and coagulase-negative staphylococci. Bacteroides fragilis accounted for a rising incidence of anaerobic bacteremia (from 0.3 to 0.7; $p < 0.05$). Clinical data were available for the 2,599 bacteremic episodes in the 20-year period 1968–87. 59% of these were hospital acquired. Of those, 38% were associated with indwelling catheters, mainly bladder catheters (28%) and i.v. lines (7%). The urinary tract dominated as source of bacteremia (46%), followed by the respiratory (11%) and the gastrointestinal tract (9%). Half of the patients had predisposing underlying diseases, most frequently malignancies (20%) and diabetes mellitus (7%). The mortality rate related to bacteremia decreased from 25% to 11% ($p < 0.001$). More than half (55%) of the fatal cases related to bacteremia occurred within the first 2 days after the first positive blood culture was obtained. Logistic regression analysis defined 7 variables that independently influenced the outcome related to bacteremia: age, source, culture verification of source, shock, body temperature, leukocyte count and empiric antibiotic treatment. A local knowledge of the most common causative microorganisms, the most common sources and the outcome of bacteremia, are of the utmost importance in the selection of the initial empirical antibiotic regimens.

M. Arpi, MD, Department of Clinical Microbiology, Frederiksberg Hospital, Ndr. Fasanvej 57, DK-2000 Frederiksberg, Denmark

INTRODUCTION

The extensive literature on bacteremia describes mainly selected aspects of the condition, such as epidemiology (1), laboratory aspects (2, 3), clinical aspects (4–6), selected patient populations (7, 8), or specific causative microorganisms (9–12). Relatively few studies have been published where a longer time span has been investigated, allowing meaningful conclusions about time trends (1, 8, 13, 14). We elucidated the epidemiological and microbiological aspects of bacteremia in 3,317 patients with 3,491 episodes of clinically significant bacteremia in the 25-year period 1968–92 at Frederiksberg Hospital, Copenhagen. In addition, clinical aspects of bacteremia were investigated in 2,470 patients with 2,599 episodes of bacteremia in the 20-year period 1968–87.

The aim of this study was to utilize the unique long investigated period to elucidate time trends of selected epidemiological, mircobiological and clinical aspects of bacteremia at a university hospital in Copenhagen. Denmark has generally the lowest per capita antibiotic consumption among the Nordic countries (15) and has a well-established hospital hygiene service that, among other things, may influence different aspects of bacteremia. Another specific purpose was to identify significant risk factors that could predict a fatal outcome related to bacteremia.

MATERIALS AND METHODS

Of 477,420 patients admitted to Frederiksberg Hospital, a university hospital in Copenhagen, in the 25-year period 1968–92, 4,177 had a positive blood culture. These patients were reviewed with regard to epidemiological and microbiological aspects of bacteremia (medical records 1968–87, laboratory charts 1988–92). In addition, clinical data were available for 2,470 patients with 2,599 bacteremic episodes in the 20-year period 1968–87 (medical records). In addition to general medical and surgical services, the hospital has special services, such as intensive care unit, orthopedics, obstetrics and gynecology, otolaryngology, nephrology (including renal dialysis, closed in 1984), neurology, psychiatry, and departments of roentgenology, pathology, clinical microbiology, clinical chemistry and clinical physiology. The hosptial has no pediatric service. During the investigated period the number of hospital beds was reduced from about 1,000 to 650 (average about 800). The majority (61%) of the bacteremic patients were ≥ 70 years, whereas only 34% of the entire hospital population belonged to this age group. For the sake of convenience the designation bacteremia in this study also includes blood stream infections with yeasts. Multiple cultures with the same species isolated from the same patient during the same bacteremic episode (positive blood cultures within 7 days) were tallied only once.

Blood culture procedure: In the period 1968–79, a 12-tube blood culture system was used (16). From 1980, a 3-bottle system was used (17), and from 1986, the Roche BCB® system was used. In 1992, a comparative study of the Roche BCB® and the BACTEC NR-860® blood culture systems was performed (18). The blood culture systems were employed according to the manufacturers. All

 ISSN 0036-5548

isolates were identified according to conventional laboratory methods (19).

Definitions

Bacteremia vs. contamination: Each positive blood culture was evaluated to determine whether the isolate represented a clinically significant bacteremia or a clinically insignificant contamination. The decision was based on multiple factors, described elsewhere (16, 20).

Hospital vs. community acquired bacteremia (HAB vs. CAB): The designation HAB was used for all patients from whom the first positive blood culture with a significant microorganism was obtained on or after the third day in hospital or following instrumentation or surgery, regardless of the length of hospitalization.

Polymicrobial bacteremia: More than 1 clinically significant organism isolated from a single blood culture, or if different significant microorganisms were isolated from different blood cultures within 7 days.

Source of bacteremia: Clinical signs of infection and isolation from a local site of the same species (with the same antibiogram) as that found in blood was ideal. Evident clinical signs of a local infection, but without culture verification, was also accepted.

Underlying diseases: Predisposing underlying diseases were stratified as rapidly fatal, ultimately fatal or non-fatal, according to criteria previously described (21).

Shock: A decrease in blood pressure to $<90/60$ mm Hg in previously normotensive patients or a ≥ 70 mm Hg decrease in systolic or diastolic pressure in hypertensive patients accompanied by tachycardia and other signs of shock (21).

Antibiotic therapy: The appropriateness of the empirical therapy (before blood culture result was known) was correlated to the in vitro susceptibility of the blood culture islolate.

Mortality: Death was related to bacteremia if it occurred within 7 days of the first positive blood culture. We distinguished between deaths related to bacteremia and deaths due to causes totally unrelated to the bacteremic episode (6, 21, 22).

Statistical analysis: The data were analysed by means of the χ^2 test or with Fisher's exact test. Differences were considered significant for p-values <0.05. A division of the 25 investigated years into 5-year periods was often used to facilitate elucidation of time trends. Risk factors found by these analyses were then entered into stepwise logistic regression analysis to determine independent predictors of a fatal outcome related to bacteremia (BMDP Statistical Soft-ware, Los Angeles, California, USA).

Table I. *Operations, instrumentations and foreign devices associated with hospital acquired bacteremia (1968–1987)*

Cause of hospital acquired bacteremia	No. of episodes	(%)[a]
Urinary tract	611	(40)
Indwelling urinary catheter (bladder catheter 433; nephrostomy catheter 38)	471	(31)
Prostatectomy	62	(4)
Cystoscopy	39	(3)
Other[b]	39	(3)
Gastrointestinal tract	181	(12)
Colon/rectum surgery	47	(3)
Biliary tract surgery	38	(2)
Esophagus/gastric surgery	32	(2)
Other[c]	64	(4)
Intravenous lines	107	(7)
Bone/joint and skin	57	(4)
Wound revision	31	(2)
Other[d]	26	(2)
Miscellaneous	67	(4)
No operation, instrumentation or foreign device	512	(33)
Total	1,535	

[a] Per cent of all episodes with a hospital-acquired bacteremia.
[b] Urethral/bladder surgery (21), miscellaneous (18).
[c] Small-bowel surgery (23), liver/pancreas surgery (17), gastrointestinal scopies (22), miscellaneous (2).
[d] Fractures/amputations/alloplastics (21), skin transplantation (5).

RESULTS

A total of 4,177 patients with positive blood cultures were identified in the 25-year period 1968–92, of whom 3,317 experienced 3,491 episodes of clinically significant bacteremia. Contaminants were isolated from 860 patients (21%), mainly coagulase-negative staphylococci (80%). The incidence of bacteremia increased from 6.0/1,000 admissions in the first to 8.5 in the last 5-year period ($p<0.001$). The incidence of blood cultures performed per 1,000 admissions increased from 85 in the first to 135 in the last 5-year period ($p<0.001$). The incidence of bacteremia was higher among men than in women (8.7/1,000 admissions vs. 5.9; $p<0.001$). The highest incidence, 36, was observed in the nephrological/dialysis service. The incidence was higher in general medical services than in general surgical services (14 vs. 11; $p<0.001$).

59% of the bacteremic episodes were HABs and 37% CABs. In 4% of the episodes, the origin of bacteremia was unknown. There was no significant change in the ratio of HAB to CAB during the investigation period. The frequency of HAB was clearly higher in surgical services, 70%, as compared with medical services, 48% ($p<0.001$). 67% of all HABs were associated with operations, instrumentations or foreign devices (Table I). Various catheters, mainly bladder catheters, accounted for 22% of all bacteremias and for 38% of all HABs.

Table II presents the microorganisms isolated from monomicrobial and polymicrobial bacteremic episodes. The rate of polymicrobial bacteremia, 8%, was fairly constant during the period. The proportions of Enterobacteriaceae and Gram-positive cocci were significantly higher in mono- than in polymicrobial bacteremia, 58% vs. 52% ($p<0.05$)

Table II. *Clinically significant blood isolates from 3,229 monomicrobial and 262 polymicrobial bacteremic episodes during the time span 1968–92*

Microorganism	Monomicrobial bacteremia no. of isolates	Polymicrobial bacteremia no. of isolates	Total no. of isolates no.	Total no. of isolates (%)
Aerobic and facultative bacteria	3,062	464	3,526	(92)
Gram-negative	1,979	343	2,322	(61)
Escherichia coli	1,214	185	1,399	(37)
Klebsiella spp.	270	45	315	(8)
Proteus mirabilis	184	38	222	(6)
Indole-positive Proteus spp.	36	22	58	(2)
Enterobacter spp.	66	9	75	(2)
Salmonella spp.	39		39	(1)
Other Enterobacteriaceae[a]	50	8	58	(2)
Subtotal Enterobacteriaceae	1,859	307	2,166	(57)
Pseudomonas aeruginosa	81	30	111	(3)
Pseudomonas spp.	8	3	11	(<1)
Haemophilus influenzae	9	2	11	(<1)
Neisseria meningitidis	8		8	(<1)
Other Gram-negative bacteria[b]	14	1	15	(<1)
Gram-positive	1,083	121	1,204	(32)
Staphylococcus aureus	459	25	484	(13)
Coagulase-negative staphylococci	112		112	(3)
Streptococcus pneumoniae	207	2	209	(5)
β-hemolytic streptococci	82	11	93	(2)
Enterococcus spp.	73	51	124	(3)
Non-hemolytic streptococci	128	31	159	(4)
Subtotal Gram-positive cocci	1,061	120	1,181	(31)
Other Gram-positive bacteria[c]	22	1	23	(<1)
Anaerobic bacteria	127	123	250	(7)
Bacteroides fragilis	64	70	134	(4)
Bacteroides spp.	21	21	42	(1)
Clostridium perfringens	15	21	36	(1)
Other anaerobic bacteria[d]	27	11	38	(1)
Yeasts	40	2	42	(1)
Candida albicans	36	2	38	(1)
Other yeasts[e]	4		4	(<1)
Total	3,229	589	3,818	

[a] Morganella morganii (18), Providencia spp. (5), Citrobacter spp. (22), Shigella spp. (2), Yersinia enterocolitica (2), Serratia spp. (3), Hafnia alvei (6).
[b] Xanthomonas maltophilia (2), Aeromonas hydrophila (5), Haemophilus parainfluenzae (3), Pasteurella multocida (1).
[c] Corynebacterium spp. (15), Listeria monocytogenes (7), Lactobacillus sp. (1).
[d] Clostridium spp. (17), Peptostreptococcus spp. (15), Peptococcus spp. (3), Eubacterium lentum (2), Veillonella parvula (1).
[e] Candida tropicalis (3), Cryptococcus neoformans (1).

and 33% vs. 20% ($p < 0.001$), respectively. By contrast, the proportion of anaerobic bacteria was significantly higher in polymicrobial bacteremia, 21% vs. 4% ($p < 0.001$). Coagulase-negative staphylococci and Enterobacter spp. had the highest rates of HAB, 100% and 78%, respectively. S. pneumoniae had the lowest rate, 22%.

Fig. 1 presents time trends in the incidence of bacteremia caused by the major bacterial groups. Enterobacteriaceae increased significantly from the first (3,7/1,000 admissions) to the third 5-year period (4.7; $p < 0.01$), and thereafter showed a decreasing tendency. At species level, this was also observed for E. coli and Proteus spp. Gram-positive

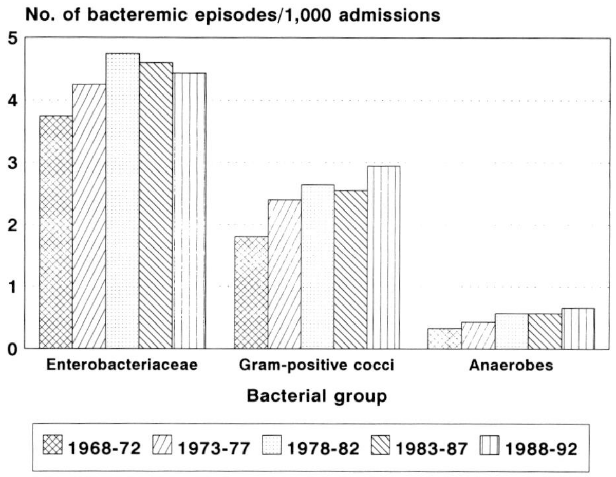

Fig. 1. Time trends in the incidence of bacteremia caused by Enterobacteriaceae, Gram-positive cocci and anaerobes in the period 1968–92 (3,289 episodes).

cocci increased throughout the period (from 1.8 to 2.9; $p < 0.001$), mainly due to increasing incidences of bacteremia caused by non-hemolytic streptococci (from 0.15 to 0.64), S. pneumoniae (from 0.15 to 0.63) and coagulase-negative staphylococci (from 0.14 to 0.31). The incidence of S. aureus bacteremia, about 1.0, remained constant during the period, as did the incidence of P. aeruginosa bacteremia, about 0.2. A rising incidence of B. fragilis bacteremia (from 0.16 to 0.36) accounted for most of the increased incidence of anaerobic bacteremia ($p < 0.05$).

Table III presents the sources of bacteremia. No significant changes in the relative proportions of different sources were observed during the investigated period. In about half of the episodes, it was possible to isolate the same species from blood and from a suspected focus. The rate of HAB was higher when i.v. line (100%), skin/wound (76%), urinary tract (68%) or gastrointestinal tract (65%) was the

Table III. *Sources of bacteremia in 2,470 patients with 2,599 bacteremic episodes (1968–1987)*

Source of bacteremia	No. of episodes	(%)
Urinary tract	1,207	(46)
Respiratory tract	279	(11)
Biliary tract	246	(9)
Gastrointestinal tract	193	(7)
Skin/wound	117	(5)
I.v. line	107	(4)
Bone, joint	34	(1)
Other[a]	102	(4)
Unknown	314	(12)
Total	2,599	

[a] Female genitalia, pancreas, peritoneal fluid, and miscellaneous.

source, than when biliary tract (45%) or respiratory tract (38%) was the source ($p < 0.001$). The rate of polymicrobial bacteremia was highest when skin/wound (26%) or biliary tract (25%) was the source. The urinary tract, followed by the biliary tract, was the most probable source when Enterobacteriaceae were isolated from the blood, whereas the respiratory tract, followed by the urinary tract, was the most probable source when Gram-positive cocci were isolated. Isolation of anaerobic bacteria implicated the gastrointestinal or the biliary tract as most probable source.

Half of the patients had predisposing underlying diseases, most frequently malignancies (solid tumours 17%, hematological malignancies 3%), diabetes mellitus (7%), liver cirrhosis (5%), and chronic renal disease (5%). These rates were fairly constant during the period. About one-fourth of the patients had a rapidly (6%) or an ultimately fatal (20%) underlying disease. Patients with serious underlying diseases had a higher rate of HAB, compared with patients without such diseases, 65% vs. 55% ($p < 0.001$). Patients with predisposing underlying diseases had a slightly higher rate of bacteremia with Gram-positive cocci, 34% vs. 28%, and a lower rate of Enterobacteriaceae bacteremia, 61% vs. 67%, compared with patients without such diseases ($p < 0.05$).

The frequency of septic shock was fairly stable in the investigation period, on average 12%. The frequency was higher in CAB than in HAB, 16% vs. 10% ($p < 0.001$). No significant difference in the rate of shock was observed between monomicrobial bacteremias caused by Enterobacteriaceae, Gram-positive cocci, and anaerobes. Polymicrobial bacteremia had a higher proportion of septic shock than monomicrobial bacteremia. The highest rate of shock was seen when the gastrointestinal tract was the source of bacteremia (25%).

Mortality related to bacteremia decreased from 25% in the first to 11% in the fourth 5-year period ($p < 0.001$). A significant decrease in mortality rate was observed for all major bacterial groups (Fig. 2). More than half (55%) of the fatal cases occurred within the first 2 days after the first positive blood culture was obtained. Logistic regression analysis showed, that age was an independent epidemiological predictor of a fatal outcome. Patients ≥ 50 years had a mortality rate of 19% vis-à-vis 8% in patients < 50 years ($p < 0.01$). The average mortality rate related to HAB was slightly higher than that in CAB, 18% vs. 14% ($p < 0.05$). The mortality rate was generally higher in medical services than in surgical services, 19% vs. 12% ($p < 0.001$). The mortality related to bacteremia depended on the source: respiratory tract 28%, gastrointestinal tract 23%, biliary tract 16%, urinary tract 14%, and i.v. line 10%. Logistic regression analysis confirmed the significantly higher mortality when bacteremia emanated from the respiratory or the gastrointestinal tract. The highest average mortality rates were observed for C. albicans (33%), Klebsiella spp. (25%), S. aureus (25%), and P. aeruginosa (23%). The mortality was generally higher in polymicrobial than in

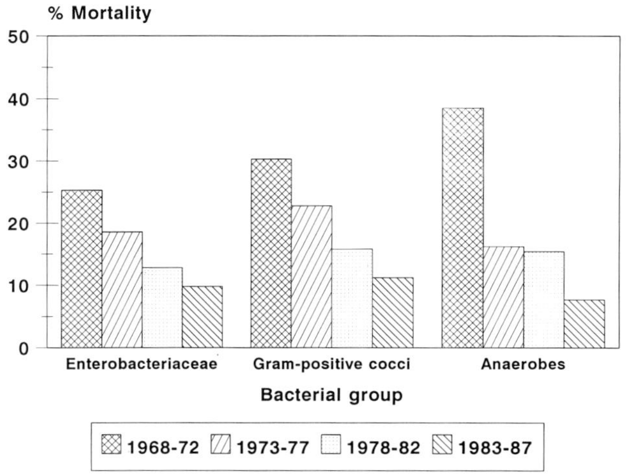

Fig. 2. Time trends in mortality rate related to bacteremia caused by Enterobacteriaceae, Gram-positive cocci and anaerobes in the period 1968–87 (2,327 patients).

monomicrobial bacteremia, 24% vs. 17% ($p < 0.05$). When a microbiological diagnosis was established from a suspected source, the mortality rate was lower for monomicrobial bacteremias caused by Enterobacteriaceae (13% vs. 29%; $p < 0.001$) and Gram-positive cocci (18% vs. 26%; $p < 0.05$), compared with episodes without a culture verification of the source. The differences were confirmed by logistic regression analysis.

The presence of shock was the overall most unfavourable independent risk factor for a fatal outcome related to bacteremia. 44% of the patients with septic shock died, compared with 13% of those without shock ($p < 0.001$). The outcome of bacteremia also depended on the underlying disease. The highest mortality rate was seen among patients with hematological malignancies (54%). In patients with chronic renal disease, connective tissue disease, liver cirrhosis, and solid malignant tumours, the average rates were 20–30%. Diabetics did not have an enhanced average mortality related to bacteremia (13%), compared with patients without underlying diseases (14%). Patients with low ($< 38°C$) and high temperatures ($\geq 40°C$) at the time when the first positive blood culture was obtained had a higher mortality, 33% and 28% respectively, than patients with temperatures between 38.0 and 39.9°C, 12% ($p < 0.05$). This was confirmed by logistic regression analysis. Total leukocyte count was available for 73% of the patients (on the day when the first blood culture was obtained). 26 patients with leukocytes $< 0.5 \times 10^9$/l had a higher mortality rate, compared with patients with counts between 0.5 and 2×10^9/l, 58% vs. 26% ($p < 0.05$). The lowest mortality rate, 11%, was observed among patients with $2–20 \times 10^9$ leukocytes/l. Patients with severe leukocytosis ($> 20 \times 10^9$/l) had a higher mortality rate than patients with counts between 2 and 20×10^9/l, 19% vs. 11% ($p < 0.01$).

Most of the patients (91%) were given empirical antibiotic therapy. A β-lactam, alone or in combination with an aminoglycoside, was included in most empirical regimens (87%). There was no difference in mortality rate between patients without empiric treatment and patients receiving therapy with inappropriate agents. These patients had a higher mortality rate than patients empirically treated with a single appropriate agent, 21% vs. 13% ($p < 0.01$). This difference was confirmed by logistic regression analysis. Patients treated with a combination of antibiotics had a higher mortality rate than patients receiving appropriate monotherapy, 26% vs. 13% ($p < 0.001$). Patients treated empirically with a combination of antibiotics had a higher rate of septic shock than patients treated with appropriate monotherapy, 19% vs. 11% ($p < 0.001$).

DISCUSSION

The incidence of bacteremia increased moderately in the present study. In other studies where ≥ 10 years were investigated, a more marked increase in the incidence, often 3–5-fold, was reported (1, 4, 21, 23). Differences in patient populations, but also the degree to which blood cultures were employed in the evaluation of febrile patients may well explain the reported variations. The rising incidence of blood cultures found in our study might partly explain the observed increase in incidence of bacteremia. The same correlation was proposed by others (23). In spite of the decreasing proportion of Enterobacteriaceae bacteremia in the last part in the present study, this bacterial group still dominated as the cause of bacteremia. This contrasted with several other investigations where Gram-positive cocci are nowadays predominant (14, 24). Among other things, explanations could be different policies with regard to antibiotic treatment, including prophylaxis, and the employment of i.v. lines.

The domination of HAB in our study was in accordance with some previous investigations (14, 20), but contrasted with several other studies where a more equal distribution between HAB and CAB was observed (1, 22, 25). As in the study by Spengler et al. (26), we could not demonstrate an increasing proportion of HABs, as was reported by McGowan et al. (1). Also as in other studies, we found that indwelling bladder catheters and i.v. lines dominated as causes of HABs. 18% of all bacteremias in our study were associated with bladder catheters, which was considerably higher than the 2–13% reported by others (6, 27), probably because of the high proportion of elderly patients in our hospital.

The significant reduction in mortality related to bacteremia caused by Enterobacteriaceae, Gram-positive cocci and anaerobes in our study was also reported by others (1). A more alert diagnostic effort to detect bacteremia, an intensification of searching the source and the accessibility of more potent antimicrobial agents could be factors that contributed to the decreasing mortality rate. In the present study, advanced age (≥ 50 years) was a risk factor for a fatal outcome of bacteremia, which confirmed previous observations (1, 22).

We found a slightly higher mortality rate in polymicrobial than in monomicrobial bacteremia, whereas a somewhat higher mortality rate in polymicrobial bacteremia was seen in other studies (28). Bacteremias caused by C. albicans, S. aureus, Klebsiella spp. and P. aeruginosa had the highest average mortality rate in the present study. This was in agreement with several other studies (1, 6, 21, 22). The mortality related to P. aeruginosa bacteremia, 23%, was considerably lower than the 36%–64% reported from other studies (21, 22, 25). Reasons could be the paucity of patients with severe leukopenia in the present study and that the majority of these bacteremias emanated from the urinary tract.

The outcome was also related to the source. Like others, we found that that a source in the respiratory tract or the gastrointestinal tract had the highest mortality (6). Bacteremia often signals the presence of a focal infection, and isolation/identification of a blood isolate was often of value in identifying the probable source of bacteremia in our study. In several reports, the source was poorly described and culture verification seldom stated. We were able to verify the source of bacteremia by culture in about half of the episodes, which was in accordance with a few other studies (13, 20). The importance of a microbiological focus diagnosis for a favourable outcome of bacteremia was clearly demonstrated in this study. In several other studies it was quite evident that the mortality rate related to bacteremia increased significantly if the source remained unknown (25, 29). This stresses the importance of finding the source.

Several studies, like ours, showed a higher mortality related to bacteremia in patients with severe underlying diseases, compared with patients without such diseases (4, 6, 14). Diabetes was a significant risk factor for a fatal outcome in several studies (6, 29), but was not confirmed in our study.

The presence of shock was the overall strongest independent predictor of a fatal outcome related to bacteremia in the present study. This was also reported by Gatell et al. (30). Also Weinstein et al. (6) analysed their data by logistic regression analysis and found shock to be an independent risk factor, but source of bacteremia and place of acquisition had a higher relative influence. Others could not significantly correlate shock to a fatal outcome (13).

The importance of appropriate empiric antibiotic therapy with respect to the outcome of bacteremia was in agreement with other investigations (4, 6, 30).

Some unfavourable risk factors are not amenable to intervention, but reduction of bacteremias emanating from indwelling catheters, more aggressive treatment of shock, and optimizing of the empirical antibiotic treatment could probably further reduce the mortality related to bacteremia. More than half of the fatalities related to bacteremia in our study occurred within the first 2 days, which was also reported by others (4). Among other things, this emphasizes the importance of employing an optimal blood culture system with respect to detection speed and yield. A local continuous surveillance of blood culture isolates is important if changes in etiology and resistance development are to be detected.

REFERENCES

1. McGowan JE, Jr, Barnes MW, Finland M. Bacteremia at Boston City Hospital: occurrence and mortality during 12 selected years (1935–1972), with special reference to hospital acquired cases. J Infect Dis 132: 316–335, 1975.
2. Reller LB, Murray PR, MacLory JD. Cumitech 1A. In: Blood Cultures II. Coordinating ed. Washington JA. Washington: American Society for Microbiology, 1–11, 1982.
3. Tilton RC. The laboratory approach to the detection of bacteremia. Ann Rev Microbiol 36: 467–493, 1982.
4. Kreger BE, Craven DE, McCabe WR. Gram-negative bacteremia. IV. Re-evalutation of clinical features and treatment in 612 patients. Am J Med 68: 344–355, 1980.
5. Svanbom M. A prospective study of septicemia. II. Clinical manifestations and complications, results of antimicrobial treatment and a report of a follow-up study. Scand J Infect Dis 12: 189–206, 1980.
6. Weinstein MP, Murphy JR, Reller LB, Lichtenstein KA. The clinical significance of positive blood cultures: a comprehensive analysis of 500 episodes of bacteremia and fungemia in adults. II. Clinical observations, with special reference to factors influencing prognosis. Rev Infect Dis 5: 54–69, 1983.
7. Sullivan NM, Sutter VL, Mims MM, Marsch VH, Finegold SM. Clinical aspects of bacteremia after manipulation of the genitourinary tract. J Infect Dis 127: 49–54, 1973.
8. Arpi M, Victor MA, Møller JK, Jønsson V, Hansen MM, Peterslund NA, Bruun B. Changing etiology of bacteremia in patients with hematological malignancies in Denmark. Scand J Infect Dis 26: 157–162, 1994.
9. Olsen H. Bacteroides bacteremia. A clinical and bacteriological study of 51 patients. Scand J Infect Dis 8: 107–111, 1976.
10. Montgomerie MB, Jeremy KO. Klebsiella bacteremia. Arch Intern Med 140: 525–527, 1980.
11. Espersen F, Frimodt-Møller N, Rosdahl VT, Skinhøj P, Bentzon MW. Changing pattern of bone and joint infections due to Staphylococcus aureus: Study of cases of bacteremia in Denmark, 1959–1988. Rev Infect Dis 13: 347–358, 1991.
12. Victor MA, Arpi M, Bruun B, Jønsson V, Hansen MM. Xanthomonas maltophilia bacteremia in immunocompromised hematological patients. Scand J Infect Dis 26: 163–170, 1994.
13. Julander I. Septicemia and endocarditis, 1965–1980, in a Swedish university hospital for infectious diseases. Infection 15: 177–183, 1987.
14. Eykyn SJ, Gransden WR, Phillips I. The causative organisms of septicaemia and their epidemiology. J Antimicrob Chemother 25 (Suppl C): 41–58, 1990.
15. Friis H, Vejlsgaard R. Antibiotikaforbrug i Norden. Ugeskr Læger 148: 2853–2855, 1986. (in Danish)
16. Bruun B, Sloth K, Bentzon MW, Frederiksen W. A study of bacteremias in Denmark from 1977–1978. Acta Pathol Microbiol Immunol Scand Sect B 90: 309–317, 1982.

17. Arpi M, Larsen SO. Comparison of detection speed and yield in agitated and non-agitated aerobic blood culture bottles. APMIS 100: 1061–1065, 1992.
18. Arpi M, Bremmelgaard A. Comparison of detection speed and yield in BACTEC NR-860® and Roche BCB® blood culture systems. APMIS 101: 545–550, 1993.
19. Balows A, Hausler WJ, Hermann KL, Isenberg HD, Shadomy HJ. Manual of clinical mircrobiology. American Society for Microbiology. Washington, D.C., 1991.
20. Weinstein MP, Reller LB, Murphy JB, Lichtenstein KA. The clinical significance of blood cultures: a comprehensive analysis of 500 episodes of bacteremia and fungemia in adults. I. Laboratory and epidemiologic observations. Rev Infect Dis 5: 35–53, 1983.
21. Kreger BE, Craven DE, Carling PC, McCabe WR. Gram-negative bacteremia. III. Reassessment of etiology, epidemiology and ecology in 612 patients. Am J Med 68: 332–343, 1980.
22. Bryan CS, Reynolds KL, Brenner ER. Analysis of 1,186 episodes of gram-negative bacteremia in non-universtiy hospitals: the effects of anitmicrobial therapy. Rev Infect Dis 5: 629–638, 1983.
23. Williams GT, Houang ET, Shaw EJ, Tabaqchali S. Bacteremia in a London teaching hospital 1966–75. Lancet 2: 1291–1293, 1976.
24. Geerdes HF, Ziegler D, Lode H, Hund M, Loehr A, Fangmann W, Wagner J. Septicemia in 980 patients at a university hospital in Berlin: Prospective studies during 4 selected years between 1979 and 1989. Clin Infect Dis 15: 991–1002, 1992.
25. Jepsen OB, Korner B. Bacteremia in a general hospital. Scand J Infect Dis 7: 179–184, 1975.
26. Spengler RF, Greenough WB, Stolley PD. A descriptive study of nosocomial bacteremias at the Johns Hopkins Hospital, 1968–1974. Johns Hopkins Med J 142: 77–84, 1978.
27. Svanbom M. Septicemia I. A prospective study on etiology, underlying factors and sources of infection. Scand J Infect Dis 11: 187–198, 1979.
28. Weinstein MP, Reller LB, Murphy JR. Clinical importance of polymicrobial bacteremia. Diagn Microbiol Infect Dis 5: 185–196, 1986.
29. Elhag KM, Bayoumi A, Johny M. Septicaemia in a teaching hospital in Kuwait. II. Factors influencing the outcome in 111 episodes. J Infect 10: 25–31, 1985.
30. Gatell JM, Trilla A, Latorre X, Almela M, Mensa J, Moreno A, Miro JM, Martinez JA, Jimenez de Anta MT, Soriano E, Garcia San Miguel J. Nosocomial bacteremia in a large Spanish teaching hospital: Analysis of factors influencing prognosis. Rev Infect Dis 10: 203–210, 1988.

Submitted June 27, 1994; accepted February 17, 1995

Antibiotika biblioteket.

Roussels uppmärksammade utbildningsserie om antibiotika- och infektionssjukdomar består nu av 5 böcker, som väckt stort intresse bland läkare. Saknar du någon del? Ring Roussel 08-775 71 00 eller faxa 08-19 29 70 så skickar vi de böcker du vill ha.

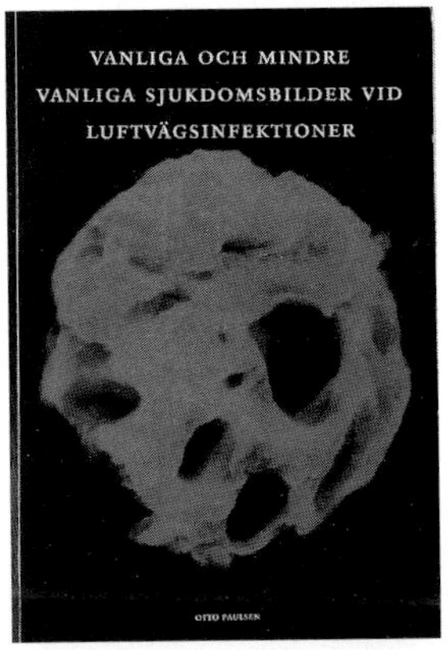

ANTIBIOTIKAMOLEKYLENS VÄG TILL FRAMGÅNG.

"Denna skrift vänder sig främst till den som i sin verksamhet kommer i kontakt med antibiotika utan att ha specialkunskaper inom området och är ett försök att kortfattat och översiktligt förklara gamla och nya begrepp rörande antibiotikas farmakokinetik och farmakodynamik."

OTTO CARS, DOCENT, CHEFSÖVERLÄKARE. INGA ODENHOLT-TORNQVIST, DOCENT, ÖVERLÄKARE.
INFEKTIONSKLINIKEN AKADEMISKA SJUKHUSET UPPSALA.

VANLIGA OCH MINDRE VANLIGA SJUKDOMSBILDER VID LUFTVÄGSINFEKTIONER.

"I denna lilla framställning presenteras några välkända sjukdomsbilder, där en klinisk undersökning, ibland med hjälp av laboratorieprov, leder till snabb diagnos och behandling. Det finns också exempel på mindre vanliga sjukdomsbilder som jag konfronterats med under många år som infektionsläkare".

OTTO PAULSEN, DOCENT/CHEFSÖVERLÄKARE.
INFEKTIONSKLINIKEN, LASARETTET HELSINGBORG

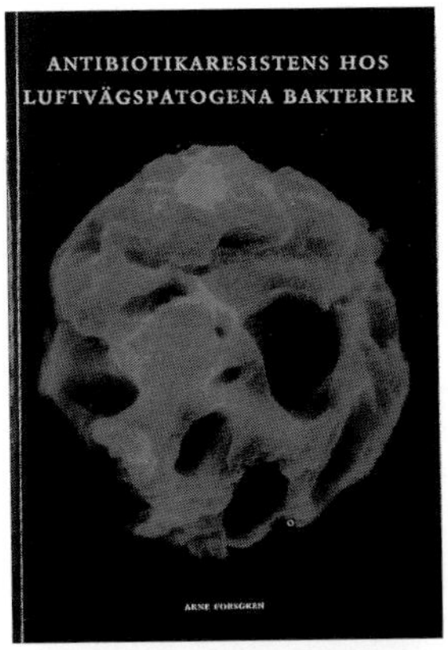

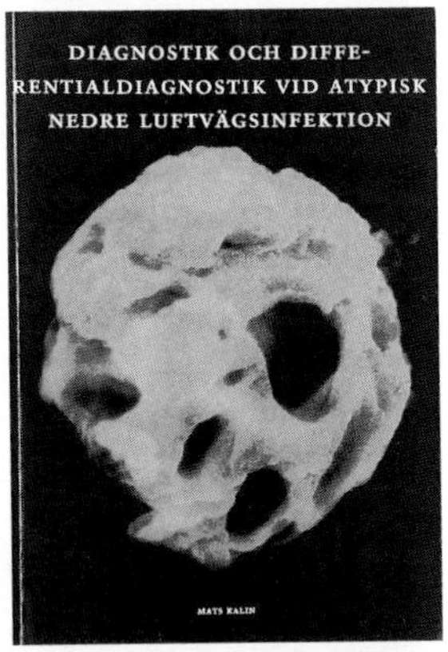

MAKROLIDERNAS PLATS I TERAPIN

Makrolider har använts i nästan 40 års tid. De senaste åren har nya makrolider tillkommit med förbättringar bl a vad gäller absorption och biverkningsprofil.

Denna bok är ett sammandrag från ett symposium i Finland under hösten 1992 där makrolidernas plats i terapin diskuterades.

ROUSSEL NORDISKA AB

ANTIBIOTIKARESISTENS HOS LUFTVÄGSPATOGENA BAKTERIER

"Denna lilla skrift vänder sig främst till dem som i sin verksamhet kommer i kontakt med antibiotika utan att ha specialkunskaper inom området och är ett försök att kortfattat förklara resistensmekanismer och omfattningen av antibiotikaresistens hos några vanliga bakterier."

ARNE FORSGREN, PROFESSOR/ÖVERLÄKARE. INSTITUTIONEN FÖR MEDICINSK
MIKROBIOLOGI/KLINISKT MIKROBIOLOGISKA LABORATORIET
LUNDS UNIVERSITET/ MALMÖ ALLMÄNNA SJUKHUS

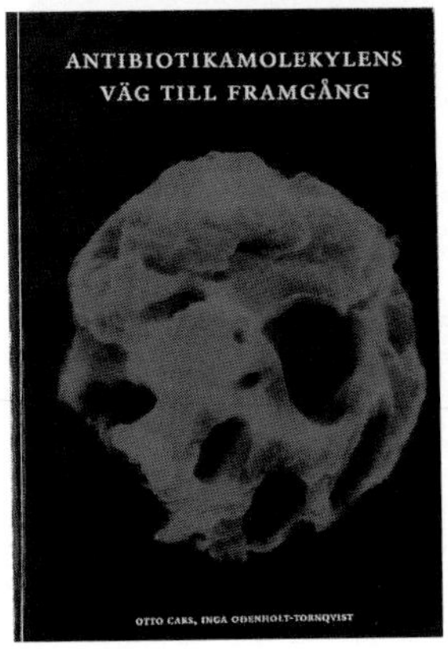

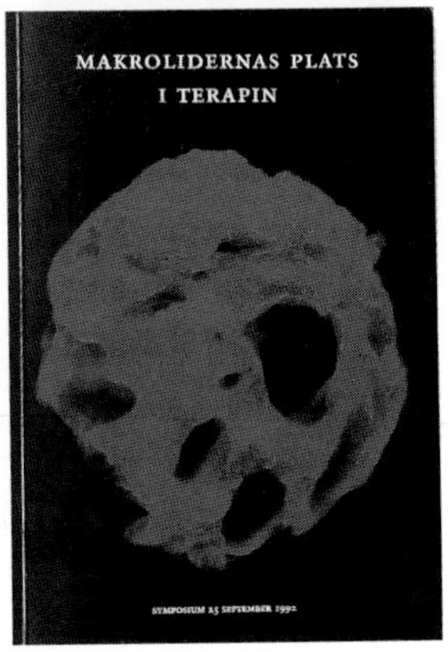

DIAGNOSTIK OCH DIFFERENTIALDIAGNOSTIK VID ATYPISK NERDRE LUFTVÄGSINFEKTION

"Gemensamt för atypiska luftvägspatogener är en viss likhet i klinisk bild samt att de inte alls är åtkomliga för behandling med betalaktamantibiotika, som annars är förstahandsmedel vid nedre bakteriella luftvägsinfektioner. Genom att ta till vara de kliniska, epidemiologiska och laboratoriemässiga indicier som kan finnas till hands kan man i ganska stor utsträckning reducera antalet möjliga etiologiska alternativ, så att en så väl riktad behandling som möjligt kan ges. I den här skriften har jag försökt sammanfatta underlaget för en sådan etiologisk sannolikhetsdiagnostik."

MATS KALIN, DOCENT INFEKTIONSENHETEN. KAROLINSKA SJUKHUSET

ROUSSEL

Roussel Nordiska AB, Box 420 58, 126 13 Stockholm. Tel 08-775 71 00. Fax 08-19 29 70.

BRUNKELL & STRÖMBERG

Scand J Infect Dis 27: 253–257, 1995 ORIGINAL ARTICLE

Bacteraemia due to Escherichia coli in a Danish University Hospital, 1986–1990

BENTE OLESEN[1,2]*, HANS JØRN KOLMOS[1], FRITS ØRSKOV[2], IDA ØRSKOV[2] and ADAM GOTTSCHAU[3]

From the [1]Department of Clinical Microbiology, Hvidovre Hospital, University of Copenhagen, and [2]International Escherichia and Klebsiella Centre (WHO) and the [3]Biostatistical Department, Statens Seruminstitut, Copenhagen, Denmark

433 episodes of E. coli bacteraemia over a 5-year period in a Danish university hospital were studied with special emphasis on possible differences between nosocomial (NO) and community-acquired (CA) cases. Data from 186 males and 247 females with ages ranging from 9 days to 94 years were recorded. The average incidence of E. coli bacteraemia was 24.4 episodes/10,000 admissions/year. Older females accounted for the largest number of cases, which reflected the composition of the background population. The highest risk of infection was in males 80–89 years of age. The highest frequency of NO infections was in the departments of Intensive Care (90%) Orthopaedic Surgery (87%) and Haematology (80%). The most common focus was the urinary tract, with 72% of the episodes with a known focus, while the biliary tract was the focus in 14%. NO bacteraemia was independently related to immunosuppressive therapy, presence of predisposing factors, polymicrobial bacteraemia and presence of a non-urinary tract focus. A urinary tract focus was associated with CA bacteraemia, monomicrobial infection, female sex and a normal or elevated total white blood cell count. Patients with NO bacteraemia had predisposing factors more often than had CA patients, especially haematological malignancies and immunosuppressive therapy. Lack of a known bacterial focus was more common in NO than CA episodes, particularly among patients with haematologic malignancies. The overall mortality was 21%. Increased mortality was independently related to leukopenia (45%), immunosuppressive therapy and NO bacteraemia.

B. Olesen, MD, The International Escherichia & Klebsiella Centre (WHO), Statens Seruminstitut, Artillerivej 5, DK-2300 Copenhagen S, Denmark

INTRODUCTION

Septicaemia is an increasingly important cause of death of hospitalized patients (1), probably due to the fact that a growing proportion of patients with severe underlying diseases are treated in hospitals.

In several studies, Escherichia coli has been reported to be the most common cause of both community-acquired (CA) and nosocomial (NO) bacteraemia (2–4). Despite this leading role in septicaemia, relatively few studies, have dealt specifically with E. coli bacteraemia, and no major Danish clinical studies exist. Moreover, the role of NO E. coli bacteraemia has not been definitively defined.

The purpose of this study was to describe clinical and epidemiological features of E. coli bacteraemia, with special emphasis on possible differences between NO and CA cases. We have therefore anlaysed retrospectively all E. coli bacteraemia episodes in a large Copenhagen hospital over a 5-year period. The main aspects studied were: time, sex and age distribution, place of acquisition, predisposing factors, primary focus, white blood cell count and mortality.

MATERIALS AND METHODS

E. coli bacteraemia was recorded in 444 patients admitted to Hvidovre Hospital over the 5-year period 1 January 1986 to 31 December 1990. Altogether 480 episodes were recorded, though only the first episode of each patient was included in this study. An episode was defined as the presence of E. coli in at least 1 blood culture set, regardless of clinical symptoms.

Blood culture was performed using a 2-bottle system ('Haemobact'), Orion, Finland). Approximately 184 blood cultures/1,000 patient admissions were obtained annually. All isolates of E. coli were identified according to standard procedures (5). Antibiotic susceptibility testing was also performed according to routine methods (6).

An episode of bacteraemia was considered NO if the first blood culture from which E. coli was isolated had been obtained >48 h after admission, given that the patient showed no clinical signs of infection at the time of admission. If a patient had been hospitalized at any hospital during the 4 weeks preceding admisssion, the episode was also considered NO. All other episodes were defined as CA.

An episode of E. coli bacteraemia was defined as polymicrobial if >1 species or 2 strains of E. coli with differing susceptibility patterns were isolated from the same blood culture or from several different blood cultures taken on the same day.

The results of the total white blood cell count were used in this study only if determined within a period from 2 days before to 2 days after the collection of the positive blood culture.

Antimicrobial therapy was considered appropriate if the patient had been treated with a drug which could reach a therapeutic concentration in blood and to which the strain had been found sensitive.

Death was related to bacteraemia if it occurred within 4 weeks after the first blood culture found positive with E. coli.

Graphic models (7, 8, 9) were used to analyse the relationship between the 9 factors: mortality, sex, age (<70, 70 years), total white blood cell count (>10, 3.8–10, $<3.8 \times 10^9 \times l^{-1}$), immunosuppressive therapy, place of acquisition (NO, CA), urinary tract focus (+, −), poly- or mono-microbial infection and presence of predisposing factors (+, −). The association between the latter 8 factors was investigated without taking mortality into account. In

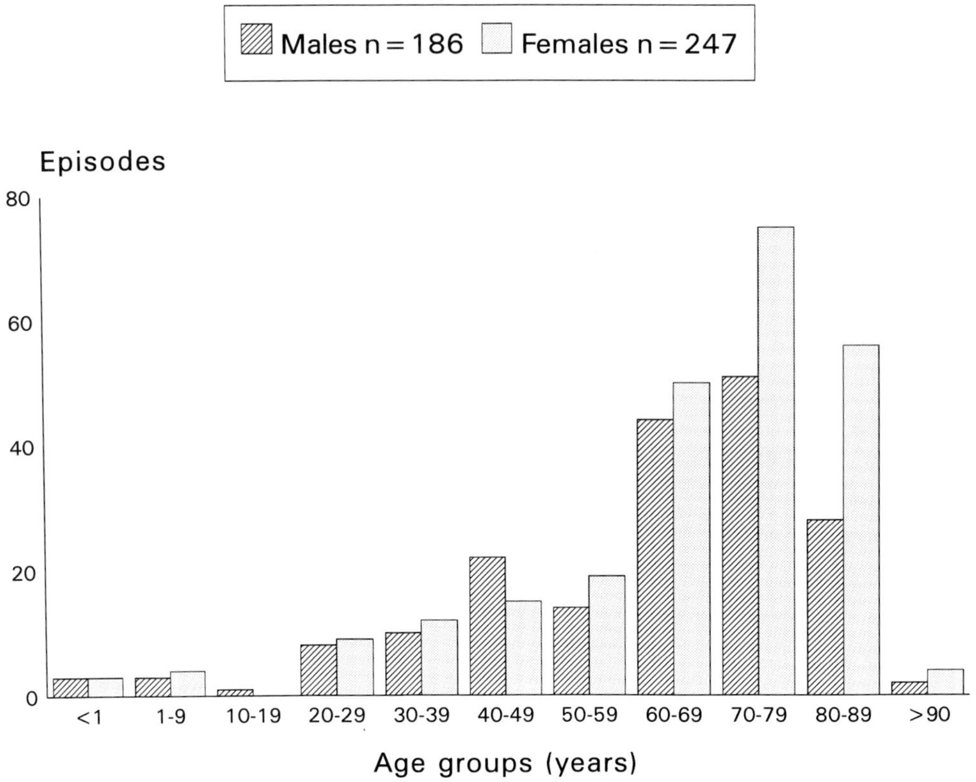

Fig. 1. Sex and age groups of patients with E. coli bacteraemia.

addition, statistical analyses were done by means of Fisher's exact test and a standard χ^2-test.

RESULTS

Bacteraemia due to E. coli was diagnosed in 444 patients. 11 records could not be located, 9 of these came from patients in the Haematological Department. Thus 433 cases of bacteraemia could be evaluated. The average incidence for the 5-year period was 24.4/10,000 admissions. 237 cases (55%) were NO; 118 (50%) of these occurred in males and 119 (50%) in females.

Age and sex distribution

Bacteraemia was diagnosed in 186 males (43%) and 247 females (57%) during the period of study. As shown in Fig. 1, older age groups predominated; the median age for all patients was 70 years (range 9 days–94 years). There was a marked predominance of females among patients over 70 years of age. This was most prominent in CA infections. Fig. 2 shows the sex and age specific incidence of E. coli bacteraemia/10,000 inhabitants in the catchment area of Hvidovre Hospital. In contrast to what might be expected from the results shown in Fig. 1, the highest incidence was found among older males, with a peak of 46.6 episodes/10,000 inhabitants/year in the age group 80–90 years. This discrepancy is due to a predominance of older women in the catchment area of the hospital. Fig. 2 also shows that the incidence of bacteraemia in patients <1 year was higher than in any of the other age groups <60 years.

Distribution according to department

283 episodes (65%) took place in the medical units, 63 of them occurring in the Haematology unit. 109 (25%) episodes were found in the Surgery Units, 15 of them in the Unit of Orthopaedic Surgery. 20 (5%) episodes were diagnosed in the Intensive Care Unit, 11 (3%) in the Paediatric Unit and 10 (2%) in the Unit of Gynaecology and Obstetrics. The highest frequencies of NO infections were found in the Departments of Intensive Care (90%), Orthopaedic Surgery (87%), and Haematology (80%) ($\chi^2 = 46.5$, DF = 6, $p < 0.0001$).

Predisposing factors

Predisposing factors for bacteraemia or underlying conditions were found in 79% of the patients. The most frequent underlying conditions were: immunosuppressive therapy (treatment with cytostatics and/or prednisolone) (21%), presence of an indwelling urinary catheter (15%), haematological malignancies (14%), alcoholism (13%), anatomic disorder in the urinary tract (12%), diabetes mellitus (12%) and cirrhosis (9%). Several patients had more than one underlying condition. NO occurred more often than CA episodes in patients with haematological malignancies (57 vs 3, $p < 0.00005$), an indwelling urinary catheter (50 vs 14,

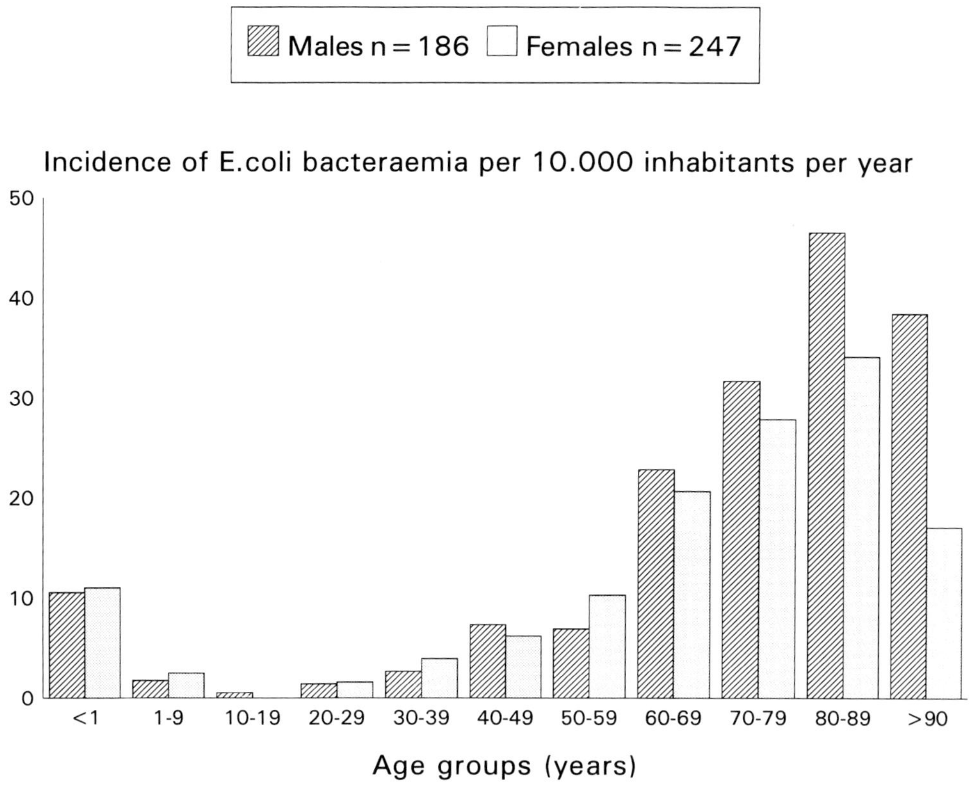

Fig. 2. Incidence of E. coli bacteraemia.

$p = 0.02$), immunosuppressive therapy (74 vs 19, $p < 0.00005$) and a permanent central venous catheter (17 vs 0, $p = 0.0001$).

Focus

A focus of the bacteraemia was found in 316 patients (73%) (Table I). 217 of these foci (69%) were microbiologically verified. The urinary tract was the predominant focus, accounting for 227/316 cases (72%). This focus was more common in CA than in NO episodes, whereas lack of a known focus was more frequent in NO than in CA cases. In 117 patients (27%) no focus was found; 37 of these were patients with haematological malignancies. Lack of focus was thus more common in this group of patients than among all others (37/60 vs. 80/373; $p < 0.00005$). Permanent central venous catheters were more common in patients with an unknown focus than in patients with a known focus, since 15/17 patients with a permanent central venous catheter had no demonstrable focus ($p < 0.00005$); 13 of them had a haematological malignancy.

Table I. *Foci of E. coli bacteraemia*

Focus	No. of episodes	
	Nosocomial	Com. acq
Urinary tract	99	128
Biliary tract	23	20
Other intra-abdominal foci	8	5
Respiratory tract	6	3
Wound/skin/soft tissue	7	2
Genital tract	0	2
Central venous catheter	3	0
Bone/joint	1	0
Meninges	0	1
Mixed foci	4	4
None (found)	86	31

Polymicrobial cases

56 (13%) episodes were polymicrobial, 46 of these were of NO origin. 19% of NO episodes and 5% of CA episodes were polymicrobial ($p < 0.00005$). The 5 most frequent microorganisms isolated together with E. coli were: Klebsiella species 15, Staphylococcus aureus 8, Enterococcus faecalis 8, coagulase-negative staphylococci 7 and E. coli with a different pattern of susceptibility 5. Eight episodes involved >2 microorganisms and were all NO ($p < 0.00005$).

Treatment

In 92% of the episodes the patients received appropriate antimicrobial chemotherapy according to definitions. There was no significant difference between the number of deaths in this group (83/400) and in the group of patients treated inappropriately or not at all (9/33).

Multivariate analysis of selected clinical and laboratory data

Fig. 3 shows statistically significant associations between the 9 variables analysed by graphic model technique. For

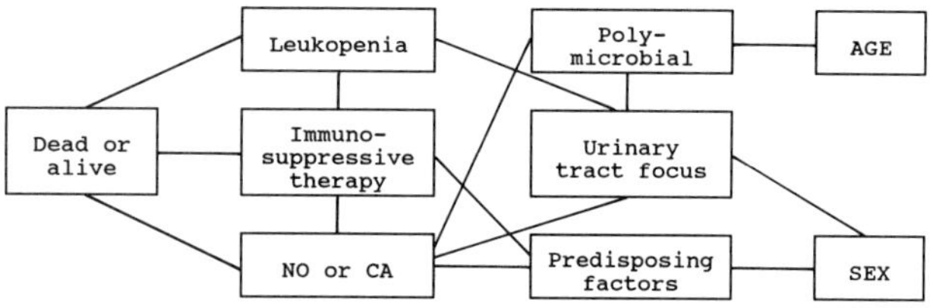

Fig. 3. Relations between selected clinical and laboratory data of E. coli bacteraemia.

related variables there is a line between the boxes. NO bacteraemia was independently related to immunosuppressive therapy, presence of predisposing factors, polymicrobial bacteraemia and presence of a non-urinary tract focus. The highest frequency of NO bacteraemia was in patients with predisposing factors treated with immunosuppressive agents and who had a non-urinary tract focus (48/55, 87%). A urinary tract focus was associated with CA bacteraemia, monomicrobial infection, female sex and a normal or elevated total white blood cell count. The highest frequency of a urinary tract focus was in females with CA bacteraemia and an elevated leukocyte count (68/88, 77%), and the lowest frequency in males with a NO bacteraemia and leukopenia (4/27, 15%). Age was related only to polymicrobial bacteraemia. Thus, the prevalence of polymicrobial infections was higher in patients <70 years of age (18%) than in older patients (8.5%). In addition to urinary tract focus, sex was related to presence of predisposing factors. In males 87% of the episodes occurred in individuals with ≥ 1 predisposing factor, whereas this was the case in only 74% of female episodes.

Outcome

The overall mortality within 4 weeks of E. coli bacteraemia was 21%. As illustrated in Fig. 3, mortality was individually related to leukopenia (45%), immunosuppressive therapy (38%) and NO bacteraemia (28%). No significant difference in mortality could be found in relation to age, sex, focus, predisposing factors, polymicrobial infection or initial appropriate therapy.

DISCUSSION

The present study of epidemiological and clinical data of 433 episodes of E. coli bacteraemia registered in the years 1986–90 showed an average incidence of E. coli bacteraemia of 24.4 episodes/10,000 admissions/year. Similar incidences were found in an English study by Gransden et al. (10) in the years 1982–85, i.e. before a CA outbreak occurred in 1986. Comparable data from other bacteriological studies are not available, though a similar incidence can be calculated from a German study by Geerdes et al. (11).

55% of the episodes were NO. Other studies have reported both higher (12, 13, 15), similar (2, 12) and lower (14) percentages of NO cases.

Most patients were on the medical wards, and the highest frequency of NO infections was found in the departments of Intensive Care, Orthopaedic Surgery and Haematology. The high frequency of NO bacteraemias in the Haematological Department reflects that many patients in this unit had recently been admitted for cytostatic treatment and thus their bacteraemia episodes were recorded as NO according to our definitions. In agreement with Gransden et al. (10) we found a female predominance among patients with E. coli bacteraemia. This was most obvious in the older age groups and in CA cases. However, a calculation of sex- and age-specific incidences on the basis of demographic data of the background population revealed that older males ran a somewhat higher risk of acquiring E. coli bacteraemia than older women. The highest risk was found in males 80–89 years of age, who had an average incidence of 46.6 episodes/10,000 inhabitants/year. We have not been able to find any earlier studies describing a similar calculation on the basis of demographic data.

Most bacteraemic patients had possibly predisposing factors for bacteraemia, perhaps because the majority were elderly. The frequency of predisposing factors differed according to sex and site of acquisition. More NO than CA bacteraemias occurred in patients with a predisposing factor. We found that males were more often predisposed to bacteraemia than were females, the difference being most obvious in the older age groups.

The predominant focus was the urinary tract, most obvious in CA bacteraemia. Like Gransden (10) we found that the age and sex distributions of patients with a urinary tract focus were similar to the distributions among patients with CA bacteraemia, while the age and sex distributions of patients with non-urinary tract focus resembled those of patients with NO bacteraemia. The female preponderance in cases with a urinary tract focus was most obvious in CA cases. 87% of the patients with CA bacteraemia and a urinary tract focus were >60 years of age.

In cases of E. coli bacteraemia the focus is sometimes not evident. It might be possible by clinical and maybe also bacteriological data to get information about the foci in those cases. In this material we have shown that some help in distinguishing between a urinary tract and a non-urinary tract or an unknown focus could be found in sex, site of acquisition, and total white blood cell count. Further investigations including a larger number of patients might clarify this and it would probably be useful to combine the clinical and the bacteriological data.

No focus was found in 27%, which is in accordance with the results of Kreger et al. (13). The lack of a known focus was most common in patients with NO bacteraemia, particularly in patients with haematological malignancies who also had a high frequency of polymicrobial bacteraemia. It has been assumed that translocation of bacteria from the intestine is the cause of bloodstream infection in these patients; another possibility might be that a permanent central venous catheter, often used in these patients, could be the focus of infection. Penner et al. (16) compiled data from 13 different studies on 1,104 patients with infected broviac catheters; 28% were caused by Gram-negative bacteria, mainly K. pneumoniae, E. coli and Enterobacter. They showed that E. coli was able to adhere extensively to silastic catheters. However, only 2/17 patients in the present study were clinically suspected to have an infected permanent intravascular catheter; this may reflect the difficulty of demonstrating a focus in catheters on the basis of retrospective data. In the majority of cases, intravascular catheters were not cultured on removal.

The overall mortality in this study was 21%, which does not differ markedly from other recent studies (10, 17), though a higher mortality rate has been reported (35% (2), 42% (15)). Like other investigators, we found that factors associated with an increased mortality rate were nosocomial acquisition (15), immunosuppressive therapy and leukopenia (2, 10). Unlike these investigators, we were unable to find a direct association between an increased mortality rate and a non-urinary tract focus, polymicrobial bacteraemia and a known underlying condition, using a multivariate analysis. Interestingly, treatment with cytostatics and/or prednisolone seemed to increase mortality, irrespective of underlying conditions and total white blood cell count. The poorest prognosis was found in leukopenic patients; this group consisted mainly of patients with haematologic malignancies. Further clinical and bacteriological investigation of E. coli bacteraemia in this patient group is under way.

We found major clinical differences between NO and CA E. coli bacteraemia regarding focus, predisposing factors, immunosuppressive therapy, polymicrobial bacteraemia and rate of mortality. An ongoing investigation for serotypes and virulence factors may reveal whether the difference in outcome between nosocomial and community-acquired bacteraemia is due only to host differences, or also to differences in the infecting bacteria.

REFERENCES

1. Increase in national hospital discharge survey rates for septicemia–United States, 1979–1987. MMWR 39: 31–33, 1990.
2. Weinstein MP, Murphy JR, Reller LB, Lichtenstein KA. The clinical significance of positive blood cultures: A comprehensive analysis of 500 episodes of bacteremia and fungemia in adults. 11. Clinical observations, with special reference to factors influencing prognosis. Rev Infect Dis 5: 54–70, 1983.
3. Eykyn SJ, Gransden WR, Phillips I. The causative organisms of septicaemia and their epidemiology. J Antimicrobial Chemotherapy 25 (Suppl C): 41–58, 1990.
4. Scheckler WE. Septicemia in a community hospital 1970 through 1973. JAMA 237: 1938–1941, 1977.
5. Kjaeldgaard P, Nissen B, Lange N, Laursen H. Evaluation of minibact, a new system for rapid identification of enterobacteriaceae. APMIS Sect. B, 94: 57–61, 1986.
6. Casals JB, Pringler N. Antibacterial-fungal sensitivity testing using neosensitabs, 9th edn. Taastrup, Denmark: Rosco Diagnostica, 1991.
7. Whittaker J. Graphical Models in Applied Multivariate Statistics. Chichester, England: John Wiley & Sons Ltd, 1990.
8. Westh H, Knudsen AM, Gottschau A, Rosdal VT. Evolution of Staphylococcus aureus resistance to erythromycin in Denmark, 1959 to 1988: Comparison with erythromycin susceptible strains. J Hosp Infect 18: 23–24, 1991.
9. Kreiner S. User Guide to Digram, a program for discrete graphical modeling. Research Report 89/10, Statistical Research Unit, University of Copenhagen, Denmark.
10. Gransden WR, Eykyn SJ, Phillips I, Rowe B. Bacteremia due to Escherichia coli: A study of 861 episodes. Rev Infect Dis 12: 1008–1018, 1990.
11. Geerdes HF, Dietmar Z, Lode H, Hund M, Loehr A, Fangmann W, Wagner J. Septicemia in 980 patients at a university hospital in Berlin: Prospective studies during 4 selected years between 1979 and 1989. Clin Infect Dis 15: 991–1002, 1992.
12. McCabe WR, Jackson GG. Gram-negative bacteremial. Etiology and ecology. Arch Intern Med 110: 847–855, 1962.
13. Kreger BE, Craven DE, Carling PC, McCabe WR. Gram negative bacteremia. 111. Reassesment of etiology, epidemiology and ecology in 612 patients. Am J Med 68: 322–343, 1980.
14. Isphani P, Pearson NJ, Greenwood D. An analysis of community and hospital-acquired bacteraemia in a large teaching hospital in United Kingdom. Q J Med 63: 427–440, 1987.
15. DuPont HL, Wesley W. Infections due to Gram-negative organisms: an analysis of 860 patients with bacteraemia at the University of Minnesota Medical Center. Medicine 48: 307–332, 1969.
16. Penner J, Allerberger F, Dierich MP, Pfaller W, Hager J. In vitro experiments on catheter-related infections due to Gram-negative rods. Experimental Chemotherapy 39: 336–354, 1993.
17. Vázquez F, Mendoza MC, Viejo G, Méndez FJ. Survey of Escherichia coli over a six-year period. Eur J Clin Microbiol Infect Dis 11: 110–117, 1992.

Submitted October 11, 1994; accepted March 15, 1995

Scand J Infect Dis 27: 259–263, 1995

Detection by Enzyme Immunosorbent Assay of Toxoplasma gondii IgG Antibodies in Dried Blood Spots on PKU-filter Paper from Newborns

MORTEN LEBECH[1,2] and ESKILD PETERSEN[1]

From the [1]Parasitology Laboratory, Department of Infection-Immunology, Biotechnology Division, Statens Seruminstitut, Copenhagen, and the [2]Department of Gynecology and Obstetrics, Frederiksberg University Hospital, Copenhagen, Denmark

Different ways of eluting IgG antibodies against Toxoplasma gondii from blood spots on PKU filter papers from newborns were examined, and the eluate was analysed by Enzyme Immunosorbent Assay (EIA). 10-mm diameter discs (method A), and 3-mm discs (method B) were eluted overnight, and 3-mm discs were eluted directly for 2 hours in the EIA wells (method C). Two groups of paired samples were tested: blood spots on the PKU card from the newborn, cord blood, and a venous blood sample from the mother collected shortly after delivery (Group 1, 191 samples); or PKU cards from the newborns and serum collected from the mother during the first trimester (Group 2, 426 samples). The best results were found for Group 1; method A, a sensitivity of 100% (63/63), and a specificity of 100% (128/128) ($r = 0.934$, $P < 0.0001$), and for Group 2; method C, a sensitivity of 100% (125/125), and a specificity of 100% (301/301) ($r = 0.822$, $P < 0.0001$). When method C, was used on 188 samples stored for 16–18 month at −20°C, a sensitivity of 100% (62/62) and a specificity of 99.2% (125/126) ($r = 0.913$, $P < 0.0001$) were found.

The PKU filter paper method is reliable and reproducible, and can be used in screening projects based on analysis of neonatal samples, and in epidemiological studies on toxoplasmosis in pregnant women.

M. Lebech, MD, Laboratory of Parasitology, Department of Infection-Immunology, Statens Seruminstitut, Artillerivej 5, DK-2300 Copenhagen S, Denmark

INTRODUCTION

Congenital toxoplasmosis is the result of intra-uterine transmission of the parasite Toxoplasma gondii from an acutely infected pregnant woman to her fetus. Intra-uterine infection can result in abortion, fetal death, or in the birth of a severely handicapped child (1). The infection is subclinical at birth in about 85–90% of children with congenital toxoplasmosis, but more than 80% of infected children develop complications such as chorioretinitis and minor cerebral disorders later in life (2–4).

In order to prevent congenital toxoplasmosis, some countries have implemented general screening programs during pregnancy (5–7), while other countries are discussing future recommendations for its prevention (8).

Serological screening for congenital toxoplasmosis involves testing of blood samples from the mother, both during pregnancy and from cord blood after delivery. Maternal IgG antibodies are transferred passively from mother to fetus, and can be detected in approximately the same concentration in the newborn (9).

In many countries, blood spots from the newborns are routinely collected on filter paper, the PKU card (Guthrie card), for use in screening newborns for phenylketonuria (PKU) and hypothyroidism. The use of dried blood on filter papers already collected routinely from all newborns for the PKU analysis would be an easy and economical solution in a neonatal screening program.

In previous studies, elution of antibodies has been compared in paired samples of filter paper blood spots and serum from adults (10–12), and antibody elution from PKU cards from newborns has been used for toxoplasma IgG screening, but without testing of paired serum samples (13–15).

The purpose of the present study was to evaluate storage conditions and different methods of elution of specific Toxoplasma gondii IgG-antibodies from blood spots on PKU filter papers from newborns, by comparison with venous and cord blood samples, in order to establish if PKU cards can be used in a neonatal screening for toxoplasmosis.

MATERIALS AND METHODS

Maternal and newborn specimens

Two sample groups were studied. Group 1 comprised of 191 paired samples of cord blood, dried blood spots from newborns collected on PKU filter papers, and blood samples from the mothers, collected after delivery.

Group 2 comprised of 426 paired samples of sera from pregnant women collected as part of the obligatory first-trimester testing for syphilis, and dried blood spots collected routinely on PKU filter papers from their babies after delivery.

For Group 1, sera from the cord blood and from the maternal blood sample were separated by centrifugation and stored at −20°C. A heel blood sample from the newborn was collected 5 to 10 days after birth on PKU filter paper. The blood spots on PKU

 ISSN 0036-5548

filter paper (Schleicher & Schuell no. 903) were collected, dried at room temperature and sent by mail according to instructions (16); they were then stored in sealed plastic bags without desiccants at −20°C until investigation. For Group 2, the maternal first-trimester serum sample was stored at −20°C until birth (on average 204 days). The PKU cards were kept at room temperature and analysed for Toxoplasma gondii antibodies within 7 days of collection.

The study was approved by the Scientific Ethics Committee of Copenhagen, Denmark (ref. no. V.100.1689/90 and L 92033).

Elution of antibodies from filter paper

Method A: a 10-mm disc of filter paper was punched into a test (NUNC cryotubes 3–63401), with 250 μl elution buffer (phosphate-buffered saline (PBS) pH 7.2 with 0.005% Triton X-100 and 1% bovine serum albumin (BSA)), and the antibodies were eluted overnight at +4°C. Before use the eluate was vortexed for 10 s, and diluted 1:4, to a final dilution of 1:64.

Method B: a 3.2-mm disc of filter paper was eluted in 200 ml elution buffer overnight at +4°C, equivalent to a 1:125 dilution of serum, and vortexed before use.

Method C: a 3.2-mm disc was punched directly into 100 μl of elution buffer in the antigen-coated EIA well, approximately to a 1:64 dilution of serum, and eluted for 2 h on a rocker board. The discs were easily removed by tapping the microtitre plates against the table. For methods A and B, 75 μl of each eluate was used for the EIA. As an elution control, a weak positive and a negative patient sample control on dried blood spots were included in each test run.

A 3.2-mm disc of blood-saturated paper contains about 3.45 μl of blood or approximately 1.6 μl of serum, and a 10-mm disc approximately 78.5 μl of serum; measured in a control procedure by ^{125}I-L-thyroxine-enriched whole blood in PKU filterpaper discs (16).

Stability of stored filter papers

Spots from group 2 were analysed from unstored PKU filter papers 3–7 days after collection (method C). Spots from group 1 were analysed from filter papers 1–3 months after collection (method A) and again after 16–18 months of storage (methods B and C). Not all samples were obtained in sufficient quantity to be analysed after storage.

EIA

All samples were analysed by an in-house EIA for specific IgG antibodies to Toxoplasma gondii. The same assay is routinely used for analysis of Toxoplasma gondii antibodies in our Department (17–18). Microtitre plates (NUNC Maxisorp) were coated with 100 μl of antigen prepared from Toxoplasma gondii (RH strain) cultured on VERO cells (18). The eluate from the blood spots, diluted or undiluted, and 75 μl of the serum samples diluted 1:100, and positive and negative control sera at a dilution of 1:100 were tested in duplicate. The microtitre plates were incubated at 26°C for 1 h, washed 3 times with PBS (pH 7.2) with 0.005% Triton X-100, and incubated for 2 h with 100 μl rabbit anti-human IgG-F(ab)$_2$ (Dakopatts cat. no. A-407) conjugated with alkaline phosphatase (Sigma cat. no. p-5521). The plates were washed 3 times, and 75 μl of the enzyme substrate (1 mg p-nitrophenyl phosphate (Sigma 104–40T) per ml of 0.1 M diethanolamine (pH 9.8) containing 0.001 M $MgCl_2$) per well were applied and incubated for 30 min before the reaction was stopped with 75 μl 1M NaOH. The Optical Density (OD) was measured at 405 nm. Results were expressed as a percentage of the OD obtained for the WHO international standard serum (TOXS, Statens Seruminstitut, Denmark). Sera with an OD percent (mean of 2 wells) above 24% were regarded as sero-positive.

Retesting of samples, and comparison of test results

If the EIA results obtained for the paired samples from the mother, the cord blood, and the blood collected on filter paper were not in agreement, all serum samples were retested, and in addition analysed by the Sabin Feldman dye test as a reference test.

The EIA results of the analysis of eluted filter paper samples and the serum samples were compared directly. The sensitivity and specificity of the different filter paper assays were calculated, using the final result of the serum sample as reference.

Correlation coefficients after $\log_{10}$ transformation of OD values were used to examine the correlation of EIA reactivity in OD% in blood spots and cord blood samples.

RESULTS

Elution method A. Group 1

33% (63/191) were IgG-positive and 128 sera seronegative. No difference in seropositivity was observed between maternal and cord blood sera. When antibodies were eluted from 10-mm paper discs overnight (method A), full consistency with the result of the reference sera was found. EIA reactivity in paired blood spots correlated closely with that in cord blood specimens ($r = 0.934$, $P < 0.0001$).

Elution method C; Group 2

There were no false-negatives in the blood spot analysis (Table I). There was close correlation in antibody level between the serum and filter paper samples ($r = 0.822$, $P < 0.0001$). The maternal serum sample was seronegative in 3 cases, but the PKU filter paper was repeatedly toxoplasma IgG seropositive. Since the samples from the mother were collected on average 204 days before birth, the difference in seropositivity between the paired mother and child samples may have been caused by an acute toxoplasma infection during pregnancy, and new blood samples from mother and child were therefore requested. Seroconversion were confirmed in 2 of the women, and congenital toxoplasmosis was diagnosed serologically by the presence of IgM antibodies in one child. The third mother was still seronegative, but the sample from her baby contained Toxoplasma gondii specific IgG antibodies, attributed to blood transfusion.

Long storage time of PKU cards, Group 1

Samples from 188 individuals (62 seropositive and 126 seronegative samples) were analysed after storage for 16–18 months. By elution of antibodies in filter papers by method B, 59 of 62 positive cases were diagnosed. For all 3 false-negative cases the cord blood serum was positive at the lowest positive dye test titre, 10. All sero-negative samples were detected.

By elution of antibodies after direct punching of blood spots into the wells of the EIA plates (method C), all seropositive samples were detected, but there was one false-

Table I. *Detection of Toxoplasma gondii IgG antibodies in paired samples of PKU cards from newborns and maternal serum from first-trimester. Group 2 sample. PKU cards not stored, and antibodies eluted by method C (3-mm paper discs)*

Maternal samples		Filter paper samples			
Result	No sera	Positive	Negative	Sensitivity	Specificity
Positive	122	122	0	100%	
Negative	304	3a	301		100%
Total	426	125	301		

[a] For all 3 patients a new blood sample was requested from mother and child. For all 3 filter paper samples, the positive result was confirmed.
For sample 1: Both mother and child seropositive, consistent with maternal seroconversion during pregnancy.
For sample 2: Both mother and child seropositive, consistent with maternal seroconversion during pregnancy.
For sample 3: Mother seronegative, but child seropositive. Concluded positive due to blood transfusions of the premature infant prior to the sampling of the blood on the PKU card.

positive case (0.53%). The antibody level was generally higher with method C than with method B. The correlation of antibody level in the blood spot samples between methods B and C for stored samples is shown in Fig. 1.

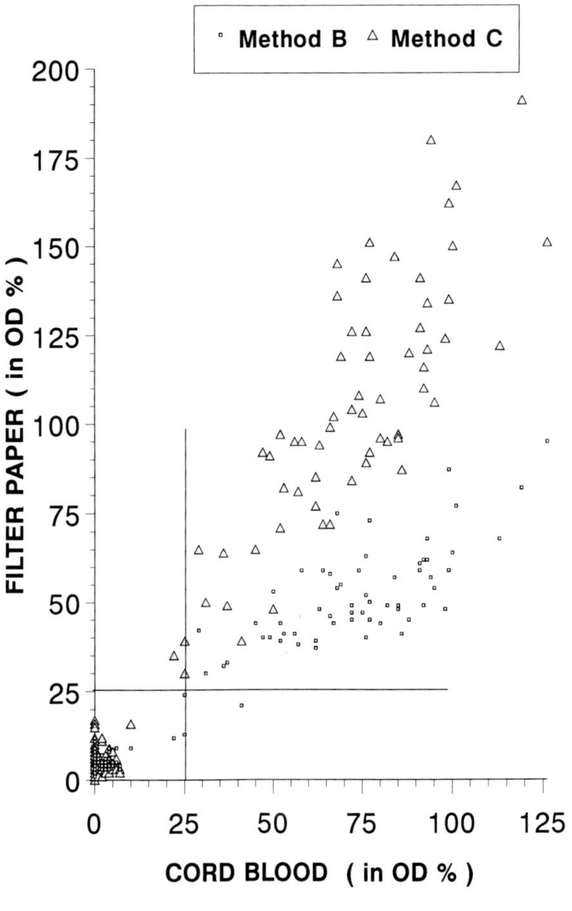

Fig. 1. Enzyme Immunosorbent Assay (EIA) reactivity for Toxoplasma gondii IgG in individually paired filter paper samples from newborns and cord blood samples after 16–18 months of storage. Two methods of antibody elution from blood spots are compared: elution in test tubes (method B), and direct elution in wells (method C). The optical density (OD) ratio (OD of specimen as a percentage of WHO reference standard OD) is plotted for each pair of samples.

The antibody levels in the blood spots eluted by method C and in the cord blood serum were closely correlated ($r = 0.913$, $P < 0.0001$). The degrees of sensitivity and specificity of the different elution methods, and after storage are shown in Table II.

Methods A and C both had 100% sensitivity and specificity for samples stored for less than 3 months.

DISCUSSION

Collection and storage of whole blood as dried blood spots on filter paper is an easy and safe way of transporting and storing blood samples, and detection of antibodies in dried blood spots on filter paper has been used for the diagnosis of several infectious diseases. There has often been close correlation between antibody reactivity in matching serum samples and blood spots on filter paper, e.g. for HIV (19), rubella (20), and syphilis (21). The method has also been used in epidemiological studies on toxoplasmosis (13, 15, 22–24). Toxoplasma IgG antibodies have been detected in dried blood spots on filter paper by IFAT (10, 12, 22, 25,

Table II. *Sensitivity and specificity of the different methods of antibody elution and storage of PKU filter-paper samples before analysis for Toxoplasma gondii IgG antibodies*

Method	Sensitivity (%)	Specificity (%)
Short storage, < 3 months		
Method A. Elution in tube of 10-mm spot	100.0	100.0
Method C. Direct elution of 3-mm spot	100.0	100.0
Long storage, 16–18 months		
Method B. Elution in tube of 3-mm spot	95.2	100.0
Method C. Direct elution of 3-mm spot	100.0	99.2

26), IHAT (24), direct agglutination (23), latex-agglutination (13–15), complement fixation (26) and by the dye test (25–27).

Parker and Cubitt reported a sensitivity of 98.8% (168/170) and a specificity of 100% (103 samples) when they compared antibody titres in serum and simulated dried blood spots, 5.5–6.0 mm in diameter, on Guthrie cards from pregnant women (15).

We found that methods A and C both gave 100% sensitivity and specificity. The use of 10-mm discs in an eluate volume of 1 ml makes it easier to confirm the testing by additional methods. However, in a screening situation the use of less material of the PKU card must be prefered. For 3-mm discs, even when used in paired tests, retesting from a new spot of material is possible before requesting a venous sample from the mother and child. The seropositive child in Group 2 whose mother was seronegative had received several blood transfusions prior to the collection of the PKU sample, and it is likely that the seropositivity resulted from transfused antibodies, i.e. it should not be regarded as a true false-positive result.

For use in epidemiological studies testing of stored filter paper samples could be of value. The feasibility of recovering IgG from blood on filter paper decreases with storage time, but less rapidly after storage at low temperatures (28). Specific antibody activity is readily demonstrated after 30 weeks (28) and even 12 months (29). One study concluded that the filter paper technique was not appropriate for a delayed assessment of toxoplasma IgG antibodies from filter paper (30).

A 3-mm disc eluted in 200 μl buffer corresponds to a serum dilution of approximately 1:125, and a degradation of antibodies with time will explain why the antibody concentration after lengthy storage is generally lower than in the serum sample. Elution directly in the EIA wells, corresponding to a dilution of approximately 1:64 gave a stronger signal and a diagnostic sensitivity of 100%, but also gave one false-positive result.

Screening of newborns for congenital toxoplasmosis by detection of specific toxoplasma IgM antibodies in PKU cards has been reported from Holland (30) and Massachusetts, USA (31). Unexpectedly few congenital infections were detected in both studies (30, 31), possibly due to a low sensitivity of the assay, but more probably related to the combination of a low incidence of congenital toxoplasmosis in the areas (14) and the fact that only a proportion of newborns with congenital toxoplasmosis have detectable IgM antibodies (1, 30). However, detection of IgM in PKU cards could help to clarify the diagnosis in cases of suspected congenital toxoplasmosis.

We conclude that the PKU filter paper routinely collected for other purposes can be used to detect specific toxoplasma IgG antibodies, and that the PKU card can replace a maternal sample or a cord blood sample if used according to method A or method C.

The methods are easy to perform; no extra venepuncture of the mother or child is needed. In addition, method C needs very little material. It can be used in screening projects based on analysis of neonatal samples, or in epidemiological studies on toxoplasmosis in pregnant women.

Method C is currently being used in a prospective study of congenital toxoplasmosis in Denmark, comparing antibodies in the PKU sample with a first-trimester sample from the mother (32).

ACKNOWLEDGMENT

The samples were kindly provided by the Department of Gynecology and Obstetrics, Frederiksberg Hospital, Copenhagen, and the study would not have been possible without the collaboration of the mothers, the midwives, nurses, and laboratory technicians. Dr Paul E. Lebech, Head of Dept. Gyn/Obstet, Frederiksberg Hospital, provided invaluable support throughout the study. We are indebted to Dr Bent Nørgaard Pedersen, Head of Department of Clinical Biochemistry, Statens Seruminstitut, and Dr Børge Jørgensen, Department of Infection-Immunology, Statens Seruminstitut, for access to the PKU cards and first-trimester serum samples. Bente Michelsen and Lise Grønbech provided skilful technical assistance throughout the study.

REFERENCES

1. Remington JS, Desmonts G. Toxoplasmosis. In: Remington JS, Klein JO, eds. Infectious diseases of the fetus and newborn infant. Philadelphia: WB Saunders, 90–190, 1990.
2. Desmonts G, Couvreur J. Toxoplasmose congenitale. Etude prospective de l'issue de la grossesse chez 542 femmes atteintes de toxoplasmose acquise en cours de gestation. Ann Pediatr 31: 805–809, 1984. [in French]
3. Koppe JG, Loewer-Sieger DH, de Roever-Bonnet H. Results of 20-year follow-up of congenital toxoplasmosis. Lancet 1: 254–256, 1986.
4. Wilson CB, Remington JS, Stagno S, Reynolds DW. Development of adverse sequelae in children born with subclinical congenital toxoplasma infection. Pediatrics 66: 767–774,1980.
5. Aspöck H. Überwachung von Toxoplasmose während der Schwangerschaft. Gynaek Rdsch 23: 57–65, 1983. [in German]
6. Desmonts G. Preventing congenital toxoplasmosis. Lancet 336: 1017–18, 1990.
7. Hengst P. Screening for toxoplasmosis in pregnant women: presentation of a screening programme in the former "East"-Germany, and the present status in Germany. Scand J Infect Dis, Suppl 84: 38–42, 1992.
8. Lebech M, Petersen E, eds. Congenital toxoplasmosis. Scand J Infect Dis, Suppl 84: 1–96, 1992.
9. Alford CA, Jr. Immunoglobulin determinations in the diagnosis of fetal infection. Pediatr Clin North Am 18: 99–113, 1971.
10. Bryce CW, Arjona J. Utilisation of whole blood specimens on filter paper for the indirect fluorescence antibody test for toxoplasmosis. J Parasitol 57: 678–680, 1971.
11. Gascon J, Torres-Rodriguez JM, Gonzalez C. Utilidad de las muestras de sangre total desecada en papel de filtro en la detección de anticuerpos antitoxoplasma. Rev Inst Med Trop Sao Paulo 31: 100–102, 1989. [in Portuguese]
12. Knaus BU von, Halpick E. Einsatz von Trockenblut zum Nachweis einer Toxoplasma-primoinfektion bei Schwangeren. Z Med Lab Diagn 28: 167–169, 1987. [in German]

13. Ades AE, Parker S, Gilbert R, Tookey PA, Berry T, Hjelm M, Wilcox AH, Cubitt D, Peckham CS. Maternal prevalence of toxoplasma antibody based on anonymous neonatal serosurvey: a geographical analysis. Epidemiol Infect 110: 127–133, 1993.
14. Hoff R, Weiblen B. Use of bloodspots for epidemiologic studies: toxoplasmosis and HIV. In: Knoppers BM, Laberge CM, eds. Genetic screening. From newborns to DNA typing. Elsevier Science Publishers BV, 67–68 and 131–132, 1990.
15. Parker SP, Cubitt WD. Modified latex agglutination test for antibodies to Toxoplasma gondii in eluates from Guthrie cards. J Clin Pathol 45: 907–909, 1992.
16. National Committee for Clinical Laboratory Standards. Blood collection on filter paper for neonatal screening programs; approved standard. National Committee for Clinical Laboratory Standards publication LA4-A, Villanova, Pa, 8: 157–182, 1988.
17. Lebech M, Olesen Larsen S, Petersen E. Prevalence, incidence and geographical distribution of Toxoplasma gondii antibodies in pregnant women in Denmark. Scand J Infect Dis 25: 751–756, 1993.
18. Pettersen EK. Investigation of two commercially available kits for determination of IgG and IgM to Toxoplasma gondii by enzyme-linked immunosorbent assay (ELISA). Acta Path Microbiol Immunol Scand 92: 325–329, 1984.
19. Hoff R, Berardi VP, Weiblen B, Mahoney-Trout L, Mitchell ML, Grady GF. Seroprevalence of human immunodeficency virus among childbearing women. Estimation by testing samples of blood from newborns. N Engl J Med 318: 525–530, 1988.
20. Punnarugsa V, Mungmee V. Detection of rubella virus immunoglubulin G (IgG) and IgM antibodies in whole blood on Whatman paper: comparison with detection in sera. J Clin Microbiol 29: 2209–2212, 1991.
21. Stevens R, Pass K, Fuller S, Wiznia A, Noble L, Duva S, Neal M. Bloodspot screening and confirmatory tests for syphilis antibody. J Clin Microbiol 30: 2353–2358, 1992.
22. Barbier D, Ancelle T, Martin-Bouyer G. Seroepidemiological survey of toxoplasmosis in la Guadeloupe, French West Indies. Am J Trop Med Hyg 32: 935–942, 1983.
23. Gascon J, Torres-Rodriguez JM, Soldevila M, Merlos AM. Sero-epidemiologia de la toxoplasmosis en dos comunidades de Rwanda (Africa Central). Rev Inst Med Trop Sao Paulo 31: 399–402, 1989. [in Portuguese]
24. Stutzin M, Contreras MC, Schenone H. Epidemiologia de la toxoplasmosis en Chile. V. Prevalencia de la infeccion humana y en mamiferos domesticos y silvestres, estudiadada mediante reaccion de hemaglutinacion indirecta, en el Archipielago de Juan Fernandez, V Region. Bol Chil Parasitol 44: 37–40, 1989. [in Portuguese]
25. Coutinho SG. Aplicacao da technica de coleta de sangue total em disco de papel para o diagnostico da toxoplasmose pelas reacoes de imunofluorescencia indireta e Sabin-Feldman. Rev Soc Bras Med Trop 4: 21–22, 1970. [in Portuguese]
26. Janitschke K, Werner H, Kolleck J. Nachweis von Toxoplasma-antikörpern in Eluaten von Trockenblutproben. Bundesgesundh Bl 22: 309–310, 1979. [in German]
27. Wallace GD. Sabin Feldman dye test for toxoplasmosis. The use of sodium citrate in accessory factor and a method for collecting and storing blood on paper disc. Am J Trop Med Hyg 18: 395–398, 1969.
28. Evengård B, Linder E, Lundbergh P. Standardization of a filter paper technique for blood sampling. Ann Trop Med Parasitol 82: 295–303, 1988.
29. Mathews HM. Parasitic disease: testing with filter paper blood spots. Laboratory Management 9: 55–62, 1981.
30. Conyn-Van Spaendonck MAE. Prevention of congenital toxoplasmosis in The Netherlands. Thesis. Rotterdam: Van Spaendonck Drukkerij B.V., Tilburg, 1991.
31. Ho-Wen H, Grady GF, Maguire JH, Weiblen B, Hoff R. Newborn screening for congenital toxoplasma infection: five years' experience in Massachusetts, USA. Scand J Infect Dis, Suppl 84: 59–64, 1992.
32. Lebech M, Petersen E. Neonatal screening for congenital toxoplasmosis in Denmark: presentation of the design of a prospective study. Scand J Infect Dis, Suppl 84: 75–79, 1992.

Submitted October 12, 1994; accepted February 19, 1995

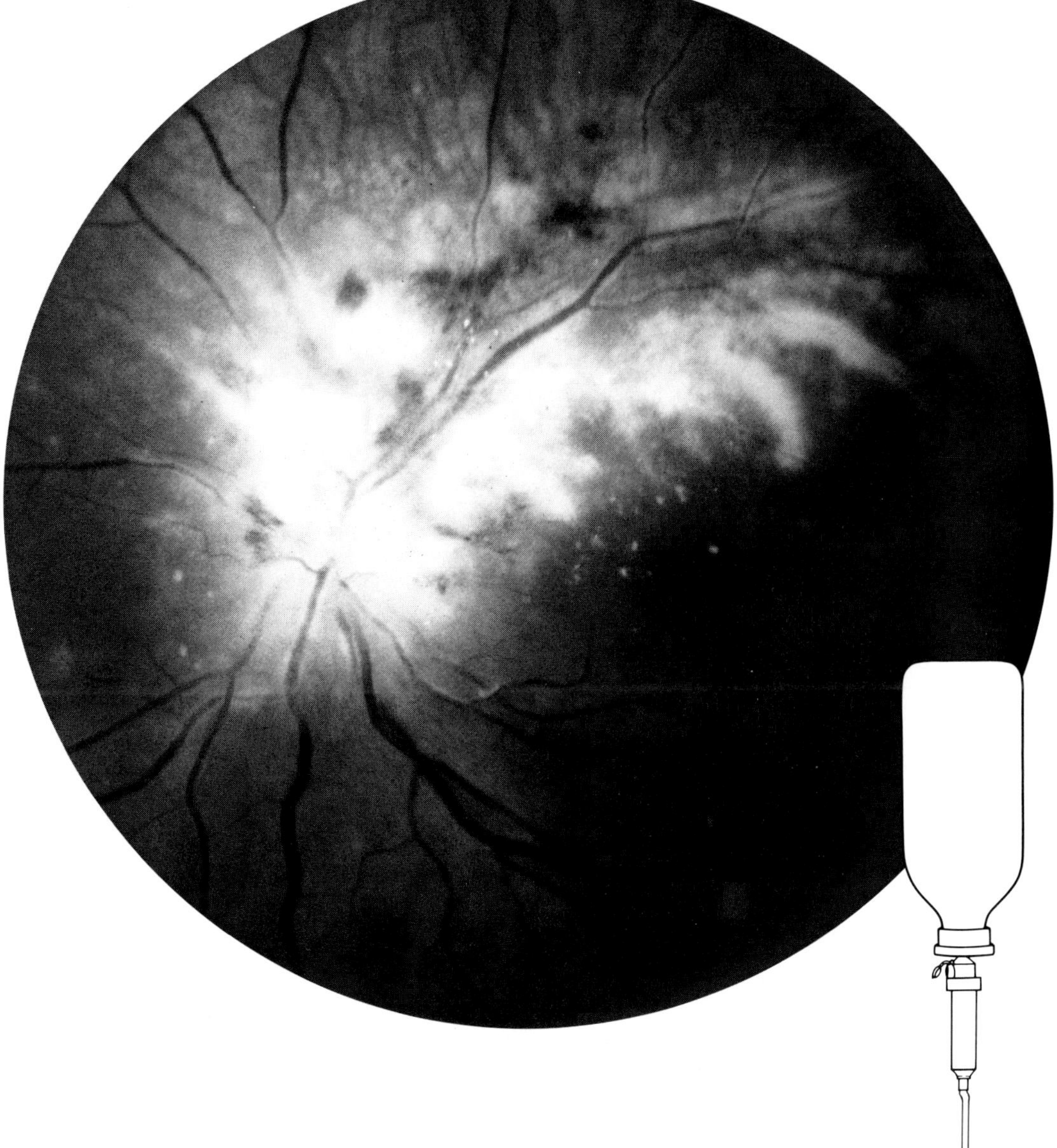

Scand J Infect Dis 27: 265–272, 1995 ORIGINAL ARTICLE

Cost-benefit Analysis of Screening for Toxoplasmosis during Pregnancy

MAIJA LAPPALAINEN[1], HARRI SINTONEN[2], MARJALEENA KOSKINIEMI[1], KLAUS HEDMAN[1], VILHO HIILESMAA[3], PIRKKO ÄMMÄLÄ[3], KARI TERAMO[3] and PENTTI KOSKELA[4]

From [1]the Haartman Institute, Department of Virology, University of Helsinki, [2]the Department of Health Policy and Management, University of Kuopio, Finland and the National Centre for Health Program Evaluation, Fairfield Hospital, Fairfield, Australia, [3]the Departments I and II of Obstetrics and Gynaecology, Helsinki University Central Hospital, University of Helsinki, Helsinki, Finland, and [4]the National Public Health Institute, Oulu, Finland

Congenital toxoplasmosis is a risk for fetus both in 'low' and 'high risk' areas. A cost-benefit analysis based on data from a Finnish prospective study (20.3% seropositivity of pregnant mothers and incidence of 2.4/1,000 seronegative pregnancies) and on Finnish cost data was performed to compare the no-screening and screening alternatives for primary toxoplasma infections during pregnancy. A maternal-feto transmission risk of 40%, effectiveness of treatment of 50%, and discount rate of 4% were used as other baseline probabilities. The calculations were carried out by decision analysis combined with sensitivity analysis.

The total annual costs of congenital toxoplasmosis without screening amount to US$ 128/pregnancy/year, and with systematic serological screening, US$ 95/pregnancy. Thus screening reduces the costs by 25%. The present value of net savings in Finland would be US$ 2.1 million every year. A one-way sensitivity analysis showed that screening together with health education is preferable to health education without screening if the incidence of maternal primary infections exceeds 1.1/1,000 and effectiveness of treatment is better than 22.1%.

Screening for toxoplasma infections during pregnancy is economically worthwhile even in a country with a low incidence. A scheme of systematic screening for maternal primary toxoplasma infections combined with health education should be considered.

M. Lappalainen, MD, The Haartman Institute, Department of Virology, Box 21, Haartmaninkatu 3, FIN-00014 University of Helsinki, Helsinki, Finland

INTRODUCTION

Thousands of children with congenital toxoplasmosis remain undetected in the USA each year (1), which is estimated to cost society several millions of dollars annually (2, 3). Prevention is the best way to tackle the problem. Applicable strategies include primary (health education of pregnant women) (4–6) or secondary (prenatal screening and treatment of maternal primary infections) (2, 7) prevention, or a combination of both. Screening also involves tertiary prevention, which means limiting the tissue damage in an infected fetus or neonate. The educational approach costs little, but the success rate is ambiguous and the fetuses at risk remain unidentified (8). Until recently, systematic serological screening has been criticised because maternal diagnosis is delayed, infections occurring around the time of conception or very early in pregnancy may be missed, and false-positive test results may be obtained, causing extra psychological burden. Furthermore, fetal diagnosis may be difficult and can result in abortion of healthy fetuses. Insufficient data on incidence, prevalence, effectiveness of treatment, and cost-benefit ratios are also factors that have discouraged systematic screening of pregnant women (9–12).

Today, the modern single-serum assays offer reliable results rapidly, and have therefore aroused new interest in serological screening. The improving results of prenatal diagnosis also make screening more inviting (13). We have recently shown that toxoplasmosis is a risk for the fetus even in a 'low risk' country (14). The purpose of this paper is to estimate, by decision analysis (15), the economic costs and benefits of toxoplasma screening combined with health education. In decision analysis, all available options and their potential outcomes are identified and structured in the form of a decision tree. The preferred choice is then subjected to sensitivity analysis to evaluate the reliability of the conclusions drawn.

METHODS

Decision tree

Decision analysis was performed using a computer-based decision tree; Fig. 1 displays its simplified version. There is 1 decision-making node with 2 alternatives. Alternative 1: Systematic serological screening is not performed, but health education is offered to pregnant women. Treatment is given only in cases diagnosed by random testing during pregnancy. Children presenting with symptomatic congenital toxoplasmosis are examined and treated. Alternative 2: Health education is provided and serological screening performed, and infected pregnant women are treated. Infected children are treated and adequate follow-up organized.

Baseline probabilities and assumptions

The baseline probabilities used for the decision analysis are shown in Table I. The expected participation rate in a screening program, prevalence measured as IgG seropositivity in pregnant women,

 ISSN 0036-5548

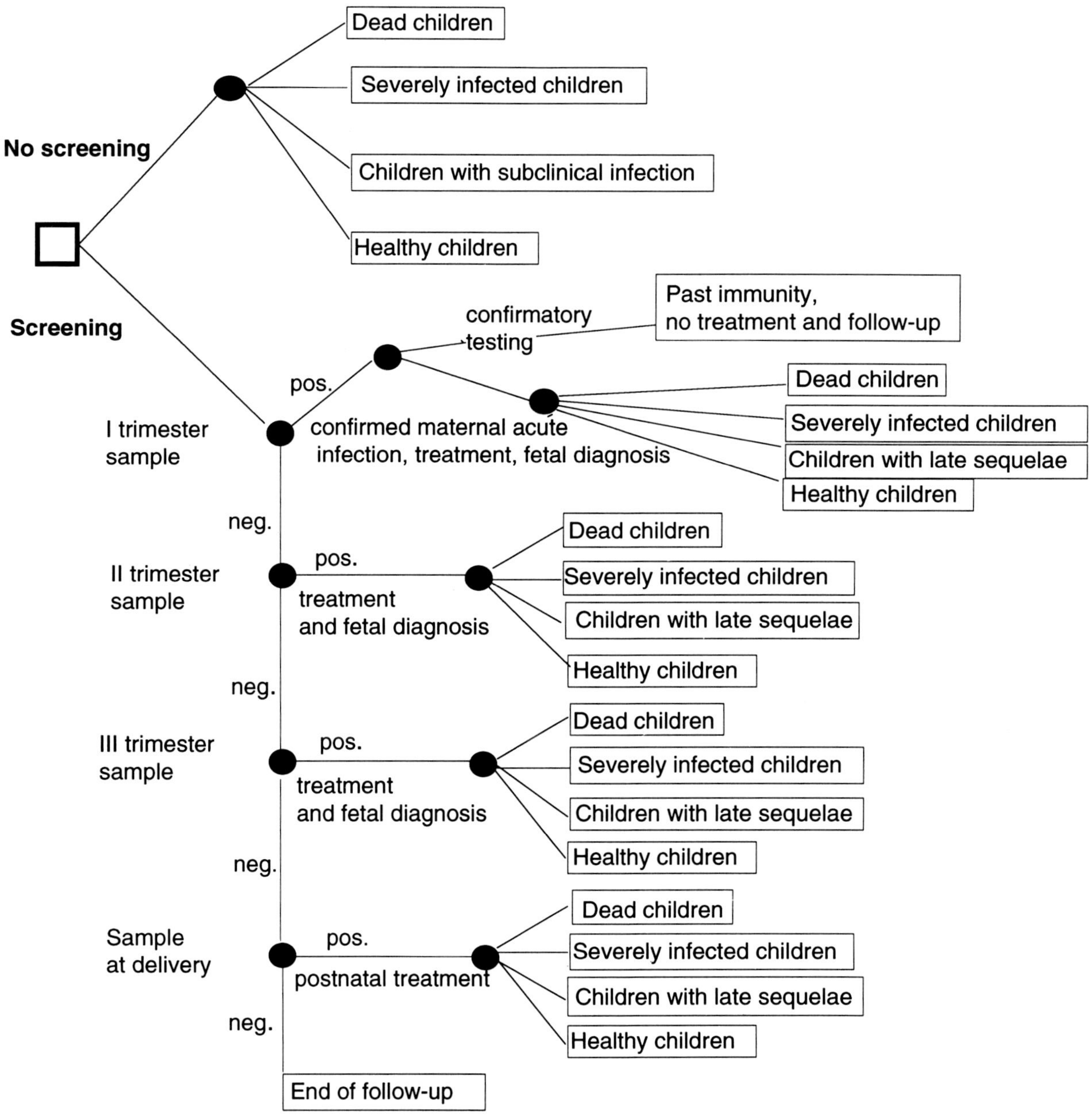

Fig. 1. Decision tree depicting outcomes of the no-screening and screening alternatives of Toxoplasma gondii in pregnant women. □, Decision node; ●, chance nodes; rectangular nodes, outcomes to be measured.

incidence measured as primary toxoplasma infections of seronegative pregnancies, and the expected number of infected offspring, were all derived from a prospective screening study (with health education) on toxoplasmosis during pregnancy, covering 16,733 pregnant women in the Helsinki area, Finland (14, 16). The maternal-feto transmission rate and effectiveness of treatment during pregnancy were earlier findings from the literature. It was assumed that there was no seasonal variation in the infection rate in the screening vs. no-screening alternative, nor any difference in the number of spontaneous abortions.

Costs

The expected total annual costs due to congenital toxoplasmosis can be divided into direct and indirect costs (17, 18). The former are those ensuing from medical and institutional care, while indirect costs refer to value of lost productivity (estimated by the loss of earnings for a presumed number of working years) and the value of the working days lost by the patients and their parents due to follow-up visits. The total costs for both alternatives were calculated according to 1990 prices. The costs in Finnmarks in various branches of the decision tree were converted into US dollars (US$) at the 1990 average exchange rate (Bank of Finland; personal communication) (19, 20). The unit costs used in decision analysis are shown in Table II. Direct costs due to special education, training and resource help were partly included, since they are being offered in institutions as an essential element of long-term care. Direct costs for behavioural disorders, minor learning disabilities and mild neurological sequelae were not included in the

Table I. *Baseline probabilities used in decision analysis*

	Probability	Reference
Prevalence	20.3%	(14)
Incidence	2.4/1,000	(14)
Participation rate	90.2%	(14)
Transmission rate	40%	(24)
Number of infected offspring ($n = 50$)		
Death	1.5[a] (3%)	(24)
Severe infection	5 (10%)	(24)
Subclinical infection	43.5[a] (87%)	(24, 35)
Effectiveness of treatment	50%	(24)
Discount rate	4%	

[a] Computational figure used in the calculations.

absence of reliable data on their prevalence. Intangible costs of a more diffuse nature, such as the value of the death of a child and the psychological burden caused by false-positive or -negative results as well as by the screening itself were also excluded. Health education costs were omitted because they were assumed to be the same in both alternatives. According to the common practice in Finland, the future costs were discounted at 4% per year.

Sensitivity analysis

For full benefit of the decision model, we applied both one-way and two-way sensitivity analyses by alternating the assumptions of incidence, transmission risk, effectiveness of treatment, participation rate and discount rate. The intersection points of the strategy lines, representing the no-screening and screening alternatives were defined as the threshold values for the variables. In addition, a two-way sensitivity analysis was performed to study the effect of various combinations of the key variables on the optimal decision. We gave different values for the effectiveness of treatment and transmission rate, while the other baseline assumptions were kept constant.

No-screening alternative

Severely infected infants, who stay alive or eventually die, require approximately 30 days of care in the neonatal intensive care unit (NICU). The average yearly or daily earnings, including the statutory social expenses, were used to estimate the indirect costs. The working life was assumed to extend from the age of 20 to 55. The estimate of average travelling costs/visit was based on a survey of health centre patients in 1981, updated by the 1990 consumer price index (21). Travelling costs/visit to hospital were estimated to be twice as high. Children were expected to visit the hospital without parents after the age of 20.

The severely ill children require permanent institutional care for the whole of their lives, i.e. 40 years (unpublished data from the Rinnekoti Foundation for the mentally disabled), and an average of three 30-day hospital periods for diagnostic and therapeutic interventions until the age of 20, due to unresolved diagnosis. The working hours lost by the parents were taken into account as well as their travelling and accommodation expenses.

Subclinically infected children were assumed to require, on average, one annual outpatient visit, and 85% of them five 10-day hospital periods at the ages of 10 to 30 at the Department of Ophthalmology due to reactivating retinochoroiditis. Travelling and accommodation costs for the patients and their parents were included. The direct costs resulting from minor neurological or psychological sequelae were excluded, as stated before.

Screening alternative

Pregnancies (after subtracting spontaneous abortions) in Finland in 1990 totalled 69,772 (Pentti Koskela, NPHI, Oulu, Finland; personal communication). With the seroprevalence of 20.3% and incidence of 2.4/1,000 (14) that would mean a total of 127 mothers with primary infection. In our prospective study, no mother requested a therapeutic abortion due to toxoplasma infection. Therefore, therapeutic abortions are included in our calculations only indirectly; the average costs of visits to the antenatal clinic for tertiary care include the costs of possible therapeutic abortion.

Table II. *Unit costs used in decision analysis*

Cost items	Unit costs, US$ 1990
1) Neonatal intensive care (Children's Hospital, HU)[a]	2,908/day
2) Short-term in-patient care (Children's Hospital, HU)[a]	771/day
3) Short-term in-patient care (Dept. of Ophthalmology, HU)[a]	343/day
4) Long-term institutionalization (Rinnekoti Foundation, Espoo, Finland)[a]	50,059/year
5) Outpatient care (Dept. of Obstetrics and Gynaecology, HU)[a]	164/visit
6) Outpatient care (Children's Hospital, HU)[a]	372/visit
7) Outpatient care (Dept. of Ophthalmology, HU)[a]	206/visit
8) Productivity lost[b]	37,875/year
9) Working time lost by parents and patients[b]	105/day
10) Travel costs of parents and patients[a]	8/visit
11) Accommodation costs of parents[a]	27/night
12) IgG-ELISA[a]	2/sample
13) IgM-ISAGA[a]	3/sample
14) IgG-avidity ELISA[a]	18/sample
15) Treatment of mothers (spiramycin)[a]	112/month
16) Treatment of exposed, non-infected children (spiramycin)[a]	31/month
17) Treatment of infected children (alternating)[a]	84/cycle

[a] Direct costs are so marked.
[b] Indirect costs.
HU = Helsinki University.

Screening program

The calculations are based on 3 serum samples during pregnancy, with 1 additional sample taken at delivery. Blood sampling was estimated to take approximately 10 min. The cost was calculated according to the average salary/h of a trained nurse, including statutory social expenses. The time required for the administration, processing, documentation and returning of the results to the practice is included in the work input of the extra staff. The extra staff needed for nationwide screening, in addition to those already employed for the syphilis and hepatitis B screening programs would comprise only 1 laboratory technician, 2 laboratory assistants and 1 office employee; their average annual earnings, including the statutory social expenses, were used in the calculations. The costs of the fetal tests (mouse inoculation and PCR of amniotic fluid, placenta and fetal blood), including the sampling and mailing were included in the costs of the tests. The costs for collecting and mailing the first-trimester samples were omitted, since the samples exist for determination of syphilis and hepatitis B. The price of spiramycin was estimated according to the retail price in Sweden, as the drug is not registered in Finland. The costs of the test reagents were calculated either from the retail (IgM-ISAGA) or wholesale prices (IgG- and IgG-avidity ELISA) of the test kits.

Follow-up and treatment of the screening alternative

We estimated that every mother with suspected primary toxoplasma infection during pregnancy requires 2–4 visits to the antenatal clinic for tertiary care. The average costs include examinations and therepeutic interventions, mainly antenatal ultrasound examinations. The costs of antenatal diagnosis are included in the costs of the tests. The costs associated with dead and severely infected children were calculated as in alternative 1, with the exception that as the cause of the handicap is known in the screening alternative (alternative 2), the repeated annual diagnostic interventions on hospital over 20 years are excluded. Normal follow-up visits as with all congenitally infected children were included: the exposed children require two outpatient visits during the first year of life (at the ages of 3 and 6 months), and the infected children are checked every fourth year, altogether 4 times (at the ages of 4, 8, 12 and 15) until the age of 15.

The costs of subclinically infected children were calculated as in alternative 1, supplemented by the normal follow-up visits of congenitally infected children were included.

Spiramycin therapy was started and continued throughout pregnancy, whenever primary toxoplasma infection of the mother was diagnosed. In verified fetal infection, spiramycin was replaced by a combination of pyrimethamine, sulfadiazine and folinic acid alternating with spiramycin (i.e. alternating therapy). Infected children were treated with the alternating therapy for 12 months, whereas exposed children without endogenous seroresponses, but born to mothers with verified primary infection, were treated with spiramycin for 1 month (22).

According to the baseline probabilities (Table I), 0.75 children will die, and 2.5 children with severe and 21.9 children with subclinical infections will be born despite screening and antenatal therapy. They will require the examinations and treatment described above. These computational figures were used in the decision analysis.

RESULTS

Costs

The annual costs of the screening and no-screening alternatives are shown in Tables IIIa–b. In the no-screening alternative (alternative 1, Table IIIa), the annual costs to the society due to death are US$ 0.7 million, due to severely injured children US$ 7.7 million, and those due to initially subclinical infection, in this case mainly retinochoroiditis, US$ 0.6 million. Average lifetime cost of congenital toxoplasmosis is US$ 0.8 million/infected child, ranging from US$ 0.01 million for a subclinically infected child to US$ 1.5 million for a severely infected one. The total annual costs without screenings are US$ 128/pregnancy, altogether US$ 8.95 million (Table IV). The corresponding direct yearly costs would be US$ 93 and US$ 6.51 million.

In the screening alternative, the costs of the tests amount to US$ 1.7 million/year with every additional sample

Table IIIa. *Annual costs in Finland of the no-screening alternative in millions of US$ in different outcomes (baseline probabilities)*

Outcome (n)	Per child	Total (127 exposed children)
Death ($n = 1.5$[a])	0.47	0.70
Severe infection ($n = 5$)	1.53	7.65
Subclinical infection ($n = 43.5$[a])	0.0137	0.60
Healthy children ($n = 77$)		
Total millions of US$/year		8.95

[a] Computational figure used in the calculations.

Table IIIb. *Annual costs in Finland of the screening alternative in millions of US$ in different outcomes (baseline probabilities)*

Outcome (n)	Per child	Total
Death ($n = 0.75$)	0.47	0.35
Severe infection ($n = 25$[a])	1.47	3.68
Subclinical infection ($n = 21.9$[a])	0.02	0.44
Healthy children ($n = 102$)	0.002	0.20
Total millions of US$/year		4.67
Costs of non participating mothers		0.88
Screening costs of healthy, uninfected mothers		1.31
Total millions of US$/year		6.86

[a] Computational figure has been used in the calculations.

Table IV. *Breakdown of annual costs per pregnancy in the screening and no-screening alternatives (US$) (baseline assumptions)*

	Screening	No screening
Screening (tests)	27.5	–
Treatment associated with screening	3.1	–
Other outpatient care	0.6	1.5
Short-term in-patient care	6.4	16.8
Long-term institutionalization	37.5	75.0
Direct costs	75.1	93.3
Indirect costs	20.0	35.0
Total costs	95.1	128.2

raising the sum by about US$ 0.4 million. The direct costs of screening amount to US$ 30.6 per pregnancy, altogether US$ 1.93 million yearly, including the costs of the tests, follow-up and treatment (Table IV). The total annual costs with systematic serological screening, including follow-up and therapy (alternative 2, Tables IIIb and IV) would be US$ 95 per pregnancy and US$ 6.86 million in all, and US$ 75 and US$ 5.36 million if only direct costs are considered, respectively. The net annual savings in the total costs would amount to US$ 2.09 million, and in direct costs to US$ 1.15 million.

Sensitivity analysis

The results of the one-way sensitivity analyses are presented graphically in Fig. 2a–e. With a transmission rate of 40% and an effectiveness of treatment of 50% the threshold value for incidence of maternal primary infection during pregnancy is 1.1/1,000 (Fig. 2c). The higher the incidence, the more favourable is the screening alternative. Also, the net savings grow with increasing transmission risk, effectiveness of treatment or participation rate, or with decreasing discount rate (Fig. 2a, b, d and e). A two-way sensitivity analysis shows the effect of transmission rate and effectiveness of treatment on the optimal decision. With the observed transmission rate of 25% (23) and according to the total costs, screening would be economically beneficial at the level of about 36% effectiveness of treatment. If only direct costs are included and the transmission rate is 25%, the threshold for effectiveness of treatment would be 50% (Fig. 3).

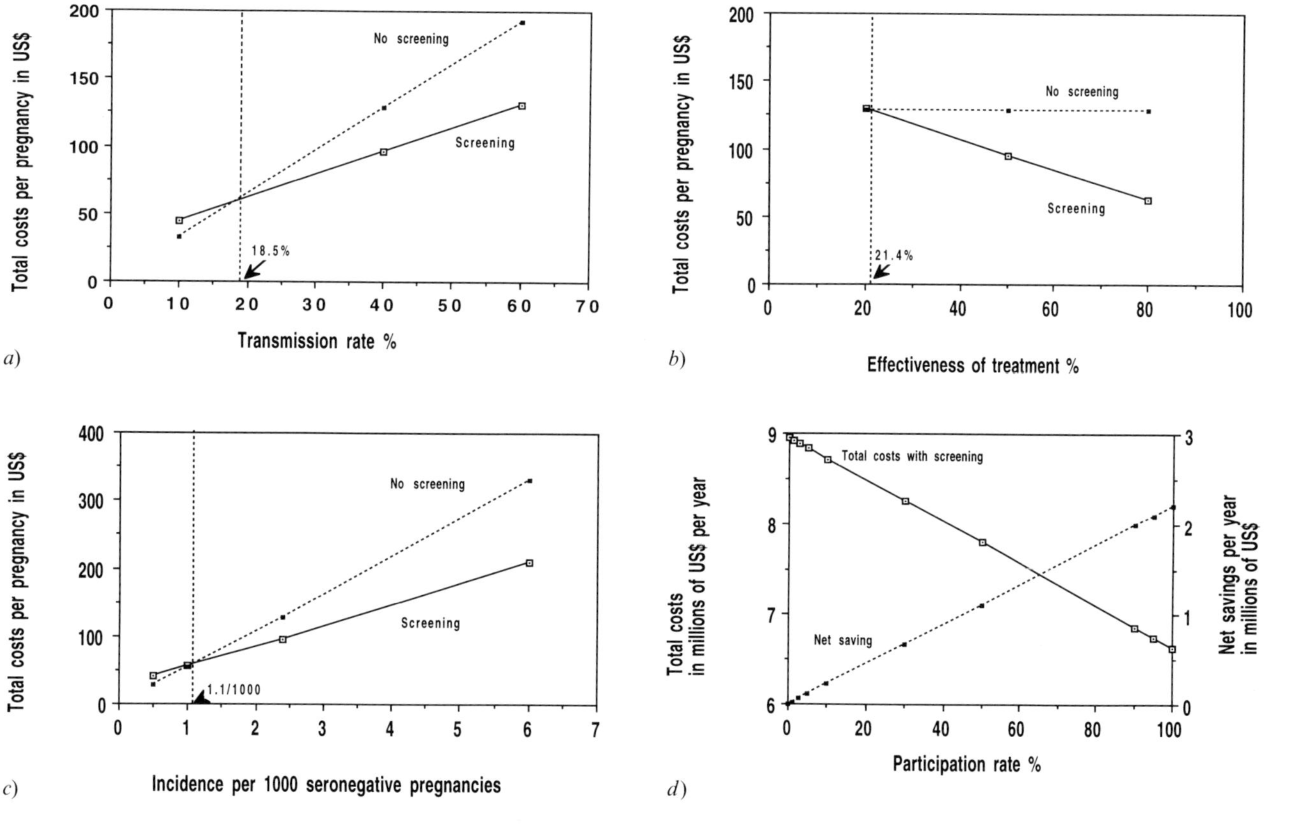

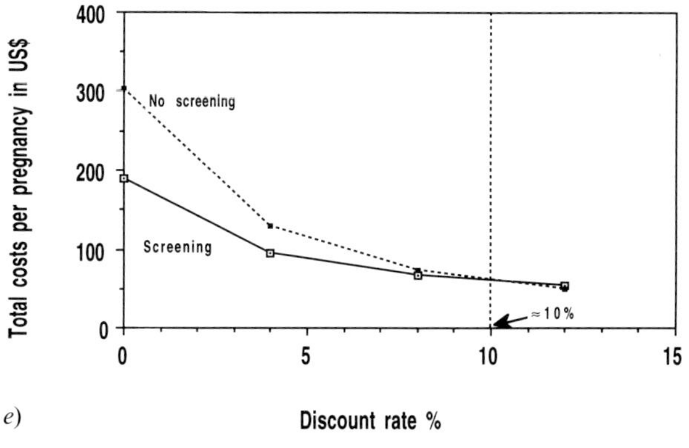

Fig. 2. One-way sensitivity analyses of annual total costs showing decision threshold values for *a*) transmission risk, *b*) efficacy of treatment, *c*) incidence of maternal primary infections, *d*) participation rate, and *e*) discount rate.

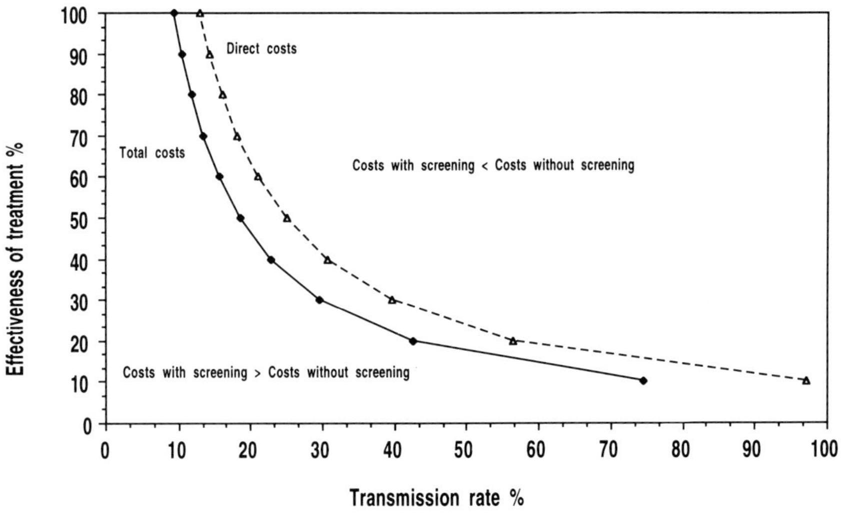

Fig. 3. Two-way sensitivity analysis with transmission rate and efficacy of treatment. On the right-hand side of the lines, the costs of the screening alternative are lower than those of the no-screening one. ————, Total costs (direct and indirect); – – – –, direct costs only.

DISCUSSION

Screening for primary toxoplasma infections during pregnancy is economically worthwhile. The present cost-benefit analysis shows that in a 'low risk' country, such as Finland with 5 million inhabitants and 70,000 pregnancies/year, the total annual costs due to congenital toxoplasmosis are US$ 8.95 million without screening and US$ 6.86 million when screening is performed. This produces annual net savings of US$ 2.1 million. A one-way sensitivity analysis gave 1.1/1,000 seronegative pregnancies as a threshold value for maternal primary infections. It is noteworthy that this figure is approximately only half of the incidence in Finland (14).

In a retrospective cost-benefit survey from Britain, the costs equalled the benefits (24), whereas in studies from the USA, Germany and Norway, screening proved more beneficial (2, 17, 18, 25, 26). Cost-benefit analysis is a helpful tool, when weighing the benefits and harms of nationwide screening. However, policy appropriate for one area may not always be appropriate for another. Since decision analysis is quantitative in nature, only financial aspects can be taken into account. Psychological and emotional factors cannot be directly measured and have to be considered separately.

In Finland, as in Sweden, Norway and Britain, the vast majority of women of childbearing age are seronegative and thus susceptible to primary toxoplasma infection (14, 22, 27, 28). In such 'low risk' countries, the majority of women of childbearing age are susceptible to primary infection, though the probability of infection for each individual is low. In 'high risk' countries, in contrast, the number of women at risk is small, but the individual risk of primary infection is high. Despite the striking differences in seropositivity, the absolute number of primary toxoplasma infections during pregnancy may eventually be the same in both cases (29).

Spiramycin appears empirically effective for treating pregnant women with primary toxoplasma infection, even though this has not been proven by placebo-controlled studies. The efficacy of antenatal treatment is generally agreen to be around 50% (24, 30, 31). A 50% reduced risk of fetal infection is assumed in this study and thereby the number of infected offspring is expected to be half of the number obtained without screening. According to a recent report, even early postnatal treatment may reduce the severe long-term sequelae of congenital toxoplasmosis (32). In screening schemes with only three samples taken during pregnancy, the effectiveness of treatment may be decreased because of the delay in diagnosis. In one-way sensitivity analysis, the 22% threshold value for effectiveness of treatment was the economic limit to justify the screening.

In decision analysis, the values of one or more parameters can be varied systematically and the calculations repeated to determine the optimal decision. The simplest approach, a one-way sensitivity analysis, examines changes in a single variable, and therefore provides only limited insight. The transmission rate is generally agreed to be 40% on average (22, 29), but was still included in our sensitivity analysis. The discount rate usually varies from 2 to 10% and alters the cost-benefit ratio (33). Our analysis showed that the optimal choice does not change until the discount rate approaches 10%. Also the participation rate influences the results; the better the compliance, the greater the net benefit. A two-way sensitivity analysis showed that even with a combination of low-effectiveness therapy and low transmission rate, screening is economically beneficial.

Direct costs caused by minor learning disabilities, behavioural disorders or mild neurological sequelae were excluded for lack of firm empirical data, even though the exclusion makes the results more favourable than the no-screening alternative. The financial costs attributable to death, psychological burden caused by the screening itself and by false-positive or -negative results were also omitted. The costs for treating subclinically infected children were consciously underestimated, as evidence of the true nature of the late sequelae of congenital toxoplasmosis is still scarce (34, 35). The calculations of the reagent costs were based on retail or wholesale prices. These costs would obviously be considerably reduced in nationwide screening. Even if loss of productivity is a difficult concept, we entered it into our analysis, as if the dead and disabled children were productive adults. However, by presenting also the direct costs alone, it was shown that optimal decision was not changed; screening was still economically worthwhile.

In screening, even a highly specific and sensitive single test produces false-positive results (12). By combining several sensitive and specific assays, false-positive diagnoses and false-negative cases become extremely rare, according to some reports the occurrence is no more than 0.02% (24, 36). The psychological burden due to screening must not be neglected, and it can be relieved by adequate counselling (10).

The benefits of prenatal education programs seem to be transient (4, 6). The impact of health education in our pilot study is difficult to estimate. Still, health education should be given to every pregnant mother irrespective of screening, because it is safe and cheap and the guidelines are simple. Austria and France have screened pregnant women systematically for years, but so far no cost-benefit analyses from these countries have been published. The British multidisciplinary working group has argued against screening, mainly due to the lack of hard data on prevalence and incidence. Their decision was additionally justified by the unavailability of a suitable screening test, uncertainty over the effectiveness of treatment, and the hazards of invasive techniques needed for fetal diagnosis (9, 37–40).

Decision analysis cannot resolve the questions of ethics, social justice or competing societal values; it merely supports conclusions concerning screening. The present cost-benefit analysis based on a prospective cohort study shows that screening together with health education can be beneficial even in a 'low risk' country. Therefore, screening for primary toxoplasma infections during pregnancy should be considered.

ACKNOWLEDGEMENTS

This study was supported by grants from the Academy of Finland, the Finnish Cultural Foundation, the Social Insurance Institution, the Finnish Medical Society Duodecim, the Orion Corporation Research Foundation, the Päivikki and Sakari Sohlberg Foundation, the Rhône-Poulenc Santé, the Rinnekoti Research Foundation, the Sigrid Jusélius Foundation, and the Swedish Medical Foundation in Finland. The language of the manuscript was revised by Ms Riitta Brelih.

REFERENCES

1. Stagno S. Congenital toxoplasmosis: marginal comment. Am J Dis Child 134: 635–637, 1980.
2. Wilson CB, Remington JS. What can be done to prevent congenital toxoplasmosis? Am J Obstet Gynecol 138: 357–363, 1980.
3. McCabe R, Remington JS. Toxoplasmosis: the time has come. N Engl J Med 318: 313–315, 1988.
4. Foulon W, Naessens A, Lauwers S, de Meuter F, Amy J-J. Impact of primary prevention on the incidence of toxoplasmosis during pregnancy. Obstet Gynecol 72: 363–366, 1988.
5. Carter AO, Gelmon SB, Wells GA, Toepell AP. The effectiveness of a prenatal education programme for the prevention of congenital toxoplasmosis. Epidemiol Infect 103: 539–545, 1989.
6. Conyn-van Spaendonck MAE, van Knapen F. Choices in preventive strategies: experience with the prevention of congenital toxoplasmosis in The Netherlands. Scand J Infect Dis Suppl 84: 51–58, 1992.
7. Ho-Yen DO, Chatterton JMW. Congenital toxoplasmosis – why and how to screen. Rev Med Microbiol 1: 229–235, 1990.
8. Desmonts G. Preventing congenital toxoplasmosis. Lancet 336: 1017–1018, 1990.
9. Anonymous. No UK prenatal toxoplasmosis screening. Lancet 339: 1291, 1992.
10. Marteau TM. Reducing the psychological costs. BMJ 301: 26–28, 1990.
11. Salmon RL. Screening for toxoplasma in pregnancy. Lancet 2: 1085–1086, 1988.
12. Thorp JM, Seeds JW, Herbert WNP, Bowes WA, Maslow AS, Cefalo RC, Chescheir N, Katz VL. Prenatal management and congenital toxoplasmosis. N Engl J Med 319: 372–373, 1988.
13. Hohlfeld P, Daffos F, Costa J-M, Thulliez P, Forestier F, Vidaud M. Prenatal diagnosis of congenital toxoplasmosis with a polymerase-chain-reaction test on amniotic fluid. N Engl J Med 331: 695–699, 1994.
14. Lappalainen M, Koskela P, Hedman K, Teramo K, Ämmälä P, Hiilesmaa V, Koskiniemi M. Incidence of primary toxoplasma infections during pregnancy in southern Finland: a prospective cohort study. Scand J Infect Dis 24: 97–104, 1992.
15. Pauker SG, Kassirer JP. Decision analysis. N Engl J Med 316: 250–258, 1987.
16. Lappalainen M, Koskela P, Koskiniemi M, Ämmälä P, Hiilesmaa V, Teramo K, Raivio KO, Remington JS, Hedman K. Toxoplasmosis acquired during pregnancy: improved serodiagnosis based on avidity of IgG. J Infect Dis 167: 691–697, 1993.
17. Roberts T, Frenkel J. Estimating income losses and other preventable costs caused by congenital toxoplasmosis in people in the United States. J Am Vet Med Assoc 196: 249–256, 1990.
18. Stray-Pedersen B, Jenum P. Economic evaluation of preventive programmes against congenital toxoplasmosis. Scand J Infect Dis Suppl 84: 86–96, 1992.
19. Statistics of activities and expenses in different branches of specialities. Helsinki: The Finnish Hospital League, 1988.
20. The Statistical Yearbook of Finland 1991. Helsinki. Central Statistical Office of Finland, 1991.
21. Ruusinen A. The use and fees of medical services in health centers. Payment policy, part 3. Helsinki. Ministry of Social Affairs and Health, Research Department, 1981.
22. Remington JS, Desmonts G. Toxoplasmosis. In: Remington JS, Klein JO, eds. Infectious Diseases of the Fetus and Newborn Infant, 3rd ed, Philadelphia: WB Saunders, 89–195, 1990.
23. Lappalainen M, Koskiniemi M, Hiilesmaa V, Ämmälä P, Teramo K, Koskela P, Lebech M, Raivio KO, Hedman L, The Study Group. Outcome of children after maternal primary toxoplasma infection during pregnancy with emphasis on avidity of specific IgG. Pediatr Infect Dis J 14: 354–361, 1995. [in press]
24. Joss AWL, Chatterton JMW, Ho-Yen DO. Congenital toxo-

plasmosis: to screen or not to screen? Public Health 104: 9–20, 1990.
25. Stray-Pedersen B. Cost-benefit analysis of different programs to prevent congenital TORCH-infections. Proceedings of the International Symposium on Progress in Perinatal Medicine, 229–37, 1983.
26. Roos T, Martius J, Gross U, Schrod L. Systematic serologic screening for toxoplasmosis in pregnancy. Obstet Gynecol 81: 243–250, 1993.
27. Forsgren M, Gille E, Ljungström I, Nokes DJ. Toxoplasma gondii antibodies in pregnant women in Stockholm in 1969, 1979, and 1987. Lancet 337: 1413–1414, 1991.
28. Stray-Pedersen B, Jenum P. Current status of toxoplasmosis in pregnancy in Norway. Scand J Infect Dis Suppl 84: 80–83, 1992.
29. Ho-Yen DO, Joss AWL, eds. In: Human Toxoplasmosis. Oxford. Oxford University Press, 1–265, 1992.
30. Couvreur J, Desmonts G, Thulliez P. Prophylaxis of congenital toxoplasmosis. Effects of spiramycin on placental infection. In: Davey P, Pechére J-C, Speller D, eds. Spiramycin reassessed. Singapore: Academic Press, 193–200, 1988.
31. Daffos F, Forestier F, Capella-Pavlovsky M, Thulliez P, Aufrant C, Valenti D, Cox WL. Prenatal management of 746 pregnancies at risk for congenital toxoplasmosis. N Engl J Med 318: 271–275, 1988.
32. Guerina NG, Hsu H-W, Meissner HC, Maguire JH, Lynfield R, Stechenberg B, Abroms I, Pasternack MS, Hoff R, Eaton RB, Grady GF, and the New England Regional Toxoplasma Working Group. Neonatal serologic screening and early treatment for congenital Toxoplasma gondii infection. N Engl J Med 330: 1858–1863, 1994.
33. Editorial. Discounting health care: only a matter of timing? Lancet 340: 148–149, 1992.
34. Wilson CB, Remington JS, Stagno S, Reynolds DW. Development of adverse sequelae in children born with subclinical congenital toxoplasma infection. Pediatrics 66: 767–774, 1980.
35. Koppe JG, Loewer-Sieger DH, de Roever-Bonnet H. Results of 20-year follow-up of congenital toxoplasmosis. Lancet 1: 254–256, 1986.
36. McCabe R, Remington JS. Prenatal management and congenital toxoplasmosis. N Engl J Med 319: 373–374, 1988.
37. Editorial. Antenatal screening for toxoplasmosis in the UK. Lancet 336: 346–348, 1990.
38. Hall SM. Congenital toxoplasmosis. BMJ 305: 291–297, 1992.
39. Henderson J, Beattie C, Hale E, Wright T. The evaluation of new services: possibilities for preventing congenital toxoplasmosis. Int J Epidemiol 13: 65–72, 1984.
40. Peckham CS, Logan S. Screening for toxoplasmosis during pregnancy. Arch Dis Child 68: 3–5, 1993.

Submitted May 11, 1994; accepted March 2, 1995

Scand J Infect Dis 27: 273–277, 1995 ORIGINAL ARTICLE

Response and Decline of Serum IgG Antibodies to Pertussis Toxin, Filamentous Hemagglutinin and Pertactin in Children with Pertussis

JERKER ISACSON[1], BIRGER TROLLFORS[1], GUNNEL HEDVALL[2], JOHN TARANGER[3] and GUNILLA ZACKRISSON[4]

From the Departments of [1]Paediatrics, East Hospital, the Paediatric Outpatient Clinics of [2]Askim and [3]Västra Frölunda, and the [4]Department of Clinical Bacteriology, Sahlgrens Hospital, University of Göteborg, Göteborg, Sweden

The serum IgG antibody response and decrease to 3 Bordetella pertussis antigens was compared in children with pertussis. Sera were obtained at the first clinical visit and 1, 3 and 12 months later from 89 children with ≥3 weeks of paroxysmal cough. IgG antibodies to pertussis toxin (PT), to filamentous hemagglutinin (FHA) and to pertactin were determined with ELISA. Of 54 children with culture-confirmed pertussis or culture-confirmed familial exposure, 45 (83%) had a significant (≥3 fold) increase in PT IgG and 40 (74%) in FHA IgG antibodies, while only 29 (54%) had a significant increase in pertactin IgG antibodies. Significant decreases in PT, FHA and pertactin IgG antibodies were found in 34 (63%), 9 (17%) and 28 (52%) children, respectively. In the remaining 35 who did not have culture-confirmed disease, significant PT and/or FHA IgG antibody increases (criteria for pertussis according to the WHO definition) were found in 17 (49%). Only 6 of these 17 children had a significant pertactin IgG antibody increase. Of the remaining 18 children (who did not fulfil WHO criteria for pertussis), significant decreases in PT and/or FHA IgG antibodies were found in 13. We conclude that a serum IgG reaction to PT and FHA occurs in almost all children with pertussis. An increase in pertactin IgG antibodies occurs less frequently than against PT and FHA. Significant decreases in PT or FHA IgG antibodies in children with clinical pertussis might be of use as a diagnostic criterion in children brought late for examination.

J. Isacson, MD, Department of Paediatrics, Östra Sjukhuset, S-416 85 Göteborg, Sweden

INTRODUCTION

Several toxins and surface antigens of Bordetella pertussis have been identified in recent years (1). Of these, pertussis toxin (PT), a protein exotoxin, plays a major role in the pathogenesis of the disease (2) and affords protection against disease (3, 4). Animal studies indicate that 2 surface proteins, filamentous hemagglutinin (FHA) and pertactin, also play a protective role (5, 6).

The difficulties of obtaining laboratory verification of the diagnosis of Bordetella pertussis infections are well known. Isolation of the organism from the nasopharynx gives a specific diagnosis, but cultures are often negative, especially if obtained in a late stage of the disease. The development of assays for determination of serum antibodies to the three above-mentioned antigens has opened up possibilities of making a serological diagnosis of pertussis. It has been convincingly shown that serum antibodies to PT and FHA develop after a symptomatic infection with B. pertussis (7–10).

Recently the World Health Organization (WHO) defined pertussis as paroxysmal cough persisting for at least 21 days, in combination with a positive culture from the patient or a household contact or serologic evidence of B. pertussis infection. An increase in IgG or IgA antibodies to PT or FHA was accepted as serologic evidence. Evaluation of the antibody response to pertactin was defined as a research priority (11).

However, the addition of serological methods to verify a serum antibody response does not solve all diagnostic problems for pertussis. The disease often has an insidious onset and many patients come late for an examination, when the antibody increase has already occurred. The possibility of diagnosing the disease by significant antibody decrease has not previously been investigated.

The aims of the present study were: 1) to compare the diagnostic sensitivity of increases in IgG antibodies to PT, FHA and pertactin in paired sera from patients with pertussis; 2) to evaluate the possibility of diagnosing pertussis according to significant decreases in antibodies against the three antigens in patients who come late for investigation.

PATIENTS AND METHODS

Study design

All children with symptoms suggestive of pertussis who were brought for medical attention at the Department of Paediatrics and at 2 paediatric out-patient clinics in Göteborg were invited to participate in the study. After informed consent had been obtained, the medical history of the child was recorded and a nasopharyngeal swab sample was obtained for culture of B. pertussis and a first serum sample (serum 1) was secured. After 1 month the parents were contacted by telephone by one of the authors (J.I.) who asked questions according to a structured questionnaire concerning the duration of the cough, whooping attacks, vomiting, exposure to pertussis, chronic disease, medication and previous vaccination against pertussis. Information about treatment with erythromycin or other antibiotics and hospitalization was obtained from the

 ISSN 0036-5548

child's medical chart. If the child at that interview had had at least 3 weeks of paroxysmal cough – as required by the WHO definition of pertussis (11) – a request was made to obtain further sera, 1, 3 and 12 months (sera 2, 3 and 4, respectively) after the initial sample. All sera were kept frozen at −60°C until analysed.

Patients

A total of 121 children were considered to have clinical pertussis and had experienced at least 3 weeks of paroxysmal cough. From 23 children, only one serum sample was obtained. These sera were not analysed. From 9 children, 2 sera were obtained, but they were not analysed because the intervals were suboptimal or because there was an insufficient amount to determine antibodies to all antigens. From the remaining 89 children, three or 4 sera were obtained. These 89 children constitute the patient material described in the present investigation. The children had a median age of 18 months (range 1 month to 7 years); 20 children (22%) were younger than 6 months. There were 37 males and 52 females. One child had bronchial asthma; the others had no known concurrent disease. 21 (24%) of the children were hospitalized because of pertussis. One, a 4-month-old boy, had pertussis encephalopathy. Erythromycin had been given to 50 (56%) of the children. None had been vaccinated against pertussis. Nasopharyngeal cultures were obtained from 76 (85%) children. In 48 (63%) of them, B. pertussis was isolated. Of the 41 children with negative or no cultures, 6 had siblings with positive culture and onset of cough less than 28 days before onset in the study child. In children with positive or negative cultures, there was no difference in the duration of symptoms before the culture was obtained.

The median duration of cough at the first visit was 2 (range 0–8) weeks. Serum 2 was obtained after a median of 7 (range 4–17) weeks, serum 3 after a median of 17 (range 12–37) weeks and serum 4 after a median of 56 (range 47–86) weeks after the onset of cough. Four sera were obtained from 52 children (58%), and 3 sera from 37.

Laboratory methods

Nasopharyngeal swabs were cultured for B. pertussis on Lacey's medium according to routine procedures in use at the laboratory at that time. Bordetella parapertussis does not grow on this medium (12). Serum IgG antibodies to PT, FHA and pertactin were determined by enzyme-linked immunosorbent assay (ELISA) (7, 8, 13). IgA and IgM antibodies to PT were analysed in one child with undetectable PT IgG antibodies in all 4 sera and with familial exposure to pertussis (8). In all assays, sera were tested in duplicate in eight 3-fold dilutions. The first dilution was 1/10. The antibody titre was expressed as the reciprocal serum dilution corresponding to an extinction of 0.2 greater than the background value. Sera with non-detectable antibodies were arbitrarily assigned a titre of 5 (half of the lowest titre detectable) for statistical calculations. All sera from an individual child were assayed on the same microtitre plate. A 3-fold increase in antibody titre against the 3 antigens was considered significant, based on determinations of intra-assay variation (10–17%) and on intra-individual variation (data on file).

Statistics

Differences in antibody titres between groups of infants were tested by Mann-Whitney U-test and within groups by Wilcoxon signed rank test. Differences in proportions were tested by the corrected χ^2-test. Calculations were performed on log10 transformed values. Two-tailed significance values were always calculated.

Ethics

The study was approved by the Ethics Committee of the University of Göteborg. The parents gave consent for the participation of their child after receiving oral and written information about the study.

RESULTS

I. Children with culture confirmed infection (n = 48) or culture confirmed familial exposure (n = 6)

Antibody response

Table I shows the median and range of IgG antibody titres in relation to time after onset of cough in 89 sera obtained within 8 weeks of onset in the 54 children. Of the 19 children from whom the first serum was obtained within 14 days of symptoms, 9 (47%) had detectable PT antibodies and 13 (68%) had detectable FHA antibodies. All had detectable pertactin antibodies (pertactin versus PT, $p < 0.001$; pertactin versus FHA, $p < 0.05$).

Of all 54 children, 45 (83%) had significant increases in PT antibodies and 40 (74%) in FHA antibodies, while only 29 (54%) had significant increases in pertactin antibodies (pertactin versus PT and FHA, $p < 0.05$). Table II shows the antibody increases against the 3 antigens and combinations of antigens. No child had a response in pertactin antibodies alone. Six children failed to respond to all 3 antigens. All had high PT IgG titres in their first sera, which were obtained 6.5 weeks (median) after onset of cough.

There were wide interindividual variations in the magnitude of the IgG antibody response and in the interval between onset of cough and its peak. In most children, the peak of antibody titres occurred 5 to 8 weeks after onset. The median values of the highest antibody titres, all obtained within 6 months of onset of cough, were as follows: PT 22,387 (range <10–100,000), FHA 1,995 (<10–14,125) and pertactin 1,318 (50–25,119). In half of the children with maximum antibody titres below 1,000, no serum samples within the optimal interval 5–8 weeks after onset of cough were available. Only 2 children had maximum PT IgG titres below 1,000, while 16 had FHA, and 25 had pertactin IgG maximum titres below 1,000. One child had undetectable PT antibodies in all 4 sera (see below) and another had undetectable FHA antibodies in the first 3 sera but a high IgG titre in the serum obtained after 1 year.

Antibody decline

Table III shows the median and range of the highest IgG antibody titres measured during the first 12 weeks after onset, compared with sera obtained after at least 50 weeks from the 39 children from whom such sera were obtained. The antibody titres against all 3 antigens decreased significantly. The decrease in median FHA IgG titre was less pronounced (1.8-fold) than that in PT and pertactin IgG titres (4–5-fold).

Table IV summarizes the pattern of significant increases and decreases in IgG titres against the three antigens.

In 6 (11%) children, a significant decrease was registered in PT IgG antibody titre without previous significant anti-

Table I. *Median serum PT, FHA and pertactin IgG titres in 89 sera obtained within 8 weeks after onset of cough from 54 children with culture-confirmed pertussis or culture-verified family exposure in relation to disease duration (from 35 children, two sera are included)*

	Median (range) antibody titres		
Disease duration. . .	<2 weeks	2–4 weeks	5–8 weeks
No. of sera . . .	19	33	37
PT-IgG	5 (<10–891)[a]	1,778 (<10–63,096)[b]	25,119 (<10–100,000)[c]
FHA-IgG	25 (<10–224)[d]	158 (<10–2,818)[e]	1,585 (71–14,125)[f]
Pertactin-IgG	112 (18–1,259)[g]	200 (11–23,442)[h]	1,413 (45–25,119)[i]

a vs. b, $p < 0.005$; b vs. c, d vs. e, e vs. f, g vs. i, h vs. i, $p < 0.001$; g vs. h = ns.

Table II. *Number of children with significant increases in PT, FHA or pertactin IgG titres, of 54 children with culture-confirmed pertussis or culture-verified family exposure*

IgG antibodies	No. of children with ≥3-fold increase
PT-FHA + Pertactin	25
PT + FHA	12
PT + Pertactin	3
FHA + Pertactin	1
PT	5
FHA	2
Pertactin	0
No response against any antigen	6

Table III. *Decrease in median IgG titres between sera obtained ≤12 and ≥50 weeks after onset of cough in 39 children with culture-confirmed pertussis or culture-verified family exposure*

If two sera were available ≤12 weeks after onset of cough, the serum with the higher titre was selected

	Median (range) antibody titre in relation to duration since first cough	
	≤12 weeks	≥50 weeks
Pertussis toxin-IgG	22,387 (<10–100,000)[a]	4,169 (224–25,704)[b]
FHA-IgG	1,995 (71–14,125)[c]	1,122 (28–12,589)[d]
Pertactin-IgG	1,259 (56–25,119)[e]	282 (22–6,607)[f]

a vs. b, e vs. f, $p < 0.0001$; c vs. d, $p < 0.01$.

Table IV. *Significant increases and decreases in pertussis toxin, FHA and pertactin IgG antibodies in 54 children with culture-confirmed pertussis or culture-verified family exposure*

	≥3 fold increase ≥3 fold decrease	≥3 fold increase <3 fold decrease	<3 fold increase ≥3 fold decrease	<3 fold increase <3 fold decrease
Pertussis toxin-IgG	28	17	6	3
FHA-IgG	6	34	3	11
Pertactin-IgG	16	13	12	13

body response. From these children the first serum was obtained after a median of 5 weeks of symptoms, 3 weeks later than from the group with initial increases in PT antibody titres. The pattern was similar for FHA antibodies in 3 children and for pertactin antibodies in 12.

One culture-negative child with a culture-positive sibling entered the study after 2 weeks of symptoms when 25 months old. This child had a significant FHA and pertactin IgG antibody response but had non-detectable PT-IgG, PT-IgA and PT-IgM antibodies in all 4 sera.

Subgroup comparisons

There were no significant and clinically relevant differences in PT, FHA or pertactin IgG titres related to age (<6 months or older), to sex, erythromycin treatment, or hospitalization.

II. Children with negative cultures (n = 25) or from whom cultures were not obtained (n = 10) and without culture confirmed familial exposure to pertussis

Antibody response

Of the 35 children, 17 (49%) had significant increases in PT IgG antibodies, FHA IgG antibodies or both, and, thus fulfilled the serological criteria for the WHO definition of pertussis. PT and FHA antibody increases were equally common, 14 (40%) and 15 (43%) children, respectively. Only 6 (17%) children had an increase in pertactin antibodies, all with concomitant increases in PT or FHA antibodies or both.

18 children did not have a significant increase in IgG antibodies to any antigen, even though their first sera were obtained after a median of 1 (range <1–22) week. Significant decreases in PT, FHA or pertactin IgG antibodies were seen in 11 (61%), 6 (33%) and 7 (39%) respectively. Four out of 5 children without significant PT or FHA antibody decrease had PT or FHA antibodies or both in all or some of their sera. All had antibodies to pertactin.

DISCUSSION

In this investigation we studied the response and decline of IgG antibodies to 3 B. pertussis antigens in children with symptoms compatible with pertussis. Most children with culture-verified pertussis or familial exposure to pertussis had low or undetectable levels of PT IgG antibodies in the first serum, followed by a pronounced response. A few more children had FHA antibodies than PT antibodies in the initial serum, but significant PT and FHA IgG responses were almost equally common. Those who did not have significant increases in PT and FHA IgG antibodies had, in most cases, higher titres in the first serum which was obtained in a later stage of the disease than in the children with a significant response. These results are consistent with previous findings (7–10, 14, 15).

Pertactin IgG antibodies could be detected in the first serum from all children in this study. Only half of those with culture-confirmed pertussis or culture-verified familial exposure had a significant increase in pertactin IgG titres. In an earlier study, paired sera from 19 infants less than 6 months of age and with pertussis according to the WHO definition were assayed with Western blot. Only 1 had detectable antibodies to pertactin in the convalescent serum (16). Thus, pertactin IgG antibody determination in paired sera is a considerably less sensitive diagnostic tool than PT and FHA IgG antibody determinations.

At least 3 explanations should be considered regarding the more frequent finding of FHA and, in particular, of pertactin IgG antibodies, than of PT IgG antibodies in early sera from patients with pertussis. First, this could be due to a swifter immune reaction to FHA and pertactin, as they are surface-associated proteins of the bacteria and not exotoxins as PT. Secondly, pre-existing antibodies could be due to an earlier contact with B. parapertussis or B. bronciseptica, both of which have FHA and pertactin surface antigens (17–19). Infection with B. pertussis despite the presence of FHA IgG serum antibodies induced by a previous infection with B. parapertussis has been reported in 3 children (20). Thirdly, there is a possibility that exposure to antigens from other organisms crossreacting with FHA and pertactin induces serum antibodies to these proteins. It has been shown recently that outer membrane proteins of non-capsulated Haemophilus influenzae crossreact with FHA (21). Asymptomatic carriage and infections caused by this organism are common in children (22–24). According to previous studies, many individuals with no history of pertussis nevertheless have FHA and pertactin serum antibodies (13, 25–27), indicating that the 2 last-mentioned possibilities are of importance.

The present and previous studies (7, 8, 10) demonstrate the importance of obtaining an early serum sample in order to establish the serological diagnosis of pertussis. Probably due to suboptimal timing of serum samples, it was not possible to detect any significant increase in IgG antibodies in some of our children. There was a considerable individual variation in the level of the IgG antibody response and also to some extent regarding how soon the increase and decline became evident. Most children showed an IgG antibody response in samples obtained after 5 to 8 weeks of cough.

In this study, 1 child exposed to culture-verified pertussis had non-detectable PT IgG, IgA and IgM antibodies in all 4 sera and the culture was negative for B. pertussis. In some rare cases of B. pertussis infection, e.g. in preterm infants, a PT antibody response has not been seen (8), but our child was 25 months old and born at term. The significant FHA and pertactin IgG antibody responses indicate an infection with a Bordetella species. Since both B. parapertussis and B. bronchiseptica have FHA and pertactin as surface antigens (17–19) it is possible that the child had been infected with 1 of these species. Only PT is considered specific for B. pertussis and crossreacting antigens have not been described.

IgG antibodies to all three antigens declined after the initial response, already within 1 to several months following the infection. The FHA IgG antibodies tended to decline less rapidly than the PT and pertactin IgG antibodies. IgG antibodies to all 3 antigens could be detected after one year in all but the child who had non-detectable PT antibodies in all 4 sera. These data indicate that a significant decrease in PT and FHA IgG antibodies can be used as a criterion for diagnosis of pertussis in patients with typical symptoms who seek medical attention at a late stage of the disease, when cultures are negative and significant antibody responses have already occurred.

In a large proportion of the infants (71/89, 80%) the clinical diagnosis of pertussis (≥ 3 weeks of paroxysmal cough) could be verified by culture or IgG serology according to the WHO criteria. This indicates that the clinical diagnosis is fairly reliable, albeit in a country with epidemic pertussis. Addition of rise in pertactin IgG as a diagnostic criterion would not have added to the number of laboratory verified cases. If significant PT and FHA IgG decreases had been regarded as criteria of pertussis, the diagnosis would have been verified in 84 of 89 (94%) children. It is remarkable that 13 out of 18 children without confirmation of pertussis according to the WHO definition had significant decreases in PT or FHA IgG titres even though their disease duration of the first serum sampling was short. Possibly, the parents had not recognized the onset of disease symptoms which is often insidious. Determinations of IgA antibodies to PT and FHA might also have increased the number of children with verified diagnosis, but these assays were not performed due to shortage of serum.

In conclusion, this study has confirmed that a serum IgG response to PT and FHA is seen in almost all children with pertussis. The diagnostic sensitivity of PT IgG serology is somewhat higher than of FHA IgG serology. Pertactin IgG antibodies are encountered in acute phase sera, even when obtained very shortly after the onset of symptoms. Fewer children have a significant increase in pertactin vis-à-vis PT and FHA IgG antibodies. The initial antibody response to all three antigens is followed by a decline and we propose that a significant decrease in PT and FHA IgG antibodies should be added to the diagnostic criteria.

ACKNOWLEDGEMENTS

We thank Anne Kinnunen for valuable technical assistance, and the Department of Paediatrics, University of Göteborg, the Göteborg Medical Society and the Petter Silfverskiöld Memorial Foundation for financial support.

REFERENCES

1. Cherry JD, Brunnell PA, Golden GS, Karzon DT. Report of the task force on pertussis and pertussis immunization – 1988. Paediatrics 81 (6 Suppl): 939–984, 1988.
2. Pittman M. The concept of pertussis as a toxin-mediated disease. Pediatr Infect Dis J 3: 467–486, 1984.
3. Ad Hoc Group for the Study of Pertussis Vaccines. Placebo controlled trial of two acellular pertussis vaccines in Sweden: protective efficacy and adverse events. Lancet 955–960, 1988.
4. Storsaeter J, Hallander H, Farrington CP, Olin P, Möllby R, Miller E. Secondary analysis of the efficacy of two acellular pertussis vaccines evaluated in a Swedish phase III trial. Vaccine 8: 457–461, 1990.
5. Roberts M, Cropley I, Chatfield S, Dougan G. Protection of mice against respiratory Bordetella pertussis infection by intranasal immunization with P.69 and FHA. Vaccine 11: 866–872, 1993.
6. Shahin RD, Amsbaugh DF, Leef MF. Mucosal immunization with filamentous hemagglutinin protects against Bordetella pertussis respiratory infection. Infect Immun 60: 1482–1488, 1992.
7. Zackrisson G, Arminjon P, Krantz I, Lagergård T, Sigurs N, Taranger J, Trollfors B. Serum antibody response to filamentous hemagglutinin in patients with clinical pertussis measured by an enzyme-linked immunosorbent assay. Eur J Clin Microbiol Infect Dis 7: 764–770, 1988.
8. Zackrisson G, Krantz I, Lagergård T, Larsson P, Sekura R, Sigurs N, Taranger J, Trollfors B. Antibody response to pertussis toxin in patients with clinical pertussis measured by enzyme-linked immunosorbent assay. Eur J Clin Microbiol Infect Dis 7: 149–154, 1988.
9. Granström M, Granström G, Lindfors A, Askelöf P. Serologic diagnosis of whooping cough by an enzyme-linked immunosorbent assay using fimbrial hemagglutinin as antigen. J Infect Dis 146: 741–745, 1982.
10. Granström G, Wretlind B, Salenstedt C-R, Granström M. Evaluation of serologic assays for diagnosis of whooping cough. J Clin Microbiol 26: 1818–1823, 1988.
11. WHO meeting on case definition of pertussis. Geneva, MIM/EPI/PERT/91.1, 10–11 January, 1991.
12. Lautrop H. Laboratory diagnosis of whooping-cough or Bordetella infections. Bull World Health Organ 23: 15–35, 1960.
13. Trollfors B, Zackrisson G, Taranger J, Lagergård T. Serum antibodies against a 69-kilodalton outer membrane protein, pertactin, from Bordetella pertussis in nonvaccinated children with and without a history of clinical pertussis. J Pediatr 120: 924–926, 1992.
14. Thomas MG, Redhead K, Lambert HP. Human serum antibody responses to Bordetella pertussis infection and pertussis vaccination. J Infect Dis 159: 211–218, 1989.
15. Thomas MG, Ashworth LAE, Miller E, Lambert HP. Serum IgG, IgA and IgM responses to pertussis toxin, filamentous hemagglutinin and agglutinogens 2 and 3 after infection with Bordetella pertussis and immunization with whole-cell pertussis vaccine. J Infect Dis 160: 838–845, 1989.
16. Guiso N, Grimprel G, Anjak I, Be'gue' P. Western blot analysis of antibody responses of young infants to pertussis infection. Eur J Clin Microbiol Infect Dis 12: 596–600, 1993.
17. Irons LI, Ashworth LAE, Wilton-Smith P. Heterogeneity of the filamentous hemagglutinin of Bordetella pertussis studied with monoclonal antibodies. J Gen Microbiol 129: 2769–2778, 1983.
18. Granström M, Lindberg AA, Askelöf P, Hederstedt B. Detection of antibodies in human serum against the fimbrial hemagglutinin of Bordetella pertussis by enzyme linked immunosorbent assay. J Med Microbiol 15: 85–96, 1982.
19. Charles IG, Li LJ, Strugnell R, Beesly K, Romanos M, Novotny P, Heron I, Jensen M, Manclark CR, Brennan MJ, Fairweather NF. Repeat sequence motifs constitute the immunodominant regions of the p. 69 protein, pertactin, from Bordetella pertussis: Comparison with repeat sequences from B. parapertussis and B. bronchiseptica. In: C. R. Manclark, ed. Proceedings of the Sixth International Symposium on Pertussis, Bethesda, Md. DHHS Publication No. (FDA) 90-1164. 136–140, 1990.
20. Taranger J, Trollfors B, Lagergård T, Zackrisson G. Parapertussis infection followed by pertussis infection. (Letter). Lancet 344: 1703, 1994.
21. Barenkamp SJ, Leininger E. Cloning, expression, and DNA sequence analysis of genes encoding nontypable Haemophilus influenzae high-molecular-weight surface-exposed proteins related to filamentous hemagglutinin of Bordetella pertussis. Infect Immun 60: 1302–1313, 1992.
22. Ingvarsson L, Lundgren K, Ursing J. The bacterial flora in the nasopharynx in healthy children. Acta Otolaryngol Suppl 386: 94–96, 1982.
23. Branefors-Helander P, Nylén O, Jeppsson PH. Acute otitis media. A bacteriological study. ORL J Otorhinolaryngol Relat Spec 34: 281–295, 1972.
24. Weiss A, Brinser JH, Nazar-Stewart V. Acute conjunctivitis in childhood. J Pediatr 122: 10–14, 1993.
25. Isacson J, Trollfors B, Taranger J, Zackrisson G, Lagergård T. How common is whooping cough in a nonvaccinating country? Pediatr Infect Dis J 12: 284–288, 1993.
26. Zackrisson G, Taranger J, Trollfors B. History of whooping cough in nonvaccinated Swedish children, related to serum antibodies to pertussis toxin and filamentous hemagglutinin. J Pediatr 116: 190–194, 1990.
27. Granström M, Granström G. Serological correlates in whooping cough. Vaccine 11: 445–448, 1993.

Submitted August 29, 1994; accepted February 21, 1995

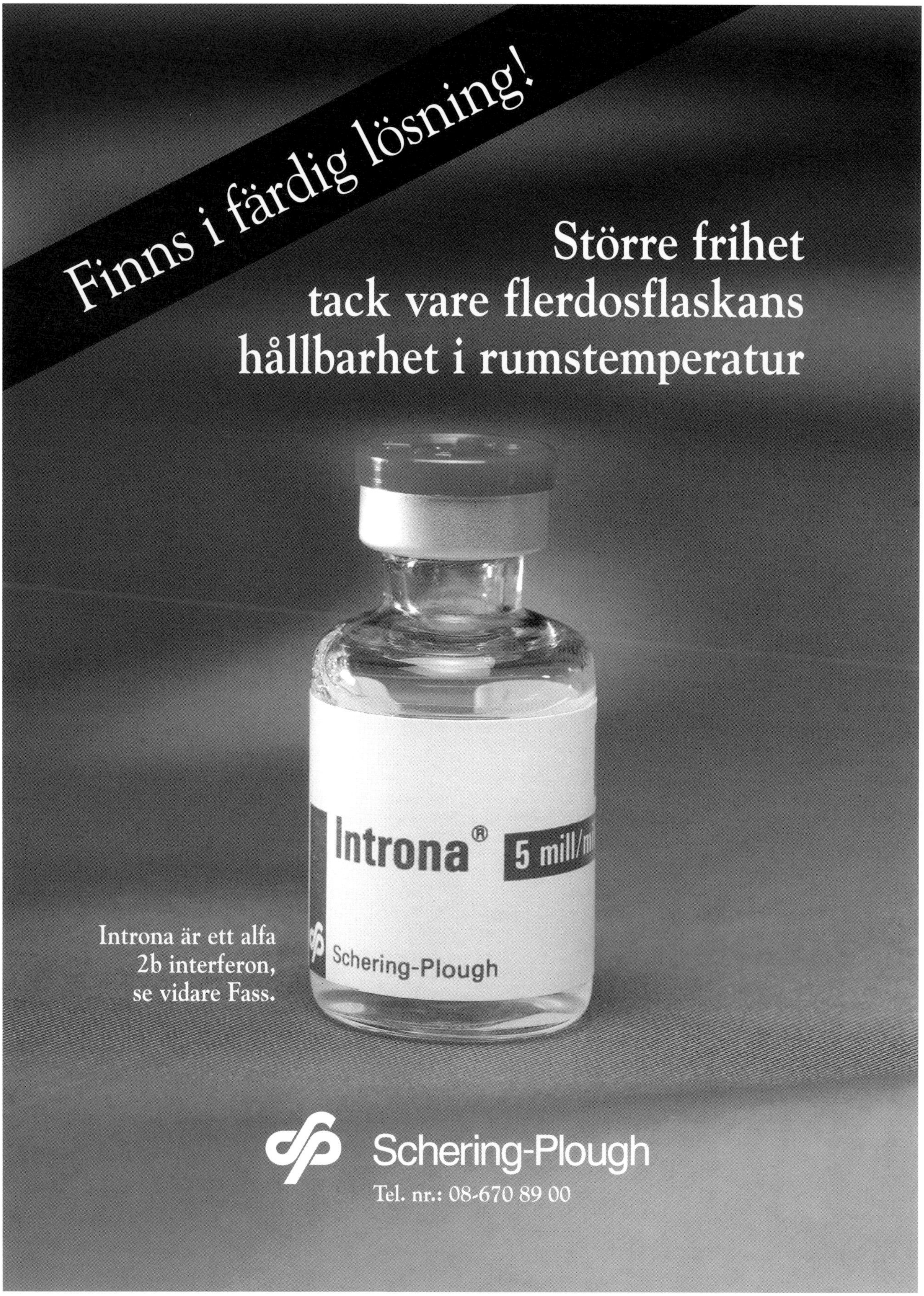
Finns i färdig lösning!
Större frihet
tack vare flerdosflaskans
hållbarhet i rumstemperatur
Introna®
Schering-Plough
Introna är ett alfa
2b interferon,
se vidare Fass.
Schering-Plough
Tel. nr.: 08-670 89 00

Scand J Infect Dis 27: 279–287, 1995 ORIGINAL ARTICLE

Safety and Immunogenicity of Two Acellular Pertussis Vaccines with Different Pertussis Toxoid and Filamentous Hemagglutinin Content in Infants 2–6 Months Old

SCOTT A. HALPERIN[1,2], BRIAN EASTWOOD[3]*, LUIS BARRETO[4], ELAINE MILLS[5], MARK BLATTER[6], KEITH REISINGER[6], GERALD BADER[7], HARRY KEYSERLING[8], E. ANN ROBERTS[9], ROLAND GUASPARINI[10], LORNA MEDD[11] and GARRY HUMPHREYS[12]

From the Departments of [1]Pediatrics, [2]Microbiology and Immunology, and [3]Community Health and Epidemiology, Dalhousie University, Halifax, [4]Connaught Laboratories Limited, Willowdale, The [5]Department of Pediatrics, McGill University, Montreal, Canada, [6]Pittsburgh Pediatric Research Incorporated, Pittsburgh, USA, The [7]Vancouver Clinic, Vancouver, Canada, The [8]Department of Pediatrics, Emory University, Atlanta, USA, [9]Calgary Health Services, Calgary, Canada, [10]Central Fraser Valley Health District, Maple Ridge, Canada, The [11]Boundary Health Unit, Surrey, Canada, and [12]Peterborough Health Unit, Peterborough, Canada

The optimal composition and antigen content of acellular pertussis vaccines is not known. Two vaccines with differrent quantities of pertussis toxoid (10 and 20 μg) and filamentous hemagglutinin (5 and 20 μg) and identical 69 kD protein (3 μg) and fimbriae 2 and 3 (5 μg) combined with diphtheria and tetanus toxoids were compared in a randomized, double-blind study in 2,050 infants undergoing their primary immunization series at 8 centers in the US and Canada. A 6:1 increased antigen to lower antigen allocation was used; 96% of infants received 3 doses and completed the study. A 'clinically significant' local reaction was reported in 3–6% of participants after each dose. Erythema was the most common reaction occurring in 3–5% of infants after the second or third dose. A clinically significant systemic adverse reaction was reported in 28–34% of vaccinees (or vacinated children) after each dose; fever (7–18%) and fussiness (12–17%) were most common. There were no differences in adverse events between the 2 vaccine formlations. Antibody responses were measured in 292 infants at 1 center. At 7 months, geometric mean anti-filamentous hemagglutinin antibody titers were higher in recipients of the higher antigen content vaccine ($p < 0.001$) whereas recipients of the lower antigen content formulation had higher anti-fimbriae antibody ($p < 0.001$) and agglutinin titers ($p < 0.05$). No differences were detected in anti-pertussis toxin or other antibody responses between the formulations. We conclude that increasing the antigen content of the acellular pertussis vaccine had a variable effect on antibody response but was not associated with increased adverse reactions.

S. A. Halperin, MD, Department of Pediatrics, Dalhousie University, Izaak Walton Killam Hospital for Children, 5850 University Avenue, Halifax, Nova Scotia B3J 3G9, Canada

INTRODUCTION

Whole-cell pertussis vaccine has been instrumental in the worldwide control of pertussis: the reported incidence of pertussis has fallen by over 90% in North America (1, 2). Resurgent disease has been reported when immunization programs have been interrupted because of poor public acceptance (3, 4) or withdrawal of the vaccine because of concerns of its safety (3) or efficacy (5). Concerns about the safety of the whole-cell vaccine have led to the development of acellular pertussis vaccines containing 1 or more antigens of the causative bacterium, Bordetella pertussis. Most acellular pertussis vaccines contain pertussis toxoid (PT) and filamentous hemagglutinin (FHA), 2 antigens which induce a protective antibody response in animal models of pertussis (6, 7). The efficacy of acellular vaccines has been demonstrated in Japan since their introduction in 1981 (8, 9) and in a Swedish clinical trial (10).

In an effort to improve their efficacy, other antigens have been considered for inclusion in acellular pertussis vaccines. Most attention has focused on fimbrial antigens (FIM; agglutinogens 2 and 3) and a 69kD membrane protein (69k, pertactin) which are also protective in animal models of pertussis (11–15). Acellular vaccines have been developed which include the 69k protein with PT and FHA (16), FIM with PT and FHA (17), PT, FHA, FIM, and 69k in fixed quantities as a result of the PT and FHA co-purification process (18, 19), and PT, FHA, FIM, and 69k protein purified separately and combined in the desired quantities (20, 21). The purpose of this study was to evaluate the safety and immunogenicity of 2 formulations of a 5-component acellular vaccine containing different quantities of PT and FHA in preparation for their use in a large efficacy study in Sweden.

MATERIAL AND METHODS

The study was a randomized, double-blind, multicenter clinical trial. The protocol was approved by the institutional review board at each study center.

* Dr. Eastwood's current affiliation is The University of Auckland, Auckland, New Zealand.

 ISSN 0036-5548

Vaccines

Two formulations of the acellular vaccine were used. The first (APV-low) contained (per 0.5 ml dose) PT (10 µg protein content), FHA (5 µg), FIM (5 µg) and 69k (3 µg). The formulation with increased antigen content (APV-high) contained the same quantity of 69k and FIM but twice the amount of PT (20 µg) and 4-fold more FHA (20 µg). The pertussis components were all individually purified (except for fimbriae 2 and 3 which were co-purified) and combined in the desired quantities; both formulations were combined with diphtheria (DIP; 15 Lf) and tetanus (TET; 5 Lf) toxoids and adsorbed to aluminum phosphate (1.5 mg per dose) with 0.6% 2-phenoxyethanol as a preservative. Vaccines were produced by Connaught Laboratories Limited (Willowdale, Ontario, Canada); a single lot of each formulation was used.

Population

The study was conducted at 5 sites in Canada (Halifax, Nova Scotia; Montreal, Quebec; Peterborough, Ontario; Calgary, Alberta; Fraser Valley, British Columbia) and three sites in the USA (Atlanta, Georgia; Pittsburgh, Pennsylvania; Vancouver, Washington). Healthy infants from 6 weeks (USA) or 2 months (Canada) to 3 months of age were eligible for enrolment. Vaccine allocation was via a computer generated table of random numbers within each center; a balanced block, 6:1 (APV-high:APV-low) allocation ratio was used in order to provide sufficient safety data on the increased antigen formulation.

Following informed consent, infants were immunized with 0.5 ml of 1 of the study vaccines by intramuscular injection into the vastus lateralis muscle of the thigh. In order to avoid disruption of the routine immunization schedule, study participants received their Haemophilus influenzae B conjugate vaccine (Act-HIB®, tetanus conjugate vaccine, Connaught Laboratories Inc., Swiftwater, USA) in the opposite thigh and oral poliovirus vaccine at the same visit.

Clinical and laboratory monitoring

Participants were monitored for local and systemic adverse reactions immediately following the immunization and by the parents for 14 days post-immunization. Data were collected via a structured telephone interview at 24 h and 14 days and by a symptom diary which was similar to the interview form at 48 h and 7 days. Local adverse reactions (erythema, swelling) were measured using a clear plastic template containing graded size markings. Tenderness and systemic reactions (irritability, decreased activity, decreased feeding) were graded as mild, moderate, or severe according to pre-established criteria by which the parent selected a severity based on structured examples. Prolonged crying, diarrhea, and vomiting were graded according to duration or number of episodes. Body temperature was measured at least once daily or whenever the child was thought by the parent to be febrile. Antipyretic use, contacts with the health care system, and hospitalizations for any reason were also monitored.

Blood samples were collected by venipuncture or by finger-prick in Montreal only at the time of the first and third vaccine dose and 1 month after the third dose. IgG antibodies to PT were measured by enzyme immunoassay (22) and PT-neutralizing antibody by Chinese hamster ovary cell cytotoxicity neutralization (CHO) (23). IgG anti-FHA, anti-FIM, an anti-69k antibodies were measured by enzyme immunoassay; unitage was calculated using the US FDA reference antiserum (no. 3) (22). Pertussis agglutinins (AGG) were also measured. Diphtheria antitoxin (DIP) was measured by microneutralization assay and tetanus antitoxin (TET) by immunoassay. Antibody titers were expressed as geometric mean titers; serum samples with titers less than the test detection limit were assigned a value of one-half the lower detection limit for the purpose of statistical calculations.

Statistical analysis

Counts of adverse reactions for each vaccine were tabulated for each reaction, any local reaction, and any general reaction. Rates of adverse reactions between vaccines were compared within each center and in a combined centers analysis. Rates of adverse reactions were compared by Mantel-Haenszel estimates of relative risk. Point estimates and 95% confidence intervals of the relative risk were estimated in each case (24); the assumption of a constant relative risk between centers (assumed in the Mantel-Haenszel estimates) was evaluated by the Breslow-Day test for homogeneity of the relative risk. Confidence intervals that do not include 1.00 are statistically significant. Rates of acetaminophen use by center and vaccine were compared by 2-way logistic regression. Country comparisons were made by a contrast of the average of the American centers compared with the average of the Canadian centers.

Geometric mean antibody titers and 95% confidence intervals were computed for each observation point and for the ratio of the 7-month to the minimum of the 2 and 6 month tests. Mean log titers at 2, 6, and 7 months and mean log-fold antibody titer rises were compared by *t*-tests and profile analysis. Proportions were compared by *t*-tests and profile analysis. Proportions were compared by Fisher's Exact test. No adjustments were made for multiple comparisons.

RESULTS

A total of 2,050 infants were enrolled in the study (47% female); 1,961 (96%) completed the 3 dose series (Table I). The mean age was 9.3 weeks at the first dose, 18.4 weeks at the second dose, and 27.6 weeks at the third dose; there were no demographic differences between recipients of

Table 1. *Study population*

	APV-low	APV-high	Total
Number enrolled (%)	291 (14)	1,759 (86)	2,050 (100)
Male (%)	156 (8)	934 (46)	1,090 (53)
Female (%)	135 (7)	825 (40)	960 (47)
Number (%) received first dose	291 (14)	1,757 (86)	2,048 (99.9)
Second dose	286 (14)	1,716 (84)	2,002 (98)
Third dose	277 (14)	1,684 (82)	1,961 (96)
Mean age (weeks) at first dose (SD)	9.3 (0.97)	9.3 (1.02)	9.3 (1.01)
Second dose (SD)	18.4 (1.40)	18.4 (1.36)	18.4 (1.37)
Third dose (SD)	27.6 (1.89)	27.5 (1.81)	27.6 (1.82)

Table II. *Proportion (%) of participants reporting an adverse event in the 14 days after immunization at 2, 4, and 6 months of age with 1 of 2 formulations of a 5-component acellular pertussis vaccine*

	2 Months			4 Months			6 Months		
Reaction	APV-low ($n = 291$)	APV-high ($n = 1,757$)	Relative risk (95% CI)[a]	APV-low ($n = 286$)	APV-high ($n = 1,716$)	Relative risk (95% CI)	APV-low ($n = 277$)	APV-high ($n = 1,684$)	Relative risk (95% CI)
Any local reaction	12	15	0.8 (0.6, 1.2)	18	22	0.8 (0.6, 1.1)	16	20	0.8 (0.6, 1.1)
Redness	4	6	0.7 (0.4, 1.3)	12	15	0.8 (0.5, 1.1)	12	16	0.8 (0.5, 1.1)
Swelling	4	4	1.0 (0.5, 2.0)	6	8	0.8 (0.5, 1.3)	5	7	0.7 (0.4, 1.2)
Tenderness	8	9	0.9 (0.6, 1.4)	8	7	1.1 (0.7, 1.7)	5	5	0.9 (0.5, 1.6)
Any systemic reaction	84	84	1.0 (0.9, 1.1)	82	78	1.0 (0.9, 1.2)	74	78	0.9 (0.8, 1.1)
Fever	40	41	1.0 (0.8, 1.2)	39	40	1.0 (0.8, 1.2)	44	44	1.0 (0.8, 1.2)
Irritability	53	52	1.0 (0.9, 1.2)	55	51	1.1 (0.9, 1.3)	50	52	0.9 (0.8, 1.1)
Crying	37	34	1.1 (0.9, 1.4)	33	31	1.1 (0.9, 1.3)	27	30	0.9 (0.7, 1.2)
Decreased activity	32	31	1.0 (0.8, 1.3)	18	18	1.0 (0.7, 1.3)	14	16	0.9 (0.6, 1.2)
Decreased feeding	30	29	1.0 (0.8, 1.3)	27	24	1.1 (0.9, 1.5)	27	26	1.0 (0.8, 1.3)
Vomiting	16	16	1.0 (0.8, 1.4)	14	12	1.2 (0.8, 1.7)	15	14	1.1 (0.8, 1.5)
Diarrhea	25	25	1.0 (0.8, 1.3)	21	20	1.0 (0.8, 1.3)	22	20	1.1 (0.8, 1.5)
Any reaction	85	85	1.0 (0.9, 1.1)	84	81	1.0 (0.9, 1.2)	79	81	1.0 (0.8, 1.1)

[a] CI = confidence interval. Intervals that do not include 1.0 are statistically significant.

APV-low and APV-high. Response rates for the telephone interviews at 2, 4, and 6 months were 99%, 97%, and 97% respectively. The corresponding response rates for diary completion were 90%, 89%, and 87%. Altogether, 89 infants were withdrawn from the study. Data from participants withdrawn from the study was included in the analysis until the time of withdrawal or exclusion. An adverse event was the cause of withdrawal in 13 participants, including Sudden Infant Death Syndrome (2 cases), hypotonic/hyporesponsive episode (2), high-pitched unusual cry (8), and prolonged cry (1). These and other severe adverse events which did not lead to withdrawal are described in greater detail below. Other reasons for withdrawal included parental request (30), sponsor request (1), family relocation or inability to contact or schedule (26) and medical conditions necessitating delay in immunization (6). Protocol violations accounted for an additional 13 exclusions to analysis including immunization with the wrong vaccine formulation or with a non-study vaccine (DTP).

Clinical reactions

An adverse reaction was reported by most participants. Overall, 85% of both APV-low and APV-high recipients reported an adverse event during the 2 weeks after the 2-month immunization, 84% and 81% respectively after the 4-month dose, and 79% and 81% respectively after the 6-month dose. At 2 months, local reactions were reported in 12% of APV-low and 15% of APV-high recipients; systemic reactions were reported in 84% of each group. After the 4-month dose, local reactions were reported in 18% of APV-low and 22% of APV-high recipients, while general reactions were reported in 82% and 78% respectively. After the third dose at 6 months, local reactions were reported in 16% of APV-low and 20% of APV-high vaccines; systemic reactions occurred in 74% and 78% respectively. None of the differences observed was statistically significant.

No differences between the 2 formulations were detected for any of the individual adverse reactions monitored after any dose (Table II). Nor were any differences found when adverse events were analysed by observation period after immunization (early: 0 to 48 h; late: 48 h to 14 days; overall: 0–14 days). Irritability was the most commonly reported reaction, reported after approximately half of the immunizations. Fever was reported after 39–44% of vaccine doses, although only 21–26% of recipients reported fever in the first 48 h after immunization. The data were also analysed for 'clinically significant' adverse reactions defined as measured local reactions ≥ 10 mm, fever ≥ 37.8°C (axillary), persistent crying >1 h, and irritability, decreased activity, anorexia, vomiting, diarrhea of at least moderate severity as elicited via the structured questionnaire. No differences were detected between the 2 vaccine formulations (Table III). Irritability (12–17%) after all 3 doses and fever after the third dose (17–18%) were the most commonly reported events.

Adverse reactions described as severe were reported by 5% of each group at 2 months, 5% of APV-low and 4% of APV-high recipients at 4 months, and 4% of both groups at 6 months (severe was defined as measured reactions

Table III. *Proportion (%) of participants reporting a 'clinically significant' adverse event in the 14 days after immunization at 2, 4, and 6 months of age with 1 of 2 formulations of a 5-component acellular pertussis vaccine*

	2 Months			4 Months			6 Months		
Reaction	APV-low ($n = 291$)	APV-high ($n = 1{,}757$)	Relative risk (95% CI)[a]	APV-low ($n = 286$)	APV-high ($n = 1{,}716$)	Relative risk (95% CI)	APV-low ($n = 277$)	APV-high ($n = 1{,}684$)	Relative risk (95% CI)
Any local reaction	4	3	1.2 (0.6, 2.2)	6	6	1.1 (0.7, 1.8)	3	4	0.7 (0.4, 1.5)
Redness	2	1	1.5 (0.6, 3.6)	5	4	1.3 (0.7, 2.3)	3	3	1.1 (0.5, 2.1)
Swelling	2	1	1.8 (0.7, 4.8)	4	3	1.4 (0.7, 2.8)	1	2	0.8 (0.3, 2.1)
Tenderness	2	1	1.3 (0.6, 3.3)	1	1	0.9 (0.3, 3.0)	1	1	1.1 (0.2, 5.1)
Any systemic reaction	34	32	1.1 (0.8, 1.3)	28	28	1.0 (0.8, 1.2)	30	31	1.0 (0.8, 1.2)
Fever	7	7	1.0 (0.6, 1.5)	8	12	0.7 (0.5, 1.1)	17	18	0.9 (0.7, 1.3)
Irritability	17	15	1.2 (0.9, 1.6)	15	13	1.2 (0.8, 1.6)	14	12	1.1 (0.8, 1.6)
Crying	7	8	0.9 (0.6, 1.4)	8	6	1.2 (0.8, 1.9)	5	6	0.9 (0.5, 1.6)
Decreased activity	9	8	1.2 (0.8, 1.8)	2	3	0.9 (0.4, 1.9)	4	3	1.4 (0.7, 2.8)
Decreased feeding	7	7	1.0 (0.6, 1.6)	4	4	0.9 (0.5, 1.7)	6	6	1.0 (0.6, 1.6)
Vomiting	2	2	1.3 (0.5, 3.1)	1	2	0.7 (0.2, 1.9)	3	2	1.4 (0.7, 2.9)
Diarrhea	7	6	1.2 (0.7, 1.8)	5	5	1.0 (0.5, 1.8)	5	5	1.0 (0.6, 1.7)
Any reaction	35	33	1.1 (0.9, 1.3)	32	32	1.0 (0.8, 1.2)	34	33	1.0 (0.8, 1.3)

[a] CI = confidence intervals. Intervals that do not include 1.0 are statistically significant.

≥35 mm, fever ≥40°C, persistent crying >3 h, other reactions graded by the parent as severe). Severely decreased activity at 2 months in 3% of APV-low and 2% of APV-high, and severe irritability in 2% of both vaccine groups at 4 and 6 months were the only severe reactions that exceeded a 1% rate. Fever ≥40°C occurred after 6/5,157 APV-high doses (0.12%) and 2/854 APV-low doses (0.23%), persistent crying ≥3 h after 4 (0.078%) APV-high and 3 (0.35%) APV-low doses, and high pitched cry after 9 (0.17%) APV-high and 2 (0.23%) APV-low doses. None of these differences was statistically significant. No seizures were reported after either vaccine formulation.

Hypotonic/hyporesponsive episodes were reported after 2/5,157 APV-high immunizations (0.039%) and 0/854 APV-low doses; both were reported after the 2-month dose. The episode in 1 child was described as a 10-min period of unresponsiveness and limpness without color change which occurred 7 h post-immunization. The participant also had fever (maximum 39.5°C), crying for $4\frac{1}{2}$ h, and fussiness, tenderness, anorexia, and decreased activity all described as severe. The child was assessed by a physician after the episode, but no abnormalities were found. The event was thought by the Health Department to be a contra-indication to further immunization. The second child reporting a hypotonic/hyporesponsive episode had a 10-min period of paleness and limpness 20 h post-immunization. Fever or other associated adverse events were not reported, except to note that the child had symptoms of an upper respiratory infection at the time of immunization. The child was not assessed by a physician and recovered uneventfully.

Adverse reactions were also analysed by time of onset (data not shown); early reactions were those reported in the first 48 h post immunization, while late reactions were collected at the 7 and 14 day contacts. Most local reactions were reported in the first 48 h; the rate of late local reactions did not exceed 3% after any dose. In contrast, late systemic sympoms were often reported, although less frequently than during the early observation period. Irritability, decreased activity, decreased feeding, and crying were more often reported in the first 48 h after the 2-month immunization, irritability, decreased feeding, and crying were reported more commonly in the first 48 h after the second dose, and decreased activity more commonly in the first 48 h after the third dose. No adverse reaction was more commonly reported in the late observation period.

Antipyretic use was variable among the study centers and reflected local custom on use of prophylactic acetaminophen. Most antipyretic use occurred in the first 24 h after immunization and was primarily for fever prevention. Prophylactic acetaminophen use was more common in Canada, ranging between 28 and 52% in Halifax and Peterborough and 90–100% in Calgary and Fraser Valley. In the USA, prophylactic acetaminophen use ranged from 3.4–1.5% in Atlanta (first dose to third dose) to 32–22% in Vancouver, Washington. Overall, prophylactic acetaminophen was used with 77%, 76%, and 71% of the first, second, and third doses respectively in Canada, compared with 20%, 14%, and 10% of doses in the USA ($p < 0.00001$ for each dose). No differences in antipyretic use were detected between recipients of the 2 vaccine formulations.

Table IV. *Antibody response in infants immunized at 2, 4, and 6 months of age with 1 of 2 formulations of a 5-component acellular pertussis vaccine*

		2 Months		6 Months		7 Months	
Test[a]	Vaccine	SS[b]	GM[c] (95% CI)[d]	SS	GM (95% CI)	SS	GM (95% CI)
PT	APV-low	41	14.3 (10.9, 18.8)	42	41.6 (33.8, 51.2)	42	105.1 (85.3, 129.4)
	APV-high	242	15.9 (14.4, 17.6)	249	46.0 (42.6, 49.6)	250	101.6 (94.1, 109.7)
CHO	APV-low	37	8.2 (5.8, 11.7)	42	13.3 (9.7, 18.4)	42	66.9 (48.9, 91.4)
	APV-high	236	9.4 (8.0, 11.1)	249	17.6 (15.5, 19.9)	250	68.7 (60.2, 78.4)
FHA	APV-low	40	4.5 (3.4, 6.1)	42	45.9 (35.1, 60.0)***	42	82.5 (63.5, 107.0)***
	APV-high	246	5.5 (4.7, 6.3)	249	89.2 (81.8, 97.4)	250	163.9 (152.1, 176.5)
69k	APV-low	41	1.5 (1.1, 2.0)*	42	8.7 (6.0, 12.6)	42	71.1 (53.9, 93.8)
	APV-high	243	2.1 (1.8, 2.4)	249	10.7 (9.2, 12.4)	250	87.6 (78.0, 98.3)
FIM	APV-low	41	10.8 (7.2, 16.2)	42	78.1 (54.8, 111.4)**	42	358.6 (283.1, 454.1)***
	APV-high	244	11.7 (10.0, 13.7)	249	45.6 (38.8, 53.6)	250	220.6 (191.0, 254.7)
AGG	APV-low	42	19.5 (12.9, 29.4)	42	57.0 (39.1, 83.2)	42	307.0 (227.8, 413.6)*
	APV-high	249	22.7 (19.4, 26.6)	249	46.6 (40.4, 53.8)	250	219.2 (192.6, 249.4)
DIP	APV-low	42	0.027 (0.016, 0.048)**	42	0.049 (0.035, 0.069)	42	0.331 (0.221, 0.496)
	APV-high	249	0.012 (0.009, 0.015)	249	0.059 (0.050, 0.068)	250	0.375 (0.323, 0.435)
TET	APV-low	42	0.048 (0.027, 0.084)	42	0.371 (0.245, 0.562)	42	1.956 (1.566, 2.442)
	APV-high	249	0.031 (0.026, 0.039)	249	0.436 (0.378, 0.503)	250	1.793 (1.643, 1.956)

[a] See text for abbreviations.
[b] Sample size.
[c] Geometric Mean; PT, FHA, 69k, and FIM in elisa units; CHO and AGG in reciprocal dilution; DIP and TET in international units/ml.
[d] 95% Confidence interval.
*$p < 0.05$, **$p < 0.01$, ***$p < 0.001$.

The differences detected in antipyretic use in the USA and Canada had no effect on the reported incidence of fever. In Canada, fever was reported by 27, 22, and 23% of APV-high participants in the first 48 h after the 2, 4, and 6 month doses, compared with 24, 25, and 24% respectively in American APV-high recipients. Similar results were demonstrated with the APV-low vaccine and for other observation periods. Differences in fever reports were also not detected when centers rarely using antipyretic prophylaxis were compared with centers using frequent prophylaxis (e.g. Atlanta and Calgary, respectively).

The effect of intercurrent respiratory infection and other infections at the time of immunization on the rates of reported adverse events were explored by stratifying participants for the reported presence or absence of a respiratory infection or use of an antimicrobial agent or remedy for common cold. Participants with an intercurrent infection were more likely to have a general reaction and a clinically significant general reaction. In the first 24 h after the 2-month immunization, 72% of APV-high recipients with infection reported a general adverse reaction, compared with 59% of uninfected APV-high recipients ($p = 0.003$) and a significant general reaction in 18% of infected compared with 13% of uninfected APV-high recipients ($p < 0.03$). Similarly, 80% of infected APV-low participants reported a general reaction, compared with 58% of uninfected vaccines ($p = 0.008$); clinically significant general reactions were reported by 30% and 12% of infected and uninfected APV-low recipients respectively ($p = 0.002$). Similar differences between infected and non-infected participants were demonstrated for the 4 and 6 month immunizations and for the 2, 7, and 14 day observation periods.

Antibody response

A significant increase in antibody titer was elicited in both vaccine groups for all antigens tested (Table IV). Pre-immunization antibody titers were equivalent except for higher anti-69k antibody in the APV-high group and higher anti-DIP antibody in the APV-low group. APV-high elicited higher antibody titers against FHA after the second and third dose. Anti-FIM and agglutinin antibody titers were higher in the APV-low group. Despite the higher PT content in the APV-high vaccine, no differences were detected between APV-low and APV-high recipients in anti-PT antibody measured by enzyme immunoassay or CHO neutralization.

The mean fold antibody rise (ratio of the 7-month antibody titer to the minimum of the 2 or 6 month titer) did not differ between the vaccine groups for anti-PT antibody by enzyme immunoassay or CHO neutralization or for anti-FIM, anti-TET, or agglutinin antibodies. A higher mean fold rise in anti-FHA antibody was found after APV-high (61.7 vs. 40.0; $p < 0.05$) and anti-DIP antibody (188.9 vs. 92.3; $p < 0.05$). The proportion of participants achieving 4-fold or greater rises in antibody titer was similar for all antigens, ranging from 64.3% in APV-low and 68% in APV-high recipients for anti-PT antibody by enzyme immunoassay to 92.9% and 95.6% respectively for

Table V. *Mean antibody increase and proportion of participants exceeding a 4-fold antibody increase or selected antibody titers after immunization at 2, 4, and 6 months of age with 1 of 2 formulations of a 5-component acellular pertussis vaccine*

			Antibody increase		Proportion (95% confidence interval) exceeding selected antibody titers		
Test[a]	Vaccine	SS[b]	Mean (SD)	Proportion 4-fold or greater (95% confidence interval)	Titer	After two doses	After three doses
PT	APV-low	42	20.2 (63.5)	64 (48, 78)	50	50 (34, 66)	93 (81, 99)
	APV-high	250[c]	10.3 (14.0)	68 (62, 74)	50	42 (36, 48)	88 (84, 92)
CHO	APV-low	42	17.9 (21.1)	69 (53, 82)	32	36 (22, 52)	81 (66, 91)
	APV-high	250[c]	24.7 (49.8)	70 (64, 75)	32	37 (31, 44)	86 (81, 90)
FHA	APV-low	42	40.0 (65.4)	86 (72, 95)	50	55 (39, 70)	83 (69, 93)
	APV-high	250[c]	61.7 (78.0)*	92 (87, 95)	50	83 (78, 88)***	96 (93, 98)**
69 kD	APV-low	42	116.8 (131.6)	93 (81, 99)	50	7 (2, 20)	69 (53, 82)
	APV-high	250[c]	111.8 (172.9)	96 (92, 98)	50	9 (6, 14)	74 (69, 80)
Fimbriae	APV-low	42	121.2 (227.6)	93 (81, 99)	50	71 (55, 84)	100 (92, 100)
	APV-high	250[c]	78.6 (157.2)	88 (83, 91)	50	51 (44, 57)*	90 (85, 93)*
Agglutinins	APV-low	42	86.5 (154.7)	81 (66, 91)	64	62 (46, 76)	98 (87, 100)
	APV-high	250[c]	37.9 (75.2)	78 (72, 83)	64	51 (44, 57)	93 (89, 96)
Diphtheria	APV-low	42	92.3 (184.4)	81 (66, 91)	0.01	95 (84, 99)	100 (92, 100)
	APV-high	250[c]	188.9 (563.0)*	88 (84, 92)	0.01	97 (94, 99)	100 (99, 100)
	APV-low	42	–	–	0.1	21 (10, 37)	83 (69, 93)
	APV-high	250[c]	–	–	0.1	28 (23, 34)	86 (82, 90)
Tetanus	APV-low	42	259.3 (446.9)	98 (87, 100)	0.01	98 (87, 100)	100 (92, 100)
	APV-high	250[c]	242.1 (367.5)	98 (95, 99)	0.01	100 (99, 100)	100 (99, 100)
					0.1	93 (81, 99)	100 (92, 100)
					0.1	89 (85, 93)	100 (99, 100)

[a] See text for abbreviations.
[b] Sample size.
[c] Except for 6 months analysis for which 249 sera were available.
$*p < 0.05$, $**p < 0.01$, $***p < 0.001$.

anti-69k antibody and 97.6% for anti-TET antibody (Table V).

After the third immunization, all participants had achieved minimum protective levels of anti-TET and anti-DIP antibodies (0.01 IU/ml) (Table V). Protective antibody levels have not been established for the pertussis antigens. There were no differences in the proportion of participants achieving arbitrarily selected antibody levels.

DISCUSSION

The acellular pertussis vaccine studied here contains more antigenic components than other products currently being evaluated. The results of this study with 2 formulations of this vaccine indicated the vaccine to be well tolerated by infants receiving their primary immunization series and that reactogenicity was not increased by doubling the quantity of PT and quadrupling the FHA content. The data derived from the large sample size of this study supports the results of earlier studies and provides additional data on the infrequency of the less commonly reported adverse effects with acellular vaccines. The low rates of fever with acellular pertussis vaccines have implications for the recommendation to administer prophylactic acetaminophen with immunization. Despite the more widespread use of prophylactic and therapeutic acetaminophen in Canada, there was no differences in the rates of fever reported. Furthermore, stratification of participants by the presence of an underlying respiratory infection provided data that a substantial proportion of adverse reactions attributed to immunization do in fact reflect the symptoms of the underlying infection.

Crying persisting >3 h was reported for 0.12% of the recipients of acellular pertussis vaccine. This compares favorably with the 1.1% rate reported after whole-cell pertussis vaccine (25). In contrast, similar rates of 'unusual crying' were reported in these recipients (0.18%) and whole-cell recipients (0.2%) (25). However, these reactions are not considered to be of pathological significance but rather a response to pain in these young infants (26). In Canada, persistent crying and unusual crying are no longer considered contra-indications to further pertussis immunization (27).

Hypotonic/hyporesponsive episodes describe an infant who becomes pale, lethargic, hypotonic, and unresponsive to the environment. The pathophysiologic mechanism of these events is not known but has been associated with diphtheria-pertussis-tetanus immunization. A recent report by the Institute of Medicine (28) concluded that the evidence was consistent with a causal relationship of diphtheria-pertussis-tetanus vaccine with hypotonic/hyporesponsive episodes but not specifically with the pertussis component. In fact, a meta-analysis performed by the committee suggested no difference in relative risk in recipients of diphtheria-tetanus-pertussis and diphtheria-tetanus vaccines. Hypotonic/hyporesponsive episodes have also been reported after acellular pertussis vaccines (29).

The optimal composition of an acellular pertussis vaccine is not known. PT is a constituent of virtually all acellular products available or under evaluation. PT is an important virulence factor of Bordetella pertussis and induces protective antibody in animal models (6, 7). FHA, another protective antigen in animal models (7), is the second antigen most commonly included in acellular vaccines. In Sweden (10), a vaccine composed of equal quantities of PT and FHA and a monocomponent PT vaccine both proved efficacious. More recently, there has been increasing interest in fimbrial antigens as a potentially useful addition to multicomponent acellular pertussis vaccines. Fimbriae 2 and 3 have been purified and proved protective in an animal model (12, 13). These antigens, also known as agglutinogens, correlate well with the agglutinating antibodies demonstrated to be the best predictors of immunity in vaccinated populations (30). Another agglutinogen, the 69k membrane protein, is protective in a mouse respiratory model of pertussis (11, 14, 15). It is similar to the 70kD protein of B. parapertussis and the 68kD protein of B. bronchiseptica; this latter protein has been used in a vaccine to protect piglets from atrophic rhinitis (31, 32).

Although other acellular vaccines contain one or more of these antigens, this is the only vaccine to contain all of the antigens in substantial quantities. At least 6 acellular products are currently in use in Japan (33). These products have been designated "B type" vaccines which contain roughly equal quantities of PT and FHA, and "T type" vaccines which are predominantly FHA vaccines with some PT and small amounts of fimbriae and 69k protein (3). Two vaccines are currently available in the USA for the booster doses (34, 35); one is the Biken vaccine marketed by Connaught Laboratories Inc. which contains PT and FHA in equal quantities (23.4 μg protein content each). The other acellular product, the Takeda vaccine marketed by Lederle Laboratories is composed of approximately 35 μg FHA, 3 μg PT, 0.7 μg fimbriae, and 4 μg 69k protein (19). This latter vaccine has the antigens in fixed quantities as a result of the co-purification method.

The 'modular' nature of the vaccine evaluated in this study in which individual components are purified and combined in the later stages of manufacture enables modification of the formulation based on the immune response and the potential identification of serologic correlates of immunity in ongoing studies. The antibody response to PT and FHA (20) in the original formulation (APV-low) which contained 10 μg PT and 5 μ FHA was lower than found after immunization with several other candidate acellular pertussis vaccines (36). Others have found improved antibody response by increasing PT content from 10 μg to 50 μg (37–39). In previous studies with APV-low and APV-high, increased immunogenicity to PT and FHA was shown in 2–6-month-old infants after a 3-dose series (21). In this study, an augmented immune response to FHA was demonstrated, but not to PT. An increased anti-PT antibody response measured by both CHO neutralization and enzyme immunoassay in APV-low recipients in this study, compared with the previous study, is the major factor accounting for the discrepant results. These differences could not be explained by differences in either the measurement of antigen content in the vaccines or the antibody assay; assay methods were not changed between studies. For the PT enzyme immunoassay, identical control sera assayed were consistent during each study. In addition, the differences in the anti-PT response between studies was found by both enzyme immunoassay and CHO neutralization. The complexity of the immune response is further demonstrated by the higher anti-fimbriae antibodies and agglutinin titers achieved in recipients of the vaccine with lower PT and FHA content, despite the identical content of fimbriae. The role of FHA or PT and FHA in interfering with the antibody response to other antigens needs further exploration.

This study demonstrated that the 5-component pertussis vaccine studied was safe and immunogenic in these 2–6-month-old children. No increased toxicity was demonstrated with increased antigen content in the acellular vaccine formulations. The APV-low vaccine formulation was part of the first phase of the second efficacy study in Sweden. Based on these data, the APV-high formulation was included in the second phase of the study. Upon completion of these studies it may be possible to make decisions on the optimal formulation of acellular pertussis vaccines, based on efficacy as well as on safety and immunogenicity data.

ACKNOWLEDGMENTS

We thank Kate Nunn and the staff of the Clinical Trials Research Center–Infectious Diseases at the IWK Children's Hospital, John Thipphawong, Sharon Wiltsey, William Schaart, Joan Bevilacqua, and Linda Young of Connaught Laboratories Ltd., Philip Hosbach, Linda Petro, and Robert Klepadlo of Connaught Laboratories Inc, and the collaborating physicians and staff at the following field sites for their indispensable assistance in performing these studies: Emory University, North Fulton Pediatrics, North Atlanta Pediatrics, Northlake Pediatrics, Lawrenceville Pediatrics, Shivers, Garner, Barfield and Wiskind, and Snapfinger Woods Pediatrics Associates in Atlanta, Georgia; Calgary Health Services in Calgary, Alberta; The Associated Study Center in the Fraser Valley Region, British Columbia; Dartmouth Medical Centre, Woodlawn Medical Clinic, Dalhousie University Health Services, Family Practice Associates, Fairview Medical Group, Quinpool Family Medicine Center, Forest Hills Medical Clinic, Albro Lake Medical Clinic, Family Health Group, Cobequid Family Practice, Sackville Medical Clinic and Sunnyside Family Practice in Nova Scotia; The Vaccine Study Center in Montreal, Quebec; The Peterborough

County–City Health Unit in Peterborough, Ontario; Pittsburgh Pediatric Research Inc. in Pittsburgh, Pennsylvania; and the Vancouver Clinic in Vancouver, Washington.

Dr Eastwood is supported by a grant from the National Science and Engineering Council of Canada.

REFERENCES

1. Centers for Disease Control. Summary of notifiable diseases, United States, 1991. MMWR 40: 35–36, 57–63, 1991.
2. Varughese P. Incidence of pertussis in Canada. Can Med Assoc J 132: 1041–1042, 1985.
3. Cherry JD, Brunell PA, Golden GS, Karzon DT. Report of the task force on pertussis and pertussis immunization – 1988. Pediatrics 81 (suppl): 939–984, 1988.
4. Cherry JD. The epidemiology of pertussis and pertussis immunization in the United States: a comparative study. Curr Probl Pediatr 14: 1–78, 1984.
5. Romanus V, Jonsell R, Bergquist SO. Pertussis in Sweden after the cessation of general immunization in 1979. Pediatr Infect Dis J 6: 364–371, 1987.
6. Sato H, Sato Y. Bordetella pertussis infection in mice: correlation of specific antibodies against two antigens, pertussis toxin, and filamentous hemagglutinin with mouse protectivity in an intracerebral or aerosol challenge system. Infect Immun 46: 415–421, 1984.
7. Oda M, Cowell JL, Burstyn DG, Manclark CR. Protective activities of the filamentous hemagglutinin and the lymphocytosis-promoting factor of Bordetella pertussis in mice. J Infect Dis 150: 823–833, 1984.
8. Aoyama T, Murase Y, Kato M, Iwai H, Iwata T. Efficacy and immunogenicity of acellular pertussis vaccine by manufacturer and patient age. Am J Dis Child 143: 655–659, 1989.
9. Mortimer EA Jr, Kimura M, Cherry JD, Kuno-Sakai H, Stout MG, Dekker CL, Hayashi R, Miyamoto Y, Scott JV, Aoyama T, Isomura S, Iwata T, Kamiya H, Kato T, Noya J, Suzuki E, Takeuchi Y, Yamaoka H. Protective efficacy of the Takeda acellular pertussis vaccine combined with diphtheria and tetanus toxoids following household exposure of Japanese children. Am J Dis Child 144: 899–904, 1990.
10. Ad Hoc Group for the Study of Pertussis Vaccines. Placebo-controlled trial of two acellular pertussis vaccines in Sweden – protective efficacy and adverse events. Lancet i: 955–960, 1988.
11. Brennan MJ, Li ZM, Cowell JL, Bisher ME, Steven AC, Novotny P, Manclark CR. Identification of a 69-kilodalton nonfimbrial protein as an agglutinogen of Bordetella pertussis. Infect Immun 56: 3189–3195, 1988.
12. Zhang JM, Cowell JL, Steven AC, Carter PH, McGrath PP, Manclark CR. Purification and characterization of fimbriae isolated from Bordetella pertussis. Infect Immun 48: 422–427, 1985.
13. Li ZM, Brennan MJ, David JL, Carter PH, Cowell JL, Manclark CR. Comparison of type 2 and type 6 fimbriae of Bordetella pertussis by using agglutinating monoclonal antibodies. Infect Immun 56: 3184–3188, 1988.
14. Shahin RD, Brennan MJ, Li ZM, Meade BD, Manclark CR. Characterization of the protective capacity and immunogenicity of the 69-kD outer membrane protein of Bordetella pertussis. J Exp Med 171: 63–73, 1990.
15. Roberts M, Tite JP, Fairweather NF, Dougan G, Charles IG. Recombinant P.69/pertactin: immunogenicity and protection of mice against Bordetella pertussis infection. Vaccine 10: 43–48, 1992.
16. Podda A, Nencioni L, Marsili I, Peppoloni S, Volpini G, Donati D, Di Tommaso A, De Magistris MT, Rappuoli R. Phase I clinical trial of an acellular pertussis vaccine composed of genetically detoxified pertussis toxin combined with FHA and 69 kDa. Vaccine 9: 741–745, 1991.
17. Miller E, Ashworth LAE, Robinson A, Waight PA, Irons LI. Phase II trial of whole-cell pertussis vaccine vs an acellular vaccine containing agglutinogens. Lancet 337: 70–73, 1991.
18. Glode M, Joffe L, The Children's Medical Center, Reisinger K, Blatter M, Plotkin S, Watson B, Grossman L, Pennridge Pediatric Associates, Asmar B, Berry M, Starobin S, Fisch G, Hackell JG, Sheip B, McKee B. Safety and immunogenicity of acellular pertussis vaccine combined with diphtheria and tetanus toxoids in 17- to 24-month-old children. Pediatr Infect Dis J 11: 530–535, 1992.
19. Blumberg DA, Mink CM, Cherry JD, Johnson C, Garber R, Plotkin SA, Watson B, Ballanco GA, Daum RS, Sullivan B, Townsend TR, Brayton J, Gooch WM III, Nelson DB, Congeni BL, Prober CG, Hackell JG, Dekker CL, Christenson PD, APDT Vaccine Study Group. Comparison of acellular and whole-cell pertussis-component diphtheria-tetanus-petussis vaccines in infants. J Pediatr 119: 194–204, 1991.
20. Halperin SA, Barreto L, Friesen B, Meekison W. Immunogenicity of a five-component acellular pertussis vaccine in infants and young children. Arch Pediatr Adolesc Med 148: 495–502, 1994.
21. Halperin SA, Barreto L, Eastwood BJ, Law B, Roberts EA. Safety and immunogenicity of a five-component acellular pertussis vaccine with varying antigen quantities. Arch Pediatr Adolesc Med 148: 1220–1224, 1994.
22. Manclark CR, Meade BD, Burstyn DG. Serological response to Bordetella pertussis. In: Rose NR, Friedman H, Fahey JL, eds. Manual of Clinical Laboratory Immunology, 3rd edn. Washington, DC: American Society for Microbiology, 388–394, 1986.
23. Gillenius P, Jäätmaa E, Askelöf P, Granström M, Tiru M. The standardization of an assay for pertussis toxin and antitoxin in microplate culture of Chinese hamster ovary cells. J Biol Stand 13: 61–66, 1984.
24. Breslow NE, Day NE. Statistical Methods in Cancer Research, vol. II. The Design and Analysis of Cohort Studies. Lyons, France: International Agency for Research on Cancer, 108–113, 1987.
25. Cody CL, Baraff LJ, Cherry JD, Marcy SM, Manclark CR. Nature and rates of adverse reactions associated with DTP and DT immunizations in infants and children. Pediatrics 68: 650–660, 1981.
26. Long SS, Deforest A, Pennridge Pediatric Associates, Smith DG, Lazaro C, Wassilak SGF. Longitudinal study of adverse reactions following diphtheria-tetanus-pertussis vaccine in infancy. Pediatrics 85: 294–302, 1990.
27. National Advisory Committee on Immunization (NACI). Statement on pertussis immunization. Can Commun Dis Rep 19: 41–45, 1993.
28. Committee to Review the Adverse Consequences of Pertussis and Rubella Vaccines. Shock and "unsual shock-like state" with hypotonicity, hyporesponsiveness, and short-lived convulsions, usually febrile. In: Howson CP, Howe CJ, Fineberg HV, eds. Adverse Effects of Pertussis and Rubella Vaccines. Washington, DC: National Academy Press, 171–177, 1991.
29. Blumberg DA, Mink CM, Lewis K, Chatfield P, Leach C, Smith LP, Christenson PD, Guravita L, Steinfeld MBJ, March SM, Levin SR, Baraff LJ, Schonfeld N, Cherry JD. Pathophysiology of reactions associated with pertussis vaccine. Dev Biol Stand 73: 289–295, 1990.
30. Medical Research Council. The prevention of whooping cough by vaccination. BMJ 1: 1463–1471, 1951.
31. Novotny P, Kobisch M, Cownley K, Chubb AP, Montaraz JA. Evaluation of Bordetella bronchiseptica vaccines in spe-

cific-pathogen-free piglets with bacterial cell surface antigen in enzyme-linked immunosorbent assay. Infect Immun 50: 190–198, 1985.
32. Kobisch M, Novotny P. Identification of a 68-kilodalton outer membrane protein as the major protective antigen of Bordetella bronchiseptica by using specific-pathogen-free piglets. Infect Immun 58: 352–357, 1990.
33. Moxon ER, Rappuoli R. Haemophilus influenzae infections and whooping cough. Lancet 335: 1324–1329, 1990.
34. Centers for Disease Control. Pertussis vaccination: acellular pertussis vaccine for reinforcing and booster use – supplementary ACIP statement. Recommendations of the Immunization Practices Advisory Committee (ACIP). MMWR 41 (No. RR-1): 1–10, 1992.
35. Committee on Infectious Diseases – American Academy of Pediatrics. Acellular pertussis vaccines: recommendations for use as the fourth and fifth doses. Pediatrics 90: 121–123, 1992.
36. Englund JA, Decker MD, Edwards KM, Pichichero ME, Steinhoff MC, Anderson EL. Acellular and whole-cell pertussis vaccines as booster doses: a multicenter study. Pediatrics 93: 37–43, 1994.
37. Sekura RD, Zhang Y, Roberson R, Acton B, Trollfors B, Tolson N, Shiloach J, Bryla D, Muir-Nash J, Koeller D, Schneerson R, Robbins JB. Clinical, metabolic, and antibody responses of adult volunteers to an investigational vaccine composed of pertussis toxin inactivated by hydrogen peroxide. J Pediatr 113: 806–813, 1988.
38. Krantz I, Sekura R, Trollfors B, Taranger J, Zackrisson G, Lagergård T, Schneerson R, Robbins J. Immunogenicity and safety of a pertussis vaccine composed of pertussis toxin inactivated by hydrogen peroxide, in 18- to 23-month-old children. J Pediatr 116: 539–543, 1990.
39. Siber GR, Thakrar N, Yancey BA, Herzog L, Todd C, Cohen N, Sekura RD, Lowe CU. Safety and immunogenicity of hydrogen peroxide-inactivated pertussis toxoid in 18-month-old children. Vaccine 9: 735–740, 1991.

Submitted September 1, 1994; accepted February 2, 1995

Scand J Infect Dis 27: 289–290, 1995 CASE REPORT

Actinobacillus actinomycetemcomitans Pneumonia with Chest Wall and Subphrenic Abscess

AN-CHYI CHEN[1], CHING-CHUAN LIU[1], WEI-JEN YAO[2], CHUN-TA CHEN[1] and JIU-YAO WANG[1]

From the Departments of [1]Pediatrics and [2]Nuclear Medicine, National Cheng Kung University Medical College and Hospital, Tainan, Taiwan

A 14-year-old girl had progressive dyspnea and right lower chest pain for about $1\frac{1}{2}$ months and a weight loss of 3 kg in 2 months. Chest X-ray revealed right pleural effusion and a round infiltration over the right lower chest, initially suspected to be malignant. Image study revealed consolidation in the right middle and lower lobes with abscess-like lesions around the right lower pleura and transdiaphrenic involvement to the subphrenic region. The lesion had also invaded the intercostal muscle. The pleural abscess was obtained by fiberoptic thoracoscopy, and culture of the pus grew typical colonies of Actinobacillus actinomycetemcomitans. After the causative microorganism had been identified, cefoxitin was given for 2 weeks followed by oral amoxicillin (250 mg/6 h) for a total period of 3 months. Follow-up chest X-ray revealed resolution of the lung lesions and the patient recovered gradually without any sequelae.

Ching-Chuan Liu, MD, Department of Pediatrics, National Cheng Kung University Hospital, 138, Sheng Li Road, Tainan, Taiwan 70428

INTRODUCTION

Actinobacillus actinomycetemcomitans is a slow-growing, capnophilic Gram-negative coccobacillus (1), which can cause endocarditis, soft tissue infection, and periodontitis. Reports of A. actinomycetemcomitans pneumonia were rare in the past, only 5 being found in the English literature before 1993 (2–5). Only one of them, an elderly woman with diabetes mellitus, had additional chest wall involvement and rib destruction (5).

We describe a case of A. actinomycetemcomitans pneumonia complicated by chest wall and transphrenic abscess formation in a previously healthy adolescent female.

CASE REPORT

A 14-year-old girl presented with progressing dyspnea and right lower chest pain for about $1\frac{1}{2}$ months. She had previously been in good health. Initially, she suffered from productive cough with yellowish sputum, then exertional dyspnea, orthopnea, and gradually developing paroxysmal nocturnal dyspnea. No definite high fever episode was noted from the beginning. Weight loss 3 kg in 2 months. At a visit to a local practitioner a chest X-ray examination revealed right pleural effusion, and she was transferred to our hospital for further management.

On physical examination at admission, she appeared subacutely ill with a body temperature of 38°C, a pulse rate of 138/min, a respiratory rate of 28/min, and blood pressure 145/95 mmHg. Her teeth showed multiple caries, and a dentist diagnosed dental caries with chronic pulpitis. There were neither palpable cervical lymph nodes nor mass. Her chest showed asymmetric expansion with obvious tenderness over the right lower chest area and diminished breathing sounds. Chest X-ray revealed consolidation of the right lower lobe, with massive right pleural effusion, and a soft tissue mass in the right lower chest wall. Thoracocentesis obtained bloody pleural effusion. The results of cytology and microbiology studies were all negative.

Other laboratory findings as follow: hemoglobin: 118 g/l; white blood cell count: 18×10^9/l; segment: 90%; platelet count 556×10^9/l; GOT: 27 U/L; GPT: 39 U/L; ALK-P: 264 U/l; LDH: 208 U/l; blood glucose: 1.2 g/l and an erythrocyte sedimentation rate of 63 mm/h. Immunology study revealed normal T-cell and B-cell functions; IgG: 10.3 g/l; IgA: 903 mg/l; IgM: 3.55 g/l; IgE: 490 mg/l; C3: 1.71 g/l; C4: 357 mg/l; and ANA: (−). Abdominal sonography revealed right pleural effusion and a hypoechoic solid mass between the diaphragm and Glirson's capsule. Colour flow images revealed hypervascularity, with high velocity in this mass.

A chest computerized tomogram demonstrated consolidation in the right middle and lower lobes with a heterogeneous hypodensity lesion extending to the subphrenic and chest wall areas. The magnetic resonance image revealed abscess-like lesions around the right lower pleura with transdiaphrenic involvement to the subphrenic region. The lesion also invaded the intercostal muscle. Fiberoptic thoracoscopy was performed, and 30 ml pus was drained from the inferior border of right anterior pleura. The Gram-stained smear disclosed Gram-negative hyphae-like organisms. The pathological finding from tissue biopsy was acute inflammation with reactive mesothelial hyperplasia without malignancy. Four days later, culture of the pus grew just typical colonies of A. actinomycetemcomitans, sensitive to ampicillin, chloramphenicol, aminoglycosides, and most cephalosporins. After the identification of the causative microorganism, cefoxitin was given for 2 weeks, followed by oral amoxicillin (250 mg/6 h) for a total period of 3 months. Follow-up chest roentgenography revealed resolution of right lung lesions. The patient recovered gradually without any sequelae.

DISCUSSION

A. actinomycetemcomitans, a small fastidious Gram-negative coccobacillus, was first isolated in 1912 by Klinger and given its distinctive name because of association with Actinomyces israelii infections (1, 2). It is a part of the normal human oral flora. The most common dental disease, periodontal disease and dental caries, is a chronic infection, and may be caused by it (6). Human pathogenicity was first reported in 1962 by King and Tatum who isolated it from pus in 32 patients suffering from actinomycosis (1). Major infections caused by A. actinomycetemcomitans include periodontitis, soft tissue abscesses, and systemic infection. The most frequently encountered systemic infection was endocarditis (4). Prior to 1993, 5 cases of A. actinomycetemcomitans pneumonia had been reported in the English literature (2–5). A. actinomycetemcomitans pleural abscess is extremely rare, and pleural infection with subphrenic involvement has never been reported in young adolescents.

In our case, the A. actinomycetemcomitans infection involved the right lower lung, invading and breaking through the visceral and parietal pleura, extending to the chest wall and subphrenic area. This feature suggests a collagenolytic activity similar to that of A. israelii (7). The pattern of invasive extension in pulmonary infection is distinct from other pathogens and may initially be misinterpreted as malignancy.

The exact portal of entry in human lung infection is unknown. Since A. actinomycetemcomitans is commonly demonstrated in humans with periodontal disease or dental caries, the infection may occur through ulcerated epithelium in diseased periodontal pockets, or follow dental manipulation (6, 8–10). Our patient had suffered from tootache for about 2 months before admission, and had dental caries with chronic dental pulpitis. This could have been the major cause of this rarely encountered pulmonary infection. The diagnosis of A. actinomycetemcomitans depends on bacterial culture. The blood cultures are frequently positive in endocarditis, while pulmonary infection rarely yields a positive blood culture.

Most cases have been diagnosed by culture of biopsy specimen or aspirate from the involved tissue (5). The fastidious and slow-growing nature of A. actinomycetemcomitans may complicate the proper diagnosis, which is frequently missed if the laboratories discard the culture specimen after 7 days of incubation (11).

A. actinomycetemcomitans is generally susceptible to cephalosporins, aminoglycosides, rifampicin, chloramphenicol, and tetracycline. Susceptibility to ampicillin and penicillin varies widely, and resistance is common (12). Treatment is governed by the results of in vitro susceptibility testing and includes adequate surgical abscess drainage. The duration of therapy in pulmonary infection varies and depends upon the clinical response of the patient.

ACKNOWLEDGEMENTS

The authors would like to thank Ay-Huey Huang for culture and identification of this organism, Dr Wu-Wei Lai for fiberoptic thoracoscopy, and Dr Yin-Tai Jin for examination of the pathological specimens. We are grateful to Dr Chao-Ching Huang for reviewing the manuscript.

REFERENCES

1. King EO, Tatum HW. Actinobacillus actinomycetemcomitans and Hemophilus aphrophilus. J Infect Dis 111: 85–94, 1962.
2. Meyer BR, Buttone E, Hirschman SZ, Schneierson SS, Gershengorn K. Infection due to Actinobacillus actinomycetemcomitans. Am J Clin Pathol 56: 204–211, 1971.
3. Carlile JR, Beckman EN, Arsensman RM. Actinobacillus actinomycetemcomitans pneumonia. Clin Pediatr 23: 578–80, 1984.
4. Kaplan AH, Weber DJ, Oddone EZ, Perfect JR. Infection due to Actinobacillus actinomycetemcomitans: 15 cases and review. Rev Infect Dis 11: 46–63, 1989.
5. Yuan A, Yang PC, Lee LN, Chang DB, Kuo SH, Luh KT. Actinobacillus actinomycetemcomitans pneumonia with chest wall involvement and rib destruction. Chest 101: 1450–1452, 1992.
6. Asikainen S., Alaluusua S. Bacteriology of dental infections. Eur Heart J 14, Suppl K: 43–50, 1993.
7. Robertson PB, Lantz M, Marucha PT, Kornman KS, Trummel CL, Holt SC. Collagenolytic activity associated with Bacteroides species and Actinobacillus actinomycetemcomitans. J Periodontal Res 17: 275–283, 1982.
8. Zambon JJ, Christersson LA, Slots J. Actinobacillus actinomycetemcomitans in human periodontal disease: prevalence in patients groups and distribution of biotypes and serotypes within families. J Periodontol 54: 707–711, 1983.
9. Hall ER, Falkler WA, Martin SA, Suzuki JB. The gingival immune response to Actinobacillus actinomycetemcomitans in juvenile periodontitis. J Periodontol 62: 792–798, 1991.
10. Aass MA, Preus RH, Gjermo P. Association between detection of oral Actinobacillus actinomycetemcomitans and radiographic bone loss in teenagers. A 4-year longitudinal study. J Periodontol 63: 682–685, 1992.
11. Grace CJ, Levitz RE, Katz-Pollak H, Brettman LR. Actinobacillus actinomycetemcomitans prosthetic valve endocarditis. Rev Infect Dis 10: 922–929, 1988.
12. Yogev R, Shulman D, Shulman ST, Glogowski WG. In vitro activity of antibiotics alone and in combination against Actinobacillus actinomycetemcomitans. Antimicrob Agent Chem Ther 29: 179–181, 1986.

Submitted September 14, 1994; accepted January 18, 1995

Scand J Infect Dis 27: 291–293, 1995 CASE REPORT

Haemophilus aphrophilus Discitis and Vertebral Osteomyelitis

JEAN C. O'DRISCOLL[1], GRAHAM S. KEENE[2], MICHAEL J. WEINBREN[1], ALAN P. JOHNSON[3], MARIE-FRANCE PALEPOU[3] and ROBERT C. GEORGE[3]

From the Departments of [1]Microbiology, RTR Healthcare NHS Trust, Queen Mary's University Hospital, Roehampton, London, and [2]Orthopaedic Surgery, Addenbrooke's Hospital, Cambridge, and the [3]Antibiotic Reference Unit, Laboratory of Hospital Infection, Central Public Health Laboratory, Colindale, London, UK

An unusual case of discitis and vertebral osteomyelitis due to Haemophilus aphrophilus is described. Infections due to this organism have usually responded to treatment with β-lactam antibiotics. However, our isolate was resistant to third-generation cephalosporins which has not been reported previously in the world literature. The patient made a good clinical response to ciprofloxacin treatment.

J. O'Driscoll, MB, Department of Microbiology, RTR Healthcare NHS Trust, Queen Mary's University Hospital, Roehampton, London SW15 5PJ, UK

INTRODUCTION

Haemophilus aphrophilus is a fastidious Gram-negative coccobacillus which is part of the normal oropharyngeal flora. It is a rare human pathogen with the most commonly reported infections reported being endocarditis (1–9). Other infections which have been reported include brain abscesses (1, 2), meningitis (1, 2, 10–13), pneumonitis (1, 2), peritonitis (1, 2), sinusitis (1, 2), and wound infections (1, 2). Osteomyelitis due to this organism is uncommon (10, 14–21).

CASE REPORT

A 53 year old gentleman was referred acutely by his General Practitioner with severe lumbar backache associated with obstructive urinary symptoms. This illness had begun 2 months previously when he developed severe backache with "shooting" pains in both legs associated with episodes of sweating. He consulted his GP who prescribed co-proxamol. The pain improved until 5 days before admission when he experienced pain of such severity that he was confined to bed.

He had attended his dentist 2 weeks prior to the onset of his illness with a sore tooth. This was considered an early infection, and ampicillin was prescribed. 10 years previously he suffered from 'sciatica' which responded to conservative treatment although he had persistent low backache.

Despite being a heavy drinker of alcohol, and a smoker, his general health was good. On examination he appeared well and not in obvious pain. There was slight lumbar spine tenderness, straight leg raising to 80° with a negative sciatic stretch test. He had normal tone and full power throughout both lower limbs, but sensation was diminished in the perianal region, although soft touch and pinprick discrimination were retained. The bladder was not palpable and anal tone was preserved. There were no signs of active dental infection.

X-rays of the lumbar spine showed some loss of the L4\L5 disc space, with surrounding sclerosis. A full blood count revealed a haemoglobin of 14.0 g/l, white cell count of 19.4×10^9/l (92% neutrophils) and an ESR of 94 mm/h. A set of blood cultures was taken.

Over the next 24 h his condition deteriorated such that he was unable to empty his bladder. An urgent myelogram was arranged which demonstrated a complete block at the level of L4. Accordingly, emergency spinal decompression was undertaken. At surgery the dura was found to be swollen and hyperaemic and 3 ml of pus was aspirated from the L4/L5 disc space and sent to the Microbiology Department. The wound was closed, with suction drainage, and IV flucloxacillin and gentamicin (a total of 6 days gentamicin therapy given) commenced.

Gram stain of the pus revealed numerous white cells with very scanty Gram-negative coccobacilli. This specimen grew an organism which was subsequently identified at the National Collection of Type Cultures, Central Public Health Laboratory, Colindale, as Haemophilus aphrophilus. The same organism was also isolated from the blood culture set taken on admission. (There was no clinical or echocardiographic evidence of endocarditis.) The organism initially appeared to show resistance to ampicillin (zone of only 2 mm compared to 7 mm for control using 2 ug disc) but sensitivity to cefotaxime (zone of 9 mm compared to 10 mm with control) on disc testing (Stokes method on DST agar containing lysed blood and NAD using H. influenzae NCTC control and incubated overnight at 37°C in CO_2). It was β-lactamase negative (nitrocefin method). In view of these results, flucloxacillin therapy was stopped and cefotaxime 1 g tds was commenced.

This dose was, however, subsequently increased to 12 g daily as the initial response was poor. In view of the disappointing clinical response to treatment with cefotaxime and the organism's unusual sensitivity pattern, it was submitted to the Antibiotic Reference Unit, Colindale, for additional antibiotic sensitivity testing.

Determination of the minimum inhibitory concentrations (MICs) of antibiotics was performed by means of an agar incorporation test using DST agar (Unipath) containing 5% (v/v) lysed blood (Tissue Culture Services) and NAD (20 mg/l). The standard bacterial inocula used in most tests, and confirmed by performing viable counts, comprised $1-3 \times 10^4$ colony-forming units (cfu)/spot. Such tests showed that the isolate was resistant to ampicillin (MIC > 8 mg/l), cefuroxime (MIC > 8 mg/l), ceftazidime (MIC > 8 mg/l) and cefotaxime (MIC > 8 mg/l). It was observed, however, that the growth on plates containing sub-inhibitory concentrations of β-lactam antibiotics was poorer than that seen with antibiotic-free medium. Resistance to ampicillin and cefotaxime was not inhibited by clavulanic acid (2 mg/l) in vitro and testing with nitrocefin failed to provide evidence of β-lactamase production. In contrast to this isolate, the type strain of H. aphrophilus (NCTC 5906) and 5 other clinical isolates of this species were found to be sensitive to ampicillin (MICs 0.25–0.5 mg/l) and cefotaxime

(MICs $\geq 0.06-0.5$ mg/l) when tested using an inoculum density of $1-3 \times 10^4$ cfu/spot.

However, a marked inoculum effect was noted in that the MICs of ampicillin and cefotaxime increased to >32 mg/l when inocula comprising $1-3 \times 10^5$ or $1-3 \times 10^6$ cfu/spot were treated.

MICs were read after 48 h (due to poor growth).

The MIC for gentamicin was <2 mg/l.

MIC results additionally showed the isolate to be sensitive to ciprofloxacin (MIC ≤ 0.25 mg/l) and therapy was therefore changed to IV ciprofloxacin 200 mg bd. The patient made a gradual clinical improvement, although his ESR and white count remained high. Magnetic resonance imaging was arranged to exclude any abscess formation. This demonstrated an osteomyelitis of lower and upper borders of L4 and L5. There was no abscess cavity.

The patient was discharged on oral ciprofloxacin and had no back pain when seen at the Out Patients Clinic 2 months later. His ESR had fallen to 12 mm/h and white cell count was 4.8×10^9/l. Radiological assessment showed no evidence of persistent osteomyelitis.

DISCUSSION

H. aphrophilus is an oropharyngeal commensal bacterium rarely associated with clinical infection. There are 7 previously reported cases of vertebral osteomyelitis due to this organism in the world literature (10, 15–20). Precipitating events were identified in 3 cases, including a traumatic lip laceration (18), the use of an epidural catheter (19) and 1 case following myelography (10).

Three cases of apparently spontaneous vertebral osteomyelitis were reported, with no obvious source of infection, although 1 patient was a diabetic (16), and diabetes is recognised as being a predisposing factor in the development of vertebral osteomyelitis. Excess alcohol consumption was not mentioned in any of these case reports. Our patient drank heavily, which may have rendered him more susceptible to infection.

The source of spread of infection by H. aphrophilus is generally accepted to be the mouth or upper respiratory tract (2). This is reflected in the types of infections caused (e.g. sinusitis, brain abscesses and infective endocarditis). In our patient it is likely that infection originated in his dental sepsis. It is possible that the short course of ampicillin which was prescribed selected for resistant strains among the oral flora.

Previous case reports have stressed the ease with which bone infections due to H. aphrophilus have been treated. However, a recent case report of H. aphrophilus endocarditis (9) described a poor clinical response to cefotaxime and netilmicin despite apparent in vitro sensitivity. There was a good response to ciprofloxacin. Our patient responded poorly to cefotaxime, which was presumably related to the finding that the isolate exhibited resistance to cefotaxime and other β-lactam antibiotics in vitro. He responded very well to ciprofloxacin, to which the organism was sensitive in vitro.

There was no evidence that the cephalosporin resistance exhibited by this isolate was due to production of extended-spectrum β-lactamases as the resistance was not inhibited by clavulanic acid in vitro, and the organisms failed to hydrolyse nitrocefin. Other possible mechanisms of β-lactam resistance, such as changes in penicillin-binding proteins or outer-membrane permeability, which have been noted in other organisms such as H. influenzae (22, 23), were not studied. Furthermore, the reason for the discrepancy between the sensitivity results obtained by disc testing and MIC determination is not clear, although it may have been related to the poor growth of the organism in the presence of β-lactam antibiotics. Interestingly, a similar problem was noted with H. influenzae when a survey of the detection of β-lactam resistance showed that resistance in non-β-lactamase producing isolates was frequently not detected in routine laboratories (24).

REFERENCES

1. Bieger RC, Brewer NS, Washington JA. Haemophilus aphrophilus: a microbiologic and clinical review and report of 42 cases. Medicine 57: 345–355, 1978.
2. Page MI, King EO. Infection due to Actinobacillus actinomycetemcomitans and Haemophilus aphrophilus. N Engl J Med 275: 181–188, 1966.
3. Root TE, Silva EA, Edwards LD, Topp JH. Haemophilus aphrophilus endocarditis with a probable primary dental focus of infection. Chest 80: 109–110, 1981.
4. Ellner JJ, Rosenthal MS, Lerner PI, McHenry MC. Infective endocarditis caused by slow growing, fastidious, gram-negative bacteria. Medicine 58: 145–158, 1979.
5. Varghese R, Melo JC, Barnum P, Chan CH, Raff MJ. Endocarditis due to Haemophilus aphrophilus: Report of a case with possible transmission from dog to man. Chest 71: 680–682, 1977.
6. Elster SK, Mattes LM, Meyers BR, Jurado RA. Haemophilus aphrophilus endocarditis: Review of 23 cases. Am J Cardiol 35: 72–79, 1975.
7. Dorf B, Kilian M. Haemophilus aphrophilus: endocarditis. Scand J Infect Dis 6: 291–294, 1974.
8. Sutter VL, Finegold SM. Haemophilus aphrophilus: infections: Clinical and bacteriologic studies. Ann N Y Acad Sci 174: 468–487, 1970.
9. Dawson SJ, White LA. Treatment of Haemophilus aphrophilus endocarditis with ciprofloxacin. J Infect 24: 317–320, 1992.
10. Petty BG, Burrow CR, Robinson RA, Bulkley GB. Haemophilus aphrophilus: meningitis followed by vertebral osteomyelitis and suppurative psoas abscess. Am J Med 78: 159–162, 1985.
11. Kim CB, King M, Dalley AK, Sandlin D. A case of meningitis with Haemophilus aphrophilus – a Case Report. J Ind State Med Assoc 255–257, 1974.
12. Maggiore G, Scotta MS, DeGiacomo C, Malfa S, Azzini M. Bacteremia and meningitis associated with Haemophilus aphrophilus infection in a previously healthy child. Infection 10: 375, 1982.
13. Miano A, Cipolloni AP, Casadei GP, Petrone M, Biasini GC. Neonatal Haemophilus aphrophilus meningitis. Helv Paediat Acta 31: 499–501, 1976.
14. Thomas E, Holden FA, Bowen CV, Silver WA. Osteomyelitis due to Haemophilus aphrophilus. Can Med Assoc J 135: 841–842, 1987.

15. Nahas RG, Cook S, Weinstern MP. Vertebral osteomyelitis due to Haemophilus aphrophilus: Treatment with ceftriaxone. J Infect Dis 159: 811–812, 1989.
16. Gribble MJ, Hunter T. Haemophilus aphrophilus vertebral osteomyelitis: A case report and literature review. Diagn Microbiol Infect Dis 8: 189–191, 1987.
17. Houssian FA, Huaux JP, Nagant de Deuxchaisnes C. Haemophilus aphrophilus: a rare pathogen in vertebral osteomyelitis. Ann Rheum Dis 46: 248–250, 1987.
18. Ho JL, Soukiasian, Oh WH, Snydman DR. Haemophilus aphrophilus osteomyelitis. Am J Med 76: 159–161, 1984.
19. Farrington M, Eykyn SJ, Walker M, Warren RE. Vertebral osteomyelitis due to coccobacilli of the HB group. BMJ 287: 1658–1660, 1983.
20. Bejuk D, Kuzman I, Soldo I, Kuzmanovic N, Popovic-Uroic T. Vertebral osteomyelitis caused by Haemophilus aphrophilus. Eur J Clin Microbiol Infect Dis 12: 643–644, 1993.
21. Sapico FL, Montgomerie JZ. Pyogenic vertebral osteomyelitis. Report of nine cases and review of the literature. Rev Infect Dis 1: 754, 1979.
22. Powell, M, Fah-YS, Seymour A, Yuan M, Williams JD. Antimicrobial resistance in Haemophilus influenzae from England and Scotland in 1991. J Antimicrob Chemother 29: 547–554, 1992.
23. Powell M, Seetulsingh P, Williams JD. In vitro susceptibility of Haemophilus influenzae to meropenem compared with imipenem, five other β-lactams, chloramphenicol and ciprofloxacin. J Antimicrob Chemother 25 (Suppl A): 175–181, 1989.
24. Powell M, Williams JD. Detection of ampicillin resistant Haemophilus influenzae in United Kingdom Laboratories. J Clin Pathol 41: 716–719, 1988.

Submitted August 4, 1994; accepted February 15, 1995

Aeromonas hydrophila Lung Abscess in a Previously Healthy Man

TAU HUR, KUO-CHEN CHENG and JUINN-MIN HSIEH

From the Pulmonary and Critical Care Section, Internal Medicine, Chi-Mei Foundation Hospital, Tainan, Taiwan, R.O.C.

We present a case of multilocular lung abscess caused by Aeromonas hydrophila, found in both sputum and bronchial washing. No aspiration or other significantly contributory medical conditions were found. We believe this to be the first report of lung abscess caused by this organism in a previously healthy individual.

T. Hur, MD, The Pulmonary and Critical Care Section, Chi Mei Foundation Hospital, 901, Chung Hwa Rd, Yung Kang Hsiang, Tainan, 71010 Taiwan, Republic of China

INTRODUCTION

In recent years, Aeromonads have been increasingly implicated as human pathogens and A. hydrophila may be the species most frequently isolated (1, 2). After reviewing the literature, we discovered a paucity of information on lower respiratory tract infections caused to this organism.

CASE REPORT

A 59-year-old farmer was admitted after 1 weeks illness with fever, chills, left-sided pleuritic chest pain, and blood-tinged purulent sputum. He appeared acutely ill, with a temperature of 39.2°C, and decreased breath sounds with moist rales over the left lower chest. Roentgenography demonstrated an area of consolidation behind the heart. Gram staining of the sputum disclosed numerous gram-negative rods. The peripheral blood white count was 4,100/μl.

Gentamicin and cephalothin therapy was started, but to no avail. Three blood cultures at admission showed no growth, but 2 sputum cultures grew pure cultures of A. hydrophila, resistant to ampicillin and cephalothin which was replaced by cefuroxime. Fiberoptic bronchoscopy revealed profuse purulent material in the left lower lobe and bronchial washes grew the same organism. Computerized tomography of the chest showed a multilocular lung abscess with air-fluid levels in the left lower lobe. Over the next few days, postural drainage removed much purulent secretion. The patient's lung abscess gradually diminished in size and he was discharged after 2 weeks, but continued with oral cefuroxime for another 2 weeks. The follow-up chest radiographs showed nearly complete resolution of his lung abscess.

DISCUSSION

The genus Aeromonas once belonged to the family Vibrionaceae, most of whom are facultative anaerobic, oxidase-positive, and Gram-negative rods. Based on molecular genetic evidence, however, it now belongs to a new family, Aeromonadaceae (3). A. hydrophila is ubiquitous and often found in natural water bodies and in the soil. They have even been recovered from tap water and distilled water, regarded as potential sources in nosocomial infections.

Generally speaking, most human infections can be divided into 3 categories: 1) water-associated traumatic wound infections in healthy subjects; 2) acute or chronic diarrhea/gastroenteritis; 3) bacteremia and/or septicemia in immunocompromised patients.

However, A. hydrophila has rarely been mentioned as causing lower respiratory tract illnesses. Among those cases reported most had a history of aspiration and most also had radiological evidence of bilateral pulmonary involvement. Pleural effusion rarely occurred. At least 3 patients progressed to adult respiratory distress syndrome and ultimately died. The mortality related to pulmonary infections with A. hydrophila was near 40% (4).

Whereas blood cultures grown from our patient proved negative, cultures from sputum and bronchial washing grew A. hydrophila. The Gram stains showed >25 polymorphonuclear leukocytes and <10 epithelial cells per low-power field. As advocated by several investigators, sputum cultures judged appropriate by initial Gram stains could support the diagnosis (5).

A large study of the minimal inhibitory concentration of 22 antimicrobial agents against 60 strains of 3 Aeromonas species revealed that most isolates were susceptible to the newer cephalosporins such as moxalactam, cefotaxime, and cefoperazone, the aminoglycosides, and chloramphenicol, tetracycline, and trimethoprim-sulfamethoxazole (6).

REFERENCES

1. Davis WA, Kane JG, Garagusi VF. Human Aeromonas infections: a review of the literature and a case of endocarditis. Medicine 57: 267–277, 1978.
2. Harris RL, Fainstein V, Elting L, Hopfer RL, Bodey G. Bacteremia caused by Aeromonas species in hospitalized cancer patients. Rev Infect Dis 7: 314–320, 1985.
3. Koneman EW, Allen SD, Janda WM, Schreckenberger PC, Winn Jr WC. The families Vibrionaceae and "Aeromonadaceae". In: Color Atlas and Textbook of Diagnostic Microbiology, 4th edn. Philadelphia: JB Lippincott Company, 258–273, 1992.
4. Baddour LM, Baselski VS. Pneumonia due to Aeromonas hydrophila complex: epidemiologic, clinical, and microbiologic features. South Med J 81: 461–463, 1988.
5. Musher DM. Gram stain and culture of sputum to diagnose bacterial pneumonia. J Infect Dis 152: 1096, 1985.
6. Motyl MR, McKinley G, Janda JM. In vitro susceptibilities of Aeromonas hydrophila, Aeromonas sobria, and Aeromonas caviae to 22 antimicrobial agents. Antimicrob Agents Chemother 28: 151–153, 1985.

Submitted September 19, 1994; accepted January 18, 1995

Scand J Infect Dis 27: 297–298, 1995 CASE REPORT

An Unusual Gastrointestinal Presentation of Leishmaniasis

MICHAEL O. McBRIDE, MARTIN FISHER, CELIA J. SKINNER, ROBERT GOLDEN and JANICE MAIN

From the Department of Genitourinary Medicine and Communicable Diseases, the Academic Department of Medicine, and the Department of Pathology, St. Mary's Hospital, London, UK

While visceral leishmaniasis (VL) generally occurs in immunocompetent subjects in endemic areas, it has been increasingly recognised as an important opportunistic infection in the immunocompromised including those infected with the human immunodeficiency virus. We report an unusual presentation of visceral leishmaniasis in a patient with the acquired immunodeficiency syndrome (AIDS) with disease which appeared to be limited to the gastrointestinal tract.

M. McBride, MB BCh, Department of Genitourinary Medicine/HIV, Royal Victoria Hospital, Grosvenor Road, Belfast BT12 8BA, Northern Ireland

CASE REPORT

A 47 year old homosexual man who was diagnosed HIV-seropositive 2 years previously when he was treated for pulmonary tuberculosis, presented with a 3 month history of epigastric pain, intermittent vomiting and weight loss. He did not describe any symptoms consistent with malabsorption. On examination he was apyrexial, with oral candidiasis, and had a postural drop in systolic blood pressure of 20 mm Hg. Medication included co-trimoxazole as prophylaxis against Pneumocystis carinii pneumonia and maintenance isoniazid and zidovudine. A synacthen test was normal and he was commenced on fludrocortisone for presumed autonomic neuropathy with symptomatic improvement. Haemoglobin at this time was 117 g/l, platelet count 103×10^9/l, neutrophils 0.6×10^9/l, CD4+ lymphocyte count 7×10^9/l. Serum alanine transferase was raised at 77 u/l (<40) and gamma glutamine transferase was 229 u/l (11–50).

Six weeks later his nausea and vomiting persisted despite cessation of zidovudine and he had developed hepatosplenomegaly, which was confirmed on abdominal ultrasound scan. Oesophagogastroduodenoscopy showed normal appearing mucosa, however multiple duodenal biopsies showed Leishmania amastigotes and these were identified on culture as L. infantum.

At review, the patient was noted to have developed Cytomegalovirus retinitis and was pancytopenic. Haemoglobin was 92 g/l, neutrophil count 0.6×10^9/l and platelet count 80×10^9/l. He was admitted for further investigation and treatment. Examination of bone marrow showed numerous Leishmania amastigotes. Serum antibodies to Leishmania were not found. The patient's retinitis was treated with intravenous foscarnet but he declined further therapeutic intervention for his leishmaniasis.

DISCUSSION

To our knowledge there have only been 2 previous reports of visceral leishmaniasis diagnosed on duodenal biopsy (1, 2). Both these patients were HIV-seropositive and both had evidence of malabsorption and disseminated disease at presentation. There has however been 1 previous report of a rectal ulcer in a patient with AIDS without evidence of visceral or cutaneous disease (3).

Visceral leishmaniasis in patients co-infected with HIV is being increasingly recognised as a not uncommon opportunistic infection not only in endemic areas, but also in patients who have lived in or travelled to endemic areas and it has been proposed that the infection be considered an AIDS-defining condition (4). These patients are unusual in many respects (5). Presentation may be atypical and in one series 20% did not have hepatosplenomegaly and 5% did not have fever (6). Antileishmanial antibodies are present in approximately 35% of cases as against 95% of immunocompetent patients. A chronic or relapsing course is seen in over 40% of cases and accompanied by a high mortality (6). It is probable that like other intracellular organisms, Leishmania species are not eradicated by drug treatment and that reactivation occurs in the immunocompromised host with impaired cell mediated immunity. While parasitological and symptomatic cure can be achieved with appropriate drug treatment it is likely that with decreasing cell mediated immunity relapse will occur (7) and longterm maintenance therapy will be required.

In this case infection probably occurred 2 years previously while the patient was on holiday in an endemic area in the Mediterranean and only became clinically expressed with progressive immunosuppression. It would appear from the initial presentation that leishmaniasis may have been confined to the gastrointestinal tract in the absence of constitutional symptoms or haematological abnormalities and only later became disseminated with the onset of pancytopenia and hepatomegaly. In the absence of initial fever and systemic symptoms there was no clinical reason to suspect VL and the findings on duodenal biopsy were entirely fortuitous.

CONCLUSION

This case emphasises the importance of endoscopy and routine biopsy in HIV-positive patients presenting with unexplained upper gastrointestinal symptoms. We are certain that visceral leishmaniasis will become an increasingly important opportunistic infection in HIV-positive patients and it is important that clinicians are familiar with its varied clinical presentation in this population.

 ISSN 0036-5548

REFERENCES

1. Datry A, Similowski T, Jais P, Rosenheim M, Katlama C, Maheu E, Kazaz S, Fassin D, Danis M. AIDS-associated leishmaniasis: an unusual gastro-duodenal presentation. Trans R Soc Trop Med Hyg 84: 239–240, 1990.
2. Sedino A, Barbado FJ, Mostaza JM, Fernandez-Martin J, Larrauri J, Vâzquez-Rodriguez JJ. Visceral leishmaniasis with malabsorption syndrome in a patient with AIDS. Am J Med 89: 673–675, 1990.
3. Rosenthal PJ, Chaisson RE, Hadley WK, Leed JH. Rectal leishmaniasis in a patient with the acquired immunodeficiency syndrome. Am J Med 84: 307–309, 1988.
4. Montalban C, Martinez-Fernandez R, Calleja JL, Garcia-Dias J de D, Rubio R, Dronda F, Moreno S, Yebra M, Barros C, Cobo J, Marinez MC, Ruiz F, Costa JR. Visceral leishmaniasis (kala-azar) as an opportunistic infection in patients infected with the human immunodeficiency virus in Spain. Rev Infect Dis 11: 655–660, 1989.
5. Peters BS, Fish D, Golden R, Evans DA, Bryceson ADM, Pinching AJ. Visceral Leishmaniasis in HIV infection and AIDS: clinical features and response to therapy. Q J Med 283: 1101–1111, 1990.
6. Montalban C, Calleja JL, Erice A, Laguna F, Clotet B, Podzamer D, Cobo J, Mallolass J, Yebra M, Gallego A, the Co-operative Group for the study of leishmaniasis in AIDS (1990). Visceral leismaniasis in patients with human immunodeficiency virus. J Infect 21: 261–270, 1990.
7. McBride MO, Linney M, Claydon E, Weber JN. Visceral leishmaniasis following treatment with liposomal amphotericin B. 19(2): 362, 1994.

Submitted November 11, 1994; accepted February 15, 1995

Scandinavian Society for Antimicrobial Chemotherapy, 12th Annual Meeting

The 12th Annual Meeting of the Scandinavian Society for Antimicrobial Chemotherapy will take place at the Royal Garden Hotel, Trondheim, Norway, Thursday October 5–Sunday October 8, 1995. The programme will include symposias on the following topics: Streptococcal Infections; Growth Factors in Infectious Diseases; Antibiotics and the Ecology of the Fecal Flora; Antiviral Chemotherapy and Viral Resistance; Impact of the Infectious Disease Epidemiology in Russia and the Baltic States on the Nordic Countries. Information about the meeting may be obtained from:

International Conference Service
Sissi P. Solberg A/S
N-0166 OSLO
Norway

Tel: +47 22 11 21 90.
Fax: +47 22 36 11 44, or

Prof. Johan N. Bruun
Dept. of Infectious Diseases
Ullevål University Hospital
N-0407 OSLO
Norway

Deadline for submission of abstracts for oral presentation and posters will be August 15, 1995.

Scand J Infect Dis 27: 299–300, 1995 SHORT COMMUNICATION

Hepatitis B in Parts of Former USSR

THOMAS O. LINGLÖF

From the Department of Infectious Diseases, University Hospital, Uppsala, and the Swedish Institute for Infectious Disease Control, Stockholm, Sweden

Hepatitis B is more frequent in many countries in eastern Europe than in the western part. In Poland the incidence is as high as 34 notified cases per 100,000 inhabitants. In the Baltic states the incidence is between 10 and 20, and in Russia 23 cases per 100,000 inhabitants. In the Baltic states the incidence has declined since 1986. This reduction has been most prominent in Lithuania, with 69%, followed by Latvia with 43% and Estonia with 23%. The infection is very often (>50%) spread by non-sterile medical instruments.

T. O. Linglöf, MD, Departmennt of Infectious Diseases, University Hospital, S-751 85 Uppsala, Sweden

INTRODUCTION

Since the emergence of new, independent states in eastern Europe, contacts have been establised between them and Sweden in the medical field. Thus more information on communicable diseases in these areas is now available. Because of the ongoing diphtheria epidemic in the former USSR, Swedish contacts were taken to discuss the situation. For this reason some of these newly independent states and certain others were visited by the author. During these contacts, other infectious diseases were also discussed.

These new states represent a high-prevalence area for hepatitis B. The annual incidences are considerably higher than in western Europe, although since 1986 the incidence has been declining in the Baltic states, Estonia, Latvia and Lithuania, as has also been shown for parts of western Europe (1).

The increase in travel from, above all, the Scandinavian countries to the Baltic states and the St. Petersburg area, has resulted in large numbers of people running the risk of infection with communicable diseases prevalent in the region. It was therefore considered of interest to report the current state of affairs regarding hepatitis B in these countries in order to give colleagues in the Scandinavian countries and elsewhere information they might need for information to people travelling there.

MATERIAL AND METHODS

All figures are based on current national statistics. In Lithuania: Republican Immunisation Centre, Vilnius. In Latvia: National Environment and Public Health Centre, Ministry of Welfare, Labour and Health of the Republic of Latvia, Riga. In Estonia: National Health Protection Center, Tallinn. In Russia: State Committee of Sanitary and Epidemiological Surveillance of the Russian Federation. In Poland: Epidemiological Department, National Institute of Hygiene, Warsaw. In the Czech Republic: Epidemiological Department, Ministry of Health, Prague.

The figures and other information were obtained during a personal visit by the author to the health authorities in the countries mentioned.

RESULTS

The incidence figures, according to notification of hepatitis B in 1993 in some East European countries, compared with those reported by Iwarson et al. (1), are given in Fig. 1. As can be seen, Poland has the highest incidence, followed by Russia. The incidence figures for 1993 correspond to a total number of cases in, for example, Poland: 13,296; Russia: 32,946; Estonia: 145; Latvia: 430; and Lithuania: 470; and Czech Republic: 732.

There has been a decline in the incidence of hepatitis B in the Baltic states over the past 7 years (Fig. 2). It is most prominent and started even earlier in Lithuania. The decline in notified cases from 1986 to 1993 was 69% in

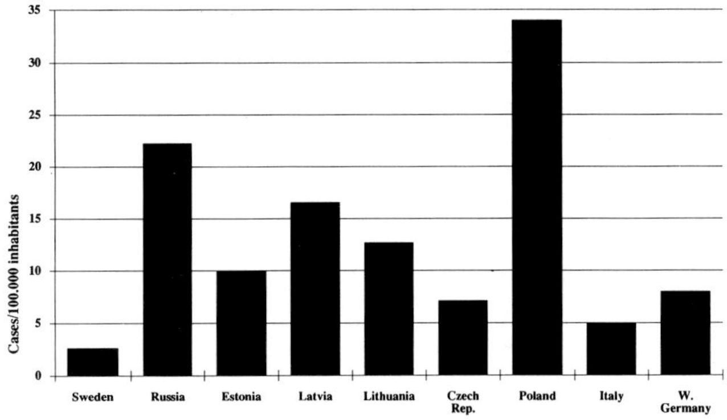

Fig. 1. Incidence of acute hepatitis B per 100,000 inhabitants in some European countries, 1993.

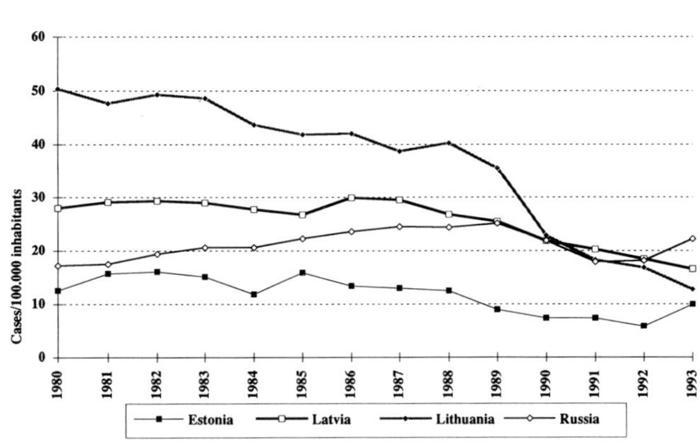

Fig. 2. Annual incidence of acute hepatitis B in some European countries 1980–93.

 ISSN 0036-5548

Lithuania, 43% in Latvia and 23% in Estonia. In Russia there has been a slight downward trend, beginning in 1989, leading to a reduction of only 12% up to 1993. It should be noted that there was an increase of 23% in Russia and 69% in Estonia between 1992 and 1993.

The source of hepatitis B infection in the former USSR is well described by the following example. In 1993, 115 patients with hepatitis B were hospitalized at the Infectious Disease Hospital in Vilnius, Lithuania. 75 of them had contracted their hepatitis through medical procedures such as operations and parenteral drug administration. Moreover 8 physicians, but only one intravenous drug abuser, were treated for hepatitis B. For the remaining 31 patients the source of infection is unknown (pers. comm. Dr Gulbiniene, Lithuania, 1994).

The incidence of medically acquired hepatitis B is high among both patients and personal. In 1993 in Latvia, 58% of all patients with hepatitis B were nosocomially infected (only 5% of them by blood transfusion). 10% are intravenous drug abusers (pers. comm. Dr I. Upmace). The incidence among health care staff is high, comprising 10–15% of all cases of hepatitis B in this category, leading to an incidence among medical staff around 100/100,000 compared with just under 20/100,000 among the general population. 30–40% of all hepatitis B cases are of unknown origin but most probably sexually transmitted, though this route of transmission has not been very well studied. In St. Petersburg, similar figures are found: 60% nosocomially infected, 5% through blood transfusion, 20% are intravenous drug abusers, 15% are of unknown origin (pers. comm. Dr S. Mukomolov, St. Petersburg, 1994).

DISCUSSION

These figures are based only upon notification to health authorities in each country and do not of course reflect the real situation. They must be interpreted with caution. Nevertheless they may give some idea of the epidemiology of hepatitis B in these countries. The reporting system for infectious diseases in all these countries is well developed and efficient. Reporting to the health authority is compulsory, but it must be understood that, as in other countries, under-reporting is not unusual. All patients with hepatitis are hospitalized and hepatitis B cases are serologically verified. There have been no changes in the reporting system or testing frequency since at least 1980.

The higher incidence in eastern Europe is probably due to the fact that sterilization and disinfection methods are sometimes old-fashioned and inadequate. Especially in Poland there has been a lack of effective sterilization methods which is considered to be the cause of the extremely high incidence. In Estonia for example, boiling of instruments was replaced by more effective sterilization methods in the 1980s.

The problem with insufficient sterilization can explain why between 50 and 60% of the hepatitis B patients have been infected through injection or instrumentation in medical settings. Despite the high incidence of nosocomially acquired hepatitis B, there are no reports of identified outbreaks. Only a few patients have contracted hepatitis B through blood transfusion or intravenous drug abuse. In Russia and the Baltic states, however, intravenous drug abuse has become an increasing problem.

It is believed that the decline of hepatitis B in the Baltic states is real. There are at least 3 possible explanations for this decline. The first is more extensive testing for HBsAg in blood donors. The second is improved sterilization methods, and the third is the introduction of disposable syringes in the late 1980s.

It is not believed that the decline has been affected by the socio-economic turmoil at the time of independence. However, a slackening affecting notifications cannot be ruled out. According to the health authorities in the Baltic states and Russia, a dramatic increase in the number of reported cases of syphilis and gonorrhea has occurred. From 1990 to 1993, syphilis has increased by over 500% and gonorrhea by 100% (2). This change in sexual behaviour has, remarkably enough, not affected the incidence of hepatitis B. This may indicate that sexual transmission is at present of less importance. The increase in sexually transmitted infections may herald a chage in this respect.

Hepatitis B vaccination has until now been little used. In the Czech Republic, vaccination of some health care staff has been going on since 1985. In Latvia all children born to HBsAg-positive mothers are vaccinated at birth. In Poland an extensive vaccination program has just started.

Two important problems must be solved in order to reduce the transmission of hepatitis B in these countries. The shortage of sterile equipment in medical care, such as syringes and other disposable material, in parts of these countries must be met, and there is an obvious need for further improvement in existing sterilization methods.

The conclusion to be drawn from this report is that there is an increased risk for visitors to these countries of contracting hepatitis B if they have to undergo medical treatment. In the near future there will also be additional risk for infection through sexual transmission.

ACKNOWLEDGEMENTS

The author wishes to thank the representatives of the Health authorities responsible for communicable diseases in each country for fruitful discussion and providing the figures. In Russia: A. Yasinski, in Estonia: A. Jõgiste, in Latvia: A. Brila, in Lithuania: V. Bakasenas, in Poland: W. Magdzik, in the Czech Republic: G. Walter.

REFERENCES

1. Iwarson S, Jilg W, Stroffolini T. Substantial decline of notified Hepatitis B in major parts of Europe after 1985. Scand J Infect Dis 26: 19–22, 1994.
2. Linglöf T. Rapid increase of syphilis and gonorrhoea in parts of the former USSR. Sex Transm Dis [in press], 1995.

Submitted August 4, 1994; accepted January 19, 1995

Scandinavian Journal of

INFECTIOUS DISEASES

Vol. 27, no. 4, 1995
pp. 301–428

SCANDINAVIAN
UNIVERSITY PRESS

Oslo - Copenhagen -
Stockholm - Boston

Scand J Infect Dis 27: 303–313, 1995 REVIEW ARTICLE

Characterization of Haemophilus influenzae Isolates from the Respiratory Tract of Patients with Primary Antibody Deficiencies: Evidence for Persistent Colonizations

ANDERS SAMUELSON[1], SILVIA BORRELLI[1], ROLF GUSTAFSON[2], LENNART HAMMARSTRÖM[2,3], C. I. EDVARD SMITH[2,3] JON JONASSON[1] and ALF. A. LINDBERG[1]

From the Department of Immunology, Microbiology, Pathology and Infectious Diseases, Karolinska Institute, Divisions of [1]Clinical Bacteriology and [2]Clinical Immunology, Huddinge Hospital, Sweden and the [3]Center for BioTechnology, Novum Huddinge, Sweden

A total of 117 consecutive patients with primary antibody deficiencies were followed for up to 5 years with regard to acute respiratory tract infections. Nontypeable Haemophilus influenzae (NTHI) was the sole pathogen in 61% (202/330) of the samples from which a potential pathogen was recovered. Common variable immunodeficiency (CVI) was the most prevalent condition (27/39 patients) in the group where H. influenzae was isolated. In patients where H. influenzae was not found only 9/78 patients had CVI. 49 of these 78 patients had isolated IgG3 or IgA deficiency. Both of these entities seemed to be associated with a lower prevalence of NTHI infections. 13 of 18 patients with at least 2 isolates of NTHI were colonized with the same strain from 3 to 43 months as shown by total genomic DNA-fingerprinting. Recurrent symptomatic infections occurred in these patients despite substitution therapy with gammaglobulins and repeated antibiotic treatments. All but 2 of the 224 H. influenzae isolates were β-lactamase negative and sensitive to ampicillin. The use of 10 lipopolysaccharide-specific monoclonal antibodies in a whole cell ELISA showed that the LPS-epitopes on the 224 H. influenzae isolates from the hypogammaglobulinemic group were very similar to 499 NTHI isolates from immunocompetent patients with respiratory infections. One may therefore conclude that i) patients with CVI, were prone to be permanently colonized with NTHI, and ii) the colonizing bacteria were ordinary strains showing the same LPS-phenotypes as those strains that cause acute respiratory tract infections in immunocompetent individuals.

A. Samuelson, MD, Division of Clinical Bacteriology, Huddinge Hospital, S-141 86 Huddinge, Sweden

INTRODUCTION

Haemophilus influenzae is a common pathogen in the human respiratory tract (1, 2). The majority of H. influenzae isolates from this environment are non-encapsulated and fall into the category of serologically non-typeable H. influenzae (NTHI), which is an important etiologic agent of acute otitis media, acute sinusitis, conjunctivitis, pneumonia and bronchitis (1, 3, 4).

Attempts to identify particular virulence traits in NTHI have so far been unsuccessful. Different parameters such as biotyping (5), lipopolysaccharide profiles (6), outer membrane protein profiles (7, 8) and antibiotic susceptibility patterns have been tested with little success. Multilocus enzyme gel electrophoresis (9, 10) and DNA techniques (11–14) have improved the ability to discriminate between isolates although the relation of observed patterns to virulence remains unknown.

Patients with primary antibody deficiency disorders, which comprise a spectrum of conditions with decreased levels of immunoglobulins ranging from absence of all immunoglobulin classes, found in common variable immunodeficiency (CVI) and X-linked agammaglobulinemia (XLA), to a selective deficiency of a single immunoglobulin subclass, often present with recurrent bacterial infections (15–18). The major symptoms in these patients originate from the sinopulmonary tract and consist of frequent recurrent and often long-lasting bacterial infections (16, 19). The most commonly found bacteria in nasopharynx and sputum specimens during disease are H. influenzae and to a lesser extent Streptococcus pneumoniae (19).

This report addresses the question whether the recurrent episodes of H. influenzae infections observed in these patients are due to persistent infection with the same bacterial strain or repeated infection with different strains. The results are based on the typing of a total of 224 isolates of H. influenzae from the respiratory tract of a consecutive series of patients with primary antibody deficiencies, using genetic fingerprinting i.e. restriction enzyme analysis of total genomic DNA – a well established method for a variety of bacterial genera (11) to study genetic relatedness between the different isolates. Monoclonal antibodies specific for H. influenzae lipopolysaccharide (LPS) were used to further characterize the isolates.

PATIENTS AND METHODS

Subjects

The 36 males and 81 females included in the study were enrolled during a 5 year period (1985–1989) because of some type of

Table I. *Type of primary antibody deficiency in relation to age, sex and bacteriological findings in nasopharyngeal and sputum cultures from 117 patients in the study group (775 samples)*

Type of Immuno-deficiency	Males (mean age) range	Females (mean age) range	Total no. of patients	Patients with Haemophilus influenzae[a]	Patients with other pathogens[b]	Patients with only negative samples[c]	Mean no. of days with antibiotics[e]	Gamma-globulin substi-tution[e]
CVI	12 (42.3) 25–64	24 (45.5) 18–79	36	27[d]	4	5	46	33/36
XLA	1 (21)	0	1	1	0	0	346	1/1
IgA	10 (41.9) 24–76	22 (47.1) 21–73	32	4	2	26	3	0/32
IgA,IgG2	0	1 (40)	1	0	0	1	0	0/1
IgA,IgG2 + 3	0	1 (54)	1	0	0	1	22	1/1
IgA,IgG3	0	3 (43.7) 20–57	3	2	0	1	55	2/3
IgG1	2 (38.5) 21–56	5 (43.4) 29–66	7	0	1	6	7	3/7
IgG1 + 2	1 (56)	2 (40.5) 37–44	3	0	0	3	20	1/3
IgG1 + 3	1 (30)	2 (48.0) 46–50	3	0	3	0	9	2/3
IgG2	1 (22)	0	1	0	0	1	0	0/1
IgG2 + 3	1 (58)	2 (55.5) 40–71	3	0	2	1	0	2/3
IgG3	7 (38.4) 25–59	19 (41.8) 22–65	26	5	1	20	13	5/26
Total	36 (40.5) 21–76	81 (45.1) 18–79	117	39	13	65	23.6	50/117

[a] Patients from whom H. influenzae were isolated in pure culture or together with other pathogens ($<10\%$ of the samples also contained M. catarrhalis or S. pneumoniae).

[b] Other pathogens of the respiratory tract (M. catarrhalis, S. pneumoniae, S. aureus, Pseudomonas spp., Enterobacteriaceae, N. meningitidis, S. pyogenes).

[c] No growth or ordinary flora of the respiratory tract (optochin negative alphastreptococci, diphtheroid rods, coagulase negative staphylococci).

[d] $\chi^2_{1\text{d.f.}} = 40.0$, $p < 0.001$ (CVI vs. all other patients excluding XLA).

[e] Jan. 1989–Jun 1990.

primary antibody deficiency (Table I). The reason for the skewed sex ratio in this group of consecutive patients remains unknown. Altogether 36 patients fulfilled the criteria of CVI: decreased levels of 2 of the Ig-classes (IgG, IgA or IgM). The majority of patients had an IgG-level < 3 g/l. One patient had X-linked agammaglobulinemia (XLA). Selective IgA deficiency (< 0.05 g/l) was seen in 32 patients. Combined IgA and IgG-subclass deficiencies were present in 5 patients. IgG-subclass deficiencies (IgG1 < 4.2 g/l, IgG2 < 1.17 g/l, IgG3 < 0.2 g/l) were found in 43 patients (Table I). 34 out of 37 patients with CVI or XLA in this study received gammaglobulin substitution therapy subcutaneously; dose and intervals as described by Gardulf et al. (20). The mean concentration of total IgG in serum using this route of administration was 8.1 g/l.

For the comparison with LPS expressed by isolates from patients with primary antibody deficiencies, 499 NTHI isolates were included from patients, suffering from acute respiratory disease without a history of abnormal gammaglobulin levels. These patients were attending the ENT-department, the outpatients clinic of the pediatric department at Huddinge hospital or were seen by a general practitioner in the nearby area during the same period.

Clinical procedures

The patients were seen by appointment at a primary antibody deficiency clinic at Huddinge hospital and managed according to standard practices. Each time they were seen by a doctor, nasopharyngeal samples were collected transnasally with a metal armed cotton swab (Biohospital, Stockholm, Sweden) which was immediately transferred to a transport medium. Sputum samples were collected when possible. All samples reached the bacteriological laboratory within 3 hours. Respiratory tract infections during the study period were treated with antibiotics prescribed according to standard practice, with due consideration given to the age of the patient, previous adverse drug reactions etc.

Bacterial strains and growth conditions

Nasopharyngeal samples were cultured on horse blood agar (Colombia II agar base, Svenska Labfab., with addition of 5% horse blood and 0.5% tryptophane), chocolate agar (Hemoglobin, BBL, 20 g; GC-agar base, BBL, 72 g; Isovitalex, BBL, 20 ml; 2000 ml distilled water) and sheep blood agar (Colombia II agarbase, Svenska Labfab., 5% sheep blood, 0.01% methylrosaniline).

The sputum samples were Gram-stained for examination by light microscopy. Only those with >5 poly-morphonuclear cells per epithelial cell were considered as representative samples from the lower respiratory tract and were cultured. The representative sputum samples were washed with tap water through a sieve and treated with sputolysin (Calbiochem®, Behring Diagnostics, La Jolla, USA) before cultivation on horse blood agar, sheep blood agar, chocolate agar and CLED agar (CLED agar base, Lab M, Stockholm, Sweden). The horse blood agar and CLED agar plates were incubated aerobically at 37°C for 16–20 h. Chocolate agar plates were incubated aerobically in humidified air with 5% CO_2 at 37°C for 16–20 h. The sheep blood agar containing methylrosaniline was incubated anaerobically at 37°C for 16–20 h.

H. influenzae was identified by colony morphology, lack of hemolysis on blood agar and growth requirements for X and V-factors (5). Isolates were stored in aliquots at −70°C in BHI-broth/glycerol 1 : 3 until studied. All strains were agglutinated with Bacto-Haemophilus influenzae antisera set (Difco) in order to determine their capsular serotype. Other bacterial specimens found were identified according to routine laboratory procedures (21).

Strains used for immunization

H. influenzae strains RM.118, Rd/b^+:01, Rd/b^+:02 (22), RM.118–26, RM.118–28 (23) were obtained from R.E. Moxon, Oxford, UK.

Preparation of DNA

Bacteria were cultivated on chocolate agar (see above) and incubated in humidified air plus 5% CO_2 at 37°C for 24–48 hours. The bacterial growth on one 100 mm diameter plate was suspended in 0.8 ml buffer (50 mM NaCl, 50 mM EDTA, 50 mM TRIS hydrochloride, pH 7.5). DNA was extracted according to Loos et al. (12). In short bacterial cells were lysed with SDS (SIGMA) and treated with RNase and proteinase K (Boehringer Mannheim, Mannheim, Germany). This was followed by three extractions with phenol-chloroform-isoamylalcohol (25 : 24 : 1) and three extractions with chloroform-isoamylalchol (24 : 1). DNA was precipitated with isopropyl-alcohol. After a short centrifugation the supernatant was discarded and the DNA pellet dried under vacuum and finally dissolved in TE (10 mM TRIS-hydrochloride, 1 mM EDTA pH 8.0).

Digestion with restriction enzymes

Purified DNA, 5–10 μg, were digested with either *Cla*I or *Eco*RI (Boehringer Mannheim) 2 units/μg DNA at a buffer-concentration of 10%, according to the recommendation by the manufacturer.

Electrophoresis

0.6% agarose was used for submerged gel electrophoresis (16 h at 0.7 V/cm) in 0.5 TBE (0.089 M Tris-borate; 0.089 M boric acid; 0.002 M EDTA). The gel was stained in ethidium bromide and left to clear in water for one hour at 22°C before being photographed in UV-light.

LPS-specific monoclonal antibodies (mabs)

A panel of 10 monoclonal antibodies, MAHI 30–39, was generated by immunization of BALB/C mice using whole bacterial cells of H. influenzae from strain RM.118 or its transductant mutants Rd/b^+:01, Rd/b^+:02, RM.118–26, RM.118–28 (heat inactivated for 60 min at 65°C) and subsequent fusions of lymphocytes with Sp2/0 cells for the production of antibody secreting hybridomas. The production of monoclonal antibodies followed the description of Lind et al. (24). The 10 monoclonal antibodies, MAHI 30–39, were selected on the basis of their reactivity with extracted LPS (25) from the RM 118 series of strains (Table II). No mab reacted with any of the LPS from the deep rough mutant of H. influenzae, I69 Rd^-/b^+ (26) or H. influenzae type b strain Eagan, Salmonella typhimurium SL1102, SL1181, SL1032, SL805, TV148, TV161, SL733, TV119, SH4809, SH1262 (24), Escherichia coli CVD73-1 or Bacteroides fragilis NCTC 9343 (27).

Whole cell ELISA

Each strain was cultured on chocolate agar plates in 5% CO_2 at 37°C overnight and suspended in PBS (superior to coating buffer for whole bacteria), and heat inactivated for 60 min at 65°C. The optical density at 595 nm was adjusted to 0.2 (approximately 10^9 bacteria/ml). Microtiter plates (Nunc, AS, Denmark) were coated with 100 μl/well of the bacterial suspension and incubated overnight at room temperature. Mabs in serumfree culture supernatant were diluted 1/10 in PBS with 0.05% Tween 20. The ELISA was then performed using antimouse polyvalent alkaline phosphatase conjugate (Sigma, St. Louis, USA) according to Carlin and Lindberg (25). The OD-values at 405 nm were read with a computerized spectrophotometer when the positive control (LPS from RM118, MAHI 30) had reached an OD-value of 1.5. Negative controls: a) S. typhimurium strain SL805-LPS, and b) PBS instead of mab.

Dot-blotting of NTHI

Each frozen isolate of NTHI was inoculated on chocolate agar plates incubated 16–20 h at 37°C in humidified air plus 5% CO_2, and 24 single colonies were picked and individually suspended in 300 μl of coating buffer in a 96-well microtiter plate (Nunc, Denmark). The top was sealed with transparent tape. The bacteria were heat inactivated for 60 min at 65°C. For the blotting a BioDot Apparatus (Bio Rad Laboratories, Richmond, USA) was used. A sheet of nitrocellulose membrane filter (Schleicher & Schuell, BA-85, 0.45 mm, Dassel, Germany) was loaded in the blotting apparatus and 20 μl of bacterial suspension added to each well using a multichannel pipette. Incubation for 60–90 min at 22°C was followed by washing with 150 μl of coating buffer per well 3 times under vacuum. The nitrocellulose membrane was removed and left to dry for 30 min. This was followed by blocking with PBS-BSA 1% overnight at +4°C. The nitrocellulose sheets were then incubated with mabs MAHI 30–39 (serumfree culture supernatant) diluted 1/10 in PBS with 0.05% Tween 20. One sheet was used for each mab. With this procedure all 24 colonies were tested against the mabs panels, MAHI 30–39. Incubation was carried out for 3 h at 22°C followed by washing 3 times in PBS with 0.05% Tween 20 and 1% bovine serum albumin (BSA). Conjugate was added (antimouse polyvalent immunoglobulin alkaline phosphatase conjugate, Sigma) diluted 1/100 and left to bind overnight at 22°C. The

Table II. *LPS-specific monoclonal antibodies (mabs) MAHI 30–39 with immunoglobulin class, immunizing strain and reactivity to LPS extracted from RM.118 series of H. influenzae*

			LPS				
Mab	Ig-class	Immunizing strain	118	Rd/b$^+$:01	Rd/b$^+$:02	118–26	118–28
MAHI 30	IgM	118–26	+ + +[a]	+ + +	+ + +	+ + +	+ + +
MAHI 31	IgM	118	+ + +	+ + +	+ + +	+	+
MAHI 32	IgG3	118	+ + +	+ + +	+	+	—
MAHI 33	IgM	118	+ + +	+ + +	+	—	—
MAHI 34	IgM	118	+ + +	+ + +	—	—	—
MAHI 35	IgM	118	+ + +	+ + +	+	—	+
MAHI 36	IgG2b	Rd/b$^+$:02	+ +	+	+ + +	+ + +	+ + +
MAHI 37	IgG3	118–26	+	+	+	+ + +	+ + +
MAHI 38	IgM	118–28	+	—	+	+ + +	+ + +
MAHI 39	IgG3	118–28	—	—	—	+ + +	+ + +

[a] OD-value in ELISA after 70 min incubation.
$OD \geq 1.2$, + + +; $0.7 \leq OD < 1.2$, + +; $0.3 \leq OD < 0.7$, +; $OD < 0.3$, –.

washing procedure was repeated with PBS-Tween-BSA and followed by extensive washing with PBS. Finally, the nitrocellulose membrane was stained for 4 min in a solution of 47.5 ml Veronal-acetate buffer (0.3 M, pH 9.6), 0.01% w/v Nitro Blue Tetrazolium (Sigma), 50 µl 0.005% v/v of 5-Bromo-4-Chloro-3-Indolylphosphate (Sigma), 200 µl of 4 mM $MgCl_2$ and distilled water up to 50 ml.

RESULTS

Bacteriological findings

Altogether 655 nasopharyngeal and 120 sputum samples were collected. H. influenzae was the dominating pathogen, and was recovered from 29% (224/775) of all specimens (34% of sputum and 28% of nasopharyngeal cultures). M. catarrhalis was found in 9% (68/775) and S. pneumoniae in 4% (28/775). In fact, H. influenzae was the sole pathogen in 61% (202/330) of the samples from which a potential pathogen was recovered. All but one of the 224 H. influenzae isolates were non-encapsulated (99.6%). The capsulated strain was type b.

Considering the type of immunodeficiency in relation to the bacterial isolates it was found that common variable immunodeficiency (CVI) was the most prevalent condition (27/39 patients) in the group where H. influenzae was isolated ($p < 0.001$, Table I). As shown in Table III the CVI and XLA patients showed a much higher proportion of isolates with H. influenzae as compared to the other three groups of patients with less complete immunodeficiencies ($\chi^2_{4d.f.} = 61.2, p < 0.0001$). As regards other bacterial pathogens no such differences were seen ($\chi^2_{4d.f.} = 3.53$, $p = 0.47$). In patients where H. influenzae was not found only 9/78 patients had CVI. 49 of these 78 patients had isolated IgG3 or IgA deficiency. Both of these entities seemed to be associated with a lower prevalence of NTHI infection (Table I). This was evident also if the bacterial findings were analysed with respect to the number of visits (Table III).

DNA-fingerprinting

Genetic relatedness between NTHI isolates was assessed through DNA-fingerprinting using whole genomic DNA

Table III. *Type of immunodeficiency in relation to mean number of visits and bacteriological findings in nasopharyngeal or sputum cultures during Jan 1989 to June 1990*

			Mean number of isolates per sampling occasion		
Type of immunodeficiency	Number of patients	Mean number of visits	Haemophilus influenzae	Other pathogens	Negative culture
CVI	36	9.0	0.38	0.12	0.50
XLA	1	21	0.71	0.05	0.24
IgA	32	0.5	0.12	0.06	0.82
IgG3	26	1.5	0.05	0.11	0.84
Other[a]	32	3.0	0.04	0.17	0.78

[a] IgA and IgG2 and IgG2 + 3; IgA and IgG3; IgG1 + 2; IgG1 + 3, IgG2; IgG2 + 3

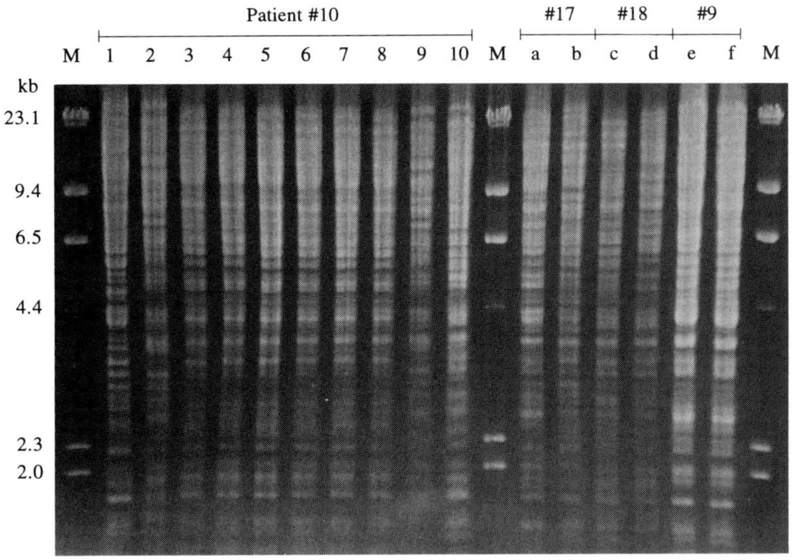

Fig. 1. Agarose gel electrophoresis of NTHI genomic DNA after digestion with the restriction enzyme EcoRI. M = DNA size marker (kb). Referring to Table IV lane 1–10 represents the isolates from patient #10. Lane 1: the genetic fingerprint designated AG-I; lane 2 and 9: AG-II, lane 3–8: AG-III and lane 10: AG-IV. From patient #17, lane a: JA-I and lane b: JA-II. Patient #18, lane c: SJ-I and lane d: SJ-II. Patient #9, lane e (the first isolate) and lane f (isolated 17 months later): LH-I.

digested with restriction enzymes and separation of the fragments by electrophoresis in agarose gels (12). The analysis was performed on 105 isolates from 18 patients selected on the basis of having 2 or more isolates of NTHI (Fig. 1 and 2, Table IV).

Identical DNA fingerprints were seen only in isolates from the same patient (Table IV). Altogether 33 different fingerprints patterns were observed. As a comparison, 5 randomly selected H. influenzae DNA digests obtained from the 499 clinical isolates in the control group, gave 5 different DNA fingerprint patterns (Fig. 2, lanes a–e).

The same strain, i.e. a patient specific strain, was repeatedly isolated in 13 of the 18 patients for periods of 3 to 43 months (Table IV). The remaining 5 patients had only 2 isolates each with different strains of NTHI on the 2 sampling occasions (Table IV). During the periods of colonization with the same strain, episodes of acute respiratory disease were common. Despite regress of symptoms and, in most instances negative cultures after antibiotic treatment, the same strain was reisolated again on several occasions (Table IV).

Characterization with LPS-specific monoclonal antibodies

Using our panel of 10 LPS-specific monoclonal antibodies, MAHI 30–39 (Table II), the 499 control H. influenzae isolates from patients with normal gammaglobulin levels gave 63 different reactivity patterns in whole cell ELISA (Table VI). The 10 most prevalent patterns accounted for almost two-thirds (63%) of the H. influenzae isolates. Only 9% of the isolates showed no reactivity with any of the 10 antibodies. Table VI also shows the results for the 224 H. influenzae isolates from patients with hypogammaglobulinemia. The similarities in antibody reactivity between the 2 patient groups were more striking than the differences. This suggests that there are no major differences in LPS epitopes between NTHI strains colonizing and infecting individuals with normal gammaglobulin levels compared to patients with hypogammaglobulinemia.

Dot blotting with 24 independent single colonies from the same isolate of NTHI revealed a greater variability than ELISA due to the possibility to visualize phase variation of the LPS epitopes. From patient #18 the one isolate giving the SJ-I DNA fingerprint gave 5 dotblot patterns: antibod-

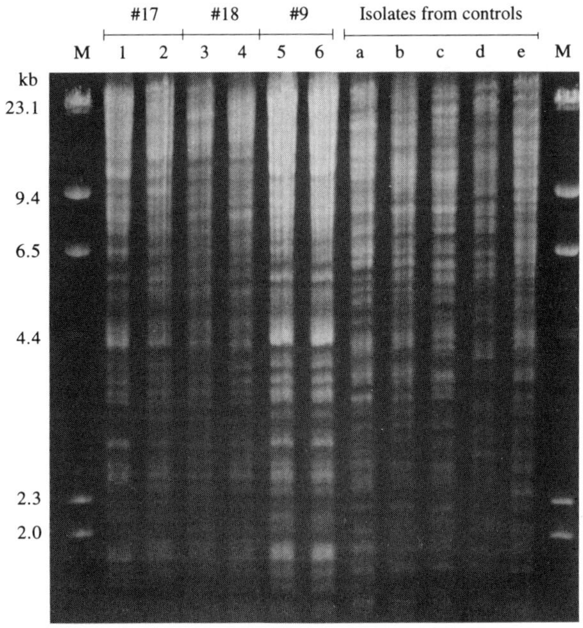

Fig. 2. Lanes 1–6: identical isolates of NTHI as in FIG 2a from the patients #17, #18 and #9, but digested with ClaI, to show that it is possible to draw the same conclusions concerning genetic relatedness between the isolates after digestion with a different restriction enzyme. Lanes a–e: 5 unrelated isolates from different patients in the control group, all 5 with different fingerprints.

Table IV. *Summary of restriction enzyme analysis of H. influenzae total genomic DNA on 105 isolates from the 18 patients with more than one NTHI isolate.*

All patients received substitution therapy with gammaglobulins. Treatment with antibiotic agents have been summarized from Jan. 1989 to June 1990 for all patients.

Patients	Time in months after the first NTHI-isolate (=0) and genetic fingerprint designation										Colonization Period with one strain in months	Type of immuno deficiency	No. of courses with antibiotics	No. of days on anti-biotics	Drugs used
1	0 BG-I	4 BG-I									4	CVI	2	18	D
2	0 IK-I	1 IK-I	1 IK-II	2 IK-II	3 IK-II	4 IK-II	5 IK-II	11 IK-III	12 IK-II		4	CVI	3	70	C, O
3	0 KL-I	12 KL-I									12	CVI	4	49	C, D, T, O
4	0 TM-I	1 TM-I	10 TM-II	13 TM-II	16 TM-III	17 TM-III	18 TM-III	21 TM-II			11	CVI	5	50	D
5	0 AJ-I	8 AJ-II									—	CVI	1	9	D
6	0 SL-I	5 SL-II									—	IgA + IgG3	10	134	A, C, O
7	0 CH-I	4 CH-II									—	IgG3	6	60	A, C, O
8	0 AH-I	11 AH-I	17 AH-II								11	CVI	2	29	A, C, O
9	0 LH-I	5 LH-I	8 LH-I	12 LH-I	17 LH-I						17	CVI	1	10	A
10	0 AG-I	39 AG-II	41 AG-III	41 AG-III	42 AG-III	47 AG-III	49 AG-III	50 AG-III	51 AG-II	69 AG-IV	12	CVI	3	27	A, O
11	0 MK-I	6 MK-I									6	CVI	2	80	A
12	0 VP-I	6 VP-II									—	CVI	3	34	A
13	0 LL-I	3 LL-I	6 LL-I	7 LL-I							7	CVI	7	220	A, C, T
14	0 BA-I	9 BA-II									—	CVI	—	—	—
15	0 AF-I	9 AF-I	17 AF-I								17	CVI	4	140	A, O
16	0 JE-I	3 JE-I	4 JE-II								3	CVI	6	87	A, C, T
17	0 JA-I	6 JA-I	39 JAI	41 JA-I	43 JA-II	43 JA-I	44 JA-II	44 JA-II	45 JA-II	45 JA-II	43	XLA	13	346	A, C, O
	47[a] JA-II	48[b] JA-II	49[c] JA-II	50 JA-II	51 JA-II										
18	0 SJ-I	3[a] SJ-II	4[d] SJ-II	5 SJ-II	5 SJ-II	6 SJ-II					3	CVI	1	9	D

[a] 4 isolates, [b] 11 isolates, [c] 4 isolates, [d] 3 isolates, A = amoxicillin, C = ciprofloxacin, D = doxycycline, T = trimethoprim-sulfamethoxazole, O = other antibotic agents

Table V. *Nasopharyngeal and sputum samples taken from patient # 17 during 1989 in relation to antimicrobial therapy and symptoms from the respiratory tract.*

This patient, suffering from XLA, was substituted with gammaglobulins during the whole study period.

Sampling date	Nasoph (n)/ sputum (s)	Bacterial isolates	Genetic fingerprint	Symptoms	Antibiotic treatment
9 Jan. 1989	s	NTHI	JA-I	Productive cough	ampicillin 2 g tid iv., 9–19 Jan. ciprofloxacin 500 mg bid, 23 Jan.–2 Feb. amoxicillin 750 mg bid, 27 Feb–19 Mar.
1 Mar.	n	NTHI	JA-I	Unchanged	amoxicillin 375 mg id, 20 Mar.–8 May amoxicillin 375 mg bid, 9–19 May
29 May	n	NTHI	JA-I	Productive cough, conjunctivitis	amoxicillin 750 mg bid, 29 May–20 June
	s	NTHI	JA-II		
14 June	n	NTHI	JA-II	Productive cough	amoxicillin 750 mg id, 21 June–3 Aug.
	s	NTHI	JA-II		
3 July	n	NTHI	JA-II	Improvement	ampicillin 2 g tid i.v., 4–7 Aug. amoxicillin 750 mg bid, 8 Aug.–3 Sep.
	s	NTHI	JA-II		
4 Sep.	n	NTHI	JA-II	Productive cough, fever	ciprofloxacin 500 mg bid, 5–26 Sep.
	s	NTHI	JA-II		
13 Sep.	n	NTHI	JA-II	Improvement	ciprofloxacin, see above
21 Sep.	n	Negative	—	Unsymptomatic	ciprofloxacin, see above
28 Sep.	n	NTHI	JA-II		amoxicillin 750 mg id, 27 Sep.–18 Oct.
12 Oct.	n	NTHI	JA-II		amoxicillin, see above
15 Oct.	n	NTHI	JA-II		amoxicillin, see above
19 Oct.	n	NTHI	JA-II	Productive cough, fever	ciprofloxacin 500 mg bid, 19 Oct.–9 Nov.
26 Oct.	n	NTHI	JA-II	Improvement	ciprofloxacin, see above
3 Nov.	n	Negative	—	Unsymptomatic	ciprofloxacin, see above
9 Nov.	n	Negative	—		ciprofloxacin, see above
16 Nov.	n	Negative	—		no treatment
23 Nov.	n	NTHI	JA-II	Productive cough, fever	ciprofloxacin 500 mg bid, 23 Nov.–13 Dec.
	s	NTHI	JA-II		
30 Nov.	n	Negative	—	Improvement	ciprofloxacin, see above cefuroxime + metronidazol i.v. because of colon surgery
22 Dec.	n	NTHI	JA-II	Productive cough	ciprofloxacin 500 mg bid, 22 Dec.–11 Jan. 1990
22 Dec. 1989	s	NTHI	JA-II		

ies MAHI 30, 35, 36 and 37 reacted with all colonies, and MAHI 31–34 and MAHI 38–39 detected phase variation (Table VII). The 11 isolates giving the SJ-II DNA fingerprint showed 15 dotblot patterns. In this case, 6 antibodies, MAHI 30–35, bound to all isolates whereas 4 antibodies, MAHI 36–39 demonstrated phase variation.

DISCUSSION

The present data show that some patients with primary antibody deficiency, predominately those with CVI or XLA, are frequently affected by respiratory tract infections with NTHI and can be colonized with the same strain for up to 43 months despite substitution therapy with gammaglobulins and antibiotic treatment. Nasopharyngeal carriage of H. influenzae as evidenced by positive swab cultures is rarely found among healthy adults. The fact that 13 of 18 immune deficient subjects in the present study harboured a specific strain for more than 3 months indicates that prolonged colonization and recurrent infections with the same strain are common among CVI patients. The analysis was based on genetic finger-printing using the ClaI or EcoRI restriction enzyme on genomic DNA (Fig. 1 and 2). This is a well established method, and probably the most sensitive, to investigate genetic relatedness. As described by other authors (12), we also found a good reproducibility on repeated typing of the same isolate. In this context it should be noted that it was unusual to find more than one fingerprint if several independent colonies were analysed from the same patient at the same sampling occasion. This confirms the findings of Groeneveld et al. (13) studying patients with chronic obstructive pulmonary disease. Furthermore, we were not able to identify the same DNA restriction pattern among isolates from different patients suggesting a great heterogeneity of NTHI. This was also evident for the isolates from patients with otitis media studied by Loos et al. (12).

In the present group of hypogammaglobulinemic patients it is still unclear where the NTHI could hide and survive

Table VI. *Reactivity patterns with LPS-specific monoclonal antibodies of 224 isolates of H.influenzae from patients with primary antibody deficiency in comparison with 499 isolates from immunocompetent patients as controls*

Reactivity patterns with MAHI 30–39 appearing in order of frequency										Frequency of the different reactivity patterns			
										224 isolates from patients with primary antibody deficiency		499 isolates from immunocompetent patients	
30	31	32	33	34	35	36	37	38	39	(*n*)	(%)	(*n*)	(%)
+[a]	—	—	—	—	—	—	—	—	—	45	20.0	80	16.0
+	+	+	+	+	+	—	—	—	—	21	9.4	36	7.2
—	—	—	—	—	—	—	—	—	—	20	8.9	47	9.4
+	+	—	—	—	—	+	+	+	+	18	8.0	6	1.2
+	—	—	—	—	—	+	—	+	—	15	6.7	41	8.2
+	—	—	—	—	—	+	—	—	—	14	6.2	17	3.4
+	+	—	+	+	+	—	—	—	—	13	5.8	8	1.6
+	+	+	+	+	+	+	—	—	—	12	5.4	15	1.4
+	—	—	—	—	—	+	+	+	+	9	4.0	29	5.8
+	+	—	—	—	—	—	—	—	—	8	3.6	24	4.8
+	+	+	+	+	+	+	+	+	+	6	2.7	0	0
+	—	—	—	—	—	+	+	+	—	6	2.7	12	2.4
+	—	—	—	—	—	—	—	+	—	5	2.2	13	2.6
+	+	—	+	+	+	+	—	+	—	5	2.2	11	2.2
+	+	—	—	—	—	+	—	—	—	4	1.8	6	1.2
+	+	—	+	+	+	+	—	—	—	3	1.3	0	0
—	+	—	—	—	—	—	—	—	—	2	0.9	12	2.4
+	+	—	+	—	—	—	—	—	—	1	0.5	8	1.6
+	—	—	—	—	—	—	—	—	+	1	0.5	13	2.6
+	+	—	—	—	—	+	—	+	—	0	0	16	3.2
+	+	—	—	—	—	+	+	+	—	0	0	5	1.0
+	+	—	+	—	+	—	—	—	—	0	0	7	1.4
+	+	+	+	—	+	—	—	—	—	0	0	7	1.4
										208 19 reactivity patterns	92.8%[b]	413 21 reactivity patterns	81.0%[c]

[a] The reactions were considered positive at OD-value >0.3 after 30 min incubation time.
[b] The remaining 7.2% consisted of 12 different reactivity patterns.
[c] The remaining 19.0% consisted of 42 different reactivity patterns.

Table VII. *Phase-variation of LPS-epitopes in relation to restriction enzyme analysis of total genomic DNA on 12 isolates from patient # 18.*
Dotblot with 24 single colonies from each isolate vs. mabs MAHI 30–39. Total genomic DNA restriction fingerprint of isolate #1, referred to as DNA-fingerprint SJ-I, differs from the isoaltes #2–12, referred to as DNA-fingerprint SJ-II. From isolate #1 it was possible to identify 5 reactivity patterns and from isolates number #2–12 a total of 15 patterns. The frames indicate positive binding common for all the colonies tested, DNA-fingerprint S-I and S-II separately.

Isolate #1 (DNA-fingerprint SJ-I)										Isolate #2–12 (DNA-fingerprint SJ-II)									
MAHI										MAHI									
30	31	32	33	34	35	36	37	38	39	30	31	32	33	34	35	36	37	38	39
+	—	—	—	—	+	+	+	—	—	+	+	+	+	+	+	—	—	—	—
+	+	+	+	+	+	+	+	—	—	+	+	+	+	+	+	+	—	—	—
+	+	+	+	—	+	+	+	—	—	+	+	+	+	+	+	+	—	+	—
+	—	+	+	—	+	+	+	+	+	+	+	+	+	+	+	+	—	+	+
+	+	+	+	+	+	+	+	+	+	+	+	+	+	+	+	+	—	—	+
										+	+	+	+	+	+	+	+	—	—
										+	+	+	+	+	+	+	+	—	+
										+	+	+	+	+	+	—	+	—	—
										+	+	+	+	+	+	—	+	+	—
										+	+	+	+	+	+	—	+	—	+
										+	+	+	+	+	+	+	+	+	—
										+	+	+	+	+	+	—	—	+	—
										+	+	+	+	+	+	—	—	+	+
										+	+	+	+	+	+	+	+	+	+
										+	+	+	+	+	+	—	—	—	+

while the patients were treated with antibiotics in doses which in theory should have been more than sufficient for eradiction of these bacteria which with few exceptions were sensitive in vitro to the drugs used (data not given). We have recently shown that viable NTHI can be found intracellularly in macrophage like cells in adenoid tissue from children (28). It is tempting to speculate that lymphoid tissue in other parts of the respiratory tract could also harbour intracellularly sequestered NTHI. Thereby, the bacteria would become less accessible to the immune defence and antimicrobial agents. The remarkably low frequency of β-lactamase producing isolates in this study (2/224, <1%, data not shown) may support the theory of intracellular escape. An additional explanation could be that the H. influenzae are harboured in other family members and that the patients with immune deficiencies acquire the same organisms repeatedly from contact with their colonized family members. However, this seems less likely since H. influenzae can not be expected to be frequently isolated with swab cultures from the nasopharynx of healthy adults (29). Furthermore, we have recently studied the nasopharyngeal turnover of H. influenzae in otitis prone children and found in many cases prolonged colonization times (up to 11 months) and recurrent infections with the same strain of NTHI (30).

It was noted during the course of these investigations that treatment with quinolones and trimethoprim-sulphamethoxazole was generally more efficient to give temporary relief of symptoms of infection in these patients compared to β-lactam antibiotics, which hardly penetrate intracellularly. Notwithstanding clinical improvement on quinolone therapy, total eradication of nasopharyngeal colonization with NTHI was usually not achieved with 10–20 day courses of oral ciprofloxacin (500 mg bid) either (data outlined in Table IV). A detailed example of this is illustrated in Table V. Longer courses or combination therapy might be required. In connection with Table V it is also worthy of note that all commerical gammaglobulin preparations (Gammonativ-Kabi, Gammagard-Baxter, Sandoglobin-Sandoz, Gammaglobulin-Kabi, Endoglobin-Immuno) tested contained high titers of IgG antibodies that would bind to strain JA-II in whole cell ELISA (data not given).

Both NTHI and capsulated H. influenzae are capable to alter their saccharide structure in the LPS through phase variation. The genetic basis for this has partly been identified for Hib (31, 32). Presumably, phase variation may allow evasion from host immune defence mechanisms. In the present study variation was demonstrated using the monoclonal antibodies MAHI 30 to 39 (Table VII). Using the panel of 10 H. influenzae LPS-specific monoclonal antibodies against H. influenzae strains RM.118 and its lipopolysaccharide mutants (Rd/b$^+$:01, Rd/b$^+$:02, RM.118–26 and RM. 118–28) we could see reactivity with more than 90% of the isolates in whole bacterial cell ELISA. This suggests that the number of epitopes expressed is restricted in spite of the extensive phase variation. The 723 isolates gave 94 recognizable mab-binding patterns (Table VI).

As seen from Table VI, no significant differences were seen between the patterns observed in the test population and those in the controls. Structural studies of the saccharide portion of H. influenzae LPS (33–35) have shown that it is highly variable which makes is difficult to interpret the basis for the LPS variation. However, we may conlcude that NTHI isolates from the hypogammaglobulinemic patient group were very similar to those NTHI that were isolated from immunocompetent patients with respiratory tract infections. These strains must therefore be considered ordinary NTHI, at least with respect to their LPS phenotype. The mapping of LPS-epitopes may eventually permit us to identify important virulence factors in NTHI. Since these epitopes are exposed on the surface of the H. influenzae cell, and the expression appears to vary both in vitro and in vivo (31) their identification would be of interest. The simple fact that specific changes in the environment can regulate the expression of specific genes coding for a surface structure is important in this context.

In conclusion, it can be inferred from the present data that patients with a more complete antibody deficiency i.e. CVI and X-linked agammaglubulinemia react fundamentally different from those with selective immunoglobulin deficiences with regard to NTHI infections although a great deal of heterogeneity was observed. With few exceptions, isolated IgA deficiency or IgG subclass deficiencies, did not seem to be associated with increased susceptibility to recurrent respiratory infection with NTHI. Brandtzaeg and coworkers (36, 37) studied patients with IgA deficiency and found that subjects who generate a compensatory secretory IgM response in the respiratory tract had less problems with recurrent infections. On the other hand, IgA-deficient individuals who failed to produce sIgM or produced sIgD antibodies instead were prone to have recurrent respiratory tract infections comparable to what is seen among CVI patients (36, 37). Local immunity due to IgA and secretory IgA classes unrelated to serum levels of antibody has been suggested to be a main defense against colonization with NTHI (13). In line with these observations, it is noteworthy that patients with CVI are known to have little or no local production of IgA and IgM antibodies in their nasal mucosa (36, 38). Patients parenterally substituted with gammaglobulins will to a variable degree leak IgG antibodies from the serum to the mucosal membranes. This will supposedly help to decrease the frequency of respiratory tract infections and subsequent development of chronic pulmonary disease.

A possible explanation for the strong predominance of non-capsulated strains of H. influenzae in comparison to capsulated strains among patients substituted with gammaglobulins in this study would be that the gammaglobulin preparations used contained sufficient amounts of anti-PRP antibodies to protect the patients from respiratory tract infections and invasive infections caused by serotype b strains (Hib). It is a well documented fact that the vast majority of healthy adults (plasma donors) are naturally well protected against Hib disease due to adequate levels of anti-PRP antibodies (1).

We speculate that the temporary improvement that is usually seen during antibiotic therapy is due to killing of extracellular bacteria but intracellularly sequestered NTHI will usually survive and eventually cause relapse. Thus, the combination of cryptic intracellular growth of NTHI and lack of specific antibodies might create a basis for the persistent NTHI infections seen in these patients.

ACKNOWLEDGEMENTS

This work was supported by the Swedish Medical Research Council grant no. B92-16X-09496-02A and the Swedish Society for Medical Research.

REFERENCES

1. Moxon R. H. influenzae. In: Mandell G, Douglas R, Bennett J, eds. Principles and practice of infectious diseases. 3rd ed. New York: Churchill Livingstone, 1722–1729, 1990.
2. Turk D. The pathogenicity of H. influenzae. J Med Microbiol 18: 1–16, 1984.
3. St. Geme III J. Nontypeable Haemophilus influenzae disease: epidemiology, pathogenesis, and prospects for prevention. Infect Agents Dis 2: 1–16, 1993.
4. Murphy TF, Apicella MA. Nontypable Haemophilus influenzae: a review of clinical aspects, surface antigens, and the human immune response to infection. Rev Infect Dis 9: 1–15, 1987.
5. Kilian M. Haemophilus influenzae. In: Lenette E, Traunt J, eds. Manual of clinical microbiology. 4th ed. Washington DC: American Society for Microbiology, 387–393, 1985.
6. Campagnari AA, Gupta MR, Dudas KC, Murphy TF, Apicella MA. Antigenic diversity of the lipooligosaccharides of nontypable Haemophilus influenzae. Infect Immun 55: 882–887, 1987.
7. Murphy TF, Apicella MA. Antigenic heterogeneity of outer membrane proteins of nontypable Haemophilus influenzae is a basis for a serotyping system. Infect Immun 50: 15–21, 1985.
8. Spinola S, Peacock J, Denny F, Smith D, Cannon J. Epidemiology of colonization by nontypable Haemophilus influenzae in children: a longitudinal study. J Infect Dis 154: 100–109, 1986.
9. Porras O, Caugant D, Lagergård T, Svanborg-Edén C. Application of multilocus enzyme gel electrophoresis to Haemophilus influenzae. Infect Immun 53: 71–78, 1986.
10. Trottier S, Stenberg K, Svanborg-Edén C. Turnover of non-typable Haemophilus influenzae in the nasopharynges of healthy children. J Clin Microbiol 27: 2175–2179, 1989.
11. Owen RJ. Chromosomal DNA-fingerprinting – a new method of species and strain identification applicable to microbial pathogens. J Med Microbiol 30: 89–99, 1989.
12. Loos BG, Bernstein JM, Dryja DM, Murphy TF, Dickinson DP. Determination of the epidemiology and transmission of nontypeable Haemophilus influenzae in children with otitis media by comparison of total genomic DNA restriction fingerprints. Infect Immun 57: 2751–2757, 1989.
13. Groeneveld K, van Alphen L, Eijk PP, Visschers G, Jansen HM, Zanen HC. Endogenous and exogenous reinfections by Haemophilus influenzae in patients with chronic obstructive pulmonary disease: the effect of antibiotic treatment on persistence. J Infect Dis 161: 512–517, 1990.
14. Groeneveld K, van Alphen L, Eijk PP, Jansen HM, Zanen HC. Changes in outer membrane proteins of nontypable Haemophilus influenzae in patients with chronic obstructive pulmonary disease. J Infect Dis 158: 360–365, 1988.
15. Björkander J, Bake B, Hanson L. Primary hypogammaglobuli-

naemia: impaired lungfunction and body growth with delayed diagnosis and inadequate treatment. Eur J Respir Dis 65: 529–536, 1984.
16. Cunningham-Rundles C. Clinical and immunological analysis 103 patients with common variable immunodeficiency. J Clin Immunol 1: 22–33, 1989.
17. Fasth A. Primary immunodeficiency disorders in Sweden: cases among children. J Clin Immunol 2: 86–92, 1982.
18. Rosen F, Wedgewood R, Eibl M. Primary immuno deficiency diseases. Report of a WHO scientific group. Immunodeficiency Rev 3: 195–236, 1992.
19. Lederman HM, Winkelstein JA. X-linked agammaglobulinemia: an analysis of 96 patients. Medicine 64: 145–156, 1985.
20. Gardulf A, Hammarström L, Smith CIE. Home treatment of hypogammaglobulinemia with subcutaneus gammaglobulin by rapid infusion. Lancet 338: 162–166, 1991.
21. Lenette E, Traunt J. Manual of clinical microbiology. 4th ed. Washington DC: American Society for Microbiology, 1985.
22. Zwalen A, Rubin LG, Moxon ER. Contribution of lipopolysaccharide to pathogenicity of Haemophilus influenzae: comparative virulence of genetically-related strains in rats. Microb Pathog 1: 465–473, 1986.
23. Weiser J, Lindberg A, Manning E, Hansen E, Moxon E. Identification of a chromosomal locus for expression of lipopolysaccharide epitopes in Haemophilus influenzae. Infect Immun 57: 3045–3052, 1989.
24. Lind SM, Carlin NIA, Lindberg AA. Production and characterization of KDO-specific monoclonal antibodies recognizing lipopolysaccharides from heptoseless mutants of Salmonella. FEMS Microbiol Lett 28: 45–49, 1985.
25. Carlin NIA, Lindberg AA. Monoclonal antibodies specific for O-antigen polysaccharides of Shigella flexneri. J Clin Microbiol 18: 1183–1189, 1983.
26. Helander IM, Lindner B, Brade H, Altmann K, Lindberg AA, Rietschel ET, Zähringer U. Chemical structure of the lipopolysaccharide of Haemophilus influenzae strain I-69 Rd^-/b^+. Eur J Biochem 177: 483–492, 1988.
27. Weintrab A, Larsson B, Lindberg A. Chemical and immunochemical analyses of Bacteroides fragilis lipopolysaccharides. Infect Immun 49: 197–201, 1985.
28. Forsgren J, Samuelson A, Ahlin A, Jonasson J, Rynnel-Dagöö B, Lindberg AA. Haemophilus influenzae resides and multiplies intracellularly in human adenoid tissue as demonstrated by in situ hybridization and bacterial viability assay. Infect Immun 62: 673–679, 1994.
29. Kuklinska D, Kilian M. Relative proportions of Haemophilus species in the throat of healthy children and adults. Eur J Clin Microbiol 3: 249–252, 1984.
30. Samuelson A, Freijd A, Jonasson J, Lindberg A. Turnover of non-encapsulated Haemophilus influenzae in the nasopharynges of otitis-prone children. J Clin Microbiol (in press) 1995.
31. Weiser J, Love J, Moxon E. The molecular mechanism of phase variation of Haemophilus influenzae lipopolysaccharide. Cell 59: 657–665, 1989.
32. Weiser J, Maskell D, Butler P, Lindberg A, Moxon E. Characterization of repetitive sequences controlling phase variation of Haemophilus influenzae lipopolysaccharide. J Bacteriol 172: 3304–3309, 1990.
33. Phillips N, Apicella M, Griffiss J, Gibson B. Structural characterization of the cell surface lipooligosaccharides from a nontypable strain of Haemophilus influenzae. Biochemistry 31: 4515–4526, 1992.
34. Phillips NJ, Apicella M, Griffiss J, Gibson B. Structural studies of the lipooligosaccharides from Haemophilus influenzae type b strain A2. Biochemistry 32: 2003–2012, 1993.
35. Schweda E, Hegedus O, Borrelli S, Lindberg A, Weiser J, Maskell D, Moxon E. Structural studies of the saccharide part of the lipooligosaccharides derived from Haemophilus influenzae strain AH13 (lic3 +). Carbohydr Res 246: 319–330, 1993.
36. Brandtzaeg P, Karlsson G, Hansson G, Petruson B, Björkander J, Hanson LÅ. The clinical condition of IgA-deficient patients is related to the proportion of IgD- and IgM-producing cells in their nasal mucosa. Clin Exp Immunol 67: 626–636, 1987.
37. Brandtzaeg P. Humoral immune response patterns of human mucosae: induction and relation to bacterial respiratory tract infections. J Infect Dis 165(suppl 1): S167–176, 1992.
38. Karlsson G. The nasal mucosa in humoral immunodeficiency – A clinical, histological and immunohistochemical study in adult patients with common variable immunodeficiency or selective IgA deficiency. PhD-thesis, University of Göteborg, 1986.

Submitted March 3, 1995; accepted June 18, 1995

Scand J Infect Dis 27: 315–318, 1995 ORIGINAL ARTICLE

Prevalence of Antibodies to Herpes Simplex Virus Types 1 and 2, Epstein–Barr Virus and Cytomegalovirus in Teenage Girls

AGNETA ANDERSSON-ELLSTRÖM[1], BO SVENNERHOLM[2] and LARS FORSSMAN[3]

From the [1]Center for Public Health Research and District Health Care Center, Gripen, Karlstad, and the Departments of [2]Clinical Virology and [3]Obstetrics and Gynecology, Östra Sjukhuset, University of Göteborg, Göteborg, Sweden

Seropositivity to herpes virus type 1 (HSV-1), herpes virus type 2 (HSV-2), cytomegalovirus (CMV) and Epstein–Barr virus (EBV) was estimated in a group of 98 16-year-old Swedish girls. Antibodies to HSV-1 were seen in 41% of the girls and to HSV-2 in 1%, and antibodies to CMV in 45 and to EBV in 82%. In girls with coitus experience, there was significantly higher prevalence of HSV-1 and EBV antibodies, compared with girls with no sexual contact. The age of coitarche or number of coitus partners did not affect the rate of seropositivity. During 2 years of follow up, 13 girls seroconverted. All but one EBV-seroconverting girl, were sexually active, and no girl converted for more than one type of virus. We conclude that transmission of herpes viruses is common in adolescence, and sexuality, even with regard to its close association with kissing, is one important determinant.

A. Andersson-Ellström, MD, Center for Public Health Research, Box 9104, S-650 09 Karlstad, Sweden

INTRODUCTION

The spread of human herpes virus infections, as caused by herpes simplex virus (HSV), cytomegalovirus (CMV) and Epstein–Barr virus (EBV), is related to socioeconomic conditions and age. As a rule, seroconversion at early ages is associated with low socioeconomic status (1–5). The prevalence of the infections varies in different populations and regions (1–5). In populations where seroconversion happens late in life, sexual activity seems to be one important determinant (5–8). Herpes simplex virus type 2 (HSV-2) is mainly associated with genital infection and antibody prevalence correlates with past sexual activity (9). Herpes simplex virus type 1 (HSV-1) is more related to facial/oral locations but genital infections also occur (10). The prevalence of antibodies to HSV-1 increases more rapidly in the teenage period, particularly in regions with a high socioeconomic level; HSV-2-antibodies appear some years later (1, 9, 11). There are at least 2 periods of increased CMV spread during life; the peri- and neonatal period, and the years of sexual maturity (2). EBV infects the vast majority of young children without clinical symptoms (3). Mononucleosis can be recognized as a primary infection in teenagers, and may be related to close contact, e.g. kissing (3).

The purpose of this study was to investigate the seroprevalence and seroincidence of HSV-1, HSV-2, CMV and EBV in a group of healthy young Swedish female teenagers, followed during 2 years, and to relate serological data to sexual experience.

MATERIAL AND METHODS

The study was carried out in Karlstad, a middle-sized Swedish city, from September 1989 until September 1990. All the girls < 18 years old, who were starting their education in the health care program of an upper secondary school, i.e. 168 girls, were invited to participate in a study about sexuality and sexually transmitted diseases. For those participating it implied 2 years of gynecological health control and access to contraceptive advice. The 98 girls who chose to participate were called to the youth clinic, every 6 months for a total of 5 visits, for blood sampling and a structural face-to-face interview with one of the investigators (A. A.-E.). A gynecological examination was carried out at the start and the end of the study, and whenever a girl reported any symptoms.

The sample was divided into 3 socioeconomic groups, according to the classification made by Statistics Sweden (12). The participants were classified according to the occupation of the father, except in 7 cases where the mother had a higher educational level, and in 2 cases where the girls related only to their mothers. Group 1 consisted of employed and self-employed professionals, higher civil servants and executives, group 2 of intermediate non-manual employees and self-employed other than professionals, and group 3 consisted of manual workers and assistant non-manual employees.

Serology. The blood samples, drawn at entry (first visit) and after 2 years (fifth visit), were used for the serological analysis. Each serum was assayed in direct enzyme-linked immunosorbent assay (ELISA) using a highly purified HSV-type common antigen, containing envelope glycoproteins (13), a HSV-2-type specific glycoprotein G (gG-2) antigen (14) and a cytomegalovirus (CMV) antigen (15). Microtiter plates (NUNC Immunoplates, Denmark), coated with antigen, were incubated with serum samples in twofold dilutions starting at 1:100. For detection, horse-radish perioxidase conjugated antihuman IgG (Jackson, USA) was used. Epstein–Barr virus specific IgG antibodies to the virus capsid antigen (VCA) were demonstrated according to standard procedures by incubation of serial twofold dilutions of sera on P3HR-1 cells in indirect immunofluorescence (16)

Samples positive against HSV-type common antigen, which were gG-2-negative, were regarded as HSV-1-positive.

Statistical analysis. The chi-square test and Fisher's exact test were used for the statistical analysis.

 ISSN 0036-5548

RESULTS

A total of 98 girls agreed to participate and 89 completed the study, but full data are available only from 88. On average each girl made 4.9 visits. Upon entry to the study the age range was 15–17 years, the mean age being 16.1 years. A total of 57 girls had grown up in a sparsely populated area, 37 in a middle-sized city and three in a big city. Nine girls belonged to socioeconomic group 1, 42 to group 2, and 46 to group 3. All but 4 girls had brothers and sisters. Of the girls, 61 had had their first intercourse before entering the study. The mean age for coitarche was 14.9 years, and it occurred 0–5 years before the start of the study. The mean number of coitus partners was 2.1. Experience of condom use was reported by 75% of these girls, and 44% had used oral contraception, but 76% also reported experience of unprotected coitus. Additionally, 9 other girls reported petting, and 28 reported no sexual contact. Nine girls who dropped out of the study were similar to the rest of the group with respect to age, socioeconomic background, age at coitarche, number of coitus partners and use of contraceptives.

The serological findings at the beginning and at the end of the study and in relation to coitarche are shown in Table I. The differences in seropositivity to HSV-1, as well as to EBV, between girls with and without coitus experience are statistically significant. There were no significant differences associated with social group, with number of coitus partners or with use of contraception, with regard to antibodies to any of the herpes viruses studied. Growing up in the town or in a sparsely populated area did not affect the rate of seropositivity.

Of the HSV-1-positive girls, 15% were aware of an oral herpes infection earlier in life, and 44% were not sure, but 41% had never recognized oral lesions. No girl reported a symptomatic genital herpes infection. No association was seen between the 4 herpes viruses with regard to seropositivity. Of the 36 girls who had no coitus experience at the first visit, 8 were seronegative for all 3 viruses (22%). The corresponding figures for girls with coitus experience were 2 out of 61 (3%, $p < 0.01$). The seroconversions which occurred during the study, are shown in Table II.

DISCUSSION

This study focuses on a group of girls preparing for future work in social care or nursing, and naturally represents a selected group of Swedish teenagers.

In accordance with Gibson et al. (5), we found that HSV-1 infections correlate to sexual activity. Recent British studies suggest increased prevalence of HSV-1 genital infections (17). We, however, found no correlation between the

Table I. *Positive herpes virus serology at the beginning and the end of the study: comparison in relation to coitus experience*

	Total		Before coitarche		After coitarche		
	n	%	*n*	%	*n*	%	*p* value
Seropositivity at first visit	98	100	37	100	61	100	
HSV	40	41	9	24	31	51	< 0.01
HSV-2	1	1	—	—	1	2	
CMV	44	45	17	46	27	44	
EBV	80	82	24	65	56	92	< 0.001
Seropositivity at fifth visit	89	100	17	100	72	100	
HSV	36	40	2	12	34	47	< 0.002
HSV-2	2	2	—	—	2	3	
CMV	44	49	9	53	35	49	
EBV	77	87	12	71	65	90	< 0.05

Table II. *Incidence of herpes virus seroconversion during 2 years of follow up with regard to sexual experience*

	Seronegative at start	Coitarche before last visit			No coitarche at last visit		
	n	*n*	Seroconverted	%	*n*	Seroconverted	%
HSV-1	56	41	3	7	15	0	0
HSV-2	88	71	1	1	17	0	0
CMV	48	40	3	8	8	0	0
EBV	18	12	5	42	6	1	17

number of coitus partners and HSV-1 positivity. Kissing, closely relating to sexual activity, may be the major cause of increasing prevalence (5, 9). The prevalence of HSV-1 antibodies found in our study is higher than previously reported. Christenson et al. reported 28–33% HSV-positivity in 15–19-year-old Swedish teenagers (11). Changing sexual behaviours (18) and/or an overrepresentation of sexually active girls may explain the higher prevalence. The frequency of HSV-2 infections was low and in agreement with previous studies (11).

In the Scandinavian countries, in spite of prosperity, the prevalence of CMV antibodies has been shown to be relatively high (2, 19), probably due to the high rate of maternal seropositivity, and the common occurrence of breast feeding and group care of infants (20, 21). According to Ahlfors, about 40% of Swedish children acquire CMV during the first year of life, and of 15–19-year-old women, considered to represent normal CMV material, 56% have been found to be CMV-positive (19). In the present study antibodies to cytomegalovirus, in contrast to HSV-1, were slightly lower than expected. No correlation was seen between CMV titers and sexual activity. The transmission of CMV occurs predominantly in early childhood (19, 20). In the early part of the 1970s when the population of our study was born, the frequency of breast-feeding in Sweden was temporarily low (22). Almost all the girls had sisters and brothers. We did not check for day care experience (20). The 3 girls who seroconverted during the study were sexually active, and sexual transmission may be assumed (2, 6, 8). At the start of the study the girls had no experience of nursing, but during the study they were attending hospitals as observers. Nursing however, seems to be a negligible risk factor for acquiring CMV (20, 23).

Evans & Niederman have reported an EBV seroprevalence of about 40% among Swedish preschool children (3). The EBV prevalence in Belgium has been shown to be 51% by the age of 4 years and 85% by the age of 19 years (4). This is in good agreement with our data. The prevalence of EBV-VCA-IgG correlated, like HSV-1-IgG, to sexual activity, probably due to the close association between sexuality and kissing. The presumed predominant mode of transmission is contact with EBV-containing oropharyngeal secretions. This contact may be direct, such as kissing (2, 23), or indirect, such as inhaling EBV-containing droplets, sharing toothbrushes, drinking cups, toys and so forth (25). Recent studies however show that both the male and female genital tract can harbour EBV and the virus is probably also transmitted genitally (7, 24). Chang emphasizes that, in spite of the high contagiousness in early childhood, there seems to be low contagiousness later on (25). It is notable in our study that five of 12 seronegative girls with experience of coitus seroconverted during the 2 years of follow up.

No difference was seen, in the prevalence of antibodies to any of the viruses, between girls growing up in the city or in the countryside. The standard of living in Sweden is generally high and great differences in illness due to standards of hygiene and housing can not be expected. Inconstancy in contraceptive habits makes it impossible to come to any conclusions about the effect of oral contraception and barrier methods on the prevalence of antibodies.

Nearly half of the infected girls were completely ignorant of their HSV infections. If the rate of asymptomatic virus excretion is high, it is of epidemiologic importance (1). Since HSV-1 infection usually occurs earlier in life than infections with HSV-2, the epidemiology of the clinical disease caused by HSV-2 may be indirectly influenced by factors important in the spread of HSV-1 (1). An initial teenage period restricted to kissing and with no genital contact, would probably promote progress to less numerous and fewer primary or symptomatic genital HSV infections (26), but increase the possibility of asymptomatic HSV-2 infections (10, 27).

We conclude that in the period around the sexual debut, HSV and EBV seem to be the most frequently transmitted herpes viruses in teenage girls. Infections are probably mainly spread by kissing. The transmission of oral HSV-1, mostly resulting in an asymptomatic infection, is probably of value for the individual and for society in counteracting the spread of genital herpes. The consequences of EBV transmission need further analysis.

REFERENCES

1. Rawls WE, Campione-Piccardo J. Epidemiology of herpes simplex virus type 1 and type 2 infections. International conference on human herpes virus Atlanta 1980. In: Nahmias AJ, ed. The human herpes viruses. New York: Elsevier, 137–152, 1981.
2. Ho M. Epidemiology of cytomegalovirus infections. Rev Infect Dis 12 (Suppl 17): 701–710, 1990.
3. Evans AS, Niederman JC. Epstein–Barr virus. In: Evans AS, ed. Viral infections in humans, 3rd edn. New York: Plenum Press 393: 265–292, 1989.
4. Schuster V, Kreth HW. Epstein–Barr virus infection and associated diseases in children. Eur J Pediatr 151: 718–725, 1992.
5. Gibson JJ, Hornung CA, Alexander GR, Lee FK, Potts WA, Nahmias AJ. A cross-sectional study of herpes simplex virus types 1 and 2 in college students: occurrence and determinants of infection. J Infect Dis 162: 306–312, 1990.
6. Collier AC, Handsfield HH, Roberts PL, DeRouen T, Meyers JD, Leach L, Murphy VL, Verdon M, Corey L. Cytomegalovirus infection in women attending a sexually transmitted disease clinic. J Infect Dis 162: 46–51, 1990.
7. Sixbey JW, Lemon SM, Pagano JS. A second site for Epstein–Barr virus shedding: the uterine cervix. Lancet 2: 1122–1124, 1986.
8. Handsfield HH, Chandler SH, Caine VA, Meyers JD, Corey L, Medeiros E, McDougall JK. Cytomegalovirus infection in sex partners: evidence for sexual transmission. J Infect Dis 151: 344–348, 1985.
9. Nahmias AJ, Lee FK, Beckman-Nahmias S. Sero-epidemiological and sociological patterns of herpes simplex virus infection in the world. Scand J Infect Dis Suppl 69: 19–36, 1990.

10. Koutsky LA, Ashley RL, Holmes KK, Stevens CE, Critchlow CW, Kiviat N, Lipinsky CM, Wölner-Hanssen P, Corey L. The frequency of unrecognized type 2 herpes simplex virus infection among women. Sex Transm Dis 17: 90–94, 1990.
11. Christenson B, Böttiger M, Svensson Å, Jeansson S. A 15 year surveillance study of antibodies to herpes simplex virus types 1 and 2 in a cohort of young girls. J Infect 25: 147–154, 1992.
12. Statistics Sweden. Swedish socioeconomic classification. Reports on statistical co-ordination 1982: 4. Stockholm, 1982.
13. Jeansson S, Forsgren M, Svennerholm B. Evaluation of solubilized herpes simplex virus membrane antigen by enzyme-linked immunosorbent assay. J Clin Microbiol 18: 1160–1166, 1983.
14. Svennerholm B, Olofsson S, Jeansson A, Vahlne A, Lycke E. Herpes simplex virus type-selective enzyme-linked immunosorbent assay with helix pomatia lectin-purified antigens. J Clin Microbiol 19: 235–239, 1984.
15. Krishna RV, Meurman OH, Zigler T, Kresh UH. Solid-phase enzyme immunoassay for determination of antibodies to cytomegalovirus. J Clin Microbiol 12: 46–51, 1984.
16. Lennette E. Laboratory diagnosis of infectious diseases. In: Lennette E, Halonen P, Murphy FA, eds. Viral, rickettsial and chlamydial diseases. Berlin: Springer-Verlag, 230–266, 1988.
17. Wilson P, Cropper L, Sharp I, Fink C. Apparent increase in the prevalence of herpes simplex virus type 1 genital infection among women. Genitourin Med 70: 228, 1994.
18. Klanger B, Tydén T, Ruusuvaara L. Sexual behavior among adolescents in Uppsala, Sweden. J Adolesc Health 14: 468–474, 1993.
19. Ahlfors K. Epidemiological studies of congenital cytomegalovirus infection. Thesis, University of Lund, Sweden, 1982.
20. Pass RF, Hutto C. Group day care and cytomegaloviral infections of mothers and children. Rev Infect Dis 8: 599–605, 1986.
21. Ahlfors K, Ivarsson SA. Cytomegalovirus in breast milk of Swedish milk donors. Scand J Infect Dis 17: 11–13, 1985.
22. National Board of Health and Welfare. Official statistics. In: Söder K, Hofvander Y, Hillervik C et al. The Swedish National Commission on baby Friendly Hospitals, Ministry of Health and Social Affairs, SOU Report 1993: 86, Stockholm, 1993.
23. Demmler GJ, Yow MD, Spector SA, Reis SG, Brady MT, Anderson DC, Taber LH. Nosocomial cytomegalovirus infections within two hospitals caring for infants and children. J Infect Dis 156: 9–16, 1987.
24. Israele V, Shirley P, Sixbey JW. Excretion of the Epstein–Barr virus from the genital tract of men. J Infect Dis 163: 1341–1343, 1991.
25. Chang RS. Infectious mononucleosis. Boston: G.K. Hall, 119–133, 1980.
26. Cheong WK et al. Clinical and laboratory study of first episode genital herpes in Singapore. Int J STD AIDS 1: 195–198, 1990.
27. Breinig MK, Kingsley LA, Armstrong JA, Freeman DJ, Ho M. Epidemiology of genital herpes in Pittsburgh: serologic, sexual, and racial correlates of apparent and inapparent herpes simplex infections. J Infect Dis 162: 299–305, 1990.

Submitted February 8, 1995; accepted March 22, 1995

Scand J Infect Dis 27: 319–324, 1995 ORIGINAL ARTICLE

Efficacy of Human Leucocyte Alpha-Interferon Treatment for Chronic Hepatitis C Virus Infection

OLA WEILAND[1], MARGARET CHEN[2], GUDRUN LINDH[1], LARS MATTSSON[1], ROBERT SCHVARCZ[1], ANDERS SÖNNERBORG[2], MARTIN WAHL[3], RUNE WEJSTÅL[3], ANDERS WIDELL[4] and GUNNAR NORKRANS[3]

From the Divisions of [1]Infectious Diseases and [2]Virology, Department of Immunology, Microbiology, Pathology and Infectious Diseases, Karolinska Institute and Huddinge Hospital, Huddinge, and the Departments of [3]Infectious Diseases, East Hospital, Göteborg and [4]Medical Microbiology, Malmö University Hospital, Malmö, Sweden

A total of 42 Swedish patients with biopsy-proven chronic hepatitis C virus (HCV) infection were treated with a natural human leucocyte alpha-interferon (HuIFN-alpha-Le), Alfanative® (BioNative AB, Umeå, Sweden) in an open uncontrolled study. Two patients were withdrawn from treatment within 2 weeks due to non-compliance and were omitted from further analysis, and 40 patients (17 females), mean age 39 years (range 24–71) completed the study. All patients were HCV RNA-positive in serum prior to treatment, with raised alanine aminotransferase (ALT) levels >1.5 times the upper normal limit known for more than 6 months. Interferon was given at a dose of 3 MU t.i.w. for an intended 24 weeks and follow-up was a further 24 weeks after treatment. Biochemical non-responders were withdrawn from treatment within 12–16 weeks but continued follow-up. Overall 21/40 (52.5%) patients had a complete biochemical response with normal ALT levels at the end of treatment. Sustained response during follow-up was seen in 8 (20%) whereas 13 (32.5%) had a non-sustained response. At the end of treatment 23 (58%) patients had undetectable serum HCV RNA and 9 (23%) at follow-up. Patients with sustained, non-sustained and non-response had a mean pretreatment HCV RNA level of 3.2×10^5, 2.5×10^6 and 3.2×10^6 genomes/ml, respectively, differences that did not reach statistical significance. Of the patients 3, 9, 10 and 14 had genotype 1b, 3a, 1a, and 2b, respectively, and 4 had mixed genotypes. Of the 23 patients with genotype 2b or 3a, 7 had a sustained response vs. none of the 13 patients with genotype 1a or 1b ($p = 0.03$). No patients with cirrhosis had a sustained response whereas 4/18 with chronic persistent and 4/18 with chronic active hepatitis had such a response. It is concluded that some 50% of patients treated with HuIFN-alpha-Le responded with normalisation of ALT levels but that only 20% had a durable response 24 weeks post-treatment, and that patients with genotypes 3a or 2b seem to respond better than patients with other genotypes.

O. Weiland, MD, Department of Infectious Diseases I 73, Karolinska Institute and Huddinge Hospital, S-141 86 Huddinge, Sweden

INTRODUCTION

Patients with chronic hepatitis C virus (HCV) infection usually have a slowly evolving disease over years and decades with few spontaneous recoveries (1–3). The long-term outcome is grave, at least in a subset with cirrhosis and hepatocellular carcinoma as end-stage outcomes (1, 2).

Interferon has, hitherto, been the only licensed treatment, to which some 50% of patients will respond with normalized alanine aminotransferase (ALT) levels during treatment, whereas the other 50% will be non-responders (4). After the end of treatment, many patients who responded during treatment will have a relapse (4). Sustained response, including eradication of the viraemia which persists after treatment cessation has thus been achieved in only 15–30% of treated patients (5, 6). A durable response after treatment cessation seems to be achieved in a higher percentage with prolonged treatment courses (5, 6). Some patients, although initially responding, will have a breakthrough of their HCV infection before completion of therapy during continued treatment, possibly caused by the evolution of neutralizing interferon antibodies (7, 8). Antibodies seem to occur more often with recombinant interferon alpha-2a than with recombinant interferon alpha-2b treatment and seem to be least common during treatment with natural interferons (9).

The factors most often claimed to predict response to interferon treatment are HCV RNA levels in serum prior to treatment and the HCV genotype (4). The aim of the present study was to evaluate the response rate (as measured by ALT normalization and eradication of HCV viraemia), tolerability and evolution of interferon antibodies during treatment with a natural interferon, Alfanative®, and to correlate the response with the pretreatment HCV RNA levels, HCV genotypes and pretreatment histological findings.

MATERIAL AND METHODS

A total of 42 Swedish patients with biopsy-proven chronic HCV infection were entered in the trial. Two men were withdrawn from treatment within 2 weeks after the start, due to non-compliance, and were omitted from further analysis. Thus 40 patients (17 females), mean age 39 years (range 24–71) were further evaluated. All these patients were positive for anti-HCV by second generation

ELISA (Ortho Diagnostic Systems, Raritan, New Jersey, USA), with positive confirmatory tests (second or third generation RIBA, Chiron, Emeryville, California, USA) and HCV RNA-positive in serum prior to entry. All the patients also had continuously raised ALT levels, > 1.5 times the upper normal limit, known for more than 6 months. No patient had antibodies against HIV or other causes of chronic liver diseases, such as hepatitis B, autoimmune hepatitis, PBC, alcohol use, haemochromatosis, Wilson's disease or alpha-1-antitrypsin deficiency. All patients gave verbal informed consent and the study was approved by the local ethics committee at the Karolinska Institute, Stockholm, Sweden. Natural human leucocyte interferon alpha (HuIFN-alpha-Le), Alfanative®, Bio-Native, Umeå, Sweden, was given at a dose of 3 MU t.i.w. for an intended 24 weeks with follow-up for another 24 weeks. Patients not responding biochemically with normalization of ALT levels within 12–16 weeks (non-responders) were withdrawn from further treatment but continued follow-up during the entire study period.

ALT levels were analysed before, during and after treatment with standard methods, normal levels being <0.6 and <0.8 μkat/l in females and males, respectively. Sera, stored frozen at −70°C and obtained prior to treatment (week 0), at treatment cessation (week 24) and at follow-up 24 weeks after treatment (week 48), were analysed qualitatively for HCV RNA. HCV RNA levels were also analysed quantitatively, and genotypes determined, in a serum obtained prior to treatment (week 0). Definitions of biochemical response were as follows: 'non-sustained response' meaning normal ALT levels at the end of treatment but relapse during follow-up; 'sustained response' meaning normal ALT levels at the end of treatment and during follow-up, and 'non-response' meaning non-normalizing ALT levels.

HCV RNA determination

HCV RNA was determined qualitatively with primers derived from the 5′-non-coding region of the genome as previously described (10). Serum (100 μl) was used for RNA extraction, which was performed with a modified guanidinium thiocyanate-phenol-chloroform method. In brief, HCV cDNA was synthesized in a total volume of 25 μl reverse transcription (RT) mixture as described earlier (10). The RT mixture was incubated at 37°C for 60 min, followed by heating at 95°C for 5 min. After the RT, one-tenth of the cDNA was amplified by double PCR. The detection limit of this PCR assay was five copies of cloned HCV genome.

Quantification of HCV RNA

The quantification of HCV RNA in pretreatment serum was performed using a method based on competitive PCR and colorimetric detection of the amplified products as described earlier (11). After reverse transcription (RT), one-tenth of the resulting cDNA, and the same volume of serially diluted cloned HCV competitor DNA, were coamplified by nested PCR. The competitive DNA consisted of the amplified regions of wild type HCV cDNA with an internal region substituted with the *lac* operator sequence. The PCR products were specifically quantitated by a colorimetric solid-phase assay. This assay reproducibly detects 10 HCV genome equivalents. The interassay variation is 10–15%, and the intra-assay variation 15–20% (11).

Genotyping of HCV

Genotyping was done with type-specific primers directed against the HCV core gene based on the principle of Okamoto et al. (12) but with several modifications (13). The typing terminology suggested by Chan et al. was used (14). Our assay also identified the important type 3a by Chan, which was never identified by the original Okamoto assay. Briefly, the typing started with a consensus amplification of bp 467–751 with primers 5′-TAGATTGGGT-GTGCGCGCGA (sense, s), 5′-ATGTACCCCATGAGGTCGGC (antisense, as); thereafter typing for each isolate was done in two different reactions under stringent conditions (annealing temperature 63°C, 25 cycles). The typing primer for type 1a was 5′-TGGGGATAGGCTGACGTCTACCT (as); for 1b 5′-CCATCC-TGCCCACCCCA (as); for 2a 5′-CCAAGAGGGACGGGAAC-CTC (as), and for 2b 5′-GCAACCCTCGTTTCC(GA)TACA-GAG (as). These primers were run against an upstream primer 5′-AGGAAGACTTCCGAGCGGTC (s). Type 3a was identified with a primer 5′-GTGTGCGCGACGCGTAAA (s) and a consensus primer 5′-GCA(TC)GT(AG)AGGGTATCGATGAC(TC)T (as). In this reaction type 1b was also confirmed with primer 5′-AACCTCGTGGAAGGCGACAA (s). (Bases within parentheses means redundant base at this position).

Determination of anti-interferon alpha antibodies in serum

Interferon-alpha-binding antibodies in serum were determined in a serum drawn before administration of the first dose of interferon-alpha and ≥48 h after the last dose. The presence of antibodies was measured by an ELISA method (BioNative AB, Umeå, Sweden) as described earlier (15). With this method, antibodies evoked both by recombinant and natural interferons can be detected.

Histological methods

All patients underwent a biopsy within 12 months prior to treatment. The biopsies were classified as chronic persistent hepatitis (CPH), chronic active hepatitis (CAH) with or without cirrhosis (Ci) as recommended by an international group (16).

Statistical methods

Statistical calculations were performed with Fisher's exact test and the Mann–Whitney U test.

RESULTS

Demographic data on the 40 patients who completed the study, according to the final biochemical outcome, are given in Table I. Before week 16, 7 patients were withdrawn from treatment due to biochemical non-response and another 2, who had achieved biochemical response, were withdrawn because of depression. All of these continued follow-up in the study.

Overall 21/40 (52.5%) patients had a complete biochemical response with normal ALT levels at the end of treatment (week 24). Of these, 13 relapsed biochemically within 24 weeks of follow-up after treatment. A sustained biochemical response with normal ALT levels at follow-up week 48 was thus seen in 8/40 (20%) patients, a non-sustained biochemical response in 13/40 (32.5%) and non-response in 19/40 (47.5%).

The number of patients with normal ALT levels and a negative HCV RNA test in serum at weeks 0, 12, 24 and 48 are given in Table II. The eradication of HCV RNA from serum exceeded the normalization rate of ALT levels at all time points during and after treatment.

The number of HCV RNA-negative patients, according to biochemical response category at week 12 during treatment, at end of treatment and at follow-up are given in Table III. All eight patients with sustained response were HCV RNA-negative at week 12 during treatment and at

Table I. *Demographic data in 40 patients with chronic hepatitis C virus infection treated with human leucocyte interferon-alpha according to biochemical response category*

	Sustained response	Non-sustained response	Non-response	Total
No. of patients	8	13	19	40
Males	4	9	10	23
Females	4	4	9	17
Age, years				
Median	35	38	39	39
Range	28–50	26–71	24–51	24–71
Mode of acquisition				
Intravenous drug use (IVDU)	2	4[a]	6	12[a]
Needle stick	—	1	1	2
Tattooing	1	—	2	3
Transfusions	0	9[a]	5	14[a]
Sporadic	5	—	5	10
Histology prior to treatment				
CPH[b]	4	5	9	18
CAH[c]	4	4	10	18
CAH/Ci[d]	—	4	—	4
Hepatitis C virus genotype				
1a	—	2	8	10
1b	—	—	3	3
2b	3	5	6	14
3a	4	3	2	9
Mixed	1	3	—	4
Pretreatment HCV RNA levels in serum, genomes/ml				
Median	3.2×10^5	2.5×10^6	3.2×10^6	2.25×10^6
Range	2.5×10^4–13×10^7	1.6×10^5–3.2×10^7	2×10^5–16×10^7	2.5×10^4–16×10^7

[a] One patient had both IVDU and blood transfusions as possible modes for acquisition.
[b] CPH = chronic persistent hepatitis.
[c] CAH = chronic active hepatitis.
[d] Ci = cirrhosis.

Table II. *The biochemical and virological response in 40 patients with chronic hepatitis C virus infection, measured as the number of patients with normal ALT levels and negative negative serum HCV RNA test before, during and after treatment with human leucocyte interferon alpha during an intended 24-week course*

	Before treatment, week 0	During treatment, week 12	End of treatment, week 24[a]	At follow-up, week 48
ALT level				
Patients with normal levels/total no. of patients	0/40 (0%)	27/40 (68%)	21/40 (53%)	8/40 (20%)
HCV RNA				
Patients testing negative/total no. of patients	0/40 (0%)	29/40 (73%)	23/40 (58%)	9/40 (23%)

[a] Patients with a biochemical non-response were withdrawn from treatment, weeks 12–16.

the end of treatment. At follow-up two (25%) had become HCV RNA-positive although they continued to have normal ALT levels. All but two non-sustained biochemical responders were HCV RNA-negative at the end of treatment. Only 2/13 non-sustained responders continued to be negative at follow-up. Also 8/19 biochemical non-responders were HCV RNA-negative at week 12 of whom 6 had normal ALT levels. During continued treatment, however, 5 of these experienced biochemical relapse (breakthrough response), and another one after prematurely ending the treatment because of depression. At follow-up only one non-responder was HCV RNA-negative. Her mean ALT level at 2, 16 and 24 weeks post-treatment, was however, in the normal range.

HCV RNA levels in serum prior to treatment according to response

The HCV RNA levels according to response category are given in Table I. Patients with a sustained biochemical response (SR) had a lower median serum HCV RNA level

Table III. *The virological response in 40 patients with chronic hepatitis C virus infection measured as the number of patients with negative serum HCV RNA test before, during and after treatment with human leucocyte interferon alpha during a 24 weeks course according to final biochemical outcome*

Response category	No.	Median HCV RNA prior to treatment	No. of patients HCV RNA negative/total no. of patients			
			Before treatment	During treatment	At end of treatment[a]	At follow-up
Sustained response	8	3.2×10^5	0/8 (0%)	8/8 (100%)	8/8 (100%)	6/8 (75%)
Non-sustained response	13	2.5×10^6	0/13 (0%)	13/13 (100%)	11/13 (85%)	2[b]/13 (15%)
Non-response	19	3.2×10^6	0/19 (0%)	8/19 (42%)	4/19 (21%)	1[c]/19 (5%)

[a] Patients with a biochemical non-response withdrawn from treatment week 12–16.
[b] Mean ALT level weeks 2, 16 and 48 after treatment, for patient GB03 1.08 μkat/l, and Gb20 0.64 μkat/l.
[c] Mean ALT level weeks 2, 16 and 48 after treatment for patient HS9 0.63 μkat/l.
Upper normal ALT level 0.6 and 0.8 μkat/l for men and women, respectively.

than those with non-sustained (NSR) or non-response (NR), the values being 3.2×10^5, 2.5×10^6 and 3.2×10^6, respectively, a difference which did not reach statistical significance (SR vs. NSR + NR, $p = 0.097$).

Genotypes according to response

The distribution of genotypes according to biochemical response is given in Table I; 10, 14, 9 and 3 patients had genotypes 1a, 2b, 3a and 1b respectively. Patients with genotypes 1a and 1b were less likely to have a sustained response than those with genotypes 2b and 3a, (0/13 vs. 7/23, respectively; $p = 0.034$). The median HCV RNA levels in patients with genotype 1a, 2b, 3a, and 1b were 2.6×10^6, 3.8×10^6, 3.2×10^5, and 8×10^5, respectively, differences that did not reach statistical significance. The median HCV RNA level in patients with genotype 3a, however, tended to be lower than that in patients with genotype 2b ($p = 0.054$).

Genotypes according to mode of acquisition

There were 4, 1, 6 and 1 patients, with post-transfusion hepatitis C, who had only genotypes 1a, 1b, 2b and 3a, respectively. The corresponding distribution for those with IVDU was 4, 1, 2 and 4, and for patients with sporadic forms it was 2, 0, 4 and 4, respectively; differences that did not reach statistical significance. One intravenous drug user who also had blood transfusions is included both among those with post-transfusion hepatitis C and those with intravenous drug use (IVDU).

Mode of acquisition according to response

The mode of acquisition of the HCV infection according to response is given in Table I. None of the 13 patients with post-transfusion hepatitis C had a sustained response vs. 8/26 (31%) of those with other routes for their infection ($p = 0.035$); the intravenous drug user who had also had blood transfusions being excluded. Five of 10 patients (50%) with sporadic hepatitis C had a sustained response, and 3/16 (19%) of those with intravenous drug use (IVDU) (including needle stick and tattooing) as their route of infection. The median serum HCV RNA levels in patients who acquired infection via transfusions, via IVDU (including tattooing and needle stick injuries) and via sporadic forms were 3.6×10^6, 1.9×10^6, and 1.65×10^6, respectively, and were not significantly different.

Histological findings prior to treatment, according to response

The distribution of histological findings according to response is given in Table I. No patient with CAH and cirrhosis responded in a sustained fashion, whereas 4/14 and 4/18 patients, with CPH and CAH respectively, did.

HCV RNA level in serum prior to treatment, according to histology

The median serum HCV RNA levels in patients with CPH, CAH and CAH with cirrhosis were 1.05×10^6, 3.25×10^6 and 1.6×10^7, respectively. Patients with CPH tended to have lower median serum HCV RNA levels than the combined group with CAH and CAH with cirrhosis ($p = 0.055$). If the 2 patients who were excluded from analysis due to non-compliance (one each with CAH and CAH with cirrhosis) are included this difference reached statistical significance ($p = 0.027$).

Interferon antibodies

No interferon-alpha-binding antibodies were detected in the patients before treatment, and no patient developed antibodies during treatment.

Adverse effects

The well known initial flu-like side-effects of interferon, such as fever, headache and muscle pains, noted earlier, were common, but tended to diminish during continued treatment. Alopecia was noted in 13 (27.5%) patients; mild in 11, but moderate with hair loss of up to 30% in 2 patients. Depression was noted by 4 patients, requiring treatment withdrawal and antidepressant therapy in 2 patients after 12 and 14 weeks treatment, respectively. Both were biochemical responders at this time point and both had a later relapse. Haematological side-effects necessitating interferon dose reduction were not noted.

DISCUSSION

The normalization of ALT levels in 52.5% of our patients at the end of treatment, sustained during follow-up in 8/40 (20%) is of the same order as that achieved in most studies utilizing lymphoblastoid and recombinant interferon alpha over 6 months (4, 17). Not all patients with a sustained biochemical response continued to show viral eradication since 2/8 (25%) were HCV RNA-positive in serum at follow-up 24 weeks after the end of treatment. A virological relapse in some patients with a continued biochemical response has been also noted in other studies (18, 19). Also one biochemical non-responder was negative for HCV RNA at follow-up. This patient, however, had very low ALT levels with a mean normal level when sampled at 2, 16 and 24 weeks post treatment. She happened to have slightly raised ALT levels at treatment cessation and at follow-up. During the follow-up after this study she had continuously normal ALT levels, and was probably miscategorized as a non-responder due to our stringent criteria. At all study points the number of patients who were HCV RNA-negative exceeded the number who had normal ALT levels, indicating that both HCV RNA testing and monitoring of ALT levels should be included in the evaluation of treatment response.

When analysing factors of possible importance for the prediction of sustained response, we found that HCV RNA levels tended to be lower in sustained responders compared to those of non-sustained and non-responders but not, however, significantly so. In an earlier study with recombinant interferon alpha we found such a difference in agreement with the findings of others (20, 21). Patients with a sustained response also tended to have HCV RNA levels more often below than above the median level (6/20 vs. 2/20, data not shown).

When analysing genotypes according to treatment response, we found that patients with genotypes 3a and 2b had a sustained response more often than patients with genotype 1a and 1b. In agreement with this, patients with genotype 1b have been found to have a poor response when compared to patients with other genotypes (4). Patients with genotype 3a tended to have the lowest median HCV RNA levels in serum prior to treatment; levels which were also somewhat lower than in patients with genotype 2b ($p = 0.054$). In line with this, 4/9 patients with genotype 3a had a sustained response whereas none of the three with genotype 1b had such a response.

The mode of HCV acquisition also seemed to influence between patients with different modes of acquisition. However, others have found that patients with post-transfusion hepatitis C seem to have higher serum levels of HCV RNA than patients with sporadic forms of HCV infection and with HCV caused by intravenous drug abuse (21).

Recently Gretch et al. have shown that the HCV RNA level in serum increases with the severity of the histological injury (22). In agreement with this, we found that patients with CPH had lower levels of HCV RNA than patients with more advanced disease. None of our 4 patients with CAH and cirrhosis responded to treatment, in line with the poorer response to treatment noted in cirrhotic patients (23). This can partly be due to high serum HCV RNA levels in cirrhotic patients (22). Our patients with cirrhosis tended to have high HCV RNA levels in serum prior to treatment, in agreement with this.

Adverse effects like alopecia and depression were noted in 27.5% and 10% of our patients respectively. In the majority of cases these were mild and did not require dose reduction. In 2 patients with depression, however, treatment had to be withdrawn after 12 and 14 weeks, respectively, when both were given antidepressant therapy. These adverse effects were fully reversible after cessation of treatment, and such effects have also been noted during recombinant interferon treatment. We have earlier noted alopecia in 15% of patients treated with recombinant interferon alpha-2b (6).

In our series 5 patients experienced a breakthrough response, with raised ALT levels after initial normalization, in spite of continued treatment. This response pattern has been claimed, at least in some patients, to be caused by the evolution of neutralizing interferon antibodies (7, 8). None of our patients with this response pattern, however, developed interferon antibodies, casting doubt on this assumption. In fact none of our patients developed interferon antibodies during or after treatment. This is in agreement with other studies showing a low incidence of interferon antibodies after treatment with lymphoblastoid interferon alpha, as compared to that seen after recombinant interferon-alpha-2a treatment (9). The observation that no interferon antibodies developed during treatment with our natural human leucocyte alpha-interferon is possibly of some importance, since high levels of neutralizing antibodies can cause lack of response according to some studies (7, 8).

In conclusion we found that a 6-month course with human leucocyte interferon-alpha induced a biochemical response in more than 50% of our patients, which was sustained in 20%. We found that patients with genotypes 3a

ACKNOWLEDGEMENTS

This study was supported by a grant from BioNative AB, Umeå, Sweden. The monitoring of patients by Katharina Engman was greatly appreciated.

REFERENCES

1. Takahashi M, Yamada G, Miyamoto R, Doi T, Endo H, Tsuji T. Natural course of chronic hepatitis C. Am J Gastroenterol 88: 240–243, 1993.
2. Kiyosawa K, Sodeyama T, Tanaka E, Gibo Y, Yoshisawa K, Nakano Y, Furuta S, Akahane Y, Nishioka K, Purcell R, Alter H. Interrelationship of blood transfusion, non-A, non-B hepatitis and hepatocellular carcinoma: Analysis by detection of antibody to hepatitis C virus. Hepatology 12: 671–675, 1990.
3. Mattsson L, Sönnerborg A, Weiland O. Outcome of acute symptomatic non-A, non-B hepatitis: a 13-year follow-up study of hepatitis C virus markers. Liver 13: 274–278, 1993.
4. Weiland O. Interferon therapy in chronic hepatitis C virus infection. FEMS Microbiol Rev 14: 279–288, 1994.
5. Shindo M, Di Bisceglie A, Cheung L, Shih W-K, Cristiano K, Feinstone S, Hoofnagle J. Decrease in serum hepatitis C viral RNA during alpha-interferon therapy for chronic hepatitis C. Ann Intern Med 115: 700–704, 1991.
6. Reichard O, Foberg U, Frydén A, Mattsson L, Norkrans G, Sönnerborg A, Wejstål R, Yun Z-B, Weiland O. High sustained response rate and clearance of viraemia in chronic hepatitis C following treatment with interferon alfa-2b for 60 weeks. Hepatology 19: 280–285, 1994.
7. Bonetti P, Diodati G, Drago C, Casarin C, Scaccabarozzi S, Realdi G, Ruol A, Alberti A. Interferon antibodies in patients with chronic hepatitis C virus infection treated with recombinant interferon alfa-2a. Hepatology 20: 416–420, 1994.
8. Milella M, Antonelli G, Santantonio T, Currenti M, Monno L, Mariano N, Angarano G, Dianzani F, Pastore G. Neutralizing antibodies to recombinant alpha-interferon and response to therapy in chronic hepatitis C virus infection. Liver 13: 146–150, 1993.
9. Antonelli G, Currenti M, Turriziani O, Dianzani F. Neutralizing antibodies to interferon-alfa: relative frequency in patients treated with different interferon preparations. J Infect Dis 163: 882–885, 1991.
10. Yun Z, Lindh G, Weiland O, Johansson B, Sönnerborg A. Detection of hepatitis C virus (HCV) RNA by PCR related to HCV antibodies in serum and liver histology in Swedish blood donors. J Med Virol 39: 57–61, 1993.
11. Yun Z, Lundeberg J, Johansson B, Hedrum A, Weiland O, Uhlén M, Sönnerborg A. Colorimetric detection of competitive PCR products for quantification of hepatitis C viremia. J Virol Methods 47: 1–14, 1994.
12. Okamoto H, Sugiyama Y, Okada S, Kurai K, Akahane Y, Sugai Y, Tanaka T, Sato K, Tsuda F, Miyakawa Y, Mayumi M. Typing hepatitis C virus by polymerase chain reaction with type-specific primers: application to clinical surveys and tracing infectious sources. J Gen Virol 73: 673–679, 1992.
13. Widell A, Shev S, Månsson S, Zhang Y, Foberg U, Norkrans G, Frydén A, Weiland O, Kurkus J, Nordenfelt E. Genotyping of hepatitis C virus isolates by a modified PCR assay using type specific primers: epidemiological applications. J Med Virol 44: 272–279, 1994.
14. Chan S, McOmish F, Holmes E, Dow B, Peutherer J, Follett E, Yap P, Simmonds P. Analysis of a new hepatitis C virus type and its phylogenetic relationship to existing variants. J Gen Virol 73: 1131–1141, 1992.
15. Ahrén B, Engman K, Lindblom A. Treatment of malignant carcinoid with a highly purified leukocyte alfa-interferon. Anticancer Res 12: 129–134, 1992.
16. International Group. Acute and chronic hepatitis revisited. Lancet 2: 914–919, 1977.
17. Tine F, Magrin S, Craxi A, Pagliaro L. Interferon for non-A, non-B chronic hepatitis. A meta-analysis of randomised clinical trials. J Hepatol 13: 192–199, 1991.
18. Lau Y, Mizokami M, Ohno T, Diamond D, Kniffen J, Davis G. Discrepancy between biochemical and virological response to interferon-alfa in chronic hepatitis C. Lancet 342: 1208–1209, 1993.
19. Saracco G, Rosina F, Abate ML, Chinadussi L, Gallo V, Cerutti E, Di Napoli A, Solinas A, Deplano A, Tocco A, Cossu P, Chien D, Kuo G, Polito A, Weiner AJ, Houghton M, Verme G, Bonino F, Rizzetto M. Long-term follow-up of patients with chronic hepatitis C treated with different doses of interferon alfa-2b. Hepatology 18: 1300–1305, 1993.
20. Yun Z, Reichard O, Chen M, Lundeberg J, Norkrans G, Fryden A, Sönnerborg A, Weiland O. Serum hepatitis C virus RNA levels in chronic hepatitis C: importance for outcome of interferon alfa-2b treatment. Scand J Infect Dis 26: 263–270, 1994.
21. Lau J, Davis G, Kniffen J, Qian K-P, Urdea M, Chan C, Mizokami M, Neuwald P, Wilber J. Significance of serum hepatitis C virus RNA levels in chronic hepatitis C. Lancet 341: 1501–1504, 1993.
22. Gretch D, Corey L, Wilson J, de la Rosa C, Willson R, carithers R, Busch M, Hart J, Sayers M, Han J. Assessment of hepatitis C virus RNA levels by quantitative competitive RNA polymerase chain reaction: high-titer viremia correlates with advanced stage of disease. J Infect Dis 169: 1219–1225, 1994.
23. Marcellin P, Boyer N, Giostra E, Degott C, Courouce A, Degos F, Coppere H, Cales P, Couzigou P, Benhamou J-P. Recombinant human alfa-interferon in patients with chronic non-A, non-B hepatitis: a multicenter randomized controlled trial from France. Hepatology 13: 393–397, 1991.

Submitted March 1, 1995; accepted May 4, 1995

Scand J Infect Dis 27: 325–329, 1995

ORIGINAL ARTICLE

Combined Alpha-interferon and Ribavirin Treatment in Chronic Hepatitis C: A Pilot Study

JEAN HENRIK BRACONIER[1], OTTO PAULSEN[2], KATARINA ENGMAN[3] and ANDERS WIDELL[4]

From the Departments of Infectious Diseases, [1]Lund University Hospital; [2]Malmö University Hospital; [4]Medical Microbiology, Malmö University Hospital and [3]BioNative AB, Umeå

16 patients with chronic hepatitis C virus (HCV) infection were treated with a combination of interferon-alpha and ribavirin for 24 weeks in an open study. One patient declined further treatment due to depression after week 16 and did not complete further follow-up. A moderate decline was observed in hemoglobin and an increase in bilirubin level both reversible after discontinuing the treatment. 24 weeks after treatment cessation 9/15 (60%) evaluable patients had complete clearance of HCV-RNA as measured with PCR. HCV genotype did not seem to be correlated with response, but patients with sustained response to treatment had a significantly reduced number of HCV RNA copies/ml serum at treatment start compared with the other patients. These findings support the promising results of this combination therapy noted in other pilot studies.

J. H. Braconier, MD, Department of Infectious Diseases, Lund University Hospital, S-221 85 Lund, Sweden

INTRODUCTION

Chronic hepatitis C (HCV) is a common disease associated with serious end-stage complications such as cirrhosis and hepatocellular carcinoma (1). The recommended treatment with interferon-alpha for 24 weeks offers a sustained normalization of serum ALT levels and a sustained clearance of the viremia in only about 10–30% of treated patients (1). Ribavirin, a nucleoside analogue with broad antiviral effect, has been used as single therapy in patients with chronic HCV. However, a non-sustained effect on ALT levels has generally been found (2, 3). Furthermore, ribavirin alone does not clear the viremia. The side effects of ribavirin treatment are generally mild (4). Since alternative treatment regimens to interferon alone are needed, a combination with ribavirin is interesting.

Here we report on the biochemical and virological outcome and adverse drug reactions seen in a pilot study when interferon-alpha therapy was combined with ribavirin for chronic HCV.

MATERIAL AND METHODS

Patients

16 patients with chronic HCV were enrolled in an open, uncontrolled, and prospective study. There were 5 females and 11 males, with a mean age of 40.2 years. All patients had had increased ALT concentrations (> 150% of upper reference level) for at least 6 months. They proved positive for antibodies to HCV (second generation HCV-ELISA, Ortho Diagnostics, Raritan, NJ, USA) with a positive confirmatory test (second or third generation RIBA, Chiron, Emeryville, CA, USA).They had no additional explanation for their liver disease and had not been given antiviral or immunomodulatory treatment within 6 months of the study. Two patients had earlier been treated with recombinant interferon-alpha alone. One had not responded, while the other had a non-sustained response after 6 months treatment.

One patient with hypertension was treated with anti-hypertensive drugs; the others had no other chronic disease. Two patients had acquired hepatitis C through blood-transfusions and 8 via previous intravenous, drug abuse (IVDU). In 6 cases, no cause for the transmission could be identified.

The present study was approved by the Ethics Committees at the University Hospitals in Lund and Malmö.

Treatment

Combination therapy was given for 24 weeks with human leukocyte interferon-alpha and ribavirin. Ribavirin (Virazole, ICN Pharmaceuticals, CA, USA) was given, 1,000 mg in 2 divided doses (1,200 mg for patients weighing > 75 kg) and HuIFN-alfaLe (Interferon Alfanative, BioNative, Umeå, Sweden) at a dose of 3 million units (MU) subcutaneously t.i.w. Adverse drug reactions were monitored by questioning, clinical examinations and by laboratory tests.

Investigations

Laboratory investigations were made before commencing treatment and at weeks 0, 1, 2, 4, and every 4th week during treatment and at weeks 4, 12 and 24 after treatment. Hemoglobin, white blood cells, differential blood cell, and platelet counts, serum creatinine, bilirubin, alkaline phosphatase, alanine amino transferase (ALT) and serum uric acid levels were determined on these occasions. HCV RNA in serum was analysed in samples drawn at weeks, 0, 12, 24 and 48.

Patients were classified as having a sustained response if they had normal ALT levels and a negative HCV RNA test at week 24 post-treatment.

Liver biopsies were done within 6 months before treatment and at week 24 post-treatment (12 patients). The biopsies were analysed under code by one experienced pathologist; no scoring system was used for the gradation of biopsies.

HCV RNA extraction

RNA extraction was performed in sera stored at −20°C or lower until testing. HCV RNA was extracted from 100 μl serum according to Chomczynski and Sacchi (5), transcribed and amplified by nested PCRs. Contamination controls (water) were included between every sample and a weak positive control between every 6 sample. These controls were carried through all subsequent steps.

Reverse transcription and the first PCR was done in the same reaction tube with all reagents present from the beginning (6). From each RNA extract, 2 aliquots corresponding to the RNA from 33 μl of serum were transcribed and amplified in parallel. Primers (slightly modified from the original publication (6)) were derived from the conserved 5′-noncoding region and were: antisense primer 5′-CATGGTGCACGGTCTACGAGAC-3′ and a mixture of sense primers 5′-GGCGACACTCCACCATAGATC-3′ and 5′-GGCGACACTCCGCCATGAA(TC)C-3′ for reverse transcription and outer PCR and antisense primer 5′-TCGCAAGCACCCTATCAGGCAG-3′ and sense primer 5′-GGAACTACTGTCTTCACGCAGA-3′ for inner PCR. 35 thermocycles were done in first PCR (94°C for 1.5 min, 50°C for 2 min and 72°C for 3 min) as well as a second PCR (94°C for 1.5 min and 55°C for 1 min). Amplification products of correct size (260 bp) were visualized on agarose gels by ethidium bromide staining and UV light.

Genotyping

Genotyping was done on HCV RNA extracted as above but amplified with PCR using type-specific primers directed against the HCV core region partly as suggested by Okamoto et al. (7), but with modifications by us as recently described (8). Genotypes 1a, 1b, 2a, 2b, and 3a were detected by the current system. The typing terminology of Chan et al. was used (9).

Quantitative HCV RNA determination

A recently introduced assay (HCV Amplicor Monitor, Roche) was used as described by the manufacturer. Viral RNA was extracted together with an added internal quantitative standard (QS) of cloned and transcribed HCV RNA. This QS shares PCR target sequences with wild type (wt) HCV but also has a short, modified internal hybridization sequence. Reverse transcription and PCR are done with one enzyme (rTth) and one of the primers is biotinylated. Amplified material is denatured and transferred to 2 sets of wells from each sample. The first set of wells (into which products are added diluted 1/1, 1/5, 1/25, and 1/625, respectively) are coated with a probe directed against the wtHCV sequence. The second set of wells into which 1/1, 1/5, 1/25 dilutions are added, are coated with a probe directed against the unique QS sequence. The biotinylated PCR products allow detection of hybridization with avidin-conjugated enzyme and substrate. Optical densities (OD) are read at 492 nm. For each sample, the weakest dilution giving a positive signal (OD > 0.25) against the wtHCV and the QS, respectively, are identified and subsequently used.The number of RNA copies per ml in the sample are calculated semiquantitatively, using the formula: $20{,}000 \times (OD_{sample} \times \text{dilution factor}_{sample})/(OD_{QS} \times \text{dilution factors}_{QS})$.

Determination of interferon-alpha antibodies in serum

Presence of interferon-alpha binding antibodies in serum before administration of the first dose of interferon-alpha and at cessation of therapy were measured by an ELISA earlier described by Ahrén et al. (10).

RESULTS

Drop-outs

One patient with chronic active hepatitis declined further treatment at week 16 due to irritability and depression, for which no specific treatment was given. She did not attend the scheduled follow-up, although she had shown initial normalization of ALT. This patient was not included in the efficacy evaluation.

Another patient, a biochemical non-responder, declined for unknown reason the final check up 24 weeks post-treatment. Although post-treatment virology is not available, this patient was considered to be a treatment failure. He never achieved normal ALT levels and was positive for HCV RNA during 24 weeks of treatment.

Biochemical response

The mean ALT level for the 15 patients at week 0 was 2.32 (reference value < 0.7 ukat/l) (Fig. 1). After therapy commenced, ALT values decreased rapidly. At the end of

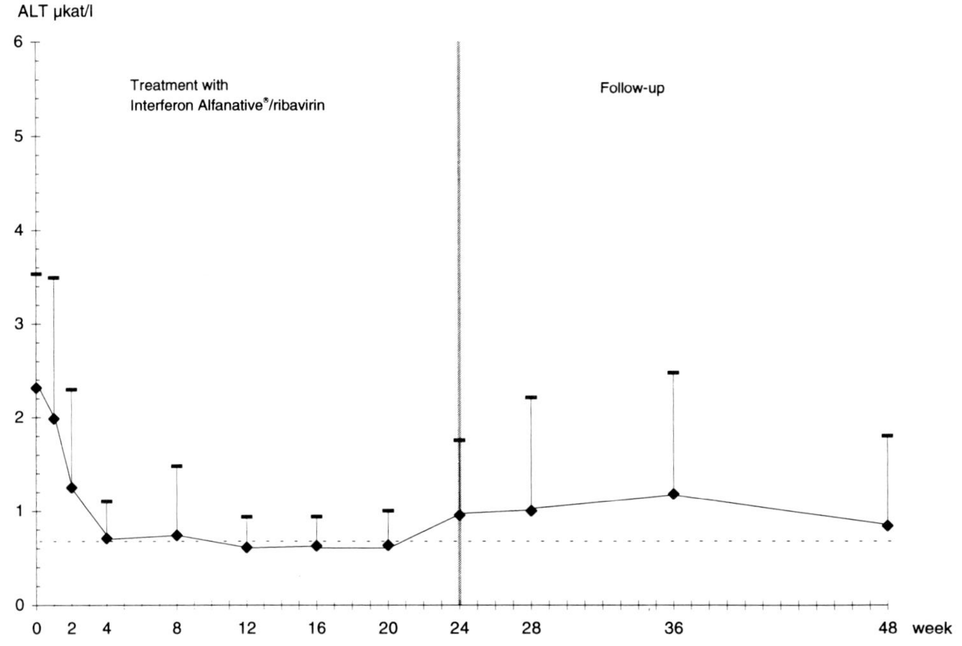

Fig. 1. ALT levels before, during and after treatment with a combination of Interferon Alfanative® and ribavirin in patients with chronic HCV. —■—, mean; ▬, SD; – – –, normal value for ALT < 0.7 µkat/l

Table I. *Demographics according to biochemical and virological response to treatment in 15 patients with chronic hepatitis C Virus (HCV) infection treated with human leukocyte interferon-alfa and ribavirin*

For the appropriate data, median values and range are presented.

Demographics	Sustained response ($n = 9$)[a]	Non-sustained response ($n = 2$)	Non-response ($n = 4$)
Age (median)	40 (28–63)	37 (30–44)	40 (32–45)
Males	7	0	4
Females	2	2	0
Mode of acquisition	IVDU = 4 Unknown = 5	Transfusion = 2	IVDU = 3 unknown = 1
HCV genotypes	1a, 1a, 1b, 2a, 2a, 2b, 3a, 3a, 3a	1a, 3a	1a, 1a, 1b, 3a
HCV-RNA number of copies/ml $\times 10^5$	0.63 (0.02–2.7)	4.55 (3.7–5.4)	2.55 (1.6–8.9)
Patients with normal ALT	7[b]	1	1
ALT[c]	0.46 (0.22–0.98)	0.9 (0.44–1.37)	1.82 (0.58–4.11)
Earlier IFN treatment	2[d]	0	0
Histology prior to treatment[e]	cirrhosis 2, CAH 1, CPH 5, lobular hepatitis 1	CPH 2	CPH 4

[a] Sustained response indicates negative HCV-RNA at treatment stop and 24 weeks later.
[b] 2 other patients with negative HCV-RNA had some increase in ALT (< 1.0 μkat/l).
[c] ALT levels 24 weeks after treatment stop.
[d] 2 patients were earlier treated with recombinant interferon-alfa; one had a non-sustained response and the other did not respond at all.
[e] CAH indicates chronic active and CPH chronic persistent hepatitis.

treatment the mean value was 1.0 and similar values were found at subsequent post-treatment check-ups. When treatment was concluded, 7/15 patients had normal ALT levels and at weeks 16 and 24 post-treatment, 9 patients had normal levels. Among patients with sustained response 2 had been treated earlier with interferon monotherapy.

Virological response

HCV RNA was detected in the pre-treatment samples from all patients and serotypes 1a, 1b, 2a, 2b and 3a were found (Table I).

Nine of 15 patients were negative for HCV RNA 24 weeks after treatment was stopped (Table I). Two of the patients with negative HCV RNA had a concomitant slight increase in ALT levels at week 24 post-treatment, while the other 7 had normal ALT levels.

Quantitative HCV RNA levels

Table I shows the median values of RNA copies before treatment start. The 9 sustained responders had median 0.63×10^5 HCV RNA copies per ml serum (range 0.02 – 2.7×10^5). The corresponding values for the other patients were 3.2×10^5 (range 1.6 – 8.9×10^5). The difference between the sustained responders and the other patients was significant (Mann-Whitney U-test, $p < 0.01$).

Liver biopises

Before treatment, cirrhosis was found in 2 patients (in 1 patient combined with chronic active hepatitis). Two and 11 patients had chronic active or chronic persistent hepatitis, respectively. Lobular hepatitis was diagnosed in one patient. A sustained response to treatment was found for both patients with cirrhosis and one with chronic active hepatitis. After treatment, improvement, mainly in the degree of inflammation, was noted in 8 biopsies. Two showed impairment, one was unchanged and in 1 the sample was too small for conclusions to be drawn.

Interferon antibodies

IFN-alpha binding antibodies were not detected in the patients before or during therapy with IFN-alpha.

Adverse drug reactions

Three patients (all women) suffered from pronounced tiredness during treatment, including both patients with cirrhosis and the young woman (excluded) who declined further treatment. In one patient (a sustained responder) the treatment was terminated after 18 weeks due to a subarachnoid hemorrhage from which he made an uneventful recovery. This patient had complained of a migraine-like headache for several years. The hemorrhage was not considered to be an adverse drug reaction. Platelet levels, bleeding time and prothrombin levels were not decreased. He completed the follow-up and was a sustained responder. The other patients completed the treatment without any dose reduction.

One non-responding patient had a flare-up like reaction. ALT levels were normal when treatment was stopped and 4 weeks later, but increased to 2.6 and 10.4 ukat/l respectively at 8 and 11 weeks after treatment. At 24 weeks post-treatment, ALT levels were normal, but the patient was still HCV-RNA positive.

As could be expected, there was a gradual decline in hemoglobin from 149 g/l at week zero to a nadir of 129.4 g/l at week 12. The largest decrease from 150 to 103 g/l, was noted in one of the patients with cirrhosis. As the protocol accepted levels down to 100 g/l, the dose of ribavirin was not changed. The dose of interferon was also kept constant during the treatment period in all patients. The hemoglobin recovered to normal levels within 4 weeks after stopping treatment.

Mean values of bilirubin (reference value < 20 μmol/l) increased from week zero (12.7 μmol/l) to a maximum of 21.7 at week 2. Bilirubin thereafter slowly decreased to 12.6 at week 24.

No changes were noticed for the other biochemical parameters.

DISCUSSION

The effect of interferon monotherapy on chronic HCV is limited, and other treatment options are clearly needed. A combination of interferon with some other antiviral agent could be advantageous. Ribavirin has the advantages of oral administration and lack of severe adverse effects (4). A mild hemolysis and a decrease in hemoglobin level was seen in this study, but there was no need to reduce the dose in any patient. There was no serious adverse reaction due to the combined drug treatment.

The present study was admittedly small and uncontrolled, but the results with the combination of interferon and ribavirin are encouraging. Our findings are in agreement with other pilot studies in small numbers of patients. Brillanti et al. have found significantly increased numbers with a sustained response after retreatment of interferon non-responders with the combination, compared to treatment with interferon alone (11). Chemello et al. (12) have compared treatment with ribavirin alone, interferon alone, and in their combination in a total of 45 patients. Among those treated with the combination, 47% had a sustained response 9 months after the end of treatment, which was significantly better than in the other groups of patients. Schvarcz et al. observed 4 sustained responders among 10 patients treated with the combination (13). These patients had earlier failed to respond in a sustained fashion to interferon alone. Brouwer et al. (14) have reported from an ongoing study on non-responders to interferon that some patients will respond to combination of interferon and ribavirin.

Highly purified native interferon-alfa together with ribavirin, as used in the present study, seems to have resulted in a high rate of sustained response (60%). Although there are no strict comparative studies on the effect of native and recombinant interferon-alfa, neither in monotherapy nor in combination therapy, it seems that native interferon-alfa is at least as effective as recombinant interferon as monotherapy for the treatment of chronic HCV infection (15).

Several host and virological factors might influence the effect of treatment (1). One of the most important may be the virus genotype. Generally speaking, genotype 1b has been reported to respond less well to treatment with interferon (16). In the present study we had sustained responders among all observed genotypes. Genotype 2a, observed in 2 patients, has not previously been found in Swedish patients.

The amount of virus may be another important factor which might influence the outcome of treatment (1). In this study the number of HCV RNA copies in serum on commencing the treatment was significantly lower among the patients with sustained response than among the other patients.

Neutralizing antibodies to interferon have been associated with diminished clinical efficacy of interferon. We did not find neutralizing antibodies to interferon in any of our patients. Various levels of antibodies to interferon have been found in patients treated with other types of interferons. Antonelli et al. (17) found antibodies in 20.2% of patients treated with recombinant interferon-alfa 2a, and in 6.9 and 1.2%, respectively in those treated with recombinant interferon-alfa 2b and lymphoblastoid interferon-alfa.

The findings in this pilot study indicate that both the spectrum of adverse drug reactions and the clinical effect on chronic HCV infection by treatment with interferon and ribavirin in combination are favourable. Large controlled studies on combination treatment are needed to confirm our promising results.

ACKNOWLEDGEMENT

This study was supported by grants from the Faculty of Medicine, University of Lund and BioNative AB, Umeå.

REFERENCES

1. Weiland O. Interferon therapy in chronic hepatitis C virus infection. FEMS Microbiol Rev 14: 279–288, 1994.
2. Reichard O, Andersson J, Schvarcz R, Weiland O. Ribavirin treatment for chronic hepatitis C. Lancet 337: 1058–1061, 1991.
3. Di Bisceglie A, Shindo M, Fong T-L, Fried M, Swain M, Bergasa N, Axiotis C, Waggoner J, Park Y, Hoofnagle JH. Pilot study of ribavirin therapy for chronic hepatitis C. Hepatology 16: 649–654, 1992.
4. Shulman NR. Assessment of hematological effects of ribavirin in humans. In: Smith R, Knight V, eds. Clinical applications of ribavirin. New York: Academic Press, 79–92, 1984.
5. Chomczyski P, Sacchi N. Single-step method of RNA isolation by acid guanidinum thiocyanate-phenol-chloroform extraction. Analytical Biochemistry 162: 156–159, 1987.
6. Widell A, Månsson AS, Sundström G, Hansson BG, Nordenfelt E: Hepatitis C virus RNA in blood donor sera detected by the polymerase chain reaction: Comparison with supplementary hepatitis C antibody assays. J Med Virol 35: 253–258, 1991.
7. Okamoto H, Sugiyama Y, Okada S, Kurai K, Akahane Y, Sugai Y, Tanaka T, Sato K, Tsuda F, Miyakawa Y, Mayummi M. Typing hepatitis C virus b polymerase chain reaction with

type-specific primers: application to clinical surveys and tracing infectious sources. J Gen Virol 73: 673–679, 1992.
8. Widell A, Shev S, Månsson S, Zhang YY, Foberg U, Weiland O, Norkrans G, Nordenfelt E. Typing hepatitis C virus using primers in a modified PCR based assay. Epidemiological applications. J Med Virol 44: 272–9, 1994.
9. Chan SW, McOmish F, Holmes EC, Dow B, Peutherer JF, Yap PL, Simmonds P. Analysis of a new hepatitis C virus type and its phylogenetic relationship to existing variants. J Gen Virol 73: 1131–1141, 1992.
10. Ahrén B, Engman K, Lindblom A. Treatment of malignant midgut carcinoid with a highly purified human leukocyte alpha-interferon. Anticancer Res 12: 129–34, 1992.
11. Brillanti S, Garson J, Foli M, Whitby K, Deaville R, Masci C, Miglioli M, Barbara L. A pilot study of combination therapy with ribavirin plus interferon alfa for interferon alfa resistant chronic hepatitis C. Gastroenterology 107: 812–817, 1994.
12. Chemello L, Cavalletto L, Bernardinello E, Silvestri E, Benvegnu L, Pontissio P, Alberti A. Response to ribavirin, alpha-interferon and to a combination of both in patients with chronic hepatitis C and its relation to HCV genotypes. Hepatology 21, abstract GS 5/29, EASL meeting, September 1994, Athens.
13. Schvarcz R, Yun Z, Sönnerborg A, Weiland O. Combined treatment with interferon alfa-2b and ribavirin for chronic hepatitis C in patients with a previous non-response or non-sustained response to interferon alone. J Virol Methods 46: 43–47, 1995.
14. Brouwer IT, Nevens F, Michielsen P, Hautekeete ML, Chamuleau RAFM, Adler M, Delwaide J, Heijtink RA, Schalm SW and the Benelux Study Group on Hepatitis C treatment. What options are left when hepatitis C does not respond to interferon? Placebo-controlled Benelux multicentre retreatment trial on ribavirin monotherapy versus combination with interferon. Hepatology 21, abstract WP2/08, EASL meeting, September 1994, Athens.
15. Weiland O, Chen M, Lindh G, Mattsson L, Schvarcz R, Sönnerborg A, Wahl M, Wejstål R, Widell A, Norkrans G. Efficacy of human leucocyte alpha-interferon treatment for chronic hepatitis C virus infection. Scand J Infect Dis 27: 319–324, 1995.
16. Constanzo A, Artini M, Ianni A, Ranone G, Martinelli R, Porcari P, Chirillo P, De Marzio E, Levrero M. Correlation between outcome of interferon therapy and HCV genotype in HCV chronic carriers. Abstract 63, IASL meeting, May 1994, Cancun, Mexico.
17. Antonelli G, Currenti M, Turriziani O, Dianzani F. Neutralizing antibodies to interferon-alpha: relative frequency in patients treated with different interferon preparations. J Infect Dis 163: 882–885, 1991.

Submitted January 18, 1995; accepted March 22, 1995

Scand J Infect Dis 27: 331–337, 1995 ORIGINAL ARTICLE

Prevalence and Determinants of Anti-HCV Seropositivity and of HCV Genotype among Intravenous Drug Users in Berlin

KLAUS STARK[1], ECKART SCHREIER[2], REINHOLD MÜLLER[3], DELIA WIRTH[1], GERHARD DRIESEL[2] and ULRICH BIENZLE[1]

From the [1]Institute of Tropical Medicine, [2]Robert Koch-Institute, and the [3]Institute of Medical Statistics, Free University, Berlin, Germany

A cross-sectional study was carried out to identify risk factors for seropositivity for antibodies against hepatitis C virus (HCV) and to assess the distribution and determinants of HCV genotypes among intravenous drug users (IVDUs). The study population consisted of 405 IVDUs. Serum specimens were tested for seromarkers for HCV, for human immunodeficiency virus (HIV), for hepatitis B virus (HBV) and for syphilis. HCV RNA determination by polymerase chain reaction (PCR) and virus typing were performed in a subsample of anti-HCV-positive specimens ($n = 135$). Of the IVDUs, 83% were anti-HCV-positive, 18% HIV-infected, and 58% HBV (anti-HBc)-positive. Longer duration of intravenous drug use, syringe sharing in prison, and higher number of IDVU sex partners were independent risk factors for anti-HCV positivity. HCV RNA was detected in 76% of anti-HCV-positive IVDUs. HCV genotypes 1 (49%) and 3 (44%) were most commonly found. All the type 3 isolates were identified as subtype 3a, and 95% of the type 1 isolates as subtype 1b. In logistic regression analysis, HCV type 3a viraemia was significantly associated with lack of HIV infection and a higher number of sex partners. The results indicate that preventive measures are needed to reduce syringe sharing among IVDUs in prisons. Sexual contacts with other IVDUs may play a role in the HCV epidemic among IVDUs. In Germany, HCV type 3a infection appears to be much more common among IVDUs than among other HCV risk groups such as transfusion recipients or haemophiliacs.

K. Stark, MD, Institute of Tropical Medicine, Engeldamm 62–64, D-10179 Berlin, Germany

INTRODUCTION

High prevalence rates of anti-hepatitis C virus (HCV)-positivity have been found among intravenous drug users (IVDUs) (1–9). Individuals infected by HCV have a high risk of progression to chronic liver disease (10, 11). Therefore, there is a need for preventive measures to reduce the transmission risk of HCV among IVDUs. The predominant route of HCV transmission is parenteral exposure. It is unclear, however, whether there are specific subgroups of IVDUs who are at a particularly high risk, or whether places can be identified, e.g. prisons or shooting galleries, where risk behaviour, such as syringe sharing, carries a particularly high risk of infection. In some studies, the seroprevalence of anti-HCV increased with longer duration of intravenous drug use (2, 3, 8). However, comparatively little is known about specific risk behaviours associated with HCV infection. The data on sexual transmission are conflicting (12–19). It is unclear whether sexual transmission plays a significant role in the spread of HCV among IVDUs.

The polymerase chain reaction (PCR) technique allows the detection and subtyping of the HCV genome in serum (20–24). At least 6 different genotypes of HCV have been identified (22). Infection by certain HCV genotypes may be associated with a more severe course of acute or chronic HCV infection and with a less favourable response to interferon treatment (25, 26). HCV genotyping may not only influence treatment options but also help to identify sources of the infection (21, 24). Little is known about the distribution of the different HCV genotypes among different populations at risk (e.g. IVDUs and haemophiliacs).

We investigated the prevalence and determinants of anti-HCV-positivity and the distribution of the genotypes among IVDUs in Berlin.

SUBJECTS AND METHODS

Study population and data collection

The study participants were recruited from October 1992 to October 1993 at 2 drug abuse treatment centres, at a storefront agency where counselling on AIDS, syringe exchange and basic medical care for IVDUs is provided free of charge, and at a hospital for infectious diseases. The different sites of recruitment were chosen to obtain a sample of the IVDU population which was as representative as possible. Individuals were eligible for participation in the study if they had injected drugs within the 3 months prior to recruitment. Participation in the study was voluntary and anonymous. The study was approved by the data protection office and was carried out in accordance with the ethical guidelines of the regional health authority and the university. Verbal informed consent was obtained from the participants who answered a standardized questionnaire, and provided a blood sample. Questionnaires and blood samples were coded by an individual number. Serum samples were stored at $-70°C$.

Of the 405 participants, 156 were recruited from the treatment centres, 197 from the storefront agency, and 52 from the hospital for infectious diseases. The corresponding response rates were 78, 75, and 87%, respectively. In order to minimize interviewer bias,

 ISSN 0036-5548

each of the specially trained interviewers was employed at all the recruitment sites. The interview included questions on sociodemographic and behavioural characteristics. Detailed information was obtained on drug-using career, injection behaviour (frequency of syringe sharing, injecting drug use and syringe sharing in prison, type of partners when sharing syringes, etc.), and on sexual behaviour (number of sexual partners, prostitution, etc.).

Laboratory methods

Serum samples were tested for antibodies against HCV, HIV and HBV infections and for syphilis. For the detection of anti-HCV, a second-generation enzyme-linked immunosorbent assay (ELISA) (Abbott, Wiesbaden, Germany) was used. The cut-off point for seropositivity was chosen according to the manufacturer's instructions. PCR and genotyping were performed in a random sample ($n = 135$) of anti-HCV-positive serum specimens, selected from the population of anti-HCV-positive specimens by a computer-based procedure using a list of random numbers. The methods, for RNA extraction, reverse transcriptase PCR, and HCV genotyping by restricted fragment length polymorphism (RFLP) analysis and sequence analysis, are described in detail elsewhere (20). The nomenclature for HCV genotypes according to Simmonds et al. is used (22).

HIV antibodies were assessed by ELISA (HIV-1/2-ELISA, Sanofi Pasteur, Freiburg, Germany). Confirmatory testing was done by Western blotting (Sanofi Pasteur) according to the WHO guidelines.

HBV seromarkers were determined in 396 IVDUs. Samples were tested for anti-HBc and HBsAg by ELISA (Abbott), and for anti-HBs by radioimmunoassay (Abbott). If any of these markers were positive, further tests (ELISA, Abbott) were performed for anti-HBc IgM, anti-HBe, and HBeAg.

Syphilis seromarkers were assessed by Treponema pallidum haemagglutination assay (Mast Diagnostika, Reinfeld, Germany) and the fluorescence treponema antibody absorption test (Biologische AG, Lich, Germany).

Statistical methods

Bivariate associations between anti-HCV-positivity and relevant sociodemographic/behavioural variables or serological characteristics (HIV, HBV, Treponema pallidum) were assessed using the chi-squared test. The associations between the outcome and explanatory variables were regarded as significant when the p value was < 0.05.

In bivariate analysis, anti-HCV-positivity was associated with a variety of demographic and behavioural variables. However, these bivariate associations could have been confounded by other variables. To adjust for confounders, logistic regression analysis was performed. All variables which were associated with the outcome in bivariate analysis, or which had to be considered as important potential confounders, such as gender or level of education, were included in the model.

The final logistic regression model was obtained by forward/backward selection based on single variables and their possible interactions. Variables were kept in the model if they improved it significantly.

The same procedures were used for assessing determinants of HCV genotypes.

RESULTS

Characteristics of the study population

Of the total study population, 70.6% were males. The median age was 29 years (interquartile range 26–33), and the median duration of injecting drug use 8 years (interquartile range 4–14). Females were significantly younger (median age 28 years, males 30 years), and had started to inject drugs at an earlier age (median 18 years, males 20 years) ($p < 0.005$), but did not differ from the males with respect to duration of injecting drug use. Of all the IVDUs, 28 (7%) originated from countries other than Germany. The commonest types of drugs used in the previous 6 months were: heroin 97% (96%), cocaine 78% (74%), benzodiazepines 70% (46%), barbiturates 41% (22%), amphetamines 21% (15%), where the data in parentheses represent use via injection.

Seroprevalence of HCV, HIV and HBV

Overall, 82.5% (334/405) of the IVDUs were anti-HCV-positive, 18.3% (74/405) were anti-HIV-positive, and 58.1% (230/396) anti-HBc-positive. HBsAg was detected in 8.4% (32/383) of the study participants. Compared to IVDUs who were receiving treatment, individuals recruited at the storefront agency had a significantly higher prevalence of anti-HCV (89.8 vs. 73.1%), anti-HIV (19.8 vs. 3.2%), and anti-HBc (63.3 vs. 48.3%) ($p < 0.001$).

Anti-HCV-positivity was significantly higher among anti-HBc-positive and HIV-infected IVDUs (Table I). It was also higher among individuals seropositive for Treponema pallidum, although this did not reach statistical significance because of the small number of syphilis-seropositive IVDUs.

In 396 individuals, serological tests for all 3 viruses (HCV, HIV, HBV) were performed. Among these IVDUs, only 48 (12%) were seronegative for all viruses and 124 (31%) had antibodies to a single virus (anti-HCV, 104; anti-HIV, 4; anti-HBc, 16). Co-infections were common: 224 (57%) were seropositive for at least 2 of the viruses, and 54 (14%) had antibodies against all 3 viruses. HCV infection, plus positive seromarkers against HIV and/or HBV, was found in 56%.

In bivariate analysis, anti-HCV-positivity was associated with several sociodemographic and behavioural characteristics, such as older age, longer duration of intravenous drug use, frequency of syringe sharing, syringe sharing with persons other than good friends, imprisonment, syringe sharing in prison, number of IVDU sex partners, and sex with HIV-positive partners (Table I). The types of drugs used and injected in the previous 6 months were not associated with HCV infection. After adjusting for potential confounding effects in the logistic regression analysis, only the variables duration of injecting drug use, syringe sharing in prison, and having had sex with more than 5 IVDU partners, were independent determinants of HCV seropositivity (Table II). Individuals who had shared syringes in prison were about 4 times more likely (95% confidence interval 1.4–11) to be anti-HCV-positive.

Fig. 1 shows the increase in HCV, HIV, and HBV seroprevalence with duration of injecting drug use. The anti-

Table I. *Associations between anti-HCV seropositivity, and demographic/behavioural and serological characteristics among intravenous drug users (IVDUs) (bivariate analysis)*

Variable	*n*	Anti-HCV-positive, % of *n*	*p* value
Gender			n.s.
Men	286	82.2	
Women	119	83.2	
Age (years)			<0.0001
<25	77	68.8	
25–29	131	77.9	
≥30	197	90.9	
Duration of injecting drug use (years)			<0.0001
<5	115	66.1	
5–9	109	84.4	
10–14	90	88.9	
≥15	91	94.5	
Syringe sharing			0.0002
No	86	72.1	
1–50 times	195	81.0	
>50 times	113	93.8	
Imprisonment			<0.0001
No	129	71.3	
Yes	276	87.7	
Syringe sharing in prison			0.0004
No	308	78.2	
1–50 times	62	95.2	
>50 times	34	97.1	
Number of IVDU sex partners			0.0007
None	75	70.7	
1–5	236	81.8	
>5	68	94.1	
History of prostitution			0.08
No	297	80.5	
Yes	108	88.0	
History of sexually transmitted disease (STD)			0.05
No	277	79.8	
Yes	124	87.9	
Anti-HIV			0.04
Negative	331	80.7	
Positive	74	90.5	
Anti-HBc			<0.0001
Negative	166	68.7	
Positive	230	91.7	
Treponema pallidum antibodies			0.10
Negative	318	82.4	
Positive	13	100.0	

n.s. = not significant.

HCV prevalence increased more rapidly than the HBV and HIV seroprevalence. Of the IVDUs who had injected for less than 1 year, 25% had already been exposed to HCV. This rose to 40% among those who had injected for 1–2 years.

HCV genotype distribution

Of the 334 anti-HCV-positive serum specimens, 135 were randomly selected for HCV RNA analysis and genotyping. They did not differ significantly by age, gender, site of recruitment, HIV status, and major behavioural character-

Table II. *Determinants of anti-HCV positivity among IVDUs (logistic regression)*

Variable	Adjusted anti-HCV prevalence odds ratio	95% CI	*p* value
Duration of intravenous drug use (years)			
<5	1.0		
5 to 9	2.2	1.1–4.3	0.021
10 to 14	2.6	1.2–5.9	0.017
≥15	5.4	2.0–14.9	0.001
Syringe sharing in prison			
No	1.0		
Yes	3.9	1.4–11.3	0.013
Number of IVDU sex partners			
None	1.0		
1–5	1.3	0.7–2.5	0.36
>5	3.0	1.0–8.9	0.047

CI = confidence interval.

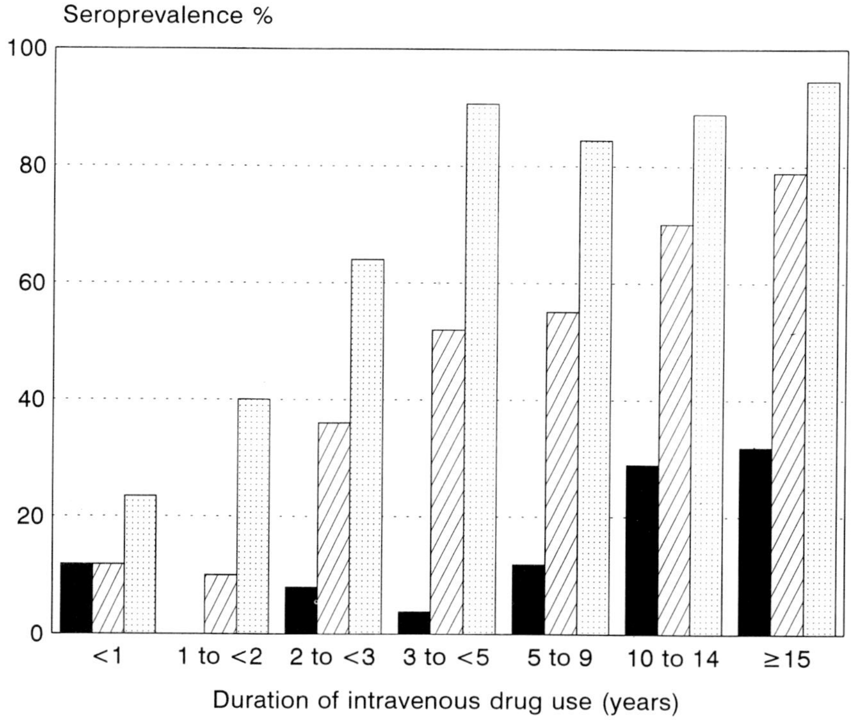

Fig. 1. Duration of intravenous drug use and HIV (■), HBV (▨) and HCV (▤) seroprevalence.

istics such as syringe sharing, imprisonment, and prostitution. HCV RNA was detected in 102 (76%) of the 135 serum samples selected for PCR analysis. In 5 samples, 2 different HCV genotypes were found, and in 9 samples it was not possible to identify specific genotypes by RFLP. A single HCV genotype could be identified in 88 HCV RNA-positive isolates: in 43 (49%) type 1, in 6 (7%) type 2, and in 39 (44%) type 3. All type 3 isolates were identified as subtype 3a, and all but 2 type 1 isolates as subtype 1b.

Since we were interested in the correlates of HCV type 3a infection, which is uncommon among non-drug injecting

Table III. *Logistic regression analysis of correlates of HCV type 3a infection among IVDUs with HCV viraemia (n = 88)*

Variable	Odds ratio for HCV type 3a infection	95% CI	*p* value
HIV serostatus			
Negative	1.00		
Positive	0.16	0.04–0.65	0.01
Number of sexual partners			
≤10	1.00		
>10	3.50	1.2–9.8	0.017

individuals in Germany, a binary outcome variable was computed (HCV genotype 3a viraemia vs. HCV genotype 1 or 2 viraemia). In bivariate analysis, compared to IVDUs with HCV type 1 or 2 viraemia, individuals with type 3a infection were less likely to have shared syringes in prison (13 vs. 26%, $p = 0.05$), to have shared with persons other than regular partners (31 vs. 55%, $p = 0.03$) or to be HIV-infected (8 vs. 31%, $p = 0.008$), and they were more likely to have had more than 10 sex partners (78 vs. 53%, $p = 0.02$). In logistic regression analysis, after adjusting for confounding effects, IVDUs with type 3a infection were significantly more likely to be HIV-negative, and to have had a higher number of sex partners (Table III).

DISCUSSION

The anti-HCV prevalence of 83% in this population of IVDUs is in the upper range of results as reported from other cities (1–9). It was much higher among IVDUs with longer injecting careers, which is in accordance with results from other studies (2, 3, 8). The duration of intravenous drug use may be regarded as a summary variable for a cumulative risk of exposure during the injecting career. HIV and HBV seroprevalence also increased significantly with a longer duration of intravenous drug use. However, of the 3 viruses, HCV seems to be spread most rapidly among new drug injectors, reaching over 80% after only a few years of injecting. If preventive measures against HCV among IVDUs are to be effective they must reach the individuals at a very early point in their injecting careers.

The use of shared syringes in prison was significantly associated with anti-HCV positivity. Since syringe sharing in prison was also found to be a strong predictor of HIV infection (27), this behaviour now appears to be a main risk factor for parenterally transmitted diseases among IVDUs in Berlin. The majority of IVDUs are well aware of the risks of virus transmission by syringe sharing, and willing and able to change their behaviour (28). However, in prisons they cannot behave according to their risk awareness because sterile injection equipment is hardly available. There is a need for preventive measures which enable IVDUs to avoid parenteral virus transmission in prison.

Our study revealed an independent effect of a high number of lifetime IVDU sex partners on anti-HCV prevalence. The association is not very strong but is in accordance with findings from other studies, suggesting that sexual transmission of HCV may occur, although infrequently (12, 15–19). Sexual transmission could partially explain the high anti-HCV prevalence (70%) among IVDUs in the study who claimed never to have shared syringes. Misclassification (i.e. underreporting of syringe sharing) is not a major problem, since the data have been shown to have good validity and reliability (27). However, apart from syringe sharing and sexual risk behaviour, other behavioural characteristics which were not assessed by the study questionnaire may have resulted in HCV transmission. In particular, these could be the practice of splitting of drug doses from a contaminated syringe (frontloading/backloading) (29), the sharing of spoons and cookers for drug preparation, or tattooing (30). Another finding suggests the possibility of sexual HCV transmission, namely that all the IVDUs who had seromarkers for previous syphilis, an indicator for sexual risk behaviour, were anti-HCV-positive, compared to 80% of the syphilis-seronegative individuals.

The main types of drugs used and injected in the previous 6 months were heroin, cocaine, benzodiazepines, and barbiturates. The type of drugs was not associated with the anti-HCV prevalence. We cannot rule out the possibility that the types of drugs used earlier may have determined risk behaviour and HCV infection rates, resulting in a confounding effect. However, multidrug use is common among IVDUs in Berlin, and it would have been difficult to assess the patterns of drug use during an entire drug-injecting career, and to separate the effects, on HCV infection rates, of the different drugs used.

HCV RNA was detected in nearly 80% of the anti-HCV-positive IVDUs. Although a few individuals may have been tested while in the postacute phase of hepatitis C, the results indicate that a high percentage of individuals infected by HCV will become chronic carriers. Similarly high rates of HCV viraemia have been reported by others (2, 31, 32). In our study where the majority of the participants were in the relatively early stages of HIV infection, HCV viraemia was not associated with the latter.

We found an interesting distribution of HCV genotypes among the IVDUs. A high percentage of HCV RNA-positive individuals were infected by HCV genotype 3a, which is detected only infrequently among non-drug-using HCV-positive individuals (e.g. haemophiliacs or transfusion recipients) in Germany (20). The isolation of type 3a was associated with a higher number of sexual partners, and with a negative anti-HIV test. The explanation for these findings is unclear. Because of the small sample size, the data must be interpreted with caution. However, we cannot rule out the possibility that HCV type 3a may be transmitted more easily by the sexual route than types 1 and 2, which would be in accordance with the predominance of the latter virus types among the parenterally infected haemophiliacs and transfusion recipients in Germany. A possible explanation for the association between HCV type 3a infection and lack of HIV infection is that HCV types 1 and 2 may be more likely to persist in HIV-infected immunocompromised individuals. To investigate these issues further, studies with larger sample sizes are needed which include IVDUs and non-drug-injecting HCV-infected individuals.

ACKNOWLEDGEMENTS

The study was funded in part by the Bundesministerium für Forschung und Technologie (Berliner Forschungsverbund Public

Health, grant: FKZ 07 PHF 01-B6). We are grateful to the staff at the institutions where the study participants were recruited.

REFERENCES

1. Chamot E, Hirschel B, Wintsch J, Robert CF, Gabriel V, Deglon JJ, Yerly S, Perrin L. Loss of antibodies against hepatitis C virus in HIV-seropositive intravenous drug users. AIDS 4: 1275–1277, 1990.
2. Crofts N, Hopper JL, Bowden DS, Breschkin AM, Milner R, Locarnini SA. Hepatitis C virus infection among a cohort of Victorian injecting drug users. Med J Aust 159: 237–241, 1993.
3. Donahue JG, Nelson KE, Munoz A, Vlahov D, Rennie LL, Taylor EL, Saah AJ, Cohn S, Odaka NJ, Farzadegan H. Antibody to hepatitis C virus among cardiac surgery patients, homosexual men, and intravenous drug users in Baltimore, Maryland. Am J Epidemiol 134: 1206–1211, 1991.
4. Esteban JI, Esteban R, Viladomiu L, Lopez-Talavera JC, Gonzalez A, Hernandez JM, Roget M, Vargas V, Genesca J, Buti M, Guardia J, Houghton M, Choo QL, Kuo G. Hepatitis C virus antibodies among risk groups in Spain. Lancet 2: 294–296, 1989.
5. Mortimer PP, Cohen BJ, Litton PA, Vandervelde EM, Bassendine MF, Brind AM, Hambling MH. Hepatitis C virus antibody [letter]. Lancet 2: 798, 1989.
6. Patti AM, Santi AL, Pompa MG, Giustini C, Vescia N, Mastroeni I, Fara GM. Viral hepatitis and drugs: a continuing problem. Int J Epidemiol 22: 135–139, 1993.
7. Roggendorf M, Deinhardt F, Rasshofer R, Eberle J, Hopf U, Möller B, Zachoval R, Pape G, Schramm W, Rommel F. Antibodies to hepatitis C virus [letter]. Lancet 2: 324–325, 1989.
8. Van den Hoek JAR, Van Haastrecht HJ, Goudsmit J, De Wolf F, Coutinho RA. Prevalence, incidence and risk factors for hepatitis C virus infection among drug users in Amsterdam. J Infect Dis 162: 823–826, 1990.
9. Westh H, Worm AM, Jensen BL, Kroon S, Kvinesdal B, Nielsen CM, Wantzin P. Hepatitis C virus antibodies in homosexual men and intravenous drug users in Denmark. Infection 21: 115–117, 1993.
10. Alter MJ, Margolis HS, Krawczynski K, Judson FN, Mares A, Alexander WJ, Hu PY, Miller JK, Gerber MA, Sampliner RE, Meeks EL, Beach MJ. The natural history of community-acquired hepatitis C in the United States. N Engl J Med 327: 1899–1905, 1992.
11. Takahashi M, Yamada G, Miyamoto R, Toshihiko D, Endo H, Tsuji T. Natural course of chronic hepatitis C. Am J Gastroenterol 88: 244–247, 1993.
12. Akahane Y, Kojima M, Sugai Y, Sakamoto M, Miyazaki Y, Tanaka T, Tsuda F, Mishiro S, Okamoto H, Miyakawa Y, Mayumi M. Hepatitis C virus infection in spouses of patients with type C chronic liver disease. Ann Intern Med 120: 748–752, 1994.
13. Bresters D, Mauser-Bunschoten EP, Reesink HW, Roosendaal G, Van der Poel CL, Chamuleau RAFM, Jansen PLM, Weegink CJ, Cuypers HTM, Lelie PN, Van den Berg HM. Sexual transmission of hepatitis C virus. Lancet 342: 210–211, 1993.
14. Everhart JE, Di Bisceglie AM, Murray LM, Alter HJ, Melpolder JJ, Kuo G, Hoofnagle JH. Risk for non-A, non-B (type C) hepatitis through sexual or household contact with chronic carriers. Ann Intern Med 112: 544–545, 1990.
15. Garcia-Bengoechea M, Cortes A, Lopez P, Vega JL, Emparanza JI, Sarriugarte A, Santos E, Arenas JI. Intrafamilial spread of hepatitis C virus infection. Scand J Infect Dis 26: 15–18, 1994.
16. Melbye M, Biggar RJ, Wantzin P, Krogsgaard K, Ebbesen P, Becker NG. Sexual transmission of hepatitis C virus: cohort study (1981–9) among European homosexual men. BMJ 301: 210–212, 1990.
17. Osmond DH, Padian NS, Sheppard HW, Glass S, Shiboski SC, Reingold A. Risk factors for hepatitis C virus seropositivity in heterosexual couples. J Am Med Assoc 269: 361–365, 1993.
18. Thomas DL, Cannon RO, Shapiro CN, Hook III EW, Alter MJ, Quinn TC. Hepatitis C, hepatitis B, and human immunodeficiency virus infections among non-intravenous drug-using patients attending clinics for sexually transmitted diseases. J Infect Dis 169: 990–995, 1994.
19. Weinstock HS, Bolan G, Reingold AL, Polish LB. Hepatitis C virus infection among patients attending a clinic for sexually transmitted diseases. J Am Med Assoc 269: 392–394, 1993.
20. Driesel G, Wirth D, Stark K, Baumgarten R, Sucker U, Schreier E. Hepatitis C virus (HCV) distribution in German isolates: studies on the sequence variability in the E2 and NS5 region. Arch Virol 139: 379–388, 1994.
21. Okamoto H, Sugiyama Y, Okada S, Kurai K, Akahane Y, Sugai Y, Tanaka T, Sato K, Tsuda F, Miyakawa Y, Mayumi M. Typing hepatitis C virus by polymerase chain reaction with type-specific primers: application to clinical surveys and tracing infectious sources. J Genet Virol 73: 673–679, 1992.
22. Simmonds P, Holmes EC, Cha TA, Chan SW, McOmish F, Irvine B, Beall E, Yap PL, Kolberg J, Urdea MS. Classification of hepatitis C virus into six major genotypes and a series of subtypes by phylogenetic analysis of the NS-5 region. J Genet Virol 74: 2391–2399, 1993.
23. Viazov S, Zibert A, Ramakrishan K, Widell A, Cavicchini A, Schreier E, Roggendorf M. Typing of hepatitis C virus isolates by DNA enzyme immunoassay. J Virol Methods 48: 81–92, 1994.
24. Widell A, Shev S, Mansson S, Zhang YY, Foberg U, Norkrans G, Fryden A, Weiland O, Kurkus J, Nordenfelt E. Genotyping of hepatitis C virus isolates by a modified polymerase chain reaction assay using type specific primers: epidemiological applications. J Med Virol 44: 272–279, 1994.
25. Pozzato G, Moretti M, Franzin F, Croce LS, Tiribelli C, Masayu T, Kaneko S, Unoura M, Kobayashi K. Severity of liver disease with different hepatitis C viral clones [letter]. Lancet 338: 509, 1991.
26. Yoshioka K, Kakumu S, Wakita T, Ishikawa T, Itoh Y, Takayanagi M, Higashi Y, Shibata M, Morishima T. Detection of hepatitis C virus by polymerase chain reaction and response to interferon-α therapy: relationship to genotypes of hepatitis C virus. Hepatology 16: 293–299, 1992.
27. Müller R, Stark K, Guggenmoos-Holzmann I, Wirth D, Bienzle U. Imprisonment: a risk factor for HIV infection counteracting education and prevention programmes for intravenous drug users. AIDS 9: 183–190, 1995.
28. Des Jarlais DC, Friedman SR, Choopanya K, Vanichseni S, Ward TP. International epidemiology of HIV and AIDS among injecting drug users. AIDS 6: 1053–1068, 1992.
29. Jose B, Friedman SR, Neaigus A, Curtis R, Grund JPC, Goldstein MF, Ward TP, Des Jarlais DC. Syringe-mediated drug-sharing (backloading): a new risk factor for HIV among injecting drug users. AIDS 7: 1653–1660, 1993.
30. Ko YC, Ho MS, Chiang TA, Chang SJ, Chang PY. Tattooing as a risk factor of hepatitis C virus infection. J Med Virol 38: 288–291, 1992.
31. Esteban JI, Lopez-Talavera JC, Genesca J, Madoz P, Viladomiu L, Muniz E, Martin-Vega C, Rosell M, Allende H, Vidal X, Gonzalez A, Hernandez JM, Esteban R, Guardia J.

High rate of infectivity and liver disease in blood donors with antibodies to hepatitis C virus. Ann Intern Med 115: 443–449, 1991.
32. Van der Poel CL, Cuypers HTM, Reesink HW, Weiner AJ, Quan S, DiNello R, Van Boven JJP, Winkel J, Mulder-Folkerts D, Exel-Oehlers PJ, Schaasberg W, Leentvar-Kuypers A, Polito A, Houghton M, Lelie PN. Confirmation of hepatitis C virus infection by second generation four-antigen recombinant immunoblot assay and polymerase chain reaction. Lancet 337: 317–319, 1991.

Submitted January 9, 1995; accepted March 30, 1995

Vilken antibiotikabehandling väljer Du vid bukinfektioner?

Kombinationsbehandling **Monoterapi**

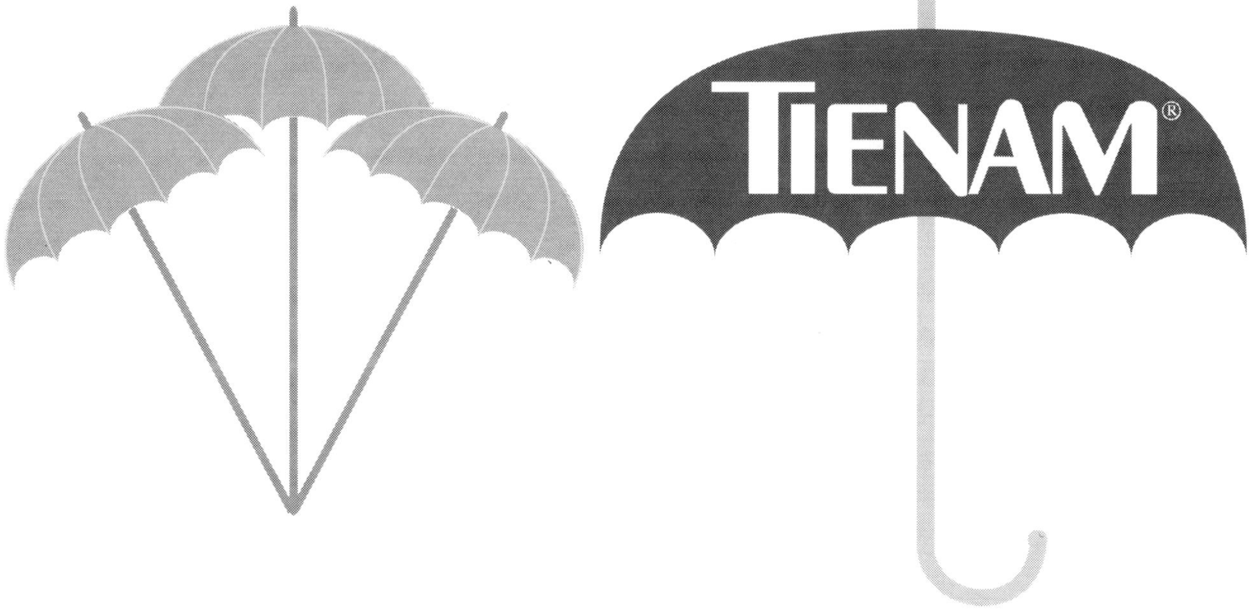

- TIENAM®* –initialterapi vid bukinfektioner
- TIENAM®* kan förkorta vårdtiden jämfört med kombinationsbehandling [1,2,3].

Ref
1 Guerra J G et al. Imipenem/cilastatin VS, gentamicin/clindamycin for the treatment of moderate to severe infections in hospitalized patients. Rev Infect Dis 1985; 7:463–470

2 Heseltine PNR et al. Imipenem therapy for perforated gangrenous appendicitis. Surg Gynecol Obstet 1986; 162: 43–48

3 Gonzenbach H R, Simmen HP, Amgwerd R. Imipenem (N–F–Thienamycin) versus netilmicin plus clindamycin:A controlled and randomized comparison in intra abdominal infections. Ann Surg 1987; 205(3): 271–275

MSD
MERCK SHARP& DOHME Merck Sharp & Dohme (Sweden) AB Tel. 08/626 14 00

*Registered trademark of MERCK & CO., Inc., Rahway, N.J., U.S.A. Ten–90–SCAN–114–J(S)

Scand J Infect Dis 27: 339–343, 1995 ORIGINAL ARTICLE

Clinical and Therapeutic Features of Childhood Neurobrucellosis

YOUSSEF A. AL-EISSA

From the Department of Pedriatics, King Khalid University Hospital, College of Medicine, King Saud University, Riyadh, Saudi Arabia

Brucellosis is a multisystem disease with diverse clinical presentations, and involvement of the nervous system is considered to be rare in childhood. Five children with meningitis ($n = 2$), meningoencephalitis ($n = 1$), meningomyelitis ($n = 1$), or cerebellar ataxia ($n = 1$) are described, all of whom had a history of exposure to a possible source of brucellosis. Examination of cerebrospinal fluid (CSF) revealed lymphocytic pleocytosis in 4 patients, high protein concentration in 5 and low glucose concentration in 3. Reciprocal brucella agglutination titers were significantly elevated in serum (≥ 160) and in CSF (≥ 80) of all patients. Brucella melitensis was isolated both from blood and CSF in one patient, from blood only in 2, and from bone marrow only in another one. All patients were treated successfully by a three-drug combination of streptomycin (4 patients) or doxycycline (one patient) with trimethoprim-sulfamethoxazole and rifampin, and in one patient dexamethasone was also added. In endemic areas, neurobrucellosis should be suspected in the evaluation of patients with unexplained neurologic symptoms.

Y. A. Al-Eissa, MD, Department of Pediatrics (39), College of Medicine, King Saud University, Box 2925, Riyadh 11461, Saudi Arabia

INTRODUCTION

Brucellosis is primarily a contagious zoonotic infection transmitted to humans through ingestion of unpasteurized milk or milk products derived from infected domestic animals and through direct contact with their tissues or secretions (1). It remains an important health problem in many parts of the world (1, 2), and the disease due to Brucella melitensis is a common infection in countries of the Middle East and Southern Europe (2).

Brucellosis is a multisystem disease with diverse clinical presentations. Involvement of the nervous system is a rare, but serious, complication and occurs primarily in adults (3–7). It may occur at the onset of the illness, during convalescence, or months after recovery from acute infection (3). The nervous system may be affected at any level simulating several neurologic diseases and neurobrucellosis may present as meningitis, encephalitis, myelitis, polyradiculoneuritis, cranial neuropathy, subarachnoid hemorrhage, or space-occupying lesion alone or in combination (3–6).

Previous descriptions of the neurologic pattern in patients with neurobrucellosis have been based mainly on studies of adult cases (3–7). A few case reports (8–11) and a small series of cases (12) of neurobrucellosis in children have been described. We report here the clinical presentations and outcome of 5 children with neurobrucellosis in order to reemphasize the diversity of neurologic abnormalities. It is particularly important to make the correct diagnosis since brucellosis is treatable by appropriate antimicrobial agents.

PATIENTS AND METHODS

Between 1988 and 1993, 5 patients presented with neurobrucellosis. Three patients were female and 2 were male, with ages ranging from 4 to 11 years. The diagnosis of nervous system involvement due to brucellosis was based on the presence of the following: neurologic abnormalities not explained by other neurologic diseases; a positive cerebrospinal fluid (CSF) culture for brucella, or significant brucella agglutination titers in the blood and CSF of ≥ 160 and ≥ 80, respectively; abnormal CSF findings of an increased protein and a lymphocytic pleocytosis, and finally, a clinical response to antibrucellar chemotherapy (3–8).

Diagnostic evaluation included complete blood count (CBC), erythrocyte sedimentation rate (ESR), blood glucose, liver and renal function profiles, blood and CSF brucella agglutination titers, blood and CSF cultures for brucella and other organisms, and CSF cell count, protein and glucose. Computed tomographic (CT) scan, myelogram, electromyography (EMG), nerve conduction studies, evoked potential audiometry (EPA) and brainstem auditory evoked potentials (BAEPs) were performed when indicated.

Brucella antibody titers were determined by the standard tube agglutination method (13) using comercially available brucella antigens (Wellcome Diagnostics, Dartford, UK). For brucella culture, blood or CSF samples were inoculated into bottles of tryptic soy broth and thioglycolate and subcultured on duplicate blood agar plates incubated with or without CO_2. Brucella isolates were identified by slide agglutination using monospecific Brucella abortus and B. melitensis antisera (Wellcome Diagnostics, Dartford, UK). Antibiotic susceptibility tests were carried out using the disc diffusion method with Isosensitest agar (Oxoid, UK).

All patients were treated with 3 antimicrobial agents. Four patients received a combination of streptomycin (20 mg/kg intramuscularly once daily for 2–3 weeks) with trimethoprim-sulfamethoxazole (TMP-SMX, 10/50 mg/kg/day orally in 2 divided doses for 12 weeks) and rifampin (20 mg/kg/day orally in 2 divided doses for 12 weeks). In one patient, doxycycline (4 mg/kg/day orally in 2 divided doses for 12 weeks) was given with TMP-SMX and rifampin. Intravenous dexamethasone was given for 5 days to case 4 because of increased intracranial pressure and papilledema.

Follow-up serology and blood cultures for brucella were performed during and after antimicrobial therapy and all patients were regularly seen for a minimum of 1 year.

RESULTS

Cases 1 and 2 presented acutely with meningitis and case 3 had impairment of consciousness and obvious features of

Table I. *Diagnostic CSF findings and brucella serology and culture in five cases of neurobrucellosis*

Case no.	Age (years)/sex	CSF findings: Cells µl (% lymphocytes)	CSF findings: Protein, g/l	CSF findings: Glucose, mmol/l	Brucella reciprocal titers: Serum	Brucella reciprocal titers: CSF	Brucella culture[a]: Blood	Brucella culture[a]: CSF	Brucella culture[a]: B. marrow	Clinical presentation	Antibiotic therapy
1	7/F	486 (90)	0.85	1.9[b]	1,280	160	+	−	ND	Meningitis	Streptomycin, TMP-SMX and rifampin
2	6/F	340 (94)	1.65	1.2[b]	10,240	320	+	−	ND	Meningitis	Streptomycin, TMP-SMX and rifampin
3	12/M	195 (92)	2.10	2.2[b]	2,560	160	+	+	ND	Meningoencephalitis	Streptomycin, TMP-SMX and rifampin
4	11/F	238 (95)	2.80	3.0	5,120	640	−	−	+	Meningomyelitis	TMP-SMX, rifampin and doxycycline
5	4/M	4 (100)	1.90	2.8	2,560	80	−	−	ND	Cerebellar ataxia	Streptomycin, TMP-SMX and rifampin

[a] All isolates were brucella melitensis

[b] CSF glucose level was < 50% of concurrent blood glucose.

CSF cerebrospinal fluid; ND not done; TMP-SMX trimethoprim-sulfamethoxazole.

meningoencephalitis. Case 4 had spastic paraplegia with deafness and urinary sphincter involvement, and case 5 had cerebellar ataxia. The initial CBC revealed mild anemia and leukopenia with relative lymphocytosis an cases 4 and 5. The ESR was 46 mm/h in case 3 and 55 mm/h in case 4, but normal in the others. Mildly elevated values of lactic dehydrogenase, alkaline phosphatase and aminotransferases were the only abnormal findings to be detected in case 5 from liver and renal function tests.

The diagnostic CSF findings together with serology and culture for brucella in the 5 cases are summarized in Table I.

All the B. melitensis isolates were susceptible to the standard antibrucellar drugs given to our patients. Brucella was not isolated from follow-up blood cultures done 7–10 days after initiation of antibiotics and at the end of therapy. Brucella titers declined gradually and became negative within 6–18 months following treatment in the 5 cases presented here.

CASE REPORTS

Case 1. A 7-year-old girl presented with a 1-week history of fever, malaise, frontal headache, photophobia, and anorexia, followed by vomiting during the last 2 days before admission. She had spent the 2-month summer holiday in a brucella-endemic area and was drinking raw goat's milk.

On examination she looked ill and had a temperature of 39°C. Her general and neurologic physical examinations were normal. Examination of CSF revealed a WBC of 510×10^6/l (56% lymphocytes and 44% neutrophils), a protein of 0.4 g/l, and a glucose of 3.0 mmol/l (60% of blood glucose). Initial brucella titers were 40 in the blood and undetectable in the CSF.

Therapy with intravenous ceftriaxone was initiated, but the patient continued to have headache and spikes of fever. A week after admission, lumbar puncture was repeated and the CSF findings are shown in Table I. At this time, her brucella titers were 1,280 and 160 in the blood and CSF, respectively. Blood cultures yielded B. melitensis, but CSF cultures grew no pathogens. Antibrucellar chemotherapy was administered and her symptoms abated within 3 days. She was treated with streptomycin for 2 weeks and TMP-SMX and rifampin for 3 months. Her EPA and BAEPs were normal. She remained asymptomatic during an 18-month follow-up.

Case 2. A 6-year-old girl was admitted with a 2-week history of intermittent fever, generalized headache, malaise, anorexia and loss of body weight. She received a 10-day course of amoxicillin without improvement. She had been drinking raw goat and camel milk regularly for several months and 2 members of her family had brucellosis for which they had received antibrucellar therapy. On examination she looked ill with a temperature of 38.6°C. Her general and neurologic physical examinations were unremarkable. The diagnosis of brucella meningitis was confirmed by the findings of brucella titers of 10,240 in the blood and 320 in the CSF, isolation of B. melitensis from blood culture, and abnormal CSF examination (Table I).

She responded well to intramuscular streptomycin for 2 weeks, and TMP-SMX and rifampin for 12 weeks. Her EPA and BAEPs were normal. She had no recurrence of her symptoms during a follow-up for 1 year.

Case 3. A 12-year-old boy presented with a 10-day history of fever, headache, arthralgia and occasional vomiting, followed by memory impairment for 2 days prior to admission. He had had brucellosis 2 months earlier, and had received rifampin and TMP-SMX for 4 weeks. He admitted to the ingestion of unpasteurized feta cheese from a friend's farm before his initial febrile illness but not after. On examination he was confused, irritable and disoriented with a temperature of 38.2°C. He had photophobia, mild papilledema, neck stiffness and a positive Kernig's sign. Muscle power was generally decreased and he was unable to stand up. The deep tendon reflexes were brisk and the plantar responses were normal. The diagnosis of neurobrucellosis was made immediately after admission (Table I). A CT scan of the head done on admission revealed mild cerebral edema.

Intravenous dexamethasone was administered for 5 days. He was treated with intramuscular streptomycin for the initial 3 weeks plus oral TMP-SMX and rifampin for 12 weeks. His confusional state and acute symptoms promptly disappeared within the first 5 days of antibrucellar chemotherapy. Both EPA and BAEPs were normal. He remained asymptomatic on subsequent follow-ups for 2 years.

Case 4. An 11-year-old female shepherd who had been regularly drinking raw goat's milk complained of intermittent fever, headache, arthralgia, generalized weakness and fatiguability for 4 months. During the month preceding admission, deterioration of bladder control, gradual loss of hearing, and progressive weakness of lower limbs were observed. The patient and her mother and two siblings had been treated at another hospital for brucellosis 1 year previously. On examination she was ill, grossly depressed and uncommunicative with a temperature of 38°C. She had intact cranial nerves except for bilateral sensorineural deafness. There were spastic paraplegia and hyperreflexia in the lower limbs. The plantar responses were extensor and the sensations were normal. The anal sphincter tone was normal. Serologic tests and CSF findings were compatible with brucellosis (Table I). Bone marrow culture yielded B. melitensis, but both blood and CSF were sterile. The EMG and the nerve conduction studies were normal. The CT scans of the head and spine were normal. A metrizamide myelogram was normal. The BAEPs confirmed sensorineural deafness.

After 3-months treatment with rifampin, TMP-SMX and doxycycline she was able to walk with assistance and bladder function had improved. When seen 2 years later she was deaf, but independently walking with a shuffling gait.

Case 5. A 4-year-old boy was admitted with a 2-month history of intermittent episodes of low-grade fever, headache, general body aches, and occasional vomiting. During these episodes he visited private clinics and received different medications. Five days prior to admission he developed difficulty in walking, progressive loss of balance with tendency to fall, and frequent vomiting. He had stayed for 2 weeks in a farm 3 weeks before the onset of his illness and had been in intimate contact with farm animals, but there was no history of raw milk ingestion. On examination there was normal temperature, mild nystagmus, ataxia, and marked intention tremor of his upper limbs. Both liver and spleen were palpable, 2 cm and 3 cm below the costal margins, respectively. Muscle power and tone were normal. Deep tendon reflexes were normal and the plantar response was equivocal. The results of laboratory investigations were consistent with brucellosis (Table I) and therapy with streptomycin, TMP-SMX and rifampin was initiated. An enhanced CT scan of the brain was normal. An EPA and BAEPs were normal.

His symptoms improved within 1 week of therapy and he was completely normal 2 weeks later. He remained asymptomatic during a 15-month follow-up.

DISCUSSION

The 5 patients whose cases are reported here had neurobrucellosis affecting various parts of the nervous system, ranging from the cerebrum to the spinal cord. Nervous system involvement is not common and the incidence has recently been estimated to be 3–5% of cases with generalized brucellosis in adult series (5, 14). The pathology of the disease is assumed to be a direct effect of the organism or its toxin on the meninges, the brain and the spinal cord (4, 5). The manifestations of neurobrucellosis are quite variable and may begin days to months after the initial infection. Despite the importance of a history of exposure in the consideration of brucellosis, unfamiliarity with the diverse clinical presentations of nervous system involvement may have led to considerable delay in the diagnosis of the 5 cases presented here. Hence, the suspicion for the diagnosis of neurobrucellosis should always be entertained in patients, living in or coming from endemic areas, who present with obscure, confusing, and often mixed constitutional or neurologic symptoms for which no obvious explanation is readily apparent (4, 8, 15, 16).

Fever, malaise, headache and vomiting were the most outstanding constitutional features of our patients' illness. If such non-specific complaints are associated with specific focal neurologic manifestations, the establishment of the diagnosis may not be difficult. The neurologic manifestations noted in our cases have suggested meningitis, meningoencephalitis, meningomyelitis and cerebellar ataxia. It is worthwhile noting that the systemic physical signs of brucellosis were inconspicuous: hepatosplenomegaly was noted in only one patient and other abnormal findings, such as arthritis and lymphadenopathy, thought to be present in patients with generalized brucellosis were not detected (2).

The most common and well defined syndrome of neurobrucellosis is meningitis (4, 5, 7, 12). It may present early and be the sole manifestation of brucellosis, as in cases 1 and 2, or the meningeal infection may extend to the cerebrum or the spinal cord and be associated with encephalitis or myelitis, as in cases 3 and 4. The clinical features of brucellar meningitis are not different from other forms of meningitis, particularly tuberculous meningitis. However, patients with meningeal brucellosis tend to be less unwell than those with tuberculous meningitis (15). Cranial nerve palsies, including the second, sixth, seventh and eighth nerve, have been reported (5, 8, 14). Sensorineural deafness and optic neuritis are the 2 most common forms of cranial nerve involvement in patients with brucella meningoencephalitis (5, 8). Case 3, with meningoencephalitis, had bilateral sensorineural deafness. Spinal cord involvement constitutes an infrequent complication of brucellosis and appears weeks or months after the onset of brucella infection (8). Brucella myelitis is postulated to occur as a complication of arachnoiditis or vasculitis (14, 17), and may present as an isolated entity or as part of meningoencephalitis (5). Brucellosis can produce spastic paraplegia as a result of cord compression by extradural abscess or granuloma secondary to brucella spondylitis (17). Cases of brucella myelopathy have previously been reported in adults (3–6, 14, 17). In case 4, radiographic studies excluded the possibilities of vertebral damage or an extradural mass. Cerebellar ataxia was seen as an isolated clinical picture in case 5 who had a normal CT scan of the head. This phenomenon occurs not infrequently in children, following the onset of a viral infection by 1–3 weeks. In our patient, the cerebellar signs developed after a latent period of a few weeks. Brucella-induced cerebellar ataxia has previously, though rarely, been described (5, 18); the pathogenesis is not clear, but a parainfectious autoimmune reaction is most probably responsible for the development of cerebellar dysfunction.

The definitive evidence of brucella infection is isolation of the organism from the patient. However, laboratory cultures of brucella species are often unsuccessful due to the slow-growing nature of these organisms and the requirement for special media (16). Brucella was isolated from the blood in 3 cases, of which one had a positive CSF culture. Culture of the aspirated bone marrow is more likely to be successful (16), as in case 4. Brucella serologic tests have proved to be invaluable in screening for the disease. One might speculate that occurrence of positive serologic studies might be frequent as a result of exposure without infection in an endemic area. However, it has been our experience (2, 11, 16) as well as that of others (4, 6, 7) that seropositivity, when the reciprocal agglutination titer is 160 or greater, represents active disease. Cholera vaccination, or infection with Vibrio cholerae, Francisella tularensis or Yersinia enterocolitica may, however, cause a false-positive brucella agglutination titer due to immunologic cross-reactivity (16). In the early period of illness, patients may fail to mount a significant serologic response, but a fourfold or greater rise in titers for sera drawn 1–4 weeks apart is indicative of recent brucella infection (16), as demonstrated in case 1. The use of the enzyme-linked immunosorbent assay (ELISA) on serum and CSF has been reported to be sensitive and specific for the rapid diagnosis of neurobrucellosis (19). Examination of the CSF generally shows a raised protein, a lymphocytic pleocytosis and reduced glucose concentration in some cases (3–7); these findings were found in our reported cases.

The efficacy of chemotherapy for any infection is largely judged by the rate of cure and the incidence of sequelae. Active generalized brucellosis always responds to antimicrobial therapy. The unpredictable relapse after treatment, however, has remained a significant problem in brucellosis, as the organisms are facultative intracellular pathogens relatively inaccessible for antibiotics (1, 2). Relapses are almost invariably associated with insufficient duration of antimicrobial treatment (2). Although the antibiotic therapy of systemic brucellosis is well established, the best drug regimen for neurobrucellosis and the duration of therapy have not been standardized. Accumulated experience favors prolonged courses of a combination of 2 or more of 4 drugs: TMP-SMX, rifampin, streptomycin, or doxycycline (1, 3, 5–7). Since aminoglycosides and tetracyclines penetrate the blood–brain barrier poorly, the additional antibiotics that achieve high levels in the CSF are needed in the treatment of neurobrucellosis. Recent reports have shown that antimicrobial regimens containing TMP-SMX and rifampin are generally effective for brucella infection of CNS (3, 5–7). Both drugs have good CNS penetration and may be synergistic (1, 3). Our patients were treated successfully by a three-drug combination of streptomycin or doxycycline with TMP-SMX and rifampin. All the patients were cured without relapses. Supplementary treatment with corticosteroids in chronic neurobrucellosis is recommended by some (1, 5, 14), but experience from controlled studies or larger series of patients is not available.

This report confirms the heterogeneous nosologic panorama of neurologic presentations of brucellosis in childhood. It underlines the need for a high index of suspicion of neurobrucellosis in patients with an unusual or unexplained neurologic illness.

REFERENCES

1. Hall WH. Modern chemotherapy for brucellosis in humans. Rev Infect Dis 12: 1060–1099, 1990.
2. AL-Eissa YA, Kambal AM, Al-Nasser MN, Al-Habib SA, Al-Fawaz IM, Al-Zamil FA. Childhood brucellosis: a study of 102 cases. Pediatr Infect Dis J 9: 74–79, 1990.
3. Bashir R, Al-Kawi MZ, Harder EJ, Jinkins J. Nervous system brucellosis: diagnosis and treatment. Neurology 35: 1576–1581, 1985.
4. Fincham RW, Sahs AL, Joynt RJ. Protean manifestations of nervous system brucellosis: case histories of a wide variety of clinical forms. J Am Med Assoc 184: 269–275, 1963.
5. Shakir RA, Al-Din ASN, Araj GF, Lulu AR, Mousa AR, Saadah MA. Clinical categories of neurobrucellosis: a report on 19 cases. Brain 110: 213–223, 1987.
6. Bahemuka M, Shemena A, Panayiotopoulos CP, Al-Aska AK, Obeid T, Daif AK. Neurological syndromes of brucellosis. J Neurol Neurosurg Psychiatr 51: 1017–1021, 1988.
7. Al-Orainey IO, Laajam MA, Al-Aska AK, Rajapakse CN. Brucella meningitis. J Infect 14: 141–145, 1987.
8. Nelson-Jones A. Neurological complications of undulant fever. Lancet 1: 495–498, 1951.
9. Strannegard I-L, Araj GF, Fattah HA. Neurobrucellosis in an eight-year-old child. Ann Trop Paediatr 5: 191–194, 1985.
10. Drutz JE. Brucellosis of the central nervous system: a case report of an infected infant. Clin Pediatr 28: 476–478, 1989.
11. Al-Eissa YA. Unusual suppurative complications of brucellosis in children. Acta Paediatr 82: 987–992, 1993.
12. Lubani MM, Dudin KI, Araj GF, Manandhar DS, Rashid FY. Neurobrucellosis in children. Pediatr Infect Dis J 8: 79–82, 1989.
13. Meyer ME. Immune response to brucellae. In: Rose NR, Friedman H, Fahey JL, eds. Manual of clinical laboratory immunology. Washington, DC: American Society for Microbiology, 385–387, 1986.

14. Pascual J, Combarros O, Polo JM, Berciano J. Localized CNS brucellosis: report of 7 cases. Acta Neurol Scand 78: 282–289, 1988.
15. Hudgson P, Al-Bunyan MA. Polyradiculoneuropathy and cranial nerve involvement in brucellosis. Ann Saudi Med 9(Suppl): 221S–223S, 1989.
16. Al-Eissa Y, Al-Zamil F, Al-Mugeiren M, Al-Rasheed S, Al-Sanie A, Al-Mazyad A. Childhood brucellosis: a deceptive infectious disease. Scand J Infect Dis 23: 129–133, 1991.
17. Ganado W, Craig AJ. Brucellosis myelopathy. J Bone Joint Surg (Am) 40: 1380–1388, 1958.
18. Gelfand MS, Kaiser AB, Dale WA. Localized brucellosis: popliteal artery aneurysm, mediastinitis, dementia, and pneumonia. Rev Infect Dis 11: 783–788, 1989.
19. Araj GF, Lulu AR, Saadah MA, Mousa AM, Strannegard I, Shaker RA. Rapid diagnosis of neurobrucellosis by ELISA. J Neuroimmunol 12: 173–182, 1986.

Submitted March 3, 1995; accepted May 7, 1995

Scand J Infect Dis 27: 344–346, 1995

ORIGINAL ARTICLE

Coxiella burnetii Infection in Subjects with HIV Infection and HIV Infection in Patients with Q Fever

MILAGROSA MONTES, GUSTAVO CILLA, JOSE M. MARIMON, JOSE L. DIAZ DE TUESTA and EMILIO PEREZ-TRALLERO

From the Servicio de Microbiología y Unidad de Epidemiología Infecciosa, Facultad de Medicina, Hospital NS Aránzazu, San Sebastián, Spain

The objective of the study was to determine whether HIV infection favors the acquisition of Coxiella burnetii infection or increases the frequency of symptomatic Coxiella infections. A total of 754 subjects were tested for Coxiella antibodies: 597 intravenous drug users (IVDUs) (306 HIV-infected IVDUs matched by age and sex with 291 non-HIV-infected IVDUs), and 157 healthy puerperal women matched to the IVDU women. A total of 520 patients with Q fever were tested for HIV antibodies. The seroprevalence of Coxiella antibodies was similar in the 2 groups of IVDUs (19.3% of HIV+ IVDUs vs 22.9% of HIV− IVDUs). Likewise, there was no difference in the prevalence of Coxiella antibodies in the groups of IVDU women and healthy women. Of the 520 subjects with acute Q fever, diagnosed between 1987 and 1992, only 4 (0.77%) had HIV infection. The proportions of HIV-infected subjects in the population of patients, with Q fever, of 20–39 years of age (the age of maximum incidence of both HIV and Coxiella infection in our region), coincided with the estimated proportions of HIV subjects in the respective general populations of the province. In conclusion, infection by Coxiella burnetii was not more frequent among HIV-infected subjects. It is not likely that Coxiella infection produces symptomatic infections more often in HIV-infected subjects.

E. Pérez-Trallero, MD, Servicio de Microbiología, Hospital NS Aránzazu, Apartado 477, E-20080 San Sebastián, Spain

INTRODUCTION

Coxiella burnetii is the causal agent of Q fever, a zoonosis distributed throughout the world, that may occur either asymptomatically or with clinical manifestations in the form of febrile syndrome with or without pneumonia and/or hepatitis (1). The infection may become chronic, most frequently in the form of endocarditis (2). C. burnetii is an obligate intracellular microorganism that grows in the phagolysosomes of eukaryote cells, particularly macrophages, where it is favored by the acid pH (3). Therefore, cellular immunity is an essential factor in the control of infection. It has been suggested recently that subjects infected with human immunodeficiency virus (HIV) may be more predisposed to C. burnetii infection than non-infected subjects. We studied the relation between HIV and Coxiella infection in a group of IVDUs and Q fever patients.

METHODS

The first part of this 2-part study was an investigation of the seroprevalence of C. burnetii infection in a group of intravenous drug users (IVDUs) with HIV infection as compared with IVDUs not infected with HIV. The second part consisted of an anonymous study of HIV antibodies in patients with acute Q fever confirmed by serology in our laboratory.

HIV-infected subjects

The study included 306 IVDUs who had HIV antibodies (83 women and 223 men) collected from 1985 to 1993. The mean age ± SD of the group was 26.6 ± 4.1 years, range 17–43. The number to be included in this group was determined on the basis of the census population aged 20–39 years, which has been found (5) to have an expected prevalence of anti-Coxiella antibodies of 28% (worst acceptable result of ± 5%, 95% confidence level) (CDC 1991 Population Survey, Sample Size & Power, Statcalc Software program, Epiinfo 5.01 b. Atlanta, Georgia, USA). As a control group for the HIV-infected IVDUs, we studied a group of IVDUs without HIV antibodies matched by age and sex (control group I) comprising 291 subjects, 70 women and 221 men, mean age ± SD 26 ± 4.3 years, range 15–42.

We also selected a second matched control group (control group II) for the HIV-infected and non-HIV-infected IVDU women (mean age 25.8 ± 3.9 years, range 16–43) consisting of 157 healthy women who underwent delivery at our hospital (mean age ± SD 26.5 ± 4.3 years, range 16–41 years). The sample was selected from a hospital that handled 65% of all deliveries in the province of Guipúzcoa during the study period.

Patients with acute Q fever studied for HIV infection

This group consisted of 520 patients (381 men and 139 women) diagnosed as having acute Q fever, at the Hospital Nuestra Señora de Aránzazu between 1987 and 1992, which represents almost all the cases of Q fever diagnosed in this period and most of the cases confirmed serologically in the province (>90%). All presented serum findings of indirect immunofluorescent seroconversion to C. burnetii and/or specific IgM at ≥1/256 titer (BioMèrieux, Marcy l'Étoile, France) after absorption with anti-IgG (RF Absorbens, Boehringwerke, Munich, Germany). In all of them, the presence of HIV antibodies was investigated anonymously by thawing an aliquot of serum from each subject and recoding it with a code that was destroyed later. Prior to this study, the immune status in relation to HIV was known in a subgroup of nine IVDUs with Q fever, 3 of whom were HIV+.

 ISSN 0036-5548

Laboratory methods

All the sera used in the study were kept at −40°C from the time of extraction. IgG against C. burnetii were detected with an indirect immunofluorescence technique using commercial slides containing C. burnetii antigen in phase II (Biomèrieux) and anti-human IgG goat immunoglobulins marked with fluorescein isothiocyanate (Fluoline-G, BioMèrieux). The sera were diluted in phosphate buffered saline (pH 7.6) from 1/16 to the maximum dilution at which a positive reaction was found. An antibody titer of ≥1/16 was considered indicative of C. burnetii infection. HIV antibodies were detected using a commercial enzymeimmunoanalysis (EIA) system (Vironostika® HIV MIXT, Organon Teknika BV, Boxtel, Holland). Serum positivity in the EIA test was confirmed using a Western blot technique (New Vav-Blot I Plus, Diagnostic Pasteur, Marnes-la-Coquette, France).

Locale

The Guipúzcoa health administration area is located in the north-eastern Basque country (1997 km^2, 675 529 inhabitants). It is bordered by the Bay of Biscay (Atlantic Ocean) and France to the north. The population stratum 20–39 years consists of 211 949 people (6). The estimated number of HIV-infected subjects in this population is 3,000–4,000, most of whom are or have been IVDUs (7).

Data analysis

The prevalence of C. burnetii antibodies was compared using the chi-squared test for independent data, using a level of significance of $p = 0.05$.

RESULTS

Seroprevalence of C. burnetii infection in HIV-infected and non-HIV-infected IVDUs

Of the HIV-infected IVDUs, 19.3% (59/306) had anti-Coxiella IgG compared with 22.9% (65/284) of the non-HIV-infected IVDUs ($\chi^2 = 1.15$, $p = 0.28$). The distribution of anti-Coxiella IgG titers was similar in the 2 groups (Table I), most Coxiella-positive subjects having titers ≤1/256. Only 8.5% of the HIV+ IVDUs and 12.3% of HIV− IVDUs had titers ≥1/512 ($\chi^2 = 0.48$, $p = 0.48$)

Seroprevalence of C. burnetii infection in IVDU women and matched healthy women

Of the IVDU women studied, 14.4% had anti-Coxiella IgG (22/153) compared to 20.4% in the group of healthy women (32/157) ($\chi^2 = 1.94$, $p = 0.1635$). No differences between groups were observed in the distribution of titers, which were generally low (Table II).

Prevalence of HIV infection in subjects diagnosed as having acute Q fever

Of the 520 subjects with acute Q fever, diagnosed in the 1987–1992 period, only 4 (0.77%) had HIV antibodies. Three of these (ages 28, 27 and 21 years) were IVDUs whose HIV infection was known before this study was made.

Of the 520 Q fever subjects, 202 were 20–39 years of age and 3 of these had HIV infection, a ratio of 1:67.

Table I. *Antibodies to Coxiella burnetii, as shown by indirect immunofluorescence in intravenous drug users (IVDUs) with HIV infection and without HIV infection*

	IVDU	HIV+	IVDU	HIV−
IgG titer	*n*	%	*n*	%
1/16	10	3.3	9	3.2
1/32	13	4.2	6	2.1
1/64	12	3.9	23	8.1
1/128	13	4.2	12	4.2
1/256	6	2.0	7	2.5
1/512	4	1.3	5	1.7
≥1/1024	1	0.3	3	1.1
Negative	247	80.7	219	77.1

Table II. *Antibodies to Coxiella burnetii, as shown by indirect immunofluorescence, in women intravenous drug users (IVDU) and healthy puerperal controls*

	IVDU		Controls	
IgG titer	*n*	%	*n*	%
1/16	2	1.3	4	2.5
1/32	4	2.6	6	3.8
1/64	5	3.3	8	5.1
1/128	7	4.6	8	5.1
1/256	3	1.9	8	5.1
1/512	0	—	1	0.6
≥1/1024	1	0.6	0	—
Negative	131	85.6	125	79.1

Estimation of cases of Q fever in subjects with HIV infection: comparison with cases detected

Considering the population of Guipúzcoa in the 20–39 years age bracket and the number of subjects with HIV infection in this age group (89.4% of the AIDS cases in Guipúzcoa are found in this age cohort (7)), the predicted proportion of HIV-infected subjects is 1 per 53–71 cases of Q fever in the normal population (3,000–4,000/211 949). These predicted figures coincide with those found in this study.

DISCUSSION

Immunosuppressed patients are more predisposed than immunocompetent persons to infection involving intracellular organisms. Human acquired immunodeficiency syndrome (AIDS) is a prototypical immunosuppression syndrome in which opportunist infections by intracellular organisms such as Pneumocystis carinii, Cytomegalovirus, Toxoplasma gondii, Mycobacterium, etc. are an important cause of morbidity and mortality (8). In recent years, studies have associated Q fever with defects in cellular immunity of different origin, i.e. organ transplantation, cancer and HIV infection (4, 9–13). Raoult et al. found that the prevalence of anti-Coxiella IgG in HIV-infected subjects was higher findings are of interest in our geographic area because of the high incidence of both HIV and C. burnetii infections. In Guipúzcoa, the 1993 incidence of new cases of AIDS was 178.86 per million inhabitants and the cumulative number of cases of AIDS by December 1993 was 977 per million inhabitants (7). This incidence is one of the highest rates of HIV infection in Europe.

Furthermore, the Basque country is the Spanish Autonomous Community with the largest number of cases of Q fever, detected as either isolated instances or epidemic outbreaks. The results obtained in our study show that the prevalence of anti-Coxiella IgG among HIV-infected subjects was similar to that among non-HIV-infected IVDUs as well as to that among IVDU women and non-IVDU women. Bélec et al., in Central African and French subjects, found no significant difference in the seroprevalence of C. burnetii among HIV-infected and non-HIV-infected subjects (13, 14). In spite of the greater susceptibility of patients with deficient cellular immunity to infections by intracellular organisms, there is no reason to think that the risk of infection by C. burnetii among HIV-infected and non-HIV-infected subjects is different.

The main route of transmission of this microorganism is by aerosol, followed at a considerable distance by intake of raw milk products. Published cases of C. burnetii transmission by other routes are exceptional (15, 16), and very little documentation exists regarding the possibility of transmission through blood transfusion (17). The extraordinary infective capacity of C. burnetii (a single microorganism may produce infection (18)) undermines the hypothesis that HIV-infected subjects may be more susceptible to Coxiella infection. In our geographic region, most subjects infected by HIV are IVDUs, but our results show that intravenous drug use does not represent a risk for infection by C. burnetii although there have been suggestions to the contrary (4, 14). Finally, our results do not support the otherwise logical hypothesis that Coxiella infection in subjects co-infected with HIV may produce more frequent or intense clinical manifestations. As most C. burnetii infections are asymptomatic, it may be that clinically manifest cases coincide with a higher percentage of HIV infections. The number of subjects with Q fever in our series, who were also infected by HIV, coincided with the number of HIV-infected subjects in the general population of that age. We do not know whether, in a more advanced phase of HIV infection or other severe immunosuppression syndrome, infection by C. burnetii may be unusually severe. However, according to published findings the form of presentation of Q fever in HIV-infected subjects does not seem to differ from that occurring in non-HIV-infected subjects (4, 9–13). In our 3 known cases of Q fever in HIV infection, the clinical manifestations of Q fever did not differ from those observed in non-HIV-infected patients. According to the CDC classification systems, their HIV status was group II. Nonetheless, the number of cases of Q fever observed in HIV-infected subjects is still small and careful surveillance of these patients is needed.

ACKNOWLEDGEMENT

This study was supported by grant FIS 93/0593.

REFERENCES

1. Reimer LG. Q fever. Clin Microbiol Rev 6: 193–198, 1993.
2. Brouqui P, Dupont HT, Drancourt M, Berland Y, Etienne J, Leport C, Goldstein F, Massip P, Micoud M, Bertrand A, Raoult D. Chronic Q fever. Ninety-two cases from France, including 27 cases without endocarditis. Arch Intern Med 153: 642–648, 1993.
3. Paretsky D. The biology of Coxiella burnetii and the pathobiochemistry of Q fever and its endotoxicosis. Ann N Y Acad Sci 590: 416–421, 1990.
4. Raoult D, Levy PI, Dupont HT, Chicheportiche C, Tamalet C, Gastaut JA, Salducci J. Q fever and HIV infection. AIDS 7: 81–86, 1993.
5. Sanzo JM, García-Calabuig MA, Audicana A, Dehesa V. Q fever: prevalence of antibodies to Coxiella burnetii in the Basque country. Int J Epidemiol 22: 1183–1188, 1993.
6. Instituto Vasco de Estadística. Habitantes, movimiento natural y migraciones. Anuario Estadístico Vasco 1992. [In Spanish]
7. Situacion del SIDA en la CAV. 1984–1993. Plan de Prevención y Control del SIDA. Departamento de Sanidad del Gobierno Vasco. Vitoria, 1994.
8. Chamberland ME, Curran JW. Epidemiology and prevention of AIDS and HIV infection. In: Mandell GL, Douglas RG, Bennett JE, eds. Principles and practice of infectious diseases. 3rd edn. New York: Churchill Livingstone, 1029–1046, 1990.
9. Kanfer E, Farrag N, Price C, MacDonald D, Coleman J, Barret AJ. Q fever following bone marrow transplantation. Bone Marrow Transplant 3: 165–166, 1988.
10. Lev BI, Shachar A, Segev S, Weiss P, Rubinstein E. Quiescent Q fever endocarditis exacerbated by cardiac surgery and corticosteroid therapy. Arch Intern Med 148: 1531–1532, 1988.
11. Raoult D, Brouqui P, Marchou B, Gastaut JA. Acute and chronic Q fever in patients with cancer. Clin Infect Dis 14: 127–130, 1992.
12. Heard SR, Ronalds CJ, Hearth RB. Coxiella burnetii infection in immunocompromised hosts. J Infect 11: 15–18, 1985.
13. Bélec L, Grésenguet G, Ekala MT, Jacob A, Vohito MD, Cotigny S, Payan C. Coxiella burnetii infection among subjects infected with HIV type 1 in the Central African Republic. Eur J Clin Microbiol Infect Dis 12: 775–778, 1993.
14. Bélec L, Ekala M-T, Gilquin J. Coxiella burnetii infection among HIV-1 infected people living in Paris, France. AIDS 7: 1136–1137, 1993.
15. Tylewska-Wierzbanowska SK, Kruszewska D. Q fever – sexually transmitted infection? J Infect Dis 161: 368–369, 1990.
16. Mann JS, Douglas JG, Inglis JM, Leitch AG. Q fever: person to person transmission within a family. Thorax 41: 974–975, 1986.
17. Q fever transmitted by blood transfusion – United States [editorial]. Can Dis Wkly Rep 3: 210, 1977.
18. Ormsbee RA, Peacock M, Gerloff R, Tallent G, Wike D. Limits of rickettsial infectivity. Infect Immun 19: 239–245, 1978.

Submitted January 9, 1995; accepted April 3, 1995

Scand J Infect Dis 27: 347–350, 1995 ORIGINAL ARTICLE

Activation of Phagocytes by Helicobacter pylori Correlates with the Clinical Presentation of the Gastric Infection

HENRIK NIELSEN[1,2] and LEIF P. ANDERSEN[2]

From the Departments of [1]Clinical Microbiology and [2]Infectious Diseases, National University Hospital (Rigshospitalet), Copenhagen, Denmark

Only a minority of subjects with Helicobacter pylori infection develop clinical gastroduodenal disease. It is unclear whether host factors or bacterial virulence properties contribute to the pathogenic mechanisms. We have previously demonstrated a 25–35-kDa protein with phagocyte stimulatory activity in bacterial sonicates. Protein preparations were made from 15 H. pylori strains isolated from patients with duodenal ulcer, chronic active gastritis or superficial gastritis. Activation of neutrophil and monocyte chemotaxis and chemiluminescence was assessed with cells from healthy donors in comparison with N-f-methionyl-leucyl-phenylalanine and C5a anaphylatoxin. The potency of bacterial protein(s) for induction of monocyte chemiluminescence was significantly higher for strains from ulcer patients (1 ± 1 μg/ml induced ≥ twofold increase of control response) and chronic active gastritis (1 ± 1 μg/ml) compared with superficial gastritis (> 1,000 μg/ml, $p < 0.05$). Neutrophil activation was also significantly more potent with strains from duodenal ulcer disease. The chemotactic activity of bacterial preparations was not significantly different between the groups. We conclude that bacterial strains with pronounced activation of phagocytes are associated with the presence of clinical ulcer disease, supporting the existence of ulcerogenic strains.

H. Nielsen, MD, Department of Clinical Microbiology 7806, Rigshospitalet, 20 Tagensvej, DK-2200 Copenhagen N, Denmark

INTRODUCTION

The association of Helicobacter pylori with gastroduodenal disease was first shown a decade ago (1), and chronic gastric infection with H. pylori is now recognized as the major cause of ulcer disease and gastritis (2). Nevertheless, most subjects with mucosal H. pylori infection will never develop clinical overt ulcer disease (3), and it remains unclear whether this can be attributed to differing virulence properties of bacterial strains or to genetically determined host factors. The possibility that certain pathogenic features of H. pylori may be responsible for ulcer development has been studied with respect to the 120-kDa antigen associated with cytotoxic activity, and a significant association between mucosal IgA recognition of 120-kDa antigen and peptic ulceration was demonstrated (4). However, based on DNA fingerprinting studies, the existence of ulcerogenic strains has been questioned and instead host factors have been emphasized (5).

A characteristic feature of chronic antral gastritis is the abundant inflammatory response closely associated with H. pylori (6). Bacterial components appear to exhibit significant influence on proinflammatory features, including neutrophil adhesion (7) and chemotaxis (8), and microvascular dysfunction (9). We have previously reported neutrophil and monocyte activation by bacterial proteins which induce a chemotactic response and release of toxic oxygen radicals (10, 11), and these properties probably play a central role in the immunopathology associated with gastroduodenal H. pylori infection. A recent study demonstrated neutrophil activation more frequently in strains from ulcer patients compared with strains from chronic gastritis only (12). We have now studied the activation of purified neutrophils and monocytes by H. pylori protein preparations made from clinical strains isolated from patients with differing gastroduodenal pathology.

PATIENTS AND METHODS

Patients

We studied 15 randomly selected clinical isolates of H. pylori obtained from dyspeptic patients attending an outpatient dyspepsia clinic (median age 53 years, range 25–74), who were undergoing routine upper gastrointestinal endoscopy. Antral biopsy samples were taken at endoscopy for histopathology and culture. The presence or absence of active gastric or duodenal ulceration was recorded. Gastritis was classified using the criteria outlined by Morson & Dawson (13). Of the patients, 10 had chronic active gastritis and of these 6 also had duodenal ulceration. No patient had gastric ulceration. Five patients had a normal endoscopy and only very slight inflammation on histopathological examination (superficial gastritis).

Bacterial preparations

Mucosal biopsy cultures were done under microaerophilic conditions for 3–4 days and H. pylori was obtained in pure culture. All isolates were confirmed to be H. pylori by standard microbiological identification and a protein profile was performed on SDS-polyacrylamide gel electrophoresis. Further antigen assessment was done by immunoblotting. Protein sonicate preparations were produced in large quantities by subcultivation and after bacterial ultrasonic disintegration, as previously described (10).

Phagocyte activation

Neutrophils and monocytes were isolated from peripheral blood by metrizoate/polysucrose separation from healthy volunteer donors,

 ISSN 0036-5548

and used for the assessment of the potency of bacterial preparations in comparison with the standard stimuli N-formyl-methionyl-leucyl-phenylalanine (fMLP) and C5a anaphylatoxin (in zymosan-activated serum). The phagocyte stimulatory activity was assessed by chemotaxis and priming for chemiluminescence as described (10, 11). The sonicate of each strain was tested in the dose range 1–3,200 μg/ml in 4–6 different experiments with both seropositive and seronegative donors. Chemotactic activity was measured in duplicate, in modified Boyden chambers, with 10^{-5} M fMLP and C5a as standard stimuli. The chemotactic activity is expressed as the mean number of cells completely migrated through a micropore filter separating the cell suspension from the sonicate preparations, after subtracting the spontaneous migration towards the medium. After preincubation for 30 min in bacterial sonicate or medium, the oxidative burst responsiveness, reflecting release of toxic oxygen radicals, was measured in duplicate in a Beckman L 8,000 scintillation counter as lucigenin-enhanced chemiluminescence after stimulation with 10^{-5} M fMLP. The activity of bacterial sonicate preparations was assessed as the priming efficacy and expressed as the phagocyte peak response of cells preincubated in sonicate proteins as a percentage of the peak response of untreated cells.

Statistical analysis

Statistical analyses were performed using the Mann–Whitney test.

RESULTS

Using conventional microbiological techniques, the strains of H. pylori tested in the present study were indistinguishable from each other. Nevertheless, the stimulatory activity for neutrophil and monocyte release of toxic oxygen radicals was significantly different between the groups (Table I). In general, monocytes were more sensitive to the priming efficacy of bacterial sonicate proteins and, from both the duodenal ulcer strains and the chronic active gastritis strains, a very low concentration of 1 μg/ml was sufficient to induce a ≥twofold increase in cell function. For neutrophils a higher concentration was required, but the group differences between duodenal ulcer strains and controls were still statistically significant (Table I and Fig. 1). The differences observed could not be linked to the previously described ulcerogenicity of 120-kDa protein-positive strains, since all but one of our isolates were positive for this characteristic protein on immunoblotting examinations (data not shown).

In contrast, the chemotactic activity of the bacterial preparations was similarly expressed in preparations from the three groups, with no difference between strains from gastritis patients and strains from duodenal ulcer patients (Table I and Fig. 2).

Table I. *Potency of bacterial sonicate proteins from clinical isolates of Helicobacter pylori for activation of human neutrophils and monocytes*

	Duodenal ulcer ($n = 6$)	Chronic active gastritis ($n = 4$)	Superficial gastritis ($n = 5$)
Chemotaxis			
Neutrophils	>1,000	>1,000	>1,000
Monocytes	365 ± 44	819 ± 112	405 ± 82
Chemiluminescence			
Neutrophils	50 ± 12[a]	183 ± 43	230 ± 78
Monocytes	1 ± 1[a]	1 ± 1[a]	>1,000

Phagocytes were tested for chemotaxis in modified Boyden chambers and for chemiluminescence in a scintillation counter. Potency for chemotaxis is expressed as mean ± SEM concentration of sonicate (μg/ml) with ≥ 50% of chemotaxis towards fMLP/C5a standard stimuli (monocytes) and ≥33% of chemotaxis towards fMLP/C5a standard stimuli (neutrophils). Potency for chemiluminescence is expressed as mean ± SEM concentration of sonicate (μg/ml) with ≥twofold priming activity upon subsequent fMLP-induced lucigenin-enhanced chemiluminescence response.
[a] $p < 0.05$.

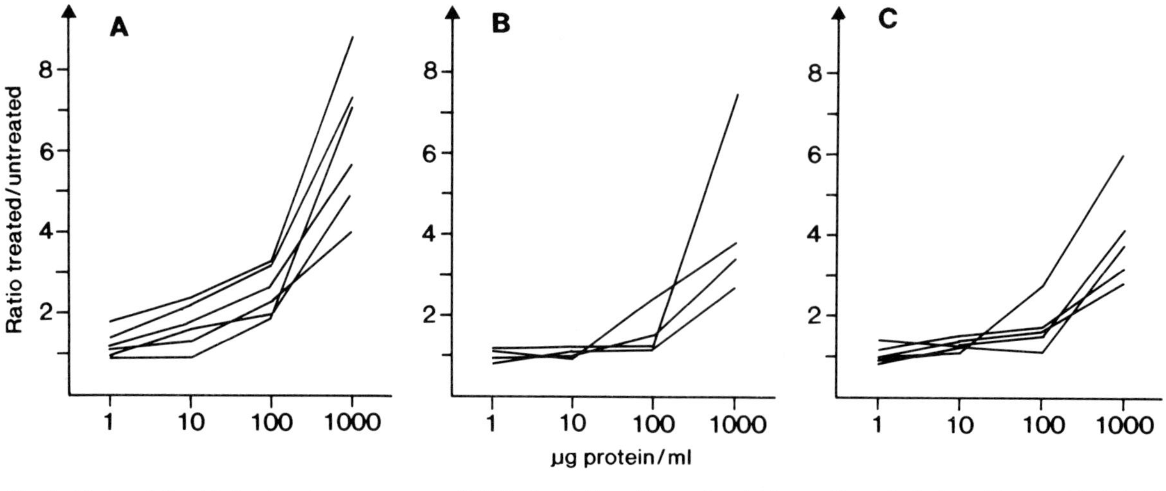

Fig. 1. Neutrophil oxidative burst response upon fMLP stimulation after preincubation with sonicate from H. pylori isolated from patients with (A) duodenal ulcer, (B) chronic active gastritis, or (C) superficial gastritis. Results are shown individually for each strain as the ratio of neutrophil response treated/untreated (i.e. after preincubation in sonicate/after preincubination in medium). Each strain was examined with 4–6 different healthy neutrophil donors, and the results expressed as the mean value for each concentration of sonicate.

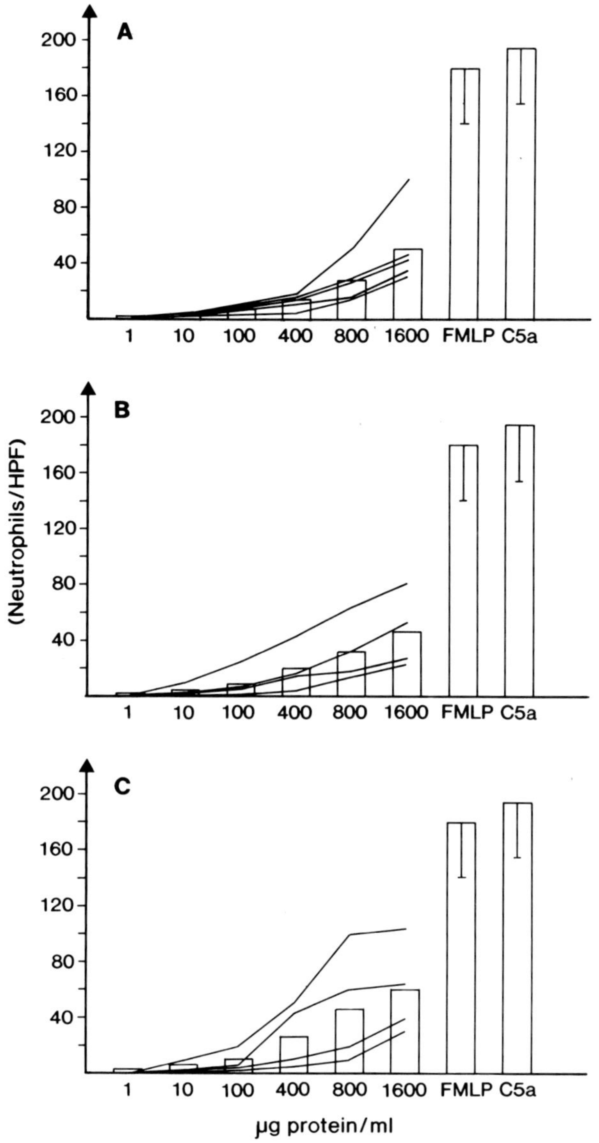

Fig. 2. Neutrophil chemotactic migration towards sonicate of H. pylori isolated from patients with (A) duodenal ulcer, (B) chronic active gastritis, or (C) superficial gastritis. Results are shown individually for each strain (and as mean) as number of neutrophils migrating per high power field. Each strain was examined with 4–6 different healthy neutrophil donors, and the results expressed as the mean value for each concentration of sonicate. The neutrophil chemotactic responsiveness to fMLP and C5a is shown for comparison.

DISCUSSION

The present findings extend our previous observations and confirm that phagocyte activation is a general feature of H. pylori. The possible association of the diverse clinical spectrum of H. pylori infection with bacterial virulence characteristics was observed to include neutrophil and monocyte stimulation for the release of detrimental oxygen radicals, whereas the chemotactic properties of the bacteria had no relation to the origin of the strains. In previous reports we have demonstrated this activity to reflect mainly a 25–35-kDa protein (10, 11) and we suggest that differing bacterial expression of this product could explain the observed differences. The study of Crabtree et al. (4) showed an association between clinical presentation and strains positive for 120-kDa protein, which could not, however, explain our results, since all strains were positive for this protein except for one strain from a control patient. Moreover, our preliminary results suggested that purified 120-kDa protein had no activity for neutrophil and monocyte stimulation (14). Therefore, we conclude that the differences in mucosal inflammation and epithelial damage between 120-kDa positive and negative strains is probably not explained by differences in neutrophil attraction.

In only one other report has the activation of neutrophil oxidative burst response been related to the clinical presentation of H. pylori infection (12), and a significantly higher percentage of strains from ulcer patients was capable of direct neutrophil stimulation compared with strains from active chronic gastritis only. A comparison with our results is difficult since the assay systems are quite different, and in the study of Rautelin et al. (12) no activation of bacterial sonicate could be observed. Most other studies have examined products released into the supernatant or on the bacterial surface (4, 11, 15). In contrast to oxidative burst responses, we observed no difference in chemoattractant activity between groups, which agrees with a previous report examining a low molecular weight soluble factor from H. pylori (15). These observations most probably reflect the fact that it is not the quantity of phagocytes in the mucosa, but their activation for release of toxic substances, which is important. The diverse clinical presentations of the infection might reflect a difference in virulence between strains, as demonstrated in this study.

ACKNOWLEDGEMENTS

We thank L. Elsborg, MD, DMSc for performing the endoscopies and S. Holck, MD, for the histopathological assessments. The expert technical assistance of Birgitte Sander Nielsen and Bente Larsen is appreciated. This study was supported by the Danish Medical Research Council (grant No. S12-9752).

REFERENCES

1. Marshall BJ, Warren JR. Unidentified curved bacilli in the stomach of patients with gastritis and peptic ulceration. Lancet 1: 1311–1315, 1984.
2. Graham DY. Treatment of peptic ulcers caused by Helicobacter pylori. N Engl J Med 328: 349–350, 1993.
3. Cullen DJE, Collins BJ, Christiansen KJ, Epis J, Warren JR, Cullun KJ. Long term risk of peptic ulcer disease in people with Helicobacter pylori infection – a community based study [abstract]. Gut 34: S72, 1993.
4. Crabtree JE, Taylor JD, Wyatt JI, Heatley RV, Shallcross TM, Tompkins DS, Rathbone BJ. Mucosal lgA recognition of Helicobacter pylori 120 kDa protein, peptic ulceration, and gastric pathology. Lancet 338: 332–335, 1991.

5. Lee A. H. Pylori-initiated ulcerogenesis: look to the host. Lancet 341: 280–281, 1993.
6. Andersen LP, Holck S, Povlsen CO, Elsborg L, Justesen T. Campylobacter pyloridis in peptic ulcer disease. I. Gastric and duodenal infection caused by C. pyloridis: histopathologic and microbiologic findings. Scand J Gastroenterol 22: 219–224, 1987.
7. Yoshida N, Granger DN, Evans DJ, Evans DG, Graham DY, Anderson DC, Wolf RE, Kvietys PR. Mechanisms involved in Helicobacter pylori-induced inflammation. Gastroenterology 105: 1431–1440, 1993.
8. Mai UEH, Perez-Perez GI, Allen JB, Wahl SM, Blaser MJ, Smith PD. Surface proteins from Helicobacter pylori exhibit chemotactic activity for human leukocytes and are present in gastric mucosa. J Exp Med 175: 517–525, 1992.
9. Kurose I, Granger DN, Evans DJ, Evans DG, Graham DY, Miyasaka M, Anderson DC, Wolf RE, Cepinskas G, Kvietys PR. Helicobacter pylori-induced microvascular protein leakage in rats: role of neutrophils, mast cells, and platelets. Gastroenterology 107: 70–79, 1994.
10. Nielsen H, Andersen LP. Chemotactic activity of Helicobacter pylori sonicate for human polymorphonuclear leucocytes and monocytes. Gut 33: 738–742, 1992.
11. Nielsen H, Andersen LP. Activation of human phagocyte oxidative metabolism by Helicobacter pylori. Gastroenterology 103: 1747–1753, 1992.
12. Rautelin H, Blomberg B, Fredlund H, Järnerot G, Danielsson D. Incidence of Helicobacter pylori strains activating neutrophils in patients with peptic ulcer disease. Gut 34: 599–603, 1993.
13. Morson BC, Dawson IMP. Gastrointestinal pathology. 2nd edn. Oxford: Blackwell Scientific Publications, 97–101, 1979.
14. Nielsen H, Andersen LP. Cellular immunity to Helicobacter pylori. In: Goodwin CS, Worsley BW, eds. Helicobacter pylori. Biology and Clinical Practice. Boca Raton: CRC Press, 257–271, 1993.
15. Craig PM, Territo MC, Karnes WE, Walsh JH. Helicobacter pylori secretes a chemotactic factor for monocytes and neutrophils. Gut 33: 1020–1023, 1992.

Submitted June 29, 1994; accepted March 31, 1995

Scand J Infect Dis 27: 351–355, 1995

ORIGINAL ARTICLE

Persistent Reduction in Lung Function after Pneumocystis Carinii Pneumonia in AIDS Patients

SUZANNE NELSING[1], BIRGITTE NYBO JENSEN[1] and VIBEKE BACKER[2]

From the Department of [1]Infectious Diseases, Rigshospitalet and the Department of [2]Pulmonary Medicine, Bispebjerg Hospital, Copenhagen, Denmark

By means of serial lung function tests we examined the changes in lung function and possible pulmonary long-term sequelae in AIDS patients with a primary episode of Pneumocystis carinii pneumonia (PCP). A total of 19 patients had lung function tests performed prospectively from the time of PCP diagnosis, at 7 days, 14 days, 1, 2, 3, 4½, 6 and 9 months after PCP. Forced vital capacity (FVC) and forced expiratory volume in 1 second (FEV1) were both reduced to a median of 61% of predicted at PCP diagnosis, and were normalized within 1 month and 1 week respectively. The median pulmonary diffusing capacity for carbon monoxide (DLCO) was severely reduced to 43% of predicted during the acute infection. Although DLCO improved significantly during the first 2 months, it remained reduced at a median DLCO of 64% of predicted 9 months after PCP. We conclude that despite a general improvement in lung function during the first 2 months following the PCP diagnosis, there was a persistent reduction in DLCO up to 9 months following PCP. The pathological mechanisms causing this reduction remain to be established.

S. Nelsing, MD, Department of Infectious Diseases, Hvidovre University Hospital, Kettegaard Allé 30, DK-2650 Hvidovre, Denmark

INTRODUCTION

Pneumocystis carinii pneumonia (PCP) is the main pulmonary infection in HIV-positive patients and is the most frequent AIDS-defining diagnosis (1–3). A morphologically verified diagnosis is obtained by means of induced sputum or fiberoptic bronchoscopy (4, 5), but several non-invasive diagnostic methods, such as chest X-ray, gallium scan and lung function test, can contribute to the diagnosis (6, 7). The pulmonary diffusing capacity for carbon monoxide (DLCO) decreases severely during acute PCP and is a very sensitive, although not specific predictor for PCP (6). Reduced values of forced vital capacity (FVC) and forced expiratory volume in one second (FEV1) have also been reported (6–9).

The reduction in lung function during acute PCP in AIDS patients is well described, but little is known about the changes in lung function and possible long-term pulmonary sequelae following PCP. To examine this issue, we conducted a 9 month follow-up study with serial lung function tests in AIDS patients with a primary episode of PCP.

MATERIALS AND METHODS

Patients

HIV-positive patients with a primary episode of morphologically verified PCP were asked to participate in the study. The study was approved by the Ethical Committee of Copenhagen, and informed consent was obtained from all participating patients. Patients were excluded if a history of drug abuse or chronic lung disease was obtained. Out of 33 consecutively eligible patients, 23 (70%) accepted. Four patients withdrew their consent and the final study population consisted of 19 patients (16 men and 3 women).

The median age (range) was 41 years (23–57). Median CD4 count at the time of enrolment was 44×10^6/L (5–260). Risk factors for HIV infection were heterosexual contacts ($n = 3$), blood transfusion ($n = 1$) and homosexual contacts ($n = 16$). Seven patients were smokers, defined as patients who smoked any amount of tobacco. One patient who stopped smoking 6 weeks before PCP was included as a smoker.

The initial chest X-ray obtained at the diagnosis was normal in six patients, showed diffuse interstitial infiltration in 10 patients, and lobar infiltration in 3 patients.

Nonparticipants were similar to participants with regard to age (36 years, 24–55) and immunological status (CD4-count 36×10^6/L, range 2–204). Two non-participants died within 2 months of the PCP diagnosis and one nonparticipant received temporary mechanical ventilation but otherwise there were no obvious differences in the severity of the acute PCP between participants and nonparticipants.

Lung function test and clinical data

It was planned that nine lung function tests, consisting of DLCO, single breath alveolar volume (Va), FVC and FEV_1, should be prospectively performed, i.e. at the time of the diagnosis (±3 days), 7 days, 14 days and 1, 2, 3, 4½, 6 and 9 months after PCP.

FVC and FEV1 were measured by a dry bellows spirometer (Vitalograph®). The best of 2 technically acceptable measurements was used for analysis. DLCO was measured by the single breath helium dilution method (PK Morgan Transfer Model 101). The transfer factor (KCO) was derived from DLCO divided by Va. The mean of 2 acceptable measurements was calculated and used for analysis. The measurements were considered acceptable if they were technically correct and if the KCO values differed less than 10% from each other. DLCO was corrected for hemoglobin concentration and body temperature (10). All values were adjusted to BTPS (body temperature pressure saturated).

At each visit the patients were questioned about intercurrent diseases and about the presence of cough, dyspnoea or fever.

Diagnosis and treatment of PCP

All patients had morphologically verified PCP, by either induced sputum or by fiberoptic bronchoscopy with bronchoalveolar lavage (BAL) and brush biopsy. The material was stained with May–Grünwald–Giemsa stain and Gomori silver stain for identification of the Pneumocystis carinii organisms. None of the patients were diagnosed as having co-infections.

PCP was treated with sulfametoxazole-trimethoprim (SMX-TMP) 100/20 mg/kg daily in 14–25 days in 18 patients. One patient was treated with SMX-TMP for 10 days and subsequently with dapsone and trimethoprim due to adverse reactions. A total of 11 patients, with arterial $PaO_2 < 9.0$ kPa or $PaCO_2 < 4.0$ Kpa at diagnosis, received adjunctive therapy with corticosteroid equivalent to 50–160 mg prednisone daily for 5–18 days. One patient received 50 mg prednisone daily for 5 days due to a drug eruption attributed to SMX-TMP.

Antiviral treatment and PCP prophylaxis

Of the patients, 16 received zidovudine (300–1200 mg/day) during the entire study period, and one patient received it during the last 3 months of the study period only. Two patients did not receive antiviral treatment. One patient received primary PCP prophylaxis with aerosolized pentamidine (AP). All patients received secondary prophylaxis with AP, 60 mg/14 days ($n = 5$) or SMX-TMP 800/160 mg daily ($n = 14$).

Statistics

All results are expressed as median (range) as a percentage of predicted (% predicted) normal values according to age, sex and height (10). FVC, FEV_1, DLCO or KCO below 80% of predicted normal value was considered abnormal. The Friedman test was employed for comparison of intraindividual changes in lung function over time. The Mann–Whitney test was used for comparison between groups. P values < 0.05 were considered significant.

RESULTS

Of 171 scheduled lung function tests, 144 (84%) were performed. Five patients were not able to perform the initial lung function test due to severe dyspnoea. Three patients were excluded after 41/2 months' follow-up, as they were unable to perform the tests due to severe diseases (toxoplasmosis cerebri, $n = 2$, or wasting syndrome, $n = 1$).

FVC, FEV_1 and FEV_1/FVC ratio

FVC and FEV1 were both reduced in the acute stage of PCP (day 0). FEV1 normalized within 1 week after the diagnosis, whereas FVC reached normal predicted values within 1 month (Table I). Smokers had a higher median FVC and FEV_1 one month after PCP ($p < 0.05$) (data not shown).

The FEV_1/FVC ratio was stable during the study period with a tendency towards a restrictive pattern (FEV_1/FVC > 80%). There was no significant difference in FEV_1/FVC ratio between smokers and non-smokers.

DLCO and KCO

DCLO was severely reduced during the acute phase of PCP to a median value of 43% predicted (Table I). There was a significant improvement in DLCO during the first 2 months after PCP ($p < 0, 001$). Following this improvement DLCO remained moderately reduced through the next 7 months and the median DLCO 9 months following PCP was 64% predicted (Table I). Smokers generally had lower values of DLCO than nonsmokers and the relative improvement of

Table I. *Median values of FVC, FEV_1, FVC/FEV_1, DLCO and KCO at different time points after Pneumocystis carinii pneumonia in Danish AIDS patients*

	Time after PCP diagnosis								
	Day 0 (± 3 days)	Day 7	Day 14	1 month	2 months	3 months	4½ months	6 months	9 months
Number	15[a]	16	16	18[a]	16	18	18[a]	14	13
FVC									
%	61	74	79	83	89	92	91	92	97
Range	28–101	49–106	67–97	64–102	52–105	56–112	39–113	69–111	79–109
FEV_1									
%	61	82	89	86	96	95	96	97	100
Range	31–100	49–111	71–106	70–107	57–108	55–117	44–118	73–114	77–117
FEV_1/FVC									
%	80	85	89	87	87	84	86	82	81
Range	67–92	58–94	68–98	72–97	68–98	68–97	60–100	70–98	69–100
DLCO									
%	43	53	60	59	67	71	67	74	64
Range	24–59	38–68	31–76	39–89	37–99	37–109	34–96	60–88	50–96
KCO									
%	64	65	71	67	78	78	72	79	72
Range	36–91	45–127	47–118	53–133	54–128	52–148	51–97	61–151	52–102

[a] One patient performed FVC and FEV_1 only.

FVC = forced vital capacity; FEV_1 = forced expiratory volume at 1 seccond; DLCO = pulmonary diffusing capacity for carbon monoxide; KCO = transfer factor. The values of FVC, FEV_1, DLCO and KCO are expressed as median (range) % of predicted normal values

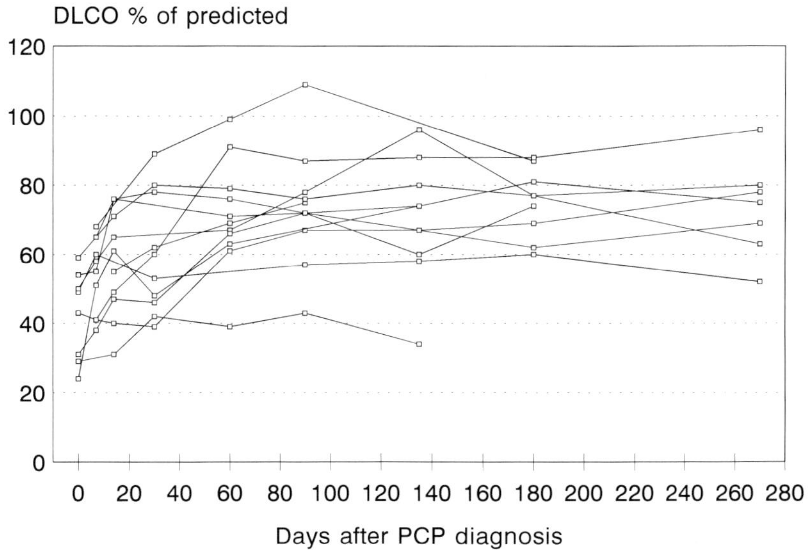

Fig. 1. Median values of pulmonary diffusing capacity for carbon monoxide (DLCO) (% of predicted normal values) in 12 non-smoking Danish AIDS patients, according to time after diagnosis of PCP.

median DLCO 9 months post PCP was less than in non-smokers (16.5 vs. 29%, data not shown). However, the difference in DLCO between smokers and nonsmokers was only significant ($p < 0.05$) at 3 months after PCP. The individual results of DLCO for nonsmokers and smokers are illustrated in Figs. 1 and 2. The lower curve in Fig. 1 presents a patient with severe weight loss who died a few months after the last lung function test. The lower curve in Fig. 2 presents a patient with severe cerebral toxoplasmosis.

The median KCO values were also reduced during the entire study period, although less markedly than DLCO values (Table I).

Corticosteroid treatment

Adjunctive corticosteroid therapy did not influence DLCO according to analysis of either the total study population or when data from smokers and nonsmokers were analysed separately.

Pulmonary complications during the study period

One patient had pneumonia diagnosed and treated by his general physician 2 weeks following the diagnosis of PCP. One patient had penicillin treatment for an episode of pneumococcal pneumonia. Secondary PCP was not diagnosed in any patient during the study period.

DISCUSSION

This prospective study describes the serial changes in lung function and long-term pulmonary sequelae following PCP.

We found a slightly longer time for restitution of FVC compared to FEV_1 and a tendency towards a restrictive

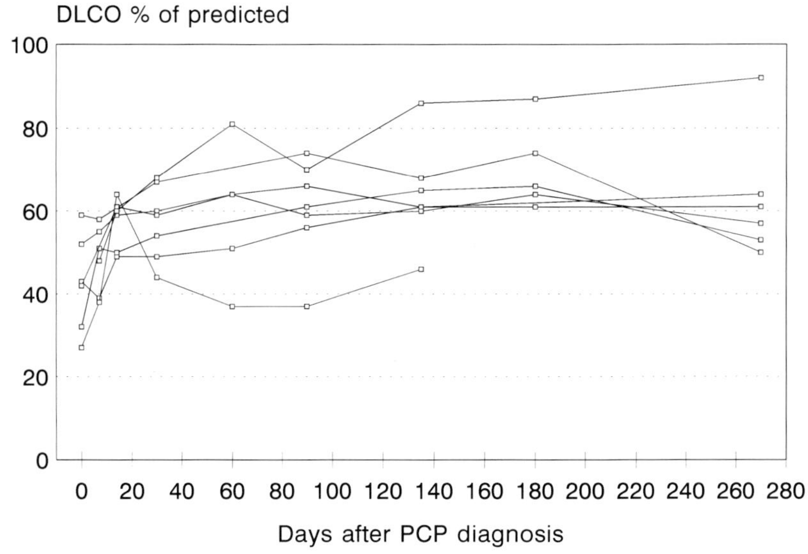

Fig. 2. Median values of DLCO (% of predicted normal values) in 7 smoking Danish AIDS patients, according to time after diagnosis of PCP.

pattern which is consistent with the alveolar location of PCP.

The persistent reduction in DLCO confirms a study by Mitchell et al., who found reduced values of DLCO up to 6 months after PCP (11). The normalization of FVC as opposed to DLCO indicates that the persistent reduction in DLCO is caused by affection of the alveolar wall, rather than by volume restriction. This is further supported by the reduced values of KCO. Our results differ from the experience with PCP in HIV-negative immunosuppressed patients, who recover to normal or near-normal values of DLCO (12, 13). This could indicate that the Pneumocystis carinii organisms interact differently with the HIV-infected host compared to a HIV-negative host. This would be consistent with the more insidious clinical course (14, 15) and atypical pathologic manifestations (15, 16) of PCP in AIDS patients. The pathogenesis of these differences however, is not known. Interstitial fibrosis, which is often diagnosed in acute PCP (15–17), would contribute to the reduced diffusing capacity. Likewise, persistence of PC organisms could adversely affect lung function, but even though PC organisms can be found in some AIDS patients months after treatment, most long term survivors are cured from PC infection during treatment (9, 17).

Previous studies indicate that PCP-independent factors affect the diffusing capacity as well. Reduced values of DLCO have been found in several groups of HIV-positive patients without PCP, i.e. in patients with persistent generalized lymphadenopathy, AIDS-related complex (ARC), or non-pulmonary Kaposi sarcoma (KS), and in AIDS patients without KS or pulmonary infection (11, 18). The nature of these pulmonary processes is unknown. HIV has been isolated from alveolar macrophages, and even though no direct correlation has been found between the presence of HIV in BAL cells and DLCO values (19), HIV might affect the diffusing capacity by causing a local inflammatory response in the lungs. Lymphocytic alveolitis, mainly comprised of CD8+ T-lymphocytes, has been found to occur very frequently in HIV-positive patients both with and without PCP (20–22), and the presence of lymphocytic alveolitis seems to be correlated to respiratory symptoms and decreased DLCO (22). These local immune responses in the lungs of HIV-positive patients, might also impair the ability of the patient to recover from PCP, causing further and persistent reduction in DLCO values.

To understand the pathological processes better, long term follow-up studies with serial pulmonary biopsies will be necessary. With the present study design we were not able to compare the lung function after recovery from PCP with the initial lung function prior to the diagnosis. Although not in the study design, seven of our patients had lung function tests performed 1–2 months prior to the diagnosis, i.e. at a time when the decline in DLCO is likely to have begun (23). Even so, only 2 of 7 patients reached their initial diffusing capacity after recovery. DLCO (% predicted) for the remaining 5 patients was 14–25% lower than the initial values, which further supports our results. In conclusion, we found that FEV_1 and FVC normalized within 1 month of the PCP diagnosis. Despite an initial improvement during the first 2 months, there was a persistent reduction in DLCO up to 9 months following PCP. The pathological mechanisms causing this reduction remain to be established.

REFERENCES

1. Murray JF, Garay SM, Hopewell PC, Mills J, Snider GL, Stover DE. Pulmonary complications of the Acquired Immunodeficiency Syndrome: an update. Am Rev Respir Dis 135: 504–509, 1987.
2. Stover D, White D, Romano P, Gellene RA, Robeson WA. Spectrum of pulmonary diseases associated with the Acquired Immune deficiency Syndrome. Am J Med 78: 429–437, 1985.
3. Jensen BN, Gerstoft J, Højlyng N, Backer V, Paaske M, Gomme G, Skinhøj P. Pulmonary pathogens in HIV-infected patients. Scand J Infect Dis 22: 413–420, 1990.
4. Kovacs JA, Ng VL, Masur H, Leoung G, Hadley WK, Evans G, Lane HC, Ognibene FP, Shelhamer J, Parrillo JE, Gill VJ. Diagnosis of Pneumocystis carinii pneumonia: improved detection in sputum with use of monoclonal antibodies. N Engl J Med 318: 589–593, 1988.
5. Chopra SK, Mohsenifar Z. Fiberoptic bronchoscopy in diagnosis of opportunistic lung infections. West J Med 131: 4–7, 1979.
6. Millar AB, Mitchel DM. Non-invasive investigation of pulmonary disease in patients positive for the human immunodeficiency virus. Thorax 45: 57–61, 1990.
7. O'Brian RF. In search of shortcuts: definitive and indirect tests in the diagnosis of Pneumocystis carinii pneumonia in AIDS. Am Rev Respir Dis 6: 1324–1327, 1989.
8. Stover DE, Meduri GU. Pulmonary function tests. Clin Chest Med 9: 473–479, 1988.
9. Coleman DL, Dodek PM, Golden JA, Luce JM, Golden E, Gold WM, Murray JF. Correlation between serial pulmonary function tests and fiberoptic bronchoscopy in patients with Pneumocystis carinii pneumonia and the Acquired Immune Deficiency Syndrome. Am Rev Respir Dis 129: 491–493, 1984.
10. Cotes JS. Lung Function, 4th edn. Oxford: Blackwell, 1979.
11. Mitchell DM, Fleming J, Pinching AJ, Harris JRW, Moss FM, Veale D, Shaw RJ. Pulmonary function in Human Immunodeficiency Virus infection. Am Rev Respir Dis 146: 745–751, 1992.
12. Sanyal SK, Mariencheck WC, Hughes WT, Parvey LS, Tsiatis AA, Mackert PW. Course of pulmonary dysfunction in children surviving Pneumocystis carinii pneumonitis. Am Rev Respir Dis 124: 161–166, 1981.
13. Suffredini AF, Owens GR, Tobin MJ, Slasky BS, Peel RL, Costa F. Long-term prognosis of survivors of Pneumocystis carinii pneumonia. Chest 89: 229–233, 1986.
14. Kovacs JA, Hiemenz JW, Macher AM, Stover D, Murray HW, Shelhamer J, Lane HC, Urmacher C, Honig C, Longo DL, Parker MM, Natanson C, Parrillo JE, Fauci AS, Pizzo PA, Masur H. Pneumocystis carinii pneumonia: a comparison between patients with the Acquired Immunodeficiency Syndrome and patients with other immunodeficiencies. Ann Intern Med 100: 663–671, 1984.
15. Gal AA, Kos MN, Strigle S, Angritt CP. Pneumocystis carinii infection in the Acquired Immune Deficiency Syndrome. Semin Diagn Pathol 6: 287–299, 1989.

16. Travis WD, Pittaluga S, Lipschik GY, Ognibene FP, Suffredini AF, Masur H, Feuerstein I, Kovacs J, Pass HI, Condron KS, Shelhamer JH. Atypical pathologic manifestations of pneumocystis carinii pneumonia in the Acquired Immune Deficiency Syndrome. Am J Surg Pathol 14: 615–625, 1990.
17. Saldana MJ, Mones JM, Martinez GR. The pathology of treated Pneumocystis carinii pneumonia. Semin Diagn Pathol 6: 300–312, 1989.
18. Camus F, de Picciotto C, Gerbe J, Matheron S, Perronne C, Bouvet E. Pulmonary function tests in HIV-infected patients. AIDS 7: 1075–1079, 1993.
19. Clarke JR, Fleming J, Donegan K, Moss FM, Nieman R, Williamson JD, Mitchell DM. Effect of HIV-1 and cytomegalovirus in bronchoalveolar lavage cells on the transfer factor for lung carbon monoxide in AIDS patients. AIDS 5: 1333–1338, 1991.
20. Jensen BN, Lisse IM, Gerstoft J, Borgeskov S, Skinhøj P. Cellular profiles in bronchoalveolar lavage fluid of HIV-infected patients with pulmonary symptoms: relation to diagnosis and prognosis. AIDS 5: 527–533, 1991.
21. Ognibene FP, Masur H, Rogers P, Travis WD, Suffredini AF, Feuerstein I, Gill VJ, Baird BF, Carrasquillo JA, Parrillo JE, Lane HC, Shelhamer JH. Nonspecific interstitial pneumonitis without evidence of Pneumocystis carinii in asymptomatic patients infected with Human Immunodeficiency Virus (HIV). Ann Intern Med 109: 874–879, 1988.
22. Guillon J, Autran B, Denis M, Fouret P, Plata F, Mayaud CM, Akoun GM. Human Immunodeficiency Virus-related lymphocytic alveolitis. Chest 94: 1264–1270, 1988.
23. Mitchell DM, Fleming J, Harris JRW, Shaw RJ. Serial pulmonary function tests in the diagnosis of P. carinii pneumonia. Eur Respir J 6: 823–827, 1993.

Submitted January 13, 1995; accepted April 16, 1995

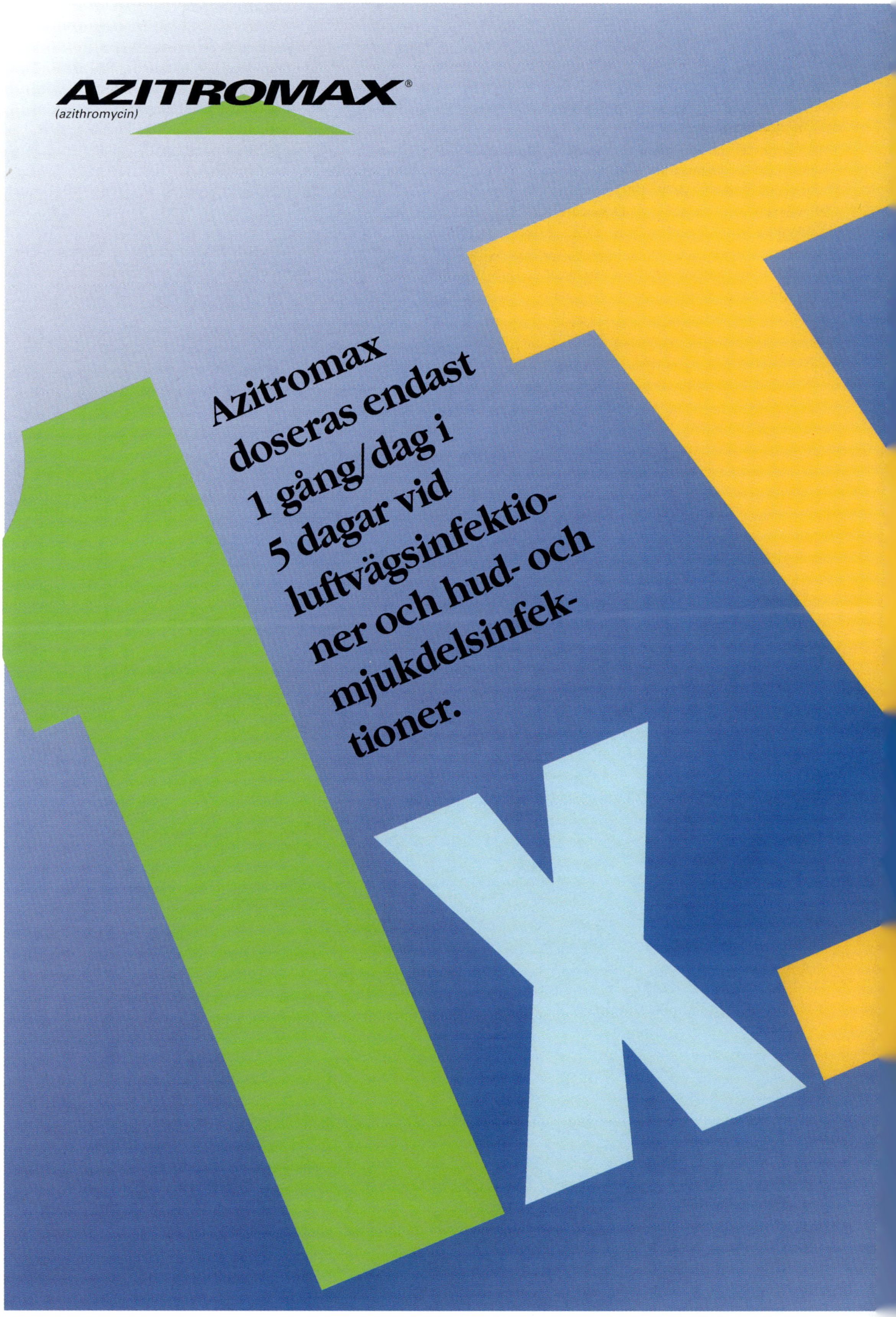
AZITROMAX®
(azithromycin)
Azitromax doseras endast 1 gång/dag i 5 dagar vid luftvägsinfektioner och hud- och mjukdelsinfektioner.
1x.

Scand J Infect Dis 27: 358–362, 1995

ORIGINAL ARTICLE

Rapid Simple and Nested Polymerase Chain Reaction for the Diagnosis of Pneumocystis carinii pneumonia

FRANÇOISE MOONENS[1], CORINNE LIESNARD[1], FRANÇOISE BRANCART[1], JEAN PAUL VAN VOOREN[2] and ELISABETH SERRUYS[1]

From the [1]Service de Microbiologie and the [2]Unite de Traitement des Immunodeficiences, Université Libre de Bruxelles, Hôpital Erasme, Brussels, Belgium

We have developed a rapid and easy extraction procedure for polymerase chain reaction (PCR) protocols. Using this simplified step, we evaluated the sensitivity and the specificity of a simple PCR using the primers of Wakefield et al, and of a nested PCR, using new internal primers selected by us, in a total of 89 bronchoalveolar lavage (BAL) fluid samples from 43 immunosuppressed patients. In 13 patients, Pneumocystis carinii pneumonia (PCP) was diagnosed by immunofluorescent antibody (IFA) staining performed on BAL cells cytospun on microscope slides. In seven of these patients we attempted to estimate the post-treatment persistence of P. carinii in BAL, by PCR. After a rapid 2-h extraction procedure, simple and nested PCR were positive in all cases of PCP. Simple and nested PCR both had a 100% sensitivity and a 98 and 84% specificity respectively, compared to IFA. After completion of treatment, BAL liquids from asymptomatic patients were no longer positive by both PCR techniques, whereas the BAL fluid of a patient who was still symptomatic was positive by simple and nested PCR. In follow-up BAL fluids of patients with proven PCP, persistence of P. carinii was detected for a longer period by nested PCR than by simple PCR. Simple PCR is a very rapid and sensitive assay for the diagnosis of PCP in BAL fluid and gives clear-cut results in the case of doubtful IFA staining results. Nested PCR seems to improve the sensitivity of the detection of P. carinii in BAL fluid, but the clinical relevance of a positive result remains to be investigated.

C. Liesnard, MD, Laboratory of Virology, Hôpital Erasme, Route de Lennik 808, B-1070 Brussels, Belgium

INTRODUCTION

Pneumocystis carinii pneumonia (PCP) is becoming more frequent because of the increasing number of immunocompromised patients susceptible to this opportunistic pathogen (1). The diagnosis of PCP has long relied only on direct examination of respiratory specimens, as culture of the organism is impossible. The sensitivity of direct examination has been improved by the introduction of immunofluorescent antibody staining techniques. Nevertheless, direct examination remains more difficult to perform in patients receiving chemoprophylaxis, such as HIV-infected patients with less than 200 CD_4 cells/µl, because P. carinii cysts are then more rarely visualized in clusters (2, 3). Recently, polymerase chain reaction (PCR) techniques have successfully been used to detect the presence of P. carinii in bronchoalveolar lavage (BAL) liquids and in induced sputum samples (4–10). However the protocols described are not convenient for a routine diagnosis. Extraction procedures are time-consuming and subject to contamination or loss of material (4, 6, 7). Post-PCR detection methods such as southern blot, dot blot and enzyme-linked immunosorbent assay add multiple steps and much time to the technique (4, 6, 10). We tested a rapid extraction step, based on a simple lysis of P. carinii organisms. We developed a nested PCR, amplifying a sequence included into the DNA sequence described by Sinclair et al. (11), and corresponding to a gene sequence of the large subunit of the mitochondrial ribosomal RNA of P. carinii. The performances of simple PCR, using the primers pAZ 102-E and pAZ 102-H (4), and nested PCR, developed by us with a simple identification of PCR products by agarose gel electrophoresis, were evaluated in comparison with IFA staining on BAL fluids of immunosuppressed patients. Finally the persistence of P. carinii, after a treated episode of PCP, was determined by simple and nested PCR in follow-up BAL samples.

MATERIALS AND METHODS

Patient population

A total of 89 BAL fluid samples were obtained from 43 immunocompromised patients. The latter included 14 HIV-infected patients, 24 organ transplant patients (13 heart–lung recipients, one liver recipient, 6 heart recipients, 2 kidney recipients and 2 lung recipients), and 5 patients undergoing long-term therapy with high doses of corticosteroids. All HIV-positive patients had <200 CD_4 cells/µl of blood and received anti-P. carinii prophylaxis consisting of pyrimethamine-sulfadoxine once a week or dapsone 50 mg/day. All BALs were performed either for follow-up of lung graft tolerance or for diagnosis or follow-up of a clinical episode of pneumonia.

A PCP was suspected in immunosuppressed patients presenting with acute respiratory illness, characterized by progressive dyspnea, cough and fever, and possibly accompanied by a diffuse interstitial infiltrate on chest X-ray, reduced PaO_2 and elevated LDH. Episodes of such acute respiratory illness were diagnosed as PCP when P. carinii cysts were demonstrated on cytospin slides of BAL samples. Patients with PCP were treated intravenously or orally for 3 weeks with high doses of trimethoprim-sulfamethoxazole, dapsone-trimethoprim or by aerosolized pentamidine. If cysts were not detected on direct examination, the patient was not considered to be infected by P. carinii, and did not receive any anti-P. carinii therapy. All BAL samples were processed for cytology and for detection of bacterial, mycobacterial, fungal and viral pathogens, using direct examinations and cultures. An alternative diagnosis was established in all patients with a clinical episode of pneumonia not attributable to P. carinii.

Immunofluorescent antibody staining for P. carinii

Cytospin slides were prepared with 2–3 drops of BAL liquid (about 30 cells/1000 × magnification field) centrifuged for 5 min at 30 g. All BAL fluids were examined on cytospin slides after fixation with acetone–ethanol 1/1, followed by direct immunofluorescent staining using a mixture of three monoclonal antibodies directed against cyst wall antigens (Cellabs Diagnostics, Brookvale, Australia).

Rapid DNA extraction procedure

BAL samples of 10 ml were centrifuged for 5 min, at 30 g. Pellets were kept frozen until processed for extraction and PCR. BAL liquid pellets of volume 200 µl were thawed and resuspended in an equal volume of lysis byffer containing 50 mM KCl, 10 mM Tris HCl pH 8.3, 1% Tween 20 and 60 µg/ml proteinase K, and digested for 1 h at 55°C. After 10 min of inactivation at 100°C, the specimens were immediately processed for PCR.

Simple PCR

Simple PCR was carried out following the protocol of Wakefield et al. (4), with the primers pAZ 102-E and pAZ 102-H, in a 50 µl reaction mixture containing 50 mM KCl, 10 mM Tris HCl pH 8.3, 5 mM $MgCl_2$, 400 mM dNTP, each primer at 1 mM and 3 units of Taq polymerase (AmpliTaq DNA Polymerase, Perkin Elmer, Roche Molecular Systems, Branchburg, New Jersey, USA). DNA was amplified in a Perkin Elmer 9600 thermocycler with a thermic program compsed of 40 cycles (30 s at 94°C for denaturation, 30 s at 55°C for annealing and 75 s at 72°C for extension), preceded by 2 min at 95°C for initial denaturation and followed by 3 min at 72°C for final extension. The products of amplification were then electrophoresed in a 1.5% agarose gel and stained with ethidium bromide to visualize the 346-bp fragment specific of P. carinii.

Nested PCR

Internal primers were selected by one of us (F.B.) in the sequence amplified by simple PCR and reported by Sinclair et al. (11) (P_1 = 5′-CTAGGATATAGCTGGTTTTC-3′ and P_2 = 5′-TCGACTATCTAGCTTATCGC-3′).

Nested PCR was performed in the same reaction mixture as for simple PCR with a first round of 30 cycles (20 s at 94°C for denaturation, 20 s at 55°C for annealing and 25 s at 72°C for extension), preceded by 2 min at 95°C for initial denaturation and followed by 3 min at 72°C for final extension, with the external primers pAZ 102-E and pAZ 102-H. A second thermic round, with the chosen internal primers P_1 and P_2 at 1 µM, was carried out in the same conditions as the first one, with 1 µl of the product amplified by the first round. After electrophoresis in 1.5% agarose, the amplified fragment of 205 bp was visualized using ethidium bromide staining.

Controls and precautions

A negative and a positive control were introduced into each simple and nested PCR run. All BAL fluids were assayed in duplicate in separate PCR reactions. PCRs were conducted on batches of BAL extracts without knowledge of individual immunofluorescence results. The standard precautions in PCR work were observed, according to accepted recommendations (12).

RESULTS

Extraction procedure

The rapid DNA extraction procedure was first compared to the technique described by Wakefield et al. (4), consisting of 16-h proteinase K digestion followed by phenol-chloroform-isoamyl alcohol extraction, on five BAL fluid samples from five patients with microbiologically proven PCP. All five specimens were correctly amplified by simple PCR. This rapid extraction procedure was then used for all the BAL samples submitted for PCR.

Simple PCR

The sensitivity and specificity of simple PCR were studied on 74 fluid samples, obtained from BAL performed for the diagnosis of an acute resiratory illness or for graft follow-up, in 43 immunocompromised patients. The results of simple PCR are compared to those of IFA staining in Table I. Of the patients, 11 presented an acute respiratory illness diagnosed as PCP. In 3 BAL fluid samples, from 3 different patients, the IFA stain was difficult to read because of the paucity of organisms. In these 3 cases the result of PCR was clearly positive. Compared to IFA staining, simple PCR had 100% sensitivity and a 98% specificity. The only result considered to be a false-positive was obtained from the BAL fluid of a patient with a recent cytomegalo-virus primo-infection. After the BAL sampling, this patient was finally

Table I. *Results of IFA staining and simple PCR in BAL fluids from 43 immunosuppressed patients*

	Simple PCR results		
IFA staining results[a]	Positive	Negative	Total
Positive	11[b]	0	11
Negative	1	62	63
Total	12	62	74

[a] A positive direct examination by IFA staining is the laboratory criteria for Pneumocystis carinii pneumonia (PCP).
[b] Corresponding to 11 patients.

Table II. *Results of IFA staining and nested PCR in BAL fluids of 18 immunosuppressed patients*

	Nested PCR results		
IFA staining results[a]	Positive	Negative	Total
Positive	7[b]	0	7
Negative	4[c]	21	25
Total	11	21	32

[a] A positive direct examination by IFA staining is the laboratory criteria for PCP.
[b] Corresponding to 6 patients.
[c] Three BAL from 1 patient.

diagnosed as having an acute graft rejection episode and reacted favorably to an increase of his immunosuppressive treatment, associated with blind anti-P. carinii prophylaxis consisting of trimethoprim-sulfamethoxazole.

Nested PCR

Nested PCR was evaluated on 32 BALs performed for the diagnosis of an acute respiratory illness or for graft follow-up, in 18 patients. The results of IFA staining and nested PCR are presented in Table II. Seven BAL samples from 6 patients with microbiologically proven PCP were positive by nested PCR.

Four BAL samples were considered as false-positives, resulting in a specificity of 84% for nested PCR. Three of these were recovered from the same HIV-positive patient who had antecedents of severe PCP and was receiving anti-P. carinii prophylaxis. He was also treated for a disseminated mycobacterial infection and a lymphoma. His general status progressively deteriorated, and he died several weeks later. No autopsy was performed. The fourth false-positive BAL sample was also positive by simple PCR and came from the patient with cytomegalovirus primoinfection and graft rejection.

Post-treatment follow-up

Three BALs were performed, with the agreement of the patients, after completion of a 3-week high dose therapy with trimethoprim-sulfamethoxazole. The 3 patients were asymptomatic at that time. The IFA stain and simple and nested PCR were negative in these three BAL samples (at days 18, 20, 24 after initiation of therapy).

On the other hand, the BAL sample from one HIV-positive patient, who remained symptomatic after a 4-week treatment with trimethoprim-sulfamethoxazole, was still positive on IFA staining by simple and nested PCR. Concomitantly this patient was suffering a progressive multifocal leukoencephalitis which rapidly led to his death. Necropsy was not permitted.

We also performed simple and nested PCR on 11 BAL samples from 3 patients who underwent successive BALs for graft monitoring or for follow-up of pneumonia in the weeks following a diagnosis of PCP. In 2 patients, a control BAL was performed, 10 and 17 days respectively after the initiation of anti-P. carinii treatment. At that time the patients were no longer symptomatic, and IFA staining and simple PCR were negative, but nested PCR was still positive. The third patient, an asymptomatic heart–lung recipient, was found positive by simple and nested PCR, but not by IFA staining, a BAL sample collected 10 days after completion of his treatment, while he had been found negative in 2 BAL samples obtained during treatment. All subsequent BAL samples investigated in these 3 patients were negative (at days 43, 44 and 46 after diagnosis). All of them recovered.

DISCUSSION

Several authors have reported the use of PCR on BAL fluids or induced sputum samples as a sensitive method for the diagnosis of PCP. However the common disadvantages of these various PCR protocols are the time-consuming extraction procedures (4–8) or, in protocols with a more simple extraction step, the laborious multiple-step procedures for PCR product detection, such as Southern-blotting (13) or enzyme-linked immunosorbent assay (10). Tamburrini et al. have developed a rapid 2-step hemi-nested PCR protocol (9) which resembles our nested PCR and performed as their previous one-step PCR (13). Compared with the 2-step PCR of Tamburini et al. (9) our simple PCR is more specific and more rapid. We have developed an extraction procedure which takes less than 2 h, compared with the 16-h protocol described by Wakefield et al. (4, 5, 14), without any loss of sensitivity. The rapidity of our extraction procedure makes simple and nested PCR, followed by electrophoresis and ethidium bromide staining, accessible for routine diagnostic purposes.

Our study demonstrated the excellent performance of simple PCR. The sensitivity was 100% and the specificity 98%. The only false-positive result of simple PCR, compared to direct examination, was obtained in the BAL liquid of a patient with a rejection episode. However, his recent primary CMV infection, which is frequently observed together with P. carinii infection, and his favourable reaction to treatment that included anti-P. carinii prophylaxis, suggested that a low-grade P. carinii infection might have been present.

Nested PCR presented a greater number of false-positive results. One was obtained in the same BAL fluid as used for simple PCR. The 3 other false-positive results were obtained in three BAL samples collected from the same HIV-positive patient, and could also indicate a subclinical P. carinii infection, as this severely immunosuppressed patient received both anti-PCP prophylaxis and antibiotics partially active on P. carinii like clarithromycin. The fact that these results were systematically obtained in the same patient also argues in favour of this hypothesis. However, we could not verify this, as no autopsy was performed after the patient's death a few weeks later.

BAL fluids sampled during the follow-up of treated patients became rapidly negative by simple PCR; no more PCR signal could be detected at days 10, 13, 17, 18, 20 and 24 after the diagnosis and initiation of treatment in 6 patients who responded to therapy. However, in the follow-up BAL samples of 2 of these patients, detection of P. carinii DNA by nested PCR occurred 4 and 17 days after the last simple PCR positive result, showing a greater sensitivity of nested PCR compared to simple PCR. The lack of detection of persistent P. carinii by a sensitive method such as nested PCR, in the BAL fluids of patients responding to therapy, suggests that they harbour only few or no microorganisms in their lungs after completion of a well-conducted anti-P. carinii therapy. Interestingly, in an

HIV-positive patient who did not respond to therapy, simple and nested PCR remained positive as long as 4 weeks after diagnosis. This has already been studied by other authors, using conventional staining techniques in follow-up BALs of HIV-infected patients treated for PCP. Positive BAL samples at 21 days of follow-up identify patients at increased risk of relapse or not responding to anti-P. carinii therapy (14). However in our series, one asymptomatic patient presented simple and nested positive results in one out of 4 BAL fluid samples, 29 days after diagnosis. This patient did not relapse. The longer persistence of positive PCR signals during anti-P. carinii therapy suggests that PCR is probably more sensitive than direct examination, even by immunofluorescence, and that false-positive results obtained by PCR could possibly be interpreted as subclinical infections.

Other studies have also reported a high sensitivity of PCR in detecting P. carinii organisms. Because of the use of both laboratory or clinical criteria to define PCP, the specificity of PCR in these studies varies from 77 to 100% (5–10, 13). It has been suggested that, because of the extreme sensitivity of PCR, the detection of P. carinii in BAL samples by this technique probably reflects P. carinii infection without clinical relevance (6, 9, 13). However, in cases of granulomatous PCP, when organisms are not easily accessible, conventional stainings of BAL samples are often negative. In these particular cases, PCR is able to detect a very small number of organisms corresponding to a clinically significant P. carinii infection (15). The sensitivity of PCR could help to avoid traumatic lung biopsy in the case of failure of conventional techniques.

In conclusion, we have successfully developed a very easy and rapid P. carinii DNA extraction method, suitable for simple and nested PCR protocols applied to BAL fluids. After this extraction step, a simple PCR followed by the detection of PCR products by ethidium bromide staining after electrophoresis is 100% sensitive and 98% specific compared to IFA staining. Nevertheless, IFA staining is more rapid and simpler to perform, and therefore remains as our standard diagnostic method for the detection of P. carinii in BAL liquids. The excellent performance of simple PCR combined with our rapid extraction procedure allows its use as a confirmation technique when direct examination is difficult to interpret. A nested PCR, using our extraction procedure and ethidium bromide staining, is probably more sensitive than direct examination. The clinical relevance of this greater sensitivity should be investigated in further studies with other clinical criteria for PCP, regardless of direct examination of IFA stain results. Nested PCR could also be useful in PCP recurrence, or to confirm a poor response to anti-P. carinii therapy. It would be interesting to test the sensitivity of our simple and nested PCR protocols on induced sputum samples compared to that of IFA staining, as these techniques could perhaps enhance the recovery of P. carinii in such samples.

ACKNOWLEDGEMENTS

We would like to thank Mr L. Debaisieux for technical advice and Ms C. Buekens for typing the manuscript.

REFERENCES

1. Hopewell PC. Pneumocystis carinii pneumonia: diagnosis. J Infect Dis 157: 1115–1119, 1988.
2. Levine SJ, Kennedy D, Shelhamer JH, Kovacs A, Feuerstein IM, Gill VJ, Stock F, Soloman D, Boylen CT, Masur H, Ognibene FP. Diagnosis of Pneumocystis carinii pneumonia by multiple lobe, site-directed bronchoalveolar lavage with immunofluorescent monoclonal antibody staining in human immunodeficiency virus-infected patients receiving aerosolized pentamidine chemoprophylaxis. Am Rev Respir Dis 146: 838–843, 1991.
3. Jules-Elysee KM, Stover DE, Zaman MB, Bernard EM, White DA. Aerosolized pentamidine: effect on diagnosis and presentation of Pneumocystis carinii pneumonia. Ann Intern Med 112: 750–757, 1990.
4. Wakefield AE, Pixley FJ, Banerji S, Sinclair K, Miller RF, Moxon ER, Hopkin JM. Detection of Pneumocystis carinii with DNA amplification. Lancet 336: 451–453, 1990.
5. Wakefield AE, Guiver L, Miller RF, Hopkin JM. DNA amplification on induced sputum samples for diagnosis of Pneumocystis carinii pneumonia. Lancet 337: 1378–1379, 1991.
6. Olsson M, Elvin K, Löfdahl S, Linder E. Detection of Pneumocystis carinii DNA in sputum and bronchoalveolar lavage samples by ploymerase chain reaction. J Clin Microbiol 31: 221–226, 1993.
7. Oka S, Kitada K, Kohjin T, Nakamura Y, Kimura S, Shimada K. Direct monitoring as well as sensitive diagnosis of Pneumocystis carinii pneumonia by the polymerase chain reaction on sputum samples. Mol Cell Probes 7: 419–424, 1993.
8. Lipschik GY, Gill VJ, Lundgren JD, Andrawis VA, Nelson NA, Nielson JO, Ognibene FP, Kovacs JA. Improved diagnosis of Pneumocystis carinii infection by polymerase chain reaction on induced sputum and blood. Lancet 340: 203–206, 1992.
9. Tamburrini E, Mencarini P, De Luca A, Antinori A, Visconti E, Ammassari A, Ortona L, Ortona E, Siracusano A, Vicari G. Simple and rapid two-step polymerase chain reaction for diagnosis of Pneumocystis carinii infection. J Clin Microbiol 31: 2788–2789, 1993.
10. Cartwright PC, Nelson NA, Gill VJ. Development and evaluation of a rapid and simple procedure for detection of Pneumocystis carinii by PCR. J Clin Microbiol 32: 1634–1638, 1994.
11. Sinclair K, Wakefield AE, Banerji S, Hopkin JM. Pneumocystis carinii organisms derived from rat and human hosts are genetically distinct. Mol Biochem Parasitol 45: 183–184, 1991.
12. Kwok S, Higuchi R. Avoiding false positives with PCR. Nature 339: 237–238, 1989.
13. Tamburrini E, Mencarini P, De Luca A, Maiuro G, Ventura G, Antinori A, Ammassari A, Visconti E, Otona L, Siracusano A, Ortona E, Vicari G. Diagnosis of Pneumocystis carinii pneumonia: specificity and sensitivity of polymerase chain reaction in comparison with immunofluorescence in bronchoalveolar lavage specimens. J Med Microbiol 38: 449–453, 1993.

14. Colangelo G, Baughman RP, Dohn MN, Frame PT. Follow-up bronchoalveolar lavage in AIDS patients with Pneumocystis carinii pneumonia. Am Rev Respir Dis 143: 1067–1071, 1991.

15. Wakefield AE, Miller RF, Guiver LA, Hopkin JM. Granulomatous Pneumocystis carinii pneumonia: DNA amplification studies on bronchoscopic alveolar lavage samples. J Clin Pathol 47: 664–666, 1994.

Submitted December 14, 1994; accepted April 3, 1995

Scand J Infect Dis 27: 363–367, 1995 ORIGINAL ARTICLE

Pneumocystis carinii in Bronchoalveolar Lavage and Induced Sputum: Detection with a Nested Polymerase Chain Reaction

JENS SKØT[1], AXEL GUSTAV LERCHE[1], HANS JØRN KOLMOS[2], JENS OLE NIELSEN[1], LARS REINHARDT MATHIESEN[1], and JENS DILLING LUNDGREN[1]

From the Departments of [1]Infectious Diseases and [2]Clinical Microbiology, University of Copenhagen, Hvidovre Hospital, Denmark

To evaluate polymerase chain reaction (PCR) for detection of Pneumocystis carinii, 117 bronchoalveolar lavage (BAL) specimens, from HIV-infected patients undergoing a diagnostic bronchoscopy, were processed and a nested PCR, followed by Southern blot and hybridization with a P_{32}-labelled probe was performed. The sensitivity and specificity were 85 and 100% (34/40 and 77/77) respectively. A non-radioactive labelling system BluGENE was evaluated on all specimens, and found to be as effective as P_{32}-labelling. To increase the speed and convenience of detection, a dot blot system was tested, but sensitivity dropped markedly with this system. A further 33 patients had both induced sputum and bronchoalveolar lavage performed and the induced sputum was analysed using PCR and routine microbiological methods. The PCR sensitivity on induced sputum was equal to that of routine methods. At present the evaluated PCR cannot replace routine microbiological methods for detection of Pneumocystis carinii, on either BAL fluid or induced sputum.

J. Skøt, MD, Department of Infectious Diseases, Hvidovre Hospital, Kettegårds Alle 30, DK-2650 Hvidovre, Denmark

INTRODUCTION

For more than a decade the problems of diagnosis and treatment of pneumonia with P. carinii, as a consequence of HIV disease, has been a challenge to the scientific world. Major progress has been made in diagnosis, but the changing pattern of the illness, mainly due to primary and secondary prophylaxis, still demands improvement of diagnostic tools (1, 2).

More recent advances in diagnosis have consisted of induced sputum examination, although the diagnostic yield has been varying (3–10), and the use of the polymerase chain reaction (PCR) to detect P. carinii DNA (11–17). Even though the diagnostic yield of the PCR is potentially high, the risk of contamination, the use of radionucleotide-labelled probes and the time-consuming procedures represent serious drawbacks. It is for the latter reasons that this procedure is still mainly a tool for research in microbiology, rather than a part of the routine diagnostic repertoire. Attempts have been made to replace gel electrophoresis and subsequent Southern blot with faster techniques, for example, dot blot (18). Non-radioactive and stable oligonucleotide-labelling systems are now widely in use.

We were interested in evaluating the efficacy of these tools, together with the fast DNA extraction method and nested PCR of Lipschik et al. (15), for the detection of P. carinii DNA in bronchoalveolar lavage (BAL) specimens. Secondly, in order to evaluate the efficacy of induced sputum for diagnosis of P. carinii pneumonia in our clinical setting, we decided to compare the diagnoses obtained from routine microbiological evaluation and PCR on induced sputum with the diagnoses obtained from the standard BAL, in all patients. This would give us a firm knowledge of the correct diagnosis. It would also make it possible to determine whether false-negative results from sputum and BAL PCR were in accordance, thus suggesting possible shortcomings of the rat P. carinii-based PCR in detecting human P. carinii.

MATERIALS AND METHODS

Patients

The population was a non-selected one of patients, seropositive for HIV, who were to undergo a fibreoptic bronchoscopy, regardless of whether the symptoms were presumptive for pneumonia with P. carinii (PCP) or other pulmonary disease. If another bronchoscopy was performed during the same episode of illness (within 6 weeks of the first bronchoscopy) this was not included in the study.

Bronchoalveolar lavage

Cell pellets obtained from bronchoalveolar lavage from 117 patients, seropositive for HIV, who had a diagnostic fibreoptic bronchoscopy performed between 9 July 1990 and 19 March 1993 were analysed for the presence of P. carinii, using routine microbiological methods and PCR. The patients included in the induced sputum part of the study were not included here.

Induced sputum

In the period from 24 September 1991 to 1 December 1992, 44 patients were included in a prospective study of combined BAL and induced sputum. Five patients were excluded because their respiratory symptoms were so severe, that it was found unethical to do both induced sputum and BAL (2 of these patients had PCP). That left 39 patients who, after giving informed consent, were enrolled in the study concerning the value of induced sputum for the diagnosis of PCP. Six of these were unable to produce sputum, and 1 of the latter 6 had PCP. A total of 33 induced sputum specimens were analysed, therefore.

 ISSN 0036-5548

Methods

Bronchoscopy was performed as described (19). For PCR analysis, 15–25 ml of BAL fluid was spun down at 500 × *G*, for 10 min. The supernatant was discarded, and the cell pellet stored at −20°C for later analysis.

Sputum induction was performed as described (7). For PCR analysis, 5 ml of sputum was treated with 3.25 mM dithiothreitol (Sputolysin, Behring Diagnostic, Somerville, New Jersey, USA) for 5 min at 37°C, and cells were spun down 500 × *G*, for 10 min, washed in PBS (SSI, Copenhagen, Denmark) and spun down again. Cell pellets were stored at −20°C for later analysis.

DNA extraction. The cell pellets were thawed and 100 μl was resuspended in 100 μl of buffer containing 2.5 mM $MgCl_2$, 10 mM Tris-HCI, 50 mM KCl, 0.5% Tween 20, pH 8.3, and 100 μg/ml proteinase K (Boehringer Mannheim, Germany), and incubated at 56°C for 1 h, and then at 99°C for 3 min to inactivate the protease. This suspension was used directly for the PCR.

Oligonucleotide primers. A nested PCR was applied (15) based on the chromosomal rRNA 16S subunit sequence of rat-derived P. carinii (20). Primers 340a (CCAGATTAGCTTTTGCTGATC-GCGGG, corresponding to position 1349–1374) and 708 (ACTT-TCCAGTAATAGGCTTATCG), complementary to position 1727–1705, amplifying a 378-bp sequence, were used in the first round. In the second round, we used primers JK1 (TGTTGGCA-TGAAGCCAATGGAA) corresponding to position 1389–1410 and JK2 (CAATAACCCATCACCAGTCCGAAG) complementary to position 1700–1677), amplifying a 312-bp sequence.

PCR

The reaction mixture for PCR contained 5 μl of proteinase-treated cells, 0.2 mM of each dNTP, 50 pM of each oligonucleotide primer, 2.5 U Taq polymerase (Amplitaq, Perkin-Elmer Cetus, Denmark) and PCR buffer (16.6 mM ammonium sulphate, 6.7 mM MgCl, 67 mM Tris Ph 8.8, 10 mM β-mercaptoethanol) to a final volume of 50 μl.

A negative (without DNA) and a positive control was included in every series. PCR was performed by heating the mixture to 94°C for 10 min, and then 36 cycles of 94°C for 1 min, 50°C for 1 min, and 72°C for 2 min were carried out and finally an incubation at 72°C for 10 min. Then, 5 μl of the reaction mixture was transferred to a fresh mixture of PCR buffer with the necessary reagents and the second primer pair. The second amplification round was performed as above.

Analysis of PCR product

The products were electrophoresed in a 3% agarose gel (Nusieve GTG Agarose, FMC Bioproducts, USA) in TAE buffer, pH 8.3 with ethidium bromide (Merck, Darmstadt, Germany), 5 μl/ml gel, 30 mA for 1 h. The bands were visualized with UV light. The gels were then blotted to a Zetaprobe Blotting membrane (Biorad, Richmond, California, USA).

The probe for PCR 372a (AAGGAAAATGAACTTGCTG-GCTCT), corresponding to position 1499–1475, was either labelled with P_{32} or with the non-radioactive nucleic acid detection system BluGENE (Gaithersburg, Maryland, USA). Briefly, in the BlueGENE system a biotin-labelled probe was hybridized to the PCR products. The membrane was then incubated with streptavidin-alakaline phosphatase conjugate, and finally the products were visualized in a colour reaction by incubation with nitroblue tetrazolium. The PCR products from BAL cells were additionally visualized in a dot blot system with probes labelled with the same systems as above. For the P_{32}-labelled specimens, an autoradiogram was produced. Reading of the results was carried out by persons unaware of the clinical diagnosis.

PCR for β-actin. Some specimens were aditionally analysed for the presence of β-actin DNA. TGACGGGGTCACCCACACT-GTGCCCATCTA, corresponding to position 1038–1067, was used as primer together with CTAGAAGCATTTGCGGTGGAC-GATGGAGGG, complementary to position 1905–1876. The PCR reaction was carried out as above except that only one amplification round was performed. The bands were visualized on agarose/ethidium bromide gel as above.

Microbiological evaluation

Cytospin slides with cells from bronchoalveolar lavage were evaluated with Giemsa stain and with a direct immunofluorescence test kit (Genetic Systems, Seattle, Washington, USA) for the detection of P. carinii. If these stains proved negative, a methenamine silver nitrate stain, according to Grocotts's modification of Gomori's stain for fungi, was also performed. Gram and Ziehl–Neelsen stains were performed to evaluate the presence of other pathogens.

The induced sputum was analysed in the same way, with the modification that the Gram and Ziehl–Neelsen stains were carried out on material not treated with dithiothreitol. With induced sputum, all three diagnostic procedures were performed for detection of P. carinii. The slides from the induced sputum test were interpreted by an investigator who was unaware of the results from PCR and from BAL cells. When slides from two out of three stains were read as positive the patient was considered to have pneumonia with P. carinii.

RESULTS

PCR for detection of P. carinii in BAL fluid

To evaluate whether a fast method of DNA extraction followed by a nested PCR, for detection of P. carinii, was superior to standard microbiological diagnosis, we performed PCR and afterwards electrophoresis of the PCR product in an ethidium bromide gel and visualized DNA bands under UV light. Where a band was found in an appropriate position, Southern blot and hybridization with a P_{32}-labelled probe was performed.

Among the 117 patients analysed, 40 (34.2%) were found to have a diagnosis of pneumonia with P. carinii after routine microbiological evaluation of BAL fluid (Table I). Of these, 34 were also identified with a band on ethidium bromide gel, and all these were afterwards confirmed with P_{32}-labelled probe. Six were not detected. No false-positive results were found. The sensitivity and specificity, with 95% confidence intervals, are 85.0% (70.2–94.3%) and 100.0% (95.3–100.0%).

To investigate false-negative results further, the nested PCR was reproduced, and a PCR with β-actin primers was also performed. This resulted in one additional positive result with PCP-PCR still recorded in Table I as a false-negative result, while the presence of β-actin DNA was confirmed in only 2 out of 6.

To investigate whether the PCR product could be detected in safer and/or faster ways, we performed Southern blot and hybridization, with probes labelled with the non-radioactive labelling system BluGENE (SB-BluGENE). A faster way of transferring the PCR product to the nylon membrane, i.e. dot blot, was also evaluated with both

Table I. *Results of PCR, on cells from bronchoalveolar lavage fluid, for detection of pneumonia with Pneumocystis carinii, compared with standard microbiological evaluation. Hybridization was done on gel-positive specimens. Number of specimens analysed = 117*

Detection method	True-positive results	False-positive results	True-negative results	False-negative results
Ethidium bromide (gel as only method)	34	0	77	6
Southern blot, with P_{32}-labelled probe	34	0	77	6
Southern blot, with BluGene-labelled probe	34	0	77	6
Dot blot with P_{32}-labelled probe	30	0	77	10
Dot blot with BluGene-labelled probe	30	0	77	10

Table II. *Results from PCR and microbiological examination of induced sputum. Southern blot and hybridization with P_{32}-labelled probe were performed only on gel-positive specimens*

Results with routine microbiological methods on BAL	PCR for Pneumocystis carinii on induced sputum			Routine microbiological evalution on induced sputum		
	Negative	Positive	Total	Negative	Positive	Total
Negative	19	1	20	20	0	20
Positive	4	9	13	4	9	13
Total	23	10	33	24	9	33

labelling systems (Table I). SB-BlueGENE proved to be as effective as SB-P_{32}. Dot blot detection (with either P_{32}- or BluGENE-labelled probes) proved to be less satisfactory, with no false-positive results, but with 4 additional false-negative results produced with these systems. Three of these patients were identical in the 2 groups.

Initially we had only hybridized specimens which had been positive on ethidium bromide gels. To evaluate the methods further, we hybridized all PCR products with probes (P_{32}-and BluGENE-labelled, on both Southern blot and dot blot) regardless whether the gel result was positive or not. This did not alter the results, except for Southern blot P_{32}, where the number of false-negative results was reduced by one, while the number of false-positive results was increased by one, and dot blot with BluGENE, where the number of false-negative results was reduced by one.

Induced sputum

A total of 33 induced sputum specimens were evaluated with PCR for P. carinii followed by Southern blot and hybridization with P_{32}-labelled probe on gel-positive specimens. Of these, 13 were found positive when cells from concomitant bronchoalveolar lavage were assessed with routine microbiological methods (Table II). One false-positive and 4 false-negative results were found, while 28 were correctly identified with the PCR.

As above, hybridization of gel-positive specimens with Blu-GENE-labelled probes was tested. The results were unchanged (data not shown). Additionally, all specimens were tested with Southern blot with the 2 labelling systems, regardless of whether the eithidium bromide gel was positive or not. The results did not change.

PCR on the corresponding BAL cells was performed on the false-positive and negative specimens. The patient with a false-positive PCR was also positive with PCR on BAL cells. The patient had a clinical course of pneumonia with P. carinii, with dyspnoea, non-productive cough, fever, and bilateral interstitial infiltrates on a chest X-ray, and responded to treatment with sulfamethoxazole–trimethoprim but the Po_2 was not decreased. This patient had been prophylactically treated with aerosolized pentamidine before the episode. One of 4 patients with a false-negative result with PCR on induced sputum, was also negative with the BAL PCR. PCR for β-actin on induced sputum was also performed, and showed a positive reaction in all 4. None of these patients had received PCP prophylaxis.

The microbiological evaluation of induced sputum produced no false-positive but 4 false-negative results (Table II). Two of these had very little columnar epithelium in the specimen. Only 1 patient was false-negative with both PCR and routine methods.

DISCUSSION

Our study has shown that the fast DNA extraction method with a nested PCR on BAL cells, is a relatively fast and safe method for detecting PCP with few false-negative and no false-positive results. The detection of P. carinii in BAL fluid using routine microbiological methods already has a very high sensitivity and specificity, so a major improvement of diagnostic power was not to be expected. Nevertheless, the problem of why the powerful technique of PCR failed to detect as many as 6 of the 40 positive specimens, when there was no doubt concerning the correct diagnosis based on microscopic findings, is intriguing, although it is in accordance with most other studies using either the same (15) or other PCRs (13, 15). The sensitivity of 95% found initially (12) was not reproduced by other groups using the same PCR (13, 15). Only 2 out of our 6 patients who were not detected, had received prophylaxis (with pentamidine). Inhibitors of PCR in the BAL fluid, or the fast technique of DNA extraction used in this study, may be the reasons for most of these false-negative results, considering that only 2 of these 6 false-negative BAL fluids could produce β-actin DNA. Concerning these 2, it might be speculated that, when the PCR primers are based on the sequences from rat P. carinii, they might have difficulties binding to possibly slightly different sequences from human-derived P. carinii. Genetic heterogeneity within rat P. carinii has been demonstrated on the chromosomal level (21), and differences between rat and human-derived P. carinii have also been described (22).

Replacing the radioactive labelling with the non-radioactive labelling system BluGENE produced exactly the same results. Reagents used for BluGENE labelling have a long life span, and thus obviate the need for continuous supplies of radioactive reagent, with less potential hazard for staff and environment.

Our attempt to make PCR more suitable for routine detection of P. carinii, by replacing the time-consuming Southern blot technique with the faster dot blot, was not a success, with sensitivity thereby dropping to a mere 75%. It could be reasoned that, when applying this technique only to gel-positive specimens, the size of the amplified DNA segment could be confirmed by gel staining, while the specificity of amplification could be supplemented by the dot blot hybridization. Our problem was, however, not decreased specificity but decreased sensitivity. The reason why 3/4 specimens not detected with the 2 dot blot systems, were identical is not clear. It might be speculated that 'contaminating' reagents could interfere with the binding of the amplified sequence of P. carinii DNA to the membrane. If much non-specific amplification had taken place, the sequences produced might compete with the amplified sequence of P. carinii DNA, while they would not represent a problem in the Southern blot system where the amplified sequences were first separated by electrophoresis.

The best results were obtained when only PCR products found positive on gel staining were hybridized. We did not find the improvement of method, which has been found by other groups (11, 12, 14, 16) when hybridizing gel-negative specimens. This may be due to the large amount of DNA produced by the nested PCR. Staining of bands found on ethidium bromide gel was usually very strong with this PCR, so hybridization in our study generally only confirmed the specificity of the PCR product, but did not produce major improvement of the strength of the signal.

We performed a prospective study of the value of PCR for PCP diagnosis, on induced sputum samples from a non-selected population of HIV-positive subjects with respiratory symptoms. In our study the correct diagnosis was always well established, based on the routine microbiological evaluation of the bronchoalveolar lavage fluid. We found equal sensitivity (69.2%) but a slightly lower specificity of PCR when comparing PCR and routine examination of induced sputum (95 and 100%), respectively). The non-radioactive labelling system was equal to P_{32}-labelling, as with the analysis of BAL cells. We have not been able to reproduce the first promising results of this nested PCR for detection of P. carinii that was found by Lipschik et al. (15) were a 100% sensitivity was found. The reason for this is clearly not only mismatch between rat P. carinii-based primers and human-derived P. carinii DNA, although this could be the case with the one patient with a false-negative PCR result on both induced sputum and BAL. Another patient was found negative with both microbiological evaluation and sputum PCR, suggesting low quality sputum induction, which could be improved, as sputum induction was not a routine procedure in our department. Finally, in the study by Lipschik et al., not all patients with negative sputum examination had a bronchoscopy done, and thus cases of PCP may have been missed.

As PCR detection did not prove to be superior to routine induced sputum examination, even though our study is small, PCR is not the method of choice, when the more time-consuming procedures involved in this procedure are also considered. When PCR is further improved, it might be applicable on induced sputum. It should be borne in mind, however, that to avoid a large number of low yield specimens, the careful selection of patients for induced sputum examination for PCR, is as important here as with routine induced sputum examination (23). The sensitivities of our methods are of course unchanged, but the positive and negative predictive values will change with the frequency of PCP in the population studied. The decreasing incidence of PCP in the HIV-infected community due to widespread prophylaxis could potentially increase the number of patients, with negative specimens, who would need a bronchoscopy afterwards. This would result in delayed diagnosis, enhanced patient discomfort and increased cost.

We conclude that the PCR, evaluated in this study for detection of P. carinii on either BAL fluid or induced sputum, has high sensitivity and specificity but not better than those of routine microbiological methods. At present this PCR for P. carinii on induced sputum can not be recommended for routine detection.

ACKNOWLEDGEMENTS

We thank Lena Hansen and Birgit Andersen for excellent technical assistance and Dr Gregg Lipschik and Dr Joseph Kovacs, NIH,

Bethesda, MD, USA for help with the PCR, and Nurse Tina Bruun and the staff at the Department of Infectious Diseases, Hvidovre Hospital, University of Copenhagen for help with sputum induction.

This study was supported by the Hartmann Foundation, the Danish Medical Research Council, the NOVO Foundation, Ingeborg Roikjers Foundation, the University of Copenhagen, the Danish National Union against Lung Diseases, Danish Hospital Foundation for Medical Research, Region of Copenhagen, The Faroe Islands and Greenland, the AIDS Foundation, Director Jacob Madsen's and his wife Olga Madsen's Foundation, and Kong Christian den Tiendes Foundation.

REFERENCES

1. Levine SH, Masur H, Gill VJ, Feuerstein I, Suffredini AF, Brown D, Lane HC, Yarchoan R, Shelhamer JH, Ognibene FP. Effect of aerosolized pentamidine prophylaxis on the diagnosis of Pneumocystis carinii pneumonia by induced sputum examination in patients infected with the human immunodeficiency virus. Am Rev Respir Dis 144: 760–764, 1991.
2. Jules-Elysee KM, Stover DE, Zaman MB, Bernard EM, White DA. Aerosolized pentamidine: effect on diagnosis and presentation of Pneumocystis carinii pneumonia. Ann Intern Med 112: 750–757, 1990.
3. Pitchenik AE, Ganjei P, Torres A, Evans DA, Rubin E, Baier H. Sputum examination for the diagnosis of Pneumocystis carinii pneumonia in the acquired immunodeficiency syndrome. Am Rev Respir Dis 133: 226–229, 1986.
4. Bigby TD, Margolskee D, Curtis JL, Michael PF, Sheppard D, Hadley WK, Hopewell PC. The usefulness of induced sputum in the diagnosis of Pneumocystis carinii pneumonia in patients with the acquired immunodeficiency syndrome. Am Rev Respir Dis 133: 515–518, 1986.
5. Zaman MK, Wooten OJ, Suprahmanya B, Ankobiah W, Finch PJP. Rapid noninvasive diagnosis of Pneumocystis carinii from induced liquefied sputum. Ann Intern Med 109: 7–10, 1988.
6. Kovacs JA, Ng VL, Masur H, Leoung G, Hadley WK, Evans G, Lane HC, Ognibene FP, Shelhamer JH, Parillo JE, Gill VJ. Diagnosis of Pneumocystis carinii pneumonia: improved detection in sputum with use of monoclonal antibodies. N Engl J Med 318: 589–593, 1988.
7. Orholm M, Holten-Anderson W, Lundgren JD. Improved detection of Pneumocystis carinii by an immunofluorescence technique using monoclonal antibodies. Eur J Clin Microbiol Infect Dis 9: 880–885, 1990.
8. O'Brien RF, Quinn JL, Miyahara BT, Lepoff RB, Cohn DL. Diagnosis of Pneumocystis carinii pneumonia by induced sputum in a city with moderate incidence of AIDS. Chest 95: 136–138, 1989.
9. Kirsch CM, Azzi RL, Yenokida GG, Jensen WA. Analysis of induced sputum in the diagnosis of Pneumocystis carinii pneumonia. Am J Med Sci 299: 386–391, 1990.
10. Miller RF, Kocjan G, Buckland J, Holton J, Malin A, Semple SJG. Sputum induction for the diagnosis of pulmonary disease in HIV positive patients. J Infect 23: 5–15, 1991.
11. Wakefield AE, Pixley FJ, Banerji S, Sinclair K, Miller RF, Moxon ER, Hopkin JM. Detection of Pneumocystis carinii with DNA amplification. Lancet 336: 451–453, 1990.
12. Wakefield AE, Guiver L, Miller RF, Hopkin JM. DNA amplification on induced sputum samples for diagnosis of Pneumocystis carinii pneumonia. Lancet 337: 1378–1379, 1991.
13. Galan F, Oliver JL, Roux P, Poirot JL, Bereziat G. Detection of Pneumocystis carinii DNA by polymerase chain reaction compared to direct microscopy and immunofluorescence. J Protozool 38: 199S–200S, 1991.
14. Schluger N, Sepkowitz K, Armstrong D, Bernard E, Rifkin M, Cerami A, Bucala R. Detection of Pneumocystis carinii in serum of AIDS patients with pneumocystis pneumonia by the polymerase chain reaction. J Protozool 38: 240S-242S, 1991.
15. Lipschik GY, Gill VJ, Lundgren JD, Andrawis VA, Nelson NA, Nielsen JO, Ognibene FP, Kovacs JA.Improved diagnosis of Pneumocystis carinii infection by polymerase chain reaction on induced sputum and blood. Lancet 340: 203–206, 1992.
16. Olsson M, Elvin K, Löfdahl S, Linder E. Detection of Pneumocystis carinii DNA in sputum and bronchoalveolar lavage samples by polymerase chain reaction. J Clin Microbiol 31: 221–226, 1993.
17. Leigh TR, Gazzard BG, Rowbottom A, Collins JV. Quantitative and qualitative comparison of DNA amplification by PCR with immunofluorescence staining for diagnosis of Pneumocystis carinii pneumonia. J Clin Pathol 46: 140–144, 1993.
18. Conway B, Adler KE, Bechtel LJ, Kaplan JC, Hirsch MS. Detection of HIV-1 DNA in crude cell lysates of peripheral blood mononuclear cells by the polymerase chain reaction and nonradioactive oligonucleotide probes. J Acquir Immune Defic Syndr 3: 1059–1064, 1990.
19. Orholm M, Lundgren JD, Nielsen TL, Iversen J. Indication for fiberoptic bronchoscopy in HIV-infected patients suspected for Pneumocystis carinii pneumonia. Dan Med Bull 37: 86–89, 1990.
20. Edman JC, Kovacs JA, Masur H, Santi DV, Elwood HJ, Sogin ML. Ribosomal RNA sequence shows Pneumocystis carinii to be a member of the fungi. Nature 334: 519–522, 1988.
21. Lundgren B, Cotton R, Lundgren JD, Edman JC, Kovacs J. Identification of Pneumocystis carinii chromosomes and mapping of five genes. Infect Immun 58: 1705–1710, 1990.
22. Wakefield AE, Pixley FJ, Banerji S, Sinclair K, Miller RF, Moxon ER, Hopkin JM. Amplification of mitochondrial ribosomal RNA sequences from Pneumocystis carinii DNA of rat and human origin. Mol Biochem Parasitol 43: 69–76, 1990.
23. Glenny RW, Pierson DJ. Cost reduction in diagnosing Pneumocystis carinii pneumonia. Sputum induction versus bronchoalveolar lavage as the initial diagnostic procedure. Am Rev Respir Dis 145: 1425–1428, 1992.

Submitted January 31, 1995; accepted March 13, 1995

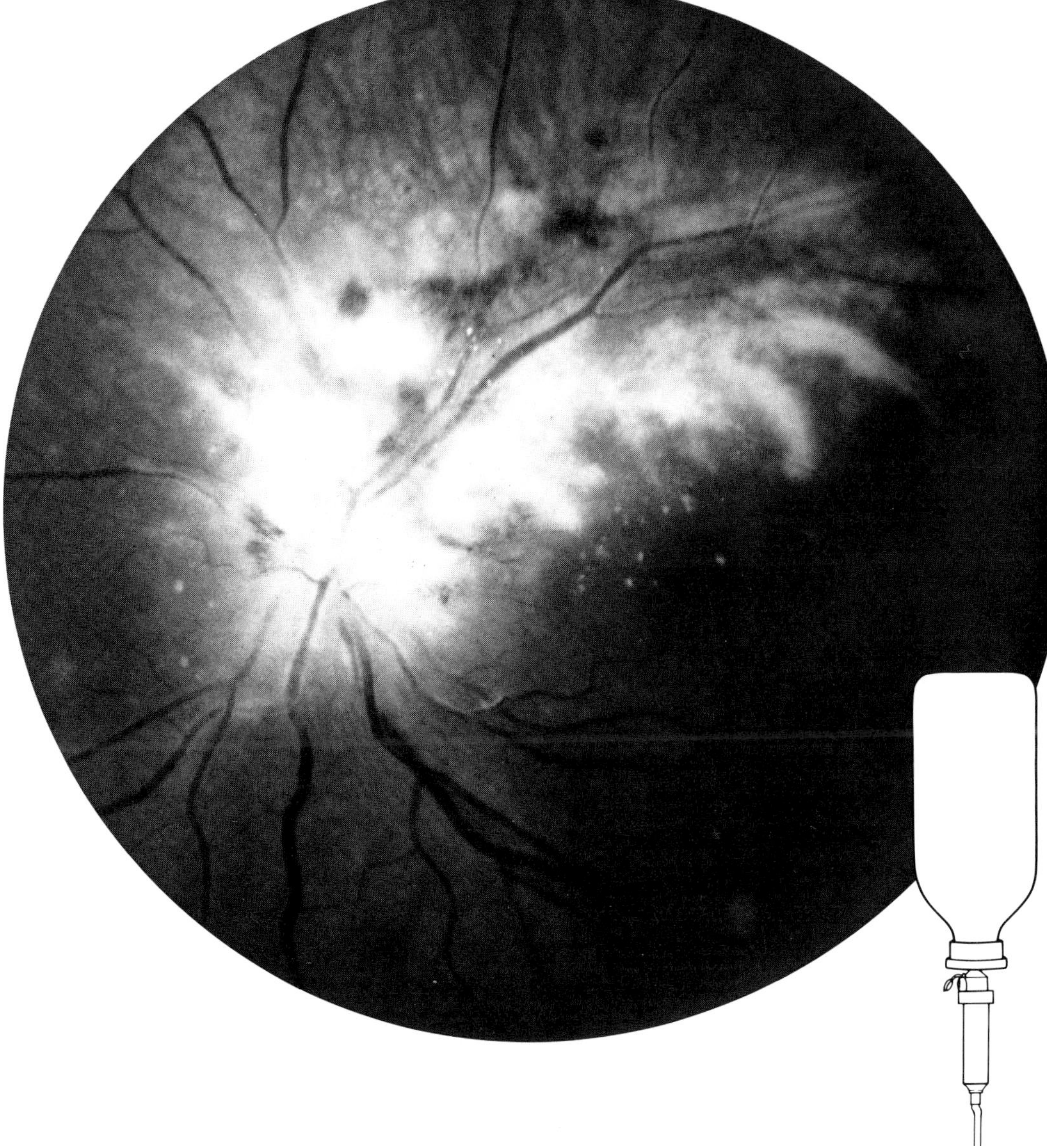

Scand J Infect Dis 27: 369–373, 1995 ORIGINAL ARTICLE

Phagocytosis and Oxidative Burst of Blood Phagocytes in Chronic Obstructive Airway Disease

GÜNTHER MÜNS[1], ISRAEL RUBINSTEIN[2] and KARL-CHRISTIAN BERGMANN[3]

From the [1]Department of Internal Medicine, University of Nebraska Medical Center, Omaha, Nebraska, [2]Department of Medicine (M/C 787), Section of Respiratory and Critical Care Medicine, University of Illinois at Chicago, Chicago, Illinois, USA, and [3]Allergie- und Asthma-Klinik Wilhelm Gronemeyer, Bad Lippspringe, Germany

Acute diseases and chronic conditions might be associated with altered blood neutrophil functions. The aim of this study was to investigate the effects of stable chronic obstructive pulmonary disease (COPD) and superimposed acute bacterial bronchopneumonia (ABP) on the phagocytosis and oxidative metabolism of blood phagocytes. The 129 participants were assigned to 6 groups: group 1, healthy controls; group 2, previously healthy controls with ABP; group 3, patients with stable COPD on inhaled corticosteroids (IC); group 4, individuals with stable COPD on IC and ABP; group 5, patients with stable COPD requiring oral corticosteroids (OC); group 6, individuals with COPD on OC and ABP. Phagocytosis and oxidative burst was measured. Both tests showed a significant difference between the groups without acute infection when compared to the patients with ABP. No differences were observed between patients with stable COPD without ABP (groups 3 and 5) and group 1. The number of phagocytized E. coli/cell was 9.1 ± 0.37, 7.9 ± 0.27 and 8.2 ± 0.28 (groups 2, 4, and 6, respectively) vs. 12.4 ± 0.33 in the control group. Incubation of cells from persons with pneumonia with plasma from healthy probands reversed the observed changes. We conclude, that acute bacterial bronchopneumonia is associated with an impairment of phagocytosis and oxidative metabolism in blood. We suggest, that stable COPD has no influence on phagocytosis and oxidative burst.

G. Müns, MD, University of Nebraska Medical Center, 600 S 42nd Street, Department of Internal Medicine, Omaha, NE 68198-2055, USA

INTRODUCTION

Granulocytes with monocytes play a central part in host defense (1), and circulating phagocytes are the first cells to reach and congregate at the sites of infection (2–4).

Inherited defects or acquired dysfunction of neutrophils secondary to chronic or acute disease affect different stages of this sequence (5–7). Recent conflicting data suggest an alteration of blood neutrophil function in chronic bronchitis (8, 9) or asthma (10). Whether the reported changes contribute to, and predispose patients with chronic bronchitis to recurrent infections, or whether they are the sequel of frequent inflammation is still contested at this time. The consequence of chronic bronchitis is destruction of airways in which neutrophils play a central role (11). However, without a sufficient attraction of functionally intact phagocytes to the lung at bacterial challenge, the result will be severe pulmonary infection. It is at present not established whether stable obstructive pulmonary disease is associated with changes in blood or pulmonary granulocyte function.

The aim of this study was to investigate the effects of stable chronic obstructive pulmonary disease (COPD) of varying severity and superimposed acute bacterial bronchopneumonia (ABP) on the phagocytosis and oxidative metabolism (oxidative burst) of whole blood granulocytes and monocytes.

MATERIAL AND METHODS

The 129 participating subjects were each assigned to one of 6 groups. Group 1 (controls) consisted of non-smoking healthy individuals; group 2 were previously healthy persons with acute bacterial bronchopneumonia (ABP); group 3 were patients with stable chronic obstructive pulmonary disease (COPD) taking inhaled corticosteroids (IC); group 4, patients with COPD on IC and ABP; group 5, patients with stable COPD on oral corticosteroids (OC); group 6 individuals meeting the criteria for group 5 and an ABP.

Patients with acute bacterial bronchopneumonia presented with fever, elevated white blood count (>11.0/nl), infiltrates on chest X-ray, and positive sputum or bronchoalveolar lavage (BAL) bacterial cultures (Table I). Sputum cultures of groups 3 and 5 were negative. In the 6 months prior to the study, the subjects in the latter groups did not experience any increase in shortness of breath, in cough or in sputum production, or report a more frequent use of metered dose inhalers or oral steroids. Furthermore they had not had any emergency room visits or hospital admissions, nor had they taken any antibiotics 6 months prior to the study. Pulmonary function tests (PFTs) were required to show that the probands of groups 3–6 had either a forced vital capacity (FVC) or a forced expiratory volume in 1 second (FEV_1) of $<80\%$ of the predicted value, in order to enter the study. PFTs were obtained the day blood was drawn, except in the ABP groups, where spirometry was performed following the patients' recovery (14–21 days after discontinuation of antibiotics). No antiinflammatory drugs were taken by any participant during the 3 weeks prior to the study, except for inhaled or oral steroids.

 ISSN 0036-5548

Table I. *Group characteristics*

Group	n	Age, years	PFT, % of predicted FVC	PFT, % of predicted FEV_1	WBC	Medication
1, controls	35	43.7 ± 5.0	110 ± 8	105 ± 9	7.5 ± 1.1	No medications, 3 weeks prior to study
2, controls with ABP	15	48.9 ± 7.1	101 ± 5	98 ± 4	13.8 ± 3.1	No medications, 3 weeks prior to study
3, COPD, on IC	21	51.1 ± 4.1	81 ± 7	67 ± 7	8.1 ± 0.9	IC (1.65 ± 0.54 mg BDP[a]/day)
4, COPD with ABP, on IC	18	46.2 ± 6.9	75 ± 5	65 ± 6	14.1 ± 3.9	IC (1.31 ± 0.37 mg BDP/day)
5, COPD, on OC	24	51.7 ± 5.6	70 ± 8	56 ± 9	7.2 ± 1.3	OC (10.5 ± 5.1 mg prednisone/day)
6, COPD with ABP, on OC	16	49.3 ± 7.0	75 ± 6	63 ± 4	18.4 ± 2.6	OC (12.3 ± 4.1 mg prednisone/day)

[a] Beclomethasone dipropionate.
All values are mean ± SD.
PFT = pulmonary function test; WBC = white blood count; ABP = acute bacterial bronchopneumonia; IC = inhaled corticosteroids; OC = oral corticosteroids.

Heparinized blood was drawn once from an antecubital vein and immediately prepared for the various tests. A cell count was performed on a Coulter counter and a differential count was obtained. Blood from patients with acute bronchopneumonia was sampled on admission, prior to changes in the maintenance dose of inhaled or oral steroids or prior to the initiation of antibiotic therapy, and 8 individuals did not enter the study when the final report of the bacterial cultures became available and was found to be negative. One sample was prepared for determination of the phagocytosis of opsonized Escherichia coli by granulocytes and monocytes following the test protocol (Phagotest, Orpegen, Heidelberg, Germany).

A second sample was processed to assess the oxidative burst by measuring the rate of oxidative conversion of the fluorogenic substrate dihydrorhodamine 123 (DHR 123) to rhodamine 123 (12), elicited by the incorporation of unlabeled opsonized E. coli by granulocytes and monocytes (Bursttest, Orpegen, Heidelberg, Germany). The ratio of bacteria to phagocyte was kept constant at 25 : 1. To eliminate autofluorescence, daily controls were run concomitantly. The cells were counted on a fluorescence-activated cell sorter utilizing blue-green light of 488 nm wavelength (FACScan, Becton Dickinson, Mountain view, California, USA). A life gate was set in the histogram of the red fluorescence (propidium iodide, PI) to include cells with DNA content of at least a human cell (to exclude bacterial aggregates). The percentage of phagocytizing or DHR 123-oxidizing cells (recruitment) was determined, and the number of ingested bacteria per phagocytizing neutrophil or monocyte was calculated from the mean fluorescence channel following the test protocol. Furthermore, the mean fluorescence channel of the subpopulation of DHR 123-oxidizing granulocytes and monocytes was measured. All tests were run in triplicate. The intraday variance of the method was 6.7 and 5.9%, and the interday variance was 8.5 and 8.9% for the Phagotest and Bursttest respectively.

Preliminary testing ruled out diurnal variations of the tested parameters. In addition, samples from eight individuals with acute pneumonia were spun down after lysis of the erythrocytes. Plasma was removed and the cells were washed three times with phosphate buffered saline (PBS). After subsequent incubation for 6 h at 4°C with plasma from healthy individuals, phagocytosis and oxidative burst was determined as described above.

Data are expressed as mean ± standard error of mean (SEM). A one-way repeated measures ANOVA was used for means of comparison, with differences being significant at $p < 0.05$.

RESULTS

Both tests showed a significant difference between the groups without acute infection (groups 1, 3, and 5) and the patients with acute bronchopneumonia (groups 2, 4, and 6). Both phagocytosis and oxidative burst activity were decreased significantly compared to the control group (Figs. 1 and 2). No differences were observed between patients with stable COPD without acute pneumonia (groups 3 and 5) and the healthy control group (group 1).

The percentage of phagocytizing granulocytes in the patients with bronchopneumonia was 80% ± 1.3 (group 2), 79% ± 1.5 (group 4) and 75% ± 1.5 (group 6) compared to 88% ± 1.6 in the healthy controls ($p < 0.05$). Similar changes were observed in the monocyte subpopulation (Fig. 1).

The burst activity of the granulocytes was also attenuated in the acute pneumonia groups, compared to the healthy controls or the COPD patients without pneumonia. The mean fluorescence channel was 270 ± 18 (group 2), 245 ± 12 (group 4) and 260 ± 15 (group 6) compared to 381 ± 21 in group 1 ($p < 0.05$).

Incubation of phagocytes from individuals with COPD and ABP with plasma from healthy controls reversed the observed changes. The number of phagocytized E. coli/granulocyte was 8.5 ± 0.36 with own plasma and 11.7 ± 0.43 with plasma from healthy individuals. Oxidative burst activity also normalized. The mean fluorescence channel was 278 ± 21 prior to substitution of the plasma and 352 ± 29 after the exchange.

DISCUSSION

From our results we conclude, that acute bronchopneumonia in COPD, but not stable COPD by itself, is associated with an impairment in phagocytic activity and frequency as well as with an attenuated oxidative burst of both blood granulocytes and monocytes. Therefore we speculate that the observed functional changes of the phagocytes in acute

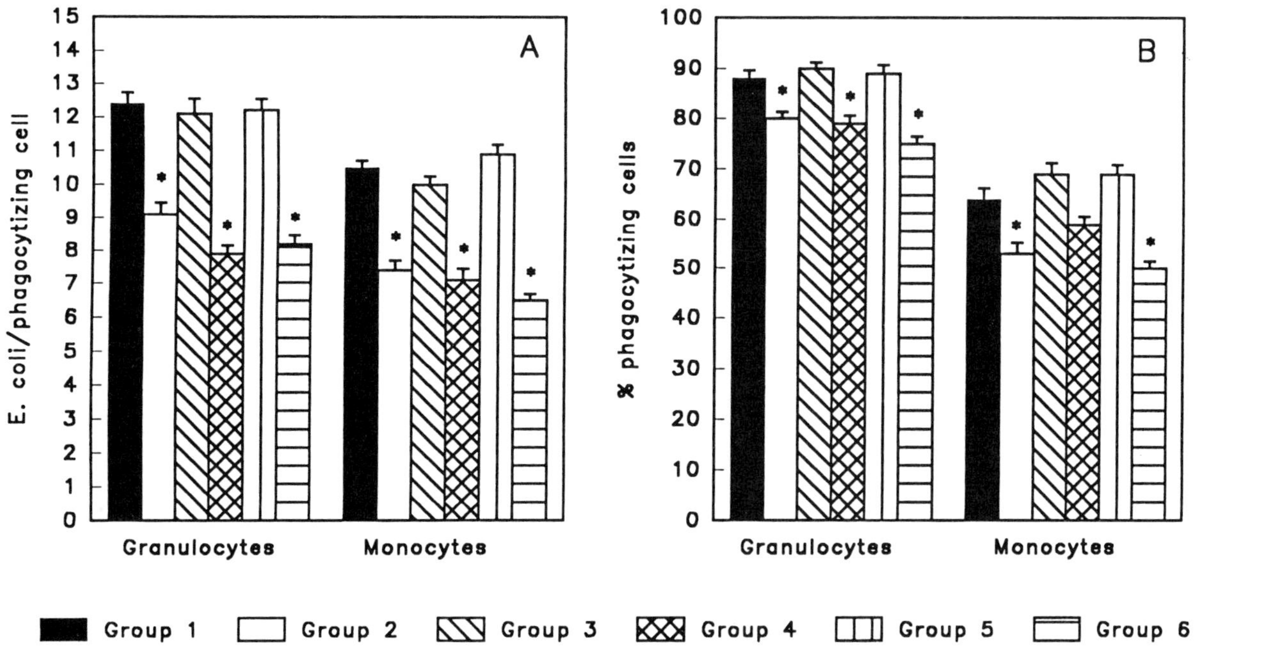

Fig. 1. Phagocytosis of opsonized E. coli by granulocytes and monocytes. Panel A represents the number of E. coli/granulocyte or monocyte of the subpopulation of phagocytizing cells. Panel B shows the percentage of phagocytizing granulocytes or monocytes (recruitment). Bars represent means ± SEM. Group 1, healthy controls; group 2, previously healthy patients with acute bacterial bronchopneumonia (ABP); group 3, patients with chronic obstructive airway disease taking inhaled corticosteroids (IC); group 4, patients with COPD taking IC and ABP; group 5, patients with COPD taking oral corticosteroids (OC); group 6, patients with COPD with ABP, taking OC. Asterisks denote significant difference ($p < 0.05$).

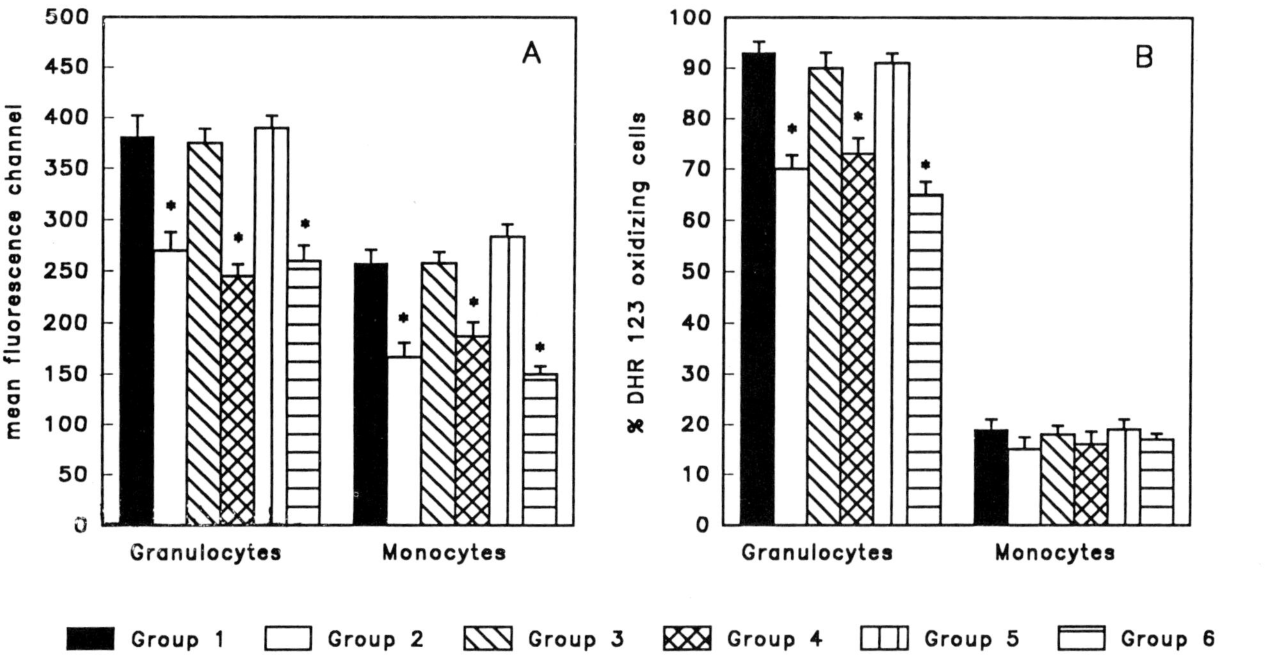

Fig. 2. Oxidative burst of granulocytes and monocytes. Panel A represents the mean fluorescence channel for granulocytes or monocytes of the subpopulation of dihydrorhodamine 123 (DHR 123)-oxidizing cells. Panel B shows the percentage of granulocytes or monocytes oxidizing DHR 123 (recruitment). Bars represent means ± SEM. Group 1, healthy controls; group 2, previously healthy patients with acute bacterial bronchopneumonia (ABP); group 3, patients with COPD taking inhaled corticosteroids (IC); group 4, patients with COPD taking ICs and ABP; group 5, patients with COPD taking oral corticosteroids (OC); group 6, patients with COPD with ABP taking OC. Asterisks denote significant difference ($p < 0.05$).

infections are due to the acute inflammation and not caused by the underlying COPD.

The total killing capacity of all mobilized blood granulocytes was, however, still slightly increased in the groups with ABP, partially because the decreased activity of each granulocyte was offset by an increase in the total number of circulating phagocytes. Incubation of phagocytes from patients with pneumonia with serum from healthy individuals reversed the observed changes. These findings suggest the presence of modulating plasma factors on phagocyte function in acute infections. The nature of these factors is not yet clear, and is the subject of current studies.

In accordance with previously published data, both tests failed to demonstrate subpopulations of granulocytes with different functional activities in acute bronchopneumonia (13). Monocytes, however, seem to incorporate E. coli at a slower rate compared to granulocytes, and the oxidative burst activity and recruitment was remarkably lower. These findings probably reflect the different biological roles of granulocytes and monocytes in inflammation (14).

Our observations are in good accordance with other studies where patients with various infections, including pneumonia, were examined, and blood neutrophil phagocytosis was found to be decreased (8, 13, 15, 16) or the oxidative burst was attenuated in bronchial bacterial infections (10). Other groups, however, observed an increase in the neutrophil oxidative metabolism in chronic bronchitis, compared to healthy controls (9), or an incease in neutrophil oxidative metabolism in acute infections (17). The discrepancies with our study can be partially explained by different study designs. Some factors crucial to phagocytosis and not addressed in our study, like adherence, opsonisation and chemotaxis, seem to be altered in chronic diseases (18), as COPD is associated with enhanced blood neutrophil chemotaxis (19).

Although no changes in the phagocytosis and oxidative burst of blood granulocytes and monocytes were detected in our study, in stable COPD without ABP, it is assumed that local tissue phagocyte function can be modulated by mediators and cytokines released by other cells involved in the inflammatory response in acute or chronic disease (20, 21). Further studies are necessary to test the effects of chronic airway disease on alveolar macrophages or on pulmonary and bronchial granulocytes.

In summary, we conclude, that acute bacterial bronchopneumonia is associated with an impairment of phagocytic functions and oxidative metabolism in blood. We speculate that the observed changes are due to the acute inflammation, are not a sequel of the chronic airway disease, and are caused by serum factors. Whether local mediators or cytokines modulate alveolar macrophage or airway granulocyte function remains to be further investigated.

ACKNOWLEDGEMENTS

This study was supported in part by Orpegen GmbH, Heidelberg, Germany, and by a grant from the American Heart Association, Nebraska Affiliate, 9304545S.

REFERENCES

1. Wardle EN. Assessment of neutrophil function. Postgrad Med J 62: 997–1000, 1986.
2. Lehrer RI, Ganz T, Selsted ME. Babior BM, Curnutte JT. Neutrophils and host defense. Ann Intern Med 19: 127–142, 1988.
3. Ho JL. Antimicrobial functions of macrophages. In: Klempner MS, Styrt B, Ho J, eds. Phagocytes and disease. Dordrecht: Kluwer Academic, 59–90, 1989.
4. Rosenberg-Arska M, Hoepelman IM, Verhoef J. Antimicrobial functions of neutrophils. In: Klempner MS, Styrt B, Ho J, eds. Phagocytes and disease. Dordrecht: Kluwer Academic, 43–55, 1989.
5. Donabedian HD. Congenital and acquired neutrophil abnormalities. In: Klempner MS, Styrt B, Ho J, eds. Phagocytes and disease. Dordrecht: Kluwer Academic, 103–118, 1989.
6. Rotrosen D, Gallin JI. Disorders of phagocytes function. Ann Rev Immunol 5: 127–150, 1987.
7. Kelly MK, Brown JM, Thong YH. Neutrophil and monocyte adherence in diabetes mellitus, alcohol cirrhosis, uraemia and elderly patients. Int Arch Allergy Immunol 78: 132–138, 1985.
8. Fietta A, Bersani C, De Rose V, Grassi FA, Mangiarotti P, Uccelli M, Grassi C. Evaluation of systemic host defense mechanisms in chronic bronchitis. Respiration 53: 37–43, 1988.
9. Venge P, Rak S, Steinholtz L, Håkansson L, Lindblatt G. Neutrophil function in chronic bronchitis. Eur Respir J 4: 536–543, 1991.
10. Laharrague P, Corberand J, Fillola G, Leophonte P, Gleizes B, Fontanilles AM, Gyrard E. Polymorphonuclear dysfunction in bronchopulmonary diseases in human adults. J Clin Lab Immunol 17: 21–24, 1985.
11. Weiss SJ. Tissue destruction by neutrophils. N Engl J Med 320: 365–376, 1989.
12. Rothe G, Oser A, Valet G. Dihydrorhodamine 123: A new flow cytometric indicator for respiratory burst activity in neutrophil granulocytes. Naturwissenschaften 75: 354–355, 1988.
13. Bassoe CF. Flow cytometric studies on phagocyte function in bacterial infections. Acta Pathol Microbiol Immunol Scand Sect C 92: 167–171, 1984.
14. Leijh PCJ, van Furth R, van Zwet TL. In vitro determination of phagocytosis and intracellular killing by polymorphonuclear and mononuclear phagocytes. In: Weir DM, Herzenberg LA, Blackwell C, eds. Handbook of experimental immunology. Oxford: Blackwell Scientific, 1–21, 1986.
15. Kolodkina LA, Shkliarevich NA, Dovnar TE. Chemotaxis phagocytosis and metabolic activation of leukocytes in patients with acute pneumonia. Ter Arkh 63: 27–30, 1990.
16. Gabrilovitch D, Ivanova L, Serebrovskaya L, Shepeleva G, Pokrovsky V. Clinical significance of neutrophil functional activity in HIV infection. Scand J Infect Dis 26: 41–47, 1994.
17. Pauksens K, Sjölin J, Venge P. Chemiluminescence of polymorphonuclear leukocytes and whole blood during acute bacterial infection. Scand J Infect Dis 21: 277–284, 1989.

18. MacGregor RR. Granulocyte adherence changes reduced by hemodialysis, endotoxin, epinephrine, and glucocorticoids. Ann Intern Med 24: 64–68, 1977.
19. Burnett D, Chamba A, Hill SL, Stockley RA. Neutrophils from subjects with chronic obstructive lung disease show enhanced chemotaxis and extracellular proteolysis. Lancet 2: 1043–1046, 1987.
20. Georgilis K, Klempner MS. Cytokinines: interaction with phagocytes and therapeutic potential. In: Klempner MS, Styrt B, Ho J, eds. Phagocytes and disease. Dordrecht: Kluwer Academic, 171–191, 1989.
21. Steppling H. Gesteigerte Sauerstoff-Radikal-Produktion von Alveolarmakrophagen und Blutmonocyten bei ARDS. Prax Klin Pneumol 40: 226–228, 1986.

Submitted December 21, 1994; accepted April 7, 1995

Scand J Infect Dis 27: 375–380, 1995 ORIGINAL ARTICLE

Interleukin-6, C-Reactive Protein, Lactoferrin and White Blood Cell Count in Patients with S. aureus Septicemia

BO SÖDERQUIST[1], KARL-GÖSTA SUNDQVIST[2], IAN JONES[3], HANS HOLMBERG[1] and TOMAS VIKERFORS[1]

From the Departments of [1]Infectious Diseases, and [3]Clinical Chemistry, Örebro Medical Center Hospital, Örebro, and [2]Clinical Immunology, Huddinge University Hospital, Huddinge, Sweden

In a prospective study of 65 patients with S. aureus septicemia, the clinical value of measuring serum IL-6 and lactoferrin levels was assessed and compared with CRP levels and WBC count. 20/65 (31%) patients had a CRP value $\leq$ 100 mg/l on admission and 10 (50%) and 11 (55%) of these had serum levels of IL-6 > 100 pg/ml or lactoferrin > 2.0 mg/l, respectively. 41/64 (64%) patients had a WBC count $\leq 15.0 \times 10^9$/l and the corresponding figures for increased IL-6 and lactoferrin values were 29 (71%) and 21 (51%) patients, respectively. The high concentrations of IL-6 and lactoferrin on admission decreased rapidly during the hospital stay, better reflecting the clinical course than CRP and WBC count. Patients with endocarditis showed higher IL-6 levels and body temperatures both on admission and during the first days of hospitalization compared with patients without endocarditis.

B. Söderquist, MD, Department of Infectious Diseases, Örebro Medical Center Hospital, S-701 85 Örebro, Sweden

INTRODUCTION

Although septicemia is a serious disease with considerable mortality, the symptoms and signs on admission may be almost identical to those of a viral infection. From a clinical point of view there is an urgent need for more sensitive and specific indicators of severe infection than those we use today, namely C-reactive protein (CRP) and white blood cell (WBC) count. Furthermore, we need parameters that tell us whether the septicemia is complicated and treatment is successful.

The early phase of inflammation releases a cascade of different cytokines. These are important for both potentiating and modulating the inflammatory response and for the recruitment and activation of neutrophils. In the initial phase of the inflammatory response, as in septicemia, IL-1 and TNF-α are the most important cytokines (1–6).

Bacterial products and early produced cytokines stimulate various cell types, particularly monocytes/macrophages, fibroblasts and endothelial cells, to produce interleukin-6 (IL-6) (7). The important effects of this pluripotent cytokine include stimulation of B-cells into antibody-producing cells (8), activation and degranulation of neutrophils (9) and stimulation of hepatocytes to produce acute-phase proteins, for instance CRP (10).

Lactoferrin is an iron-binding glycoprotein present in specific (secondary) granules of neutrophils. These granules have been shown to be the exclusive source of circulating lactoferrin (11) and the serum levels reflect the activation of neutrophils in vivo (12). Lactoferrin contributes to the host defence by promoting neutrophil adhesiveness (13) and displaying antibacterial effects (14–16).

The aim of the present study was clinically to evaluate the information obtained by measuring serum IL-6 and lactoferrin levels in patients with S. aureus septicemia and to compare this information with that of routine diagnostic parameters.

PATIENTS AND METHODS

Patients admitted to the Department of Infectious Diseases of the Örebro Medical Center Hospital between 1988–92 with a suspected clinical diagnosis of S. aureus septicemia on admission were included in this prospective study. During the study period, S. aureus septicemia was diagnosed in 140 patients.

Patients

A total of 339 serum samples from 65 consecutive patients with S. aureus septicemia were further analysed. The characteristics of the patients have been described in detail elsewhere (17). The median age of the total study population was 71 years (range 10–91 years) and 59% were men. Patients with staphylococcal septicemia not suspected at the time of admission were not included. These patients were in no respect intentionally selected. Their age distribution was almost identical (median 73 years) with that of the study group.

Antibiotic treatment was instituted not later than the day after admission. In most cases the therapy was switched to cloxacillin when the results of the blood cultures became available.

Complicated septicemia, defined as a complicated clinical course with septic metastasis, such as acute osteomyelitis, septic arthritis or extensive abscesses (long-standing, insufficiently drained) was found in 45 patients. 15 patients with endocarditis (1 definite, 6 probable and 8 possible) according to the strict case definitions given by von Reyn et al. (18) were included. Five patients (8%) died soon after the acute septicemic event (3–15 days after admission to hospital). Uncomplicated septicemia, i.e. septicemia without any evident complicating foci was present in 20 patients.

The patients served as their own controls, as they were followed throughout the complete clinical course of the disease and serum samples were collected sequentially. As negative controls, serum IL-6 and lactoferrin concentrations were analysed in serum samples from blood donors (n = 20).

Laboratory methods

IL-6 analyses were performed with a commercial enzyme immunoassay [IL-6 EASIA (enzyme amplified sensitivity immunoassay), Medgenix Diagnostics, Fleurus, Belgium]. IL-6 was not detectable (< 3 pg/ml) in the blood donor population.
CRP was analysed by an immunoturbidometric method in routine use (BM/Hitachi 911, Boehringer Mannheim GmbH, Germany). The reference range was < 5 mg/l.
Peripheral WBC count was determined by a method in routine use at the Department of Clinical Chemistry. The reference range was 4.0–9.0 × 10^9/l.
Lactoferrin Polystyrene microplates were coated overnight with sheep anti-human lactoferrin (The Binding Site, Birmingham, England) in a 0.05 mol/l $NaHCO_3$ buffer, pH 9.5. The antibody concentration was 12 mg protein/l. The wells were then washed 5 times with a washing solution (19). The standard curve (2.0–100 μg/l) was based upon human lactoferrin (cat. no. L3770, Sigma Chemical Company, St Louis, USA). The serum samples were diluted 1:60 in most cases, 1:100 and 1:200 dilutions being used for the few highly concentrated samples. The patient samples and the standard curve were diluted in a buffer described by Antonsen et al. (20). Samples and standards (100 μl) were pipetted into the wells in duplicate and the plate was incubated for 60 min. The plate was then washed 4 times before the second 60 min incubation with a horseradish peroxidase labelled sheep anti-human lactoferrin (The Binding Site, Birmingham). This antibody was diluted in the wash solution to a concentration of 5 mg protein/l. The plate was then washed 4 times before the substrate incubation step. The substrate consisted of freshly prepared orthophenylenediamine (OPD tablets, Dakopatts A/S, Copenhagen, Denmark) dissolved in 0.1 mol/l citrate-phosphate buffer, pH 5.0 (12 mg OPD + 18 ml buffer + 8 μl 30% hydrogen peroxide). The incubation time was 5–10 min and the absorbance read at 490 nm after the reaction was stopped with 1 mol/l sulphuric acid. The recovery of a serum sample spiked with 1 mg/l lactoferrin was 85%. The within- and between-series imprecision was 6.9% ($n = 15$) and 8.7% ($n = 11$) respectively at a level of 1.9 mg/l. In the blood donors ($n = 20$), the mean lactoferrin value (± S.D.) was 0.86 ± 0.43 mg/l. The upper limit of normal lactoferrin values was defined as mean value + 2 S.D. = 1.72 mg/l.
Erytrocyte sedimentation rate (ESR) was determined by routine laboratory procedure (Westergren method). Normal ESR is defined as < 15 mm/l h.

The following levels of routine acute-phase parameters, generally regarded as indicative of a bacterial infection, were in this study assigned as CRP > 100 mg/l, WBC count > 15.0 × 10^9/l, and ESR ≥ 50 mm/l h. The corresponding limits for IL-6 and lactoferrin were set to > 100 pg/ml and > 2.0 mg/l, respectively.

Statistical analysis

IL-6 values < 3 pg/ml were treated as 0 and values > 1,000 pg/ml were truncated at 1,000. The Mann-Whitney U test was used when

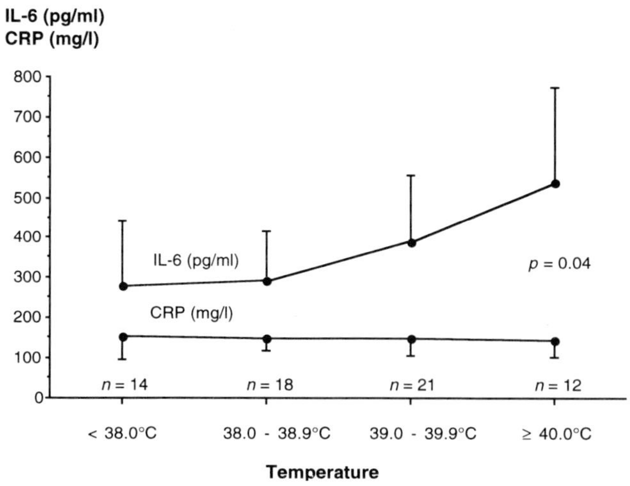

Fig. 1. Mean IL-6 and mean CRP serum concentrations (95% confidence intervals) related to body temperature on admission in 65 patients with S. aureus septicemia.

comparing various parameters in different groups, since these parameters were not normally distributed. Correlations between parameters were made using Spearman's rank correlation test. Fisher's exact test was used when comparing proportions. A p-value of < 0.05 was considered as significant. The statistical packages StatView II™ and InStat were used for the calculations.

RESULTS

The acute-phase parameters were elevated on admission in most of the 65 patients with S. aureus septicemia, as shown in Table I.

The number of patients with an increased lactoferrin level (> 2.0 mg/l) was 41/65 (63%) and significantly higher than in those with an increased (> 15.0 × 10^9/l) WBC count 23/64 (36%) ($p = 0.003$). Elevated serum IL-6 concentrations (> 100 pg/ml) were found in 50/65 (77%) patients on admission and elevated CRP values (> 100 mg/l) in 45/65 (69%) cases (ns).

Correlations between lactoferrin levels and WBC counts ($r_s = 0.55$, $p = 0.0001$) as well as IL-6 concentrations were noted. CRP correlated with all the other parameters. Body temperature on admission correlated only with serum IL-6 concentrations on admission, as illustrated in Fig. 1.

The mean IL-6 and CRP concentrations on admission in relation to the delay (number of days between onset of

Table I. *Acute-phase parameters at the time of hospital admission in 65 patients with S. aureus septicemia*

	IL-6[a] (pg/ml)	CRP[a] (mg/l)	WBC count[a] (× 10^9/l)	Lactoferrin[a] (mg/l)	ESR[a] (mm/l h)	Temp[a] (°C)
Elevated levels No (%)	50/65 (77%)	45/65 (69%)	23/64 (36%)	41/65 (63%)	47/61 (77%)	42/65 (65%)
Mean (± S.D.)	366 ± 326	149 ± 83	13.4 ± 6.9	3.0 ± 2.4	77 ± 35	38.9 ± 1.1
Median	220	143	11.95	2.5	82	39.0

[a] Elevated levels were defined as IL-6 > 100 pg/ml, CRP > 100 mg/l, WBC count > 15.0 × 10^9/l, Lactoferrin > 2.0 mg/l, ESR ≥ 50 mm/l h, Temp ≥ 38.5°C.

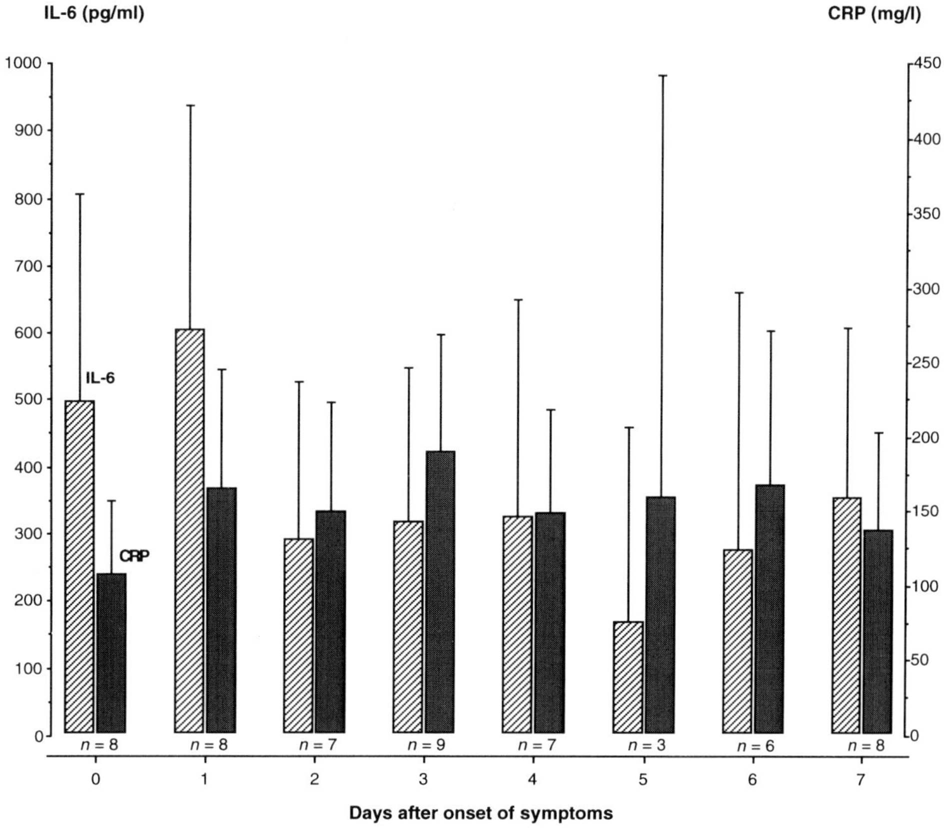

Fig. 2. Mean IL-6 (▨) and mean CRP (■) serum concentrations (95% confidence intervals) on admission related to days after onset of symptoms in 56 patients with S. aureus septicemia (n = number of patients analysed at indicated time).

symptoms and admission to hospital) are illustrated in Fig. 2. The highest serum IL-6 values were seen in patients with a short delay. However, IL-6 values were still elevated in patients with a delay of one week. The CRP values were elevated to the same level, regardless of the number of days between onset of symptoms and admission, except in patients with a very short delay (< 1 day) in whom the mean CRP value was lower.

The kinetics of the acute-phase parameters are illustrated in Fig. 3. A rapid decrease in the acute-phase reactants was seen, being most pronounced for IL-6 and lactoferrin. 25/31 patients with a short delay (≤ 3 days) showed gradually decreasing IL-6 concentrations during the first 3 days after admission (1 patient was followed up for less than 3 days), whereas an additional increase in CRP values during the first 3 days after admission was seen in 14/31 patients ($p = 0.008$).

No statistically significant differences regarding the levels of the acute-phase parameters were found on admission between the patients with complicated and uncomplicated S. aureus septicemia.

Patients with endocarditis had higher serum IL-6 concentrations on admission than had patients without endocarditis ($p = 0.0275$). No such differences were found for the other acute-phase parameters. A higher mean temperature, 39.6°C, was recorded in patients with endocarditis, than in those without endocarditis (mean 38.6°C) ($p = 0.0025$). The kinetic profiles of serum IL-6 levels and body temperature were also different in these 2 groups during the first days after admission.

No differences were found concerning the acute-phase parameters on admission when comparing non-survivors ($n = 5$) with survivors ($p > 0.05$).

A CRP value ≤ 100 mg/l on admission was found in 20/65 (31%) patients and in those cases a serum IL-6 value > 100 pg/ml or a lactoferrin value > 2.0 mg/l was found in 10 (50%) and 11 (55%) cases, respectively. An increase in either IL-6 or lactoferrin was found in 15 (75%) patients.

A WBC count $\leq 15.0 \times 10^9$/l was found in 41/64 (64%) patients and in those cases an increased IL-6 or lactoferrin value was found in 29 (71%) and 21 (51%) patients, respectively. An increase in either IL-6 or lactoferrin was found in 35 (85%) patients. In patients with a WBC count $\leq 15.0 \times 10^9$/l or CRP < 100 mg/l on admission ($n = 46$) increased IL-6 (> 100 pg/ml) was found in 33 (72%) cases, increased lactoferrin (> 2.0 mg/l) in 25 (54%) patients, and either increased IL-6 or increased lactoferrin was found in 39 (85%) cases. If both a WBC count $\leq 15.0 \times 10^9$/l and a CRP ≤ 100 mg/l were present, the corresponding figure for increased IL-6 or lactoferrin was 11/16 (69%).

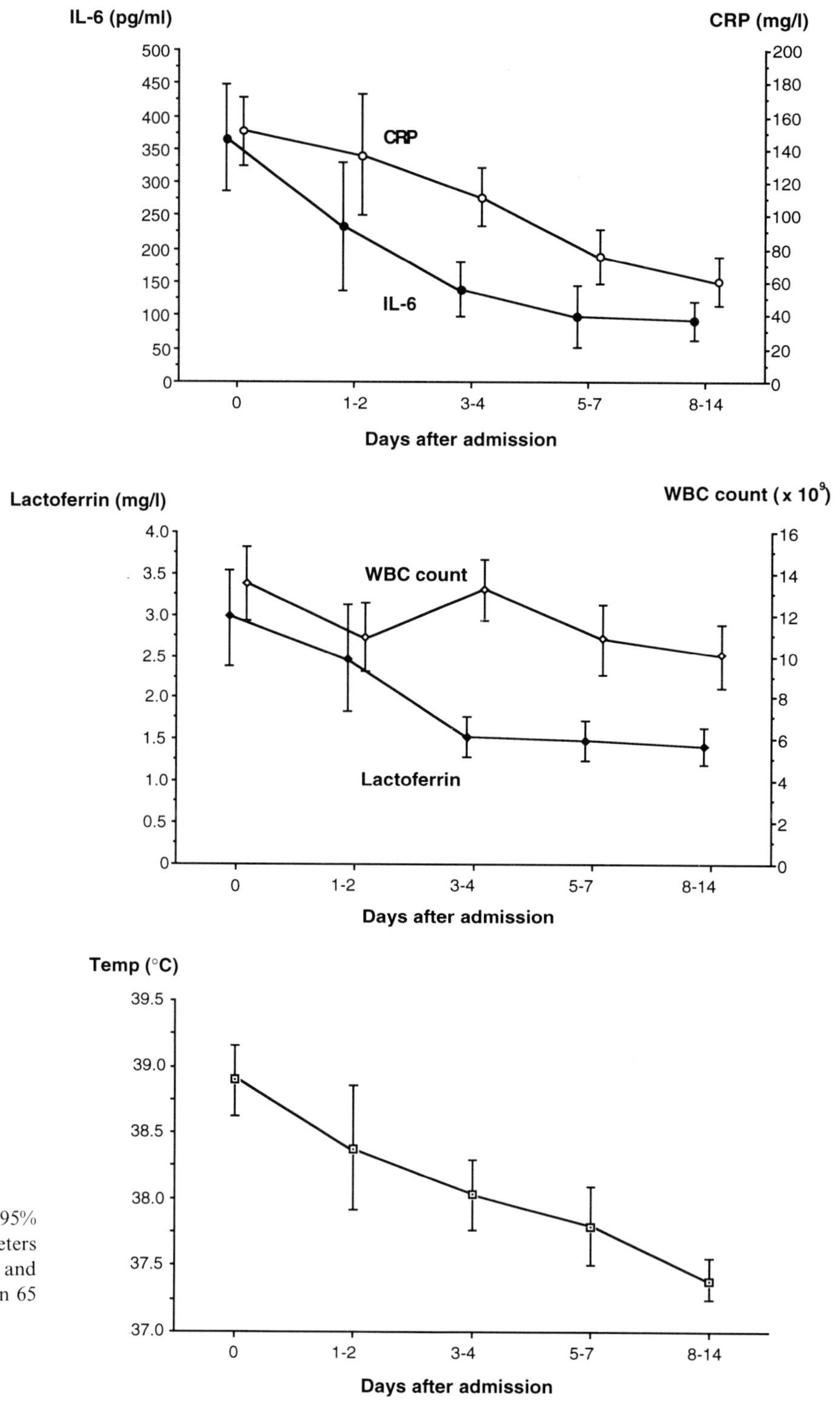

Fig. 3. The kinetics (mean values and 95% confidence intervals) of acute-phase parameters (IL-6, CRP, lactoferrin and WBC count) and body temperature during the first 14 days in 65 patients with S. aureus septicemia.

DISCUSSION

In the present study, we found that most of the patients with septicemia due to S. aureus had high IL-6 and CRP levels on admission. Patients with a short delay (≤ 3 days) between onset of symptoms and admission to hospital had in most cases rapidly decreasing serum IL-6 levels, whereas an ongoing increase in serum CRP levels was seen in about half the cases during the first 3 days after admission. This finding is probably due to the differing kinetics of IL-6 and CRP, as CRP is induced by IL-6 in a dose- and time-dependent manner (10). Since IL-6 elevation during infections precedes the CRP increase in serum by hours to days (21) it may be diagnostically beneficial to determine IL-6 levels rather than CRP on admission. This could also be demonstrated in the present study. The diagnostic benefit of IL-6 vis-à-vis CRP, based on the different kinetics of IL-6 and CRP may, however, be diminished due to localized persistent subclinical infections, which in some cases give rise to increased CRP values before the patient develops septicemia and arrives at the hospital.

The IL-6 concentrations were elevated on admission to rather high levels even 1 week after onset. Conceivably, the initial IL-6 elevation during the early phase of infection is followed by a sustained IL-6 production as long as the infection is present. Complications such as osteomyelitis, septic arthritis or extensive abscesses might stimulate further cytokine production by the release of toxins or degraded bacterial components, resulting in long-lasting elevation of cytokine concentrations (17).

The neutrophils play an important role in the initial phase of the bacterial infection. Several cytokines are involved in this process. IL-6 has been shown to activate neutrophils and induce secretion of granule markers, including lactoferrin, in a dose-dependent manner (9). In our study we found a significant correlation between the IL-6 and lactoferrin concentrations on admission, but not between IL-6 and WBC. A significantly larger proportion of the patients (63%) had increased lactoferrin levels as compared with those with increased WBC counts (36%). As an indicator of the degree of neutrophil activation in an acute bacterial infection, the determination of lactoferrin seems to give additional diagnostic information, compared with analysing WBC count only.

The kinetics of lactoferrin in plasma have been studied (22) in 8 patients with acute bacterial infections (meningitis and pneumonia). Increased lactoferrin levels on admission were found in 50% of the patients and these quickly returned to normal during the clinical course. Patients with sepsis have been reported to have increased lactoferrin concentrations on admission (23) and the levels are similar to those found in our study. Children with localized bacterial infections and septicemia (24) as well as elderly patients with infections (25) had significantly higher lactoferrin levels than corresponding controls. Correlations between lactoferrin and CRP (25), IL-6 (23) and WBC count (22, 23) have been reported.

Patients with endocarditis had higher levels of acute-phase parameters and body temperature, than patients without endocarditis during the first days after admission. Consequently, a S. aureus septicemia complicated by endocarditis may be indicated by the kinetics of the acute-phase parameters and the pattern of body temperature during the clinical course.

Correlations between the serum IL-6 level and body temperature and between IL-6 and CRP have been reported (26), i.e. consistent with the results of the present study. This emphasizes the importance of monitoring body temperature as an indicator of the course of the disease.

A recurrent diagnostic problem is the patient with septicemia, despite normal or only slightly increased concentrations of acute-phase reactants on admission. This finding could be explained by a very short delay between onset of symptoms and admission to hospital but there may also be an inability of the host to respond to various inflammatory inducers. We found in our study that patients who upon admission did not show an elevation of WBC counts or of CRP values had increased IL-6 or lactoferrin concentrations in 85% of the cases. When neither the WBC count nor the CRP level was elevated, the corresponding figure for increased IL-6 or lactoferrin was 69%. Low IL-6 and/or low lactoferrin values were related to increased WBC counts and/or increased CRP values in only a few cases, apart from the 18/33 cases with either low IL-6 or low lactoferrin values, where increased CRP values or WBC counts were found.

These findings indicate that measurement of serum IL-6 and lactoferrin concentrations might add important diagnostic information, but since we lack a control group of patients with other infections, this statement remains to be verified by further studies.

It was concluded that in patients with S. aureus septicemia, the levels of serum IL-6 on admission give additional diagnostic information, compared with CRP only. Serum lactoferrin levels more accurately reflect neutrophil activation than does the WBC count. During hospitalization, IL-6 and lactoferrin concentrations better reflect the clinical course than do CRP levels and WBC counts and should be of clinical value.

ACKNOWLEDGEMENTS

We thank Ewa-Lena Sjöberg for skilful laboratory assistance, Assistant Professor Lennart Bodin for statistical advice, and the Research Committee of Örebro County Council for financial support.

REFERENCES

1. Bone RC. The pathogenesis of sepsis. Ann Intern Med 115: 457–469, 1991.
2. Dinarello CA. Interleukin-1 and interleukin-1 antagonism. Blood 77: 1627–1652, 1991.
3. van Deuren M, Dofferhoff ASM, van der Meer JWM. Cytokines and the response to infection. J Pathol 168: 349–356, 1992.
4. Beutler B, Grau GE. Tumor necrosis factor in the pathogenesis of infectious diseases. Crit Care Med 21 (Suppl): S423–S435, 1993.
5. Bone RC. Gram-positive organisms and sepsis. Arch Intern Med 154: 26–34, 1994.
6. Kunkel SL, Lukacs NW, Kasama T, Strieter RM. Chemotactic cytokines. In: Griffin GE, ed. Cytokines in Infection. London: Baillière Tindall, WB Saunders, 25–36, 1994.
7. Van Snick J. Interleukin-6: an overview. Ann Rev Immunol 8: 253–278, 1990.
8. Heinrich PC, Castell JV, Andus T. Interleukin-6 and the acute phase response. Biochem J 265: 621–636, 1990.
9. Borish L, Rosenbaum R, Albury L, Clark S. Activation of neutrophils by recombinant interleukin 6. Cell Immunol 121: 280–289, 1989.

10. Castell JV, Gómez-Lechón MJ, David M, Fabra R, Trullenque R, Heinrich PC. Acute-phase response of human hepatocytes: regulation of acute-phase protein synthesis by interleukin-6. Hepatology 12: 1179–1186, 1990.
11. Bennett RM, Kokocinski T. Lactoferrin turnover in man. Clin Sci 57: 453–460, 1979.
12. Lash JA, Coates TD, Lafuze J, Baehner RL, Boxer LA. Plasma lactoferrin reflects granulocyte activation in vivo. Blood 61: 885–888, 1983.
13. Oseas R, Yang H-H, Baehner RL, Boxer LA. Lactoferrin: a promoter of polymorphonuclear leukocyte adhesiveness. Blood 5: 939–945, 1981.
14. Arnold RR, Cole MF, McGhee JR. A bactericidal effect for human lactoferrin. Science 197: 263–265. 1977.
15. Bullen JJ, Armstrong JA. The role of lactoferrin in the bactericidal function of polymorphonuclear leucocytes. Immunology 36: 781–791, 1979.
16. Appelmelk BJ, An YQ, Geerts M, Thijs BG, de Boer HA, MacLaren DM, de Graaff J, Nuijens JH. Lactoferrin is a lipid A-binding protein. Infect Immun 62: 2628–2632, 1994.
17. Söderquist B, Sundqvist K-G, Vikerfors T. Kinetics of interleukin-6, tumor necrosis factor-α and interleukin-1β in patients with Staphylococcus aureus septicemia. Immun Infect Dis 4: 235–242, 1994.
18. von Reyn CF, Levy BS, Arbeit RD, Friedland G, Crumpacker CS. Infective endocarditis: an analysis based on strict case definitions. Ann Intern Med 94: 505–518, 1981.
19. Gutteberg TJ, Slørdal L, Kolmannskog S. Lactoferrin and C-reactive protein in response to cytostatic drugs with emphasis on methotrexate. Pediatr Hematol Oncol 4: 315–322, 1987.
20. Antonsen S, Wiggers P, Dalhøj J, Blaabjerg O. An enzyme-linked immunosorbent assay for plasma-lactoferrin. Concentrations in 362 healthy, adult blood donors. Scand J Clin Lab Invest 53: 133–144, 1993.
21. Heney D, Lewis IJ, Evans SW, Banks R, Bailey CC, Whicher JT. Interleukin-6 and its relationship to C-reactive protein and fever in children with febrile neutropenia. J Infect Dis 165: 886–890, 1992.
22. Hansen NE, Karle H, Andersen V, Malmquist J, Hoff GE. Neutrophilic granulocytes in acute bacterial infection. Sequential studies on lysozyme, myeloperoxidase and lactoferrin. Clin Exp Immunol 26: 463–468, 1976.
23. Nuijens JH, Abbink JJ, Wachtfogel YT, Colman RW, Eerenberg AJM, Dors D, Kamp AM, Strack van Schijndel RJM, Thijs LG, Hack CE. Plasma elastase α_1-antitrypsin and lactoferrin in sepsis: evidence for neutrophils as mediators in fatal sepsis. J Lab Clin Med 119: 159–168, 1992.
24. Tegtmeyer FK, Maacks S, van Wees J, Wood WG. Elastase-α_1-proteinasinhibitorkomplex (Eα_1PI) und Lactoferrinplasmakonzentrationen bei viralen und bakteriellen Infektionen. Monatsschr Kinderheilkd 139: 96–101, 1991. [in German]
25. Adeyemi EO, D'Anastasio C, Impallomeni MG, Hodgson HJ. Plasma lactoferrin as a marker of infection in elderly individuals. Aging Clin Exp Res 4: 135–137, 1992.
26. Damas P, Ledoux D, Nys M, Vrindts Y, De Groote D, Franchimont P, Lamy M. Cytokine serum level during severe sepsis in human IL-6 as a marker of severity. Ann Surg 215: 356–362, 1992.

Submitted January 16, 1995; accepted March 22, 1995

Scand J Infect Dis 27: 381–384, 1995 ORIGINAL ARTICLE

High IL-6 Serum Levels are Associated with Septic Shock and Mortality in Septic Patients with Severe Leukopenia due to Hematological Malignancies

MASSIMO ANTONELLI[1], GIAN MARCO RAPONI[2], PIETRO MARTINO[3], GIOVANNI ROSA[1], GIORGIO CONTI[1], J. JALOUK[3] and ALESSANDRO GASPARETTO[1]

From the [1]Institute of Anesthesiology and Intensive Care, [2]First Department of Microbiology and [3]Department of Hematology, 'La Sapienza' University of Rome, Rome, Italy

The serum levels of immunoreactive interleukin-6 (IL-6) and tumor necrosis factor (TNF) were analyzed in 14 leukopenic patients with documented sepsis, at 60 min (T0), 24 h (T1), 48 h (T2) and 1 week (T3) after the onset of sepsis syndrome. Sera from 10 leukopenic patients without sepsis (controls) were also tested. All septic patients had high IL-6 levels at T0. These levels persisted only in the seven patients who died of septic shock, presenting a 30-fold increase ($p < 0.001$) as compared to the survivors and the controls. At T3, 7 survivors had recovered from sepsis and showed low IL-6 serum levels. The TNF serum concentration always <30 pg/ml in both the subjects and in the controls. The C-reactive protein (CRP) and clinical parameters appeared to be less specifically associated with shock and mortality than IL-6.

M. Antonelli, MD, Istituto di Anestesiologia e Rianimazione, Università 'La Sapienza', Policlinico Umberto I, Viale del Policlinico, 155, I-00161 Rome, Italy

INTRODUCTION

Cytokines such as tumor necrosis factor (TNF) and interleukin 6 (IL-6) are believed to exert a crucial pathophysiological role in acute sepsis, and septic shock (1). It has been suggested that TNF may be essential in eliciting the complete spectrum of acute hemodynamic and metabolic disruption associated with bacterial sepsis (2). Moreover, TNF may also induce a shock-like condition when administered to animals at 10–100 mg/kg (3). Interleukin-6 has been considered to be a mediator of a variety of diseases when overexpressed in vivo or when produced in an unbalanced fashion during trauma, surgery and all states of infection (4).

Patients with hematological malignancies are at the highest risk of dying of sepsis because of their underlying disease and immunosuppressive treatment. It is still not clear whether cytokines, such as TNF and IL-6, may play a role during sepsis and septic shock, when one of the major sources of cytokine production, i.e. white blood cells (WBC) is seriously depleted, as in leukopenic conditions. Moreover, the steroids currently administered in these clinical settings, have the well known property of down-regulating cytokines, making the picture more complicated.

The aim of the present study was, therefore, to investigate whether TNF and IL-6 are released into the bloodstream of leukopenic patients with sepsis syndrome, and if these levels can be correlated with the onset of septic shock and mortality.

MATERIAL AND METHODS

A total of 14 leukopenic patients (age 40 ± 10 years) with sepsis syndrome and 10 leukopenic subjects (age 41 ± 9 years) without sepsis (controls) were studied. Nine of the septic patients had acute myeloid leukemia, 3 had non-lymphoid acute leukemia and 2 non-Hodgkin's lymphoma. All the controls had actue myeloid leukemia.

Leukopenia was defined as a total WBC count $< 1000/\mu l$. All the subjects were leukopenic as a consequence of their underlying disease and immunosuppressive therapy. All the septic patients were already leukopenic before the onset of the sepsis.

Being aware that signs of infection are often scarce in leukopenic patients, we decided to enrol only patients meeting all the criteria for sepsis syndrome, as described by Bone (5). Patients were considered to have developed septic shock when the hypotension lasted for >1 h, despite volume resuscitation, and required vasopressors or doses of dopamine $> 6\ \mu g/kg/min$ (5). The severity of illness was evaluated by means of the APACHE II score. All patients and controls had been receiving low doses of methylprednisolone (20 mg/day), as part of the immunosuppressive therapy, for at least 10 days before the onset of sepsis.

All the subjects or their next of kin gave informed consent under a protocol approved by the ethics committee of the institutions involved.

Blood cell counts, routine laboratory tests and blood gas analyses were evaluated daily. Sample collection for the determination of TNF, IL-6 and C-reactive protein (CRP) was performed over 1 week. On the first day (within 1 h from enrolment), (T0 or basal), a venous blood sample (10 ml) was drawn. The sample collection was then repeated 24 h (T1), 48 h (T2) and 1 week (T3) after T0. The serum samples were clotted and then harvested by centrifugation at $1500 \times g$ for 10 min at 4°C and immediately stored at −80°C until analysis.

 ISSN 0036-5548

Table I. *Clinical parameters and cytokine levels of leukopenic patients*

	Patients with sepsis							
	Survivors ($n = 7$)				Non-survivors ($n = 7$)			
	T0 (basal)	T1 (24 h)	T2 (48 h)	T3 (1 week)	T0 (basal)	T1 (24 h)	T2 (48 h)	Controls ($n = 10$)
APACHE score	20 ± 3.8	—	—	—	19.8 ± 3	—	—	12 ± 3
Mean arterial pressure, mmHg	59.4 ± 8.2	73.3 ± 12.6	83 ± 11*	86 ± 10	65 ± 9	62 ± 7	62 ± 3*	90 ± 5
Pulse	129 ± 6	93 ± 10*	87 ± 13**	77 ± 12	112 ± 23	130 ± 14*	126 ± 6**	88 ± 11
Temperature, °C	39.6 ± 8	37.8 ± 1.4	37.4 ± 1	36.5 ± 0.3	39.4 ± 0.5	38.2 ± 1.4	37.8 ± 1.2	36.3 ± 0.2
WBC/μl	420 ± 260	491 ± 446	948 ± 879	9713 ± 992	496 ± 271	570 ± 447	956 ± 323	580 ± 123
Patients with organ failure/type	—	—	—	—	1/liver	1/kidney	2/kidney, liver	—
TNF, pg/ml	11 ± 3	12 ± 4	13 ± 5	13 ± 4	20 ± 10	13 ± 5	11 ± 2	14 ± 6
IL-6, pg/ml	751 ± 626	65 ± 25**	23 ± 42**	10 ± 6	1281 ± 901	1561 ± 920**	1065 ± 785**	21 ± 13
CRP, mg/L	3.2 ± 0.4	2.7 ± 1.2	4.5 ± 1.7	3.6 ± 1.6	3.2 ± 1	3.3 ± 0.5	3.5 ± 0.7	1.6 ± 0.2

*$p < 0.05$; **$p < 0.001$.
All the data are expressed as mean ± SD.
All non-survivors died within the first 72 h after T0, developing septic shock. Organ failure was the clinical picture at onset in only one patient. In another 3, organ failure was a terminal event. IL-6: survivors, basal vs. T1, T2 and T3 and controls $p < 0.001$; basal survivors vs. non-survivors p = ns. T1, T2 and T3 of survivors vs. T1 and T2 of no-survivors $p < 0.001$. TNF never differed between the survivors, the non-survivors and the controls over the study period. In the surviving group, patient no. 3 at basal time and patient no. 4 at T1 had TNF slightly below the detection limit for the assay (8 and 9 pg/ml respectively); for means calculation their values were considered as missing in both cases. The CRP levels were always within normal range for both the patients and the controls.

The samplings for the cytokine determinations were performed once daily for ethical reasons in order to limit the drawing of blood in already pancytopenic patients. Blood cultures and cultures from other sites were taken when needed in all subjects over the study period.

The CRP was determined by means of the standard turbidometric method; the normal range was 1–5 mg/l.

The TNF and IL-6 levels were determined on the collected samples using the enzyme immunobsorbent assay (ELISA) (Endogen, Massachusetts and R&D System, Minnesota, USA). The detection limit for TNF was 10 pg/ml and for IL-6, 3 pg/ml. TNF alpha values were confirmed by bioassay by using the L-929 TNF-sensitive murine fibrosarcoma cell line, as previously reported for non-leukopenic patients (6).

The t-test, non-parametric tests (median, rank and Kolmogrof tests), linear regression and calculation of correlation coefficients were utilized for the statistical analyses.

RESULTS

All the routine clinical controls (including ECG and echocardiography) performed just prior to the septic episode, excluded cardiomyopathy linked to cardiotoxicity of antineoplastic drugs.

None of the controls (APACHE 12 ± 3) developed sepsis over the study period. The WBC counts did not differ from those of the septic patients (Table I). Of the patients, 50% (7/14), died during the study period. All these patients developed refractory septic shock between T0 and the third day of observation. In all of these subjects, the blood samples, drawn at 24 or 48 h, also corresponded to a time interval ranging between 2 and 6 h after the onset of septic shock.

One of the non-surviving patients had negative cultures, but had disseminated exantema with papulomacular lesions and highly positive serology (indirect immunofluorescene ≥1 : 320) for Herpes-6 virus; another presented fungemia from Candida tropicalis. Another four non-survivors had bacteremias (one Escherichia coli and Enterococcus faecalis, one Pseudomonas aeruginosa, one Acinetobacter anitratus and one Staphylococcus aureus) and another had a bronchoalevolar lavage which was positive for Klebsiella pneumoniae ($> 10^6$ cfu/ml). Five survivors had bacteremias (one Escherichia coli, one Streptococcus mitis, one Staphylococcus epidermidis and Candida albicans, one Pseudomonas aeruginosa and one Staphylococcus epidermidis and Streptococcus). The other 2 survivors had positive urinary cultures for Enterobacter cloacae. All of the surveillance cultures from the controls were negative.

There were no statistical differences between the survivors and the non-survivors in terms of either the APACHE scores or the WBC count (Table I). In addition, the laboratory parameters of these 2 groups were also similar for the entire study period (data not shown). All the control subjects showed normal clinical parameters, with the exception of the WBC count. The CRP, always within the normal range for all the 24 subjects, showed only a slight increase in the 14 septic patients, as compared to the controls.

The TNFα amounts, which never exceeded 30 pg/ml, did not differ between the survivors and the non-survivors nor with regard to the controls. However, the IL-6 levels differed significantly ($p < 0.001$) both after 24 and 48 h after T0 (1561 ± 920 pg/ml for the non-survivors vs. 65.7 ± 25.8 pg/ml for the survivors at T1; 1065 ± 785 pg/ml vs. 23 ± 42 pg/ml at T2) (Table I and Fig. 1).

After 1 week, IL-6 was almost undetectable in all the survivors. As compared to the controls, the non-surviving patients presented significantly higher IL-6 levels at all times. On the other hand, the IL-6 levels measured in the survivors significantly differed from those of the controls only at the admission to protocol, when all of them manifested a sepsis syndrome; however, these were not significantly different after 24 h, 48 h and after one week (Fig. 1). No statistical correlation could be found between individual serum IL-6 levels and heart rate, temperature, mean blood pressure or WBC count by means of calculation of the correlation coefficient.

DISCUSSION

Some studies have demonstrated the role of cytokines in the pathophysiology of septic shock (2, 7). However, data concerning cytokines in leukopenic patients with sepsis and in patients developing refractory septic shock are, to our knowledge lacking. In the present study, TNF did not reach high serum concentrations in the leukopenic septic patients, even when they developed septic shock.

The timing of our sampling could have missed some TNF spikes due to the short half-life of this cytokine.

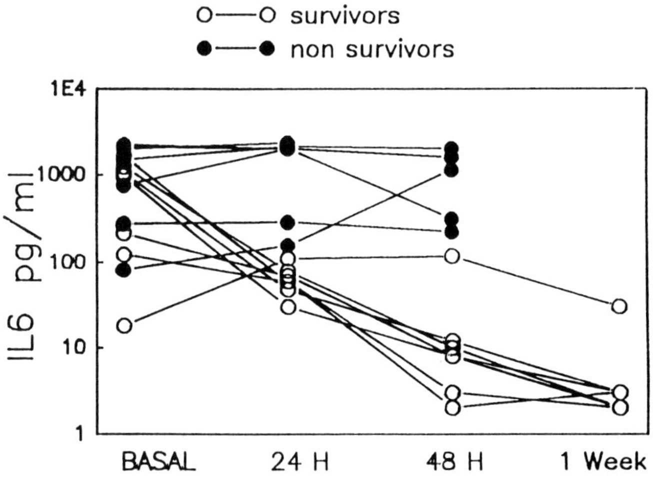

Fig. 1. Individual serum levels of IL-6 and time evolution in all 14 leukopenic septic patients. Note logarithmic scale. The open circles represent the survivors ($n = 7$), while the closed circles represent the non-survivors ($n = 7$). All non-survivors died within the third day of the study, developing refractory septic shock. After 48 h, 2 patients had already died. After 1 week from the onset of sepsis, all survivors had serum IL-6 levels similar to the controls (21 ± 13 pg/ml). The IL-6 levels differed significantly between the 2 groups 24 and 48 h after basal time (see text).

However, the detection of TNF over a prolonged period has been reported in some patients who died of septic shock (8).

On the other hand, the frequency with which this cytokine can be detected in the bloodstream varies greatly in the populations studied (1, 2), and the administration of immunosuppressive therapy may have had a significant influence. Indeed, it is known that steroids block TNF synthesis (9). In contrast, high IL-6 levels in all the 14 neutropenic patients with sepsis syndrome were observed. However, only the 7 patients who died of refractory septic shock maintained high serum levels of IL-6.

These data, showing an association between both septic shock and mortality, seem to be consistent with that reported in critically ill patients without leukopenia (7). No correlation between the IL-6 levels and the CRP concentrations was found and the latter inflammatory protein was always within a normal range and failed to reflect the clinical evolution of sepsis in our patients.

The data presented in the present paper are in conflict with those reported by other authors (10–12). Indeed, the CRP levels in our leukopenic septic patients were lower than those observed in similar groups of patients, but these discrepancies may be due to various factors: the administration of steroids down-regulating the TNF may inhibit one of the most powerful stimuli to CRP production, with a response of less amplitude. Unfortunately cytokine levels were not measured in those studies and data regarding steroid therapy are lacking, preventing a valid comparison with our data. Another possible interfering factor might be the heterogeneity of the sepsis syndrome. The pathogenesis is, in fact, variable and comprises not only Gram-negative but also Gram-positive bacteria and fungi. During these natural infections, the cytokine patterns are somewhat different from those observed after the classical acute endotoxin challenge. Nevertheless, in our group of leukopenic patients with sepsis, CRP values were higher than those found in leukopenic patients without sepsis, even though this was not statistically significant.

Other data reported in the literature are conflicting. Good correlations between the plasma concentrations of TNF or IL-6 and CRP have been found in severely septic patients without leukopenia (13). On the other hand, IL-6 concentrations have been shown, in children with febrile neutropenia, to be a more sensitive marker of acute infection than CRP (14).

Interleukin-6 is produced by phagocytes, fibroblasts endothelial cells and other tissues (15). It is well known that the sepsis syndrome and septic shock induce severe hypoperfusion with widespread and generalized damage (15). It is possible that in an environment where white blood cells are scarce, IL-6 generation could be sustained by several perturbed tissues other than WBC, for example endothelial cells. In part, this could also explain the high IL-6 levels, notwithstanding the daily administration of low-dose steroids. Conversely, in more advanced infections, IL-6 increase may represent a futile host defense response. Cause and effect can only be demonstrated by showing a better outcome in association with neutralizing IL-6.

The bacteriologic analyses of blood cultures have confirmed that endotoxin, Gram-positive or yeast cell wall products and viral or fungal agents can initiate the septic cascade. We believe that further clinical studies and laboratory studies on experimental animals could be helpful for better understanding of the role of cytokines, i.e. IL-6, in the pathophysiology of sepsis, the sepsis syndrome and septic shock in neutropenic patients.

REFERENCES

1. Fong Y, Moladawer LL, Shires GT, Lowry SF. The biological characteristics of cytokines and their implications in surgical injury. Surg Gynecol Obstet 170: 363–378, 1990.
2. Debets JHM, Kampmejer R, van der Linden MPMH, Buurman WA, van der Lined CJ. Plasma Tumor Necrosis Factor and mortality in critically ill septic patients. Crit Care Med 17: 489–494, 1989.
3. Dinarello CA. The proinflammatory cytokines interleukin-1 and tumor necrosis factor and the treatment of septic shock syndrome. J Infect Dis 163: 1177–1184, 1991.
4. Bauer J, Herrmann F. Interleukin-6 in clinical medicine. Ann Hematol 62: 203–207, 1991.
5. Bone R. The pathogenesis of sepsis. Ann Intern Med 115: 457–469, 1991.
6. Raponi GM, Antonelli M, Gaeta A, Bufi M, DeBlasi RA, Conti G, D'Errico RR, Mancini C, Filadoro F, Gasparetto A. Tumor necrosis factor in serum and in bronchoalveolar lavage of patients at risk for the adult respiratory distress syndrome. J Crit Care 7: 183–188, 1992.
7. Hack CE, de Groot ER, Felt-Bersma RJF, Nuijens JH, Strack Van Schijindel RJ, Eerenberg Belmer AJ, Thijs LG, Aarden LA. Increased plasma levels of interleukin-6 in sepsis. Blood 74: 1704–1710, 1989.
8. Calandra T, Baumgartner JD, Grau GE, Wu MN, Lambert PH, Schelleke NSJ, Verhoef J, Glauser MP. Prognostic values of tumor necrosis factor/cachectin, interleukin-1, interferon alpha and interferon gamma in the serum of patients with septic shock. J Infect Dis 161: 982–987, 1990.
9. Beutler B, Krochin N, Milsark IW, Luedke C, Cerami A. Control of cachectin (tumor necrosis factor) synthesis: mechanism of endotoxin resistance. Science 232: 977, 1986.
10. Rose PE, Johnson SA, Meakin M, Mackie PH, Stuart J. Serial study of C-reactive protein during infection in leukaemia. J Clin Pathol 34: 263–266, 1981.
11. Gozzard DI, French FA, Blecher TE, Powell RJ. C-reactive protein levels in neutropenic with pyrexia. Clin Lab Haematol 4: 307–316, 1985.
12. Starke ID, deBeer FC, Donnelly JP, Catovsky D, Goldman JM, Galton DA, Pepys MB. Serum C-reactive protein levels in the management of infection in acute leukaemia. Eur J Cancer Clin Onco 3: 319–325, 1984.
13. Dofferhoff AS, Bom VJ, de Vries Hosper, Van Ingen J, Van de Meer J, Hazenberg BP, Mulder PO, Weist J. Patterns of cytokines, plasma endotoxin, plasminogen inhibitor and acute phase proteins during the treatment of severe sepsis in humans. Crit Care Med 20: 185–192, 1992.
14. Heney D, Lewis JJ, Evans SW, Banks R, Bayley CC, Wicher JT. Interleukin 6 and its relationship to C reactive protein and fever in children with febrile neutropenia. J Infect Dis 165: 886–890, 1992.
15. Van Snick J. Interleukin-6: an overview. Ann Rev Immunol 8: 253–278, 1990.

Submitted October 26, 1994; accepted April 21, 1995

Scand J Infect Dis 27: 385–389, 1995 ORIGINAL ARTICLE

Effect of Supplementation with an Iron-Fortified Milk on Incidence of Diarrhea and Respiratory Infection in Urban-Resident Infants

GLORIA HERESI[1], FERNANDO PIZARRO[2], MANUEL OLIVARES[2], MARISOL CAYAZZO[2], EVA HERTRAMPF[2], TOMAS WALTER[2], JAMES R. MURPHY[3] and ABRAHAM STEKEL[2]

From the [1]Division of Infectious Diseases, Department of Pediatrics, University of Texas Medical School at Houston, Texas, USA, the [2]Hematology Unit, Institute of Nutrition and Food Technology, University of Chile, Santiago, Chile, and the [3]Center of Infectious Diseases, University of Texas, Schools of Medicine and Public Health, Houston, Texas, USA

To address the hypothesis that increased infectious morbidity is associated with iron supplementation, 783 randomly selected infants were provided with a powdered full fat cow's milk (non-fortified group) and 872 with a powdered acidified full fat cow's milk fortified with 15 mg of iron as ferrous sulfate (fortified group). All infants were followed from birth to 15 months of age with a monthly home visit by a nurse who recorded morbidity occurring during the previous 30 days. At 9 months of age, 15% of infants in each cohort were receiving breast milk only; data for these infants were segregated to make the third group. Episodes (mean $\pm$ SD) of diarrhea/infant/year were 1.06 $\pm$ 1.29, 1.14 $\pm$ 1.37, and 0.82 $\pm$ 1.04 for the fortified, non-fortified and breast-fed groups, respectively; the fortified and non-fortified bottle-fed groups had a very similar incidence of respiratory illness; 2.66 $\pm$ 2.07 and 2.74 $\pm$ 2.24 episodes/infant/year, respectively. The incidence of respiratory illness for both bottle-fed groups was significantly higher than that for the breast-fed group (2.22 $\pm$ 1.84 respiratory espisodes/infant/year). We conclude that for the infants the tested form of iron fortified milk, which is sufficient to lower iron deficiency anemia, does not result in an increased incidence of diarrhea or respiratory illness.

G. P. Heresi, MD, Department of Pediatrics, Pediatric Infectious Diseases, 6431 Fannin, JFB 1739, Houston, TX 77030, USA

INTRODUCTION

The effect of supplemental iron on infectious morbidity is controversial. Decreased incidence of bronchitis and gastroenteritis (1, 2), reduction in hospitalization for infectious diseases (3) and lowered frequency of bacterial infections in infants receiving iron have been described. However, other data suggest that iron therapy may aggravate infectious processes (4–7).

Because Chile has been considering the introduction of iron-fortified milk into its National Program of Supplementary Feeding, we made a study within the infrastructure of the National Supplementary Food Program in order to determine, whether dietary iron supplementation is associated with increased incidence of infections, specifically diarrhea and respiratory illness.

SUBJECTS AND METHODS

The study population was resident in an urban area of Santiago, Chile, in an area served by 7 outpatient clinics of the National Health System (NHS), with a population of approximately 400 000, and where 15 000 infants per year are born in NHS hospitals in the area. The population was of relatively low socioeconomic status, but had good access to public utilities, with 100, 70 and 70% of homes having electricity, running water and sewage connections, respectively. In Chile, about 85% of infants are eligible to receive free milk distribtued by the NHS through a National Program of Supplementary Feeding.

The study employed unblinded sequential cohorts in order to ensure distribution and monitoring of distribution of the formulas. Infants born during June–July ($n = 783$) received a powdered cow's milk (26% fat). Those born in the following 2 months ($n = 872$) received a powdered full fat milk; biologically acidified (total acidity = 2.5 g lactic acid/100 g), fortified with 15 mg of iron (as ferrous sulfate) and 100 mg of ascorbic acid per 100 g. Previous studies of absorption showed that the iron in this milk had a bioavailability of 11% (8). Each infant received 3 kg of powdered milk monthly from birth to 6 months of age, and then 2 kg monthly until 2 years of age. The powdered milk was diluted 1 : 10 (wt/vol) in boiled water and 5% sucrose and 3% cornflour were added. The consumption of the milk by study-enrolled infants was evaluated at 9 months of age; 79 and 84% of the fortified and non-fortified groups, respectively, reported consumption of all milk provided. Solid foods were introduced in accordance with the usual practise in Chile: fruits and juices at 3 months, meat–vegetable soup at 4 months, legumes at 6 months and table food at 9 months.

The trial was designed to follow all the infants prospectively from birth to 15 months of age, with home visits every month by a nurse who recorded gastrointestinal, respiratory and other morbid episodes recalled by the mother. One episode of diarrhea was defined as the presence of liquid stools for >24 h, and one episode of respiratory infection as cough and/or wheezing for a duration ≥ 5 days. Episodes were considered separate when they occurred after 7 or more symptom-free days. At each visit the nurse adminis-

 ISSN 0036-5548

tered a 24-h recall questionnaire about the food intake of the infant and counselled the mother concerning infant care. The breast-feeding habits of the population were not interfered with.

Additionally, every month, infants were seen at the outpatient clinics where anthropometric measurements were performed. Subsamples of randomly selected infants from both groups, at 9 and 15 months of age, were evaluated for nutritional status. In this randomization those babies who had been breast-fed after 6 months were excluded. The following measures were performed: hemoglobin (Hb) (9), transferrin saturation (Fe/TIBC) (10), free erythrocyte protoporphyrin (FEP) (11) and serum ferritin (SF) (Gamma Dab 125-I ferritin radioimmunoassay kit, Travenol, Cambridge, Massachusetts, USA). A socioeconomic questionnaire was also completed using standard methods (12).

The informed consent of parents was obtained prior to inclusion of a child in the study, and the protocol was approved by the Ethics in Human Research Committee of the Institute of Nutrition and Food Technology of the University of Chile.

Statistical analysis was carried out by ANOVA, the Bonferroni test, and chi-square evaluation.

RESULTS

Data from 515 of the 1,655 enrolled infants were excluded from analysis because of change in address (316) poor protocol compliance (127); mother working outside of household (62); and hemoglobin levels < 90 g/l at 9 months of age (10). (The latter 10 infants were placed in therapy for iron deficiency.) Additionally, it was found that mothers of 173 infants had chosen to provide these children with breast milk as the sole source of milk through 9 months of age. Data from children who had received breast milk as their sole milk source were segregated. Thus, the study comprised three groups: recipients of fortified milk (458), recipients of non-fortified milk (509) and breast-fed children (173). Comparison of selected anthropometric, socioeconomic and behavioural characteristics established that the two bottle-fed groups were similar in composition (Table I). The breast-fed group differed from both the fortified and non-fortified groups in mean birth weight and percentage of infants above 2.5 kg at birth: both measures were significantly increased in the breast-fed group. In each

Table I. *Selected characteristics of studied group*

	Iron-fortified	Non-fortified	Breast-fed
n	458	509	173
Male, %	52	49	51
Birth weight <2.45 kg, %	10.2	8.9	2.9[a]
Mean birth weight ±SD, kg	3.10 ± 0.56	3.12 ± 0.61	3.32 ± 0.46[a]
Mean socioeconomic score ± SD	26.4 ± 10.1	25.7 ± 10.2	24.9 ± 10.8

[a] $p < 0.01$ compared to both fortified and non-fortified groups.
Statistical significance was tested using χ^3 for differences in rates and ANOVA followed by the Bonferroni test for differences between means.

Table II. *Incidence of diarrhea and respiratory illness by groups*

Group	No. of children	Diarrhea[a]	Respiratory illness[a]
Iron-fortified	458	1.06 ± 1.29	2.66 ± 2.07
Non-fortified	509	1.14 ± 1.37	2.74 ± 2.24
Breast-fed	173	0.82 ± 1.04*,**	2.22 ± 1.84***

[a] (mean ± SD/infant/year).
Differences in means were tested for statistical significance by ANOVA followed by Bonferroni test.
* $p < 0.01$ compared to fortified group.
** $p < 0.001$ compared to non-fortified group.
*** $p < 0.001$ compared to fortified and non-fortified group.

of the bottle-fed groups 80% had received some cow's milk before 3 months of age. The pattern of introduction of solid foods was similar for the 3 groups.

Dietary supplementation with fortified milk did not significantly influence the incidence of diarrhea or respiratory infection (Table II). In contrast, the solely breast-fed group had significantly fewer episodes of diarrhea and respiratory infection than the bottle-fed groups.

The efficacy of the applied iron fortification was established by determining the incidence of iron deficiency when infants reached 9 and 15 months of age. Iron deficiency anemia was defined as hemoglobin level < 110 g/l. At 9 and 15 months, the incidence of anemia was 11.8 vs. 32.5% and 5.5 vs. 29.9% for fortified compared to non-fortified groups respectively, (χ^2, $p < 0.001$).

The effect on morbidity of iron deficiency anemia at 9 months of age was evaluated. Infants with iron deficiency anemia had a higher mean number of episodes of diarrhea than infants with normal iron nutritional status (Table III). Iron deficiency was not a contributing factor in the incidence of respiratory illness.

The effect of fortification on nutritional status was determined. An infant was classified as undernourished when the weight/age (W/A) ratio was below 90% of the 50th percentile for W/A ratio of NCHS standards, in two or more consecutive antropometrical evaluations. Eutrophic infants had W/A ratio >90% in all evaluations. Undernutrition was found at the statistically similar rates of 23.4 and 29.1% for infants in the fortified and non-fortified groups, respectively. Breast-fed infants had a 15.7% incidence of undernutrition (χ^2, $p < 0.03$ or $p < 0.001$ compared with non-fortified or fortified groups, respectively). Undernourished infants had a significantly ($p < 0.01$) higher number of diarrheal episodes than eutrophic infants (Table IV). Nutritional status was not reflected in changed incidence of respiratory infection.

DISCUSSION

A powdered cow's milk-based supplementary feeding program in Chile, which is well established, was modified in

Table III. *Influence of iron deficiency anemia at 9 months of age on morbidity*

Group	Iron	No. of children	Diarrhea[a]	Respiratory illness[a]
Iron-fortified	Normal[b]	62	0.95 ± 1.31	2.86 ± 2.28
	Deficient			
	Non-anemic[c]	19	1.39 ± 1.19	3.15 ± 2.14
	Anemic[d]	10	1.59 ± 1.83	1.26 ± 0.85
Non-fortified	Normal	44	0.79 ± 0.92	2.50 ± 2.00
	Deficient			
	Non-anemic	28	1.00 ± 1.14	2.78 ± 2.67
	Anemic	37	1.47 ± 1.61*	2.52 ± 2.09

[a] Mean ± SD episodes/infant/year.
[b] Iron normal = Hb > 110 g/l, FEP < 1200 μg/l RBC, Fe/TIBC > 10% and SF > 10 μg/l.
[c] Iron-deficient, non-anemic = Hb > 110 g/l and ≥2 biochemical parameters altered (FEP > 120 μg/l RBC, Fe/TIBC < 10% and SF < 10 μg/l).
[d] Iron-deficient anemic = Hb < 110 g/l.
Differences in means were tested for statistical significance by ANOVA followed by Bonferroni test.
* $p < 0.1$ as compared with iron normal group.

Table IV. *Influence of undernutrition on morbidity*

Group	Nutrition	No. of children	Diarrhea[a]	Respiratory illness[a]
Iron-fortified	Eutrophic	101	0.93 ± 1.17	2.59 ± 2.16
	Undernourished	60	1.10 ± 1.42	3.08 ± 2.21
Non-fortified	Eutrophic	121	0.80 ± 1.06	2.76 ± 2.28
	Undernourished	64	1.37 ± 1.45*	3.07 ± 2.34

[a] Mean ± SD episodes/infant/year).
Differences in means were tested for statistical significance by ANOVA followed by Bonferroni test.
* $p < 0.01$ as compared with eutrophic group.

order to address iron deficiency anemia, which is known to be prevalent in the studied population (13), by incorporation of ferrous sulfate into the powdered milk (8). This iron supplementation was effective in reducing iron deficiency anemia; a result which is consistent with that of previous studies of this regime (14). The 15 months of follow up, directed to determining the influence of iron-fortified milk on infectious morbidity, showed that there were no significant differences in diarrhea or respiratory illnesses between groups or infants provided with powdered milk or with powdered milk fortified with iron. Given this result, and the clear demonstration that iron fortification reduced iron deficiency anemia (14, 15), it is concluded that there is advantage in provision of iron-fortified milk.

Although the results of the present study show no increase in infectious morbidity with iron fortification, there is not a consensus in the literature on the effect of iron therapy on infectious morbidity. Considerations which might explain why the result of this study agrees with those which show no increase in infectious morbidity in association with iron supplementation, include route of delivery of the medicinal iron, the dose, and the frequency of encounters with pathogens. In the present study iron was delivered *per os* and the total iron/day provided was much lower than the standard doses used in iron therapy. Parental delivery of iron for therapeutic purposes, which usually results in delivery of much higher doses than those used in this study, seem more associated with increased infectious morbidity (4, 5).

The low-income population studied is somewhat atypical for developing country residents, in its relatively low rates of diarrheal and respiratory illnesses. The observed low rates of infectious morbidity are similar to those reported for previous studies of this population (16, 17) and studies made in other areas of Santiago (18). There exists one report of a higher rate of diarrhea (2.2 episodes/infant/year) for the studied population (19). However, the definition of diarrhea employed for that study was less stringent than employed for the others. Even this higher rate is significantly below what is found for similar populations in most developing countries (20–23). The possibility that the cumulative debits (nutritional, immunological etc.) from more frequent infections might influence the infectious disease morbidity associated with an iron supplementation program deserves study.

Previous studies have established that entreotoxigenic E. coli (24) and Shigella (19) are prevalent causes of diarrhea in the studied population. By inference, our results suggest that the tested iron supplementation did not enhance the virulence of these pathogens.

Two potentially confounding variables which can influence morbidity are breast-feeding and malnutrition. In the present study an exclusively breast-fed group was segregated and found to have a lower incidence of diarrhea and respiratory illness compared to both bottle-fed groups. The breast-feeding behavior in both formula-fed groups, was documented to be similar.

This study demonstrated, as expected from previous work (20, 25, 26), that malnutrition was associated with higher rates of diarrhea. It was shown that both the iron-fortified and non-iron-fortified bottle-fed groups had a similar number of undernourished infants. Thus, the composite result is that both breast-feeding and undernutrition had the expected associations with morbidity, and both formula-fed (iron-fortified and non-fortified) groups were similar with respect to breast-feeding and malnutrition variables. Therefore, differences in breast-feeding and nutritional status between the bottle-fed groups did not cause the observed result.

In contradiction to the hypothesis that iron supplementation might increase infectious morbidity, data were obtained supporting the view that iron fortification is associated with reduced infectious morbidity. However, this trend did not reach statistical significance. The same trend was also found in a precursor study where consumption of formulas was closely monitored and where household visits were performed twice weekly (16). Although this trend seems rational, and consistent with demonstrations of increased infectious morbidity in iron-deficient children, formal proof of its validity is lacking.

We interpret this study, and a previous pilot study (16), as supporting the incorporation of the evaluated iron-fortified regimen into the Chilean National Program of Supplemental Feeding and into possible similar programs elsewhere. Iron fortification, as provided in this study, was associated with reduced anemia and trends towards reduced diarrheal morbid episodes. No evidence of an adverse effect on morbidity of the provided iron supplementation was found.

REFERENCES

1. MacKay HMM. Anemia in infancy: its prevalence and prevention. Arch Dis Child 3: 117–144, 1928.
2. Andelman MB, Sered BR. Utilization of dietary iron by term infants. A study of 1,048 infants from a low socio-economic population. Am J Dis Child 111: 45–55, 1966.
3. Cantwell RJ. Iron deficiency anemia of infancy: some clinical principles illustrated by the response of Maori infants to neonatal parenteral iron administration. Clin Pediatr (Phila) 11: 443–449, 1972.
4. Barry DM, Reeve AW. Increased incidence of gram negative neonatal sepsis with intramuscular iron administration. Pediatrics 60: 908–912, 1977.
5. Farmer K, Becroft DM. Administration of parenteral iron to newborn infants. Arch Dis Child 51: 486, 1976.
6. Murray MJ, Murray AB, Murray MB, Murray CJ. The adverse effect of iron repletion on the course of certain infections. BMJ 2: 1113–1115, 1978.
7. Masawe AE, Muindi JM, Swai GBR. Infections in iron deficiency and other types of anaemia in the tropics. Lancet 2: 314–317, 1974.
8. Stekel A, Olivares M, Pizarro F, Chadud P, Lopez I, Amar M. Absorption of fortification iron from milk formulas in infants. Am J Clin Nutr 43: 917–922, 1986.
9. International Committee for Standardization in Haematology. Recommendations and requirements for haemoglobinometry in human blood. Clin Pathol 18: 353–355, 1965.
10. Fischer DS, Price DC. A simple serum iron method using the new sensitive chromogen tripyridyl-S-triazine. Clin Chem 10: 21–30, 1964.
11. Heller SR, Labbe RF, Nutter JA. A simplified assay for porphyrins in whole blood. J Clin Pathol 18: 353–355, 1965.
12. Alvarez ML, Wurgaft F, Salazar ME. Measurements of the urban low socioeconomic level in families with malnourished infants. Arch Latinoam Nutr 32: 650–662, 1982.
13. Rios E, Olivares M, Amar M, Chadud P, Pizarro F, Stekel A. Evaluation of iron status and prevalence of iron deficiency in Chile. In: Underwood BA, ed. Nutrition interventions strategies in national development. New York: Academic Press, 315–323, 1983.
14. Stekel A, Olivares M, Cayazzo M, Chadud P, Llaguno S, Pizarro F. Prevention of iron deficiency by milk fortification. II. A field trial with a full fat acidified milk. Am J Clin Nutr 47: 265–269, 1988.
15. Stekel A, Pizarro F, Olivares M, Chaudud P, Llaguno S, Cayazzo M, Hertrampf E, Walter T. Prevention of iron deficiency by milk fortification. III. Effectiveness under the usual operational conditions of a nation-wide food program. Nutr Rep Inter 38: 1119–1128, 1988.
16. Heresi G, Olivares M, Pizarro F, Cayazzo M, Stekel A. Effect of an iron fortified milk on morbidity in infancy. A field trial. Nutr Res 7: 915–922, 1987.
17. Cayazzo M, Pizarro F, Olivares M, Hertrampf E, Vega V, Walter T, Heresi G. Comparison of the morbidity registered at clinics and in the field. Prospective study in infants. Rev Chil Pediatr 58: 485–489, 1987.
18. Espinoza J, Figueroa G, Araya M, Spencer E, Pacheco I, Brunser O. Acute diarrhea in infants. A field study. XXIIth Annual Meeting of the Latinoamerican Pediatric Research Society (SLAIP). Los Andes, Chile, 1984 [Abst 72].
19. Ferreccio C, Prado V, Ojeda A, Cayyazo M, Abrego P, Guers L, Levine M. Epidemiologic patterns of acute diarrhea and endemic Shigella infections in children in a poor periurban setting in Santiago, Chile. Am J Epidemiol 134: 614–627, 1991.
20. Mata LJ. The children of Santa Maria de Cauque: prospective field study of health and growth. Cambridge, Massachusetts: MIT Press, 1978.
21. Guerrant RL, Kirchoff LV, Shields DS, Nations MK, Leslie J, De Sousa M, Araujo MJ, Correia LL, Saver KT, McCelland KE, Trowbridge FL, Hughes JM. Prospective study of diarrheal illnesses in northeastern Brazil: patterns of disease, nutritional impact, etiologies, and risk factors. J Infect Dis 148: 986–997, 1983.
22. Zaki AW, Dupont HL, El-Alamy MA, Arafat RR, Amin K, Awad MM, Bassiounni L, Imam IZ, El Malish GS, El Marsafie TA. The detection of enteropathogens in acute

diarrhea in a family cohort population in rural Egypt. Am J Trop Med Hyg 35: 1013–1022, 1986.
23. Black RE, Lopez de Romana G, Brown KH, Bravo N, Bazalar OG, Kanashiro HC. Incidence and etiology of infantile diarrhea and major routes of transmission in Huascar, Peru. Am J Epidemiol 129: 785–799, 1989.
24. Figueroa G, Troncoso M, Galeno H, Faundez G. Oral iron supplementation and diarrhoeal disease in infants: a prospective bacteriological study. Microb Ecol Health Dis 3: 139–143, 1990.
25. Trowbridge FL, Newton LH, Campbell CC. Nutritional status and severity of diarrhea. Lancet 1: 1374–1375, 1981.
26. Keusch JT. Nutritional and infection. In: Remington JS, Swartz MN, eds. Current clinical topics in infectious diseases. New York: McGraw-Hill, 106–123, 1984.

Submitted June 4, 1994; accepted March 22, 1995

Scand J Infect Dis 27: 391–395, 1995 ORIGINAL ARTICLE

Oral Candida albicans Isolates with Reduced Susceptibility to Fluconazole in Swedish HIV-infected Patients

ERJA CHRYSSANTHOU[1], JAN TORSSANDER[2] and BJÖRN PETRINI[1]

From the Departments of [1]Clinical Microbiology, Karolinska Hospital, and [2]Dermatology, Stockholm Söder Hospital, Stockholm, Sweden

A total of 62 patients with HIV-related conditions were examined for clinical and mycological oral findings. Cultures from 51 patients were positive for yeasts and included 49 Candida albicans and 8 non-albicans isolates. Of patients with positive culture, 35% had pseudomembraneous thrush. In vitro susceptibility testing of 49 C. albicans isolates revealed that the minimal inhibitory concentration for 50% of the strains (MIC_{50}) was 2.0 mg/l for fluconazole, and the MIC_{50} was ≤ 0.125 mg/l for both ketoconazole and itraconazole. Fluconazole resistance (MIC ≥ 32.0 mg/l) was found for 14% of the C. albicans isolates tested. Two C. albicans isolates showed cross-resistance to ketoconazole and itraconazole. Associations between reduced susceptibility to fluconazole and low CD4+ cell counts, the length of time since the first AIDS-defining illness and the interval from the first fluconazole treatment, indirectly reflecting the total fluconazole exposure, were observed.

E. Chryssanthou, MD, Department of Clinical Microbiology, Karolinska Hospital, S-171 76 Stockholm, Sweden

INTRODUCTION

Pseudomembraneous candidosis (thrush) is a typical presentation of oral candidosis in the HIV-infected patient. Fluconazole is highly effective against C. albicans, and has proved to be a useful and well tolerated drug for treatment of oropharyngeal candidosis in HIV-infected patients (1–3). A common approach has been to use fluconazole as secondary prophylaxis for oral candidosis. Recently, several reports have described the increasing recognition of fluconazole-resistant C. albicans strains isolated from HIV-infected patients (4–8). An increased prevalence of C. krusei and C. glabrata has also been observed in HIV-associated oral candidosis (7). Moreover, fluconazole-resistant oropharyngeal candidosis was observed in patients with HIV infection which was more advanced in terms of the interval since the diagnosis of AIDS and of CD4+ cell counts (5). The present study of oral thrush in HIV-infected individuals was undertaken to evaluate the occurrence of fluconazole-resistant strains and a possible association with resistance to other azoles. Furthermore, the objective was to determine the prevalence of non-albicans strains in this patient population.

MATERIALS AND METHODS

Patients and controls

A total of 62 homosexual males with HIV-related conditions, hospitalized in an HIV medical unit, were consecutively examined for clinical and mycological oral findings. The median age was 42 years (range 26–73). Of the patients, 47 (76%) had AIDS. The mean $\pm$ SE CD4+ cell count for the 62 patients was $69 \pm 16 \times 10^6$/l. Oral C. albicans strains had previously been collected from 20 apparently healthy HIV-seronegative homosexual males (median age 47 years, range 30–58) attending a screening program for venereal diseases. These subjects had no signs of oral candidosis and had never been treated with oral azoles. The antimycotic susceptibility of these virgin strains served as a comparison to the patients' strains.

Sampling procedure and yeast identification

Oral specimens for the culture of yeasts were obtained by sampling the surfaces of the buccal mucosa and the tongue with cotton-stick swabs as described before (9). The specimens were inoculated onto Sabouraud dextrose agar plates containing penicillin (0.01 g/l) and streptomycin (0.03 g/l). Plates were incubated at room temperature and all cultures positive for yeast were transported to the mycological laboratory. Strains were identified as C. albicans by development of germ tubes in horse serum. Germ tube negative strains were identified by their assimilation pattern with the ID 32 C identification system for yeasts (BioMérieux, Marcy-l'Étoile, France). The yeast strains were grown on Sabouraud dextrose agar at 35°C prior to testing.

Antifungal agents

Four antifungal agents were used in this study: fluconazole (Pfizer, New York, USA), ketoconazole and itraconazole (Janssen Pharmaceutica, Piscataway, New York, USA) and amphotericin B (Squibb Institute for Research, Princeton, New Jersey, USA). Fluconazole was dissolved in 0.85% saline, ketoconazole in dimethyl sulfoxide (DMSO) and amphotericin B, with 0.41% deoxycholate, in sterile water, and these were stored in the dark at −20°C as stock solutions of 5 g/l. Itraconazole was dissolved in 50% acetone–50% 0.2 M HCl (10) and stored at 4°C as a stock solution of 10 g/l.

Determination of minimal inhibitory concentrations (MICs)

Susceptibility testing of yeasts was performed according to the broth macrodilution method proposed by the National Committee for Clinical Laboratory Standards (NCCLS) (11) with some modifications. RPMI 1640 medium (Sigma) buffered to pH 7.0 with 0.165 M morpholinepropanesulfonic acid (MOPS) buffer (Sigma), with L-glutamine and sodium bicarbonate was used. The range of drug concentrations tested was: 0.125–32 mg/l for fluconazole and

 ISSN 0036-5548

itraconazole; 0.125–8 mg/l for ketoconazole, and 0.125–4 mg/l for amphotericin B. The yeast inoculum was prepared by suspending yeast cells in 5 ml of 0.85% saline, and the cell density was adjusted to (1–5) × 10^6 colony-forming units (CFU)/ml by a spectrophotometric method (12), and further diluted 100-fold in RPMI 1640 medium. The tubes with 100 μl of drug dilutions were inoculated by adding 900 μl of the cell suspension to each tube. For itraconazole susceptibility testing the yeast inoculum was prepared in saline and the cell density was adjusted to (5–6) × 10^5 CFU/ml. The tubes containing 1 ml of itraconazole dilutions were inoculated with 50 μl of the cell suspension. The growth control tubes contained yeast inoculum and drug-free medium.

After incubation at 35°C for 48 h, the growth in the tubes was measured spectrophotometrically at 530 nm for azole susceptibility testing. The minimal inhibitory concentration (MIC) end-point was defined as the first drug concentration exhibiting 50% (or more) reduction of growth compared with the growth control tube. The MIC end-point for amphotericin B was defined as the lowest drug concentration inhibiting growth.

The MIC_{50} and the MIC_{90} values were defined as concentrations which inhibited the growth in 50 and 90% of the strains, respectively.

Candida kefyr ATCC 28838 and Saccharomyces cerevisiae ATCC 36375 were included as control organisms for susceptibility testing of azoles and amphotericin B, respectively (13).

RESULTS

Clinical and mycological findings

Mycological assessment was carried out for 62 patients. Of the 18 patients with thrush, none had a negative culture, 17 had C. albicans and one had C. albicans + non-albicans. Of the 44 without thrush, 11 had a negative culture, 26 had C. albicans, 5 had C. albicans + non-albicans and 2 had non-albicans only. Eight out of the 11 patients with negative oral culture were being treated with fluconazole. The mean ± SE of CD4+ cell counts were $67 \pm 28 \times 10^6$/l in culture-negative patients, $71 \pm 19 \times 10^6$/l in those with C. albicans in pure culture and $29 \pm 12 \times 10^6$/l in patients with mixed culture.

Antifungal susceptibility testing: controls

Azole susceptibility testing was performed on 20 C. albicans strains isolated from HIV-seronegative homosexual men (azole-MIC control group). The following MICs were obtained: fluconazole ≤0.125–0.25 mg/l, ketoconazole ≤0.125 mg/l and itraconazole ≤0.125–0.25 mg/l.

C. kefyr ATCC 28838, a control organism for the susceptibility testing of fluconazole and ketoconazole, had fluconazole MICs in the range ≤0.125–0.25 mg/l. The ketoconazole and itraconazole MICs were both ≤0.125 mg/l. Saccharomyces cerevisiae ATCC 36375 had amphotericin B MICs in the range 0.25–0.5 mg/l. Control organisms were tested 15 times during the study period.

Antifungal susceptibility testing: patients

The results of the in vitro susceptibility testing of the 49 C. albicans isolates from HIV-infected patients with regard to fluconazole, ketoconazole and itraconazole are shown in Fig. 1a, b, c. The MIC_{50} and the MIC_{90} for fluconazole were 2.0 mg/l and ≥32.0 mg/l, respectively. All fluconazole-resistant strains were susceptible (MIC 0.125–0.25 mg/l) to amphotericin B. Two of these fluconazole-resistant strains showed cross-resistance to ketoconazole and itraconazole.

The MIC_{50} was ≤0.125 mg/l for both ketoconazole and itraconazole. The MIC_{90} was 0.5 mg/l for ketoconazole and 1.0 mg/l for itraconazole, respectively.

Nine out of 49 patients with a positive culture for C. albicans had no history of fluconazole exposure. The MICs of fluconazole for these isolates were in the range 0.125–0.25 mg/l.

Azole susceptibility was also tested on 8 non-albicans isolates: 3 C. krusei, 2 C. glabrata, 1 C. famata, 1 Tr. capitatum and 1 S. cerevisiae. The MICs of fluconazole ranged from 4.0 to >32.0 mg/l (MIC_{50} 32.0 mg/l). The MICs of ketoconazole ranged from ≤0.125 to 8.0 mg/l (MIC_{50} 1.0 mg/l), and the MICs of itraconazole ranged from 0.25 to 32.0 mg/l (MIC_{50} 0.5 mg/l).

Mean intervals, in months, from the first fluconazole treatment to oral sampling could be determined from data from 36 patients. These data, and the fluconazole MICs of the 36 C. albicans strains collected from the patients, are shown in Table I. MICs gradually increased with time, resulting in MICs of 16.0–≥32.0 mg/l for C. albicans strains sampled from patients with a mean interval of 25 months after their first exposure to fluconazole. The relation between the fluconazole MICs of the 49 C. albicans isolates and CD4+ cell counts, are also shown in Table I.

Table I. *Relation between fluconazole MICs and interval from first treatment to sampling, CD4+ cell counts, and oral thrush in HIV-infected patients*

No. of patients	Fluconazole MIC (mg/l)	Mean interval from first treatment, months (range)	CD4+ cells × 10^6/l Mean ± SE	Oral thrush
9–21	0.125–0.5	10 (1–35)	119 ± 40	1
6	1.0–2.0	10 (2–16)	37 ± 12	2
10	4.0–8.0	19 (0–49)	58 ± 23	6
11–12	16.0–≥32.0	25 (6–48)	9 ± 3	9

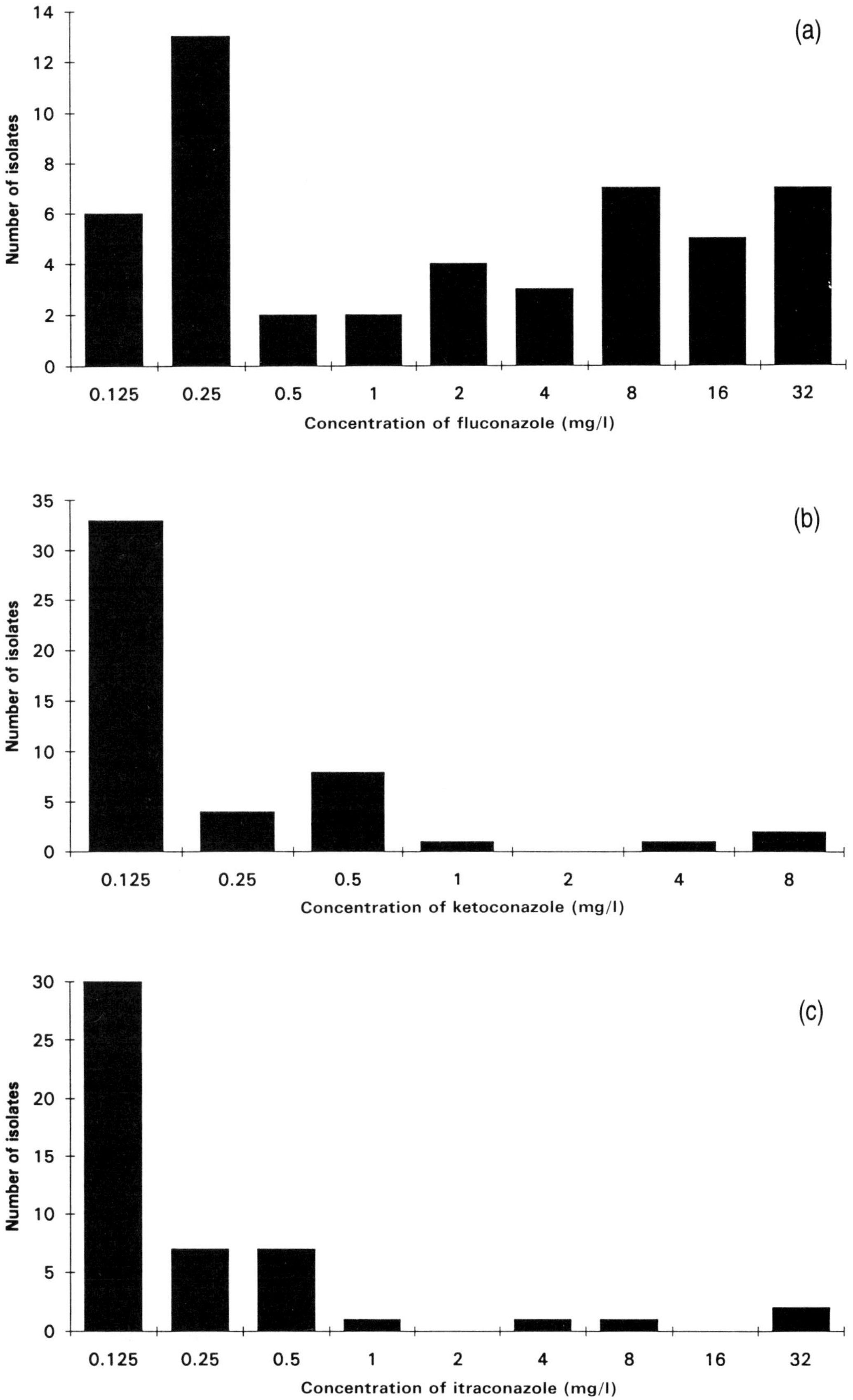

Fig. 1. MICs for 49 Candida albicans strains isolated from 49 HIV-infected patients: a, fluconazole; b, ketoconazole; c, itraconazole.

In summary, decreased susceptibility to fluconazole was seen in parallel with decreasing CD4+ cell counts and increasing occurrence of oral thrush.

Patients with susceptible strains (MICs 0.125–0.5 mg/l) had a mean interval of 2 months (range 0–24) after the first AIDS-defining illness and yeast sampling, as compared with a mean of 18 months (range 3–39) in patients with isolates with reduced susceptibility (MICs 16.0– ≥32.0 mg/l).

DISCUSSION

Oral candidosis is often the first clinical symptom of HIV infection, and is a predictor of a decline in immune function. Thrush is typically seen at CD4+ cell counts $\leq 400 \times 10^6$/l, or and recurrent oral candidosis occurs at 300×10^6/l. In advanced HIV infection, relapse of oral candidosis tends to occur within 1–2 months after treatment (14).

A permanent elimination of Candida from the mucous membranes cannot be achieved in these immunologically depressed patients. Repeated and long-term azole treatment is therefore regularly needed. This has also been typically seen in our patients. Following initiation of fluconazole treatment, this drug has been used for the treatment of all recurrences or as a prophylactic agent, in varying dosages, until a clinically evident fluconazole resistance has developed.

We consider the length of the period from the first fluconazole treatment episode as a measure which reflects the magnitude of the individual exposure to fluconazole in our patients. Patients infected with the least sensitive C. albicans strains had a mean duration of 25 months since the first fluconazole treatment.

Long-term use of fluconazole was associated with the occurrence of resistant strains of C. albicans and a minor shift to less susceptible Candida species such as C. krusei and C. glabrata. Only 1 out of 8 patients carrying non-albicans strains had symptoms of oral thrush, and this patient had a dual infection involving C. albicans as well. The occurrence of fluconazole-resistant strains might provide a basis for transmission of these strains to other individuals. However, only patients with a history of previous fluconazole exposure carried less susceptible C. albicans strains.

The development of clinical resistance is well correlated with in vitro resistance to fluconazole (4, 5, 7, 15). Clinical resistance to fluconazole has been defined as a failure to respond to 100 mg fluconazole given daily for 7 days. In vitro susceptibility testing with azoles, using the proposed reference method of the NCCLS, can identify resistant strains and provide a reliable basis for individualized and effective therapy. Redding et al. (15) have shown that C. albicans isolates with fluconazole MICs of 0.25–8.0 mg/l responded clinically to standard therapy (100 mg/day) but isolates with MICs of 32.0– >64.0 mg/l responded poorly or not at all. Resistance to fluconazole appeared in our most immunodeficient HIV patients (9×10^6 CD4+ cells/l), which is similar to the results obtained in other studies (7, 15).

The fluconazole-resistant organisms may show cross-resistance to ketoconazole and itraconazole (7, 16) but this is not always found (6). In our study, the in vitro resistance to fluconazole occurred on its own, not generally associated with resistance to ketoconazole and itraconazole.

In summary, there was a correlation between reduced in vitro susceptibility to fluconazole and low CD4+ cell counts, length of time living with AIDS and the length of time from the first fluconazole treatment, indirectly reflecting the total fluconazole exposure. Thus, in patients with advanced HIV infection and prolonged fluconazole exposure, consideration should be given to the possibility of emergent fluconazole-resistant C. albicans strains. In vitro susceptibility testing can identify these strains, which is of significant clinical importance.

REFERENCES

1. Meunier F, Aoun M, Gerard M. Therapy for oropharyngeal candidiasis in the immunocompromised host: a randomized double-blind syudy of fluconazole vs. ketoconazole. Rev Infect Dis 12 Suppl 3: 364–368, 1990.
2. Viscoli C, Castagnola E, Fioredda F, Ciravegna B, Barigione G, Terragne A. Fluconazole in the treatment of candidiasis in immunocompromised children. Antimicrob Agents Chemother 35: 365–367, 1991.
3. Dupont B, Drouet E. Fluconazole in management of oropharyngeal candidosis in a predominantly HIV antibody-positive group of patients. J Med Vet Mycol 26: 67–71, 1988.
4. Bart-Delabesse E, Boiron P, Carlotti A, Dupont B. Candida albicans genotyping in studies with patients with AIDS developing resistance to fluconazole. J Clin Microbiol 31: 2933–2937, 1993.
5. Troillet N, Durussel C, Bille J, Glauser MP, Chave JP. Correlation between in vitro susceptibility of Candida albicans and fluconazole-resistant oropharyngeal candidiasis in HIV-infected patients. Eur J Clin Microbiol Infect Dis 12: 911–915, 1993.
6. Phaffer MA, Rhine-Chalberg J, Redding SW, Smith J, Farinacci G, Fothergill AW, Rinaldi MG. Variations in fluconazole susceptibility and electrophoretic karotype among oral isolates of Candida albicans from patients with AIDS and oral candidiasis. J Clin Microbiol 32: 59–64, 1994.
7. Millon L, Manteaux A, Reboux G, Drobacheff C, Monod M, Barale T, Michel-Briand Y. Fluconazole-resistant recurrent oral candidiasis in human immumodeficiency virus-positive patients: persistence of Candida albicans strains with the same genotype. J Clin Microbiol 32: 1115–1118, 1994.
8. Ruhnke M, Eigler A, Tennagen I, Geiseler B, Engelmann E, Trautmann M. Emergence of fluconazole-resistant strains of Candida albicans in patients with recurrent oropharyngeal candidosis and human immunodeficiency virus infection. J Clin Microbiol 32: 2092–2098, 1994.
9. Torssander J, Morfeldt-Manson L, Biberfeld G, Karlsson A, Putkonen P-O, Wasserman J. Oral Candida albicans in HIV infection. Scand J Infect Dis 19: 291–295, 1987.
10. Denning DW, Hanson LH, Stevens DA. In vitro activity of saperconazole (R66 905) compared with amphotericin B and

itraconazole against Aspergillus species. Eur J Clin Microbiol Infect Dis 9: 693–697, 1990.
11. National Committee for Clinical Laboratory Standards. Reference method for broth dilution antifungal susceptibility testing for yeasts. Proposed standard M27-P. Villanova, Pennsylvania: National Committee for Clinical Laboratory Standards, 1992.
12. Phaffer MA, Burmeister L, Bartlett MS, Rinaldi MG. Multicenter evaluation of four methods of yeast inoculum preparation. J Clin Microbiol 26: 1437–1441, 1988.
13. Espinel-Ingroff A, Kerkering TM, Goldson PR, Shadomy S. Comparison study of broth macrodilution and microdilution antifungal susceptibility tests. J Clin Microbiol 29: 1089–1094, 1991.
14. Marriott DJE, Jones PD, Hoy JF, Speed BR, Harkness JL. Fluconazole once a week as secondary prophylaxis against oropharyngeal candidiasis in HIV-infected patients. Med J Aust 158: 312–316, 1993.
15. Redding S, Smith J, Farinacci G, Rinaldi M, Fothergill A, Rhine-Chalberg J, Phaller M. Resistance of Candida albicans to fluconazole during treatment of oropharyngeal candidiasis in a patient with AIDS: documentation by in vitro susceptibility testing and DNA subtype analysis. Clin Infect Dis 18: 240–242, 1994.
16. Hitchcock CA, Pye GW, Troke PF, Johnson EM, Warnock DW. Fluconazole resistance in Candida glabrata. Antimicrob Agents Chemother 37: 1962–1965, 1993.

Submitted February 1, 1995; accepted April 3, 1995

Liver Abscess: An Unusual Manifestation of Pneumococcal Infection

STEIN LUND-TØNNESEN

From the Medical Department, Haukeland Hospital, Norway

A 50-year old male with a history of alcohol abuse, recurrent pancreatitis and insulin-dependent diabetes mellitus, with a liver abscess caused by Streptococcus pneumoniae is reported.

S. Lund-Tønnesen, MD, Medical Department Haukeland Hospital, N-5021 Haukeland sykehus, Norway

INTRODUCTION

Streptococcus pneumoniae is a common cause of otitis media, sinusitis, pneumonia and meningitis. Pleural effusion and pericarditis may also develop. Other extrapulmonary manifestations such as endocarditis, arthritis and osteomyelitis, which may occur in the course of a bacteremia, have become unusual. An equally rare manifestation is the primary pneumococcal peritonitis reported in patients with liver cirrosis (1). To the best of our knowledge there has been no previous report of a liver abscess caused by S. pneumoniae.

CASE REPORT

A 50-year-old male was admitted in February 1994 with a 4–5 week history of loss of weight and variable abdominal pain. His pre-morbid history included periodic alcohol abuse and several admissions to the surgical department for acute and chronic pancreatitis. Liver decompensation or ascites had previously not been noted. Since 1992 he had been treated with insulin for diabetes mellitus.

On admission he was without fever, pale, and had signs of moderate dehydration. No further abnormalities were found on physical examination, in particular no hepatomegaly or ascites. The results of laboratory examinations were: hemoglobin 82 g/l; peripheral white blood cell count 7.7×10^9/l; erythrocyte sedimentation rate 115 mm/h; C-reactive protein 0.134 g/l. Bilirubin and liver function tests were normal. There was no growth of microorganisms in three sets of blood cultures. Chest X-ray was normal. ACT scan of the abdomen revealed a $7 \times 7 \times 6$ cm large abscess in the right liver lobe (Fig. 1). A Gram stain of aspirated pus from the abscess yielded Gram positive cocci. S. pneumonia in pure culture was isolated from the pus. Drainage of the abscess was performed with a percutaneous catheter and benzylpenicillin 3 g t.i.d. was given intravenously for 14 days. A CT scan 12 days later showed considerable reduction in the size of the abscess. When seen in the outpatient clinic 5 weeks after admission, the patient felt well and routine laboratory tests were normal.

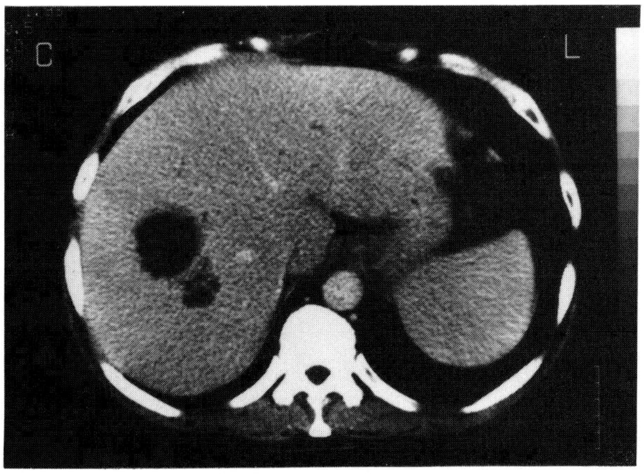

Fig. 1. CT scan of the abdomen in a 50-year-old man showing a large $7 \times 7 \times 6$ cm abscess in the right liver lobe.

DISCUSSION

Of patients with pneumococcal pneumonia, 25–30% have bacteremia. However, patients with pneumococcal infections outside the respiratory tract often have no sign of pulmonary infection (1). Whether the bacteremia in such patients arises from a subclinical pulmonary focus or directly from the nasopharynx is not known (2). Our patient had neither signs nor symptoms of respiratory tract infection.

Patients with liver abscesses often have positive blood cultures. In earlier studies blood cultures were found to be positive in one-half of the patients with pyogenic abscesses (3, 4). In our patient no bacterial growth was observed in the blood.

Most often, pyogenic liver abscesses have polymicrobial etiology with enteric Gram-negative bacilli and anerobic bacteria, including anerobic Gram-positive cocci, Bacteroides spp, Fusobacterium spp and Actinomyces spp, as the most prevalent findings. Group A streptococci, enterococci and S. milleri are the most common streptococci associated with liver abscess (5). To the best of our knowledge a liver abscess caused by S. pneumoniae has not been reported previously.

Liver abscesses are prevalent in patients with disorders of the biliary tract and pancreas (5). Our patient had a history of relapsing pancreatitis, but also had predisposing factors for pneumococcal infection such as alcohol abuse and diabetes mellitus.

He had not been vaccinated against pneumococci. This has a bearing on the current discussion about a more liberal vaccination policy in patients who are at increased risk of pneumococcal infections.

Liver abscesses, if large, should be treated with percutaneous drainage combined with systemic antibiotic administration. Direct Gram stain of aspirated pus is a useful guideline to antibiotic therapy. As long as the isolates are susceptible to penicillin, benzylpenicillin is the drug of choice for invasive pneumococcal infections in any location.

REFERENCES

1. Mufson MA. Streptococcus pneumoniae. In: Mandell GL, Douglas RG, Bennett JE, eds. Principles and practice of infectious diseases. Edinburgh: Churchill Livingstone, 1539–1550, 1990.
2. Greenwood BM. Pneumococcal Infection. In: Weatherall DJ, Ledingham JGG, Warrel DA, eds. New York; Oxford Textbook of Medicine, 49–158, 1984.
3. Sabbaj J, Sutter VL, Finegold SM. Anaerobic pyogenic liver abscess. Ann Intern Med 77: 629–638, 1972.
4. Lazarchick J, De Souza E, Silva NA, Nichols DR, Washington JA. Pyogenic liver abscess. Mayo Clin Proc 48: 349–355, 1973
5. Hansen N, Vargish T. Pyogenic hepatic abscess: a case for open drainage. Am J Surg 59: 219–222, 1993.

Submitted December 9, 1994; accepted April 16, 1995

Scand J Infect Dis 27: 399–400, 1995 CASE REPORT

Atypical Cellulitis due to Group B Streptococcus

RINUS A. DOEDENS, CARIEN J. MIEDEMA, SIDARTO BAMBANG OETOMO and JAN L. L. KIMPEN

From the Beatrix Children's Hospital, University Hospital Groningen, Groningen, The Netherlands

In a minority of late-onset Group B streptococcal (GBS) cases in neonates, facial or buccal cellulitis has been described. We report a case of sepsis with GBS, in which an atypical cellulitis in the inguinal area was seen as presenting symptom.

J. L. L. Kimpen, MD, Beatrix Children's Hospital, University Hospital Groningen, Oostersingel 59, 9713 EZ Groningen, The Netherlands

INTRODUCTION

Group B streptococci are an important cause of neonatal infections. Early-onset disease is evident within the 1st week of life, characterized by symptoms of sepsis/meningitis and respiratory distress. Late-onset disease occurs after a median of 3–4 weeks, with meningitis as the most usual feature. Facial cellulitis has been described as a presenting symptom of invasive Group B streptococcal disease in 4–6% of cases with late-onset disease (1).

CASE REPORT

We present the case of a patient with late onset disease, with a peculiar cellulitis in a 'diaper-shaped' pattern. The patient, a boy, was born at a gestational age of 29 weeks as the first of twins. Delivery was uneventful, with Apgar scores of 8, 9 and 9 after 1, 5 and 10 min, respectively. Amoxicillin and amikacin administration was started shortly after birth, because of a leucopenia. There were no clinical symptoms of infection. Blood cultures were negative, and antibiotics were stopped after 5 days. He was transferred, 2 weeks later, to a regional hospital in good clinical condition.

After 2 weeks the boy was readmitted with tachycardia, abdominal distension, and progressive respiratory insufficiency. He was intubated and ventilated. On physical examination, he had a temperature of 37°C rectally, a heart rate of 180/min, and a blood pressure of 60/35 mmHg. The abdomen was painful and distended, without peristaltic activity. A diaper-shaped cellulitis was seen (Fig. 1). The lesion extended without interruption on the back and thighs. It was slightly elevated with sharp margins, and indurated.

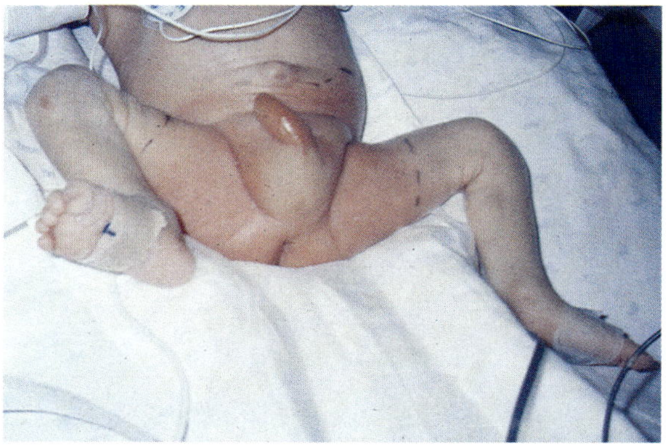

Fig. 1. Diaper-shaped cellulitis.

An abdominal X-ray showed intestinal distension. The chest X-ray was normal. Cultures of blood, urine, faeces and skin were obtained, and intravenous antibiotic therapy was started with amikacin and amoxicillin/clavulanic acid. A blood culture grew Gram-positive cocci, identified as group B streptococci. The same organism was found in a faecal sample. Antibiotic therapy was switched to amoxicillin monotherapy.

In conclusion, the patient suffered from a sepsis and cellulitis, preceding a paralytic ileus, due to Streptococcus agalactiae. After 2 days he improved, and could be weaned from the ventilator. The redness started to fade. After 4 days it was possible to detubate the patient; the redness had disappeared completely, although the induration persisted longer. He was discharged in good health, after 14 days of antibiotic therapy.

DISCUSSION

Cellulitis, as a presenting symptom of Group B streptococcal disease, has been described previously. However, the pattern of the cellulitis presented in this case, has not been hitherto reported. Most reports describe facial cellulitis, in submandibular or submental areas (1, 2, 4–6), possibly related to otitis media. Only Rand et al. (2) and Baker et al. (6) have reported Group B streptococcal inguinal cellulitis.

Cellulitis must be differentiated from erysipelas, panniculitis and erythema nodosum/induratum. The latter was very unlikely considering the age of the patient. Panniculitis is more usually characterized by the appearance of crops of subcutaneous nodules, while erysipelas is usually associated with lymphangitis or wounds in the diaper area.

In conclusion, cellulitis can be an important clue to an underlying sepsis/bacteraemia, with Group B streptococci, in the neonatal period.

REFERENCES

1. Yagupsky P, Menegus M, Powell K. The changing spectrum of the GBS-disease in infants; an eleven-year experience in a tertiary care hospital. Pediatr Infect Dis J 10: 801–808, 1991.

2. Rand TH. GBS-cellulitis in infants: a disease modified by prior antibiotic therapy or hospitalization? Pediatrics 81: 63–65, 1988.
3. Bonadio WA, Jurec W, Anderson Y, Smith D. Systemic infection due to group B beta-hemolytic streptococcus in children. Clin Pediatr: 230–233, 1992.
4. Hauger SB. Facial cellulitis: an early indicator of GBS-bacteremia. Pediatrics 67: 376–377, 1981.
5. Patamasucon P, Siegel JD, McCracken GH Jr. Streptococcal submandibular cellulitis in young infants. Pediatrics 67: 378–379, 1981.
6. Baker CJ. GBS-cellulitis-adenitis in infants. Am J Dis Child 136: 631–633, 1982.

Submitted January 13, 1995; accepted March 22, 1995

Scand J Infect Dis 27: 401–403, 1995 CASE REPORT

Increased Bactericidal Activity as Documented by Serum Bactericidal Titers for a Triple Combination of Cell Wall Active Agents against Gentamicin-resistant Enterococci

SURESH J. ANTONY[1,3], PETER MATHERIN[1] and CHARLES STRATTON[1,2,3]

From the Departments of [1]Medicine, [2]Pathology and the [3]Division of Infectious Diseases, Vanderbilt University School of Medicine, Nashville, Tennessee, USA

Infections caused by enterococci have become increasingly difficult to treat because these bacteria are becoming increasingly resistant to commonly used antibiotics such as ampicillin, gentamicin and vancomycin. A consensus for an optimal therapy of enterococcal infections caused by resistant isolates has not yet been determined. We present a patient with prolonged enterococcal sepsis in whom a combination of ampicillin, vancomycin and imipenem was ultimately sucessfull in suppressing enterococcal bacteremia. The enhanced activity of this triple combination was documented by the results of serial serum bactericidal titers.

S. J. Antony, MD, Division of Infectious Diseases, Vanderbilt University School of Medicine, A-3310 Medical Center North, Nashville, TN 37232, USA

INTRODUCTION

The treatment of patients with serious enterococcal infections has become a therapeutic dilemma due to the emergence of resistance to beta-lactam agents, aminoglycosides and, most recently, vancomycin. Various antimicrobial combinations have been studied in vitro and have proven synergy against enterococci. However, little if any clinical data has so far become available with which to assess and corroborate such syngergistic combinations in vivo.

We present a patient with Cushing's Syndrome who had enterococcemia with high-level gentamicin-resistant enterococcus from a perinephric abscess against which the combination of ampicillin, vancomycin and imipenem was used successfully to clear the bacteremia. In addition, serum bactericidal titers were used to document increased bactericidal activity as each of these cell wall active agents was sequentially added.

MATERIAL AND METHODS

To determine the serum bactericidal titers in this patient we used the broth microdilution method, in which the serum is diluted geometrically and a standard inoculum of the patient's organism is added to each tube or well, after which it is incubated for 24 h at 35°C. The serum inhibitory titer is the highest dilution of the serum that inhibits the visible growth. A sample from each tube showing no growth is then plated on agar and allowed to incubate for 24–72 h. The serum bactericidal titer is defined as the maximum dilution of the serum that can reduce the concentration of the patient's organism by 99.9% (1).

CASE REPORT

A 41-year-old female with no significant medical history was admitted to Vanderbilt University Hospital for evaluation of severe Cushing's Syndrome. On admission she was found to be afebrile, with a blood pressure of 187/102 mm/Hg and pulse rate of 89/min. Physical examination revealed central obesity, 'a buffalo hump', prominent facial/truncal hirsutism, a large right supraclavicular lymph node and proximal wasting. The rest of the examination was unremarkable. The admission laboratory tests were also unremarkable. A chest/abdominal CT scan revealed extensive mediastinal and supraclavicular lymphadenopathy with multiple lesions in the liver and bilateral adrenal hyperplasia. Biopsy of the right supraclavicular lymph node revealed a poorly differentiated neuroendocrine tumor with some carcinoid features. Chemotherapy with VP-16 and cisplatin was begun. She did well on this regimen and was subsequently discharged home.

One week later the patient was readmitted with diffuse abdominal pain. She was noted to be afebrile but was somnolent and hypotensive (BP 90/70 mmHg) with generalized weakness. Significant laboratory tests included a white blood cell count of 30,000 cells/μl, a hematocrit of 26% and potassium 2.6 mmol/l. Blood cultures were obtained and empiric therapy with ceftazidime and gentamicin initiated for presumed sepsis. The blood cultures obtained on admission were sterile; however, repeat cultures on days 6, 7 and 9 all grew Enterococcus fecalis. This isolate exhibited high-level resistance to gentamicin (MIC > 2000 mg/l), intermediate susceptibility to ampicillin (MIC = 1 mg/l) and low-level resistance to vancomycin (MIC = 8 mg/l). Gentamicin and ceftazidime were discontinued and, on day 7, vancomycin (500 mgIV q 6 h) was initiated; serum bacericidal titers on day 9 revealed a peak inhibitory titer of 1:8 and a trough inhibitory titer of 1:4. The peak and trough bactericidal titers were both 1:4. The similarities of these values are due in part to giving the vancomycin with a 6 h half-life every 6 h as evidence by peak and trough vancomycin levels of 40 mg/l and 12 mg/l respectively. Because of these low bactericidal titers for vancomycin as well as a positive blood culture for Enterococcus fecalis 2 days into therapy, ampicillin was added (2 g q 6 h) on day 14. A transthoracic echocardiogram done at this time was normal. However, an abdominal CT scan revealed a fluid collection in the perinephric space of the left kidney. When aspirated, this grew Enterococcus fecalis. Antibiotic concentrations

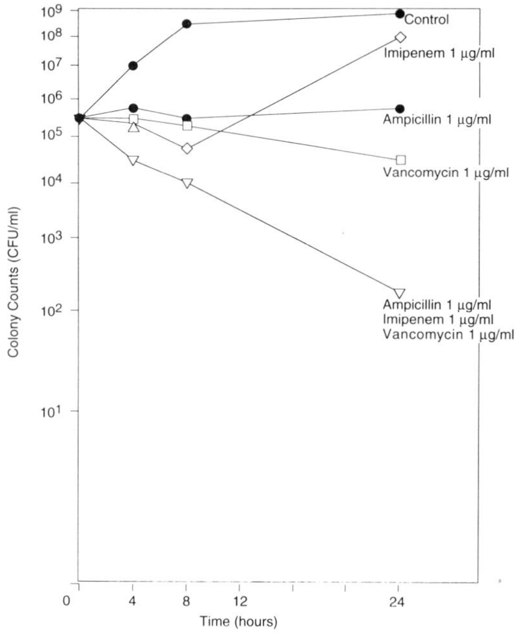

Fig. 1. In vitro time-kill curves using the triple combination of antibiotics.

were not determined in the aspirate from the abscess. At this time, peak inhibitory and bactericidal titers were 1 : 32 and 1 : 2, while trough inhibitory and bactericidal titers were 1 : 16 and 1 : 2. The MIC of this strain to vancomycin was 8 mg/l, while that for ampicillin was 1 mg/l.

Dosing schedules were selected to maximize the time during which the concentration exceeded the MICs, although vancomycin was changed to 1 g every 12 h. The patient continued to do poorly despite drainage and antimicrobials. On day 20, due to a continued low serum bactericidal titers with this combination therapy, imipenem (500 mg q 6 h) was added. The MIC of the patient's enterococcal strain to imipenem was 2 mg/l. With this triple regimen, serum bactericidal titers increased markedly; the peak was 1 : 256 and the trough was 1 : 64. Peak and trough vancomycin levels were 32 mg/l and 24 mg/l. Repeat serum bactericidal titers on day 30 were 1 : 256 (peak) and 1 : 128 (trough). Time-kill studies on this isolate were also performed (Fig. 1).

On this regimen the patient showed defervescence, with resolution of the leukocytosis. Repeat CT scan of the left renal area revealed no fluid collection. Chemotherapy with etoposide was initiated in order to reduce the tumor mass. However, this had to be discontinued due to the development of severe neutropenia. The antibiotics were discontinued on day 40. Blood cultures obtained after day 40 remained sterile. Chemotherapy with octreotide and aminoglutethmide also proved unsuccessful. On day 45 the patient showed symptoms and signs of an acute abdomen. Her underlying condition precluded surgical intervention and on day 46, the patient died of a presumed bowel perforation.

DISCUSSION

Enterococci have become the third most common cause of nosocomial infections in the USA (2), with E. fecalis causing 80–85% of all infections and E. fecium the remainder (3). Enterococci are known to cause endocarditis, intra-abdominal abscesses, cystitis/pyelonephritis, post-partum infection/endometritis and sepsis.

The enteroccoci are commensals of the gutu, vagina and urethral meatus (4–6) and thus may cause urinary tract infections (62%), intra-abdominal/pelvic infections (25%) as well as sepsis/bacteremia (10%) (7).

Despite the recent availability of many new classes of antimicrobial agents, enterococci continue to pose a therapeutic problem, as demonstrated by clinical failures such as that seen with penicillin therapy of endocarditis (8, 9) as well as the use of normally synergistic combinations such as the beta-lactam agent and an aminoglycoside (10, 11). The latter failures are of significant concern, as the therapy for serious enterococcal infections routinely had been an aminoglycoside combined with penicillin in order to achieve bacterial synergy (12, 13). Such synergistic activity against enterococci is lacking when strains exhibit high-level gentamicin resistance (MIC > 2000 mg/l) (14).

The reason for this emerging resistance of enterococci appears to be multifactorial, including indiscriminate use of antibiotics – especially cephalosporins (15) – and an increasing incidence of both intrinsic and acquired resistance. Enterococcal spp. demonstrate intrinsic resistance to penicillin, cephalosporin, clindamycin and aminoglycosides. The resistance to beta-lactam agents may be due to low affinity of penicillin-binding proteins, (PBPs, primarily PBP-5), which allows inhibition but not killing of the organism. Repeated exposure to beta-lactams appears to produce tolerance/resistance related to altered PBPs (16–19).

Acquired resistance may be due to acquisition of plasmids/transposons having resistance mechanisms. This is seen in high-level gentamicin resistance (20, 21) beta-lactamase resistance and vancomycin resistance (22, 23).

Enterococci with high-level resistance to gentamicin need to be tested for streptomycin resistance, because a small percentage of gentamicin-resistant isolates may be susceptible to this drug. We were unable to test for streptomycin resistance. This isolate was not a beta-lactamase producer according to a prolonged nitrocefin test (24); patients with serious enterococcal infections are usually treated with a beta-lactam (penicillin) or vancomycin in combination with an aminoglycoside (25). Instead of ampicillin, vancomycin is recommended for patients with penicillin allergy (26) and is used in combination with gentamicin (27, 28). With ampicillin- or penicillin-resistant strains due to altered PBPs, teicoplannin (Synercid RP 59500) or imipenem have been recommended as alternatives to vancomycin (25). Imipenem has been used against gentamicin-resistant enterococci as well as against strains moderately resistant to ampicillin in heroin addicts (29). A rabbit endocarditis model found imipenen to be just as effective as penicillin for reducing E. fecalis titers within vegetations (30). The serum bactericidal titers are used to determine the lethal activity of antibiotics in a patient's serum against the patient's own infecting organism. The test integrates both the pharmokinetic and pharmodynamic properties of the antimicrobial agents that the patient is receiving. Standardized methods for this test are available (1). Our laboratory uses broth without added serum, as well as the patient's serum, rather than an ultrafiltrate. In this case, three cell wall active agents were used with a step-wise addition of ampicillin to vancomycin therapy, and then imipenem added to the ampicillin/vancomycin therapy to increase the serum bactericidal levels.

Drainage of the abscess was undoubtedly important in the resolution of this bacteremia. The serum bactericidal titers obtained (peak 1 : 256, trough 1 : 128) on day 30 were high (or higher) than the usual peak and trough levels achieved with gentamicin and ampicillin therapy against a susceptible strain of enterococcus (4, 5).

Combinations of cell wall active agents have been evaluated in-vitro and have been suggested as an alternative therapy for enterococcal strains with high-level gentamicin resistance (24). It is possible that the addition of imipenem to ampicillin and vancomycin was useful due to differences in PBP affinity, as compared with ampicillin, with the combination resulting in increased saturation (30).

In conclusion, this case highlights the therapeutic use of serum bactericidal titers to document increased serum bactericidal activity. The SBTs thus guided therapy for cell wall active agents used against a high-level gentamicin-resistant enterococcus. Further clinical studies with this triple combination are needed in order to assess its clinical efficacy before definitive recommendations can be made for such therapy.

REFERENCES

1. National Committee for Clinical Laboratory Standards. Methodology for the Serum Bactericidal Test. Tentative guidelines. NCCLS document. M21-T (ISBN-1 56238-143-1). NCCLS, Villanova, PA 1992.
2. Centers for Disease Control. Nosocomial infection surveillance: 1984. MMWR 35: 17–29, 1986.
3. Lewis MC, Zervos MJ. Clinical manifestations of enterococcal infections. Eur Clin Microbiol Infect Dis 9: 111–117, 1990.
4. Noble CJ. Carriage of group D streptococci in the human bowel. J Clin Pathol 31: 1182–1186, 1978.
5. Mandell GI, Kaye D, Levison ME. Enterococcal endocarditis: an analysis of 38 patients observed at the New York Hospital–Cornell Medical Center. Arch Intern Med 125: 258–264, 1970.
6. Kaye E. Enterococci: biological and epidemiological characteristics and in vitro susceptibility. Arch Intern Med 142: 2006–2009, 1982.
7. Jones RN. The clinical impact of enterococcal resistance. Challenges in Infectious Disease 1: 1–6, 1993.
8. Christie RV. Penicillin in subacute endocarditis. BMJ 1: 381–386, 1976.
9. Tompsett R, Pizette M. Enterococcal endocarditis: Lack of correlation between therapeutic results and antibiotic sensitivity tests. Arch Intern Med 109: 146–150, 1962.
10. Horodniceanu T, Bougueleret L, El-Solh N, Bieth G, Delbos F. High level plasmid borne resistance to gentamicin in Streptococcus fecalis subspecies zymogenes. Antimicrob Agents Chemother 16: 686–689, 1979.
11. Hoffman SA, Moellering RC. The enterococcus: "Putting the bug in our ears". Ann Intern Med 106: 757–761, 1987.
12. Boulanger JM, Lee FJ, Matlow AG. Enterococcal bacteremia in a pediatric institution: a four year review. Rev Infect Dis 13: 847–856, 1991.
13. Gullberg RM, Homann SR, Phair JP. Enterococcal bacteremia: analysis of 75 episodes. Rev Infect Dis 11: 74–85, 1989.
14. Sahm DF, Torres C. Effects of medium and inoculum variation on screening for high level aminoglycoside resistance in Enterococcal faecalis. J Clin Microbiol 26: 250–256, 1988.
15. Whiteside M, Moore J, Ratzan K. An investigation of enterococcal bacteremia: Am J Infect Contrl 11: 125–129, 1983.
16. Storch GA, Krogstad DJ, Parquette AR. Antibiotic induced lysis of enterococci. J Clin Invest 68: 639–645, 1981.
17. Malouin F, Bryan LE. Modification of penicillin binding proteins as mechanisms of beta-lactam resistance. Antimicrob Agents Chemother 30: 1–5, 1986.
18. Williamson R, Calderwood SB, Moellerring RC, Tomasz A. Studies on the mechanism of intrinsic resistance to beta-lactam antibiotics in group D streptococci. J Gen Microbiol 129: 813–822, 1983.
19. Fontana R, Cerini R, Longini P, Grossoto A, Canpari P. Identification of streptococcal penicillin binding protein that reacts very slowly with penicillin. J Bacteriol 155: 1343–1350, 1983.
20. Zervos MJ, Kauffman CA, Therasse PM, Bergman AG, Mikessell TS, Schaberg DR. Nosocomial infection by gentamicin resistant Streptococcus faecalis: an epidemiological study. Ann Intern Med 106: 687–691, 1987.
21. Schaberg DR. Resistant nosocomial enterococal infections. Infectious Disease Newsletter 7: 1–5, 1988.
22. Uttley AHC, Collins CH, Naidoo J, George RC: Vancomycin resistant enterococci. Lancet 1: 57–58, 1988.
23. Leclereq R, Derlot E, Duval J, Courvalin P. Plasmid mediated resistance to vancomycin and teicoplanin in Enterococcal faecium. N Engl J Med 319: 157–161, 1988.
24. Stratton CW, Cooksey RC: Susceptibility tests: Special tests. In: Balows A, Hansler WJ, Hermann KL, et al., eds. Manual of Clinical Microbiology, 5th edn. Washington, D.C.: American Society of Microbiology, 1153–1157, 1991.
25. Leclercq R, Bingen E, Su QH, Lambert-Zechovski N, Courvalin P, Duval J. Effects of combinations of B lactams, daptomycin, gentamicin, and glycopeptides resistant enterococci. Antimicrob Agents Chemother 35: 92–98, 1991.
26. Bisno AL, Dismukes WE, Durack DT, Kaplan EL, Karchmer AW, Kaye D, Rahimitoola SH, Sande MA, Sandford JP, Watankunakorn C, Wilson WR. Antimicrobial treatment of infective endocarditis due to viridans streptococci, enterococci and staphylococci. JAMA 261: 1471–1477, 1989.
27. Cook FV, Coddington CC, Wadland WC, Farrar WE. Treatment of bacterial endocarditis with vancomycin. Am J Med Sci 276: 153–158, 1978.
28. Fernandez-Guerrero ML, Barro C, Rodrigues Tudela JL. Aortic endocarditis caused by gentamicin resistant Enterococcal faecalis. Eur J Clin Microbiol 7: 525–527, 1988.
29. Reiner NE, Gopalkrishna KV, Lerner PI. Enteroccal endocarditis in heroin addicts. JAMA 235: 1861–1863, 1976.
30. Auckenthaler GM, Wilson WR, Wright AJ, Washington AJ, Durack DT, Geraci JE. Lack of an in vivo and in vitro bactericidal activity of N-formimidoyl thienamycin against enterococcus. Antimicrob Agents Chemother 22: 448–452, 1982.

Submitted December 13, 1994; accepted March 16, 1995

Scand J Infect Dis 27: 405–407, 1995 CASE REPORT

Progressive Intractable Actinomycosis in Patients with AIDS

ROBERTO MANFREDI[1], ALDO MAZZONI[2], GINEVRA MARINACCI[1], ANNA NANETTI[2] and FRANCESCO CHIODO[1]

From the Institute of [1]Malattie Infettive and [2]Microbiologia, Università di Bologna, Bologna, Italy

Two rare cases of progressive oropharyngeal actinomycosis, characterized by a subacute and invasive course despite seemingly appropriate antibiotic and surgical treatment, have been observed in patients with AIDS. A brief review of previously reported cases of actinomycosis in HIV-infected patients is presented. Clinical, diagnostic and therapeutic problems dealing with actinomycosis in the immunocompromised host are discussed.

R. Manfredi, MD, Istituto Malattie Infettive, Università di Bologna, Via Massarenti 11, I-40138 Bologna, Italy

INTRODUCTION

Actinomycosis is a rare human disease caused by anaerobic bacteria belonging to the genus Actinomyces, which frequently colonize the oropharyngeal cavity and the gastrointestinal tract.

Cervicofacial localization is usually found in more than 50% of cases of actinomycosis. A progressive, indurated granulomatous infiltration, slowly spreading to contiguous tissues, with multiple abscesses and fistulas, often follows dental disease, chronic sinusitis, oral surgery or trauma, all local conditions supporting tissue necrosis and a microaerophilic environment (1–7). The microorganism is susceptible to penicillin and other antimicrobial agents; resistant strains have not been reported (8, 9). In more than 90% of treated patients, the outcome of actinomycosis is favourable, and a complete or partial response to chemotherapy and surgical treatment is obtained, even when the diagnosis is established late in the course of the disease (1–4, 6, 7, 10).

Two cases of severe oropharyngeal actinomycosis, characterized by a subacute and invasive course and by a poor response to antibiotics and surgery are described in patients with AIDS.

CASE REPORTS

Two patients aged 25 and 36 years, with a previous diagnosis of AIDS, developed a subacute, invasive inflammatory process, initially characterized by ulcerative, necrotizing lesions of the soft and hard palate, 2–3 cm in diameter, associated with an indurated infiltration of the adjacent soft tissues. Both patients were severely immunocompromised, showing a total leukocyte count of 1,780 and 2,450/μl, and a CD4+ cell count of 9 and 2/μl, respectively. No gingivodental disease, oral surgery or trauma were recorded in the weeks preceding hospitalization.

Since multiple bacterial and fungal organisms were initially isolated from pharyngeal swabs and biopsy specimens (Candida spp. and Staphylococcus aureus in both cases, associated with Pseudomonas aeruginosa in the first patient), treatment with fluconazole, ceftriaxone and netilmicin, followed by itraconazole and ceftazidime was started in the first patient, while the second received fluconazole, ceftriaxone and netilmicin, and subsequently itraconazole, piperacillin and clindamycin. After surgical debridement had been performed, an unequivocal histopathological diagnosis of actinomycosis was established by recognition of the typical sulphur-like granules with radiating Gram-positive filamentous bacteria in the affected tissue, in the absence of a significant inflammatory infiltrate (Fig. 1). Unfortunately, biopsy specimens were not cultured for actinomycosis in the early phase of the disease, and cultures were repeatedly negative in subsequent attempts, performed after confirmation of the diagnosis by histological examination.

Surprisingly, both cases presented a very similar clinical picture and disease course. Despite antibiotic treatment (including benzyl penicillin 7.2 g/day for 45 days in the second patient), the ulcerative necrotizing process spread during the following weeks to the rhinopharynx, maxillary sinuses and nasal cavity, with extensive soft tissue and bone necrosis (as evaluated by radiological and CT scan studies). This led to the formation of a large oronasal fistula, causing severe dysphagia and rhinolalia. Our patients died, due to respiratory failure following an interstitial pneumonia in the first case, and the development of other AIDS-related complications in the second case (Mycobacterium kansasii disseminated infection and toxoplasmic encephalitis).

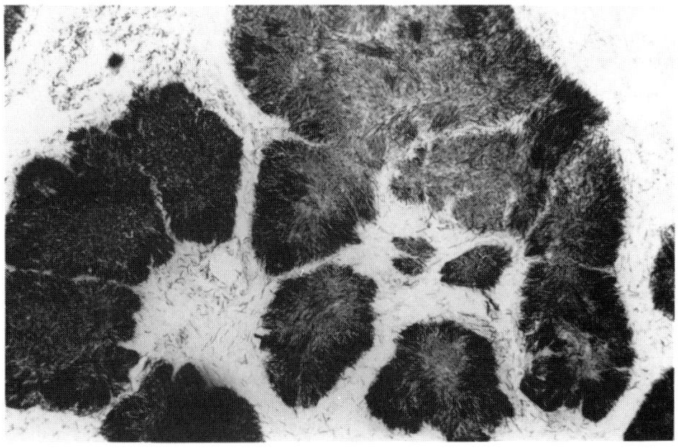

Fig. 1. Tissue Gram stain from the second patient, demonstrating colonies of Actinomyces. Branching filamentous Gram-positive bacteria with clubbed ends form round colonies, with a characteristic shape. Original magnification 400 ×.

 ISSN 0036-5548

DISCUSSION

Even though some studies have raised the possibility that cancer, immunosuppression, diabetes and malnutrition may act as risk factors for this disease (2, 3, 7, 11), and an effective T-lymphocyte and monocyte-macrophage function seems responsible for an adequate immune defence against these pathogens (5), actinomycosis is not considered as an opportunistic infection affecting immunocompromised individuals.

In fact, despite the spread of the HIV epidemic during the last decade, actinomycosis associated with AIDS has remained an exceedingly rare finding. To our knowledge, only 10 cases of actinomycosis have been reported up to now in HIV-infected subjects (11–19). In particular, an oral or cervicofacial localization was found in only 3 cases (12–14), all of them presumably secondary to dental extraction. Pulmonary disease has been recognized in 2 patients (15, 16), as well as perianal and anorectal involvement in 2 others (11, 17). More rare disease localizations occurred in the remaining 3 patients, with multiple cutaneous abscesses in 1 case (18), and oesophageal involvement in 2 (19). Among cases showing cervico-facial localization, only 1 suffered from extensive soft tissue and bone involvement (12), resembling the clinical picture of our patients.

Moreover, 7 of 8 evaluable HIV-infected patients with actinomycosis have been successfully treated by specific antibiotic therapy, and surgical drainage when necessary (11, 12–15, 17, 18). The case of pulmonary disease reported by Cendan et al. (16) showed a good clinical response, but only a partial resolution of endobronchial lesions, on bronchoscopic examination. In the remaining 2 cases information about treatment and outcome is lacking (19).

Unlike previously described cases, our patients with HIV-associated actinomycosis suffered from a severe and progressive clinical course of infection with extensive involvement of bone and soft tissues and craniofacial spread. They also showed a very poor response to specific antimicrobial treatment with benzyl penicillin G or cephalosporins, semisynthetic penicillins, and clindamycin (8, 9), administered at full doses for prolonged periods. The deep HIV-related immunodeficiency and neutropenia may have caused a more aggressive clinical course and a limited responsiveness to antimicrobial treatment.

Furthermore, both our cases were characterized by late recognition, confirmed by histological examination of tissue specimens obtained by surgical debridement. Especially in immunocompromised subjects, many factors may contribute to delay the diagnosis of actinomycosis: the low degree of suspicion due to the relative rarity of the disease; a clinical picture often consistent with that of other infectious or neoplastic disorders, and the reduced chances of successful laboratory isolation (because of the demanding culture requirements, the frequent overgrowth of other associated microbial agents and the widespread use of broad-spectrum antibiotics potentially effective against Actinomyces) (1–6). Diagnostic difficulties were even more evident in our patients, because of the absence of local predisposing conditions supporting entrance of microorganisms to deeper tissue, the concomitant isolation of other bacterial and fungal pathogens from the site of infection, and the absence of a granulomatous reaction (attributable to the severe HIV-related immunosuppression and granulocytopenia).

In conclusion, subacute invasive actinomycosis, although remaining a rare infectious complication, should be carefully considered in the wide spectrum of disorders possibly involving the oropharyngeal and craniofacial regions in patients with AIDS, because of the diagnostic difficulties, the potentially severe clinical course, and the poor responsiveness to specific antimicrobial treatment.

REFERENCES

1. Brown JR. Human actinomycosis. A study of 181 subjects. Hum Pathol 4: 319–330, 1973.
2. Weese WC, Smith IM. A study of 57 cases of actinomycosis over a 36-year period. A diagnostic failure with good prognosis after treatment. Arch Intern Med 135: 1562–1568, 1975.
3. Bartels LD, Vrabec DP. Cervicofacial actinomycosis: a variable disorder. Arch Otolaryngol 104: 705–708, 1978.
4. Rankow RM, Abraham DM. Actinomycosis: masquerader in the head and neck. Ann Otolaryngol 87: 230–237, 1978.
5. Burden P. Actinomycosis. J Infect 19: 95–99, 1989.
6. Benhoff DF. Actinomycosis: diagnostic and therapeutic considerations and a review of 32 cases. Laryngoscope 94: 1198–1217, 1984.
7. Feder HM Jr. Actinomycosis manifesting as an acute painless lump of the jaw. Pediatrics 85: 858–864, 1990.
8. Lerner PI. Susceptibility of pathogenic Actinomycetes to antimicrobial compounds. Antimicrob Agents Chemother 5: 302–309, 1974.
9. Holmberg K, Nord C, Dornbusch K. Antimicrobial in vitro susceptibility of Actinomyces israelii and Arachnia propionica. Scand J Infect Dis 9: 40–45, 1977.
10. Lad SD, Chandy MJ. Cranio-facial actinomycosis. Br J Neurosurg 5: 361–370, 1991.
11. Fry RD, Birnbaum EH, Lacey DL. Actinomyces as a cause of recurrent perianal fistula in the immunocompromised patient. Surgery 111: 591–594, 1992.
12. Yeager BA, Hoxie J, Weisman RA, Greenberg MS, Bilaniuk LT. Actinomycosis in the acquired immunodeficiency syndrome-related complex. Arch Otolaryngol Head Neck Surg 112: 1293–1295, 1986.
13. Watkins KV, Richmond AS, Langstein IM. Nonhealing extraction site due to Actinomyces naeslundii in patient with AIDS. Oral Surg Oral Med Oral Pathol 71: 675–677, 1991.
14. Molina M, Ortega G, De Paco M, Montoya JJ. Actinomicosis cervical en un portador de anticuerpos antivirus de la inmunodeficiencia humana. Rev Clin Esp 189: 301–302, 1991. [In Spanish]

15. Klapholz A, Talawera W, Rorat E, Salsitz E, Widrow C. Pulmonary actinomycosis in a patient with HIV infection. Mt Sinai J Med 56: 300–303, 1989.
16. Cendan I, Klapholz A, Talawera W. Pulmonary actinomycosis. A cause of endobronchial disease in a patient with AIDS. Chest 103: 1886–1887, 1993.
17. Smith TR. Actinomycosis of the distal colon and rectum. Gastrointest Radiol 17: 274–276, 1992.
18. Gresser U, Preac-Mursic V, Dörfler H, Spengel FA, Zöllner N. Actinomikose der Haut bei HIV-Infektion. Klin Wochenschr 66: 651–653, 1988. [In German]
19. Spencer GM, Roach D, Skucas J. Actinomycosis of the esophagus in a patient with AIDS: findings on barium esophagograms. Am J Roentgenol 161: 795–796, 1993.

Submitted January 9, 1995; accepted March 26, 1995

Cefrom®. Cefalosporinet med mycket brett spektrum.

(cefpirom)

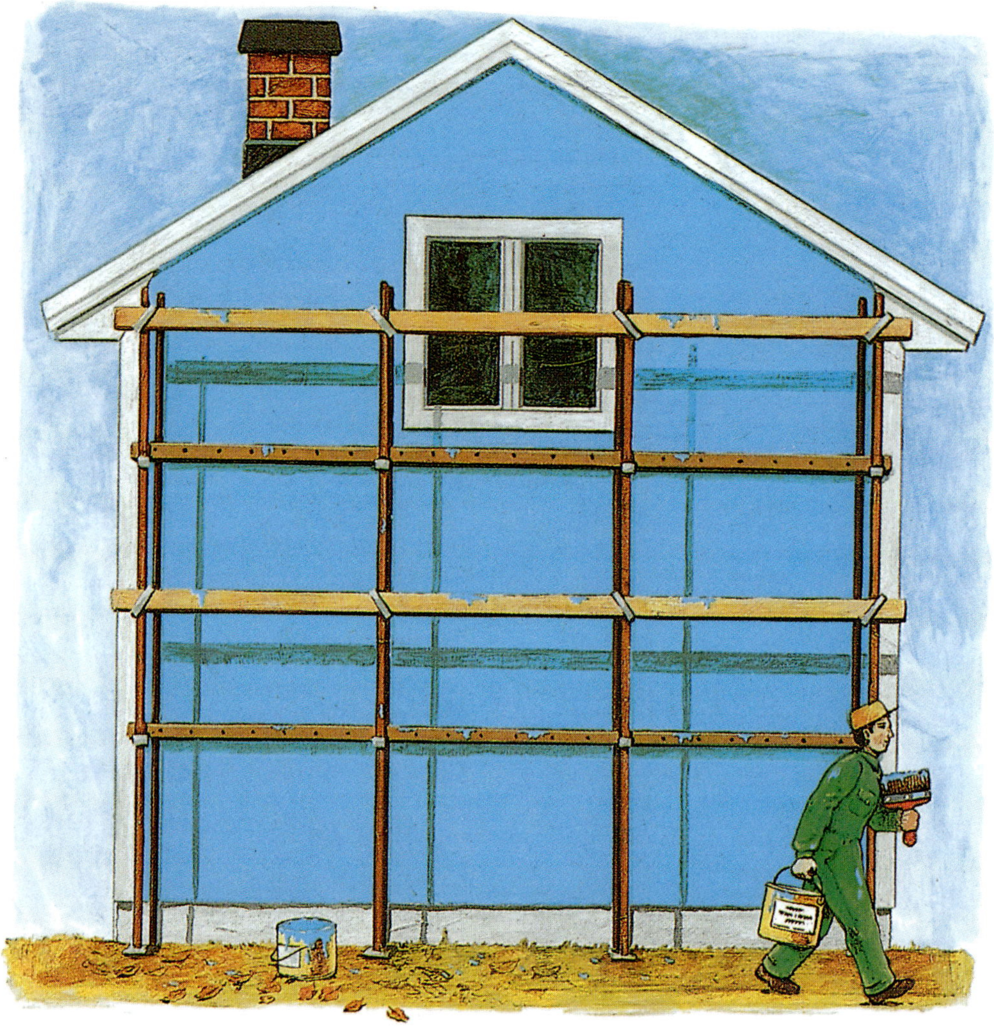

Rosell & Hansson, Gbg

Cefrom vidgar möjligheten till snabb och effektiv behandling med cefalosporiner. Cefrom kännetecknas av:

- **3:e generationens effekt på Gramnegativa bakterier**
- **1:a generationens effekt på stafylokocker**
- **effekt på enterokocker**

Praktiskt för empirisk terapi!

Cefrom®

cefpirom

Först av 4:e generationens cefalosporiner.

__Indikationer:__ Komplicerade eller livshotande infektioner i luft- och urinvägar. Septikemi utgången från urinvägar eller tarm med eventuellt tillägg av anaerobmedel.

__Förpackningar:__ Injektionvätska 5 x 0,5 g, 5 x 1,0 g, 5 x 2,0 g. Infusionsvätska 5 x 1,0 g, 5 x 2,0 g.

Svenska Hoechst AB
Läkemedelsdivisionen
Box 42026, 126 12 Stockholm
Telefon 08-775 70 00

Scand J Infect Dis 27: 409–410, 1995

CASE REPORT

Yersinia Enterolitica Bacteremia with Intracranial Extension

LYNE COPPENS, BERNARD SZTERN, DOMINIQUE KORMAN and FRANÇOIS LUSTMAN

From the Department of Internal Medicine, Centre Hospitalier Molière-Longchamp, Université Libre de Bruxelles, Bruxelles, Belgium

We report an unusual observation of Yersinia enterolitica (YE) bacteremia with subcutaneous abscesses on the scalp and, by gradual extension, cerebritis in a diabetic patient. All clinical signs disappeared after surgical drainage of the abscesses and protracted antibiotherapy. The well-known affinity of YE for iron led us to demonstrate an unrecognized hemochromatosis.

F. Lustman, MD, Centre Hospitalier Molière-Longchamp, rue Marconi 142, B–1180 Bruxelles, Belgium

INTRODUCTION

In Western Europe, Yersinia enterolitica (YE) has become as common as Salmonella sp. and Campylobacter as a cause of acute gastro-enteritis (1). Severe disease in adults due to YE mostly occurs in patients with cirrhosis, iron overload, immunodepression, and diabetes, Bacteremias are rare, and the mortality in these cases is high (2, 3).

The tendency of YE to exploit siderophores can explain its proliferation in the digestive tract where it benefits from those in other enterobacteria and can thus cause acute enterocolitis or a pseudo-appendicular syndrome (2). This is also a proposed explanation for the potential virulence of this bacteria in patients with an iron overload and, in particular, in those who have been treated with desferrioxamine (4, 5). We describe here an unusual case of YE bacteremia with subcutaneous abscesses and extension of the infection to the brain.

CASE REPORT

A 42-year-old diabetic woman was admitted with fever, headache, polydipsia, and confusion. Three weeks previously, she had stopped her insulin therapy. In 1983, gastrectomy, splenectomy, and caudal pancreatectomy had been performed. In 1986, diabetes was discovered and insulin treatment instituted. Physical examination gave normal results, except for fever (38.8°C) and confusion. The patient's serum glucose concentration was 402.8 mmol/l, the erythrocyte sedimentation rate (ESR) 92 mm/h, white-cell count $31{,}700 \times 10^9$/l (89% PMN), C Reactive Protein 314 mg/l (N < 5), total LDH 758 UI/l (N 230–460), γ-glutamyl transferase 167 UI/l (N 98–279), hemoglobin A1C 9.6% (N 5.6–7.5) of total Hb, and serum ferritin 5,269 mg/l (N 20–500). HbS, HIV, and syphilis serology were normal. A chest X-ray, brain CT scan, and abdominal echography all gave negative results.

Bacteremia was suspected and treatment with insulin and piperacillin + netilmicin was instituted. Dramatic improvement followed within 48 h except for the headache, which persisted. Palpation of the scalp revealed painful masses, clearly visible after the scalp was shaved (Fig. 1).

Puncture of one of these masses released pus containing Yersinia enterolitica, biotope 4, sero group 0:3, also present in the blood cultures from day 1.

The antibiotics were then replaced by pefloxacin 2 × 400 mg/d from day 3 on. However, the abscesses had to be drained on day 8. Meanwhile , on day 4, a heart echography gave normal results. On day 7, an isotopic MDP-Tc-99 m bone scintigraph showed an enhanced uptake in the skull. On day 12, an isotopic DTPA-Tc-99 m brain scan showed signal increase hyperfixation suggestive of cerebritis. On days 13 and 14, myoclonic seizures occurred, with paresis of the upper left arm. On day 13, brain CT scan and blood cultures were normal. Cerebritis was suspected, and pefloxacin was replaced by glazidim (4 g i.v./8 h). Diphenylhydantoin was also added to the treatment.

Magnetic resonance imaging (MRI) of the head on day 13 (Fig. 2, left) showed increased signal in the skull underlying a subcutaneous abscess, and after i.v. gadolinium injection (Fig. 2, right), enhancement of the meninges. In view of the risk of thrombophlebitis of the lateral sinus, the patient was treated with heparin from day 13 until day 51. The paresis of the left arm gradually disappeared. MRI of the brain remained unchanged on day 29. Antibiotic treatment was discontinued on day 43, but insulin was continued.

The clinical evolution was excellent, and all the laboratory test results became normal except ferritin, which remained too high (1,332 mg/l). Given the great affinity of YE for iron, an MRI of the liver was performed on day 30; it suggested hemochromatosis. A liver biopsy performed on day 55 was consistent with primary hemochromatosis.

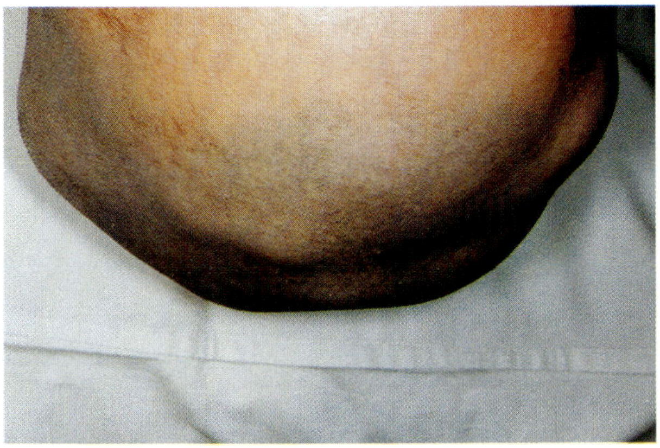

Fig. 1. Scalp masses corresponding to the subcutaneous abscesses.

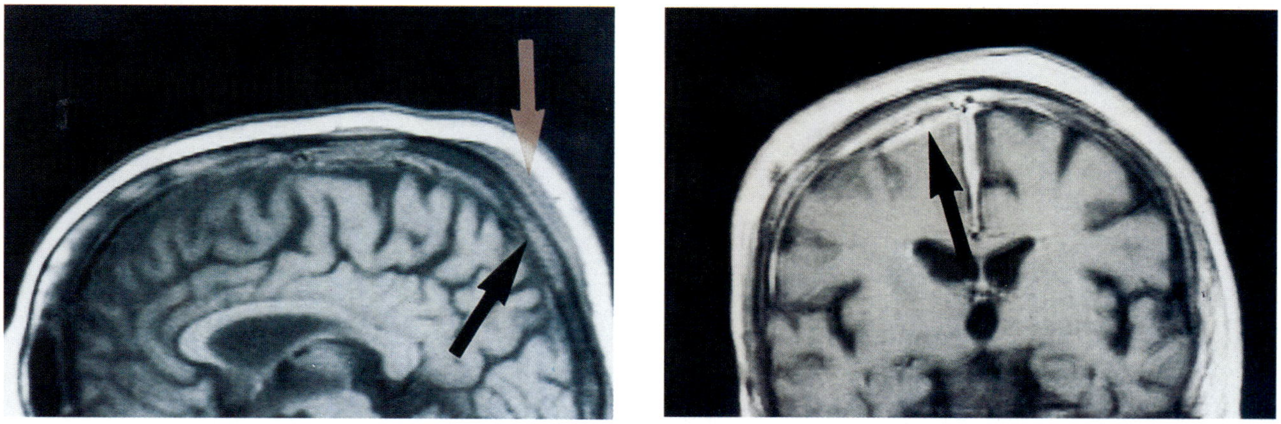

Fig. 2. Magnetic resonance imaging of the head. Left, sagittal section, showing increased signal (T2-weighted image) of the skull, underlying a subcutaneous abscess (*arrows*). Right, coronal section, showing after i.v. Gadolinium injection (T1-weighted image), enhancement of the meninges (*arrow*).

DISCUSSION

Numerous complications of YE have been described, including meningitis, osteitis, and erythema nodosum (the most common cutaneous effect) and bullous lesions of the skin, but subcutaneous abscesses are generally associated even with minor traumas, both surgical and non-surgical (6). The pathogenicity of YE as regards the subcutaneous tissues could be due to a membrane protein called invasine (6). Although bullous lesions of the skin associated with bacteremia have been described (7), we have not found in the literature any report of multiple subcutaneous abscesses in a patient with bacteremia, nor the development of cerebritis consecutive to a gradual invasion via the skull. This is why our observation seemed to us to be completely unusual.

Finally, as various authors stress, it was the identification of YE that led us to look for and demonstrate a primary hemochromatosis in this diabetic patient and not be satisfied with the diabetes as the only risk factor (5, 8).

ACKNOWLEDGEMENT

We thank Veronique Vleminckx for her help in preparing the manuscript.

REFERENCES

1. Jarvis WR. Yersinia enterolitica: A new or unrecognized nosocomial pathogen? Infect Control Hosp Epidemiol 13: 137–138, 1992.
2. Cover TL, Aber RC. Yersinia enterolitica. N Engl J Med 321: 16–24, 1989.
3. Abbott M, Galloway A, Cunningham JL, Politis D. Haemochromatosis presenting with a double yersinia infection. J Infection 13: 143–145, 1986.
4. Chiu HY, Flynn DM, Hoffbrand AV. Infection with Yersinia enterolitica in patients with iron overload. BMJ 292: 97, 1986.
5. Henrion J, De Neve A, Heller F. Septicémie bactérienne: une complication méconnue de l'hémochromatose idiopathique. Acta Clini Belg 41: 10–17, 1986. [in French]
6. Krogstadt P, Mendelman PM, Miller VL, et al. Clinical and microbiologic characteristics of cutaneous infection with Yersinia enterolitica. J Infect Dis 165: 740–743, 1992.
7. Le Paih MF, Pigney F, Fremaux A, Estrangin E, Cohen R, Geslin P. Yersiniose systémique à point de départ cutané. Presse Méd 19: 1767, 1990. [in French]
8. Bories C, Mezieres P, Courouble Y, Marche C, Gislon J. Hémochromatose idiopathique découverte à la suite d'une infection à Yersinia: deux nouvelles observations. Gastroenterol Clin Biol 10: 184–191, 1986. [in French]

Submitted December 28, 1994; accepted March 15, 1995

Scand J Infect Dis 27: 411–413, 1995 CASE REPORT

Tuberculous Pericarditis in an HIV-Infected Patient

SURESH J. ANTONY and DAVID W. HAAS

From the Department of Medicine, Division of Infectious Diseases, Vanderbilt University School of Medicine, Nashville, Tennessee, USA

Persons co-infected with mycobacterium tuberculosis (MTB) and HIV are at increased risk for developing active tuberculosis. While extrapulmonary tuberculosis is particularly common in patients with AIDS, tuberculous pericarditis is a very uncommon complication of AIDS in the United States. We present a case of tuberculosis involving the pericardium and review the current literature on this topic.

S. J. Antony, MD, Division of Infectious Diseases, Vanderbilt University School of Medicine, A-3310 Medical Center North, Nashville, Tennessee 37232-2605, USA

INTRODUCTION

HIV infection causes progressive immunodeficiency and increased susceptibility to opportunistic infections (1–3). In developing countries where HIV infection and tuberculosis are prevalent, tuberculosis is a relatively common cause of pericardial disease in HIV-infected patients (4). However, tuberculous pericarditis as a complication of AIDS in the United States has rarely been described (5–7). We report such a case and review the relevant clinical aspects of this disease.

CASE REPORT

In July 1994, a 25-year-old black male with AIDS was admitted to Vanderbilt University Hospital with a 2-week history of night sweats, fever, weight loss, anorexia and progressive dyspnea. His past medical history was significant for injection drug use, a remote episode of bacterial pneumonia, and oral candidiasis.

On physical examination he was in moderate distress with a temperature of 39°C, pulse of 103/min, respiratory rate of 24/min, and a blood pressure of 130/70 mmHg. Lung examination revealed fine bibasilar crackles and a left pleural friction rub. The cardiac apical impulse was displaced to the left sixth intercostal space in the midaxillary line. A pericardial knock, distant heart sounds and elevated jugular venous pressure were noted.

Initial laboratory tests were significant for a hematocrit of 36%, white blood cell count of 7.4×10^9/l with a normal differential, an LDH of 340 IU/l, an alkaline phosphatase of 223 IU/l, and a CD4 cell count of 76×10^6/l. Sputum acid fast stains and blood cultures were negative. The chest roentgenogram revealed an enlarged cardiac silhouette with small bilateral pleural effusions (Fig. 1). Electrocardiography showed non-specific ST-T wave changes and electrical alternans, and echocardiography demonstrated a large pericardial effusion with right atrial ventricular collapse. The patient was anergic to tuberculin, mumps and candida skin tests antigens.

Because of progressive dyspnea, a pericardiocentesis was performed, which yielded 1600 ml of serosanguinous fluid. A pigtail catheter was placed for continued drainage. The pericardial fluid had a glucose of 85 g/dl, a protein 5.4 g/dl, and a white blood cell count of 12.6×10^9/l, with 44% polymorphonuclear leukocytes, 46% lymphocytes, and 10% monocytes. A presumptive diagnosis of tuberculous pericarditis was made and isoniazid, rifampin, and pyrazinamide were begun. The patient defervesced within 48 h. The pericardial fluid subsequently grew Mycobacterium tuberculosis which was sensitive to all first-line anti-tuberculous agents. The patient's subsequent course was uncomplicated except for an episode of atrial fibrillation. An echocardiogram performed 6 days following drainage and initiation of antituberculous therapy showed resolution of the pericardial effusion, and a chest roent-genogram showed decreased size of the cardiac silhouette (Fig. 2).

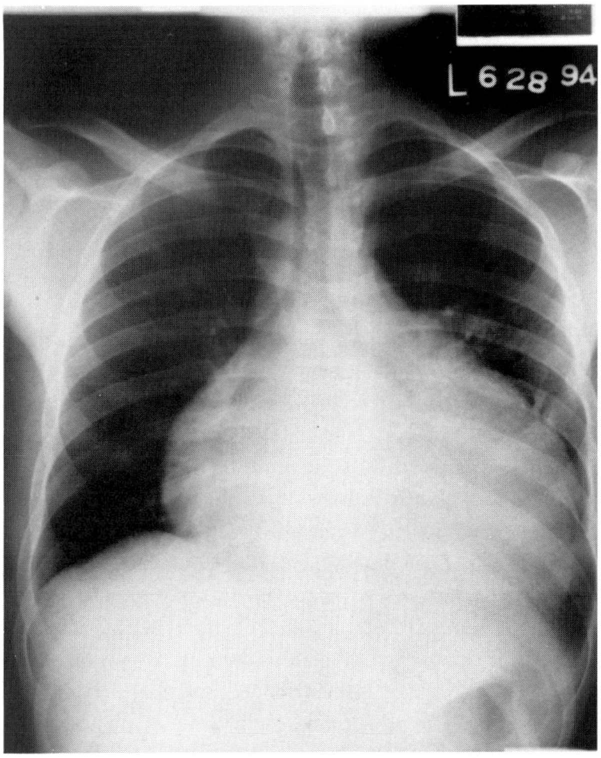

Fig. 1. Chest roentgenogram before pericardiocentesis.

 ISSN 0036-5548

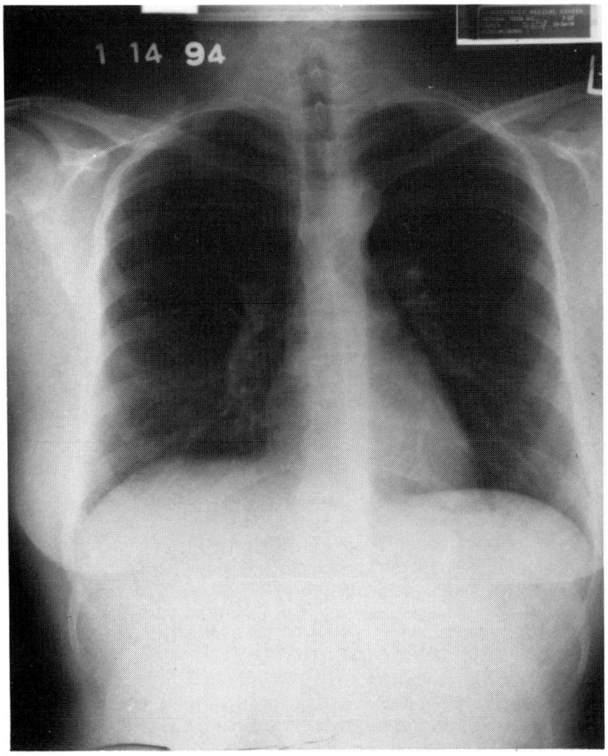

Fig. 2. Chest roentgenogram following pericardiocentesis.

DISCUSSION

Prior to 1981, the incidence of pulmonary tuberculosis had demonstrated a yearly decline but the incidence of extrapulmonary tuberculosis had remained relatively constant at about 4000 cases per year (8). However, since the AIDS epidemic, the incidence of extrapulmonary tuberculosis has been between 37 to 70% in the USA (9). Among AIDS patients in the United States, extrapulmonary tuberculosis commonly involves the genitourinary tract, musculoskeletal system and lymph nodes. The heart is involved infrequently (5, 10–12). Among 330 patients described in 4 large studies in the United States, only 3 (0.9%) out of 333 HIV-positive patients with tuberculosis were noted to have pericardial involvement (13–16). This appears to be in contrast to reports from Africa, where tuberculous pericarditis is a relatively frequent finding among HIV-infected patients (4, 17).

Tuberculous pericarditis appears to occur more often in the black population with a low incidence of pulmonary infiltrates and high incidence of pleural effusion (18, 19).

Studies which predated the AIDS epidemic showed tuberculous pericarditis to occur most commonly following contiguous spread from adjacent lymph nodes and, less often, to be due to hematogenous seeding. Common symptoms include dyspnea and orthopnea, and signs of elevated right heart pressure are commonly present. A pleural rub is apparent in one-third of patients (18, 19). The diagnosis of tuberculous pericarditis is best established by pericardiocentesis and/or pericardial biopsy (19, 20). The pericardial fluid may be turbid or hemorraghic, with a white blood cell count which ranges from 5–10 × 10^9/l, consisting predominantly of lymphocytes. There may be an elevation of the protein and glucose. Agner & Gallis (21) noted in their series that the pericardial effusion had a mean WBC, lymphocyte, and monocyte count of 12.6 × 10^9/l, 46.3 × 10^9/l and 9.2 × 10^9/l respectively. The mean glucose was 85 g/dl (21). Culture of the pericardial fluid fails to grow M. tuberculosis in approximately 50% of cases (22). However, pericardial biopsies have been positive in for granulomas in 87 to 100% of cases (7, 18, 23). Echocardiography readily demonstrates a pericardial effusion in active cases. Constrictive pericarditis is commonly seen in patients who are untreated and survive the acute disease.

Clinical manifestations of tuberculous pericarditis are probably a result of the acute inflammatory response or due to fluid accumulation in the pericardium. It is uncertain to as to what extent, if at all, that concomitant HIV infection affects the clinical manifestations of tuberculous pericarditis. A study performed in Africa failed to demonstrate any significant differences in the clinical features (chest pain, shortness of breath, leg edema, orthopnea), frequency of tamponade, duration of hospital stay or morbidity from tuberculous pericarditis between HIV-positive and HIV-negative patients (4). However, this may reflect the fact that the patients reported had relatively intact immunologic function, as evidenced by preserved tuberculin reactivity. However, it may be hypothesized that in these patients there may be a greater likelihood of finding granulomas in a biopsy, having a positive culture or developing constriction.

The fact that most reported cases of tuberculous pericarditis have been from Africa may reflect the very high incidence of both tuberculosis and HIV infection, and may also be due to other factors, such as the prolonged interval between infection and medical management and lack of clinical findings in the early stage of the disease.

Extrapulmonary involvement has been documented in almost 70% of AIDS patients with tuberculosis, the frequency increasing at lower CD4 cell counts (10). It is unclear why tuberculous pericarditis is so uncommon in this country, despite a large proportion of patients with advanced HIV disease.

Reported causes of pericardial effusion in patients with AIDS include early diagnostic pericardiocentesis. If negative, pericardial biopsy may be diagnostic. Controversy exists regarding the utility of pericardiectomy to prevent constrictive pericarditis (24). Measurement of pericardial fluid adenosine deaminase levels (normal level < 40 IU/l) is relatively sensitive and specific for tuberculosis (25), but this test has not been extensively studied in the United States. Furthermore, the effect of HIV infection on the diagnostic utility of adenosine deaminase measurement is not known.

Corticosteroids given concomitantly with antituberculous medications have been shown to increase survival, to reduce the need for surgical intervention, and to reduce the incidence of late pericarditis by 51% (26). In early HIV infection the pathologic manifestations of tuberculosis in other organ systems are much like those in HIV-negative persons, and steroids may be useful. However, their potential benefit in more immunocompromised patients must be balanced against the risk of further immunosuppression. If both rifampin and corticosteroids are used, relatively high doses of corticosteroids are indicated because rifampin induces steroid metabolism. In non-AIDS patients, untreated tuberculous pericarditis has a mortality of greater than 80%, with constrictive pericarditis eventually occurring in many survivors. The mortality of TB pericarditis in AIDS when untreated is not known but would probably be very high.

In conclusion, tuberculous pericarditis is uncommon among patients with AIDS in the United States. Tuberculosis should be included in the differential diagnosis of HIV-related pericarditis. Such patients appear to respond well to standard chemotherapy. Corticosteroids are likely to be of benefit when pericarditis complicates early HIV infection, but their role in advanced AIDS is uncertain.

REFERENCES

1. Scott PJ, Conway SP, Dacosta P. Cardiac tamponade complicating cytomegalovirus pericarditis in a patient with AIDS. J Infect Dis 20: 92–93, 1990.
2. Freedberg RS, Gindea AJ, Dietrich DT, Greene JB. Herpes simplex pericarditis in AIDS. N Y J Med 87: 304–306, 1987.
3. Schuster M, Valentine F, Holzman R. Cryptococcal pericarditis in an intravenous drug abuser [letter]. J Infect Dis 152: 182, 1985.
4. Cegielski JP, Ramaiya K, Lallinger GJ, Mtulia IA, Mbaga IM. Pericardial disease and human immunodeficiency virus in Dar-es-Salaam, Tanzania. Lancet 335: 209–212, 1990.
5. D'Cruz IA, Sengupta EE, Abrahams C, Reddy HK, Turlapi RV. Cardiac involvement including tuberculous pericardial effusion complicating acquired immunodeficiency syndrome. Am Heart J 112: 1100–1102, 1986.
6. Reynolds M, Berger M, Hecht S, Kolokathis A, Horowitz SF. Large pericardial effusion in the acquired immunodeficiency syndrome. Chest 102: 1746–1747, 1992.
7. Dalli E, Quesda A, Juan G, Navarro R, Paya R, Tormo V. Tuberculous pericarditis as the first manifestation of acquired immunodeficiency syndrome. Am Heart J 114: 905–906, 1987.
8. Mehta JB, Dutt A, Harvill L, Mathews KM. Epidemiology of extrapulmonary tuberculosis: a comparative analysis with the pre-AIDS era. Chest 99: 1134–1138, 1991.
9. Weir MR, Thoerton GF. Extrapulmonary tuberculosis: experience of a community hospital and review of the literature. Am J Med 79: 467–469, 1985.
10. Slutsker L, Castro KG, Ward JW, Dooley SW. Epidemiology of extrapulmonary tuberculosis among persons with AIDS in the United States. Clin Infect Dis 16: 513–518, 1993.
11. Reider HL, Snider DE, Cauthen GM. Extrapulmonary tuberculosis in the United States. Am Rev Respir Dis 141: 347–351, 1990.
12. Horn DL, Hewlett D, Alfalla C, Peterson S. Fatal hospital acquired multidrug resistant tuberculous pericarditis in two patients with AIDS. N Eng J Med 17: 1816–1817, 1992.
13. Shafer RW, Kim DS, Weiss JP, Quale JM. Extrapulmonary tuberculosis in patients with human immunodeficiency syndrome. Medicine 70: 384–397, 1991.
14. Hill RA, Premkumar S, Brustein S, Vaidya K, Powell S, Li PW, Suster B. Disseminated tuberculosis in the acquired immunodeficiency syndrome era. Am Rev Respir Dis 144: 1164–1170, 1991.
15. Theuer CP, Hopewell PC, Elias D, Schecter GF, Rutherford GW, Chaisson RE. Human immunodeficiency virus infection in tuberculosis patients. J Infect Dis 162: 8–12, 1990.
16. Handwerger S, Mildvan D, Serrie R, McKinely FW. Tuberculosis and the acquired immunodeficiency syndrome at a New York City Hospital. Chest 91: 176–182, 1987.
17. Taelman H, Kagame A, Batungwanayo J, Nyiralareja A, Abdel AM, Blanch P, Bogaerts J, Vandeperre P. Pericardial effusion and HIV infection. Lancet 14: 924, 1990.
18. Schepers GW. Tuberculosis pericarditis. Am J Cardio 9: 248–276, 1962.
19. Fowler NO. Tuberculous pericarditis. J Am Med Assoc 266: 99, 1991.
20. Ortbals DW, Marr JJ. A comparative study of tuberculosis and other mycobacterial infections and their association with malignancy. Am Rev Respir Dis 117: 39–45, 1978.
21. Agner RC, Gallis HA. Pericarditis. Differential diagnostic considerations. Arch Intern Med 139: 407–412, 1979.
22. Rooney JJ, Croco JA, Lyons HA. Tuberculous pericarditis. Ann Inter Med 72: 73–78, 1970.
23. Reynolds M, Berger M, Hecht S, Kolokathis A, Horowitz SF. Large pericardial effusions in the acquired immunodeficiency syndrome. Chest 102: 1746–1747, 1992.
24. Carson TJ, Murray GF, Wilcox BR. The role of surgery in tuberculous pericarditis. Ann Thorac Surg 17: 163, 1974.
25. Koh KK, Kim JE, Cho HC, Choi JM, Cho KS, Kim SS, Kim HM, Lee JC, Kim MJ, Nam SH, Lee HY. Adenosine deaminase and carcinoembryonic antigen in pericardial effusion diagnosis, especially in suspected tuberculosis pericarditis. Circulation 89: 2728–2734, 1994.
26. Strang JG, Gibson DG, Mitchison DA, Girling DJ, Kakasa HS, Allen BW, Evans DJ, Nunn AJ, Fox W. Controlled clinical trial of complete surgical drainage and use of prednisolone in the treatment of tuberculous pericardial effusion in Transkei. Lancet 2: 759–764, 1988.

Submitted January 30, 1995; accepted April 16, 1995

Scand J Infect Dis 27: 415–417, 1995 CASE REPORT

Hepatobiliary Tuberculosis Presenting as a Gall Bladder Tumor

REN-JY BEN[1], TZUUGUANG YOUNG[2] and HERNG-SHENG LEE[3]

From the Departments of Medicine,[1] 802 Army General Hospital, Kaohsiung, [2]Division of Infectious Diseases, and [3]Department of Pathology, Tri-Service General Hospital, Taipei, Taiwan, Republic of China

A 64-year-old married female was admitted with a presentation of anorexia, easy fatiguability, skin discoloration, tea-colored urine and weight loss of 1 month's duration. After a series of clinical and laboratory examinations including radiological image studies, a diagnosis of gall bladder tumor was presumed. A final diagnosis of tuberculosis of the liver and gall bladder was established by histopathological examination of tissue specimens obtained during exploratory laparotomy. Hepatobiliary tuberculosis presenting as a gall bladder tumor is rare and no pathognomonic diagnostic characteristics can be relied upon. It is necessary to confirm the diagnosis by histopathology, polymerase chain reaction (PCR), or microbiological studies on biopsy specimens in order to make possible appropriate, early therapy.

R.-J. Ben, MD, Division of Infectious Diseases, Department of Medicine, Tri-Service General Hospital, No. 8, Sec 3, Ting-Chow Road, Taipei, Taiwan, Republic of China

INTRODUCTION

The incidence of gall bladder tuberculosis is very low in extrapulmonary tuberculosis, and is much rarer than local tuberculosis of the liver (1). Hepatobiliary tuberculosis is uncommon and the diagnosis is difficult because of the lack of characteristic symptoms and signs. Exploratory laparotomy or autopsy has often been required in the past, to establish the diagnosis (1). Recently, the use of abdominal sonography, computed tomography (CT) or radionuclide scan has made it possible to localize abnormal lesions in the liver and gall bladder. However, tissue biopsy with microbiological confirmation and/or polymerase chain reaction (PCR) is often needed to verify the diagnosis of tuberculosis.

CASE REPORT

A 64-year-old housewife had been well until 8 months before admission when she developed intermittent nausea and dizziness. At 1 month prior to admission she began to experience decreased appetite and excessive fatigue, with yellowish skin discoloration, dark-colored urine and weight loss of 11 kg. At a local hospital, the patient was found to have elevated serum alkaline phosphatase and serum bilirubin. Because of the persistence of her symptoms, she was referred to the Tri-Service General Hospital for further evaluation.

Past medical history revealed a diagnosis of a goiter which was operated on when she was 44 years of age, and the patient had been on diet management for non-insulin-depenent diabetes mellitus for the 2–3 years prior to admission.

On admission, her vital signs were within normal limits. Her skin was slightly yellowish and the sclerae were mildly jaundiced. The liver and spleen were not palpable and there was no localized abdominal tenderness. The remaining physical examination was unremarkable.

Initial laboratory examinations revealed a platelet count of 139×10^9/l, a serum glucose of 7.97 mmol/l, an aspartate transaminase of 116 U/l (normal range, 0–42 U/l), an alanine transaminase of 142 U/l (normal range, 0–42 U/l), an alkaline phosphatase of 725 U/l (normal range, 65–270 U/l) and a total bilirubin of 34 μmol/l (3.4–17.1 μmol/l). She tested negative for HIV.

Chest X-ray disclosed no abnormality. Abdominal sonography showed hyperechoic materials surrounded by an anechoic ring with near total occupation of the entire lumen of the gall bladder. A hyperechoic nodule with a halo ring about 2 cm in diameter was located over the right lobe of the liver just abutting the gall bladder. Another hyperechoic nodule, about 1 cm in diameter over the left lobe of the liver, was also identified. A CT scan demonstrated an abnormally high CT value, around 20–30 Hounsfield units (HU), in the lumen of the gall bladder. The liver nodules detected by sonography showed hypodensity on CT scan (Fig. 1). Endoscopic retrograde cholangiopancreatography (ERCP) showed negative findings.

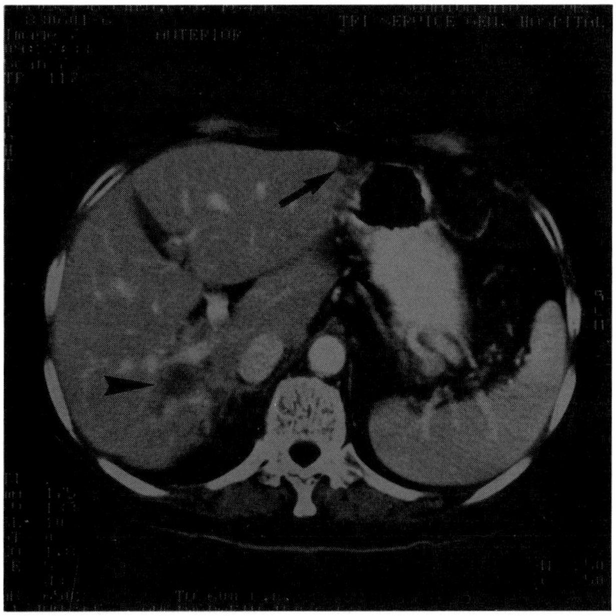

Fig. 1. Abdominal computed tomography demonstrated an ill-defined hypodense lesion (2 × 2 × 2 cm) near the gall bladder fossa (arrowhead), and a further small hypodense lesion (1 × 1 × 1 cm) in the lateral segment of the left lobe of the liver (arrow).

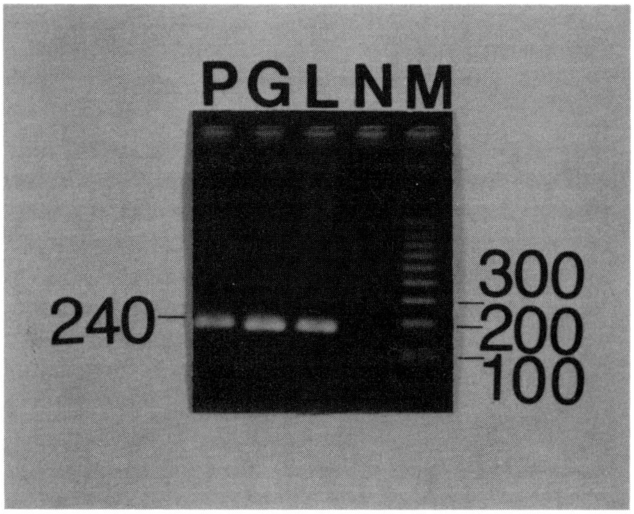

Fig. 2. Electrophoresis of the PCR product showing a positive 240 bp band from the formalin-fixed paraffin-embedded liver and gall bladder tissue. (M, marker; L, liver; G, gall bladder; N, negative control; P, positive control).

As a gall bladder tumor was suspected, a laparotomy with cholecystectomy and wedge resection of the left lobe of liver were performed. Grossly, the gall bladder contained a conspicuous yellowish-colored substance, and the liver tissue was firm and gray in color. Microscopically, the sections of the gall bladder and liver showed caseating granulomas composed of Langhans' giant cells, and epithelioid histiocytes and lymphocytes in the granulomatous wall. Acid-fast bacilli were demonstrated by Ziehl–Neelsen stain only in the gall bladder lesion. Culture for mycobacteria was not performed. Extraction of DNA samples from the formalin-fixed paraffin-embedded tissues of liver and gall bladder granulomas, for PCR using primers with 5′-TCC GCT GCC AGT CGT CTT CC-3′ and 5′-GTC CTC GCG AGT CTA GGC CA-3′, showed a positive 240 base pair band in a 1% agarose gel (Fig. 2).

Anti-tuberculous drugs consisting of isoniazid, ethambutol and rifampin were given after surgery. A PPD skin test (5TU) was positive with 14 mm of induration at 48 h. The patient developed fever 2 days after the operation and cefazolin plus gentamicin was given, but the fever persisted. T-tube drainage fluid on the 14th postoperative day yielded Acinetobacter anitratus. On the basis of the sensitivity test, piperacillin and amikacin were given and her fever resolved. The patient was discharged on the 106th hospital day to continue antituberculous treatment at home.

DISCUSSION

Following the first published report of gall bladder tuberculosis by Simmonds in 1908, this theme was comprehensively discussed by Rankin & Massie in 1926 (2) and more case reports were described (3, 4). The incidence of gall bladder tuberculosis remains low (4), but the reason for the rarity of occurrence is unknown. It may be due to a failure in diagnosis, or to a particular resistance of the gall bladder to the Mycobacterium tuberculosis (2). Tuberculoma is a conglomerate of granulomas with caseation necrosis from which the organism may frequently be identified by staining procedures (5). In our case, cultures for mycobacteria were not obtained due to the presumptive diagnosis of gall bladder tumor, without consideration of an infectious etiology.

Tuberculosis of the gall bladder is more common in women over 30 years of age and is frequently associated with gallstones (1). Gallstones may be of pathogenic significance for the development of tuberculosis in the gall bladder (4). Tuberculous infection of the gall bladder is probably caused by hematogenic or lymphogenic spread (2); direct involvement or secondary involvement from a preexisting infection in the liver may also play a role. Mycobacterium tuberculosis can ascend from the pylorus or duodenum and pass through the diaphragm by way of the lymphatics (3). Involvement of portal lymph nodes may occur via direct spread from the gall bladder, or by hematogenic or lymphogenic spread (6).

Hepatic granulomas are usually associated with an elevated alkaline phosphatase level. Larger granulomas with caseation are associated with more pronounced hepatic dysfunction (7). Obstructive jaundice, secondary to lymphadenopathy in the portal tract, and peripancreatic area has been reported as a rare complication of tuberculosis (6, 8). In our case, we may speculate that the transient jaundice was a result of obstruction of bile flow by tuberculomas in the portal tract.

Two different ultrasonic patterns of liver tuberculomas have been described, which seem to represent 2 pathogenic forms corresponding to evolutionary stages of the disease. The first pattern shows hypoechoic and low-density lesions without a distinct wall resulting from conglomeration of numerous small tubercles. The second shows hypoechoic and low-density lesions with hyperechoic rims related to a tuberculous abscess (9). However, in the case presented here, the sonographic examinations showed a distinctive sonographic picture which might have given a clue for the diagnosis. In tuberculosis, presumably the low-density nature of the involved nodes is secondary to caseation necrosis which has a characteristic feature on the abdominal CT scan. Nevertheless, there are no CT findings, alone or in combination, that are pathognomonic for tuberculosis (10).

All reported cases of tuberculosis of the gall bladder have been diagnosed intraoperatively or postmortem (3). Postoperative complications include permanent fistula formation, tuberculous peritonitis or both (2). In the past, surgery was considered mandatory because there was no satisfactory non-invasive method of diagnosing intra-abdominal lesions, and no way of observing the response to treatment. The development of radionuclide scan, ultrasonography, and CT has had a major impact on the diagnosis and treatment of intra-abdominal lesions.

Diagnosis of intra-abdominal tuberculosis is difficult because of a paucity of symptoms, and because of non-specific signs and inconclusive clinical tests (10). In many cases, the diagnosis was achieved by Ziehl–Neelsen staining of involved tissues or, more commonly, by the microscopic appearance of caseating granulomas (11). Although there may be a number of reasons for failure to culture (12), isolation of M. tuberculosis remains the most sensitive and specific diagnostic method and is the hallmark for diagnosis of all types of tuberculosis (13). The organisms are slow-growing, and hence laboratory diagnosis by conventional methods can take as long as 10 weeks. The PCR method can be used as a rapid screening method for the presence of M. tuberculosis (14). The oligonucleotide primers used amplify a 240 base pair fragment from the gene encoding for the immunogenic protein MPB64, cloned from M. bovis BCG (15). In PCR, the specificity is ensured by the choice of the amplified sequence. The gene sequence coding for the MPB64 protein seems to be specific for the M. tuberculosis complex (16). As demonstrated in our patient, PCR may be particularly suitable for the detection of pathogens which are present in small numbers, or which are difficult to culture (15).

ACKNOWLEDGEMENT

We thank Dr. Mein-Kai Gueng, radiology specialist, for kindly interpreting the image study.

REFERENCES

1. Leader SA. Tuberculosis of the liver and gall bladder with abscess formation: a review and case report. Ann Intern Med 37: 594–606, 1952.
2. Rankin FW, Massie FM. Primary tuberculosis of the gall bladder. Ann Surg 83: 800–806, 1926.
3. Lazarus JA, Eisenberg AA. Tuberculosis of the gall bladder: report of a case of primary tuberculous cholecystitis. Am J Med 24: 166–173, 1934.
4. Bergdahl L, Boquist L. Tuberculosis of the gall bladder. Br J Surg 59: 289–292, 1972.
5. Harrington PT, Gutierrez JJ, Ramirez-Rona CH, Quinones-Soto R, Bermudez RH, Chaffey J. Granulomatous hepatitis. Rev Infect Dis 4: 638–653, 1982.
6. Kohen MD, Altman KA. Jaundice due to a rare cause: tuberculous lymphadenitis. Am J Gastroenterol 59: 48–53, 1973.
7. Korn RJ, Kellow WF, Heller P, Chomet B, Zimmerman HJ. Hepatic involvement in extrapulmonary tuberculosis Am J Med 27: 60–71, 1959.
8. Murphy TF, Gray GF. Biliary tract obstruction due to tuberculous adenitis. Am J Med 68: 452–454, 1980.
9. Brauner M, Buffard MD, Jeantils V, Legrand I, Gotheil C. Sonography and computed tomography of macroscopic tuberculosis of the liver. J Clin Ultrasound 17: 563–568, 1989.
10. Hulnick DH, Megibow AJ, Naidich DP, Hilton S, Cho KC, Balthazar EJ. Abdominal tuberculosis: CT evaluation. Radiology 157: 199–204, 1985.
11. Zipser RD, Rau JE, Ricketts RR, Bevans LC. Tuberculous pseudotumors of the liver. Am J Med 61: 946–951, 1976.
12. Cutler RR, Baithun SI, Doran HM, Wilson P. Association between the histological diagnosis of tuberculosis and microbiological findings. Tuber Lung Dis 75: 75–79, 1994.
13. Alvarez S, McCabe WR. Extrapulmonary tuberculosis revisited: a review of experience at Boston City and other hospitals. Medicine 63: 25–55, 1984.
14. Cousins DV, Wilton SD, Francis BR, Gow BL. Use of polymerase chain reaction for rapid diagnosis of tuberculosis. J Clin Microbiol 30: 255–258, 1992.
15. Cormican MG, Barry T, Gannon F, Flynn J. Use of polymerase chain reaction for early identification of Mycobacterium tuberculosis in positive cultures. J Clin Pathol 45: 601–604, 1992.
16. Shankar P, Manjunath N, Lakshimi R, Aditi B, Seth P, Shriniwas. Identification of Mycobacterium tuberculosis by polymerase chain reaction. Lancet 335: 423, 1990.

Submitted December 15, 1994; accepted May 7, 1995

Scand J Infect Dis 27: 419–420, 1995

Candida albicans Meningitis in a 27 Weeks Premature Infant Treated with Liposomal Amphotericin-B (AmBisome^R)

JENS OTTO JARLØV[1], PETER BORN[2] and BRITA BRUUN[1]

From the Departments of Clinical Microbiology [1] and Neonatology [2], The National University Hospital (Rigshospitalet), Copenhagen, Denmark

We report a case of Candida albicans meningitis in a neonate born after 27 weeks of gestation. To the best of our knowledge this is the first report of a premature infant with Candida-meningitis treated with liposomal amphotericin B (AmBisome^R). The patient did not respond well to conventional Amphotericin B, but was successfully cured wtih AmBisome^R. Liposomal amphotericin B was well tolerated and the baby recovered with a postinfectious hydrocephalus which necessitated a permanent ventriculo-peritoneal shunt. Six months after the infection the baby appears to have a near-normal cerebral development.

J. O. Jarløv, MD, Department of Clinical Microbiology, Afsnit 9301, Rigshospitalet, Juliane Maries vej 22, DK-2100 Copenhagen Ø, Denmark

INTRODUCTION

Fungal infections, especially Candida infections, are often fatal in immunocompromised patients, including neonates with a very low birth weight (1–6). The keystone in systemic treatment of these infections has been amphotericin B, despite its adverse effects, most serious of which is dose-dependant kidney damage. Moreover, some patients do not respond to treatment with amphotericin B. Liposomal preparations of amphotericin B are currently being investigated (1, 7, 8), and liposomal amphotericin B (AmBisome^R, Vestar inc., San Dimas, CA, USA) is commercially available. With this preparation it is possible to give higher doses than with conventional amphotericin B, but without its severe side effects (1). AmBisome^R has been used successfully in infants (4–6), including very low-birth weight infants, suffering with systemic candidiasis (4, 6). We report here a case of Candida albicans meningitis in a premature infant treated with AmBisome^R with a favourable outcome.

CASE REPORT

A male infant, weighing 1,060 g, was born after 27 weeks' gestation by acute cesarean section due to premature rupture of membranes and maternal pyrexia. The infant's condition was stable but because of the premature rupture of the membranes, antibiotic treatment was inititated with ampicillin and gentamicin. On the third day of life, the infant developed bradycardia and increasing abdominal distension; roentenography of the abdomen revealed pneumoperitoneum. Mechanical ventilation was started and a laparotomy performed, revealing a perforating, necrotizing enterocolitis with large amounts of intraperitoneal meconium, necessitating an ileostomy.

The immediate postoperative course was uncomplicated. The antibiotics were replaced by cefuroxime, gentamicin and metronidazole. During the following days the infant's general condition improved, mechanical ventilation was stopped on day 7 and antibiotics on day 9. When 13 days old, the infant's condition again became unstable and cefuroxime, gentamicin and mechanical ventilation were reintroduced, and one day later metronidazole was added. The C-reactive protein (CRP) concentration was 200 mg/l (range 0–200, normal level < 10). Direct microscopy of pus from a pea-sized abscess on the right wrist disclosed numerous yeast cells. As the patient was considered septicemic, a blood and cerebrospinal fluid (CSF) cultures were set up and antifungal treatment was immediately initiated, with amphotericin B 1 mg/kg once daily and flucytosine 3.8 mg/kg 4 times daily. CSF biochemistry revealed 155×10^6 leukocytes/l, glucose 2.0 mmol/l; plasma-glucose 4.6 mmol/l. After 2 days the blood cultures grew Candida-like yeast and after another 2 days, yeast was grown from the CSF. The patient's condition was now stabilized, mechanical ventilation and antibacterial antibiotics were stopped. Because of the low serum concentrations of amphotericin B (< 0.33 μg/ml), the dosage was increased to 1.5 mg/kg after 8 days and to 1.8 mg/kg after a further 4 days. The CRP was 100 mg/l and did not decline further. The yeasts were identified as Candida albicans susceptible to amphotericin B (MIC $= 0.1$ μg/ml), but resistant to flucytosine (MIC > 15 μg/ml). Flucytosine was therefore replaced with fluconazole 6 mg/kg daily on day 25. Moreover on day 25, as Pseudomonas aeruginosa was isolated from a tracheal aspirate and from an abscess in the lachrymal canal, ceftazidime and gentamicin were started and the patient again required mechanical ventilation. There was no clinical improvement, however, and CRP remained elevated. On day 30, cerebral ultrasound revealed ventriculomegaly. CSF obtained from a ventricular tap contained $1{,}600 \times 10^6$ leukocytes/l, but there was no growth of microorganisms. Therefore, after 16 days of conventional amphotericin B therapy, this was replaced with liposomal amphotericin B (AmBisome^R) 3 mg/kg daily. Fluconazole was continued. The infant's clinical condition improved over the next days and the CRP declined to <10.

The situation was complicated by progressive ventriculomegaly and repeated ventricular taps were performed during the following weeks, showing a rapid decline in CSF leukocyte count. The patient improved clinically, gaining weight, and the antifungal therapy was stopped after 28 days of AmBisome^R and 33 days of fluconazole therapy. During antifungal therapy, liver and kidney function were assessed regularly and urea, creatinine, alanine-aminotransferase, basic phosphatase and bilirubin all remained within normal limits. During the next month the ileostomy was

 ISSN 0036-5548

closed and a permanent ventriculo-peritoneal shunt was established. The patient was discharged on day 100. At subsequent check-ups the patient appeared to follow a near-normal cerebral development.

DISCUSSION

Systemic Candida albicans infection is a life-threatening condition, especially for infants with a very low birth weight (2–4), like the patient described in this case report. It is of great importance to institute the most effective treatment as soon as there is evidence of systemic candidiasis. In the present case, conventional amphotericin B therapy improved the patient's condition to some extent, but total regression of the infection was not achieved. Addition of fluconazole to amphotericin B, which is controversial (9), did not result in any immediate improvement. After AmBisome[R] was initiated, the CRP was normalized within a few days, the patient improved and gained weight, and repeated ventricular taps showed a rapid decline in the CSF leukocyte count. AmBisome[R] was well tolerated and the favourable outcome we noted has also been documented in reports of systemic candidiasis without meningitis in neonates (4, 6). To the best of our knowledge, the present patient is the first very low birth-weight infant with documented Candida meningitis treated with AmBisome[R].

Some controversy persists over the activity of liposomal amphotericin B versus conventional amphotericin B. It is generally believed that the antifungal activity of the drugs is the same (7), and that the advantage of the liposomal preparation is its much lower toxicity, allowing higher doses, which raises the therapeutic index (1). However, Pahls and Schaffner (8) were recently unable to find a raised therapeutic index for liposomal amphotericin B compared with the conventional amphotericin B in an animal model, demonstrating that although liposomal Amphotericin B was less toxic, it also appeared to possess less antifungal activity. It is noteworthy that in the present case there was no renal or liver impairment, even when very high doses of conventional amphotericin B were used. The reason for changing over to liposomal amphotericin B was the poor response to the conventional amphotericin B. Nevertheless, many reports concerning therapy with liposomal amphotericin B are clearly in favour of this drug (1, 4–6). In the future we shall not hesitate to consider AmBisome[R] for the treatment of Candida meningitis in infants with very low birth weights.

REFERENCES

1. Chopra R, Blair S, Strang J, Cervi P, Patterson KG, Goldstone AH. Lipsomal amphotericin B (AmBisome) in the treatment of fungal infections in neutropenic patients. J Antimicrob Chemother 28 Suppl B: 93–104, 1991.
2. Johnson DE, Thompson TR, Green TP, Ferrieri P. Systemic Candidiasis in very low birth weight infants (< 1500 grams). Pediatrics 73: 138–143, 1984.
3. Butler KM, Baker CJ. Candida: An increasingly important pathogen in the nursery. Pediatr Clin North Am 35: 543–563, 1988.
4. Vincent M, Webster MH, Pether JVS. Lancet 339: 374–375, 1992.
5. Tollemar J, Duraj F, Ericzon BG. Liposomal amphotericin B treatment in a 9-month-old liver recipient. Mycoses 33: 251–252.
6. Lackner H, Schwinger W, Urban C, Müller W, Ritschl E, Retterer F, Kuttnig-Haim M, Urlesberger B, Hauer C. Liposomal amphotericin B (AmBisome) for treatment of disseminated fungal infections in two infants of very low birth weight. Pediatrics 89: 1259–1261, 1992.
7. Anaissie E, Paetznick V, Proffitt R, Adler-Moore J, Bodey GP. Comparison of the in vitro antifungal activity of free and liposome-encapsulated amphotericin B. Eur J Clin Microbiol Infect Dis 10: 665–668, 1991.
8. Pahls S, Schnaffner A. Comparison of the activity of free and liposomal amphotericin B in vitro and in a model of systemic and localized murine candidiasis. J Infect Dis 169: 1057–1061, 1994.
9. Walsh TJ, Pizzo A. Treatment of systemic fungal infections: Recent progress and current problems. Eur J Clin Microbiol Infect Dis 7: 460–475, 1988.

Submitted November 27 1994; accepted March 14, 1995

Scand J Infect Dis 27: 421–424, 1995 CASE REPORT

Fluconazole Failure in Two Cases of Disseminated Candidosis

LENA JAHNSON[1], ERJA CHRYSSANTHOU[2], BJÖRN PETRINI[2] and TOMAS VIKERFORS[1]

From the [1]Department of Infectious Diseases, Örebro Medical Center, Örebro, and the [2]Department of Clinical Microbiology, Karolinska Hospital, Stockholm, Sweden

Amphotericin B has been the standard treatment of disseminated candidosis although the less toxic fluconazole tends to be used more frequently. In a recent report, no significant difference in the efficacy of candidaemia treatment was observed between fluconazole and amphotericin B. However, we report on 2 cases of invasive candidosis where fluconazole failed to eradicate Candida albicans although the isolates were susceptible to fluconazole in vitro. Pulsed-field gel electrophoresis was used to confirm the persistence of the same C. albicans strain after therapy failure in both patients.

L. Jahnson, MD, Department of Medicine, Örebro Medical Center, S-70185 Örebro, Sweden

INTRODUCTION

Fluconazole is, in contrast to amphotericin B, a well tolerated antifungal drug with few adverse effects, and is easy to administer. Therefore, fluconazole is an attractive alternative for the treatment of invasive candidosis and tends to be used as primary therapy in these infections. However, few clinical or experimental studies have evaluated the efficacy of fluconazole in the treatment of invasive candidosis (1). We here report on two cases of therapy failure in spite of in vitro susceptibility of the candida isolates to fluconazole.

CASE REPORTS

Case 1

A previously healthy 72-year-old woman weighing 52 kg was admitted to hospital for gross macroscopic haematuria. An abdominal computerized tomographic (CT) scan demonstrated a large tumour in the left kidney. Pulmonary X-ray and bone scan showed no metastases.

A nephrectomy was performed although the tumour was adherent to the mesocolon, the pancreas and the psoas muscle. There was a postoperative leakage of pancreatic fluid from the abdominal drainage.

The patient developed a temperature of 39.7°C and chills 9 days after the operation. Treatment with imipenem 0.5 g × 3 was given. Fluconazole, 400 mg × 1 intravenously, was added 2 days later on suspicion of invasive candidosis. Two sets of blood cultures drawn on day 9 after the operation yielded C. albicans and another 2 sets drawn 2 days later grew the same pathogen.

The patient was reoperated for intestinal obstruction with resection of 25–30 cm of jejunum, 11 days after the first operation. The central venous catheter inserted at the first operation was replaced. The patient's condition gradually improved and the body temperature slowly normalized.

The patient again developed fever (39.5°C) 7 days after fluconazole was initiated, while she was still on imipenem treatment, and therefore piperacillin 4 g × 3 was added. A CT scan showed no abdominal abscess. Serum C-reactive protein (CRP) was 81 mg/l (normal < 5); ESR 46 mm (2–15); WBC 11.3 × 10^9/l (4–9); Hb 110 g/l (115–165), and serum creatinine 95 μmol/l (60–115).

The patient's general condition worsened 10 days after fluconazole was initiated. She still had fever (39.2°C), tachycardia (140), and hypotension (70/50 mmHg). Bilateral infiltrates compatible with adult respiratory distress syndrome were detected on chest radiographs. As arterial oxygen saturation fell to 88% despite maximal oxygen administration, she was put on mechanical ventilation and inotropic support was given. The central venous catheter was replaced once again. Indirect fundoscopy revealed lesions in both eyes consistent with candidal endophtalmitis. Imipenem and piperacillin were discontinued. Fluconazole was, after 10 days of treatment, replaced by amphothericin B in escalating doses to 40 mg/d (0.8 mg/[kg × d]) and flucytosine 2.5 g × 2, intravenously. C. albicans was reisolated from 2 sets of blood cultures drawn 7 days after fluconazole was initiated. A culture from the tip of the central venous catheter yielded C. albicans in abundance. Serum CRP was 289 mg/l, WBC 34 × 10^9/l, Hb 95 g/l and serum creatinine 141 μmol/l.

During the following week the patient's condition improved temporarily and the fever diminished. She received a total of 0.81 g of amphotericin B. As renal function deteriorated, amphotericin B was replaced by liposomal amphotericin B, (14 days after fluconazole was initiated) in escalating doses to 100 mg × 1. Flucytosine was discontinued. Subsequently her condition deteriorated gradually. On CT scan a suspect fluid collection (diameter about 4 cm) was observed near tha tail of the pancreas, 20 days after fluconazole was initiated. Drainage was not attempted as the patient was in poor general condition and the renal cell carcinoma was not radically operated. She died 24 days after fluconazole was initiated. Autopsy was not performed.

Susceptibility testing using the National Committee for Clinical Laboratory Standards (NCCLS) method (2) of the 2 C. albicans isolates in blood, obtained immediately before fluconazole treatment and 7 days later showed identical results. The minimum inhibitory concentration (MIC) for fluconazole was 0.25 mg/l (susceptible, performed at the Department of Clinical Microbiology, Karolinska Hospital, Stockholm, Sweden). In addition the isolates were susceptible to amphotericin B and flucytosine. Molecular epidemiological studies, employing pulsed-field gel electrophoreses, confirmed the persistence of the same C. albicans strain.

Case 2

A previously healthy 55-year-old man weighing 92 kg was admitted to hospital with haemorrhagic shock after a car accident. The spleen was injured with massive intra-abdominal haemorrhage

 ISSN 0036-5548

and a splenectomy was performed. A fracture of the left ulna was stabilized and a right pneumothorax was drained. He was put on mechanical ventilation due to pulmonary contusion and fractured ribs. Treatment with benzylpenicillin 3 g × 4 and cefuroxime 1.5 g × 3 was given at admission. The former was discontinued after 2 days and the latter was replaced by cefotaxime 1 g × 2, 6 days later. Infiltrates consistent with adult respiratory distress syndrome were detected on chest radiographs.

The body temperature rose to 39.4°C 10 days after admission, and treatment with fluconazole 400 mg × 1 intravenously was started on suspicion of disseminated candidosis. The central venous catheter inserted at admission was changed at the same occasion. Two sets of blood cultures drawn 8 days after admission yielded C. albicans and the same pathogen was isolated in abundance from the tip of the central venous catheter, 2 days later. The patient's general condition improved gradually over the following days and his temperature was around 38°C.

The fever increased to 39.0°C 4 days after fluconazole was initiated, and cefotaxime was replaced by imipenem 1 g × 3 2 days later. Serum CRP was 164 mg/l, WBC 27 × 10^9/l and Hb 98 g/l.

The patient became critically ill 9 days after fluconazole was initiated, in spite of this modified therapy. He developed septic shock with tachycardia (165), hypotension (90/45 mmHg) and fever (40.5°C). Fluconazole was replaced the following day by amphotericin B in escalating doses to 80 mg/d and flucytosine 3 g × 4 intravenously. Imipenem was discontinued. The central venous catheter was removed. Indirect fundoscopy revealed no lesions consistent with candidal endophtalmitis in the eyes.

Thereupon the patient's general condition improved and his temperature quickly normalized. A culture from the tip of the central venous catheter yielded moderate growth of C. albicans 9 days after fluconazole treatment was initiated. The same pathogen was reisolated in 1 of 2 sets of blood cultures, after 10 days of fluconazole treatment. However, 2 sets of blood cultures, after 6 days of fluconazole treatment were negative.

Susceptibility testing using the NCCLS method (2) of the 2 C. albicans isolates from blood, obtained immediately before fluconazole treatment and 10 days later showed identical results. MIC for fluconazole was 0.25 mg/l (susceptible). In addition the isolates were susceptible to amphotericin B and flucytosine. Molecular epidemiological studies employing pulsed-field gel electrophoresis confirmed the persistence of the same C. albicans strain. The patterns of the 2 sets of C. albicans strains from case 1 and case 2 were not identical.

MATERIAL AND METHODS

Blood cultures

The Bactec® (Becton Dickinson, USA) blood culture system was used.

Antifungal agent

Fluconazole (Pfizer, New York, USA) was dissolved in 0.85% saline and stored at − 20°C as stock solution of 5 g/l.

Fluconazole susceptibility testing

The broth macrodilution method for susceptibility testing of yeasts was performed according to the NCCLS guidelines (2) with some modifications. The range of fluconazole concentrations tested was 0.125–32 mg/l. The yeast inoculum was adjusted to 1–5 × 10^6 CFU/ml by a spectrophotometric method (3) and further diluted 100-fold in RPMI 1640 medium. The growth in the tubes was measured spectrophotometrically at 530 nm, after 48-h incubation at 35°C. The MIC end point was defined as the first drug concentration exhibiting 50% (or more) reduction of growth compared with the growth control tube.

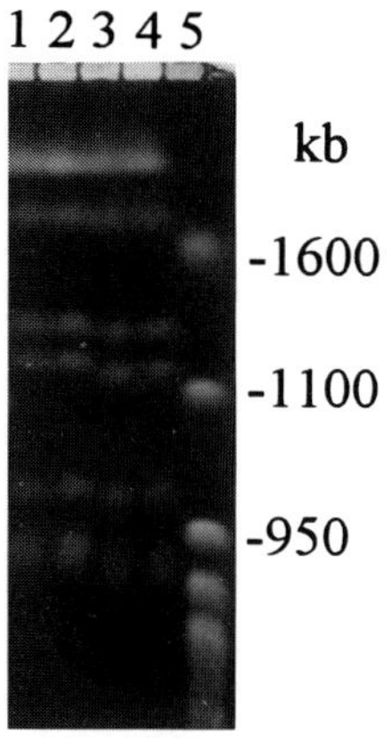

Fig. 1. Electrophoretic karyotypes (the patterns of chromosome-sized DNAs) of C. albicans. Chromosomal DNAs were separated by PFGE at 4 V/cm with a ramp of 90–325 s for 48 h. Lanes 1 to 4: C. albicans DNA from strains 497/93 and 518/93, isolated from patient 1, and C. albicans DNA from strains 498/93 and 528/93, isolated from patient 2, respectively; Lane 5: Saccharomyces cerevisiae DNA.

Pulsed-field gel electrophoresis

DNA plugs were prepared as described previously (4) with minor modifications. Yeast chromosomes were separated by contour-clamped homogeneous electric field electrophoresis on 0.8% agarose gel with the CHEF-DRII system (Bio-Rad Laboratories, Richmond, California, USA). The electrophoresis was performed with a ramp of 90–325 s at 4.0 V/cm for 48 h, using TBE (0.045 M Tris, 0.045 M boric acid, 1 mM EDTA) as a running buffer.

RESULTS

Four C. albicans strains were isolated from blood cultures from 2 patients; strains 497/93 and 518/93 from patient 1, and strains 498/93 and 528/93 from patient 2, respectively. The fluconazole MIC for the 4 strains was 0.25 mg/l. The patients were colonized by different strains of C. albicans as defined by electrophoretic karyotypes (EK). For each patient, the EK of both isolates showed identical banding patterns (Fig. 1).

DISCUSSION

These 2 cases illustrate the problem of clinical and microbiological failure in the antifungal treatment of disseminated candidosis with fluconazole. Similar experiences have been reported by others. In 1 patient with invasive oesophageal candidosis both C. albicans and C. glabrata were reisolated from blood despite intravenous fluconazole therapy for 3 days (1). In another case, failure of fluconazole therapy for sternal osteomyelitis caused by C. albicans was described (5). However, no susceptibility testing was performed on the isolates in these cases. Persistence of the same C. albicans strain in sputum and urine cultures, despite fluconazole therapy for 12 days, was reported in a patient with fungaemia. Pulsed-field gel electrophoresis was used to confirm the persistence of the same C. albicans strain in this case (6).

In spite of low MIC values in our isolates the fluconazole full dose therapy failed to eradicate C. albicans in the patients. This might be explained by the fact that there is a poor correlation between the results of in vitro susceptibility testing of some antifungal agents and the clinical response (7–9). The fluconazole and itraconazole MIC values derived in vitro for yeasts are often considered to be unreliable and subject to variation (10). This is attributable, in part, to the variations in test methods, size of inoculum, length of incubation, temperature of incubation, composition of the medium and determination of the end points. The latter is an important source of interlaboratory variability of susceptibility testing for azole agents such as fluconazole. For these agents, inhibition does not develop abruptly over a small concentration range but merely as a slowly ascending curve (11). Recent advances in antifungal susceptibility testing have, however, been achieved, particularly through the efforts of the NCCLS (2).

Other possible causes of therapeutic failure with fluconazole, in our cases, could be poor drug penetration into affected tissue, lack of fungicidal activity or host immunosuppression (10). The serum concentrations of the antifungal agents were not determined but should have been high with the doses given.

The central venous catheter may be an important source of persistent candidaemia (12, 13), although in the present cases relapse of candidaemia was demonstrated despite replacement of catheters.

Only a few reports have been published on the efficacy of fluconazole in the treatment of systemic fungal infections in non-neutropenic and non-AIDS patients. A premature infant was treated successfully for a C. albicans septicaemia with orally administered fluconazole for 20 days (14). A comparative study of the efficacy of fluconazole versus amphotericin B/flucytosine in 40 surgical patients with systemic mycoses showed no difference in cure rates (15). In an open non-comparative study evaluating the efficacy of fluconazole 200–400 mg/d in the treatment of systemic fungal infections in 40 patients, clinical and microbiological response was achieved in 62% of the C. albicans infections. This pathogen was reisolated from blood cultures in two patients, 5 and 13 days, respectively, after fluconazole treatment was discontinued (16). Recently a randomized study comparing fluconazole with amphotericin B for the treatment of candidaemia in non-neutropenic patients showed no statistically significant difference in outcome between the two study groups, each consisting of 103 patients (13).

Fluconazole was as effective as the combination of amphotericin B and flucytosine when used for early treatment of acute and subacute disseminated candidosis in granulocytopenic rabbits. However, when treatment was delayed 6 days after established infection, fluconazole was less effective than amphotericin B plus flucytosine (17). Other studies in immunocompetent and immunosuppressed animals have shown fluconazole to be effective in the treatment of disseminated candidosis (18, 19).

Although our 2 patients were treated at the same intensive care unit during the same period, a nosocomial spread could be excluded, as pulsed-field gel electrophoresis revealed different electrophoretic karyotypes of the C. albicans strains in their respective blood cultures.

We would like to draw attention, with these case reports, to the fact that the correlation between in vitro antifungal susceptibility testing of fluconazole and therapeutical outcome may be poor. Therefore, in spite of low MIC values for fluconazole, a therapeutic failure should be suspected in a patient with disseminated candidosis who does not improve clinically on fluconazole treatment.

REFERENCES

1. Evans TG, Mayer J, Cohen S, Classen D, Carroll K. Fluconazole failure in the treatment of invasive mycoses. J Infect Dis 164: 1232–1235, 1991.
2. National Committee for Clinical Laboratory Standards. Reference method for broth dilution antifungal susceptibility testing of yeasts: proposed standard. NCCLS document M 27-P. Villanova, PA. 12: 1992.
3. Pfaller MA, Burmeister L, Bartlett MS, Rinaldi G. Multicenter evaluation of four methods of yeast inoculum preparation. J Clin Microbiol 26: 1437–1441, 1988.
4. Wickes B, Staudinger J, Magee BB, Kwon-Chung KJ, Magee PT, Scherer S. Physical and genetic mapping of Candida albicans: several genes previously assigned to chromosome 1 map to chromosome R, the rDNA-containing linkage group. Infect Immun 59: 2480–2484, 1991.
5. Dan M, Priel I. Failure of fluconazole therapy for sternal osteomyelitis due to Candida albicans. Clin Infect Dis 18: 126–127, 1994.
6. Blumberg HM, Hendershot EF, Lott TJ. Persistence of the same Candida albicans strain despite fluconazole therapy. Diagn Microbiol Infect Dis 15: 545–547, 1992.
7. Sheehan DJ, Espinel-Ingroff A, Moore LS, Webb CD. Antifungal susceptibility testing of yeasts: a brief overview. Clin Infect Dis 17(Suppl 2): 494–500, 1993.
8. Pfaller MA, Dupont B, Kobayashi GS, Müller J, Rinaldi MG, Espinel-Ingroff A, Shadomy S, Troke PF, Walsh TJ, Warnock DW. Standardized susceptibility testing of fluconazole: an international collaborative study. Antimicrob Agents Chemother 36: 1805–1809, 1992.
9. Boken DJ, Swindells S, Rinaldi MG. Fluconazole-resistant Candida albicans. Clin Infect Dis 17: 1018–1021, 1993.
10. Kobayashi GS, Spitzer ED. Testing of organisms for susceptibility to triazoles: is it justified? Eur J Clin Microbiol Infect Dis 8: 387–389, 1989.
11. Rex JH, Pfaller MA, Rinaldi MG, Polak A, Galgiani JN. Antifungal susceptibility testing. Clin Microbiol Rev 6: 367–381, 1993.
12. Lecciones JA, Lee JW, Navarro EE, Witebsky FG, Marshall D, Steinberg SM, Pizzo PA, Walsh TJ. Vascular catheter-associated fungemia in patients with cancer: analysis of 155 episodes. Clin Infect Dis 14: 875–883, 1992.

13. Rex JH, Bennett JE, Sugar AM, Pappas PG, van der Horst CM, Edwards JE, Washburn RG, Scheld WM, Karchmer AW, Dine AP, Levenstein MJ, Webb CD. A randomized trial comparing fluconazole with amphotericin B for the treatment of candidemia in patients without neutropenia. N Engl J Med 331: 1325–1330, 1994.
14. Bodé S, Pedersen-Bjergaard L, Hjelt K. Candida albicans septicemia in a premature infant successfully treated with oral fluconazole. Scand J Infect Dis 24: 673–675, 1992.
15. Kujath P, Lerch K, Kochendörfer P, Boos C. Comparative study of the efficacy of fluconazole versus amphotericin B/flucytosine in surgical patients with systemic mycoses. Infection 21: 376–382, 1993.
16. Milatovic D, Voss A. Efficacy of fluconazole in the treatment of systemic fungal infections. Eur J Clin Microbiol Infect Dis 11: 395–402, 1992.
17. Walsh TJ, Aoki S, Mechinaud F, Bacher J, Lee J, Rubin M, Pizzo PA. Effects of preventive, early and late antifungal chemotherapy with fluconazole in different granulocytopenic models of experimental disseminated candidiasis. J Infect Dis 161: 755–760, 1990.
18. Van't Wout JW, Mattie H, van Furth R. Comparison of the efficacies of amphotericin B, fluconazole and itraconazole against a systemic Candida albicans infection in normal and neutropenic mice. Antimicrob Agents Chemother 33: 147–151, 1989.
19. Troke PF, Andrews RJ, Brammer KW, Marriott MS, Richardson K. Efficacy of UK-49,858 (fluconazole) against Candida albicans experimental infections in mice. Antimicrob Agents Chemother 28: 815–818, 1985.

Submitted February 13, 1995; accepted May 14, 1995

Scand J Infect Dis 27: 425–426, 1995

SHORT COMMUNICATION

Short-term Quinolones for Successful Eradication of Multiply Resistant Vibrio Cholerae in Adult Patients

LEVENT DOĞANCI[1], HÜSEYIN GÜN[1], MEHMET BAYSALLAR[1], ALI ALBAY[1], EŞREF ÇINAR[2] and TUNCER HAZNEDAROĞLU[1]

From the Departments of [1]Clinical Microbiology and [2]Infectious Diseases, Gülhane Military Medical Academy, Etlik Ankara, Turkey

There has been an increasing multiple drug resistance problem in Vibrio cholerae biotype Eltor, the causative agent of 7th pandemic. The aim of this study was to show in vitro and in vivo susceptibility and effectiveness of quinolones in the treatment of endemic cholera cases. Excellent results were obtained in 53 bacteriologically confirmed cholera patients treated with short-term ofloxacin and ciprofloxacin. To our knowledge, there has been no previous report on this subject in the international medical literature. Our results show that quinolones can be an alternative drug for the treatment of multiply resistant V. cholerae infections.

L. Doğanci, MD, Department of Clinical Microbiology, Gülhane Military Medical Academy, 06018 Etlik-Ankara, Turkey

INTRODUCTION

The seventh pandemic of Vibrio cholerae 01 Eltor continued in all regions of the world in 1994. As of 22 September 1994, a total of 234, 578 cases and 7,392 deaths associated with cholera were reported to the World Health Organization (WHO) (1). Vibrio cholerae 01 Eltor had no antibiotic resistance problem until recently. Consequently common and inexpensive first-line antibiotics as tetracyclines, chloramphenicol and trimethoprim sulfamethaxazole (TMP/SMX) were recommended by many centres for these infections (2). However, beginning in 1980, V. cholerae 01 Eltor has been developing a multiple resistance pattern due to widespread misuse of these first-line antibiotics all over the world (3, 4). Our purpose in this study was to investigate the clinical and bacteriological outcome of endemic cholera cases treated with short-term quinolones (ofloxacin and ciprofloxacin) at our centre in the summer of 1994.

MATERIAL AND METHODS

Between July and September 1994 altogether 53 young adult males (median age: 21.7, range 21–27) with bacteriologically confirmed V. cholerae biotype Eltor, serotype Ogawa diarrhea received 2 days of quinolone therapy at the Special Center of Gülhane Military Academy (G.M.M.A) in Ankara. All patients showed the WHO criteria of 'some dehydration' (2). They received oral rehydration solutions (ORS) plus peroral quinolones (42 patients received ofloxacin 400 mg/day and 7 ciprofloxacin 1000 mg/day) for 2 days in the Centre. Patients with severe dehydration ($n = 4$) were referred for hospitalization and treated with i.v. solution and i.v. ofloxacin elsewhere. Fecal specimens from all patients were inoculated into alkaline peptone water (APW) and taken to the Department of Clinical Microbiology of GMMA where the final bacteriological isolation and identification procedures were carried out. In addition to conventional identification, 11 randomly selected isolates were tested for antibiotic susceptibility by the Kirby Bauer Disc Diffusion test (2, 5). API sytem (Bio-Merieux/France) microdilution technique was also used for 6 samples to confirm the results obtained by disc diffusion method. Serotyping was performed with Bacto V. cholerae polyvalent and monovalent antisera (Difco Laboratories, USA) at our centre (5). Final fecal samples were cultured for V. cholerae from pooled-fecal specimens (approximately 5–6 samples in a pool) 3 days after the last quinolone dose. Clinical outcome was followed by checking the hydration level and the daily number and volume of liquid stools.

RESULTS

V. cholerae biotype Eltor serotype Ogawa were isolated from 53 stool samples of the patients seen at our specialist centre. 11 of the randomly selected isolates showed uniform resistance to tetracyclines, chloramphenicol, TMP/SMX and ampicillin, but showed sensitivity to ofloxacin and ciprofloxacin. These susceptibility patterns were confirmed by API microdilution technique. No V. cholerae were isolated in pooled fecal specimens collected 3 days after the last quinolone dose. There was an exact correlation between the clinical outcome of the diarrheal illness illustrated by a significant decrease in the number and volume of liquid stools and the bacteriological results within 72 h of therapy in 49 patients treated at the specialist centre. There was no difference between the ofloxacin and ciprofloxacin treatment groups.

DISCUSSION

Cholera caused by V. cholerae Eltor has struck many countries since 1961 and has reached pandemic proportions (6). It is quite evident that the spread of cholera into a country cannot be prevented by any kind of measure, but that the epidemic status is closely related to the level of development. In the beginning of the 7th pandemic of V. cholerae Eltor, economic embargo and administrative limitations led many developing countries to under reporting the number of cholera cases to WHO. Thus, the cumulative statistical data at the WHO Diarrheal Disease Centre are not realistic (1, 6). Rapid, global international travel and trade increases the need for true and effective exchange of medical information. On the other hand, V. cholerae biotype Eltor serotype Ogawa has been developing in vitro and in vivo resistance to tetracyclines, chloramphenicol and TMP/SMX which are all highly recommended for travellers' diarrhea all over the world (7). In our study, these multidrug-resistant V. cholerae isolates are higly susceptible to quinolones and only 2 days treatment clearly stopped all the clinical manifestations and eradicated the fecal carriage phase in all 49 bacteriologically confirmed cases. Comparative susceptibility analyses at different European centres indicated good in vitro activity of quinolones against V. cholerae 01 (8–10). To our knowledge, no data have been published on quinolones for the treatment of endemic cholera in the international medical literature (11). Quinolones may seem more expensive as the first-line anitbiotic, but the short-term dosage and a sharp decrease in the need for hospitalization and intraveneous fluid therapy make this regime an economic alternative. A shorter duration of fecal carriage also decreases the possibile cholera impact on public health. Thus, especially in poor environmental conditions, the increase in costs may be motivated. On the other hand, V. cholerae is closely related to other members of the Enterobacteriaceae and antibiotic resistance can easily be transferred between these. The possibility of the emergence of quinolone resistance in other enteric pathogens (7) as well as in V. cholerae should be considered. The WHO recommendations for antibiotic use in cholera are of value, especially for developed countries where sanitation is good, but the recognition and treatment of cholera at some western centres could also be suboptimal (12). Most cholera centres do not recommend routine final cultures after antimicrobial therapy, but in this study final cultures were performed earlier because of the very short clinical course and also for early detection of possible fecal shedding. Post-antibiotic effects of quinolones were considered to be minimal after 72 h and no relapse of diarrhea was noted in any of the groups within the study period.

In conclusion, because of the high fecal concentrations, longer plasma half-life and the high degree of biological activity and low MIC values (13), short-term quinolone seems to be a good alternative treatment for multiply drug resistant V. cholerae infections.

REFERENCES

1. WHO. Global cholera update, 22 September 1994.
2. WHO. Guidelines for cholera control. Geneva, pp: 1–63, 1993.
3. Threlfall EJ, Said B, Rove B. Emergence of multiple drug resistance in Vibrio cholerae 01 Eltor from Equador. Lancet 342: 1173, 1993.
4. Ross A, Glas M, Binztein N, Rivas M, Caffer MI, Corso A, Radice M, Gutkind G. Unusual multiresistant Vibrio cholerae 01 Eltor in Argentina. Lancet 342. 1172–1173, 1993.
5. Baron EJ, Firegold SM. Vibrio and related species. In: Diagnostic Microbiology, 8th edn. CV Mosby Company, Baltimore, 431–444, 1990.
6. WHO. Cholera in 1993 WHO Wkly Epidem Rec 29: 213–216, 1994.
7. Akalin E. Quinolones in the treatment of acute bacterial diarrhoeal diseases. Drugs (Suppl 3) 45: 114–118, 1993.
8. O'Hare MD, Felmingham D, Ridgeway GL, Gruneberg RN. The comparative in vitro activity of twelve 4-quinolone antimicrobials against enteric pathogens. Drugs Exp Clin Res 11: 253–257, 1985.
9. Bergan T, Lolekha S, Cheong MK, Poh CL, Doencham S, Charoenpipop D. Effect of recent antibacterial agents against bacteria causing diarrhoea. Scand J Infect Dis Suppl 56: 7–10, 1988.
10. Habiyaremye T, Verbist L, Vandepitte J. Comparative in vitro activity of 10 new 4-quinolones against enteropathogenic bacteria. Pathol Biol Paris 35: 800–804, 1987.
11. MEDLINE EXPRESS. Silver Platter 1990–1995 January.
12. Besser RE, Feikin DR, Eberhart-Philips JE, Mascola L, Griffin PM. Diagnosis and treatment of cholera in the United States: Are we prepared? JAMA 272: 1203–1205, 1994.
13. Altay G, Willke A, Tulunay FC: Ofloxacin in cholera. In: Selected Proceedings from the International Congress for Infectious Diseases, Rio de Janeiro, Brazil, April 17–21, 1988. Excerpta Medica: 65–66, 1988.

Submitted January 16, 1995; accepted March 15, 1995

Scand J Infect Dis 27: 427–428, 1995 SHORT COMMUNICATION

Infrequent Finding of Verotoxin-Producing Escherichia coli in Diarrheal Stools in Belgrade, Serbia

MILOJE ČOBELJIĆ, ZORICA LEPŠANOVIĆ and SLOBODANKA VELIMIROVIĆ

From the Institute of Preventive Medicine, Military Medical Academy, Belgrade, Serbia

Out of 2,638 patients, with acute diarrhea, verotoxin-producing Escherichia coli (VTEC) was isolated from the stools of 8 (0.3%). There was no visible blood in their stools and none of them developed other syndromes associated with VTEC infection. None of the isolated VTEC agglutinated with O157 E. coli antiserum, while only 3 strains hybridized with the DNA probe CVD 419, designed to detect VTEC. The data obtained suggest that VTEC is not an important causative agent of acute diarrhea in Belgrade.

M. Čobeljić, MD, Institute of Preventive Medicine, Military Medical Academy, Crnotravska 17, 11000 Belgrade, Serbia

INTRODUCTION

Data on the presence of verotoxin (VT)-producing Escherichia coli (VTEC) in diarrheal stools in different parts of the world are variable, with strong evidence that serogroup O157 predominates among strains isolated in North America (1). Since the frequency of isolation of this pathogen has not so far been investigated in the Balkan region, we carried out this study to determine the isolation rate of VTEC in stools of persons with acute diarrhea.

MATERIAL AND METHODS

Stool samples from patients with acute diarrhea were collected in 1993, in the city of Belgrade (1.5 million inhabitants), from May through December. After incubation on MacConkey agar, growing cultures were tested for cytotoxicity to Vero and HeLa cells according to the method of Karmali (1). The identification of VT-producing strains, their serogrouping with comercially available E. coli antisera (including O157), and the susceptibility to antimicrobials were investigated by conventional methods. Enterohemolysin and alpha-hemolysin detection and the expression of the biotype of VTEC by a numerical code were carried out as described by Beutin et al. (2). The test for adhesiveness of these strains was carried out using a 6 h incubation period (3). Plasmids in VTEC were detected by the method of Birnboim & Doly, modified by Ish-Horowitz (4). For the detection of virulence plasmid, a probe consisting of a 3.4 kilobase Hind III fragment of this plasmid, cloned into pCVD 419, was used (5).

RESULTS AND DISCUSSION

Out of 2,638 sporadic cases with acute diarrhea, VTEC was found in 8 (0.3%). No other pathogens were detected in the stools, except in 1 male (75 years) from whom Campylobacter jejuni was isolated. Macroscopic examination of VTEC-positive stools did not reveal the presence of blood. Repeated physical examination (10–20 days from the beginning of illness) revealed that all the patients with VTEC infection had fully recovered. The age and sex of patients with VTEC infection and the properties of the isolated strains are shown in Table I.

None of the isolated VTEC strains agglutinated with O157 or with the other antisera available, but all of them fermented sorbitol promptly. Only 1 strain exhibited diffuse adherence to HEp-2 cells.

Table I. *Properties of verotoxin-producing Escherichia coli isolated from patients with acute diarrhea in Belgrade, Serbia*

Strain no.	Patient age in years, sex	Biotype[a]	Drug resistance	Hemolysin production[b]	Cytoxicity to cells		Hybridization with pCVD 419	Plasmid mol. weight[c]			
					Vero	HeLa					
7	10, M	314	None	Alpha hly	+	+	+	60	2.2		
154	14, M	611	None	None	+	+	−	60			
183	28, F	715	None	Ent hly	+	+	+	60	9	3.9	3.6
199	43, F	771	None	None	+	+	−	60			
956	7, F	611	Tetracycline	None	+	−	−	60			
1694	54, F	771	None	Ent hly	+	+	+	60	35		
2558	75, M	775	Tetracycline	None	+	−	−	60	40	3.6	2.8
2981	23, F	715	Tetracycline	None	+	+	−	60	40	3.6	2.8

[a] Expressed according to Beutin et al. (2).

[b] Production of alpha-hemolysin (alpha hly) and enterohemolysin (ent hly).

[c] Molecular weight expressed in megadaltons.

This investigation showed that VTEC is not a frequent cause of acute diarrhea in Belgrade. The reported detection rates of this pathogen in European populations are: 0% in the Netherlands (6); 0.9% in the United Kingdom (7), and 1.2% in Switzerland (8). Biotypes of our VTEC isolates were different from the biotypes of the strains of Beutin et al. (2). Also, the association between enterohemolysin and VT production, described by those authors, could not be confirmed in this, as in the study of Burnens et al. (8). Localized adherence to HEp-2 cells has been registered among VTEC (3), but none of our strains expressed this type of adhesion. A substantial proportion of non-O157 VTEC in this and in other studies (3, 8) did not hybridize with the CVD 419 DNA probe constructed for the detection of VTEC (5).

ACKNOWLEDGEMENTS

We thank Dr R. Trbojević, Institute of Public Health, Belgrade, Dr M. Čanić-Radojlović, Dr Kosta Todorović Institute for Infectious and Tropical Diseases, Belgrade, and Dr M. Marković and Dr L. Sarjanović, Institute for Mother and Child Health Care of Serbia, Belgrade, for providing patient stool specimens and clinical data.

REFERENCES

1. Karmali MA. Laboratory diagnosis of verotoxin-producing Escherichia coli infections. Clin Microbiol Newslett 9: 65–70, 1987.
2. Beutin L, Montenegro MA, Ørskov I, Ørskov F, Prada J, Zimmermann S, Stephen R. Close association of verotoxin (Shiga-like toxin) production with enterohemolysin production in strains of Escherichia coli. J Clin Microbiol 27: 2559–2564, 1989.
3. Scotland SM, Willshaw GA, Smith HR, Rowe B. Properties of strains of Escherichia coli O26:Hll in relation to their enteropathogenic or enterohemorrhagic classification. J Infect Dis 162: 1069–1074, 1990.
4. Maniatis T, Fritsch EF, Sembrook J. Molecular cloning: a laboratory manual. Cold Spring Harbor, New York: Cold Spring Harbor Laboratory, 368–369, 1982.
5. Levine MM, Xu JG, Kaper JB, Lior H, Prado V, Tall B, Nataro J, Karch H, Wachsmuth K. A DNA probe to identify enterohemorrhagic Escherichia coli of O157:H7 and other serotypes that cause hemorrhagic colitis and hemolytic uremic syndrome. J Infect Dis 156: 175–182, 1987.
6. Rademaker CM, Fluit AC, Jansze M, Jansen WH, Glerum JH, Werhoef J. Frequency of enterovirulent Escherichia coli in diarrhoeal disease in the Netherlands. Eur J Clin Microbiol Infect Dis 12: 93–97, 1993.
7. Chapman PA, Wright DJ, Norman P. Verotoxin-producing Escherichia coli infections in Sheffield: cattle as a possible source. Epidemiol Infect 102: 439–445, 1989.
8. Burnens AP, Boss P, Ørskov I, Ørskov F, Schaad UB, Müller F. Occurrence and phenotypic properties of verotoxin producing Escherichia coli in sporadic cases of gastroenteritis. Eur J Clin Microbiol Infect Dis 11: 631–634, 1992.

Submitted February 7, 1995; accepted May 8, 1995

Dear Subscriber,

Due to a printing error in the last issue we have enclosed a reprint of the article Scand J Infect Dis 27: 319–324, 1995 "Efficacy of Human Leucocyte Alpha-Interferon Treatment for Chronic Hepatitis C Virus Infection".

Please accept our apology for any inconvenience this may have brought you.

The Publisher

Scand J Infect Dis 27: 319–324, 1995 ORIGINAL ARTICLE

Efficacy of Human Leucocyte Alpha-Interferon Treatment for Chronic Hepatitis C Virus Infection

OLA WEILAND[1], MARGARET CHEN[2], GUDRUN LINDH[1], LARS MATTSSON[1], ROBERT SCHVARCZ[1], ANDERS SÖNNERBORG[2], MARTIN WAHL[3], RUNE WEJSTÅL[3], ANDERS WIDELL[4] and GUNNAR NORKRANS[3]

From the Divisions of [1]Infectious Diseases and [2]Virology, Department of Immunology, Microbiology, Pathology and Infectious Diseases, Karolinska Institute and Huddinge Hospital, Huddinge, and the Departments of [3]Infectious Diseases, East Hospital, Göteborg and [4]Medical Microbiology, Malmö University Hospital, Malmö, Sweden

A total of 42 Swedish patients with biopsy-proven chronic hepatitis C virus (HCV) infection were treated with a natural human leucocyte alpha-interferon (HuIFN-alpha-Le), Alfanative® (BioNative AB, Umeå, Sweden) in an open uncontrolled study. Two patients were withdrawn from treatment within 2 weeks due to non-compliance and were omitted from further analysis, and 40 patients (17 females), mean age 39 years (range 24–71) completed the study. All patients were HCV RNA-positive in serum prior to treatment, with raised alanine aminotransferase (ALT) levels >1.5 times the upper normal limit known for more than 6 months. Interferon was given at a dose of 3 MU t.i.w. for an intended 24 weeks and follow-up was a further 24 weeks after treatment. Biochemical non-responders were withdrawn from treatment within 12–16 weeks but continued follow-up. Overall 21/40 (52.5%) patients had a complete biochemical response with normal ALT levels at the end of treatment. Sustained response during follow-up was seen in 8 (20%) whereas 13 (32.5%) had a non-sustained response. At the end of treatment 23 (58%) patients had undetectable serum HCV RNA and 9 (23%) at follow-up. Patients with sustained, non-sustained and non-response had a mean pretreatment HCV RNA level of 3.2×10^5, 2.5×10^6 and 3.2×10^6 genomes/ml, respectively, differences that did not reach statistical significance. Of the patients 3, 9, 10 and 14 had genotype 1b, 3a, 1a, and 2b, respectively, and 4 had mixed genotypes. Of the 23 patients with genotype 2b or 3a, 7 had a sustained response vs. none of the 13 patients with genotype 1a or 1b ($p = 0.03$). No patients with cirrhosis had a sustained response whereas 4/18 with chronic persistent and 4/18 with chronic active hepatitis had such a response. It is concluded that some 50% of patients treated with HuIFN-alpha-Le responded with normalisation of ALT levels but that only 20% had a durable response 24 weeks post-treatment, and that patients with genotypes 3a or 2b seem to respond better than patients with other genotypes.

O. Weiland, MD, Department of Infectious Diseases I 73, Karolinska Institute and Huddinge Hospital, S-141 86 Huddinge, Sweden

INTRODUCTION

Patients with chronic hepatitis C virus (HCV) infection usually have a slowly evolving disease over years and decades with few spontaneous recoveries (1–3). The long-term outcome is grave, at least in a subset with cirrhosis and hepatocellular carcinoma as end-stage outcomes (1, 2).

Interferon has, hitherto, been the only licensed treatment, to which some 50% of patients will respond with normalized alanine aminotransferase (ALT) levels during treatment, whereas the other 50% will be non-responders (4). After the end of treatment, many patients who responded during treatment will have a relapse (4). Sustained response, including eradication of the viraemia which persists after treatment cessation has thus been achieved in only 15–30% of treated patients (5, 6). A durable response after treatment cessation seems to be achieved in a higher percentage with prolonged treatment courses (5, 6). Some patients, although initially responding, will have a breakthrough of their HCV infection before completion of therapy during continued treatment, possibly caused by the evolution of neutralizing interferon antibodies (7, 8). Antibodies seem to occur more often with recombinant interferon alpha-2a than with recombinant interferon alpha-2b treatment and seem to be least common during treatment with natural interferons (9).

The factors most often claimed to predict response to interferon treatment are HCV RNA levels in serum prior to treatment and the HCV genotype (4). The aim of the present study was to evaluate the response rate (as measured by ALT normalization and eradication of HCV viraemia), tolerability and evolution of interferon antibodies during treatment with a natural interferon, Alfanative®, and to correlate the response with the pretreatment HCV RNA levels, HCV genotypes and pretreatment histological findings.

MATERIAL AND METHODS

A total of 42 Swedish patients with biopsy-proven chronic HCV infection were entered in the trial. Two men were withdrawn from treatment within 2 weeks after the start, due to non-compliance, and were omitted from further analysis. Thus 40 patients (17 females), mean age 39 years (range 24–71) were further evaluated. All these patients were positive for anti-HCV by second generation

ELISA (Ortho Diagnostic Systems, Raritan, New Jersey, USA), with positive confirmatory tests (second or third generation RIBA, Chiron, Emeryville, California, USA) and HCV RNA-positive in serum prior to entry. All the patients also had continuously raised ALT levels, > 1.5 times the upper normal limit, known for more than 6 months. No patient had antibodies against HIV or other causes of chronic liver diseases, such as hepatitis B, autoimmune hepatitis, PBC, alcohol use, haemochromatosis, Wilson's disease or alpha-1-antitrypsin deficiency. All patients gave verbal informed consent and the study was approved by the local ethics committee at the Karolinska Institute, Stockholm, Sweden. Natural human leucocyte interferon alpha (HuIFN-alpha-Le), Alfanative®, Bio-Native, Umeå, Sweden, was given at a dose of 3 MU t.i.w. for an intended 24 weeks with follow-up for another 24 weeks. Patients not responding biochemically with normalization of ALT levels within 12–16 weeks (non-responders) were withdrawn from further treatment but continued follow-up during the entire study period.

ALT levels were analysed before, during and after treatment with standard methods, normal levels being <0.6 and <0.8 µkat/l in females and males, respectively. Sera, stored frozen at −70°C and obtained prior to treatment (week 0), at treatment cessation (week 24) and at follow-up 24 weeks after treatment (week 48), were analysed qualitatively for HCV RNA. HCV RNA levels were also analysed quantitatively, and genotypes determined, in a serum obtained prior to treatment (week 0). Definitions of biochemical response were as follows: 'non-sustained response' meaning normal ALT levels at the end of treatment but relapse during follow-up; 'sustained response' meaning normal ALT levels at the end of treatment and during follow-up, and 'non-response' meaning non-normalizing ALT levels.

HCV RNA determination

HCV RNA was determined qualitatively with primers derived from the 5′-non-coding region of the genome as previously described (10). Serum (100 µl) was used for RNA extraction, which was performed with a modified guanidinium thiocyanate-phenol-chloroform method. In brief, HCV cDNA was synthesized in a total volume of 25 µl reverse transcription (RT) mixture as described earlier (10). The RT mixture was incubated at 37°C for 60 min, followed by heating at 95°C for 5 min. After the RT, one-tenth of the cDNA was amplified by double PCR. The detection limit of this PCR assay was five copies of cloned HCV genome.

Quantification of HCV RNA

The quantification of HCV RNA in pretreatment serum was performed using a method based on competitive PCR and colorimetric detection of the amplified products as described earlier (11). After reverse transcription (RT), one-tenth of the resulting cDNA, and the same volume of serially diluted cloned HCV competitor DNA, were coamplified by nested PCR. The competitive DNA consisted of the amplified regions of wild type HCV cDNA with an internal region substituted with the *lac* operator sequence. The PCR products were specifically quantitated by a colorimetric solid-phase assay. This assay reproducibly detects 10 HCV genome equivalents. The interassay variation is 10–15%, and the intra-assay variation 15–20% (11).

Genotyping of HCV

Genotyping was done with type-specific primers directed against the HCV core gene based on the principle of Okamoto et al. (12) but with several modifications (13). The typing terminology suggested by Chan et al. was used (14). Our assay also identified the important type 3a by Chan, which was never identified by the original Okamoto assay. Briefly, the typing started with a consensus amplification of bp 467–751 with primers 5′-TAGATTGGGT-GTGCGCGCGA (sense, s), 5′-ATGTACCCCATGAGGTCGGC (antisense, as); thereafter typing for each isolate was done in two different reactions under stringent conditions (annealing temperature 63°C, 25 cycles). The typing primer for type 1a was 5′-TGGGGATAGGCTGACGTCTACCT (as); for 1b 5′-CCATCC-TGCCCACCCCA (as); for 2a 5′-CCAAGAGGGACGGGAAC-CTC (as), and for 2b 5′-GCAACCCTCGTTTCC(GA)TACA-GAG (as). These primers were run against an upstream primer 5′-AGGAAGACTTCCGAGCGGTC (s). Type 3a was identified with a primer 5′-GTGTGCGCGACGCGTAAA (s) and a consensus primer 5′-GCA(TC)GT(AG)AGGGTATCGATGAC(TC)T (as). In this reaction type 1b was also confirmed with primer 5′-AACCTCGTGGAAGGCGACAA (s). (Bases within parentheses means redundant base at this position).

Determination of anti-interferon alpha antibodies in serum

Interferon-alpha-binding antibodies in serum were determined in a serum drawn before administration of the first dose of interferon-alpha and ≥48 h after the last dose. The presence of antibodies was measured by an ELISA method (BioNative AB, Umeå, Sweden) as described earlier (15). With this method, antibodies evoked both by recombinant and natural interferons can be detected.

Histological methods

All patients underwent a biopsy within 12 months prior to treatment. The biopsies were classified as chronic persistent hepatitis (CPH), chronic active hepatitis (CAH) with or without cirrhosis (Ci) as recommended by an international group (16).

Statistical methods

Statistical calculations were performed with Fisher's exact test and the Mann–Whitney U test.

RESULTS

Demographic data on the 40 patients who completed the study, according to the final biochemical outcome, are given in Table I. Before week 16, 7 patients were withdrawn from treatment due to biochemical non-response and another 2, who had achieved biochemical response, were withdrawn because of depression. All of these continued follow-up in the study.

Overall 21/40 (52.5%) patients had a complete biochemical response with normal ALT levels at the end of treatment (week 24). Of these, 13 relapsed biochemically within 24 weeks of follow-up after treatment. A sustained biochemical response with normal ALT levels at follow-up week 48 was thus seen in 8/40 (20%) patients, a non-sustained biochemical response in 13/40 (32.5%) and non-response in 19/40 (47.5%).

The number of patients with normal ALT levels and a negative HCV RNA test in serum at weeks 0, 12, 24 and 48 are given in Table II. The eradication of HCV RNA from serum exceeded the normalization rate of ALT levels at all time points during and after treatment.

The number of HCV RNA-negative patients, according to biochemical response category at week 12 during treatment, at end of treatment and at follow-up are given in Table III. All eight patients with sustained response were HCV RNA-negative at week 12 during treatment and at

Table I. *Demographic data in 40 patients with chronic hepatitis C virus infection treated with human leucocyte interferon-alpha according to biochemical response category*

	Sustained response	Non-sustained response	Non-response	Total
No. of patients	8	13	19	40
Males	4	9	10	23
Females	4	4	9	17
Age, years				
Median	35	38	39	39
Range	28–50	26–71	24–51	24–71
Mode of acquisition				
Intravenous drug use (IVDU)	2	4[a]	6	12[a]
Needle stick	—	1	1	2
Tattooing	1	—	2	3
Transfusions	0	9[a]	5	14[a]
Sporadic	5	—	5	10
Histology prior to treatment				
CPH[b]	4	5	9	18
CAH[c]	4	4	10	18
CAH/Ci[d]	—	4	—	4
Hepatitis C virus genotype				
1a	—	2	8	10
1b	—	—	3	3
2b	3	5	6	14
3a	4	3	2	9
Mixed	1	3	—	4
Pretreatment HCV RNA levels in serum, genomes/ml				
Median	3.2×10^5	2.5×10^6	3.2×10^6	2.25×10^6
Range	2.5×10^4–13×10^7	1.6×10^5–3.2×10^7	2×10^5–16×10^7	2.5×10^4–16×10^7

[a] One patient had both IVDU and blood transfusions as possible modes for acquisition.
[b] CPH = chronic persistent hepatitis.
[c] CAH = chronic active hepatitis.
[d] Ci = cirrhosis.

Table II. *The biochemical and virological response in 40 patients with chronic hepatitis C virus infection, measured as the number of patients with normal ALT levels and negative negative serum HCV RNA test before, during and after treatment with human leucocyte interferon alpha during an intended 24-week course*

	Before treatment, week 0	During treatment, week 12	End of treatment, week 24[a]	At follow-up, week 48
ALT level				
Patients with normal levels/total no. of patients	0/40 (0%)	27/40 (68%)	21/40 (53%)	8/40 (20%)
HCV RNA				
Patients testing negative/total no. of patients	0/40 (0%)	29/40 (73%)	23/40 (58%)	9/40 (23%)

[a] Patients with a biochemical non-response were withdrawn from treatment, weeks 12–16.

the end of treatment. At follow-up two (25%) had become HCV RNA-positive although they continued to have normal ALT levels. All but two non-sustained biochemical responders were HCV RNA-negative at the end of treatment. Only 2/13 non-sustained responders continued to be negative at follow-up. Also 8/19 biochemical non-responders were HCV RNA-negative at week 12 of whom 6 had normal ALT levels. During continued treatment, however, 5 of these experienced biochemical relapse (breakthrough response), and another one after prematurely ending the treatment because of depression. At follow-up only one non-responder was HCV RNA-negative. Her mean ALT level at 2, 16 and 24 weeks post-treatment, was however, in the normal range.

HCV RNA levels in serum prior to treatment according to response

The HCV RNA levels according to response category are given in Table I. Patients with a sustained biochemical response (SR) had a lower median serum HCV RNA level

Table III. *The virological response in 40 patients with chronic hepatitis C virus infection measured as the number of patients with negative serum HCV RNA test before, during and after treatment with human leucocyte interferon alpha during a 24 weeks course according to final biochemical outcome*

Response category	No.	Median HCV RNA prior to treatment	No. of patients HCV RNA negative/total no. of patients			
			Before treatment	During treatment	At end of treatment[a]	At follow-up
Sustained response	8	3.2×10^5	0/8 (0%)	8/8 (100%)	8/8 (100%)	6/8 (75%)
Non-sustained response	13	2.5×10^6	0/13 (0%)	13/13 (100%)	11/13 (85%)	2[b]/13 (15%)
Non-response	19	3.2×10^6	0/19 (0%)	8/19 (42%)	4/19 (21%)	1[c]/19 (5%)

[a] Patients with a biochemical non-response withdrawn from treatment week 12–16.
[b] Mean ALT level weeks 2, 16 and 48 after treatment, for patient GB03 1.08 µkat/l, and Gb20 0.64 µkat/l.
[c] Mean ALT level weeks 2, 16 and 48 after treatment for patient HS9 0.63 µkat/l.
Upper normal ALT level 0.6 and 0.8 µkat/l for men and women, respectively.

than those with non-sustained (NSR) or non-response (NR), the values being 3.2×10^5, 2.5×10^6 and 3.2×10^6, respectively, a difference which did not reach statistical significance (SR vs. NSR + NR, $p = 0.097$).

Genotypes according to response

The distribution of genotypes according to biochemical response is given in Table I; 10, 14, 9 and 3 patients had genotypes 1a, 2b, 3a and 1b respectively. Patients with genotypes 1a and 1b were less likely to have a sustained response than those with genotypes 2b and 3a, (0/13 vs. 7/23, respectively; $p = 0.034$). The median HCV RNA levels in patients with genotype 1a, 2b, 3a, and 1b were 2.6×10^6, 3.8×10^6, 3.2×10^5, and 8×10^5, respectively, differences that did not reach statistical significance. The median HCV RNA level in patients with genotype 3a, however, tended to be lower than that in patients with genotype 2b ($p = 0.054$).

Genotypes according to mode of acquisition

There were 4, 1, 6 and 1 patients, with post-transfusion hepatitis C, who had only genotypes 1a, 1b, 2b and 3a, respectively. The corresponding distribution for those with IVDU was 4, 1, 2 and 4, and for patients with sporadic forms it was 2, 0, 4 and 4, respectively; differences that did not reach statistical significance. One intravenous drug user who also had blood transfusions is included both among those with post-transfusion hepatitis C and those with intravenous drug use (IVDU).

Mode of acquisition according to response

The mode of acquisition of the HCV infection according to response is given in Table I. None of the 13 patients with post-transfusion hepatitis C had a sustained response vs. 8/26 (31%) of those with other routes for their infection ($p = 0.035$); the intravenous drug user who had also had blood transfusions being excluded. Five of 10 patients (50%) with sporadic hepatitis C had a sustained response, and 3/16 (19%) of those with intravenous drug use (IVDU) (including needle stick and tattooing) as their route of infection. The median serum HCV RNA levels in patients who acquired infection via transfusions, via IVDU (including tattooing and needle stick injuries) and via sporadic forms were 3.6×10^6, 1.9×10^6, and 1.65×10^6, respectively, and were not significantly different.

Histological findings prior to treatment, according to response

The distribution of histological findings according to response is given in Table I. No patient with CAH and cirrhosis responded in a sustained fashion, whereas 4/14 and 4/18 patients, with CPH and CAH respectively, did.

HCV RNA level in serum prior to treatment, according to histology

The median serum HCV RNA levels in patients with CPH, CAH and CAH with cirrhosis were 1.05×10^6, 3.25×10^6 and 1.6×10^7, respectively. Patients with CPH tended to have lower median serum HCV RNA levels than the combined group with CAH and CAH with cirrhosis ($p = 0.055$). If the 2 patients who were excluded from analysis due to non-compliance (one each with CAH and CAH with cirrhosis) are included this difference reached statistical significance ($p = 0.027$).

Interferon antibodies

No interferon-alpha-binding antibodies were detected in the patients before treatment, and no patient developed antibodies during treatment.

Adverse effects

The well known initial flu-like side-effects of interferon, such as fever, headache and muscle pains, noted earlier, were common, but tended to diminish during continued treatment. Alopecia was noted in 13 (27.5%) patients; mild in 11, but moderate with hair loss of up to 30% in 2 patients. Depression was noted by 4 patients, requiring treatment withdrawal and antidepressant therapy in 2 patients after 12 and 14 weeks treatment, respectively. Both were biochemical responders at this time point and both had a later relapse. Haematological side-effects necessitating interferon dose reduction were not noted.

DISCUSSION

The normalization of ALT levels in 52.5% of our patients at the end of treatment, sustained during follow-up in 8/40 (20%) is of the same order as that achieved in most studies utilizing lymphoblastoid and recombinant interferon alpha over 6 months (4, 17). Not all patients with a sustained biochemical response continued to show viral eradication since 2/8 (25%) were HCV RNA-positive in serum at follow-up 24 weeks after the end of treatment. A virological relapse in some patients with a continued biochemical response has been also noted in other studies (18, 19). Also one biochemical non-responder was negative for HCV RNA at follow-up. This patient, however, had very low ALT levels with a mean normal level when sampled at 2, 16 and 24 weeks post treatment. She happened to have slightly raised ALT levels at treatment cessation and at follow-up. During the follow-up after this study she had continuously normal ALT levels, and was probably miscategorized as a non-responder due to our stringent criteria. At all study points the number of patients who were HCV RNA-negative exceeded the number who had normal ALT levels, indicating that both HCV RNA testing and monitoring of ALT levels should be included in the evaluation of treatment response.

When analysing factors of possible importance for the prediction of sustained response, we found that HCV RNA levels tended to be lower in sustained responders compared to those of non-sustained and non-responders but not, however, significantly so. In an earlier study with recombinant interferon alpha we found such a difference in agreement with the findings of others (20, 21). Patients with a sustained response also tended to have HCV RNA levels more often below than above the median level (6/20 vs. 2/20, data not shown).

When analysing genotypes according to treatment response, we found that patients with genotypes 3a and 2b had a sustained response more often than patients with genotype 1a and 1b. In agreement with this, patients with genotype 1b have been found to have a poor response when compared to patients with other genotypes (4). Patients with genotype 3a tended to have the lowest median HCV RNA levels in serum prior to treatment; levels which were also somewhat lower than in patients with genotype 2b ($p = 0.054$). In line with this, 4/9 patients with genotype 3a had a sustained response whereas none of the three with genotype 1b had such a response.

The mode of HCV acquisition also seemed to influence the response to interferon. Thus none of our post-transfusion cases had a sustained response, whereas 31% of patients with other routes for their infection responded in a sustained fashion ($p = 0.035$). This was neither caused by different serum HCV RNA levels in patients with different routes for their infection, nor was it explained by the distribution of genotypes which did not differ significantly between patients with different modes of acquisition. However, others have found that patients with post-transfusion hepatitis C seem to have higher serum levels of HCV RNA than patients with sporadic forms of HCV infection and with HCV caused by intravenous drug abuse (21).

Recently Gretch et al. have shown that the HCV RNA level in serum increases with the severity of the histological injury (22). In agreement with this, we found that patients with CPH had lower levels of HCV RNA than patients with more advanced disease. None of our 4 patients with CAH and cirrhosis responded to treatment, in line with the poorer response to treatment noted in cirrhotic patients (23). This can partly be due to high serum HCV RNA levels in cirrhotic patients (22). Our patients with cirrhosis tended to have high HCV RNA levels in serum prior to treatment, in agreement with this.

Adverse effects like alopecia and depression were noted in 27.5% and 10% of our patients respectively. In the majority of cases these were mild and did not require dose reduction. In 2 patients with depression, however, treatment had to be withdrawn after 12 and 14 weeks, respectively, when both were given antidepressant therapy. These adverse effects were fully reversible after cessation of treatment, and such effects have also been noted during recombinant interferon treatment. We have earlier noted alopecia in 15% of patients treated with recombinant interferon alpha-2b (6).

In our series 5 patients experienced a breakthrough response, with raised ALT levels after initial normalization, in spite of continued treatment. This response pattern has been claimed, at least in some patients, to be caused by the evolution of neutralizing interferon antibodies (7, 8). None of our patients with this response pattern, however, developed interferon antibodies, casting doubt on this assumption. In fact none of our patients developed interferon antibodies during or after treatment. This is in agreement with other studies showing a low incidence of interferon antibodies after treatment with lymphoblastoid interferon alpha, as compared to that seen after recombinant interferon-alpha-2a treatment (9). The observation that no interferon antibodies developed during treatment with our natural human leucocyte alpha-interferon is possibly of some importance, since high levels of neutralizing antibodies can cause lack of response according to some studies (7, 8).

In conclusion we found that a 6-month course with human leucocyte interferon-alpha induced a biochemical response in more than 50% of our patients, which was sustained in 20%. We found that patients with genotypes 3a and 2b responded better than those with genotypes 1a and 1b, and that patients with lower pretreatment HCV RNA levels tended to respond better than those with higher levels. We also found that patients who had acquired their infection via blood transfusions responded less well than those with other routes for their infection, and that none of our patients with cirrhosis responded.

ACKNOWLEDGEMENTS

This study was supported by a grant from BioNative AB, Umeå, Sweden. The monitoring of patients by Katharina Engman was greatly appreciated.

REFERENCES

1. Takahashi M, Yamada G, Miyamoto R, Doi T, Endo H, Tsuji T. Natural course of chronic hepatitis C. Am J Gastroenterol 88: 240–243, 1993.
2. Kiyosawa K, Sodeyama T, Tanaka E, Gibo Y, Yoshisawa K, Nakano Y, Furuta S, Akahane Y, Nishioka K, Purcell R, Alter H. Interrelationship of blood transfusion, non-A, non-B hepatitis and hepatocellular carcinoma: Analysis by detection of antibody to hepatitis C virus. Hepatology 12: 671–675, 1990.
3. Mattsson L, Sönnerborg A, Weiland O. Outcome of acute symptomatic non-A, non-B hepatitis: a 13-year follow-up study of hepatitis C virus markers. Liver 13: 274–278, 1993.
4. Weiland O. Interferon therapy in chronic hepatitis C virus infection. FEMS Microbiol Rev 14: 279–288, 1994.
5. Shindo M, Di Bisceglie A, Cheung L, Shih W-K, Cristiano K, Feinstone S, Hoofnagle J. Decrease in serum hepatitis C viral RNA during alpha-interferon therapy for chronic hepatitis C. Ann Intern Med 115: 700–704, 1991.
6. Reichard O, Foberg U, Frydén A, Mattsson L, Norkrans G, Sönnerborg A, Wejstål R, Yun Z-B, Weiland O. High sustained response rate and clearance of viraemia in chronic hepatitis C following treatment with interferon alfa-2b for 60 weeks. Hepatology 19: 280–285, 1994.
7. Bonetti P, Diodati G, Drago C, Casarin C, Scaccabarozzi S, Realdi G, Ruol A, Alberti A. Interferon antibodies in patients with chronic hepatitis C virus infection treated with recombinant interferon alfa-2a. Hepatology 20: 416–420, 1994.
8. Milella M, Antonelli G, Santantonio T, Currenti M, Monno L, Mariano N, Angarano G, Dianzani F, Pastore G. Neutralizing antibodies to recombinant alpha-interferon and response to therapy in chronic hepatitis C virus infection. Liver 13: 146–150, 1993.
9. Antonelli G, Currenti M, Turriziani O, Dianzani F. Neutralizing antibodies to interferon-alfa: relative frequency in patients treated with different interferon preparations. J Infect Dis 163: 882–885, 1991.
10. Yun Z, Lindh G, Weiland O, Johansson B, Sönnerborg A. Detection of hepatitis C virus (HCV) RNA by PCR related to HCV antibodies in serum and liver histology in Swedish blood donors. J Med Virol 39: 57–61, 1993.
11. Yun Z, Lundeberg J, Johansson B, Hedrum A, Weiland O, Uhlén M, Sönnerborg A. Colorimetric detection of competitive PCR products for quantification of hepatitis C viremia. J Virol Methods 47: 1–14, 1994.
12. Okamoto H, Sugiyama Y, Okada S, Kurai K, Akahane Y, Sugai Y, Tanaka T, Sato K, Tsuda F, Miyakawa Y, Mayumi M. Typing hepatitis C virus by polymerase chain reaction with type-specific primers: application to clinical surveys and tracing infectious sources. J Gen Virol 73: 673–679, 1992.
13. Widell A, Shev S, Månsson S, Zhang Y, Foberg U, Norkrans G, Frydén A, Weiland O, Kurkus J, Nordenfelt E. Genotyping of hepatitis C virus isolates by a modified PCR assay using type specific primers: epidemiological applications. J Med Virol 44: 272–279, 1994.
14. Chan S, McOmish F, Holmes E, Dow B, Peutherer J, Follett E, Yap P, Simmonds P. Analysis of a new hepatitis C virus type and its phylogenetic relationship to existing variants. J Gen Virol 73: 1131–1141, 1992.
15. Ahrén B, Engman K, Lindblom A. Treatment of malignant carcinoid with a highly purified leukocyte alfa-interferon. Anticancer Res 12: 129–134, 1992.
16. International Group. Acute and chronic hepatitis revisited. Lancet 2: 914–919, 1977.
17. Tine F, Magrin S, Craxi A, Pagliaro L. Interferon for non-A, non-B chronic hepatitis. A meta-analysis of randomised clinical trials. J Hepatol 13: 192–199, 1991.
18. Lau Y, Mizokami M, Ohno T, Diamond D, Kniffen J, Davis G. Discrepancy between biochemical and virological response to interferon-alfa in chronic hepatitis C. Lancet 342: 1208–1209, 1993.
19. Saracco G, Rosina F, Abate ML, Chinadussi L, Gallo V, Cerutti E, Di Napoli A, Solinas A, Deplano A, Tocco A, Cossu P, Chien D, Kuo G, Polito A, Weiner AJ, Houghton M, Verme G, Bonino F, Rizzetto M. Long-term follow-up of patients with chronic hepatitis C treated with different doses of interferon alfa-2b. Hepatology 18: 1300–1305, 1993.
20. Yun Z, Reichard O, Chen M, Lundeberg J, Norkrans G, Fryden A, Sönnerborg A, Weiland O. Serum hepatitis C virus RNA levels in chronic hepatitis C: importance for outcome of interferon alfa-2b treatment. Scand J Infect Dis 26: 263–270, 1994.
21. Lau J, Davis G, Kniffen J, Qian K-P, Urdea M, Chan C, Mizokami M, Neuwald P, Wilber J. Significance of serum hepatitis C virus RNA levels in chronic hepatitis C. Lancet 341: 1501–1504, 1993.
22. Gretch D, Corey L, Wilson J, de la Rosa C, Willson R, carithers R, Busch M, Hart J, Sayers M, Han J. Assessment of hepatitis C virus RNA levels by quantitative competitive RNA polymerase chain reaction: high-titer viremia correlates with advanced stage of disease. J Infect Dis 169: 1219–1225, 1994.
23. Marcellin P, Boyer N, Giostra E, Degott C, Courouce A, Degos F, Coppere H, Cales P, Couzigou P, Benhamou J-P. Recombinant human alfa-interferon in patients with chronic non-A, non-B hepatitis: a multicenter randomized controlled trial from France. Hepatology 13: 393–397, 1991.

Submitted March 1, 1995; accepted May 4, 1995

Scandinavian Journal of

INFECTIOUS DISEASES

Vol. 27, no. 5, 1995
pp. 429–540

SCANDINAVIAN
UNIVERSITY PRESS

Oslo - Copenhagen -
Stockholm - Boston

Adjunctive Corticosteroid Therapy in Bacterial Meningitis

ANNE LAURITSEN and BJARNE ØBERG

From the Department of Anaesthesia and Intensive Care, Copenhagen University Hospital, Herlev, Denmark

Experimental studies of bacterial meningitis have shown that components of bacterial cell walls stimulate the local production of inflammatory cytokines in the cerebrospinal fluid, leading to inflammation and alterations in the cerebral microvasculature. Animal studies and clinical trials have demonstrated that adjunctive corticosteroid therapy reduces the production of cytokines in the CSF. This results in decreased severity of the inflammatory process and fewer neurologic sequelae. These data support the use of adjunctive dexamethasone in infants and children with S. pneumoniae and H. influenzae type B (HiB) meningitis. There is not sufficient evidence supporting the use of adjunctive corticosteroid therapy in children with meningitis caused by N. meningitidis. Also, the routine use of dexamethasone in adult meningitis cannot presently be recommended. When using dexamethasone timing is crucial. Administration before or with antibiotics is optimal for attenuating the subarachnoid space inflammatory response. Patients receiving the therapy need careful monitoring for the possibility of gastrointestinal bleeding. Future studies of the pathogenesis and pathophysiology of bacterial meningitis may lead to the development of other adjunctive treatment strategies, improving the outcome of this serious disease.

B. Øberg, MD, Hans Jensensvej 12, DK-2900 Hellerup, Denmark

INTRODUCTION

Bacterial meningitis remains a relatively common and serious disease with an overall attack rate in Denmark of approximately 8 cases per 100 000 inhabitants. Mortality rates associated with the 3 most common causative agents of bacterial meningitis, Haemophilus influenzae, Neisseria meningitidis and Streptococcus pneumoniae were <2, 8 and 17%, respectively, during the period 1989–1992 (1). Also, the occurrence of long-term neurologic sequelae in surviving children and adults remains high. The overall incidence of sensorineural hearing loss in surviving children is 10%, but is 31% following S. pneumoniae meningitis (2). It now appears that further improvements in outcome will not come from better bactericidal agents but from early diagnosis and new treatments based on a better understanding of basic disease mechanisms (3). Also, in most industrialized countries the occurrence of HiB meningitis has been reduced considerably due to mass vaccination.

During the last 6–7 years several investigations have indicated that both morbidity and mortality may be reduced by administration of dexamethasone as adjunctive therapy in bacterial meningitis. In particular, the occurrence of sensorineural hearing loss, but also other neurologic sequelae, may be reduced in children, especially following H. influenzae type B (HiB) meningitis (4–10).

This overview focuses on the potential advantages in using corticosteroids as adjunctive therapy in bacterial meningitis, reviewing both experimental animal studies and clinical trials.

EXPERIMENTAL STUDIES

In bacterial meningitis the infected cerebrospinal fluid (CSF) contains approximately 10^5–10^7 bacteria/ml. When adequate antibiotic treatment is instituted, rapid bacteriolysis will release high concentrations of inflammatory bacterial fragments (e.g. cell walls from S. pneumoniae and lipopolysaccharides from H. influenzae), thereby potentially exacerbating the inflammation and abnormalities in the cerebral microvasculature (3). The bacterial fragments stimulate the production and release into the CSF of numerous cytokines, for example tumor necrosis factor (TNF) and interleukin-1 (IL-1), which are crucial mediators of the inflammatory response (11–15). Many experimental animal studies have been performed in order to investigate the possible benefits of modifying the host response to infection (16–20). Most of these studies have compared animals treated with an antibiotic with animals receiving antibiotics plus corticosteroids. In general, these studies have demonstrated effects of the adjunctive treatment on the CNS that are considered beneficial to the host. Decreases in brain edema, CSF pressure, CSF white blood cell count and decreased concentrations of CSF lactate have been observed in animals receiving anti-inflammatory agents.

In experimentally induced pneumococcal meningitis in rabbits, Täuber et al. found that, although ampicillin plus dexamethasone or methylprednisolone sterilized the CSF and reversed brain edema within 24 h, only the combination of ampicillin plus dexamethasone resulted in a significant reduction of CSF lactate levels and CSF pressure (16).

In another study, treatment with the antibiotic ceftriaxone was compared with treatment with ceftriaxone plus dexamethasone in an experimental rabbit model of HiB meningitis (17). Combination therapy consistently reduced the water content of the brain, the CSF pressure, and the lactate concentration in the CSF to a greater degree than ceftriaxone alone, although the differences were not statistically

 ISSN 0036-5548

significant. The authors proposed that one of the reasons for the less convincing effect of the combination treatment was that dexamethasone was given too late, and they suggested that dexamethasone might be more beneficial if administered early during antibiotic therapy after (or even before) antibiotic-induced lysis and release of microbial products.

In 1989 Kadurugamuwa et al. demonstrated that concomitant administration of ampicillin and dexamethasone to rabbits with meningitis caused by S. pneumoniae reduced the massive influx of serum albumin into the CSF, compared with animals treated only with the antibiotic (18). The death rate was also reduced. Reversion to normal CSF protein patterns was fastest in the group receiving the combination therapy.

The same year an experimental study, utilizing a rabbit model of HiB, demonstrated a significant increase in concentrations of endotoxin in CSF 2 h after ceftriaxone administration (19); this increase was followed by a rise in TNF concentrations in CSF. Simultaneous administration of ceftriaxone and dexamethasone did not affect the appearance of endotoxin in CSF, but there was a marked attenuation in concentrations of TNF in CSF 8 h later. If dexamethasone was given 1 h *after* the start of antibiotic treatment, TNF production was hardly affected, and the reduction of meningeal inflammation was limited. Adjunctive dexamethasone therapy resulted in a significant decrease in CSF leukocytosis and a trend towards earlier improvement in concentrations of glucose, lactate and protein in CSF.

In conclusion, adjunctive dexamethasone therapy appears to improve a number of parameters of subarachnoid space inflammation in experimental animal models of bacterial meningitis. These parameters improve without any apparent adverse effects such as a decrease in the rate of bacterial killing in the CSF by the antibiotic.

Dexamethasone administration before or with antibiotics is optimal for attenuating the inflammatory response.

CLINICAL TRIALS

The experimental studies described above indicate that adjunctive dexamethasone therapy diminishes the CSF inflammatory response and its subsequent pathophysiological consequences, specifically elevated water content in the brain and elevated CSF pressure. On the basis of these observations, several controlled clinical trials have been undertaken to examine the effects on outcomes of adjunctive corticosteroids in patients with bacterial meningitis (Table I).

Early clinical trials performed in the 1960s failed to show any benefit for adjunctive therapy with dexamethasone or methylprednisolone (21, 22). However, it may be objected that in the first study (21) insufficient doses of dexamethasone were applied, and in the second study (22) a glucocorticoid with suboptimal effect (methylprednisolone) was used. A Danish study from 1968 included 85 children and adults with S. pneumoniae meningitis (23). One group of patients were treated with antibiotics alone (sulfonamide, penicillin and streptomycin); in the other group an initial injection of intramuscular hydrocortisone was added followed by oral prednisone for at least 7 days. Even though the difference might not have been statistically significant, the lowest mortality was found in the group receiving the combination treatment. However, neither the corticosteroids used nor the study design were optimal.

Recent investigations have produced more promising results. In 1988 a double-blind, placebo-controlled trial including 200 infants and children with meningitis was published (4). In 77% of the patients, where the causative agent was HiB, dexamethasone reduced the incidence of sensorineural hearing loss. The patients received ceftriaxone or cefuroxime with either dexamethasone (0.15 mg/kg every 6 h for the first 4 days of therapy) or placebo. Moderate or more severe bilateral hearing loss was reported in 13/84 patients in the placebo group (15%) and in 3/92 (3%) of the dexamethasone-treated children ($p < 0.01$). There was also a more rapid increase in CSF glucose concentrations and reduction in lactate and protein concentrations in the dexamethasone group than in the placebo group. Two patients in the dexamethasone group (but none in the placebo group) had gastrointestinal bleeding. Bleeding developed in these 2 infants during the 2nd and 3rd days of steroid therapy and blood transfusions were necessary. It is uncertain, however, whether the bleeding was the result of dexamethasone therapy, of the infants' central nervous system disease, or of both. It was concluded that dexamethasone is beneficial in the treatment of infants and children with bacterial meningitis, particularly in preventing deafness.

In 1989 Girgis et al. studied 429 children and adults in Egypt with bacterial meningitis caused by S. pneumoniae, N. meningitidis, or H. influenzae (6). The majority of these patients (370/429) had received inadequate therapy for the 3–5 days prior to hospitalization, and 273 were comatose when included in the study. The patients were randomly assigned to receive either standard therapy (ampicillin and chloramphenicol) alone or in combination with a 3-day course of intramuscular dexamethasone (8 mg to children <12 years and 12 mg to adults, every 12 h). Patients treated with dexamethasone had a reduction in case fatality rate and permanent neurologic sequelae, but these differences reached statistical significance only in patients with S. pneumoniae meningitis.

In a study from 1991 infants and children with bacterial meningitis were randomized in a placebo-controlled, double-blind fashion to receive cefotaxime with or without adjunctive dexamethasone therapy (7). Of these patients 78% had HiB meningitis. In the study dexamethasone was administered 15–20 min before the first antibiotic dose in an effort to attenuate the CSF inflammatory response associated with administration of bacteriolytic antibiotics. By

Table I. *Controlled clinical trials investigating the effects of adjunctive corticosteroid therapy in bacterial meningitis*

Reference	Organism	Adjunctive agent	Patients		Variable
			n	Age group	
Roshdahl et al. 1968 (23)	S. pneumoniae	Initial hydrocortisone i.m., then prednisone p.o. for 7 days	85	Children and adults	Lower mortality, but not significant
Belsey et al. 1969 (21)	> 50% HiB	Dexamethasone 0.8 mg/m^2 every day for 4 days	102	Infants and children	Fewer neurologic sequelae, but not significant
Delemos & Haggerty 1969 (22)	> 50% HiB	Methylprednisolone 40 mg every 6 h for 4 days	117	Infants and children	No change
Lebel et al. 1988 (4)	77% HiB	Dexamethasone 0.15 mg/kg every 6 h for 4 days	200	Infants and children	Reduction in sensorineural hearing loss follow-up ($p < 0.01$)
Girgis et al. 1989 (6)	S. pneumoniae N. meningitidis HiB	Dexamethasone for 3 days; 8 mg to children < 12 years and 12 mg to adults, every 12 h	429	Children and adults	Reduction in case fatalities and neurologic sequelae. Significant in S. pneumoniae
Odio et al. 1991 (7)	78% HiB	Dexamethasone 0.15 mg/kg every 6 h for 4 days, 15–20 min *before* first antibiotic dose	101	Infants and children	Significantly lower rate in one or more neurologic or audiologic sequelae ($p = 0.007$)
Kennedy et al. 1991 (10)	S. pneumoniae	Dexamethasone 0.15 mg/kg every 6 h for 4 days	97	Infants and children	Significantly lower adverse neurologic long-term outcome ($p = 0.025$)
Schaad et al. 1993 (5)	58% HiB	Dexamethasone 0.40 mg/kg every 12 h for 2 days 10 min *before* first antibiotic dose	115	Infants and children	Lower rate of one or more neurologic or audiologic sequelae ($p = 0.066$)

12 h after the beginning of therapy, the patients receiving adjunctive dexamethasone (0.15 mg/kg every 6 h for 4 days) had lower mean CSF pressure, improved indices of CSF-inflammation, and lower concentrations of the cytokines TNF-α and platelet-activating factor compared to the control group. At 24 h the clinical condition and mean prognostic score were significantly better among those treated with dexamethasone than among controls. At follow-up examination, after a mean of 15 months, 7 of the surviving 51 dexamethasone-treated children (14%) and 18/48 surviving controls (38%) had one or more neurologic or audiologic sequelae ($p = 0.007$); the relative risk of sequelae for a child receiving placebo as compared with a child receiving dexamethasone was 3.8 (95% confidence interval: 1.3–11.5). Mortality rates were similar in the two groups, no significant adverse effects attributable to dexamethasone therapy were noted, and corticosteroid treatment did not delay sterilization of the CSF.

Also in 1991, a study was published, where 97 infants and children with S. pneumoniae meningitis were evaluated in a double-blind, placebo-controlled manner to determine whether corticosteroid therapy improved disease outcome (10). A total of 32 patients were given steroid therapy (dexamethasone 0.15 mg/kg every 6 h for 4 days) within 24 h of initiating parenteral antibiotic therapy. Four patients each in the steroid- and non-steroid-treated groups had clinically evident gastrointestinal bleeding, and 3 patients in each group required blood transfusion. The survivors were examined 6 weeks and 6 months after discharge, and the percentage with any adverse neurologic long-term outcome, including hearing impairment, was markedly smaller in those given steroid therapy compared with the patients who never received steroid therapy (9% vs. 33%; $p = 0.025$).

Finally, in a clinical, double-blind, placebo-controlled trial from 1993 (5) 115 children with bacterial meningitis were included. In 58% the causative agent was HiB, in 24% it was N. meningitidis and in 10% S. pneumoniae. One group received either placebo ($n = 55$) or dexamethasone ($n = 60$) in addition to antibiotic treatment with ceftriaxone. Dexamethasone therapy (0.4 mg/kg) was started 10 min before the first dose of ceftriaxone and given every 12 h for 2 days. After 24 h of treatment meningeal inflammation, as shown by CSF glucose concentration was significantly less with dexamethasone than with placebo ($p = 0.008$). Other indices of inflammation showed similar changes in both groups. Clinical and laboratory monitoring for possible adverse effects of dexamethasone revealed no abnormalities, no gastrointestinal bleeding was recorded and addition of dexamethasone did not affect the rate at which CSF became sterile. At follow-up examinations 3, 9 and 15 months after hospital discharge 9 (16%) of 55 placebo recipients and 3 (5%) of 60 dexamethasone recipients had 1 or more neurologic or audiologic sequelae ($p = 0.066$); the relative risk of sequelae was 3.27 (95% confidence limits: 0.93–11.47).

Although there are not sufficient data to demonstrate, with statistical significance, a beneficial effect of dexamethasone treatment in children with pneumococcal meningitis (24, 25), recent investigations generally support the use of adjunctive dexamethasone in infants and children with S. pneumoniae and H. influenzae type B (HiB) meningitis.

REFERENCES

1. Holk K. Purulent meningitis og meningokoksepsis 1989–92. EPI-NYT 17. Statens Seruminstitut, 1993.
2. Dodge PR, Davis H, Feigin RD, Holmes SJ, Kaplan SL, Jueblirer DP, Stechenberg BW, Hirsh SK. Prospective evaluation of hearing impairment as a sequela of acute bacterial meningitis. N Engl J Med 311: 869–874, 1984.
3. Quagliarello V, Scheld WM. Bacterial meningitis: pathogenesis, pathyphysiology, and progress. N Engl J Med 327: 864–872, 1992.
4. Lebel MH, Freij BJ, Syrogiannopoulos GA, Chrane DF, Hoyt MJ, Stewart SM, Kennard BD, Olsen KD, McCracken GH. Dexamethasone therapy for bacterial meningitis. N Engl J Med 319: 964–971, 1988.
5. Schaad UB, Lips U, Gnehm HE, Blumberg A, Heinzer Ivo, Wedgwood J. Dexamethasone therapy for bacterial meningitis in children. Lancet 342: 457–461, 1993.
6. Girgis NI, Farid Z, Mikhail IA, Farrag I, Sultan Y, Kilpatrick ME. Dexamethasone treatment for bacterial meningitis in children and adults. Pediatr Infect Dis J 8: 848–851, 1989.
7. Odio CM, Faingezicht I, Paris M, Nassar M, Baltodano A, Rogers J, Sáez-Llorens X, Olsen KD, McCracken GH. The beneficial effects of early dexamethasone administration in infants and children with bacterial meningitis. N Engl J Med 324: 1525–1531, 1991.
8. Lebel MH, Hoyt MJ, Waagner DC, Rollins NK, Finitzo T, McCracken GH. Magnetic resonance imaging and dexamethasone therapy for bacterial meningitis. Am J Dis Child 143: 301–306, 1989.
9. Mustafa MM, Ramilo O, Sáez-Llorens X, Olsen KD, Magness RR, McCracken GH. Cerebrospinal fluid prostaglandins, interleukin 1β, and tumor necrosis factor in bacterial meningitis. Am J Dis Child 144: 883–887, 1990.
10. Kennedy WA, Hoyt MJ, McCracken GH. The role of corticosteroid therapy in children with pneumococcal meningitis. Am J Dis Child 145: 1374–1378, 1991.
11. Dinarello CA. Interleukin-1 and its biologically related cytokines. Adv Immunol 44: 153–205, 1989.
12. Waage A, Halstensen A, Shalaby R, Brandtzæg P, Kierulf P, Espevik T. Local production of tumor necrosis factor α, interleukin 1, and interleukin 6 in meningococcal meningitis. J Exp Med 170: 1859–1867, 1989.
13. Tunkel AR, Scheld WM. Pathogenesis and pathyphysiology of bacterial meningitis. Clin Microbiol Rev 6: 118–136, 1993.
14. Saukkonen K, Sande S, Cioffe C, Wolpe S, Sherry B, Cerami A, Tuomanen E. The role of cytokines in the generation of inflammation and tissue damage in experimental gram-positive meningitis. J Exp Med 171: 439–448, 1990.
15. Jacobs RF, Tabor DR. The immunology of sepsis and meningitis – cytokine biology. Scand J Infect Dis, Suppl 73: 7–15, 1990.
16. Täuber MG, Khayam-Bashi H, Sande MA. Effects of ampicillin and corticosteroids on brain water content, cerebrospinal fluid pressure, and cerebrospinal fluid lactate levels in experimental pneumococcal meningitis. J Infect Dis 151: 528–534, 1985.
17. Syrogiannopoulos GA, Olsen KD, Reisch JS, McCracken GH. Dexamethasone in the treatment of experimental haemophilus influenzae type b meningitis. J Infect Dis 155: 213–219, 1987.
18. Kadurugamuwa JL, Hengstler B, Zak O. Cerebrospinal fluid protein profile in experimental pneumococcal meningitis and its alteration by ampicillin and anti-inflammatory agents. J Infect Dis 159: 26–34, 1989.
19. Mustafa MM, Ramilo O, Mertsola J, Risser RC, Beutler B, Hansen EJ, McCracken GH. Modulation of inflammation and cachectin activity in relation to treatment of experimental hemophilus influenzae type b meningitis. J Infect Dis 160: 818–825, 1989.
20. Tuomanen E, Hangstler B, Rich R, Bray MA, Zak O, Tomasz A. Non-steroidal anti-inflammatory agents in the therapy for experimental pneumococcal meningitis. J Infect Dis 155: 985–990, 1987.
21. Belsey MA, Hoffpauir CW, Smith MHD. Dexamethasone in the treatment of acute bacterial meningitis: the effect of study design on the interpretation of results. Pediatrics 44: 503–513, 1969.
22. DeLemos RA, Haggerty RJ. Corticosteroids as an adjunct to treatment in bacterial meningitis: a controlled clinical trial. Pediatrics 44: 30–34, 1969.
23. Rosdahl N, Jensen K, Ranek L. Kortikosteroidbehandling af pneumokokmeningitis. Nord Med 79: 146–150, 1968.
24. Schuster V, Kreth HW. Dexamethasone in childhood meningitis [letter]. N Engl J Med 325: 1654, 1991.
25. McCracken GH. Dexamethasone in childhood meningitis [reply]. N Engl J Med 325: 1654–1655, 1991.

Submitted January 30, 1995; accepted May 23, 1995

Scand J Infect Dis 27: 435–440, 1995

ORIGINAL ARTICLE

Diagnostic Markers and Risk Factors of Cytomegalovirus Infection and Disease in Renal Allograft Recipients

INGEGERD HÖKEBERG[1], BRITT MARIE ERIKSSON[1], BENITA ZWEYGBERG-WIRGART[2], GUNNAR TUFVESSON[3], ELISABETH OLDING-STENKVIST[1] and LENA GRILLNER[2]

From the Departments of [1]Infectious Diseases, [3]Urology, University Hospital of Uppsala, Uppsala and [2]Clinical Microbiology, Section of Virology, Karolinska Hospital, Stockholm, Sweden

In a prospective study, the incidences of CMV infection and disease were 56 and 23%, respectively, during the first 6 months following kidney transplantation. Viremia was found in all patients with CMV disease and arthralgia was present in 71% prior to the development of CMV disease. The positive predictive value for CMV disease reached up to 90% for viremia and arthralgia in combination. Viruria was poorly correlated to viremia and hence CMV disease. The majority of patients (93%) who developed CMV disease had a seropositive donor, and viremia was significantly more common in patients who received CMV-seropositive kidneys. CMV disease was more common in CMV-seronegative recipients than in seropositive recipients. The 1-year graft survival rate was 75% in the entire study group. In patients with CMV viremia and disease, the survival rates were 61 and 60%, respectively. The patient survival rate 1 year after transplantation was 91% in the entire study group. In patients with CMV viremia and CMV disease the rates were 78 and 73%, respectively. Antiviral treatment was initiated within 3 weeks of viremia detection in the 6 patients with CMV disease who survived. We found that the combination of arthralgia and viremia was a useful predictor of CMV disease and that recipients of CMV-seropositive allografts were at a greater risk of developing CMV disease. To obtain an early diagnosis and commence an early treatment of CMV disease, patients prone to develop CMV disease should be identified and clinical examination and viremia surveillance should be performed regularly

I. Hökeberg, MD, Department of Infectious Diseases, Uppsala University Hospital, S-751 85 Uppsala, Sweden

INTRODUCTION

During the last decades herpes viruses have been recognized as important causes of severe infections in patients with impaired immune defence. In particular, cytomegalovirus has been identified as a major agent of morbidity and mortality. In kidney transplant patients, cytomegalovirus is considered to be the single most important infectious cause of mortality (1–3). Since drugs like forscarnet and ganciclovir have become available, the need for early diagnosis of CMV infection and disease has become essential (4, 5). It is therefore of importance to recognize clinical signs and laboratory parameters associated with cytomegalovirus disease to facilitate an early diagnosis.

The purpose of this study was to identify early symptoms and laboratory parameters of CMV infection and disease and to correlate these to virological findings. Furthermore, the role of donor and recipient pretransplant CMV antibodies in the development of CMV disease was studied and also the consequences of CMV disease and CMV viremia for graft and patient survival.

MATERIALS AND METHODS

Patients

From February 1987 to August 1988, 79 kidney allograft recipients were followed prospectively at the Department of Urology, University Hospital, Uppsala.

A total of 73 patients received kidney allografts and 6 received kidney and pancreas allografts. Of these 79 patients, 61 (77%) were CMV-seropositive before transplantation. Out of the 79 patients, 66 (84%) were followed for more than 6 weeks and were therefore included in the study. The average follow-up time was 23 weeks (range 9–26). The average number of occasions for sampling was 12 (range 3–22). The mean age of the 66 eligible patients was 44.7 years (range 16–71), and 42 patients were men and 24 women. Of the patients, 60 received a kidney transplant and 6 both a kidney and a pancreas. The underlying causes of renal failure were glomerulonephritis (21 patients), diabetes nephropathy (20 patients), polycystic kidney disease (7 patients), pyelonephritis (5 patients), IgA-nephritis (3 patients), nephrosclerosis (1 patient) and miscellaneous causes (9 patients). The CMV antibody status of donors and recipients is shown in Table I.

The patients were interviewed and tested once a week during the first 1–4 weeks following transplantation. Thereafter, the patients were examined once or twice a month and when admitted to hospital during the first 6 months. Clinical symptoms associated with CMV infection such as fever (>38°C), cough, sore throat, arthralgia, diarrhea and impaired vision were enquired about using a questionnaire. Heparinized blood, throat swab and urine were sampled on each occasion for viral detection and a serum sample was drawn. A total of 834 samples each of blood, urine and throat swabs were analysed. Routine laboratory tests, i.e. leukocyte count, thrombocyte count, serum creatinine and serum alanine aminotransferase (s-ALT) were performed.

Immunosuppressive treatment

Prednisolone (Prednisolon, ACO, Sweden) was initially given at a dose of 30 mg per day, later reduced to 5–10 mg per day. Pred-

 ISSN 0036-5548

Table I. *The impact of donor (D) and recipient (R) CMV antibody status on CMV viremia and disease in 66 renal transplant patients. Percentages are shown in parentheses*

	Donor/recipient CMV antibody status[a]					
	Cadaveric kidney				Living donor kidney	
	D+/R+	D+/R−	D−/R+	D−/R−	D?/R+	D?/R−
No. of patients	34	10	10	1	6	5
Viremia ($n = 23$)	17/34 (50)	5/10 (50)	1/10 (10)	0/1 (0)	0/6 (0)	0/5 (0)
Non-viremia ($n = 43$)	17/34 (50)	5/10 (50)	9/10 (90)	1/1 (100)	6/6 (100)	5/5 (100)
CMV disease ($n = 15$)	8/34 (24)	6/10 (60)	1/10 (10)	0/1 (0)	0/6 (0)	0/5 (0)
No CMV disease ($n = 51$)	26/34 (76)	4/10 (40)	9/10 (90)	1/1 (100)	6/6 (100)	5/5 (100)

[a] + CMV positive; − CMV negative, ? unknown.

nisolone was combined initially with 8 mg/kg of cyclosporine A (Sandimmun, Sandoz, Switzerland) which was later reduced to a maintenance dose. Azathioprine (Imuran, Wellcome, United Kingdom) was given at an initial dose of 2.0 mg/kg and later as a maintenance dose of 1–1.5 mg/kg.

Therapy for CMV disease

Patients with symptomatic CMV infection were treated with foscarnet (Foscavir, Astra, Södertälje, Sweden). A few patients were also treated with ganciclovir (Cymevene, Astra-Syntex, Södertälje, Sweden) and/or human monoclonal CMV antibodies, as described elsewhere (6).

Virus isolation

The leukocyte fraction was prepared from 10 ml of heparinized blood using Ficoll Paque. The leukocytes, urine specimens and throat swabs, were inoculated into two tubes on a monolayer of human embryonic lung fibroblasts. The tubes were observed weekly for 6 weeks for a typical cytopathic effect. All CMV isolates were identified by immunofluorescence, using the monoclonal CMV antibody, CCH2 (7).

Detection of CMV early antigen in cell culture after short incubation

The detection of CMV early antigen in cell culture after a short incubation of urine samples was performed according to Zweygberg-Wirgart et al. (7). After incubation for 18 h the cells were fixed and CMV was detected with the CCH2 monoclonal antibody and indirect immunofluorescence.

Serology

CMV IgM and IgG antibodies in serum were determined by an indirect ELISA technique using a nuclear CMV antigen (8). All sera were tested in 2 dilutions against a positive and a negative antigen. Sera with a positive IgM reaction were retested by a μ-capture technique (9).

Laboratory investigations

Leukocytes (LPK), thrombocytes (TPK), s-alanine-aminotransferase (s-ALT) and s-creatinine were analysed according to the routines at the hospital. LPK $< 4 \times 10^9$/l, TPK $< 100 \times 10^9$/l, s-ALT $<$ 0.7 μkat/l and s-creatinine $>$ 106 μmol/l were considered pathological.

Definitions

Asymptomatic CMV infection after transplantation was defined as the isolation of cytomegalovirus from any site, and/or detection of IgM antibodies, and/or the appearance of a significant rise of IgG antibodies, and included only asymptomatic patients. The asymptomatic CMV infection was defined as *primary* in patients who were CMV seronegative prior to transplantation and *secondary* in those with CMV antibodies prior to transplantation.

CMV disease described virological findings which were the same as those found in asymptomatic CMV infection, and additionally, symptoms associated with CMV disease. CMV disease was considered mild when the following criteria were met; fever >38°C on two or more consecutive days without any other explanation and abnormal laboratory parameters, i.e. s-ALT increase and/or leucopenia and thrombocytopenia. Severe CMV disease included organ manifestations such as pneumonitis, colitis, or retinitis. CMV pneumonitis comprised dyspnoea, cough, a pattern of interstitial infiltrations on chest X-ray and CMV isolated from bronchoalveolar lavage. Gastrointestinal CMV disease, including colitis, comprised protracted diarrhea with or without intermittent bleeding and a CMV isolation from the mucous membrane of the intestine.

CMV disease due to primary and secondary infection was defined as primary and secondary CMV disease, respectively.

Statistics

Comparison of groups were performed using the chi-square test with Yates' correction. Statistical significance was considered as $p < 0.05$.

RESULTS

Of the eligible patients 24% (16/66) were CMV-seronegative before transplantation and 76% (50/66) were CMV-seropositive. CMV disease developed in 23% (15/66) of the patients and 56% (37/66) developed asymptomatic CMV infection. Of the CMV-seropositive patients 92% (46/50) developed CMV disease or asymptomatic CMV infection. The virological findings are summarized in Table II.

CMV disease

In all, 15 patients (23%) developed CMV disease. All 6 patients with a primary infection developed disease (100%). Mild CMV disease was observed in 5, and CMV pneumonitis in 1, of the 6 patients. In the group of patients with secondary infection ($n = 46$), 9 developed disease (20%). Four patients had a mild CMV disease, 4 pneumonitis and 1

Table II. *CMV findings from different sites and serological response in 52 of 66 kidney transplanted patients with CMV disease and asymptomatic infection; percentages shown in parentheses*

	CMV disease (n = 15)[a]			Asymptomatic CMV infection (n = 37)[b]			Total
Site of CMV isolation	Isol. of CMV	CMV IgM	CMV IgG	Isol. of CMV	CMV IgM	CMV IgG	No. of patients/total no
Blood	14 (93)	8 (53)	14 (93)	9 (24)	0 (0)	8 (22)	23/66 (35)
Throat	13 (87)	7 (47)	12 (80)	12(32)	0 (0)	12 (32)	25/66 (38)
Urine	15 (100)	8 (53)	14 (93)	27 (73)	3 (8)	25 (68)	42/66 (64)
Blood, throat and urine	12 (80)	6 (40)	11 (73)	6 (16)	0 (0)	6 (16)	18/66 (27)
Blood and urine	2 (13)	1 (7)	2 (13)	3 (8)	0 (0)	3 (8)	5/66 (8)
Throat and urine	1[c] (6)	1[c] (6)	1[c] (6)	6 (16)	0 (0)	4 (11)	7/66 (11)
Throat or urine alone	0 (0)	0 (0)	0 (0)	12 (32)	3 (8)	12 (32)	12/66 (18)
Total no of patients	15 (100)	8 (53)	14 (93)	27 (73)	3 (8)	35 (95)	52/66 (79)

[a] Primary CMV, $n = 6$; secondary CMV, $n = 9$.
[b] Primary CMV, $n = 0$; secondary CMV, $n = 37$.
[c] In one patient no blood samples were taken during 3–7 weeks after transplantation.

patient had CMV colitis. Primary CMV disease developed 5–12 weeks (median 6 weeks) and secondary CMV disease 6–23 weeks (median 9 weeks) following transplantation. The frequency of clinical symptoms and laboratory findings in all patients in comparison to the findings in those with CMV disease are presented in Table III. The positive predictive values for CMV disease are given for single or for combinations of parameters. Many of the clinical symptoms, and virological and laboratory parameters investigated were more frequent in patients with CMV disease, but were also common in asymptomatic patients and had low positive predictive values for CMV disease.

Table III. *Frequency of symptoms and laboratory parameters in patients with CMV disease in comparison to the whole group of kidney transplant patients; percentages are shown in parentheses*

	CMV disease n = 15	All patients n = 66	Positive predictive value
Clinical symptoms			
Arthralgia	10 (66)	21 (32)	10/21 (48)
Cough	9 (60)	32 (48)	9/32 (28)
Diarrhea	5 (33)	10 (15)	5/10 (50)
Virological findings			
CMV IgM positive	7 (47)	11 (17)	7/11 (64)
CMV IgG titer rise	14 (93)	49 (74)	14/49 (29)
CMV in blood	14 (93)	23 (35)	14/23 (61)
CMV in urine	15 (100)	42 (64)	15/42 (36)
CMV in throat	13 (87)	25 (38)	13/25 (52)
Laboratory findings			
Leucopenia	4 (27)	12 (18)	4/12 (33)
Thrombocytopenia	1 (7)	9 (14)	1/9 (11)
S-ALT > 0.7 μkat/l	14 (93)	37 (56)	14/37 (38)
Combinations			
Viremia and arthralgia	9 (60)	10 (15)	9/10 (90)
CMV in throat and CMV IgM antibodies and IgG titer rise	6 (40)	7 (47)	6/7 (86)

The most common symptom associated with CMV disease was arthralgia, which was present in 10 (66%) of the patients with CMV disease. Arthralgia was first registered 2–11 weeks (median 6.5 weeks) following transplantation. In 9 of the 10 patients arthralgia appeared prior to CMV disease or at the same time as diagnosis. Arthralgia was noticed 1 week after diagnosis of the disease in only 1 patient. The positive predictive value for arthralgia was 48%.

Viremia was found to be a prerequisite for CMV disease and was detected 2–17 weeks (median 7 weeks) following transplantation. CMV IgM antibodies, viremia and CMV excretion in throat swabs had positive predictive values above 50%. The combination of CMV excretion in throat swabs and serological signs (IgM antibodies and a significant IgG titer rise) had a positive predictive value of 86% whereas CMV excretion in urine and serological signs had a positive predictive value of 72%.

CMV was detected in 261 urine samples either by conventional virus isolation and/or with early detection with immunofluoresence after short incubation in cell culture using the monoclonal antibody CCH2. The sensitivity for short incubation of urine samples was 74% compared with virus isolation. The correlation of CMV excretion in urine with viremia had sensitivity, specificity and negative and positive predictive values below 50%.

By combining symptoms and virological parameters associated with CMV disease, a more accurate diagnosis could be attained. The positive predictive values for arthralgia and viremia were 48% and 61%, respectively, whereas the positive predictive value for the combination was 90%.

Eight patients with CMV disease were treated with drugs, commencing therapy 6–36 weeks following transplantation (median 10.5 weeks). Treatment was initiated in 6 patients within 3 weeks of viremia detection; all 6 patients recovered. Two patients started treatment at 6 and 36 weeks after viremia was detected, respectively; both of these patients died. The causes of death were CMV pneumonia with multiorgan failure and protracted CMV disease and Staphylococcus aureus septicaemia.

Asymptomatic CMV infection

In all, 37 patients developed a secondary CMV infection without symptoms (56%). None of the asymptomatic patients had a primary CMV infection.

CMV was isolated from blood, urine or throat swabs in 27 of the 37 patients with asymptomatic secondary CMV infection; 9 of them (24%) had viremia. Viremia appeared 2–26 weeks after transplantation (median 6 weeks). All patients with viremia had viruria. In 7 patients viremia was diagnosed simultaneously or later than viruria.

IgM antibodies were found in only 3 patients with secondary asymptomatic CMV infection, 5–9 weeks after transplantation. A significant increase of CMV IgG antibodies occurred in most patients (35/37, 95%) with CMV excretion, irrespective of viremia, and was the only sign of secondary CMV infection in 10 patients.

CMV infection and disease in relation to the CMV status of donor and recipient

The impact of donor and recipient CMV antibody status on CMV viremia and disease is shown in Table I for the 66 renal transplant patients. CMV disease was more common in CMV-seronegative recipients than in seropositive recipients (38 vs. 18%). The difference was, however, not statistically significant. The majority of patients who developed CMV disease or viremia had received a kidney allograft from a seropositive donor, 96 and 93%, respectively. Irrespective of the CMV status of the recipient, viremia was significantly more common in patients who received CMV-seropositive allografts compared with seronegative ones ($p < 0.05$). CMV-seropositive recipients were also more likely to develop viremia if the donor was seropositive ($p < 0.05$).

Graft survival rate

Among the 66 eligible patients the 6-month graft survival rate was 88% (58/66) and the 1-year survival rate was 77% (51/66). The reasons for transplantectomy were rejection (5 patients), unspecified infection (2 patients), kidney failure (2 patients), CMV infection (1 patient), renal artery thrombosis (1 patient) and unknown cause (1 patient). Three patients died during the first 6 months following transplantation. Among the patients with CMV viremia and disease, the frequency of transplantectomy was 6/23 for CMV viremia, and 5/15 patients for CMV disease at 6 months after transplantation, and after 1 year it was 9/23 patients (CMV viremia) and 6/15 patients (CMV disease). This gives a 1-year transplant survival rate of 61% in patients with viremia and 60% in patients with CMV disease.

In the entire study group the 6-month graft survival rate was 84% (66/79) and the 1-year survival rate was 75% (59/79).

Patient survival rate

The 6-month patient survival rate was 95% (63/66), and the 1-year rate was 91% (60/66). The causes of death were myocardial infarction (3 patients), cytomegalovirus disease (2 patients, 1 in combination with septicemia) and heart and pulmonary failure after untreated CMV pneumonitis (1 patient). Among the 23 patients with CMV viremia, 5 died during the first postoperative year and of patients with CMV disease, 4/15 died during the same period, survival rates of 78 and 73%, respectively.

The 6-month patient survival rate in the entire group was 94% (74/79) and the 1-year patient survival rate was 91% (72/79).

DISCUSSION

CMV infection is common among renal transplant patients. The incidence of CMV infection and disease is, however, dependent on different factors, such as the criteria used for the diagnosis of infection and disease, the type of immunosuppressive treatment given and the CMV seroprevalence in the study group. We could not find any significant difference in the risk of developing CMV disease among patients with different immunosuppressive treatment regimens.

CMV disease usually develops during the first 6 months following transplantation, but late onset of fatal CMV disease has also been reported (10). In this study, 79% of the patients showed virological signs of asymptomatic CMV infection or disease, a result that is in accordance with several other studies (11, 12). A total of 23% of the patients developed CMV disease. The outcome in patients with CMV disease is dependent on early treatment, and hence the early detection of CMV disease is important. This is stressed by a recent report that showed almost 100% recovery after ganciclovir treatment (13). It is also in accordance with our own findings. The 2 patients in our study who started treatment at a late stage of the disease died, whereas the 6 patients who received early treatment survived.

We confirmed earlier findings showing that a primary CMV infection is more likely to proceed to symptomatic disease than a secondary infection (14); all our patients with primary infection developed disease. Therefore, in a population with a smaller proportion of CMV-seronegative recipients, there is a decreased risk of primary CMV infection and disease. In Sweden the CMV-seroprevalence is high, i.e. 72% among women of childbearing age (15), as compared with only 30% in parts of the United States (2). In our study, the CMV seroprevalence was as high as 76%, which may explain in part, why only 23% of the patients developed CMV disease (16).

CMV disease is difficult to recognize in renal transplant patients because the symptoms are often vague and resemble those of rejection episodes and other infections. When we analysed symptoms and virological parameters in our patients, we found a strong correlation between arthralgia and CMV disease. Furthermore, all the patients with CMV disease were viremic except 1. Viremia alone had a positive predictive value of 61% for CMV disease. This is a considerably higher value than was found in a previous study among renal transplant patients (17) but agrees with findings in bone marrow transplant patients (i.e. 60%) (18).

An even better predictor of CMV disease was achieved when arthralgia and viremia were combined, giving a positive predictive value of 90%. To our knowledge, the strong association between CMV disease and the combination of viremia and arthralgia has not been recognized previously. Furthermore, arthralgia as well as viremia appeared in close relation to CMV disease. It is of importance that questions about arthralgia are addressed because this symptom can easily be overlooked.

Viremia was found to be the most reliable virological predictor of CMV disease. CMV excretion in throat and urine was a common finding in patients both with and without CMV disease, and is often found to persist for months to years after a primary CMV infection (19). In 74% of the urine samples which were CMV positive by virus isolation, CMV was also detected by immunofluorescence and monoclonal antibodies. However, surveillance for CMV excretion in urine after kidney transplantation is inappropriate, since the correlation to CMV disease was low. In the early phase of the study, we used virus isolation only to detect CMV in blood. In the latter part of the study, when the importance of viremia was clarified, a rapid technique for detection of CMV matrix protein (pp65) in leukocytes was developed (20). CMV antigenemia has been proven to be a specific and early marker of CMV infection in renal allograft recipients (21) and the earliest laboratory indicator of an active CMV infection (22).

In the present study, all patients with primary CMV infection developed CMV disease in contrast to only 50% of patients with secondary infections and viremia. Viremia was significantly more common in a seropositive recipient if the donor was CMV-seropositive. This finding is in agreement with the findings of Grundy et al. (23), who also found a significant increase in the rate of CMV infection in seropositive renal recipients when the donor was seropositive. This indicates that CMV reinfection might be of greater importance than reactivation in kidney transplant recipients. In contrast, the donor serology had no influence in seropositive allogenic bone marrow recipients (18).

Patients with CMV viremia and disease showed an increased risk of losing their renal allograft and increased mortality. However, the increase in mortality was not clearly associated with CMV disease, but with myocardial infarction. Whether CMV can play an etiological part in arteriosclerosis and myocardial infarction is a matter of debate. In a recent report (24), it was suggested that CMV might be a causative agent in restenosis after coronary angioplasty.

Because CMV disease is a risk factor in renal transplant recipients, concerning morbidity, survival and organ survival, a surveillance program for patients at risk for developing CMV disease is important during the first 3 months after transplantation. This should include recipients with CMV-seropositive donors and especially those recipients who are seronegative. The surveillance should include clinical symptoms with special reference to arthralgia and weekly surveillance for viremia using a rapid method.

REFERENCES

1. Rubin RH. Impact of cytomegalovirus on organ transplant recipients. Rev Infect Dis 12: 754–766, 1990.
2. Glenn J. Cytomegalovirus infections following renal transplantation. Rev Infect Dis 3: 1151–1178, 1981.
3. Fiala M, Payne JE, Berne TV, Moore TC, Henle W, Montgomerie JZ, Chatterjee SN, Guze LB. Epidemiology of cytomegalovirus infection after transplantation and immunosuppression. J Infect Dis 132: 421–433, 1975.
4. Reed EC, Bowden RA, Dandliker PS, Lilleby KE, Meyers JD, Treatment of cytomegalovirus pneumonia with ganciclovir and intravenous cytomegalovirus immunoglobulin in patients with bone marrow transplants. Ann Intern Med 109: 783–788, 1988.
5. Balfour HH Jr. Management of cytomegalovirus disease with antiviral drugs. Rev Infect Dis 12: 849–860, 1990.
6. Skarp Örberg I, Hökeberg I, Olding-Stenkvist E, Tufveson G. Use of a human monoclonal anti-cytomegalovirus antibody for the treatment of severe cytomegalovirus infection after renal transplantation. Transplant Proc 22: 234, 1990.
7. Zweygberg-Wirgart B, Landqvist M, Hökeberg I, Eriksson BM, Olding-Stenkvist E, Grillner L. Early detection of cytomegalovirus in cell culture by a new monoclonal antibody. CCH2. J Virol Meth 27: 211–220, 1990.
8. Grillner L. Screening of blood donors for cytomegalovirus (CMV) antibodies: an evaluation of different tests. J Virol Meth 17: 133–139, 1987.
9. Schmitz H. Improved detection of virus-specific IgM antibodies. Elimination of non-specific IgM binding. J Gen Virol 40: 459–463, 1978.
10. Boehler A, Schaffner A, Salomon F, Keusch G. Cytomegalovirus disease of late onset following renal transplantation: a potential fatal entity. Scand J Infect Dis 26: 369–373, 1994.
11. Arnfred J, Möller Nielsen C, Spenser ES, Andersen HK. A prospective study on infections with cytomegalovirus in renal allograft recipients immunosuppressed with cyclosporine A and low dose prednisone. Scand J Infect Dis 19: 297–302, 1987.
12. Gadler H, Sundqvist V, Tillegård A, Wahren B. Studies of cytomegalovirus infections in renal allograft recipients. II. Serological response to various viral antigens. Scand J Infect Dis 14: 89–94, 1982.
13. Sawyer MD, Mayoral JL, Gillingham KJ, Kramer MA, Dunn DL. Treatment of recurrent cytomegalovirus disease in patients receiving solid organ transplants. Arch Surg 128: 165–170, 1993.
14. Smiley ML, Wlodaver CG, Grossman RA, Barker CF, Perloff LJ, Tustin NB, Starr SE, Plotkin SA, Friedman HM. The role of pretransplant immunity in protection from cytomegalovirus disease following renal transplantation. Transplant 40: 157–161, 1985.
15. Ahlfors K, Ivarsson S-A, Johnsson T, Svanberg L. Primary and secondary cytomegalovirus infections and their relation to congenital infection. Analysis of maternal sera. Acta Pediatr Scand 71: 109–113, 1982.

16. Rubin RH, Cosimi AB, Tolkoff-Rubin NE, Russell PS, Hirsch MS. Infectious disease syndromes attributable to cytomegalovirus and their significance among renal transplant recipients. Transplant 24: 458–464, 1977.
17. Pillay D, Ali AA, Liu SF, Kops E, Sweny P, Griffiths PD. The prognostic significance of positive CMV cultures during surveillance of renal transplant recipients. Transplant 56: 103–108, 1993.
18. Meyers JD, Ljungman P, Fisher LD. Cytomegalovirus excretion as a predictor of cytomegalovirus disease after marrow transplantation: importance of cytomegalovirus viremia. J Infect Dis 162: 373–380, 1990.
19. Chessman SH, Stewart JA, Winkle S, Cosimi AB, Tolkoff-Rubin NE, Russel PS, Baker GP, Herrin J, Rubin RH. Cytomegalovirus excretion 2–14 years after renal transplantation. Transplant Proc 11: 71–4, 1979.
20. Zweygberg-Wirgart B, Hökeberg I, Landqvist M, Grillner L. Detection of cytomegalovirus directly in blood leucocytes and evaluation of a new monoclonal antibody, AAC10. Serodiagn Immunother Infect Dis 4: 419–426, 1990.
21. van der Bij W, van Son WJ, van der Berg APM, Tegzess AM, Torensma R, The TH. Cytomegalovirus antigenimia: rapid diagnosis and relationship with CMV-associated clinical syndromes in renal allograft recipients. Transplant Proc 21: 2061–2064, 1989.
22. van den Berg AP, van den Bij W, van Son WJ, Anema J, van der Giessen M, Schirm J, Tegzess AM, The TH. Cytomegalovirus antigenemia as a useful marker of symptomatic cytomegalovirus infection after renal transplantation – a report of 130 consecutive patients. Transplant 48: 991–995, 1989.
23. Grundy J, Super M, Sweny P, Moorhead J, Lui SF, Berry NJ, Fernando ON, Griffiths PD. Symptomatic cytomegalovirus infection in seropositive kidney recipients: reinfection with donor virus rather than reactivation of recipient virus. Lancet ii: 132–135, 1988.
24. Speir E, Modali R, Huang ES, Leon MB, Shawl F, Finkel T, Epstein SE. Potential role of human cytomegalovirus and p53 in coronary restenosis. Science 265: 391–394, 1994.

Submitted October 17, 1994; accepted June 16, 1995

Scand J Infect Dis 27: 441–444, 1995 ORIGINAL ARTICLE

Beauty Treatments and Risk of Parenterally Transmitted Hepatitis: Results from the Hepatitis Surveillance System in Italy

ALFONSO MELE[1], ROSAMARIA CORONA[1,2], M. ELENA TOSTI[1], FILIPPO PALUMBO[3], ANGELA MOIRAGHI[4], FRANCESCA NOVACO[5], CLAUDIO GALANTI[6], ROSSANA BERNACCHIA[7] and PLACIDO FERRARO[8]

From the [1]Laboratory of Epidemiology and Biostatistics, Istituto Superiore di Sanità, Roma, Italy; [2]Epidemiology Department, Istituto Dermopatico dell'Immacolata IRCCS, Roma, Italy; [3]Regional Epidemiology Service, Regione Campania, Napoli, Italy; [4]Department of Hygiene and Community Medicine, University of Torino, Italy; [5]Regional Health Authority Office, Regione Emilia Romagna, Bologna, Italy; [6]Regional Health Authority Office, Regione Toscana, Firenze, Italy; [7]Regional Health Authority Office, Regione Marche, Ancona, Italy; [8]Regional Health Authority Office, Regione Veneto, Venezia, Italy

The role of ear-piercing, tattooing, attendance at chiropodist or manicurist and barber shop shaving in transmitting hepatitis B and hepatitis non-A, non-B was evaluated. Data reported here were collected from 1985 to 1993 by the National Viral Hepatitis Surveillance System. The association between parenterally transmitted hepatitis and the considered risk factors was estimated, comparing 6,395 hepatitis B and 2,558 hepatitis non-A, non-B cases with 4,789 hepatitis A cases, using the case–control method. Of the non-A, non-B cases tested from 1991 to 1993, 56.6% were anti-HCV positive. The incidence of parenterally transmitted hepatitis cases reporting specific beauty treatments was also evaluated. Tattooing, ear-piercing and barber shop shaving were associated with both parenterally transmitted hepatitides, while attendance at a chiropodist or manicurist was associated only with hepatitis B. During the study period the incidence of acute hepatitis B and non-A, non-B cases reporting beauty treatments declined by 49%. In spite of this decline, considering that a large part of the general population is exposed to the considered risk factors, the role of beauty treatments in transmitting hepatitis B and hepatitis non-A, non-B should not be underestimated.

A. Mele, MD, Reparto di Epidemiologia Clinica, Istituto Superiore di Sanità, Viale Regina Elena 299, I-00161 Rome, Italy

INTRODUCTION

Ear-piercing, tattooing, attendance at chiropodists or manicurists and barber shop shaving are widely used beauty treatments. During these procedures, instruments can very often become contaminated by blood from the treated subjects and hence, if not properly sterilized, can act as a route of transmission for parenterally transmitted hepatitis viruses. The Surveillance of Acute Viral Hepatitis System (SEIEVA, Sistema Epidemiologico Integrato dell'Epatite Virale Acuta) in Italy has shown as association between other percutaneous exposures, including beauty treatments, and hepatitis B and hepatitis non-A, non-B (1, 2). SEIEVA was begun in 1984 and since then 241 local health departments (LHDs), covering 41% of the Italian population, have joined the system.

The aim of this paper was to evaluate the role of specific beauty treatments in the transmission of hepatitis B and non-A, non-B and the changes over time in exposure to the risk factors considered.

MATERIALS AND METHODS

Data from the National Viral Hepatitis Surveillance System (SEIEVA) (3) were used.

The SEIEVA method is described in detail elsewhere (1). Briefly, following notification of an acute viral hepatitis case, each patient is interviewed by a public health officer or physician, using a standard questionnaire, and the results of the hepatitis marker tests are recorded. The exposure to parenteral and fecal/oral risk factors within 6 weeks and 6 months before the onset of disease is investigated. Copies of completed questionnaires are forwarded to the National Coordinating Centre at the National Institute of Health in Rome. To estimate the incidence of notified hepatitis B and non-A, non-B cases the population of each participating LHD was ascertained from the 1991 census records.

A hepatitis B case is defined as a subject with clinical and laboratory findings of acute illness with HBsAg in the absence of anti-HAV IgM or whose anti-HAV status is unknown. Hepatitis A cases are defined by the presence of anti-HAV IgM in the serum. Cases negative for HBsAg and anti-HAV IgM are defined as non-A, non-B. From 1991 data on the anti-HCV positivity were also collected.

To estimate the association between parenterally transmitted hepatitis and beauty treatments, hepatitis B, non-A, non-B and anti-HCV positive non-A, non-B cases were compared with hepatitis A cases, using the case–control method. Crude odds ratios (OR) with 95% confidence intervals (95% CI) for considered risk factors were computed. Multiple logistic regression was used for estimating adjusted odds ratios. Age, sex, education (in case of children, the father's education), place of residence, surgical interventions, dental therapy, number of sexual partners in the previous year as well as all the exposure variables considered in the crude analysis were included in the model. Blood transfused cases and intravenous drug users were excluded from the study.

To evaluate the incidence trend, we calculated rates by year for hepatitis B and hepatitis non-A, non-B cases reporting specific beauty treatments, considering as the nominator the notified cases and as denominator the population of the 69 LHDs

 ISSN 0036-5548

Table I. *Description of the study population and prevalence of risk factors considered. SEIEVA, 1985–1993*

	Hepatitis B (n = 6,395)			Hepatitis non-A, non-B (n = 2,558)			Anti-HCV + ve hepatitis non-A, non-B (n = 363)			Hepatitis A (n = 4,879)		
	n	%	Total[a]	n	%	Total[a]	n	%	Total[a]	n	%	Total[a]
Sex												
Males	4,251	66.6		1,493	58.5		229	63.4		2,971	61.0	
Females	2,133	33.4		1,059	41.5		132	36.6		1,896	39.0	
Age, years												
0–14	468	7.4		157	6.2		3	0.8		1,648	33.9	
15–24	2,181	34.4		790	31.1		98	27.1		1,458	30.0	
25–34	1,537	24.2		529	20.8		86	23.8		1,027	21.1	
≥35	2,161	34.0		1,065	41.9		175	48.3		726	14.9	
Length of education, years												
≤5	1,515	23.7		716	28.0		104	28.7		1,046	21.4	
>5, ≤13	3,477	54.4		1,323	51.7		189	52.1		2,813	57.7	
>13	1,403	21.9		519	20.3		70	19.3		1,020	20.9	
Geographic area												
North	4,800	75.1		1,802	70.4		291	80.2		2,706	55.5	
South	1,595	24.9		756	29.6		72	19.8		2,173	44.5	
No. of sexual partners in the previous year												
0–1	2,975	71.9		1,415	80.6		231	74.8		1,937	84.2	
≥2	1,161	28.1		340	19.4		78	25.2		363	15.8	
Risk factors[b]												
Tattooing	90	1.5	6,146	30	1.2	2,456	6	1.7	343	16	0.3	4,612
Ear-piercing	205	3.3	6,146	58	2.4	2,457	12	3.5	343	74	1.6	4,610
Manicure/chiropody	297	4.9	6,096	95	3.9	2,430	17	5.0	340	102	2.2	4,581
Electrolysis[c]	22	1.2	1,882	11	1.2	932	1	0.8	126	26	2.4	1,069
Barber[d]	838	23.5	3,568	272	21.1	1,282	48	23.3	206	275	16.1	1,711

[a] Discrepancies between the totals are due to missing values.
[b] Cases may have more than one risk factor.
[c] Women of age ≥15 years.
[d] Men of age ≥18 years.

participating in SEIEVA since 1986. Of the latter LHDs, 63 are located in Northern-Central Italy and 6 in the South and they cover 13.1% of the Italian population. For the specific aim of trend evaluation, hepatitis B and non-A, non-B were considered both jointly and separately.

The BMDP statistical software package, version 1990 (4), was used for statistical analysis.

RESULTS

A total of 3,124 subjects reporting intravenous drug use and/or blood transfusion in the 6 months before onset of the disease were excluded from the study. A total of 6,395 hepatitis B, 2,558 hepatitis non-A, non-B and 363 anti-HCV positive non-A, non-B cases were compared with 4,879 hepatitis A cases, to evaluate the association with each beauty treatment. The proportions of the exposed cases are reported in Table I. Of hepatitis B and hepatitis non-A, non-B cases, 22.8 and 19.0%, respectively, reported at least one of the exposures considered compared with 11% of hepatitis A cases. The proportion of exposed cases varied from 20.3% in 1986 to 27.2% in 1993 for hepatitis B, and from 16.3% in 1988 to 22.2% in 1989 for non-A, non-B hepatitis.

During the period 1991–1993, 363 out of 641 (56.6%) non-A, non-B cases tested were anti-HCV positive. Among the anti-HCV positive cases, 21.5% reported exposure to at least one beauty treatment.

Tables II and III show the crude odds ratios of the risk factors considered and the adjusted odds ratios, respectively. Ear-piercing and barber shop shaving were significantly associated with both hepatitis B and non-A, non-B, while attendance at a chiropodist or manicurist was associated only with hepatitis B. The association between tattooing and hepatitis non-A, non-B was nearly significant (OR, 2.04; 95% CI, 0.93–4.46).

When anti-HCV positive hepatitis non-A, non-B cases were considered, the magnitude of the estimated ORs for tattooing and ear-piercing, although more imprecise, was slightly higher.

Between the years 1986–1993 the incidence of both acute hepatitis B and non-A, non-B case reporting beauty treatments declined overall by 49%, from 2.05 per 100,000 per

Table II. *Crude odds ratios (OR) and 95% confidence intervals (CI) obtained by comparing parenterally transmitted hepatitis cases to hepatitis A cases. SEIEVA, 1985–1993*

	Hepatitis B		Hepatitis non-A, non-B		Anti-HCV + ve non-A, non-B hepatitis	
	OR	95% CI	OR	95% CI	OR	95% CI
Tattooing	4.27	2.50–7.28	3.55	1.93–6.53	5.11	1.99–13.2
Ear-piercing	2.12	1.62–2.77	1.48	1.05–2.10	2.22	1.20–4.13
Manicure/chiropody	2.25	1.79–2.83	1.79	1.34–2.37	2.31	1.37–3.91
Electrolysis[a]	0.47	0.27–0.84	0.48	0.24–0.98	0.32	0.04–2.39
Barber[b]	1.60	1.38–1.86	1.41	1.17–1.70	1.59	1.12–2.25

[a] Women of age ≥15 years.
[b] Men of age ≥18 years.

Table III. *Adjusted[a] odds ratios (OR) and 95% confidence intervals (CI) obtained by comparing parenterally transmitted hepatitis cases to hepatitis A cases. SEIEVA, 1985–1993*

	Hepatitis B		Hepatitis non-A, non-B		Anti-HCV + ve non-A, non-B hepatitis	
	OR	95% CI	OR	95% CI	OR	95% CI
Tattooing	2.12	1.10–4.09	2.04	0.93–4.46	2.50	0.80–7.79
Ear-piercing	2.20	1.51–3.22	1.57	0.97–2.55	2.76	1.31–5.82
Manicure/chiropody	1.30	0.99–1.70	0.81	0.57–1.16	0.99	0.53–1.84
Electrolysis[b]	0.56	0.28–1.12	0.60	0.23–1.57	N.D.	—
Barber[c]	1.61	1.35–1.92	1.27	1.02–1.58	1.32	0.89–1.96

[a] Adjusted for age, sex, education level, geographic area, surgical interventions, dental therapy, sexual exposure and the other listed variables.
[b] Women of age ≥15 years.
[c] Men of age ≥18 years.

Table IV. *Incidence (rates × 100,000) of hepatitis B and non-A, non-B cases associated with bequty treatments[a] in 69 local health districts participating in the SEIEVA since 1986[b]*

	Hepatitis B	non-A, non-B	Total
1986	118 (1.61)	32 (0.44)	150 (2.05)
1987	140 (1.91)	38 (0.52)	178 (2.43)
1988	86 (1.17)	21 (0.29)	107 (1.46)
1989	71 (0.97)	37 (0.50)	108 (1.47)
1990	67 (0.91)	24 (0.33)	91 (1.24)
1991	66 (0.90)	26 (0.35)	92 (1.25)
1992	58 (0.79)	26 (0.35)	84 (1.14)
1993	67 (0.91)	10 (0.14)	77 (1.05)

[a] Tattooing, ear-piercing, manicure/chiropody, electrolysis, barber shop shaving.
[b] The total population of the 69 LHD is 7,340,639 people (13.1% of the Italian population).

year to 1.05 per 100,000 per year (Table IV). The decline was most noticeable in the 15–24 years age group (from 7.13 to 2.85 per 100,000 per year).

During the same period the incidence of hepatitis A cases associated with beauty treatments varied from 0.23 per 100,000 in 1989 to 0.91 per 100,000 in 1993.

DISCUSSION

Hepatitis B and hepatitis non-A, non-B are a significant public health problem in Italy because both infections produce thousands of deaths from liver cirrhosis and/or hepatocellular carcinoma (5). The identification of specific risk factors and prevention measures are the main purposes of the SEIEVA.

The present study shows that tattooing, ear-piercing, attendance at a chiropodist's or manicurist's and shaving at barber shops are independent risk factors for parenterally transmitted hepatitis. Their role in transmitting hepatitis B and non-A, non-B is not negligible. Although the precise number is not known, it may be expected that a large proportion of the general population will be exposed to these risk factors.

Fortunately, as already stated (6, 7), there is a decreasing trend in the incidence of hepatitis B and non-A, non-B in Italy and, as reported in the present paper, there is also a decreasing incidence of both hepatitis B and non-A, non-B cases reporting exposure to beauty treatments. The overall incidence of acute hepatitis cases notified during the study period was 30 per 100,000 in 1985 vs. 12 per 100,000 in 1993. The ongoing campaign against AIDS has probably played a role in decreasing the incidence of parenterally transmitted hepatitis attributable to beauty treatments. Nevertheless, beauty treatments are still risk factors for hepatitis B and non-A, non-B, and the importance of enforcing effective sterilization of instruments, coupled with recommendations for an increased use of disposable materials is emphasized.

The potential biases of the present study must be considered. Hepatitis A cases were used as controls. Hepatitis A virus has different modes of transmission from hepatitis B and parenterally transmitted hepatitis non-A, non-B. However, since the abovementioned viruses occasionally share the same risk factors such as blood transfusion and intravenous drug use, an underestimate of the odds ratios may occur (8). On the other hand, all the hepatitis cases considered were notified cases, identified through the same surveillance system and were therefore exposed to similar selective factors, if any. As far as the validity of the study is concerned, comparability is a very important issue in case–control design. In addition, after excluding blood-transfused and intravenous drug-using patients, in our logistic regression model we took into account potential cofounders such as age, sex, education, geographical area, and other variables associated with parenterally transmitted hepatitis (surgical interventions, dental therapy and sexual exposure).

Finally, although patients who acknowledged the use of intravenous drugs were not included in the analysis, we cannot rule out that some hepatitis B and non-A, non-B cases untruthfully denied the use of intravenous drugs. If this occurred, it could lead to an overestimate of the risk associated with tattooing and ear-piercing which may be linked to certain lifestyles. On the other hand, an association between the use of intravenous drugs and our reference group, hepatitis A, also exists (9) and we have no reason to hypothesize a differential reporting bias.

Regarding our estimate of trends over time in the incidence of hepatitis B and non-A, non-B, the notification system was not modified throughout the period considered.

ACKNOWLEDGMENTS

The authors thank Monica Fucci for help in editing the manuscript.

This study was partially supported by the Assessorato alla Sanità della Regione Campania, Naples, Italy.

REFERENCES

1. Mele A, Stazi MA, Gill ON, Pasquini P, SEIEVA Collaborating Group. Prevention of hepatitis B in Italy: lessons from surveillance of type-specific acute viral hepatitis. Epidemiol Infect 104: 135–141, 1990.
2. Mele A. Epidemiologia delle epatiti virali in Italia. Atti del Convegno: La Regione Marche nel Controllo delle Malattie Infettive: Epatiti Virali e Morbillo, Ancona 5 giugno 1992. [in Italian]
3. Mele A, Stazi MA, Corona R, Ferrigno L, Sagliocca L, Palumbo F, Falasca P, Galanti C, Moiraghi A, Rosmini F, Gill ON, Pasquini P, SEIEVA Collaborating Group. Decline of incidence of A, B and nonA-nonB hepatitis in Italy. Results of four years surveillance (1985–88). Ital J Gastroenterol 22: 274–280, 1990.
4. BMDP Statistical Software Manual. Berkeley, California: University of California Press, 1990.
5. Stroffolini T. The descriptive epidemiology of primary liver cancer in Italy. Ital J Gastroenterol 23: 443–447, 1991.
6. D'Amelio R, Matricardi PM, Biselli R, Stroffolini T, Mele A, Spada E, Chionne P, Rapicetta M, Ferrigno L, Pasquini P. Changing epidemiology of hepatitis B in Italy: public health implications. Am J Epidemiol 135: 1012–1018, 1992.
7. Mele A, Ferrigno L, Marzolini A, Catapano R, Cialdea L, Pasquini P. SEIEVA Sistema epidemiologico integrato dell'epatite virale acuta. Rapporto annuale 1992. ISTISAN 94/12. [in Italian]
8. Mannucci PM, Gdovin S, Gringeri A, Colombo M, Mele A, Schinaia N, Ciavarella N, Emerson SU, Purcell RH, Italian Collaborating Group. Transmission of hepatitis A to patients with hemophilia by factor VIII concentrates treated with organic solvent and detergent to inactivate viruses. Ann Intern Med 120: 1–7, 1994.
9. Sagliocca L, Mele A, Ferrigno L, Palumbo F, Converti F, Tosti ME, Amoroso P, Manzillo G. Case control study of risk factors for hepatitis A: Naples 1990–1991. Ital J Gastroenterol 27: 181–184, 1995.

Submitted March 6, 1995; accepted July 18, 1995

Scand J Infect Dis 27: 445–448, 1995 ORIGINAL ARTICLE

The Seroprevalence of Hepatitis B and C in Hospitalized Danish Patients

SUZANNE NELSING[1], PER WANTZIN[2], JENS SKØT[1], ELIZABETH KRARUP[1], THYGE L. NIELSEN[1], HENRIK B. KRARUP[3] and JENS O. NIELSEN[1]

From the Departments of [1]Infectious Diseases and [2]Clinical Immunology, Hvidovre University Hospital, Copenhagen, Denmark, and [3]Biochemistry, Aalborg Hospital, Denmark

Health care workers are at risk of acquiring blood-borne infections. To assess the risk of exposure to hepatitis B or C in the case of occupational blood exposure, we determined the seroprevalence of these infections in 466 patients admitted to a Copenhagen university hospital. Serological markers for hepatitis B or C were detected in 56 patients (12.0%). The seroprevalence of HBsAg and anti-HCV was 0.9% and 1.5% respectively. HCV RNA, indicating ongoing hepatitis C, was found in five of seven anti-HCV-positive patients by polymerase chain reaction. The serological findings had not previously been diagnosed in 4 of 10 potentially infectious patients and only 6 of 10 patients belonged to high-risk groups. In conclusion, health care workers should be aware of the potential the occupational risk of hepatitis B and C even in a low-prevalence country like Denmark. Management of health care workers after blood exposure should include serological testing for both hepatitis B and C. Strict adherence to universal precautions is recommended and vaccination against hepatitis B should be encouraged.

S. Nelsing, MD, Department of Infectious Diseases, Hvidovre Hospital, Kettegaard allé 30, DK-2650 Hvidovre, Denmark

INTRODUCTION

Hepatitis B and C are among the most serious occupationally acquired infections. To ensure appropriate counselling, serological testing and prophylactic vaccination of health care workers who experience exposure to blood, it is important to know the prevalence of these infections in the patient population.

The hepatitis C virus was discovered only a few years ago (1). Since then, the prevalence of hepatitis C in Denmark has been determined in voluntary blood donors (P. Wantzin, unpublished data) and in various high risk groups such as patients undergoing dialysis (2), multi-transfused patients (3) and intravenous drug users (IVDUs) (4), but not in a general patient population. Previous 20-year-old studies have determined the prevalence of hepatitis B in hospitalized patients in Copenhagen (5, 6). However, since the laboratory techniques for detection of serological markers are more sensitive today and the incidence of hepatitis B has declined during the last decades (7), new data are required.

In this study, we determined the seroprevalence of hepatitis B and C in 466 patients admitted to a Copenhagen university hospital.

MATERIAL AND METHODS

Study design

The study was performed from March to April 1994 in Hvidovre hospital, a 1000-bed inner-city university hospital in Copenhagen, Denmark. The point prevalence of serological markers for hepatitis B virus (HBV) and hepatitis C virus (HCV) was determined in a cross-sectional design. One or 2 wards were surveyed a day. Participation was not anonymous, hence no double-testing of patients, due for example to transfer to other wards occurred.

The wards for infectious medicine, rheumatology, endocrinology, cardiology, neurology, nephrology, medical gastroenterology, orthopaedics, plastic surgery, surgical gastroenterology, urology, neurosurgery, ophthalmology, gynaecology and obstetrics were surveyed. During 1994, 23 905 patients were admitted at least once to these wards. Emergency care, day-care units and outpatient clinics including the dialysis unit were not surveyed.

The inclusion criterias were age 18 years or above, and informed written consent. The exclusion criterias were confusion, dementia or psychosis, or a reduced level of consciousness, and critical psychological or physical conditions, e.g. terminal illness or severe emotional distress.

HBsAg-positive and anti-HCV-positive patients were interviewed and their medical records were reviewed to establish the possible source of the infection, if a medical history of the infection or hepatitis serology was present in the medical record and if the patient belonged to a high-risk group.

Patients

A total of 578 out of 696 patients were eligible, of whom 466 (81%) participated. Informed consent was not given by 75 patients, phlebotomy was not obtained in 5 patients and 32 patients were not present in the ward at inclusion or at the time of the phlebotomy. Of the 118 excluded patients, 106 were excluded due to their psychological or physical condition, 4 patients were below 18 years of age and 8 patients were unable to give informed written consent due to language barriers.

Serology

A 10-ml venous blood sample was taken from each patient. After centrifugation a serum aliquot was frozen immediately at 20°C for later HCV RNA testing by polymerase chain reaction (PCR). The remaining serum was tested for anti-HBc (Ortho™ HBc ELISA Test System, Chiron). Positive samples were tested for HBsAg (Ortho™ HBsAg ELISA Test System 3) and anti-HBs (IMx HBe Reagent Pack No. 2227-20, Abbott). HBsAg-positive samples were tested for HBeAg (IMx AUSAB Reagent Pack No. 2262-20, Abbott). Serum was also tested for anti-HCV with a third-generation test (Ortho HCV ELISA Test System). Anti-HCV-positive samples were tested further by a third generation recombinant immunoblot assay (RIBA) (Chiron RIBA HCV Test System) and for HCV RNA by PCR.

Seropositive samples were retested and considered positive if the result was confirmed in the second test.

HCV virology

All samples that were anti-HCV-positive in ELISA were tested for HCV RNA twice by single PCR. The following synthetic oligonucleotides, selected from the 5′-non-coding region of the virus were used: primer A (sense) 5′GTGAGGAACTACTGTCTTCA (nucleotide position 30–49); primer B (antisense) 5′GGCTGCACGACACTCATACT (nucleotide position 95–76), and for detection probe (sense) 5′-biotine-CGCAGAAAGCGTCTAGCCAT (nucleotide position 50–69). For the internal amplification standard, 5′GTGAGGAACTACTGTCTTCATATGACCCATACTCGATTGCAATACCAGTATGAGTGTCGTGCAGCC, was used, and the internal amplification standard probe was 5′-biotin-CCATAACGTTAGCTCATACC. HCV RNA was isolated from 100 μl of serum by a standard procedure (8).

Amplification was performed for 45 cycles at 92°C for 30 s for denaturing, and at 58°C for 60 s for annealing and primer extension. After the final cycle elongation was continued for 5 min. PCR products were hybridized to a biotin-labelled probe and then captured to an avidin-coated microtitre plate. The amount of captured PCR product was detected by a sensitive fluoroimmunoassay. An internal amplification standard was used to assure that amplification had taken place.

Statistical analysis

Results are expressed as prevalences in per cent, with 95% binomial confidence intervals (95% CI).

RESULTS

The prevalence of anti-HBc- and anti-HCV in the participating patients, according to sex, age, country of birth and ward, is shown in Table I. The distribution of sex in non-participants (non-eligible plus non-participating eligible patients, $n = 230$) was the same as that in the participating patients (percentage of women 65.2% vs. 62.2%). The median age among non-participants was 74 years (range 1–105) compared to 65 years (range 18–96) among participants. The percentage of patients born in countries with a high prevalence for HBV was higher among non-participants than among participants (7.8% vs. 5.6%).

Serological markers for hepatitis B or C were present in 56 of 466 patients (12.0%; 95% CI, 9.2–15.3). Anti-HBc was found in 55 patients (11.8%; 95% CI, 9.0–15.1) of whom 44 were anti-HBs-positive. HBsAg was found in 4 patients (0.85%; 95% CI, 0.23–2.18). One of these patients was also positive for HBeAg and another was anti-HCV-positive and HBsAg-positive. Seven patients were anti-HCV-positive (1.5%; 95% CI, 0.6–3.1). HCV RNA indicating ongoing hepatitis was detected by PCR in 5/7 anti-HCV positive patients. Two other patients were anti-HCV positive in ELISA, but anti-HCV-negative in RIBA and HCV RNA-negative. Thus a total of 10 patients (2.1%) were potentially infectious due to HBV or HCV.

These patients are described further in Table II. Hepatitis B or C had not been diagnosed prior to the study in four of these patients and only 6 belonged to high-risk groups. Patient no. 6 had probably acquired hepatitis C from a blood transfusion in 1972. Patient no. 10 had a serum aspartate-amino-transferase (ASAT) value of 158 U/l (normal range 10–40 U/l) and a liver biopsy showing chronic active hepatitis, but despite repeated hepatitis serology including HCV RNA analysis by PCR, no aetiology for her hepatitis was disclosed. She had an IVDU sexual partner but denied belonging to any high-risk group herself.

Table I. *Prevalence of anti-HBc and anti-HCV according to sex, age, country of birth and ward in hospitalized Danish patients. (Percentages are shown in parentheses)*

	n	Anti-HBc-positive	Anti-HCV-positive
Total	466	55 (11.8)	7 (1.5)
Sex			
Male	176	19 (10.8)	2 (1.1)
Female	290	36 (12.4)	5 (1.7)
Age, years			
18–40	113	12 (10.6)	4 (3.5)
41–60	98	6 (6.1)	1 (1.0)
61–80	182	32 (17.6)	2 (1.1)
>80	73	5 (6.8)	0 (0.0)
Country of birth			
Denmark	422	43 (10.2)	6 (1.4)
Other countries with low HBsAg prevalence[a]	18	5 (27.8)	0 (0.0)
Countries with intermediate/high HBsAg prevalence[b]	26	7 (26.9)	1 (3.8)
Ward			
Medical	193	24 (12.4)	2 (1.0)
Surgical	194	26 (13.4)	4 (2.1)
Obstetrics and gynaecology	79	5 (6.3)	1 (1.3)

[a] Northern, Central and Western Europe, and North America.

[b] Greenland, Mediterranean countries, Eastern Europe, former USSR, South America, Middle East, South-west Asia and North-east Africa.

Table II. *Characteristics of HBsAg-positive and anti-HCV-positive Danish hospitalized patients*

Patient	Sex	Age, years	Country of birth	Ward	Anti-HBc	HBsAg	Anti-HCV	HCV-RNA	High-risk group	Status[a]
1	M	58	Denmark	Infectious diseases	+	+	−	NA[b]	HIV-positive homosexual	Known
2	M	36	Yemen	Infectious diseases	+	+	−	NA	HIV-positive homosexual	Known
3	F	49	Austria	Nephrology	+	+[c]	−	NA	None	Known
4	M	35	Iran	Orthopaedic surgery	+	+	+	+	IVDU	Unknown[d]
5	F	74	Denmark	Orthopaedic surgery	+	−	+	+	None	Unknown
6	F	74	Denmark	Orthopaedic surgery	−	NA	+	+	None	Known
7	F	30	Denmark	Maternity	+	−	+	+	IVDU	Unknown
8	M	41	Denmark	Plastic surgery	+	−	+	+	IVDU	Unknown
9	F	30	Denmark	Infectious diseases	+	−	+	−	HIV-positive, IVDU	Known
10	F	40	Denmark	Infectious diseases	+	−	+	−	None	Known

[a] Status was considered known if hepatitis serology or a medical history of hepatitis was present in the medical record.
[b] NA, not analysed.
[c] Both HBsAg and HBeAg were detected.
[d] Hepatitis B status known; hepatitis C status unknown.
IVDU, intravenous drug use.

DISCUSSION

Denmark is considered to be an area of low prevalence for hepatitis B and C. The estimated prevalence of HBsAg in the general population is 0.25% (9). Nevertheless, previous studies have shown a significantly increased prevalence of HBV-markers among Danish surgeons (10) and dentists (11) compared to that in the general population. Despite the declining incidence of hepatitis B over the last decade (7), we found a HBsAg-prevalence of 0.9%. Considering that the estimated risk of infection following percutaneous exposure to HBsAg-positive blood is 6% (12), hepatitis B still seems to constitute an occupational risk in Denmark for health care workers. Serological tests should be performed in health care workers after blood exposures, and hepatitis B vaccination should be encouraged.

The HBc antibodies were most frequent among patients aged 61–80 years and in patients born in countries where hepatitis B is highly endemic. Since a relatively larger proportion of non-participants compared to participants belonged to these groups, our figures are probably a slight underestimation.

We found a relatively high prevalence of anti-HCV- and HCV RNA-positive hospitalized patients. In comparison, only 0.08% of voluntary blood donors in the Copenhagen area are anti-HCV-positive (P. Wantzin, unpublished data). HCV infection has been reported following percutaneous as well as mucocutaneous blood exposures (13–15). Japanese estimations of the risk for an infection after percutaneous exposure to HCV RNA-positive blood range from 1.4 to 10% (13, 14). Scandinavian studies (16, 17) and other European studies (18, 19) have found an increased, though not significantly higher, anti-HCV prevalence in health care workers compared to that found in blood donors, while studies among New York dentists (20) and health care workers in Japan (21) found a significantly increased prevalence of anti-HCV compared to that in age-matched blood donors.

Our results indicate, that hepatitis C should not be overlooked as an occupational risk even in this low-prevalence area and that serological tests for HCV markers should be included in the management of health care workers who are exposed to blood. Only 6 out of 10 potentially infectious patients belonged to a known high-risk groups like IVDUs, where 98% are anti-HCV-positive (4), or HIV-positive homosexuals (22). The risk of sexually transmitted hepatitis C is very low (23), and other risk factors could be suspected in patient no. 10. The fact that several patients with potentially infectious hepatitis did not belong to any known high-risk group or did not have a prior diagnosis of the infection, underlines the importance of strict adherence to the principle of universal precautions.

In conclusion health care workers should be aware of the occupational risk of hepatitis B and C even in a low-prevalence country like Denmark. Management of health care workers after blood exposures should include serological testing for both hepatitis B and C and vaccination against hepatitis B should be encouraged.

REFERENCES

1. Choo Q, Kuo G, Weiner AJ, Overby LR, Bradley DW, Houghton M. Isolation of a cDNA clone derived from a blood-borne non-A, non-B viral hepatitis genome. Science 244: 359–362, 1989.
2. Bukh J, Wantzin P, Krogsgaard K, Knudsen F, Purcell RH, Miller RH and the Copenhagen Dialysis HCV Study Group. High prevalence of hepatitis C (HCV)RNA in dialysis patients: failure of commercially available antibody tests to identify a significant number of patients with HCV infections. J Infect Dis 168: 1343–1348, 1993.
3. Lund BV, Korsgaard N, Peterslund NA. Hepatitis C antistof hos multitransfunderede hæmatologiske patienter. Ugeskr Læger 153: 3084–3086, 1991.
4. Westh H, Worm AM, Jensen BL, Kroon S, Kvinesdal B, Nielsen CM, Wantzin P. Hepatitis C virus antibodies in homosexual men and intravenous drug users in Denmark. Infection 21: 115–117, 1993.
5. Lous P, Skinhøj P, Olesen H. Hepatitis-associated (AU/SH) antigen determination in 10,000 patients in a Copenhagen general hospital. Lancet, 119–121, 1970.
6. Skinhøj P. Epidemiology of hepatitis B antigen and antibody in hospital patients in Copenhagen. Scand J Infect Dis 7: 85–89, 1975.
7. Statens Seruminstitut, Copenhagen, Denmark. Epidemiologisk afdeling. EPI-NYT uge 50, 1994.
8. Chomczynski P, Sacchi N. Single-step method of RNA isolation by acid guanidinium thiocyanate-phenol-chloroform extraction. Analyt Biochem 162: 156–159, 1987.
9. Statens Seruminstitut, Copenhagen, Denmark. Epidemiologisk afdeling. EPI-NYT uge 37, 1991.
10. Hardt F, Aldershvile J, Dietrichson O, Juhl E, Nielsen JO, Schlichting P, Skinhøj P, Tage-Jensen U. Hepatitis B virus infections among Danish surgeons. J Infect Dis 140: 972–974, 1979.
11. Scheutz F, Melbye M, Esteban JI, Aldershvile J, Ebbesen P, Alter HJ. Hepatitis B virus infection in Danish dentists. A case-control and follow-up study. Am J Epidemiol 128: 190–196, 1988.
12. Centers for Disease Control MMWR. Atlanta, Georgia: Centers for Disease Control, 313–324, 329–335, 1985.
13. Sodeyama T, Kiyosawa K, Urushihara A, Matsumoto A, Tanaka E, Furuta S, Mizokami M, Akahane Y. Transmission of hepatitis C virus through needlestick accidents in health care workers. In: Viral hepatitis and liver disease. Tokyo: Springer-Verlag, 459–462, 1994.
14. Mitsui T, Iwano K, Masuko K, Yamazaki C, Okamoto H, Tsuda F, Tanaka T, Mishiro S. Hepatitis C virus infection in medical personnel after needlestick accident. Hepatology 16: 1109–1114, 1992.
15. Sartori M, La Terra G, Aglietta M, Manzin A, Navino C, Verzetti G. Transmission of hepatitis C via blood splash into conjunctiva. Scand J Infect Dis 25: 270–271, 1993.
16. Norrgren H, Flodman-Norrlund IG, Lindholm T, Hansson BG, Nordenfelt E. Prevalence of antibodies against hepatitis B and C viruses among different groups of medical staff. Scand J Infect Dis 24: 553–554, 1992.
17. Struve J, Aronsson B, Frenning B, Forsgren M, Weiland O. Prevalence of antibodies against hepatitis C virus infection among health care workers in Stockholm. Scand J Gastroenterol 29: 360–362, 1994.
18. Thomas DL, Factor SH, Kelen GD, Washington AS, Taylor E, Quinn TC. Viral hepatitis in health care personnel at the Johns Hopkins Hospital. Arch Intern Med 153: 1705–1712, 1993.
19. Campello C, Majori S, Poli A, Pacini P, Nicolardi L, Pini F. Prevalence of HCV antibodies in health-care workers from northern Italy. Infection 20: 224–226, 1992.
20. Klein RS, Freeman K, Taylor PE, Stevens CE. Occupational risk for hepatitis C virus infection among New York dentists. Lancet 338: 1539–1542, 1991.
21. Kiyosawa K, Sodeyama T, Tanaka E, Furuta S. Hepatitis C infection in health care workers. Viral hepatitis and liver disease. Tokyo: Springer-Verlag, 479–482, 1994.
22. Hofmann B, Kryger P, Pedersen NS, Nielsen JO, Oehlenschlager J, Koerner EA, Van Den Berg T, Sprechler HH, Nielsen CM, Gerstoft J, Ryder LP, Faber V, Svejgaard A. Sexually transmitted diseases, antibodies to Human Immunodeficiency Virus, and subsequent development of Acquired Immunodeficiency Syndrome. Sex Transm Dis 15: 1–4, 1988.
23. Alter HJ. Transmission patterns in hepatitis C virus infection. Viral hepatitis and liver disease. Tokyo, Springer-Verlag, 445–449, 1994.

Submitted February 24, 1995; accepted May 22, 1995

Scand J Infect Dis 27: 449–452, 1995 ORIGINAL ARTICLE

Transmission of Hepatitis C Virus by Transfusion in Örebro County, Sweden, 1990–1992

RUT NORDA[1,3], ANN-SOFIE DUBERG[2], ANDERS SÖNNERBORG[4], and PER OLCÉN[3]

From the Departments of [1]Transfusion Medicine and Immunohemotherapy, [2]Infectious Diseases and [3]Clinical Microbiology and Immunology, Örebro Medical Center Hospital, Örebro, and [4]Division of Clinical Virology, Karolinska Institutet, Huddinge University Hospital, Huddinge, Sweden

A retrospective study of hepatitis C virus (HCV) transmission by transfusion was conducted in Örebro county. Out of the 7 900 active, registered blood donors, 21 repeatedly anti-HCV reactive (RIBA 2 positive or indeterminate) donors were diagnosed. Their 84 recipients from January 1990 through June 1992 were identified and 41 (49%) were alive in December 1992. A total of 13 anti-HCV reactive (RIBA 2 positive or indeterminate) were diagnosed in 39 investigated recipients. Of these 11 were previously undiagnosed, and seven were HCV RNA-positive. In the donor population 1.03% were anti-HCV-positive by ELISA, but only 0.09% were RIBA and HCV RNA-positive. In 1990, 0.06% of the blood components came from the HCV RNA-positive donors, and none during the first 6 months of 1992. In order to identify transfusion-transmitted HCV infections that took place before the introduction of tests for anti-HCV antibodies, patients with a history of transfusion and symptoms and signs of liver dysfunction or damage should be thoroughly tested.

R. Norda, MD, Department of Transfusion Medicine and Immunohemotherapy, Örebro Medical Centre Hospital, S-701 85 Örebro, Sweden

INTRODUCTION

Blood donation in Sweden is voluntary and non-commercial. Prior to registration as a donor, the applicant's general health and possible exposure to hepatitis viruses, HIV, HTLV or blood-borne parasites by way of life or risk behaviour is assessed during an individual interview. Laboratory investigation includes "surrogate markers" (ALAT and anti-HBc) as well as specific antigens and antibodies besides hematology parameters. Prior to any blood or plasma donation from an accepted donor recent exposure to blood-borne infection is again assessed. Before tests for hepatitis C virus (HCV) became available any blood donor involved in post-transfusion hepatitis (PHT) non-A, non-B investigations, involving less than 12 donors, was dismissed from further blood donation. Assays for the demonstration of hepatitis C virus antibodies (anti-HCV) have offered the possibility of preventing PTH C as effectively as PTH B. According to the recommendations of the Swedish Board of Health (1), screening for anti-HCV was to be implemented in the transfusion services during 1991 and mandatory on all units of blood and plasma by 1 January 1992. Prior to the publication of the recommendations, it was discussed whether the donors or the donated blood and plasma units should be tested and what the cost-benefit would be (2).

In Örebro County, few cases of PTH non-A, non-B have been reported via the Infectious Diseases Surveillance system to the Local Board of Health (3). It was decided to perform a retrospective survey of transfusion-transmitted HCV infections in Örebro County in order to determine the number of transmitted cases of HCV infection, and to identify patients in need of referral for medical follow-up and/or treatment.

MATERIAL AND METHODS

In Örebro County (275 000 inhabitants) approximately 7 900 registered donors are active and about 16 000 units of blood are collected annually. Screening for anti-HCV was introduced on the 27 August 1991. Previously registered donors with a repeated positive reaction for anti-HCV by ELISA (Ortho HCV ELISA 2.0) and positive or indeterminate reaction in recombinant immunoblot assay (RIBA 2, Ortho) during the period 27 August 1991 to 30 June 1992 were defined as the index donors.

Patients transfused with erythrocytes, plasma or platelets from the index donors from 1 January 1990 until the positive anti-HCV (ELISA) test were the study group of recipients. In December 1992 those recipients, who were alive, were contacted and asked to supply a blood sample for analysis of liver enzymes and anti-HCV. Sera with repeatedly positive anti-HCV results were further investigated with RIBA and polymerase chain reaction (PCR) for HCV RNA. Serum samples, stored at $-20°C$ were assayed with a nested PCR using primers for the 5′non-coding region, as described earlier (4). Product detection was performed by agarose gel electrophoresis. HCV RNA analysis of the index donors was performed on the first anti-HCV positive serum sample.

Permission to collect information regarding the transfusion history and concomitant therapy from the recipients, medical records was requested from the Chief Medical Officers of the appropriate departments. Consent from the Ethical Committee of Örebro County Council was obtained before the start of the study.

RESULTS

Identified anti-HCV positive indexdonors

In 1990 there were 7886 registered active blood donors, in 1991 there were 7847, and in 1992, 8272. In 1990 19

 ISSN 0036-5548

Table I. *RIBA and HCV RNA reactivity in the recipients (R) as correlated with the RIBA reactivity and HCV RNA pattern in the RIBA-positive index donors (D)*

Index donor	RIBA pattern	HCV RNA	Investigated recipient	RIBA pattern	HCV RNA	ALAT (<0.70 μkat/l)	At transfusion	
							Age, years	Diagnosis
D1	C22, C33	pos	R1	C22	neg	0.19	68	Laparotomy (abscess)
			R2	pos	pos	0.80–0.62	39	Hip arthroplasty
			R3	C22	neg	1.08–0.32	48	Systemic vasculitis
D2	C22, C33	pos	R4	C22	pos	1.35–0.40	33	Systemic lupus erythematosus
			R5	pos	pos	1.34–0.21	83	Femoral fracture
D3	C22, C33	pos	R6	pos	neg	1.54–0.22	19	Inflammatory bowel disease Reconstructive surgery
D4	C22, C33, C100, 5-1-1	pos	R7	C22	pos	0.40	72	Ca colli uteri
D5	C22, C33	pos	R8	C22	pos	0.84	67	Ca ovarii
D6	C22, C33	pos	R9	C22	neg	0.27	74	Coronary by-pass Aortic valvuloplasty
			R10	pos	neg[a]	0.26	45	Acute myelogenous leukemia
D7	C22, C33 C100, 5-1-1	pos	[b]					
D8	C100, 5-1-1	neg	[c]					

[a] While on alpha-interferon therapy.
[b] All recipients deceased.
[c] Recipient not investigated.

(0.24%) index donors were active. In 1991, these 19 donors and 2 new index donors, registered in February 1991, were active (0.27%). In 1992, only 1 of these donors (0.01%) was active, but was excluded at the second donation. In 1990 23 331 blood components were transfused in Örebro County of which 48 (0.21%) came from the index donors. Of these 48 blood components, 13 came from the RIBA- and HCV RNA-positive donors. In 1991, 24 159 components were transfused, of which 42 (0.17%) came from indexdonors. Of these 42, 15 came from the RIBA and HCV RNA-positive donors. In 1992 2 components came from 1 index donor and comprised 0.008% of the 24 802 transfused components. This donor was anti-HCV-positive by ELISA, RIBA-indeterminate (C33 pos) in the first HCV-test and anti-HCV-negative by ELISA in the second screening. The second blood unit was processed into components and transfused.

Eight of 21 index donors were RIBA-positive, of whom seven were HCV RNA-positive (Fig. 1). All had antibodies against the C22 and C33 antigens in the RIBA test. The HCV RNA-negative donor showed antibodies againts the 5-1-1 and C100 antigens only (Table I). Of the index donors 13 were indeterminate in RIBA, and they were all HCV RNA-negative by PCR (Fig. 1).

Characterization of the recipients

The 21 index donors had donated 58 units of whole blood from which 92 components were produced and transfused to 84 recipients, 47 men and 37 women. A total of 41 recipients were alive in December 1992, and 39 of them supplied blood samples for the study. The mean age of the deceased was 57.3 years and for the living 57.1 years. On an average, 25.9 months passed from the transfusion to the time of anti-HCV testing of the recipient, with a range of 8–36 months. Follow-up information was available for 34 of the 41 living recipients. A total of 19 patients were transfused in connection with surgical procedures, 13 during therapeutic plasma exchange, and 2 due to severe anemia or thrombocytopenia. Of the recipients 10 received <4 components, 13 received 5–12 components and 11 >12 during the studied time, and 11 of the recipients had more than 1 series of transfusions.

Determination of anti-HCV and HCV RNA in the recipients

Of the 39 tested recipients, 13 were anti-HCV positive by ELISA. Four recipients were RIBA-positive and had received components from RIBA and HCV RNA-index donors. Two were HCV RNA-positive (Fig. 1). Nine recipients exhibited an indeterminate RIBA pattern, all with antibodies against the C22 antigen only (Table I). Seven had received components from the RIBA and HCV RNA-positive index donors. Four of these 7 were HCV RNA-positive. Two recipients of blood components obtained from ELISA-positive, RIBA-indeterminate (C22-positive) and HCV RNA-negative donors were positive in ELISA and C22 reactive in RIBA (Fig. 1). One of them was HCV RNA-positive. This patient had received 278 blood components of which half came from other transfusion centers. Two seronegative recipients had been iden-

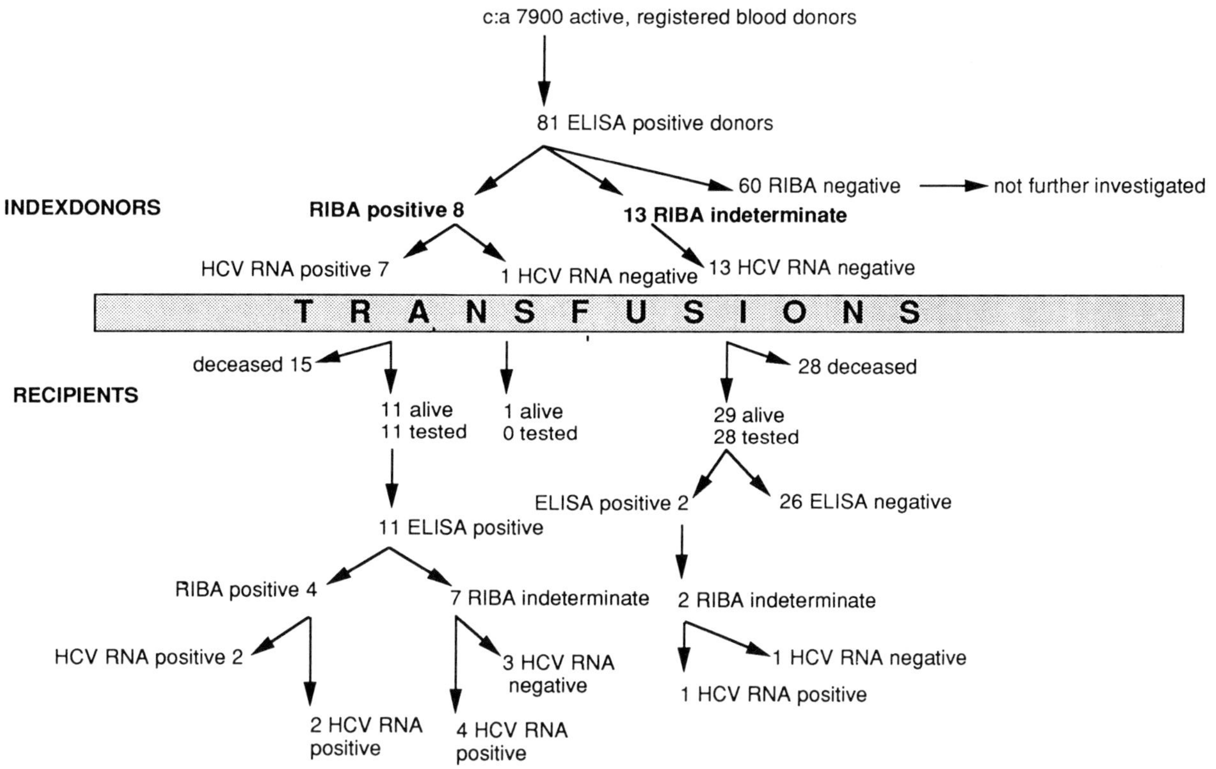

Fig. 1. Anti-HCV and HCV RNA results for the active, registered donors, index donors (RIBA 2-positive or indeterminate) and their recipients.

tified from this same index donor. The other recipient was HCV RNA-negative and the sole living recipient from this particular index donor. The patient had received transfusions in 1978 and 1983, but no blood samples from these periods were available for testing.

Outcome of the present study

A total of 13 patients with serological signs of past or present HCV infection were found. Most probably these were all cases of PTH C. In 2 of them the diagnosis of PTH C had been made prior to the present study. The two patients who required regular clinical and laboratory follow-up due to their chronic disease and cytotoxic drug treatment had been identified due to increased liver enzyme concentrations and by subsequent anti-HCV testing. Two other recipients were not investigated with respect to HCV serology when increased liver enzyme concentrations were found. Thus, 11 new cases of transfusion-transmitted HCV infections were discovered during the present study. Recipients who were RIBA- or HCV RNA-positive were offered referral to a specialist in infectious diseases.

DISCUSSION

The present study shows that approximately 1 in 1100 registered donors (0.09%) probably was contagious concerning HCV when screening was introduced. In 1990 and 1991, 0.06% of the transfused components came from these donors and were probably contagious for HCV. The previously shown correlation between RIBA 2-positivity and HCV RNA positivity was confirmed (5, 6). The RIBA-positive but HCV RNA-negative donor had no antibodies to C22 or C33. This antibody pattern has been claimed to be associated with lower infectivity (7, 8). Donors with indeterminate RIBA 2 were HCV RNA-negative and probably not infectious. Two recipients from these donors, however, showed serological evidence of HCV-infection. In 1 case probably a component other than the index donors' was infectious, since 2 other seronegative recipients were found. In the other recipient an infection with the index component cannot be excluded, but HCV-transmission by previous transfusions is also possible. Transmission of HCV from a C22-positive, RIBA-2 indeterminate donor has been reported, but this donor was HCV RNA-positive (9).

The real number of transfusion transmitted HCV infections is most probably 26, including all recipients to the 7 HCV RNA-positive donors. This would correspond to 16 cases per year in Örebro County (275 000 inhabitants) before the introduction of the screening of anti-HCV, a figure that agrees well with the calculations made by Bäck in 1991 (2). All but 1 index donor, who was RIBA-indeterminate and HCV RNA-negative, were identified at the first donation after screening was introduced. In Örebro County one registered donor converted during 12 months 1993/94, a conversion of 0.012% of the donor population. Retrospective investigation of the recipients from this donor did not reveal HCV transmission.

Altogether 13 cases of transfusion transmitted HCV infections were found. Six of the 13 (45%) HCV-infected recipients were HCV RNA-negative upon follow-up, one during alpha-interferon treatment. They were transfused in 1990 with products from three donors. This may represent resolved infection although intermittent viremia cannot be excluded. All recipients from 1991 were still HCV RNA-positive. For the 7 younger HCV-infected recipients (< 50 years of age at the transfusion) the risk for development of significant HCV-related liver disease during the expected lifetime has to be considered. Five of them have underlying diseases and potential hepatotoxic treatment and alpha-interferon therapy is therefore less easily undertaken, if and when indicated. Thus, so far only two recipients are potential candidates for anti-viral therapy. A 75% rate of chronic infection has been reported in another study (10). The follow-up time in the latter study was up to 17 years, and it may be difficult to control other possible sources of infection. In another study, chronic hepatitis developed in 61% of patients with acute PTH C (11). The reasons why some recipients resolve their HCV infection are not known. Although it has been shown that the recovery rate from HCV infection increases with time (12), it is less likely that a difference of only 1 year should be of such importance. Thus, it is possible that other factors, such as the amount of the virus transfused, the HCV strain of the donor and the clinical status of the recipients may influence the development of chronicity. Our material is small, but unselected and primarily investigated with a second generation test system and a sensitive PCR, suggesting reliable data. Follow-up of our patient group and other unselected patients from the time before screening will give us more knowledge about the natural course of clinically silent hepatitis C infections.

The performance of retrospective studies of transfusion-transmitted HCV infections is controversial. However, in the Netherlands, blood bank regulations provide for a continual survey system (13), which is recommended by them. The mortality rate in the studied recipients is comparable to ours, and no clinical data on the recipients have so far been provided. Foberg and co-workers have conducted a retrospective study in their region of Sweden (unpublished data) and cannot recommend a general Swedish survey going back to before the introduction of the screening. However, a prospective survey of the recipients of seroconverted registered active donors is worth considering, as a tool for identifying infected individuals, for measuring infectivity and for evaluating the cost-effectiveness of the screening in the present donor population.

ACKNOWLEDGEMENTS

This study was supported by grants from the Research Committee of Örebro County Council. The hard and enthusiastic work performed by Carina Ragnemyr, RN, in manually retrieving the transfusion records was highly appreciated.

REFERENCES

1. SOFS. 1990: 25 §2
2. Bäck E. Skall vi göra kostnad-nytta bedömningar vid införandet av nya rutiner? Läkartidningen 88: 720–723, 1991.
3. Epidemiology statistics. Örebro County Council 1991.
4. Yun ZB, Lindh G, Weiland O, Johansson B, Sönnerborg A. Detection of hepatitis C virus (HCV) RNA by PCR related to HCV antibodies in serum and liver histology in Swedish blood donors. J Med Virol 39: 57–61, 1993.
5. Garson JA, Clewley JP, Simmonds P, Zhang LQ, Mori J, Ring C, Follett EA, Dow BC, Martin S, Gunson H. Hepatitis C viraemia in United Kingdom blood donors. A multicentre study. Vox Sang 62: 218–223, 1992.
6. Shev S, Foberg U, Fryden A, Hermodsson S, Lindh G, Lindholm, A, Månsson AS, von Sydow M, Weiland O, Widell A, Norkrans G. Second-generation hepatitis C Elisa antibody tests confirmed by the four-antigen recombinant immunoblot assay correlate well with hepatitis C viremia and chronic liver disease in Swedish blood donors. Vox Sang 65: 32–37, 1993.
7. Bresters D, Zaaijer HL, Cuypers HT, Reesink HW, Winkel IN, van Exel-Oehlers PJ, van Drimmelen AA, Jansen PL, van der Poel CL, Lelie PN. Recombinant immunoblot assay reaction patterns and hepatitis C virus RNA in blood donors and non-A, non-B hepatitis patients. Transfusion 33: 634–638, 1993.
8. Zaaijer HL, Cuypers HT, Reesink HW, Lelie PN. Should the c100 antigen be removed from HCV antibody assays? Vox Sang 66: 150, 1994.
9. Watanabe M, Ohkoshi S, Tawaraya H, Miyajima T, Shimotohno K, Kamimura T, Asakura H. Hepatitis C viral markers in patients who received blood that was positive for hepatitis C virus core antibody, with genetic evidence of hepatitis C transmission. Transfusion 34: 125–129, 1994.
10. Skaug K, Li H, Jonassen TO, Larsen J, Figenschau KJ. Hepatitis C (HCV) RNA among anti-HCV-positive blood donors and their recipients. Vox Sang 64: 215–219, 1993.
11. Mattson L, Grillner L, Weiland O. Seroconversion to hepatitis C virus antibodies in patients with acute posttransfusion non-A, non-B hepatitis in Sweden with a second generation test. Scand J Infect Dis 24: 15–20, 1992.
12. Dittman S, Roggendorf M, Durkop J, Wiese M, Lorbeer B, Deinhardt F. Long-term persistance of hepatitis C virus antibodies in a single source outbreak. J Hepatol 13: 323–327, 1991.
13. Vrielink H, van der Poel CL, Reesink HW, Zaaijer HL, Scholten E, Kremer LCM, Cuypers HT, Lelie PN, van Oers MH. Look-back study of infectivity of anti-HCV ELISA-positive blood components. Lancet 345: 95–96, 1995.

Submitted February 7, 1995; accepted June 14, 1995

Scand J Infect Dis 27: 453–456, 1995 ORIGINAL ARTICLE

Increased Production of Nitric Oxide in Patients Infected with the European Variant of Hantavirus

PAUL H. P. GROENEVELD[1], PAUL COLSON[2], KITTY M. C. KWAPPENBERG[1] and JAN CLEMENT[3]

From the [1]Department of Infectious Diseases, University Hospital Leiden, Leiden, The Netherlands, the [2]Centre de Santé des Fagnes, Chimay, and the [3]Queen Astrid Military Hospital, Brussels, Belgium

Serum nitrate levels, a measure of nitric oxide (NO) production in vivo, were very high (95 ± 14 μM) in 13 patients infected with Puumala virus, the European variant of Hantavirus (HTV), as compared to those in healthy subjects (33 ± 3 μM). Serum nitrate levels showed a high and significant correlation with scores on the Acute Physiological And Chronic Health Evaluation (APACHE II) scale and with serum creatinine, and an inverse correlation with platelet counts. Serial serum measurements of nitrate in 2 severe cases showed very high levels at the onset of arterial hypotension and acute renal failure. We conclude that excessive amounts of NO are produced in patients infected with Puumala virus and that this reactive nitrogen intermediate could play an important role in the pathogenesis of the disease.

P. H. P. Groeneveld, MD, Department of Infectious Diseases, Building 1-C5, Academic Hospital Leiden, Rijnsburgerweg 10, NL-2333 AA Leiden, The Netherlands

INTRODUCTION

The rodent-borne disease caused by the European variant of hantavirus (HTV), typically presents with sudden onset of high fever, chills, and with thrombocytopenia as 1 of the characteristic laboratory abnormalities (1). Although the disease is usually self-remitting within a few weeks, the clinical course may be complicated by arterial hypotension, oliguric acute renal failure (ARF), capillary leak syndrome and exceptionally also by diffuse intravascular coagulation (DIC) and adult respiratory distress syndrome (ARDS) (2). The pathogenesis of HTV diseases is still unclear, but several factors contributing to these complications have been postulated (1). ARF may be caused by congestion and excessive dilatation of medullary renal arteries, compromising local blood flow, which could lead to ischemia and injury of tubular cells. Decreased peripheral vascular resistance and increased vascular permeability are also considered to be important factors in the development of arterial hypotension, ARF and possibly ARDS (1). Thrombocytopenia could be due to the adherence and aggregation of platelets to damaged vascular endothelium and subendothelial connective tissue in HTV-infected patients (1). Recent findings indicate that extensive activation of the cellular immune response could be involved in the development of inflammation and pathologic lesions of patients with HTV (3). The production of proinflammatory cytokines, as part of the cellular immune response, are thought to play an important role in the pathogenesis of this disease; however, these data are limited (1, 3).

Nitric oxide (NO), a highly reactive nitrogen intermediate, is produced by the enzyme NO-synthase (NOS), and at least two major isoforms of NOS can be distinguished (4). The constitutive (cNOS) isoform produces low amounts of NO, while the cytokine-inducible (iNOS) isoform gives rise to large amounts of NO. Endothelial cells express cNOS activity and are able to synthesize iNOS after stimulation with endotoxin or proinflammatory cytokines, such as interferon-γ (IFN-γ) or tumor necrosis factor-α (TNF-α) (4). In human septic shock, peripheral vasodilation is now considered to be due to the production of nitric oxide (NO) by endothelial cells, which causes relaxation of smooth muscle cells in the vessel wall (4–7). Other biological effects of NO include inhibition of platelet and leucocyte adherence to vascular endothelium and platelet aggregation (4). This reactive nitrogen intermediate has also been implicated in the murine host defense during bacterial and viral infections (8–10), but the role of NO in the host defense of humans to bacterial or viral infections is unknown.

The aim of the present study was to determine the production of NO in patients infected with *Puumala* virus, the European variant of HTV. Therefore, we measured serum nitrate levels, as a parameter of NO production in vivo, in patients during the acute phase of the disease. In order to determine the correlation between NO production and the development of complications, we also measured nitrate levels in serial serum samples of two severe cases.

PATIENTS AND METHODS

The patients ($n = 13$, age 47 ± 5 years) were cases from the 1993 HTV outbreak in Belgium, serologically proven by capture enzyme-linked immunosorbent assay (ELISA) for IgM and immunofluorescent assay (IFA) for IgG antibodies against the Puumala strain CG 18–20 (11). They were selected on the basis of acute fever for less than 2 weeks (onset of fever 6 ± 1 days). Healthy subjects recruited from laboratory personnel without restriction in diet, relevant medication or evidence for an active infection served as controls ($n = 19$, age 36 ± 3 years).

Serum samples (250 μl) were stored at −20°C after sampling. Immediately before analysis, the samples were diluted 1 : 1 with distilled water and then deproteinized with 50 μl 30% (w/v) $ZnSO_4$ for 20 min at room temperature. Next, deproteinized serum was incubated with HCl-activated spongy cadmium, prepared by overnight incubation of a zinc rod in cadmium sulfate (20%; Sigma, St Louis, Missouri, USA) and subsequently activated by incubation with 2% HCl for 15 min, in order to reduce nitrate to nitrite (6, 12). Nitrite was then determined using Griess reagens and the absorbance of the reaction product measured at 550 nm. The serum concentrations of nitrate were calculated from a standard curve using serial dilutions of sodium nitrate (0–200 μM).

Interassay variability was low with a coefficient of variation of 8%. Values are expressed as means ± SEM. Differences between the groups were analysed using the Mann–Whitney *U* test. The correlation between different parameters was calculated using Spearman's rank test; two-tailed analysis was performed with the level of significance set at $p < 0.05$.

CASE REPORTS

The clinical data and serial serum measurements of nitrate in 2 severe cases of HTV disease are summarized in Table I.

Case A

The first case (A) was a 69-year-old male hospitalized because of fever (38.2°C), cold chills, myalgia, headache and diarrhoea for 5 days. Arterial hypotension (65/40 mmHg), lactic acidosis (lactate 2.6 mM) and marked thrombocytopenia (36×10^9/l) developed during a period of high NO production (serum nitrate 147–162 μM). Treatment with vasoactive drugs was given from day 6 to day 28 because of arterial hypotension and decreased systemic vascular resistance, as confirmed by haemodynamic monitoring. Oliguric ARF necessitated peritoneal dialysis for 10 consecutive days (day 8–18). Non-cardiogenic pulmonary oedema (pulmonary capillary wedge pressure ≤15 mmHg) with bilateral interstitial infiltrates, typical for ARDS, developed and severe hypoxaemia (arterial P_{O_2} of 40 mmHg and P_{CO_2} of 30 mmHg) prompted mechanical ventilation from day 8 to day 20. Furthermore, purpura and intestinal bleeding developed on day 7 due to severe thrombocytopenia (platelet count 12×10^9/l) and DIC.

The patient recovered eventually without sequelae with normalization of serum nitrate levels from day 35 on.

Case B

This patient was a 50-year-old male hospitalized because of high fever (39.4°C), cold chills, headache, nausea, vomiting, diarrhoea and severe muscle pain. On admission, blood pressure was slightly decreased to 120/60 mmHg, the platelet count was 49×10^9/l, serum creatinine was 292 μM, and the nitrate level 186 μM (Table I). Arterial blood gas analysis revealed hypoxaemia (P_{O_2} was 70 mmHg with 3.1 of oxygen) and hypocapnia (P_{CO_2} was 30 mmHg). Bilateral interstitial pulmonary infiltrates on X-ray were compatible with ARDS. Oliguric ARF peaked on day 10 (Table I). No dialysis, mechanical ventilation or vasoactive treatment was required in this case. The relatively high nitrate level on day 17 can only be explained by excessive dietary intake of nitrate before his visit to the outpatient department, and was excluded in further analysis. Serum nitrate levels returned to normal at day 20.

RESULTS

The serum concentration of nitrate in patients during the acute phase of HTV infection was 95 ± 14 μM (range 35–186 μM, $n = 13$), which was significantly higher ($p < 0.0001$) than in control subjects (33 ± 3 μM; range 21–67 μM, $n = 19$) (Fig. 1). The serum nitrate levels were significantly higher ($p < 0.05$) in HTV patients with creatinine levels about 200 μM (serum nitrate 127 ± 17 μM, $n = 6$), compared with those in patients with creatinine values below 200 μM (serum nitrate 69 ± 17 μM, $n = 7$). Serum nitrate determinations correlated with creatinine levels ($r = 0.47$, $p < 0.05$; $n = 21$) and showed an inverse correlation with platelet counts ($r = -0.46$, $p < 0.05$; $n = 21$). Creatinine levels and platelet counts were also inversely

Table I. *Clinical and laboratory parameters in two patients infected with Puumala virus, the European variant of hantavirus*

Day of illness	Severity of disease APACHE II score	Haemodynamic parameter Arterial blood pressure mmHg	Renal function creatinine, μM	Haematology platelet counts, $\times 10^9$/l	Nitric oxide production Serum nitrate, μM
Case A[a]					
6	23	65/40	513	36	147
10	33	100/50	742	32	162
16	30	140/60	610	89	83
17	32	170/80	548	89	93
28	13	120/60	124	193	87
35	10	160/90	97	324	28
Case B					
6	16	120/60	292	49	186
10	11	140/80	902	248	78
13	10	140/80	221	465	61
17	2	150/70	115	326	120[b]
20	2	140/80	115	247	36

[a] Treatment of case A: peritoneal dialysis from day 8 to 18; mechanical ventilation from day 8 to 20 and from day 22 to 30; vasoactive treatment, dopamine 2 μg/kg/min from day 6 to 22, dopamine 1 μg/kg/min from day 22 to 28, dobutamine 5–6 μg/kg/min from day 6 to 12.

[b] High serum nitrate probably due to excessive dietary intake of nitrate.

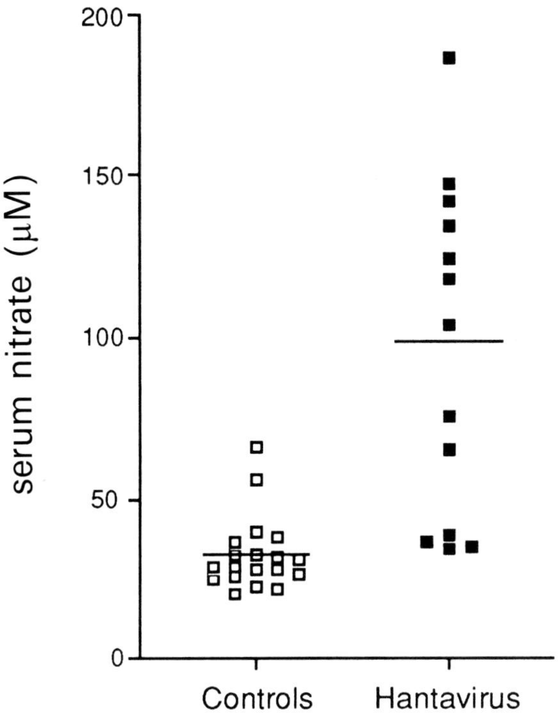

Fig. 1. Individual values of serum nitrate levels in patients infected with Puumala virus, the European variant of hantavirus, during the acute phase of the disease ($n = 13$), and of healthy subjects ($n = 19$). The horizontal lines indicate mean values of serum nitrate.

correlated ($r = -0.43$, $p < 0.05$; $n = 22$). Serial measurements in two severe cases revealed that serum nitrate levels correlated highly with scores on the Acute Physiological And Chronic Health Evaluation (APACHE II) scale ($r = 0.78$, $p < 0.01$; $n = 10$) (13). A good correlation between APACHE II scores and creatinine levels ($r = 0.68$, $p < 0.05$; $n = 10$), and an inverse correlation between APACHE II scores and platelet counts ($r = -0.82$, $p < 0.005$; $n = 10$) was also demonstrated.

DISCUSSION

The main finding of this study is that serum nitrate levels are much higher in patients with an acute infection of the European variant of HTV, than in control subjects. Serum nitrate levels have been used as an indirect parameter for NOS activity in vivo, especially in sepsis and septic shock (5–7). In septic patients, increases in serum nitrate concentrations have been demonstrated that are comparable with those found in patients with HTV infection; Ochoa et al. (5) and Evans et al. (6) showed serum nitrate levels of 63 ± 7 μM and a mean value of 124 μM, respectively, in patients with sepsis, while Gómez-Jiménez et al. detected 53 ± 10 μM of nitrate in serum samples of patients with septic shock (7).

However, serum nitrate levels reflect a balance between dietary intake of nitrate and endogenous production of NO on the one hand, and urinary excretion of nitrate on the other. The possibility that renal insufficiency is responsible for the elevated serum nitrate levels in our patients is unlikely, because high nitrate levels have been demonstrated without renal impairment and vice versa in patients with septic shock (5, 6, 14) and after surgery (15). Therefore, we conclude that the very high nitrate levels in serum of our patients with HTV are due to an excessive production of NO in vivo; its cellular origin remains to be determined. Since the vascular endothelium is considered to be the most important cellular target, as demonstrated by the widespread deposition of viral antigen in endothelial cells throughout the body (1), HTV-infected vascular endothelium is the most likely source for the excessive NO production in patients with HTV, although other cellular sources cannot be excluded. Excessive NO production is probably due to the induction of iNOS in response to HTV itself, viral proteins and/or indirectly through the production of pro-inflammatory cytokines.

Our results indicate that NO could play a major role in the pathogenesis of HTV disease because serum nitrate levels correlated positively with APACHE II scores and serum creatinine and negatively with platelet counts. Serial determinations of serum nitrate in one of the severe cases also suggest that arterial hypotension could be due to the production of NO by endothelial cells during the acute phase of the disease. NO-induced arterial hypotension and excessive dilation of renal medullary arteries could explain the strong correlation between serum nitrate and creatinine, indicating that NO is, at least to some extent, involved in the pathogenesis of ARF in HTV-infected patients.

The potentially beneficial roles of NO in this viral disease, besides its antiviral properties, include an inhibitory effect on vascular permeability, platelet aggregation and adherence of platelets to endothelial cells. It has been shown that NO decreases the permeability of endothelial cell monolayers by relaxing these cells and narrowing the width of endothelial junctions (16). In vivo studies demonstrated that inhibition of NO induced microvascular albumin leakage in the mesenteric postcapillary venules of rats and promoted the adhesion of leucocytes to vascular endothelium (17). These findings suggest that NO could act as a feedback inhibitor, attenuating the increased vascular permeability often present in patients with HTV. In addition, NO also reduces platelet aggregation and the adherence of platelets to vascular endothelium (4), which may counteract HTV-induced thrombocytopenia.

We conclude that NO is produced at high levels in patients with the European variant of HTV, and that this reactive nitrogen intermediate could have both beneficial and detrimental effects in the pathogenesis of the disease.

REFERENCES

1. Cosgriff TM. Mechanisms of disease in Hantavirus infection: pathophysiology of hemorrhagic fever with renal syndrome. Rev Infect Dis 13: 97–107, 1991.
2. Clement J, Colson P, McKenna P. Hantavirus pulmonary syndrome in New England and Europe. N Engl J Med 331: 545–546, 1994.
3. Huang C, Jin B, Wang M, Li E, Sun C. Hemorrhagic fever with renal syndrome: relationship between pathogenesis and cellular immunity. J Infect Dis 169: 868–870, 1994.
4. Moncada S, Higgs A. The L-arginine-nitric oxide pathway. N Engl J Med 329: 2002–2012, 1993.
5. Ochoa JB, Udekwu AO, Billiar TR, Curran RD, Cerra FB, Simmons RL, Peitzman AB. Nitrogen oxide levels in patients after trauma and during sepsis. Ann Surg 214: 621–626, 1991.
6. Evans T, Carpenter A, Kinderman H, Cohen J. Evidence of increased nitric oxide production in patients with sepsis syndrome. Circ Shock 41: 77–81, 1993.
7. Gomez-Jimenez J, Salgado A, Mourelle M, Martin MC, Segura RM, Peracaula R, Moncada S. L-arginine: nitric oxide pathway in endotoxemia and human septic shock. Crit Care Med 23: 253–258, 1995.
8. Nathan CF, Hibbs JB. Role of nitric oxide synthesis in macrophage antimicrobial activity. Curr Opin Immunol 3: 65–70, 1991.
9. Karupiah G, Xie Q, Mark R, Buller L, Nathan C, Duarte C, MacMicking JD. Inhibition of viral replication by interferon-induced nitric oxide synthase. Science 266: 1445–1448, 1993.
10. Croen KD. Evidence for an antiviral effect of nitric oxide. Inhibition of herpes simplex type 1 replication. J Clin Invest 91: 2446–2452, 1993.
11. Clement J, McKenna P, Colson P, Damoiseaux P, Penalba C, Halin P, Lombart D. Hantavirus epidemic in Europe, 1993. Lancet 343: 114, 1994.
12. Hegesh E, Shiloah J. Blood nitrates and infantile methemoglobinemia. Clin Chim Acta 125: 107–115, 1982.
13. Knaus WA, Draper EA, Wagner DP, Zimmerman JE. APACHE II: a severity of disease classification system. Crit Care Med 13: 818–829, 1985.
14. Groeneveld PHP, Ringers J, van Dissel JT. Effect of nitric oxide on renal function in septic shock. N Engl J Med 330: 1620, 1994.
15. van Dissel JT, Groeneveld PHP. Serum nitric oxide and morbidity in postoperative patients. Lancet 344: 888–889, 1994.
16. Oliver JA. Endothelium-derived relaxing factor contributes to the regulation of endothelial permeability. J Cell Physiol 141: 505–511, 1992.
17. Kurose I, Kubes P, Wolf R, Anderson DC, Paulson J, Miyasaka M, Granger DN. Inhibition of nitric oxide production. Mechanisms of vascular albumin leakage. Circ Res 73: 164–171, 1993.

Submitted February 23, 1995; accepted June 5, 1995

Scand J Infect Dis 27: 457–462, 1995 ORIGINAL ARTICLE

Diagnostic and Prognostic Value of Interleukin-6 and C-reactive Protein in Community-acquired Pneumonia

ÅKE ÖRTQVIST[1], JONAS HEDLUND[1], BENGT WRETLIND[2], ANDERS CARLSTRÖM[3] and MATS KALIN[4]

From the [1]Department of Infectious Diseases, Danderyd Hospital, the [2]Division of Bacteriology, Huddinge Hospital, the [3]Department of Clinical Chemistry, Danderyd Hospital, and the [4]Department of Medicine, Division of Infectious Diseases, Karolinska Hospital, Karolinska Institute, Stockholm, Sweden

The diagnostic and prognostic value of admission serum levels of interleukin-6 (IL-6) and C-reactive protein (CRP) was investigated in 203 hospital-treated patients with community-acquired pneumonia (CAP). In serum samples obtained during the first 24 h after admission, IL-6 was detectable in 198 patients (98%), with a median value of 50 ng/l. Ten % of the patients had IL-6 values of 1000 ng/l. A clear positive correlation between IL-6 and CRP was found ($r = 0.29$, $p < 0.0001$). Patients with high IL-6 or CRP levels had longer duration of fever, longer hospital stay, and had less often recovered clinically or radiographically on follow-up weeks after discharge. A high IL-6, but not a high CRP, also seemed to be associated with a higher mortality. Bacteremic pneumococcal pneumonia had the highest levels of IL-6 (mean 2852 and median 420 ng/l) and CRP (mean 292 and median 285 mg/l). High IL-6 values were also seen in patients with non-bacteremic pneumococcal pneumonia, while all patients with pneumonia due to other bacterial, or viral, aetiology had IL-6 levels of ≤300 ng/l. In conclusion, IL-6 and CRP are promising diagnostic and prognostic tools in the management of CAP. Further studies are needed to establish the usefulness of repeated measurements early in the hospital course of the disease.

Å. Örtqvist, MD, Department of Infectious Diseases, Karolinska Institute, Danderyd Hospital, S-182 88 Danderyd, Sweden

INTRODUCTION

Community-acquired pneumonia (CAP) remains a common cause of hospital admission (1), as well as a potentially fatal disease even in previously healthy persons (2–6). A large number of factors have been associated with higher death rates in pneumonia (2–4, 7). However, although often specific, the positive predictive value of these factors, alone or in combination, has generally been low (19–29%) (1, 8–9). It is therefore of interest to seek better indicators for identifying patients with severe pneumonia, including those who are at a high risk of a complicated course.

In studies of CAP, an aetiologic diagnosis is seldom identified in more than 50–70% of cases (2, 4), and in the hospital routine this figure becomes much lower (10). Since appropriate, early, antibiotic therapy may improve diagnosis of CAP (2), new rapid tests for identifying, or indicating, the major respiratory pathogens are needed. Furthermore, identification of factors of importance in the pathogenesis of pneumonia could possibly provide alternative means for intervention.

The release of inflammatory mediators from activated mononuclear phagocyte cells constitutes an important part of the host response to infection (11). Of these mediators, interleukin-6 (IL-6) is a major inducer of acute-phase proteins, including the C-reactive protein (CRP) (12–13). Plasma IL-6-levels on admission have been shown to correlate to the severity of the disease in sepsis and septic shock (13–18), and recent data indicate that this might be valid also for patients with pneumonia (19). Further, data from experimental pneumococcal sepsis in pigs indicate that pretreatment with a monocyte activator prevents a strong IL-6 increase and reduces mortality (20). CRP has been shown in some studies (21–22), but not all (23), to be a useful tool for differentiating between bacterial and viral disease in pneumonia and meningitis. Similarly, it is possible that plasma IL-6 levels may have a differential-diagnostic potential in patients with pneumonia (24).

The aim of the present study was to investigate the potential of CRP and IL-6 plasma levels on admission as early indicators of the aetiology and outcome in CAP in hospitalized patients.

PATIENTS AND METHODS

The patient population has been described in detail earlier (4). In brief, during a 10-month period in 1987, all patients ≥18 years old with CAP admitted to the Department of Infectious Diseases at Danderyd Hospital were included in a prospective study of the aetiology and prognosis of CAP. CAP was defined as an acute lower respiratory tract disease with onset before admission to hospital and radiological signs of acute pneumonia. In total, 277 patients with CAP were included in the study. An aetiologic diagnosis was established in 68% of the patients. The diagnostic methods and definitions used have been described earlier (4). A bacteremic pneumonia was defined as CAP with growth of a potential respiratory tract pathogen in blood cultures. Growth of pneumococci in pleural fluid, bronchial secretions, or sputum ($\geq 10^5$ cfu/ml), or detection of pneumococcal antigen in sputum or urine, or a 2-fold or greater rise of pneumolysin antibody titre, or a single pneumolysin titre in either sample above the 99th percentile upper limits for healthy adults, was considered diagnostic for a non-bacteremic S. pneumoniae pneumonia. For M. pneumoniae

 ISSN 0036-5548

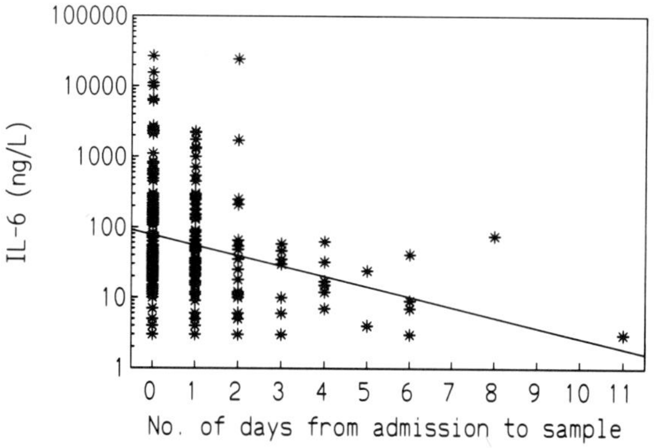

Fig. 1. Correlation between the serum IL-6 (ng/l) level and the number of days after admission to hospital before the serum sample was obtained in 247 patients with CAP.

and respiratory viruses a significant rise of antibody titres in an enzyme immunoassay on paired sera was required for the diagnosis. The outcome variables studied were death, duration of fever, length of hospital stay and clinical radiological recovery at follow-up 8 weeks earlier after discharge. Duration of fever was defined as the number of days from admission until the temperature reached a stable level below 37.5°C. One patient who had an extremely long hospital stay (95 days) was excluded from the analysis of the length-of-stay parameter.

In 247 of the 277 patients a serum sample from the hospital period was available for the present study. In these 247 samples the IL-6 level was analysed using a commercial enzyme immunoassay technique (Quantiking, R&D Systems, Inc., Minneapolis, USA), with a detection limit of ≥3 ng/l. CRP was analysed on the same sera with a turbidimetric assay on a Paramax instrument (Baxter, USA) using antibodies from Dako, Copenhagen, Denmark.

IL-6- and CRP-levels were then correlated to the major aetiologic agents: S. pneumoniae (bacteraemic and non-bacteraemic), M. pneumoniae, and respiratory viruses, and also to non-pneumococcal bacteraemic pneumonia. The IL-6 and CRP levels were also correlated to the five outcome variables mentioned above.

Statistical analysis

Statistical calculations were done using Instat® (Version 2.0, GraphPad Software, San Diego, California, USA). For analysis of categorical variables Fisher's exact test (2-tailed) or the Mann-Whitney U-test (2-tailed) was used. If >2 groups were being compared the Kruskal-Wallis non-parametric ANOVA test was used. Linear regression was used to determine whether there were correlations between variables. Logarithmic IL-6 values were used for linear regression.

Table I. *Serum IL-6 values in 247 patients with CAP correlated to when the sample was obtained after admission to hospital*

	IL-6 (ng/l)[a]			
	Day 0 ($n = 130$)	Day 1 ($n = 73$)	Day 2 ($n = 21$)	Day ≥3 ($n = 23$)
Median	52.5[b]	47	18	17
Range	0–27 000	0–2260	0–24 500	0–75

[a] Variation among columns greater than expected by chance, $p < 0.0001$.
[b] Day 0 vs. day 1 (NS), day 0 vs. day 2 ($p < 0.05$), day 0 vs. day 3 ($p < 0.001$)
Kruskal-Wallis non-parametric ANOVA test.

RESULTS

The serum sample for analysis of IL-6 and CRP was obtained immediately on admission (day 0) in 130/247 patients, within 24 h (day 1) in 73 patients, on day 2 in 21 patients, and on day 3 or later in 23 patients. There was a significant decrease ($p < 0.0001$) of the IL-6 levels with time, from admission to when the sample was obtained (Fig. 1 and Table I). Since this decrease was most evident from day 2 and onwards, only patients in whom the sample was drawn within 24 h ($n = 203$) were considered for the remaining analyses. However, in these 203 patients, the total duration of illness according to the patient was not associated with the admission IL-6 level (Table II).

The 203 patients were 59.5 years of age on average, and 57% were female. The median value of IL-6 was 50 ng/l (range 0–27 000) and the mean was 616 ng/l. IL-6 was non-detectable in 5 patients (2%) and a further 37 patients (18%) had low levels (3–19 ng/l). In 82 patients (40%) the IL-6 level was between 50 and 999 ng/l, and in 21 (10%) ≥1000 ng/l.

CRP values on admission could be analysed in 196/203 patients. In 7 patients the amount of serum available was not enough for running both tests. The mean CRP was 167 (±108) mg/l (range 0–493). There was a positive correlation between serum levels of (log) IL-6 and CRP ($r = 0.29$, $p < 0.0001$). Antibiotic treatment prior to admission resulted in significantly lower levels of both IL-6 and CRP.

Table II. *Serum IL-6 in 201[a] patients with CAP in relation to the duration of illness, from onset of disease to the time for the IL-6 serum sample*

	IL-6 (ng/l)[b]					
	0–1 days ($n = 23$)	2 days ($n = 33$)	3 days ($n = 36$)	4–5 days ($n = 42$)	6–7 days ($n = 31$)	>7 days ($n = 36$)
Median	115	50	79	55	54	29
Mean	533	484	395	1434	308	353
SD	883	1199	1146	4965	623	1659

[a] In 2 of the 203 patients the duration of illness before admission was unknown.
[b] $p = 0.10$ for variation among columns, Kruskal-Wallis non-parametric ANOVA test.

Table III. *Serum IL-6 values on admission to hospital in 203 patients in relation to the outcome of CAP*

	IL-6 (ng/l) Median (first quartile, third quartile)	p
Survived		0.069
Yes ($n = 196$)	48 (20, 180)	
No ($n = 7$)	77 (70, 2700)	
Follow-up after 2 months		0.005
Healthy ($n = 142$)	44 (20, 151)	
Not healthy ($n = 44$)	121 (34, 480)	
Chest X-ray at 2 months		0.054
Normal ($n = 142$)	48 (19, 163)	
Pathologic ($n = 27$)	90 (32, 240)	

The median IL-6 value was 27.5 ng/l in patients who had received antibiotics compared to 73 ng/l ($p < 0.0004$) in those who were untreated, and the corresponding figures for CRP were 127 mg/l vs. 172 mg/l ($p < 0.0007$).

IL-6 and CRP levels correlated both with the in-hospital duration of fever ($r = 0.22$, $p < 0.01$ and $r = 0.21$, $p < 0.01$, respectively) and with the length of hospitalization ($r = 0.16$, $p < 0.05$ and $r = 0.22$, $p < 0.01$, respectively). Patients who died seemed to have higher IL-6 levels, than those who survived (Table III). Significantly higher admission IL-6 levels were seen in patients who had not recovered subjectively or objectively (according to chest X-ray) at follow-up 2 months after discharge, than in those who had recovered (Table III). The CRP levels in patients who

Table IV. *CRP values on admission to hospital in 196 patients in relation to the outcome of CAP*

	CRP (mg/l)			
	Mean ($\pm$SD)	CI_{95}	Median	p
Survived				0.269
Yes ($n = 189$)	172 (106)	157, 187	159	
No ($n = 7$)	204 (77)	132, 275	215	
Follow-up after 2 months				0.001
Healthy ($n = 135$)	160 (100)	143, 177	148	
Not healthy ($n = 44$)	223 (118)	187, 259	216	
Chest X-ray at 2 months				0.002
Normal ($n = 135$)	162 (104)	144, 180	148	
Pathologic ($n = 27$)	233 (102)	193, 273	217	

Table V. *Admission serum levels of IL-6 and CRP in 109 patients with CAP in relation to the aetiologic diagnosis of pneumonia*

	Aetiologic diagnosis					
	S. pneumoniae (bacteraemic) ($n = 18$)	S. pneumoniae (non-bacteraemic) ($n = 57$)	Other[a] bacteraemic pneumonia ($n = 5$)	Mycoplasma pneumoniae ($n = 16$)	Viruses ($n = 13$)	p
IL-6 ng/l						<0.0001[b]
Mean	2852	679	112	40	53	
CI_{95}	533, 5170	−270, 1629	−15, 239	4, 77	9, 97	
Median	420	54	53	20	26	
Range	13–15 500	0–27 000	33–260	4–290	0–280	
CRP mg/l						<0.0001[c]
Mean	292[c]	173[d]	111	100	123	
CI_{95}	232, 351	145, 201	−30, 247	63, 138	84, 163	
Median	285	172	41	103	138	
Range	32–407	10–410	26–482	1–225	30–242	

[a] H. influenzae (1), S. aureus (1), K. pneumoniae (2), E. coli (1).
[b] Variation among columns, Kruskal-Wallis non-parametric ANOVA test.
Bacteraemic- vs. non-bacteraemic pneumococcal pneumonia $p < 0.01$, bacteraemic pneumococcal pneumonia vs. mycoplasmal pneumonia $p < 0.001$, bacteraemic pneumococcal pneumonia vs. viral pneumonia $p < 0.001$.
[c] Serum available for CRP analysis in 13 patients.
[d] Serum available for CRP analysis in 56 patients.
[e] Variation among columns, Kruskal-Wallis non-parametric ANOVA test.
Bacteraemic- vs. non-bacteraemic pneumococcal pneumonia $p < 0.01$, bacteraemic pneumococcal pneumonia vs. "other" bacteraemic pneumonia $p < 0.01$, bacteraemic pneumococcal pneumonia vs. mycoplasmal pneumonia $p < 0.001$, bacteraemic pneumococcal pneumonia vs. viral pneumonia $p < 0.001$.

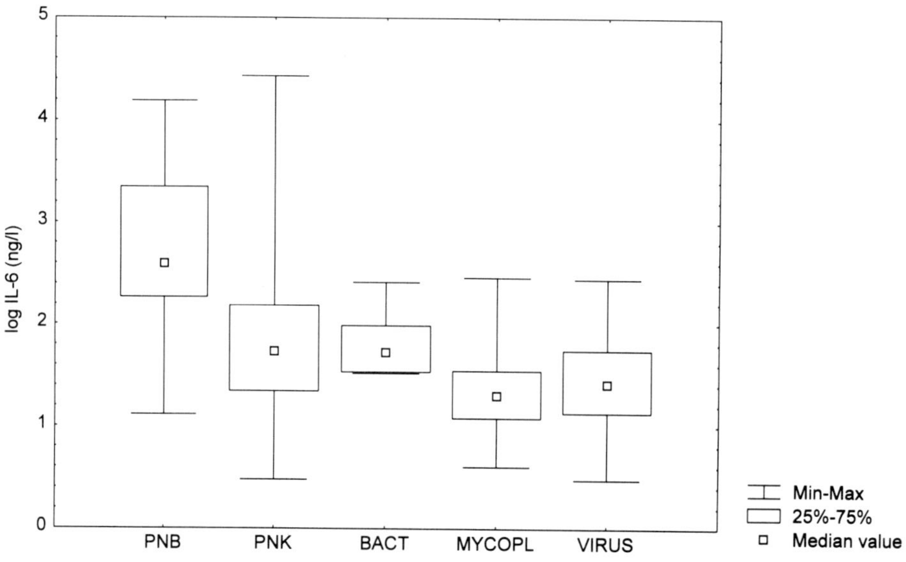

Fig. 2. Admission serum (log) IL-6 levels (median, first and third quartiles, and range) in patients with bacteraemic pneumococcal pneumonia (PNB, $n = 18$), non-bacteraemic pneumococcal pneumonia (PNK, $n = 57$), bacteraemic non-pneumococcal pneumonia (BACT, $n = 5$), mycoplasmal pneumonia (MYCOPL, $n = 16$), and in viral pneumonia (VIRUS, $n = 13$).

died during the hospitalization and in those who survived were similar (Table IV). However, admission CRP levels were significantly higher in patients who had not recovered clinically or radiographically after 2 months follow-up, than in those who had recovered (Table IV).

Bacteraemic pneumococcal pneumonia (Pnb) was present in 18 patients, and bacteraemic pneumonia with other pathogens in 5 (Table V). In 86 patients with non-bacteraemic pneumonia a single organism was identified as the causative agent; S. pneumoniae in 57, M. pneumoniae in 16, and a virus in 13 patients. The highest levels of IL-6 and CRP were seen in patients with pneumococcal pneumonia, especially in those with bacteraemia (Table V, Fig. 2). Seven of 18 (39%) Pnb patients and 4/57 (7%) of those with non-bacteraemic pneumococcal pneumonia had IL-6 levels of 1000 ng/l, or more, while no patients in the other 3 groups had an admission value above 300 ng/l. Only 2/5 patients with bacteraemic pneumonia due to agents other than pneumococci had IL-6 values >100 ng/l, and the corresponding figures were 1/16 and 1/13 for those with mycoplasmal or viral pneumonia.

DISCUSSION

The principal finding of this study was that pneumonia caused by S. pneumoniae, especially when bacteraemic, elicited a much more marked host response, characterized by elevation of plasma IL-6 and CRP, than pneumonia caused by the other pathogens. Furthermore, admission levels of both IL-6 and CRP seemed to correlate to outcome.

Eighty percent of our patients had plasma IL-6 levels of ≥20 ng/l on admission, with a median value of 50 ng/l. IL-6 levels >300 ng/l were seen only in patients with pneumococcal pneumonia (9 bacteraemic and 9 non-bacteraemic patients). If the third quartile (≥188 ng/l) of all IL-6 values was used as a cut-off level, 14/18 patients with bacteraemic pneumococcal pneumonia were identified, corresponding to a sensitivty of 78% and a specificity of 80% (data not shown). The same IL-6 level was found in 14/57 patients with non-bacteraemic pneumococcal pneumonia, in 1/5 of patients with "other bacteraemic pneumonia", and in 1 patient each in the mycoplasmal and viral groups. Our findings are in accordance with those of Kragsbjerg et al. (24), who showed that a majority of CAP patients with a well-defined aetiology had IL-6 levels >75 ng/l, and that the highest IL-6 levels are seen among patients with pneumococcal pneumonia and the lowest among those with mycoplasmal or viral pneumonia. In contrast, Moussa et al. (25) found elevated IL-6 levels in only 23% of 46 consecutive CAP patients. The latter is somewhat surprising, since the patients in Moussa's study, compared with the present material, seemed to be more severely ill and since prior antibiotic treatment was equally common in both studies.

In pneumonia, higher levels of TNF-α and IL-8 have been found intrapulmonary than in plasma (26). It is probable that also the production of IL-6 is compartmentalized, as indicated by studies of bacterial meningitis (27) and of urinary tract infection (28). The higher plasma IL-6 levels in bacteraemic than in non-bacteraemic pneumococcal pneumonia may thus reflect a more intense local inflammation, with a subsequent systemic release of both bacterial antigens and cytokines (28–29). However, the reason for the more intense IL-6 response in pneumococcal pneumonia, compared with other bacterial pathogens, and the role of IL-6 in the pathogenesis of this disease should be investigated further.

Significantly lower IL-6 levels were found in patients where the sample was obtained >24 h after admission to hospital (Table I, Fig. 1), and in patients who had received antibiotics prior to admission. However, in accordance with earlier findings (24), we found no correlation between the duration of illness and the admission IL-6 level (Table II).

High IL-6 levels may persist for several days until the patient spontaneously recovers (30), or until antimicrobial treatment is begun. Further, the time for the onset of pneumonia is often difficult to establish clearly, e.g. when a primary viral bronchitis is complicated by a bacterial pneumonia.

High IL-6 levels on admission have been associated with a poor prognosis in sepsis (13–15, 17–18). In a recent study of 12 ICU-treated pneumonia patients, 8 less severely ill pneumonia patients and 2 groups of uninfected controls, there was a strong association between IL-6 levels and the APACHE II score (19). This finding suggests that plasma IL-6-level may reflect the severity of disease also in patients with pneumonia. That none of the previous pneumonia studies (19, 24–15) have demonstrated any association between IL-6 concentration and outcome may be due to the small number of patients studied. However, our findings confirmed the association between high admission IL-6 levels and the severity of pneumonia, characterized by the duration of fever, length of hospital stay and the recovery rate 2 months after discharge, and possibly also by the risk for in-hospital death. Six of the 7 patients with a fatal outcome had an IL-6 level of ≥ 70 ng/l on admission. If this IL-6 level is used as a cut-off, 6/87 (7%) patients above this level died, compared with 1/116 (0.9%) of those who had lower IL-6 values ($p = 0.044$, odds ratio 8.5 with CI_{95} [1.01, 72.15]), corresponding to a sensitivity of 86% and a specificity of 59%. However, the positive predictive value (7%) of this single IL-6 level for a fatal outcome was low.

Since IL-6 is a major inducer of CRP (12, 13), it is not surprising that there was a positive correlation between the levels of these on admission. As for IL-6, a high CRP level was associated with the presence of a bacteraemic pneumococcal pneumonia, a longer duration of fever, a longer hospital stay and a lower recovery rate on follow-up 2 months after discharge. In contrast, there was no association between CRP levels on admission and death in pneumonia.

In conclusion in patients with CAP admitted to hospital a high plasma level of IL-6 (>180 ng/l) probably indicates a pneumococcal aetiology. Furthermore, the IL-6 level seems to be correlated to the prognosis of pneumonia. CRP seems to offer similar information as IL-6 does, with the important exception that no association between CRP and death was found. Further studies are needed to establish the potential diagnostic and prognostic usefulness of IL-6. Measurements at repeated times in the hospital course, especially during the first 24 h (15–17, 241), may increase the usefulness.

ACKNOWLEDGEMENTS

We thank Dr Bengt Gårdlund for helpful comments on the manuscript. This work was supported by the Swedish Heart Lung Foundation and by the Karolinska Institute.

REFERENCES

1. Macfarlane J. An overview of community-acquired pneumonia with lessons learned from the British Thoracic Society study. Semin Resp Infect 9: 153–165, 1994.
2. British Thoracic Society. Community-acquired pneumonia in adults in British hospitals in 1982–1983: a survey of aetiology, mortality, prognostic factors and outcome. Q J Med, NS 62: 195–220, 1987.
3. Marrie TJ, Durant H, Yates L. Community-acquired pneumonia requiring hospitalisation: 5 year prospective study. Rev Infect Dis 11: 586–599, 1989.
4. Örtqvist Å, Hedlund J, Grillner L, Jalonen E, Kallings I, Leinonen M, Kalin M. Aetiology, outcome and prognostic factors in community-acquired pneumonia requiring hospitalisation. Eur Respir J 3: 1105–1113, 1990.
5. Fang G-D, Fine M, Orloff J, Arisumi D, Yu VL, Kapoor W, Grayston JT, Wang SP, Kohler R, Muder RR, Yee YC, Rihs JD, Vickers RM. New and emerging etiologies for community-acquired pneumonia with implications for therapy. Medicine 69: 307–316, 1990.
6. Örtqvist Å, Julander I, Kalin M, Mufson M. Deaths in bacteremic pneumococcal pneumonia: a comparison of two populations – Huntington, USA, and Stockholm, Sweden. Chest 103: 710–716, 1993.
7. Fine MJ, Orloff JJ, Arisumi D, Fang GD, Arena VC, Hanusa BH. Prognosis of patients hospitalized with community-acquired pneumonia. Am J Med 88: 5-1N–5-8N, 1990.
8. Karalus NC, Cursons RT, Leng RA, Mahood CB, Rothwell RP, Hancock B, Cepulis S, Wawati M, Coleman L. Community acquired pneumonia: aetiology and prognostic index evaluation. Thorax 46: 413–418, 1991.
9. Farr BM, Sloman AJ, Fisch MJ. Predicting death in patients hospitalized for community-acquired pneumonia. Ann Intern Med 115: 428–436, 1991.
10. Woodhead MA, Arrowsmith J, Chamberlain-Weber R, Wooding S, Williams I. The value of routine microbial investigation in community-acquired pneumonia. Resp Med 85: 313–317, 1991.
11. Molloy RG, Mannick JA, Rodrick ML. Cytokine, sepsis, and immunomodulation. Br J Surg 80: 289–297, 1993.
12. Castell JV, Gómez-Lechón MJ, David M, Andus T, Geiger T, Trullenque R, Fabra R, Heinrich PC. Interleukin-6 is the major regulator of acute phase protein synthesis in adult hepatocytes. FEBS Lett 242: 237–239, 1989.
13. Hack CE, De Groot ER, Felt-Bersma RJF, Nuijens JH, Strack Van Shiijndel RJM, Eerenberg-Balmer AJM, Thijs LG, Aarden LA. Increased plasma levels of interleukin-6 in sepsis. Blood 74: 1704–1710, 1989.
14. Waage A, Brandtzaeg P, Halstensen A, Kierulf P, Espevik T. The complex pattern of cytokines in serum from patients with meningococcal septic shock. J Exp Med 169: 333–338, 1989.
15. Damas P, Ledoux D, Nys M, Vrindts Y, de Groote D, Franchimont P, Lamy M. Cytokine serum level during severe sepsis in human IL-6 as a marker of severity. Ann Surg. 215: 356–362, 1992.
16. Pinsky MR, Vincent J-L, Deviere J, Alegre M, Kahn RJ, Dupont E. Serum cytokine levels in human septic shock. Chest 103: 565–575, 1993.
17. Fisher CJ, Opal SM, Dhainaut J-F, Stephens S, Zimmerman JL, Nightingale P, Harris SJ, Schein RM, Panacek EA, Vincent J-L, Foulke GE, Warren EL, Garrard C, Park G, Bodner MW, Cohen J, Van der Linden C, Cross AS, Sadoff JC, the CB0006 sepsis study group. Influence of an anti-tumor necrosis factor monoclonal antibody on cytokine levels in patients with sepsis. Crit Care Med 21: 318–327, 1993.
18. Casey LC, Balk RA, Bone RC. Plasma cytokine and endotoxin levels correlate with survival in patients with the sepsis syndrome. Ann Intern Med 119: 771–778, 1993.
19. Puren AJ, Feldman C, Savage N, Becker PJ, Smith C. Patterns of cytokine expression in community-acquired pneumonia. Chest 107: 1342–1349, 1995.

20. Ziegler-Heitbrock HW, Passlick B, Käfferlein E, Coulie PG, Izbicki JR. Protection against lethal pneumococcal septicemia in pigs is associated with decreased levels of interleukin-6 in blood. Infect Immun 60: 1692–1694, 1992.
21. Kerttula Y, Leinonen M, Koskela M, Mäkelä PH. The aetiology of pneumonia. Application of bacterial serology and basic laboratory methods. J Infect 14: 21–30, 1987.
22. Hansson LO, Axelsson G, Linné T, Aurelius E, Lindqvist L. Serum C-reactive protein measurement in the differential diagnosis of acute meningitis. Scand J Infect Dis 25: 625–630, 1993.
23. Burman LÅ, Trollfors B, Andersson B, Henrichsen J, Juto P, Kallings I, Lagergård T, Möleby R, Norrby R. Diagnosis of pneumonia by cultures, bacterial and viral antigen detection tests, and serology with special reference to antibiotics against pneumococcal antigens. J Infect Dis 163: 1087–1093, 1991.
24. Kragsbjerg P, Vikerfors T, Holmberg H. Serum levels of interleukin-6, tumour necrosis factor-α, interleukin-γ and C-reactive protein in adults with community-acquired pneumonia. Serodiagn Immunother Infect Dis 5: 156–160, 1993.
25. Moussa K, Michie HJ, Cree IA, McCafferty AC, Winter JH, Dhillon DP, Stephens S, Brown RA. Phagocyte function and cytokine production in community acquired pneumonia. Thorax 49: 107–111, 1994.
26. Chollet-Martin S, Montravers P, Gibert C, Elbim C, Desmonts JM, Fagon JY, Gougerot-Pocidalo MA. High levels of interleukin-8 in the blood and alveolar spaces of patients with pneumonia and adult respiratory distress syndrome. Infect Immun 61: 4553–4559, 1993.
27. Helfgott DC, Tatter SB, Santhanam U, Clarick RH, Bhardwaj N, May LT, Sehgal PB. Multiple forms of IFN-β2/IL-6 in serum and body fluids during acute bacterial infection. J Immunol 142: 948–953, 1989.
28. Benson M, Jodal U, Andreasson A, Karlsson Å, Rydberg J, Svanborg C. Interleukin-6 response to urinary tract infection in childhood. Pediatr Infect Dis J 13: 612–616, 1994.
29. Marik R, Kraus P, Sribante J, Havlik I, Lippman J, Johnson DW. Hydrocortisone and tumor necrosis factor in severe community-acquired pneumonia. Chest 104: 389–392, 1993.
30. Bauer J, Herrmann F. Interleukin-6 in clinical medicine. Ann Hematol 62: 203–210, 1991.

Submitted February 16, 1995; accepted July 11, 1995

Scand J Infect Dis 27: 463–468, 1995 ORIGINAL ARTICLE

Ampicillin plus Mecillinam vs. Cefotaxime/Cefadroxil Treatment of Patients with Severe Pneumonia or Pyelonephritis: a Double-Blind Multicentre Study Evaluated by Intention-to-Treat Analysis

STIG CRONBERG[1], STAFFAN BANKE[2], ANNE-MARIE BRUNO[3], MIKAEL CARLSSON[4], HENRIK ELMRUD[2], SÖREN ELOWSSON[5], KAJ JOSEFSSON[3], ANN-CHARLOTTE LINDHOLM[6], HENNING MONTELIUS[6], RUNE NERINGER[7], BJÖRN ODE[1], GÖRAN STENLUND[6], BIRGITTA SVANTESON[1], ANDERS THORÉN[1], MATS WALDER[8] and EWA WALLMARK[1]

From the Departments of Infectious Diseases at Central Hospitals in [1]Malmö, [2]Kristianstad, [3]Halmstad, [4]Jönköping, [5]Skövde, [6]Eskilstuna and [7]Karlskrona and the [8]Bacteriological Laboratory, Malmö, Sweden

In this double-blind multicentre study, using the intention-to-treat approach, a total of 293 patients with fever (≥38.5°C), symptoms of sepsis and signs of pneumonia or pyelonephritis were randomly assigned to treatment with ampicillin and mecillinam (A + M) or cefotaxime followed by cefadroxil. In the febrile phase, treatment was given intravenously twice daily, either with 1,200 mg ampicillin together with 600 mg mecillinam or with 2 g cefotaxime alone. When the patients stayed afebrile, the intravenous administration was replaced by oral treatment twice daily for 14 days, either with 500 mg pivampicillin and 400 mg pivmecillinam or 1 g cefadroxil. In the A + M group, 33% (48/144) of the patients did not complete the full course of treatment as compared with 32% (47/149) in the cephalosporin group, the reasons being treatment failure in 27 and 29, respectively, or adverse effects ($n = 16$ in both groups). The median duration of fever was 47 h in the A + M group and 50 h in the cephalosporin group. Of 135 patients with pneumonia, 68% were completely cured in the A + M group, and 65% in the cephalosporin group, the main reasons for treatment failure being Mycoplasma pneumonia or ornithosis. Of 136 patients with pyelonephritis, 63% were cured in each group. The main reason for failure was bacteriological relapse. Side-effects were reported by 32 patients (22%) of the A + M group, as compared with 41 (28%) of the cephalosporin group. Epigastric complaints were equally frequent in both groups, but there was a tendency for a higher frequency of exanthema in the A + M group, and for antibiotic-associated diarrhoea and fungal superinfections in the cephalosporin group.

S. Cronberg, MD, Department of Infectious Diseases, Malmö General Hospital, S-214 01 Malmö, Sweden

INTRODUCTION

Mecillinam is highly active against Gram-negative enterobacteria (1–3), and is excellent for the treatment of acute pyelonephritis (4, 5). Acute septicaemia requires empirical therapy with antibiotics that also cover Gram-positive bacteria. This can be achieved by using a combination of ampicillin with mecillinam which provides broad spectrum coverage and acts synergistically against many Gram-negative organisms. Cephalosporins are also indicated in these situations. We therefore compared the combination of ampicillin and mecillinam (A + M), first given intravenously and later orally, with intravenous cefotaxime followed by oral cefadroxil, for treatment of patients with symptoms of sepsis, high fever, and signs of pneumonia or pyelonephritis.

We wanted to enrol patients with suspected pneumonia or pyelonephritis whom we would normally treat with beta-lactam antibiotics, and to avoid the inclusion of patients with influenza not complicated with pneumonia. We also wanted to avoid inclusion of cases of Mycoplasma pneumonia infection, Legionnaire's disease, or ornithosis which all fail to respond to treatment with beta-lactam antibiotics. Since ampicillin and mecillinam exert no effect on staphylococci, we also tried to avoid including patients in whom the febrile disease was associated with osteomyelitis, septic arthritis or soft tissue infection.

For unbiased evaluation, a double-blind design was adopted. To detect relapse, the last follow-up was to be 2 weeks after the end of treatment. To simulate routine clinical conditions, where empirical treatment is started on a presumptive diagnosis, all the results were to be evaluated according to an intention-to-treat approach. To obtain a sufficiently large series, the trial was performed as a multicentre study.

METHODS

Study design

This was a multicentre, prospective, randomized, double-blind, parallel group comparison, at the departments of infectious diseases in 7 Swedish hospitals. Each centre provided a mean of 42 patients (range 20–54).

Sample size

We aimed to enrol at least 270 patients in the trial to detect a difference of 15% with a power of 80% (type II error, beta = 0.20) and a 5% level of significance (type I error, alpha = 0.05), with a presumptive curve rate of 80%.

Randomization

Randomization was performed with a computer-generated, random numbers table. Each participating centre received trial medication in blocks of 6, each block containing 3 treatments with Miraxid® and 3 treatments with cefotaxime/cefadroxil.

Inclusion criteria

The inclusion criteria were symptoms of sepsis with fever ≥38.5°C, and clinical signs and symptoms suggestive of acute pneumonia or pyelonephritis, in patients ≥18 years of age and with no history of impaired renal function, HIV infection, leukopenia or treatment with cytotoxic drugs. Patients known to be infected with bacteria resistant to the A + M combination or cefotaxime were excluded.

Withdrawal

Voluntary withdrawal. Patients were informed that they were free to withdraw from the study at any time and for any reason.

Treatment failure. Treatment could be changed at the discretion of the investigator when an unsatisfactory therapeutic response made treatment with an alternative antibiotic desirable.

Adverse effect. Treatment could be interrupted or changed at the discretion of the investigator in the event of an unacceptable side-effect attributable to the test drugs.

Treatment

Patients were randomly assigned to treatment with either ampicillin + mecillinam given intravenously followed by oral treatment with pivampicillin + pivmecillinam for 14 days, or intravenous treatment with cefotaxime followed by oral treatment with cefadroxil for 14 days. Drug administration was double-blind.

Intravenous phase. Miraxid, 900 mg (600 mg ampicillin plus 300 mg mecillinam, Leo, Copenhagen, Denmark) or 1,000 mg cefotaxime (Claforan®, Hoechst, Stockholm, Sweden) packed in indistinguishable vials.

Oral phase. This was Miraxid tablets of 450 mg (250 mg pivampicillin plus 200 mg pivmecillinam) or cefadroxil capsules of 400 mg (Cefamox®, Bristol-Myers, Stockholm, Sweden) and matching placebos (double-dummy technique).

Administration. In the intravenous phase, 2 vials were given twice daily until the patient's rectal temperature stayed normal (≤37.5°C in the morning and ≤38°C in the afternoon) for a full 30-h period. In the oral phase, 2 tablets of Miraxid or 2 capsules of cefadroxil were given twice daily for a fixed period of 14 days.

Evaluation of efficacy and safety

All decisions concerning classification and evaluation of efficacy and safety were made before the randomization code was broken. We used an intention-to-treat approach. All patients were included in the evaluation of safety. Efficacy was evaluated both in the series as a whole and in pneumonia and pyelonephritis subgroups. Acute pneumonia was defined as symptoms of sepsis accompanied by fever with symptoms and signs of acute respiratory infection and radiographic signs of infiltrates in the lung compatible with pneumonia. Acute pyelonephritis was defined as fever, symptoms and signs suggestive of pyelonephritis, and bacteriuria (≥10^7 colony forming units (cfu). Patients whose treatment was interrupted because of adverse events were still evaluated for efficacy if they had received no other antibiotic.

Patients were followed daily during hospitalization, once during the oral phase and 14 days after the end of oral treatment.

The variables of particular interest were as follows: in the series as a whole, the number of patients who stopped treatment due to side effects or therapeutic failure, and the number of intravenous doses actually given (as the duration of i.v. therapy was dependent on febrile response); in the pneumonia subgroup, duration of fever, clinical and radiographic cure, and any relapse; and in the pyelonephritis subgroup, duration of fever, clinical cure, and recurrence of bacteriuria.

Safety criteria. Knowledge of adverse events was obtained from spontaneous reports and by asking the patients for any complaints.

Laboratory variables. The laboratory variables followed were haemoglobin, WBC count, platelet count, and the serum concentrations of bilirubin (total), alkaline phosphatase, aspartate aminotransferase (ASAT), alanine aminotransferase (ALAT), and creatinine. All changes from baseline (admission) values were noted.

Bacteriological evaluation

Urine culture. Clean, voided midstream urine samples were examined at admission, during treatment and 2 weeks after the end of treatment. Examination included identification of pathogens, quantification and susceptibility testing. Only cultures ≥10^7 cfu/l were considered significant.

Blood culture. Three blood cultures were performed at admission, and in the event of treatment change because of therapeutic failure. All aerobic and anaerobic pathogens were identified and tested for susceptibility to ampicillin, mecillinam, Miraxid, cefotaxime, co-trimoxazole, gentamicin and VBD 2085 (pivampicillin plus brobactam) using Biodisk equipment, Stockholm, Sweden).

Resistant isolates were tested for beta-lactamase production using the nitrocefin test.

Chest X-ray

A chest X-ray was performed at admission and, in the case of abnormality, was repeated after the end of treatment.

Temperature

Body temperature was recorded on admission, and every morning and afternoon during hospitalization. Temperature was measured rectally. If any other measurement was used, the temperature was converted to rectal temperature.

Statistics

Group and sub-group differences in sex distribution, suspected diagnosis, and clinical signs of septicaemia were analysed using the chi-squared test, differences in age with the ANOVA F-test, and differences in duration of the present episode and in temperature at initiation of treatment with the Kruskal–Wallis test. Efficacy variables were analysed with the Wilcoxon test or Fisher's exact test, as appropriate. Duration of fever was analysed by comparison of Kaplan–Meier curves for the 2 treatment groups, using the log-rank test.

RESULTS

Patients characteristics

Of 293 patients presenting with fever (≥38.5°C, mean 39.4°) (1 patient from the original series was excluded

Table I. *Treatment summary for 293 patients*[a]

	Ampicillin plus mecillinam	Cephalosporin
Assigned to treatment	144	149
Interrupted course because of therapeutic failure	27	29
Interrupted course because of adverse events	16	16
Interrupted course for other reasons	5	2
Completed course	96	102

[a] One patient of the original 294 was excluded because of absence of fever.

owing to absence of fever), 144 were randomly assigned to treatment with the ampicillin plus mecillinam combination (A + M) and 149 to treatment with cephalosporins (cefotaxime and cefadroxil) (Table I). The 2 groups were well matched with regard to mean age (61 years in both), and mean body weight (70 vs. 72 kg). The frequency of concomitant disorders was similar in the 2 groups (diabetes mellitus 8 vs. 9%; cardiovascular disease 39 vs. 36%), as was previous treatment for malignancy (8 vs. 10%). Also 63 vs. 54% were on concomitant drug treatment, 28 vs. 22% had undergone antibiotic treatment within the preceding 4-week period, and there was a similar preponderance of women inboth groups (56 vs. 57%).

Pneumonia was diagnosed in 135 cases and pyelonephritis in 136 cases; 15 patients with clinical symptoms, pulmonary infiltrates and bacteriuria suggesting the coexistence of the 2 diseases were included in both groups. In 37 patients, neither pneumonia nor pyelonephritis was diagnosed. Bacteraemia was present in 29 patients in the A + M group and in 34 patients in the cephalosporin group. The bacteria most frequently found were Escherichia coli (32 cases overall, 13 vs. 19) and Streptococcus pneumoniae (15 cases overall, 9 vs. 6). The remaining patients with suspected pneumonia manifested no radiological evidence of pulmonary infiltration, because some of them might have had influenza. In some patients with suspected pyelonephritis, significant bacteriuria was not found. A few patients had tonsillitis, erysipelas, cholecystitis, or diverticulitis. Two patients had lung cancer, and 1 had lung embolus.

Duration of fever

The median duration of fever was 47 h (mean 2.8 days) in the A + M group and 50 h (mean 2.8 days) in the cephalosporin group (Fig. 1). The mean number of intravenous doses given was 7.5 in the A + M group and 7.9 in the cephalosporin group. Neither of these differences was significant.

Interrupted treatment

Treatment was interrupted (Table I) in 33% (48/144) of the patients in the A + M group and in 32% (47/149) of the cephalosporin group (odds ratio, OR, 1.09, 95% confidence interval, CI, 0.66–1.77), due to therapeutic failure ($n = 27$ vs. $n = 29$, OR 0.96, 95% CI 0.53–1.71), or side-effects ($n = 16$ in each group, OR 1.04, 95% CI 0.50–2.17), or for other reasons ($n = 2$).

Deaths

Two patients in each group died, postmortem being performed in all four cases. A 46-year old woman with systemic lupus erythematosus died of myocardial infarction on the third day of A + M treatment for pneumonia and (S. pneumoniae) septicaemia; an 87-year old woman died of

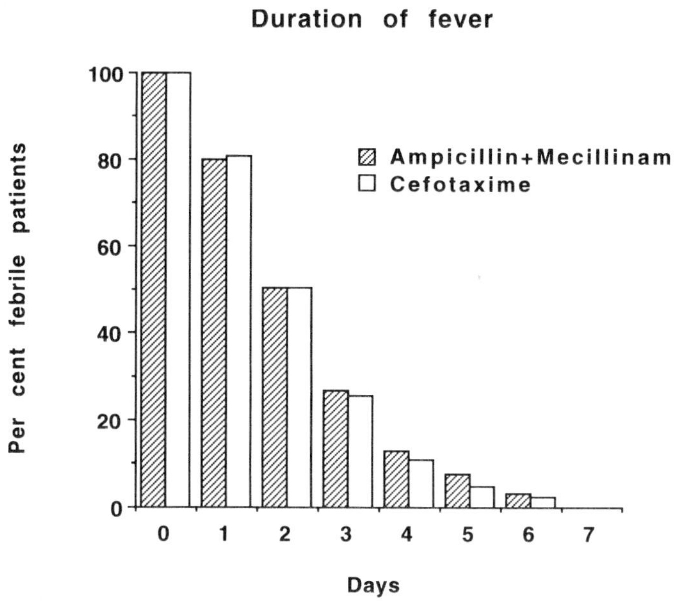

Fig. 1. Duration of fever in patients with pneumonia and pyelonephritis.

Table II. *Adverse events*

	Ampicillin plus mecillinam (n = 144)	Cephalosporin (n = 149)
Exanthema	12	6
Nausea, vomiting, epigastric pain	11	10
Diarrhoea	4	11
(Interrupted treatment	1	6)
Stomatitis, vulvovaginitis urethritis,	3	6
Thrombophlebitis	2	4
Other events	0	4
Total	32	41

myocardial infarction and heart failure while on oral A + M treatment 8 days after inclusion for pneumonia; an 85-year old man with a previous myocardial infarction died on the 3rd day of cefotaxime treatment for pneumonia; and an 88-year old man died of myocardial infarction on the 4th day of cefotaxime treatment for pneumonia.

Adverse events

Adverse events were reported (Table II) by 73 patients (25%), 32 in the A + M group and 41 in the cephalosporin (OR 0.75, 95% CI 0.44–1.28).

Exanthema occurred in 12 and 6 patients, respectively (OR 2.17, 95% CI 0.79–5.94). Antibiotic-associated bacterial or fungal superinfection tended to be more frequent in the cephalosporin group, diarrhoea being reported by 11 patients of whom 6 stopped medication, as compared with only 4 patients in the A + M group (OR 0.36, 95% CI 0.11–1.15) of whom one stopped treatment. Clostridium difficile diarrhoea was diagnosed in three patients, all in the cephalosporin group. Fungal superinfection giving rise to stomatitis, vulvovaginitis or urethritis occurred in 6 patients in the cephalosporin group, but with only 3 in the A + M group (OR 0.51, 95% CI 0.12–2.07). The frequency of nausea, vomiting or epigastric pain was similar in the 2 groups (7 vs. 8%). Thrombophlebitis occurred in 4 patients in the cephalosporin group, and in 2 of the A + M group.

In each group abnormal laboratory values were normalized to the same extent.

Table III. *Treatment results in pneumonia (135 patients)*

	Ampicillin plus mecillinam	Cephalosporin
n	73	62
Failure because of mycoplasma or ornithosis	7	5
Non-evaluable	3	2
Failure	10	10
Relapse	3	5
Complete cure	50	40

Table IV. *Urine culture*

Pathogen	Ampicillin plus mecillinam (n = 144)	Cephalosporin (n = 149)
Escherichia coli	49	58
Klebsiella spp.	5	3
Proteus mirabilis	2	6
Pseudomonas aeruginosa	2	1
Unspecified Gram-negative rods	5	6
Enterococci	2	3
Staphylococcus spp.	4	3
Citrobacter	0	1
Enterobacter	2	2
Proteus vulgaris	1	0
Salmonella	1	0

Pneumonia

In the patient with pneumonia (Table III), complete cures were obtained in 68% of those treated with A + M and in 64% of those treated with cephalosporins (OR 1.20, 95% CI 0.58–2.45). S. pneumoniae was a frequent cause of pneumonia, and those so affected were cured equally well in both treatment groups, whereas treatment failed in all 12 patients with ornithosis or Mycoplasma pneumoniae infections.

The median duration of fever was 48 h (mean 3.1 days) among those treated with A + M, and 42 h (mean 2.7 days) among those treated with cephalosporins, and the mean total number of i.v. injections was 8.5 and 7.5, respectively.

Pyelonephritis

E. coli was the commonest pathogen in urine cultures, being present in 107 patients (Table IV). Complete cures were obtained in 63% of both treatment groups (OR 0.99, 95% CI 0.49–1.98); treatment failure occurred in 3 of those treated with A + M and in 6 of those treated with cephalosporins, and bacteriological relapse occurred in 16 and 29 cases, respectively (OR 0.89, 95% CI 0.41–1.93) (see Table V).

The median duration of fever was 51 h in both treatment groups (mean 2.7 days in the A + M group vs. 2.9 days in the cephalosporin group), and the mean total number of i.v. injections was 7.4 and 7.9, respectively.

Table V. *Treatment results in pyelonephritis (136 patients)*

	Ampicillin plus mecillinam	Cephalosporin
n	65	71
Non-evaluable	5	1
Failure	3	6
Relapse	16	20
Complete cure	41	45

Table VI. *Blood culture*

Pathogen	Ampicillin plus mecillinam ($n = 144$)	Cephalosporin ($n = 149$)
Streptococcus pneumoniae	9	6
Staphylococcus epidermidis	4	3
Staphylococcus aureus	1	1
Escherichia coli	13	19
Haemophilus influenzae	1	1
Klebsiella pneumoniae	1	0
Proteus mirabilis	0	1
Acinetobacter spp.	0	2
Corynebacterium	0	1
Total	29	34

Relapse with fully sensitive E. coli occurred in 23% of the A + M group and in 25% of the cephalosporin group. Only 5 beta-lactamase-producing strains were found, 2 in the A + M group and 3 in the cephalosporin group, one patient being cured in each group. In only a few patients were radiological lesions found which might have predisposed to recurrence.

In patients who had fever for only 1–2 days (treated with a mean of 5.9 intravenous doses), treatment was successful with eradication of bacteria without relapse in 58%, whereas in patients with fever for ≥ 3 days without change of therapy (treated with a mean of 9.0 intravenous doses), 78% were completely cured ($p = 0.02$).

Septicaemia

Bacteraemia was present in 63 patients (22%) (Table VI). S. pneumonia was a common pathogen in patients with pneumonia, being present in 9 patients on A + M treatment (8 cures and 1 treatment failure) and in 6 patients on cephalosporins (4 cures and 2 treatment failures). Mean duration of fever was 3.0 days in the A + M group and 3.3 days in the cephalosporin group; the mean number of i.v. injections given was 9.3 and 17, respectively

E. coli was grown from blood cultured from 32 patients, 12 in the A + M group (7 cures and 2 treatment failures or recurrences), and 20 in the cephalsporin group (13 cures and 6 treatment failures or relapse). Mean duration of fever was 3.6 days in the A + M group and 4.0 days in the cephalosporin group, the mean number of i.v. injections given being 9.6 and 10.3, respectively

Other diagnoses

Of the 37 patients with diagnoses other than pneumonia or pyelonephritis, 19 completed the course of treatment, which was successful in 17 cases, 5 stopped treatment owing to adverse events, and 13 discontinued because of treatment failure or rediagnosis.

Some patients with respiratory tract infection had only influenza and healed rapidly. Cures were obtained in most of the patients with suspected urinary tract infection who might have had pyelonephritis, though there was no significant growth of bacteria in cultures of the urine. Two patients with cholecystitis were cured, whereas treatment was changed in 2 patients with diverticulitis, in 2 with tonsillitis and in 2 with erysipelas.

DISCUSSION

The purpose of this trial was not to show the superiority of the ampicillin plus mecillinam combination over the cephalosporins, cefotaxime and cefadroxil, but to create test conditions favouring the detection of differences between the 2 regimens in therapeutic effect and adverse events. Thus, treatment was discontinued owing to treatment failure or adverse events in as many as 1/3 of our patients, in contrast to other trials of new antibiotics where cure rates of 80–90% are obtained. In many investigations, only patients infected with susceptible organisms are included, patients are excluded from evaluation in the event of changes in antibiotic treatment, and the patients are assessed only during treatment and immediately afterwards, before relapse has had time to develop. In earlier studies by our group, a similarly high incidence of bacterial relapse to that in the present study was found in patients with acute septic pyelonephritis (5, 6). Sandberg et al. (7) found, however, a higher bacteriological cure rate with norfloxacin than with cefadroxil.

Our aim was to enrol patients in the acute septic phase and follow them under clinical conditions which were as realistic as possible. As pneumonia and pyelonephritis are the two most fequent causes of septicaemia in the elderly, and may be difficult to distinguish at admission, initial treatment must cover both conditions, a criterion satisfied both by the ampicillin plus mecillinam combination and cefotaxime.

Whereas many investigations designed to compare the efficacy of antibiotics have included such readily cured conditions as uncomplicated bronchitis and cystitis, we wanted to study patients with symptoms of sepsis and high fever. Of the 293 patients, not less than 22% were found to have a positive blood culture, and were thus suffering from severe infections.

According to the study design, overall analysis of the series as a whole was to be based on crude variables, such as the number of treatment courses completed or of treatment discontinued owing to adverse events, therapeutic failure or for other reasons. Patient groups with pneumonia or pyelonephritis were then to be analysed, using more subtle variables. In the event, both types of analysis yielded similar results, suggesting that the findings were clinically valid.

Both regimens were equally efficient in the treatment of acute pneumonia or pyelonephritis. The duration of fever was comparable in both treatment groups, as was the number of patients who discontinued treatment owing to adverse events.

As expected, the A + M group was associated with more cases of exanthema, whereas in the cephalosporin group there were more cases of antibiotic-associated diarrhoea, often due to C. difficile, and more cases of fungal superinfection causing stomatitis, vulvovaginitis and urethritis. Diarrhoea and fungal infections taken together gave an OR of 0.40 (95% CI 0.16–0.99). The findings are consistent with those reported by others (8).

Although pivmecillinam and pivampicillin have been reported to reduce the serum carnitine concentrations (9), none of our patients reported any symptoms compatible with carnitine deficiency.

Pneumonia and septicaemia caused by S. pneumoniae responded just as well in both treatment groups, as did pyelonephritis and septicaemia caused by susceptible strains of E. coli. However, bacteriological relapse was also quite common in both treatment groups, affecting 25% of patients.

As mecillinam is highly active against E. coli but less stable than cefotaxime against beta-lactamases of the TEM type, we wanted to ascertain whether mecillinam cures infections caused by beta-lactamase-producing strains. Unfortunately, however, only 5 such strains were isolated, 3 in the A + M group and 2 in the cephalosporin group, 1 case in each group being cured.

ACKNOWLEDGEMENT

The study was supported by a grant from Leo Pharmaceuticals.

REFERENCES

1. Neu HC. Synergy of mecillinam, a beta-amidinopenicillanic acid derivative, combined with beta-lactam antibiotics. Antimicrob Agents Chemother 10: 535–542, 1976.
2. Spratt BG. The mechanism of action of mecillinam. J Antimicrob Chemother 3: 13–19, 1977.
3. Kramer MJ, Mauriz YR, Timmes MD, Robertson TL, Cleeland R. Morphologic changes produced by amidinocillin alone in combination with beta-lactam antibiotics: in vitro and in vivo. Am J Med 75: 30–41, 1983.
4. Ekwall E, Scheja A, Cronberg S, Ganrot-Norlin K, Jonsson M, Juhlin I, Kahlmeter G, Thorén A, Thulin KE, Tunevall G. Mecillinam and ampicillin separately or combined in gram-negative septicemia. Infection 8: 37–40, 1980.
5. Ode B, Flamholc L, Walder M, Cronberg S. Intravenous mecillinam, trimethoprim and ampicillin in acute pyelonephritis. Drugs Exper Clin Res 9: 337–343, 1981.
6. Ode B, Cronberg S, Bröms M, Walder M. Failure of excessive doses of ampicillin to prevent bacterial relapse in the treatment of acute pyelonephritis. Acta Med Scand 207: 305–307, 1980.
7. Sandberg T, Englund G, Lincoln K, Nilsson L-G. Randomised double-blind study of norfloxacin and cefadroxil in the treatment of acute pyelonephritis. Eur J Clin Microbiol Infect Dis 9: 317–323, 1990.
8. de Lalla F, Privitera G, Ortisi G, Rizzardini G, Santoro D, Pagano A, Rinaldi E, Scarpellini P. Third generation cephalosporins as a risk factor for Clostridium difficile-associated disease: a four-year survey in a general hospital. J Antimicrob Chemother 23: 623–631, 1989.
9. Holme E. Carnitine deficiency induced by pivampicillin and pivmecillinam therapy. Lancet 2: 469–473, 1989.

Submitted October 25, 1994; accepted June 22, 1995

In Vivo and In Vitro Study of Several Pharmacodynamic Effects of Meropenem

F. FUENTES, M. M. MARTÍN, J. IZQUIERDO, M. L. GOMEZ-LUS and J. PRIETO

From the Department of Microbiology, Faculty of Medicine, Complutense University of Madrid, Madrid, Spain

Several pharmacodynamic parameters are being studied and applied to the design of dosage regimens. The thigh infection model in neutropenic mice has been used in this study to investigate the in vivo postantibiotic effect (PAE) of meropenem against S. aureus, E. coli and P. aeruginosa. The sub-minimum inhibitory concentration (sub-MIC) postantibiotic effect (PA SME) of 1/2, 1/4 and 1/8 × MIC was also determined in vitro on S. aureus and E. coli after pre-exposure of these microorganisms to 10 × MIC of meropenem. The in vitro PAE was also determined. In vivo killing curves using 2 different short dosage regimens were also studied to relate the lethal effect to the time that serum levels were above the MIC. No significant in vivo and in vitro PAEs were observed. The PA SMEs were higher for S. aureus than for E. coli. The 2 short dosage regimens, in vivo, were equally effective in killing S. aureus, but not E. coli. These results suggest that the pharmacodynamics of meropenem on Gram-negative strains may need further study to elucidate the mechanisms and characteristics of these parameters. On the other hand, we need to standardize a reliable in vitro method to monitor regrowth with a good correlation with the in vivo conditions.

J. Prieto Prieto, MD, Department of Microbiology, Faculty of Medicine, Complutense University, Ciudad Universitaria, Av. Complutense s/n, E-28040 Madrid, Spain

INTRODUCTION

The postantibiotic effect (PAE) has been studied since Bigger observed a delay in the growth of microorganisms which had been exposed to penicillin (1). This phenomenon has an obvious clinical interest, since the antibacterial agents which induce high PAEs would allow longer intervals between administrations without a loss in effectiveness. These effects depend on the type of microorganism and the kind of antimicrobial agent.

The PAE has been studied both in vitro and in vivo. Only 6 animal models have been much employed to determine the duration of the in vivo PAE: experimental endocarditis in rats (2); the tissue cage model in rabbits (3); the thigh infection model in neutropenic mice (4); pneumonia in mice (5); meningitis in rabbits (6), and infected subcutaneous threads in mice (7). The thigh infection model in neutropenic mice is widely employed in the investigation of this phenomenon, and it is faster and less laborious than others. In this technique the thigh muscle can be easily removed and homogenized, and the levels of the antimicrobial agent in the muscle have been found to closely approximate those observed in serum (8). The immunological system is usually suppressed by cyclophosphamide.

We have previously reported a significant PAE for aminoglycosides using this model (9), and other authors have also observed long values for other groups of antimicrobial agents, such as quinolones or macrolides (10). In the group of β-lactam antibiotics only imipenem has shown a significant in vitro or in vivo PAE against Gram-negative strains (4, 11–13), although absence of this effect has also been reported (2). Meropenem is a new carbapenem and as well as imipenem, it has also induced longer in vitro PAEs than other new β-lactams (14–17). However, other authors have reported non-significant values using different methods to determine the in vitro PAE (18, 19). We have previously pointed out an absence of this effect both in vivo and in vitro (20). The in vivo PAE has been studied only with Staphylococcus aureus (21) and Pseudomonas aeruginosa (22), but significant values were only observed with the latter strain.

Another pharmacodynamic effect related to the PAE has also been described. The in vitro effect of sub-minimum inhibitory concentrations (sub-MICs) on bacteria pre-exposed (PA SME) or not pre-exposed (SME) to supra-MIC concentrations (3, 23) has been invoked, together with the PAE, to explain the success of some intermittent dosing regimens (18). The effect of sub-inhibitory concentrations of meropenem on several strains has also been reported, but sub-MICs only had significant effects on P. aeruginosa in the PAE phase (18).

We have studied the in vivo PAE of meropenem against standard strains of S. aureus, Escherichia coli and P. aeruginosa using the thigh infection model in neutropenic mice. The in vitro PA SME and PAE of E. coli and S. aureus were performed using the viable counting method. In vivo killing curves with E. coli and S. aureus using 2 different dosing regimens of meropenem were also investigated to evaluate whether bactericidal activity is related to the length of time above MIC, as other authors have reported for other β-lactams (24).

The study of these pharmacodynamic parameters could affect the dosing design of this antibiotic, since longer dosing intervals could be used if the PAE and the sub-MIC activity prevent bacterial regrowth.

 ISSN 0036-5548

MATERIALS AND METHODS

Antimicrobial agent and microorganisms

Meropenem was obtained from ICI-Pharma SA (Madrid, Spain) as reference powder with known potency. Stocks were made on the day of experiments by dilution in distilled water. The MICs of all strains were determined by the broth macrodilution method (25) in Mueller–Hinton (MH) broth. The determination of minimum bactericidal concentrations (MBCs) were performed on MH agar the day after the experiment, using standard methods (25).

The microorganisms used in this study were S. aureus, Escherichia coli and P. aeruginosa (ATCC 25923, 25922 and 27853, respectively).

Animals

Female BALB-c mice, weighing 26–28 g were used for pharmacokinetic and thigh infection studies. Mice were rendered neutropenic by injecting cyclophosphamide (Funk Laboratories, Spain), 150 and 100 mg/kg ip 1 and 3 days prior to infection (4).

In vitro postantibiotic sub-MIC effect (PA SME) and in vitro PAE

These experiments were performed in triplicate only for E. coli and S. aureus. The microorganisms (10^7 cfu/ml in MH broth) were exposed for 1 h to meropenem (10 × MIC) at 37°C in a shaking incubator. Since a high initial number of microorganisms was required to re-expose them to the sub-MICs, the antimicrobial agent was removed by centrifugation (5 min at 1,200*g*). Unexposed control cultures were also centrifuged. Then the treated cultures were divided into 4 tubes, and meropenem at concentrations of 1/2 × MIC, 1/4 × MIC and 1/8 × MIC were added to 3 of them. The fourth tube was not re-exposed to sub-MICs (PAE curve). All these cultures (including the unexposed control) were incubated at 37°C for another 7 h, and samples were withdrawn every h for counting. The PA SME values were calculated using the formula (18):

$$\text{PA SME} = T_{PA} - C$$

where T_{PA} is the time for the pre-exposed cultures, exposed to different sub-MICs, to increase by 1 $\log_{10}$ above the number of cfu present immediately after drug removal, and C is the corresponding time for the unexposed control cultures.

The in vitro PAEs were calculated using this formula, and the growth curves of pre-exposed cultures not exposed to sub-MICs.

Pharmacokinetics

After a subcutaneous administration of meropenem (10 × MBC mg/kg) to the mice (3 mice/group), the blood was collected from the retroorbital sinus at 5, 15, 30, 45, 60 and 75 min. The possible serum activity was assayed using a group of 3 control mice to which saline solution was administered.

Plasma drug levels were determined by using a standard agar well diffusion assay, with E. coli (ATCC 25922) as indicator microorganism (26). The area under the curve, concentration–time, and the half-life, as well as the length of time that serum levels exceeded the MIC were calculated with a BASIC subroutine, on the basis of a one-compartment open model. All assays were performed at least 3 times, and the arithmetic mean and its standard error were used as statistical parameters.

In vivo postantibiotic effect

The in vivo PAEs were determined for E. coli, P. aeruginosa and S. aureus, in accordance with the experimental procedure of Gudmundsson et al. (4), as follows. On the day of the experiment (day 4) 0.1 ml of MH broth with a bacterial suspension in a log phase of growth were injected into one thigh in all neutropenic mice. The inoculum was standardized by using a spectrophotometer (model U.1100, Hitachi) to give a $T_{580\ nm}$ value of 85–90% corresponding to 10^6–10^7 cfu/ml. At time 0, 2 h later, 0.2 ml of saline solution with 10 × MBC mg/kg of meropenem were injected s.c. into the treated group. Saline solution was administered to the control group in the same conditions. Three or 4 animals of the treated and control groups were then killed, every h for the first 4 h, and then every 2 h up to 10 h after drug administration. At each sampling time thigh muscles were removed and immediately homogenized in 9 ml of ice-cold 0.85% NaCl, and the viable counts were determined on MH agar plates.

The in vivo PAE was calculated using the formula:

$$\text{PAE} = T - C$$

according to Renneberg & Walder (7), where T is the time required for the mean count of cfu in the thighs of treated mice to increase by one $\log_{10}$ above its value at the time that the antibiotic concentration in serum fell below the MIC. C is the time required for the mean count of cfu in the thighs of control mice to increase by one $\log_{10}$ above the viable count at time 0.

In vivo killing curves

These assays were performed only with E. coli and S. aureus. On the day of the experiment, the mice were infected as described above. At time 0, 2 h later, they were divided in 3 groups with 3 different treatments.

Treatment A: This comprised 20 mg/kg of meropenem s.c., every 3 h in the E. coli assay (at 0, 3, 6 and 9 h), and every 2.5 h with S. aureus (at 0, 2.5, 5 and 7.5 h). These periods were the times that the serum levels of meropenem exceeded the MICs of these microorganisms.

Treatment B: This was 40 mg/kg every 6 h in the E. coli assay (at 0 and 6 h), and every 5 h with S. aureus (at 0 and 5 h). These periods were twice those used in treatment A.

Controls: These were allowed to grow without antimicrobial treatment.

Procedure: At each sampling time during the next 10 h, the thigh muscles were removed and immediately homogenized as described above, and viable counts were determined on MH agar plates. The in vivo lethal effect (LE) was expressed as the $\log_{10}$ difference between each treatment curve and non-treated control, at the end of the experiment.

RESULTS

Minimal inhibitory and bactericidal concentrations

The MICs and MBCs of meropenem against the 3 strains are shown in Table I. The MBC was the same for E. coli and S. aureus, and the highest value (2 mg/l) corresponded to P. aeruginosa.

In vitro postantibiotic sub-MIC effect (PA SME) and in vitro PAE

The PA SME values of several sub-MIC concentrations of meropenem for E. coli and S. aureus are shown in Table II. The highest value corresponds to 1/2 × MIC against S. aureus (2.85 h), decreasing to 1.14 h for 1/8 × MIC. A low value was observed for E. coli with 1/2 × MIC, smaller than those with 1/4 or 1/8 × MIC, and significantly lower than for S. aureus.

Table I. *Dose, pharmacokinetic parameters (AUC, half-life and time above MIC) and in vivo PAEs of meropenem against E. coli, S. aureus and P. aeruginosa*

Microorganism	MIC mg/l	MBC mg/l	Dose mg/kg	AUC mg h/l	Half-life h	Time above MIC h	In vivo PAE h
E. coli, ATCC 25922	0.03	0.06	0.60	0.11	0.32	0.90	0.30 ± 0.2
S. aureus, ATCC 25923	0.06	0.06	0.60	0.11	0.32	0.77	0.10 ± 0.5
P. aeruginosa, ATCC 27853	2	2	20	6.50	0.41	0.92	0.10 ± 0.4

MIC = minimum inhibitory concentration; MBC = minimum bactericidal concentration; AUC = area under the curve; PAE = postantibiotic effect.

Table II. *Time and concentration of pre-exposure, in vitro PAE, fraction of MIC added and postantibiotic sub-MIC effect (PA SME) of meropenem against E. coli and S. aureus*

Microorganism	Time of pre-exposure h	Concentration of pre-exposure mg/l	In vitro PAE h	Fraction of MIC added	PA SME h
E. coli, ATCC 25922	1	0.30	−0.1 ± 0.3	1/2	0.18 ± 0.3
				1/4	0.50 ± 0.4
				1/8	0.29 ± 0.3
S. aureus, ATCC 25923	1	0.60	0.3 ± 0.2	1/2	2.85 ± 0.5
				1/4	1.40 ± 0.4
				1/8	1.14 ± 0.6

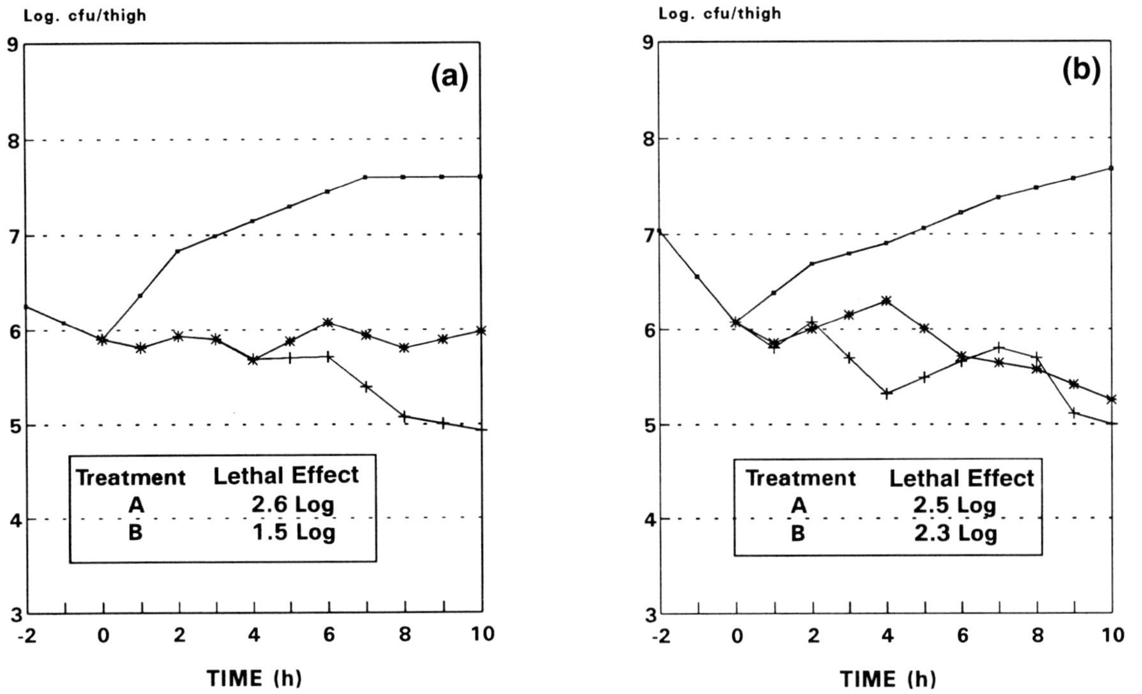

Fig. 1. In vivo killing curves and lethal effects of meropenem with 2 different dose schedules, against: a. E. coli (□ = control; + = treatment A, 20 mg/kg/3 h; * = treatment B, 40 mg/kg/6 h); b. S. aureus (□ = control; + = treatment A, 20 mg/kg/2.5 h; * = treatment B, 40 mg/kg/5 h).

The in vitro PAE values are also shown in Table II. No significant values were obtained against E. coli and S. aureus (<0.5 h).

In vivo postantibiotic effect

The PAE values of meropenem against E. coli, S. aureus and P. aeruginosa, and the pharmacokinetic parameters, are shown in Table I. No significant PAEs were observed against any microorganism, although all values were positive. The times that serum levels exceeded the MIC were around 45–55 min, giving a half-life of meropenem, in mice, of approximately 20–25 min. The greatest area under the curve (AUC) corresponds to the higher dose (20 mg/kg).

In vivo killing curves

The in vivo killing curves and the values of lethal effect (LE) are shown in Fig. 1. Treatment B was significantly less effective than treatment A for E. coli (Fig. 1A), with a difference of 1.1 $\log_{10}$. For S. aureus (Fig. 1B), treatments A and B were both significantly effective, with LE values of 2.3–2.5 $\log_{10}$. The total dose of meropenem was the same, but T > MIC was longer in treatment A than in treatment B.

DISCUSSION

Meropenem has been reported to induce significant PAEs in vitro against Gram-negative microorganisms, as well as imipenem (12, 14–17, 27). In vivo PAE studies of meropenem have also been reported, but with only 2 microorganisms: S. aureus (21) and P. aeruginosa (22). All these studies have been performed using the thigh infection model in neutropenic mice. Tanio & Fukasawa (22) found an in vivo PAE of 1.9 h with P. aeruginosa, while Mattie & Li-Chen (21) were only able to find a minimal delay in growth, which was not attributed to a true PAE. Our studies with P. aeruginosa were performed using the same dose as Tanio & Fukusawa but no significant PAE (0.1 h) was observed, even though our time of serum levels above the MIC (T > MIC) were similar to theirs. Meropenem also induced minimal and non-significant values with E. coli (0.3 h) and S. aureus (0.1 h) in our study, as Mattie & Li-Chen (21) also obtained with this latter strain. However, all these in vivo studies have been performed in mice, where there is a shorter half-life than in humans, and very short times of exposure to the antimicrobial agent (T > MIC) have been obtained with all the microorganisms assayed (Table I). It would be expected that the PAE would be increased in humans since the exposure would be longer.

The low number of in vivo studies makes comparison of in vivo and in vitro data difficult. On the other hand, it has recently been reported (28) that the viable count method should not be employed in the study of the PAE of this antimicrobial agent, owing to the inability to detect the growth of aberrant forms (spheroplasts) induced by meropenem. This would lead to an underestimation of the PAE values when this method is used, because these spheroplasts appear to have some clinical relevance (28). Other techniques to monitor bacterial growth kinetics are being offered, such as the use of the morphological technique, the bioluminescence assay of bacterial ATP or the measure of impedance (29), although further studies are required to determine how accurately these methods quantify the bacterial growth (28). However, when in vivo PAE studies are performed, these last 2 methods cannot be applied to monitor bacterial growth kinetics because they would measure the ATP of the animal tissue cells in which we have performed the assay or the impedance of metabolites produced by these same tissue cells. In addition, we have employed the thigh infection model to study the morphology of several microorganisms and have hardly any positive results (unpublished observations). A thorough purification of the sample would be required to ensure a correct level of bacterial cells when these methods were used, making the process very long and laborious. On the other hand, almost all the in vivo PAE results, including other β-lactam antibiotics, have been obtained using this standard technique (10) and this would increase its relevance in the study of this phenomenon.

Another parameter that can affect the duration of the in vivo PAE is the possible action of subinhibitory concentrations of the antimicrobial agent. The effect of sub-MICs on the growth of bacteria pre-exposed or not to suprainhibitory concentrations has been widely studied, in vitro and in vivo, with a variety of antimicrobial agents (aspoxicillin, vancomycin, roxithromycin, sparfloxacin, amikacin) (30–32). Antimicrobial agents with long PAEs and high bactericidal effects appear to have longer sub-MIC effects (23). The in vitro SMEs (sub-MIC effects) of some antibiotics are very low when comparing with PA SME (postantibiotic sub-MIC effects (23, 30). Meropenem has been reported to show a long in vitro PA SME and SME against some Gram-negative strains, such as P. aeruginosa, but only a small effect has been observed with E. coli (18). In our study we observed no in vitro PA SME with E. coli and a significant effect against S. aureus (1.14 h with 1/8 × MIC), which partly supports these results. No explanation has been given about the action of sub-MICs on these microorganisms, although differences between species may be involved (with new synthesis of PBPs, etc.) (32).

The in vivo action of these sub-MICs has been reported by Oshida et al. (30), who found that these residual concentrations would prolong the PAE in the case of aspoxicillin. We have previously reported that these sub-MICs would not be responsible for the long PAEs found with some aminoglycosides (9). However, these 2 studies have been performed using different models, and we think that a more standardized technique would be necessary to determine the in vivo relevance of this parameter.

The delay in the growth of microorganisms could also be affected by another important phenomenon. The bactericidal action of all antimicrobial agents appears to be related to one or several pharmacokinetic parameters (33). The activity of imipenem has been reported to be related to the time that serum levels exceed the MIC, and not to the total dose or high peak concentrations (24). In the present study, we have investigated this phenomenon with meropenem. The in vivo killing curves against S. aureus and E. coli were investigated using 2 different short dosing schedules, with the same total dose but different T > MIC. The lethal effect of treatment A (in which meropenem was always above the MIC) was significantly more effective when E. coli was assayed, but no important differences were observed with S. aureus (Fig. 1). We think that more than one pharmacokinetic parameter, such as T > MIC and high peak concentrations, would be related to the activity against this strain, but further studies with longer treatments would be necessary.

In conclusion, it seems from the data of the present study that meropenem would require a continuous administration against the microorganisms assayed to maintain serum levels above the MIC, because of its short in vivo PAE and PA SME, and the possible relation of activity to this pharmacokinetic parameter. On the other hand, the study of the PAE of this antibiotic is very method-dependent. As the viable counting method is not recommended for studying this phenomenon in vitro, but is necessary to determine the in vivo PAE, we think that the nature of the PAE of meropenem needs further consideration, to establish a reliable in vitro technique which best correlates with the in vivo conditions. Only when we find accurate methods to quantify these pharmacodynamic effects, can we use these phenomena to decide the dosage design of this antimicrobial agent.

REFERENCES

1. Bigger JW. The bactericidal action of penicillin on Staphylococcus pyogenes. Irish J Med Sci 227: 533–568, 1944.
2. Hesen MT, Pitsakis PG, Levison ME. Absence of postantibiotic effect in experimental Pseudomonas endocarditis treated with imipenem, with or without gentamicin. J Infect Dis 158: 542–548, 1988.
3. Odenholt I, Holm SE, Cars O. Effects of supra and sub-MIC benzylpenicillin concentrations on group A β-haemolytic streptococci during the postantibiotic phase in vivo. J Antimicrob Chemother 26: 193–201, 1990.
4. Gudmundsson S, Vogelman B, Craig WA. The in vivo postantibiotic effect of imipenem and other new antimicrobials. J Antimicrob Chemother 18 (Suppl E): 67–73, 1986.
5. Craig WA, Redington J, Ebert SC. Pharmacodynamics of amikacin in vitro and in mouse thigh and lung infections. J Antimicrob Chemother 27 (Suppl C): 29–40, 1991.
6. Sande MA, Korzeniowski OM, Allegro GM, Brennan RO, Zak O, Scheld WM. Intermittent or continuous therapy of experimental meningitis due to S. pneumoniae in rabbits: preliminary observations on the postantibiotic effect in vivo. Rev Infect Dis 3: 98–109, 1981.
7. Renneberg J, Walder M. Postantibiotic effects of imipenem, norfloxacin and amikacin in vitro and in vivo. Antimicrob Agents Chemother 33: 1714–1720, 1989.
8. Ryan D, Cars O. Antibiotic assays in muscle: are conventional tissue levels misleading as indicators of the antibacterial activity? Scand J Infect Dis 12: 307–309, 1980.
9. Minguez F, Izquierdo J, Martin MM, Fuentes F, Prieto J. In vivo postantibiotic effect of isepamicin and other aminoglycosides in a thigh infection model in neutropenic mice. Chemotherapy 38: 179–184, 1992.
10. Craig WA, Gudmundsson S. The postantibiotic effect. In: Lorian V, ed. Antibiotics in laboratory medicine, 3rd edn. Baltimore: Williams and Wilkins, 403–431, 1991.
11. Bustamante CI, Drusano GL, Tatem BA, Standiford HC. Postantibiotic effect of imipenem on P. aeruginosa. Antimicrob Agents Chemother 26: 678–682, 1984.
12. Nadler HL, Pitkin DH, Sheikh W. The postantibiotic effect of meropenem and imipenem on selected bacteria. J Antimicrob Chemother 24 (Suppl A): 225–232, 1989.
13. Odenholt I, Isaksson B, Nilsson L, Cars O. Postantibiotic and bactericidal effect of imipenem against Pseudomonas aeruginosa. Eur J Clin Microbiol Infect Dis 8: 136–141, 1989.
14. Ferrara A, Dos-Santos C, Pirina P. Postantibiotic effect of meropenem alone or in combination with gentamicin or sparfloxacin. Recent advances in chemotherapy. Proceedings of the 18th International Congress of Chemotherapy, Stockholm 1993, 170–171, 1994.
15. Hanberger H, Nilsson LE, Svensson E, Nilsson M. Pharmacodynamic effects of imipenem and meropenem on non-growing and growing gram-negative bacteria: initial killing and postantibiotic effect. J Chemother 5 (Suppl 1): 119–120, 1993.
16. Debbia EA, Molinari G, Pesce A, Schito GC. Antibacterial activity of meropenem in combination with other drugs and postantibiotic effect. J Chemother 5 (Suppl 1): 114–117, 1993.
17. Nadler HL, Sheikh W. A comparison of the in vitro postantibiotic effect of meropenem and imipenem versus selected Enterobacteriaceae and other pathogens. Diagn Microbiol Infect Dis 17: 71–73, 1993.
18. Odenholt-Tornqvist I. Studies on the postantibiotic sub-MIC effect of meropenem. J Antimicrob Chemother 31: 881–892, 1993.
19. Wu PJ, Livermore DM. Response of chemostat cultures of Pseudomonas aeruginosa to carbapenems and other β-lactams. J Antimicrob Chemother 25: 901–902, 1990.
20. Martín MM, Fuentes F, Izquierdo J, Gómez-Lus ML, Prieto J. In vivo and in-vitro study of the postantibiotic effect of meropenem [Letter]. J Antimicrob Chemother 32: 917–918, 1993.
21. Mattie H, Li-Chen Z. Antibiotic and postantibiotic effect (PAE) of meropenem (MP) and cloxacilin (CX) against S. aureus in vitro and in an experimental infection. Clin Infect Dis 17: 550, 1993.
22. Tanio T, Fukasawa M. In vitro and in vivo postantibiotic effect of meropenem. Chemotherapy (Japan) 40: 103–107, 1992.
23. Odenholt I, Holm SE, Cars O. Effects of benzylpenicillin on Streptococcus pyogenes during the postantibiotic phase in vitro. J Antimicrob Chemother 24: 147–156, 1989.
24. Flückiger U, Segessenmann C, Gerber U. Integration of pharmacokinetics and pharmacodynamics of imipenem in a human-adapted mouse model. Antimicrob Agents Chemother 35: 1905–1910, 1991.
25. Jones RN, Barry AL, Gavan RL, Washington II JA. Susceptibility tests: microdilution and macrodilution broth procedures. In: Lennette EH, Balows, A, Hausler WJ, Shadomy HJ, eds. Manual of clinical microbiology. Washington DC: American Society for Microbiology, 972–977, 1985.

26. Roosendaal R, Bakker-Woudenberg IAJM, van der Berghe-van Raffe M, Michel MF. Continuous versus intermittent administration of ceftazidime in experimental Klebsiella pneumoniae pneumonia in normal and leukopenic rats. Antimicrob Agents Chemother 30: 403–408, 1986.
27. Majcherczyck PA, Livermore DM. Penicillin-binding Protein (PBP) 2 and the post-antibiotic effect of carbapenems. J Antimicrob Chemother 26: 593–594, 1990.
28. MacKenzie FM, Gould IM, Chapman DG, Jason D. Postantibiotic effect of meropenem on members of the family Enterobacteriaceae determined by five methods. Antimicrob Agents Chemother 38: 2583–2589, 1994.
29. MacKenzie FM, Gould IM. The postantibiotic effect. J Antimicrob Chemother 32: 519–537, 1993.
30. Oshida T, Onta T, Nakanishi N, Matsishita T, Yamaguchi T. Activity of subminimal inhibitory concentrations of aspoxicillin in prolonging the postantibiotic effect against Staphylococcus aureus. J Antimicrob Chemother 26: 29–38, 1990.
31. Odenholt-Tornqvist I, Löwdin E, Cars O. Postantibiotic sub-MIC effects for vancomycin, roxithromycin, sparfloxacin and amikacin. Antimicrob Agents Chemother 36: 1852–1858, 1992.
32. Odenholt-Tornqvist I, Löwdin E, Cars O. Pharmacodynamic effects of subinhibitory concentrations of β-lactams antibiotics in vitro. Antimicrob Agents Chemother 35: 1834–1839, 1991.
33. Vogelman B, Gudmundsson S, Leggett J, Turnidge J. Correlation of antimicrobial pharmacokinetic parameters with therapeutic efficacy in an animal model. J Infect Dis 158: 831–847, 1988.

Submitted February 20, 1995; accepted June 19, 1995

Scand J Infect Dis 27: 475–479, 1995 ORIGINAL ARTICLE

Testing of Methicillin Resistance by in vitro Susceptibility and the Presence of the mecA Gene in Clinical Staphylococcus aureus Isolates in Finland

PIRKKO KOTILAINEN[1,2], JUKKA HYVÄRINEN[1], HELINÄ JÄRVINEN[1], LINNEA LINKO[3], ERKKI EEROLA[4], OLLI-PEKKA LEHTONEN[5], AULIKKI SIVONEN[6], PENTTI HUOVINEN[1] and JAANA VUOPIO-VARKILA[7]

From the [1]Antimicrobial Research Laboratory, National Public Health Institute, Turku, and the Departments of [2]Medicine, and [4]Medical Microbiology, Turku University, Turku, and [3]Meltola Hospital, Meltola, and [5]Laboratory of Medical Microbiology, Turku University Central Hospital, Turku, and the Departments of [6]Bacteriology and Immunology, Helsinki University, and [7]Special Bacterial Pathogens, National Public Health Institute, Helsinki, Finland

A total of 140 epidemiologically unrelated Staphylococcus aureus strains collected in Finland between 1983 and 1994 were sent to the reference laboratory with verified or suspected methicillin resistance. These strains and 37 S. aureus strains previously identified as methicillin-susceptible were retested using 5 different susceptibility test methods including agar screening, disc diffusion, growth around methicillin (25 µg) test strips and minimal inhibitory concentration (MIC) determinations by an agar dilution method and E-test. The isolates were also analyzed for the presence of the mecA gene by the polymerase chain reaction (PCR). Based on in vitro susceptibility, 69 strains were identified as methicillin-resistant and were positive for the mecA gene in PCR, while 84 strains were methicillin-susceptible and negative for this gene. Susceptibility testing gave conflicting results for 24 (14%) strains. When the tests were repeated in triplicate for each isolate, discrepant results were still achieved with 18 of the 24 strains in at least 2 different tests. Thus, based on in vitro susceptibility, these strains could not be definitely classified as resistant or susceptible to methicillin. Yet 7 of them were positive for the mecA gene as an indication of genetic resistance to methicillin. Corroborating earlier studies, these results illustrate the difficulty of detecting methicillin resistance/susceptibility based only on susceptibility testing and underscore the importance of confirming methicillin resistance in S. aureus in specialized laboratories.

P. Kotilainen, MD, Department of Medicine, Turku University Central Hospital, Kiinamyllynkatu 4–8, FIN-20520 Turku, Finland

INTRODUCTION

Testing Staphylococcus aureus for resistance to methicillin by in vitro methods is a complicated and unreliable procedure, since within each resistant strain different subpopulations often exist which are capable of growing at different antibiotic concentrations (1). Moreover, culture conditions can alter the phenotypic expression of methicillin resistance (2). However, all methicillin-resistant S. aureus (MRSA) strains are known to produce a unique penicillin binding protein (PBP), called PBP2a or PBP2′, which has a relatively low affinity to betalactam antibiotics (3–5). This MRSA-specific PBP is encoded by the mecA gene on the chromosome (6–8). At the present time, the most reliable method for detecting truly methicillin-resistant S. aureus strains is to demonstrate the presence of the mecA gene.

During recent years, major efforts have been made to contain the spread of MRSA in Finland and in the other Scandinavian countries. In this respect, rapid and accurate identification of MRSA in clinical specimens is of vital importance. The purpose of this study was to evaluate the reliability of identification of methicillin resistance by in vitro susceptibility testing in clinical microbiology laboratories in Finland. To do so, we have retested S. aureus isolates sent from diagnostic laboratories to the reference laboratory on account of verified or suspected methicillin-resistance and compared the results of in vitro susceptibility testing with analysis of these strains for the presence of the mecA gene by the polymerase chain reaction (PCR).

MATERIALS AND METHODS

Bacterial strains

We included in this study a total of 177 epidemiologically unrelated S. aureus strains present in the culture collections of the National Public Health Institute, Helsinki, Finland and the Department of Medical Microbiology, Turku University, Turku, Finland. These strains, recovered from various clinical settings, had originally been tested for methicillin susceptibility in clinical microbiology laboratories in different parts of Finland and sent to the reference laboratory for further analysis. The strain collection consisted of 96 isolates previously classified as methicillin-resistant [minimal inhibitory concentration (MIC) of oxacillin >4 mg/l], 44 isolates previously classified as borderline or low-level resistant to methicillin (MIC of oxacillin 2–4 mg/l) and 37 isolates previously classified as susceptible to methicillin (MIC of oxacillin <2 mg/l oxacillin). The resistant and borderline isolates from the National Public Health Institute Culture Collection included 11 isolates collected between 1983 and 1990 and 98 isolates collected between 1991 and 1994. The resistant isolates from the Turku University Culture Collection included 10 isolates collected between 1988 and

 ISSN 0036-5548

1990 and 21 isolates collected between 1991 and 1994. The methicillin-susceptible isolates had been collected in 12 clinical microbiology laboratories during the years 1992–1993. Stock cultures of the strains were stored at −70°C in skimmed milk or tryptone soya broth (Oxoid Ltd., Basingstoke, England) containing glycerol.

All staphylococcal isolates were gram-positive clustering cocci which were catalase- and coagulase-positive and identified as S. aureus by the API Staph-Trac system (Analytab, Plainview, NY). The MRSA population contained 14 epidemic strains and 82 sporadic isolates. For each individual MRSA outbreak recognized in Finland during the 1990s, only one isolate representing the epidemic strain was included. When the strains were typed by the International phage set at RTD, 100 × RTD and 1000 × RTD, a total of 39 S. aureus isolates were non-typable. Of the epidemic MRSA strains, 10 were of different phage types and 4 non-typable. Of the sporadic isolates, 61 were of different phage types and 21 non-typable. Of the borderline resistant isolates, 35 were of different phage types and 9 were non-typable with phages. The methicillin-susceptible S. aureus population consisted of 32 isolates of different phage types and 5 isolates non-typable with phages. There was no evident epidemiological linkage between any of the S. aureus isolates studied.

Testing for methicillin resistance

The staphylococcal isolates were tested for methicillin resistance following the guidelines recommended by the National Committee for Clinical Laboratory Standards (NCCLS) (9); 5 different methods were used. First, the isolates were screened for methicillin resistance by growth on Mueller-Hinton agar (Becton Dickinson Microbiology Systems, USA) supplemented with 4% NaCl and 6 mg oxacillin/l. The plates were inoculated with 1 μl of a bacterial suspension (10^8 cfu/ml, 0.5 McFarland) and examined for the presence of growth after incubation for 24–48 h at 35°C. Second, the susceptibility was tested using the disc diffusion test by plating bacteria (inoculum adjusted to 10^5 cfu/ml) onto Mueller-Hinton agar (no salt added) together with oxacillin discs containing 1 μg of oxacillin (AB Biodisk, Sweden). The plates were evaluated after incubation at 35°C for 24 h; isolates with the diameter of the inhibition zone ≤10 mm were considered resistant and those with the inhibition zone ≥13 mm susceptible. Third, all isolates were tested for growth around methicillin test strips (METHI TEST, Medical Wire and Equipment Co., Wiltshire, UK) containing 25 μg of methicillin. The bacteria were streaked onto Mueller-Hinton agar supplemented with 5% NaCl on a vertical line with the methicillin strip; three test strains together with a methicillin-resistant and -susceptible control strain were streaked onto 1 plate. According to the manufacturer's guidelines, strains exhibiting a measurable inhibition zone around the methicillin strip were considered susceptible and strains with no inhibition zone were considered resistant. Finally, the MICs of oxacillin for the isolates were determined both by an agar dilution method and by E-test. When using the agar dilution method, 1 μl of bacterial suspension adjusted to 10^4 cfu/ml was inoculated on Mueller-Hinton agar supplemented with 2% NaCl (9); the concentration range was 0.5–512 mg/l of oxacillin. When using the E-test, bacterial inoculum was plated on Mueller-Hinton agar supplemented with 2% NaCl together with an E-test strip (Ab Biodisk, Solna, Sweden) with the oxacillin concentration range from 0.016 to 256 mg/l. After incubating the plates in 35°C for 24 h, the MIC value was read at the point of the intersection between the growth zone edge and the E-test strip (10). Strains with an MIC of oxacillin ≥4 mg/l were considered resistant; those with an MIC of oxacillin ≤2 mg/l were considered susceptible. In susceptibility testing, S. aureus ATCC 29213 was used as a methicillin-susceptible control strain and S. aureus R1 (11) as a methicillin-resistant control strain.

Detection of mecA gene with PCR

Detection of the presence of the mecA gene in the isolates was performed following the procedure previously described by Predari et al. (12). Briefly, whole-cell lysates were prepared from 3 bacterial colonies grown over-night on blood and suspended in 1 ml of aqua. Cells from the suspension were harvested by centrifuging for 10 min in a microcentrifuge (14,000 *g*) and resuspended in 100 μl of 50 mM Tris (pH 8) containing 50 mM NaCl, 25% sucrose, 10 μl of lysostaphin (Sigma Chemical Co., St. Louis, MO.) and 100 μg of lysozyme (Sigma). After incubation at 37°C for 60 min, 0.5 mg of proteinase K (Sigma) in 100 μl of 50 mM Tris was added and the lysate was incubated at 50°C for 30 min and then placed in a boiling water bath for 5 min. The lysate was centrifuged for 10 min (14,000 *g*) to remove cellular debris and the supernatant used as a source of DNA in PCR.

Two oligonucleotide primers used were based on the published sequence of the PBP 2a gene (13) and were 5′-d GGGATCATAGCGTCATTATTC-3′(nucleotides 516 to 536) and 5′-dAACGATTGTGACACGATAGCC-3′(nucleotides 1024 to 1044). The amplification reaction was carried out in a total volume of 100 μl of amplification buffer containing 200 μmol deoxynucleoside triphosphates, 100 p-mol of primers, and 2.5 U of *Taq* DNA polymerase (Perkin-Elmer Cetus). An amount of 20 μl of crude cell lysate was used as a source of template DNA. The first cycle consisted of 5 min of denaturation at 96°C, 3 min of annealing at 55°C, and 5 min of extension at 72°C. The next 25 cycles consisted of denaturation at 96°C for 30 s, annealing at 55°C for 30 s, and extension at 72°C for 30 s and were concluded with a final extension at 72°C for 5 min. The amplification products were separated on 1% agarose (Seakem, LE; FMC BioProducts, Rockland, Maine) in TBE buffer (0.089 M Tris-borate, 0.089 M boric acid, 0.002M EDTA [pH 8]) at 30 V/cm for 15 min. The gels were stained with ethidium-bromide and photographed under UV illumination. In the PCR examinations, S. aureus 27r kindly provided by Dr A. Tomasz, USA (7) and S. aureus R1 (11) were used as mecA gene-positive control strains and S. aureus 27s as a mecA gene-negative control strain (7).

RESULTS

Susceptibility testing

All 5 methods used to detect methicillin susceptibility or resistance provided analogous results for 153 (86%) of the 177 S. aureus strains studied. Based on in vitro susceptibility, 69 strains were identified as resistant and 84 strains as susceptible to methicillin. The MICs of oxacillin were ≥32 mg/l for 66 strains including 34 strains with MICs ≥256 mg/l. Of the 14 MRSA epidemic strains, 9 had MICs ≥256 mg/l. Only 3 resistant strains had MICs between 4 and 16 mg/l of oxacillin. For the methicillin-susceptible S. aureus strains, the MICs were <1 mg/l for all except one isolate with an MIC of 1 mg/l.

The results of the susceptibility tests were discrepant for the remaining 24 (14%) S. aureus strains. This means that within the set of all 5 tests, the result of at least 1 test in the first assay was in discordance with the others. Thus, based on in vitro susceptibility these strains could not be definitely classified as resistant or susceptible to methicillin. The complete set of 5 tests was then repeated on each strain. The results were congruent in the second and third test sets for 6 strains but only in the third test set for 8 strains. However, for the remaining 10 strains, all 3 test sets yielded discrepant results. Moreover, interassay variation was observed in 3 (13%) of 24 strains in the agar screening tests, 4 (17%) of 24 strains in the disc diffusion and E-tests, in 6 (25%) of 24 strains in the MIC determination by the plate dilution method and in 13 (54%) of 24 strains in the testing with the methicillin test strips. The agreement between the results of the 360 in vitro assays performed on these 24 strains is presented in Table I.

MecA gene

Of all clinical S. aureus strains, 76 were positive for the mecA gene by PCR and 101 isolates were negative for this gene. Of the control strains, S. aureus R1 and 27r were positive and 27s negative for the mecA gene. A total of 69 clinical mecA gene-positive S. aureus strains were identified as methicillin-resistant based on susceptibility testing. For the remaining 7 mecA gene-positive S. aureus strains, the results of the susceptibility testing were discrepant. All 84 S. aureus strains identified as methicillin-susceptible based on susceptibility testing were shown to be negative for the mecA gene. For the remaining 17 mecA-negative strains, the results of the susceptibility testing were discrepant. Comparative results of classifying these strains by the presence of the mecA gene and based on in vitro susceptibility are shown in Table I.

Agreement between the present and earlier classification

The previous classification of these strains as methicillin-resistant or -susceptible in clinical microbiology laboratories was compared with their definition in our laboratory. Of the 96 strains previously characterized as methicillin-resistant, 69 (72%) were here characterized as methicillin-resistant based on in vitro susceptibility. These strains were also positive for the mecA gene. Further, 11 strains were characterized as methicillin-susceptible and were negative for the mecA gene, while 16 strains (7 positive and 9 negative for the mecA gene) yielded discrepant results in susceptibility testing.

Of the 44 strains previously classified as borderline-resistant to methicillin, 36 were here classified as methicillin-susceptible based on in vitro susceptibility; they were also mecA-negative. The remaining eight strains yielded discrepant results in susceptibility testing but were mecA-negative. Of the MIC determinations either by the E-test or plate dilution method for these strains, 50% were ≤ 1 mg/l and 50% between 2 and 8 mg/l of oxacillin. The 37 S.

Table I. *Comparative analysis of results of susceptibility testing of 24 clinical Staphylococcus aureus strains as methicillin-resistant (R) or -susceptible (S) by the presence of the mecA gene and five different in vitro susceptibility test methods. Strains positive for the mecA gene were designated as R and those negative for this gene as S. The phenotypic assays were repeated in triplicate for each isolate; the total number of assays for each test was 72*

			Agreement between the results (%)									
			Agar screening[a]		Disc diffusion[a] test		Methicillin[a] strip test		MIC[b] by the E test[a]		MIC by the plate dilution method[a]	
		No. of tests	R	S	R	S	R	S	R	S	R	S
MecA[c]	R	7	24	76	71	29	95	5	81	19	100	
MecA	S	17	8	92	27	73	57	43	6	94	41	59
Agar screening	R	9			67	33	89	11	67	33	89	11
	S	63			37	63	65	35	22	78	52	48
Disc diffusion test	R	25	20	80			84	16	56	44	92	8
	S	47	9	91			57	43	13	87	40	60
Methicillin strip test	R	49	10	90	49	51			39	61	78	22
	S	23	4	96	17	83			4	96	30	70
MIC by the E test	R	20	30	70	80	20	80	20			100	
	S	52	6	94	25	75	58	42			44	56
MIC by the plate dilution method	R	42	19	81	64	36	86	14	48	52		
	S	30	3	97	7	93	43	57		100		

[a] The test was carried out and interpreted as described in the Materials and Methods section.

[b] MIC indicates minimal inhibitory concentration of oxacillin.

[c] The presence of the mecA gene was determined by the polymerase chain reaction (PCR) technique as described in the Materials and Methods section.

aureus strains previously characterized as methicillin-susceptible were characterized susceptible also in this study and were negative for the mecA gene.

All 76 S. aureus strains hybridizing with the mecA gene had been characterized as MRSA in clinical microbiology laboratories. Of the 101 mecA gene-negative strains, 20 had been originally characterized as methicillin-resistant, 44 strains as borderline resistant to methicillin and 37 strains as susceptible to methicillin.

DISCUSSION

The results of this study illustrate the complicated nature of the laboratory diagnosis of MRSA. Of those S. aureus strains characterized in our laboratory as susceptible to methicillin both by phenotypic methods and by absence of the mecA gene, 11 had been previously characterized as MRSA in clinical microbiology laboratories. The majority of these strains had been collected from different hospitals in Finland before the year 1990. At that time, MRSA did not belong to the predominant resistant pathogens to be recognized in hospitals, and one can hypothesize that this incorrect classification might have been due to insufficient experience in detecting MRSA. During the 1990s, however, the number of yearly isolated new MRSA strains has continuously increased in our country, and the importance of controlling MRSA is now generally accepted. Every routine laboratory should aim at reliable primary identification of MRSA by carefully following the guidelines recommended to enhance the expression of methicillin resistance. These techniques include adding salt to the growth medium and incubating for up to 48 h at a temperature of 35°C or lower (2).

Despite the best efforts and the use of recommended methods in susceptibility testing, results with some strains may be undeterminable. These strains can appear to be susceptible in 1 test and be borderline or resistant in others. Of all the 177 S. aureus strains in this study 24 (14%) fell into this category. Even when the tests were repeated in triplicate for each isolate, discrepant results were still achieved with 18 of these strains in at least 2 different tests. When the results were compared with the strain classification by the presence of the mecA gene, all 5 susceptibility testing methods used proved unsatisfactory for these specific S. aureus strains. Admittedly, the agar dilution method was sensitive and correctly recognized all 7 mecA gene-positive strains as MRSA. Yet the specificity of this method was poor: the results indicated methicillin resistance also in as many as 41% of the assays performed on the 17 mecA-gene negative S. aureus strains. Similarly, while 95% of the methicillin strip tests correctly identified mecA-positive S. aureus as MRSA, mecA-negative S. aureus strains were falsely identified as MRSA in 57% of these assays. Further, agar screening correctly classified 92% of the susceptible but only 24% of the resistant S. aureus strains. Finally, S. aureus strains were correctly classified in less than 74% of the disc diffusion tests and in less than 95% of the MIC determinations by the E-test. These results clearly show that an accurate in vitro determination of methicillin resistance/susceptibility can be seriously affected by variability in the expression of resistance.

Phenotypic expression of methicillin resistance can be either heterogeneous or homogeneous. Under routine culture conditions, most MRSA strains express heterogeneous resistance. This means that the majority of the cells in these strains are susceptible to low concentrations of beta-lactam antibiotics (1, 8). Identification of heterogeneous MRSA strains may be a great problem, especially if they contain very rare resistant clones. In contrast, virtually all bacterial cells among MRSA strains expressing homogeneous methicillin resistance show resistant phenotype (1, 8). Identification of the homogeneous, highly resistant MRSA strains usually poses no problems: these strains invariably grow at high drug concentrations, even without modified culture conditions. Consistently in this study, as many as 66 of those 69 mecA gene-positive MRSA isolates which were uniformly resistant in all 5 in vitro susceptibility tests had MICs ≥ 32 mg/l.

Conditions used to favour the expression of methicillin resistance may result in slightly higher MICs also for some low-level resistant strains. Thus, S. aureus strains with MICs between 2 and 4 mg/l of oxacillin present a special problem for clinical microbiology laboratories. Some of these strains are actually methicillin-resistant but with an extremely small subpopulation of the cells being resistant (8). Like all truly methicillin-resistant strains, they possess the mecA gene and produce PBP2a. Another mechanism behind consistently elevated MIC values may be overproduction of beta-lactamases (14, 15) or, alternatively, modification of normal PBPs (16). These particular borderline strains do not possess the mecA gene nor produce the PBP2a. In this study, the S. aureus strains characterized as borderline-resistant in clinical microbiology laboratories were all collected during or after the year 1992. Finnish laboratories were then generally aware of the fact that borderline-resistant S. aureus strains may represent true MRSA. These borderline-resistant strains initially caused considerable confusion in some hospitals, prompting clinicians to implement hygienic precautions and, moreover, to use vancomycin instead of a beta-lactam antibiotic. Therefore, the finding that none of these strains possessed the mecA gene was significant. Experimental data suggest that infections caused by borderline-resistant mecA-negative S. aureus strains can be treated with beta-lactam antibiotics (17). The strains of this phenotype have perhaps no special clinical importance except that they must be differentiated from truly methicillin-resistant strains. This can be accomplished by verifying that those strains do not contain the mecA gene.

Detection of the mecA gene is the most reliable and fundamental method of identifying MRSA. The mecA gene can be demonstrated by DNA hybridization or in vitro amplification of DNA by PCR (12, 18–20). Of these two methods, the PCR technique is easier to perform. Yet it is technically too demanding to be adopted for routine laboratory use. On the other hand, isolation of MRSA from a clinical specimen has a major clinical importance on the patient, as well as epidemiological importance on the hospital. Therefore, it is recommended that every new MRSA strain be sent to a specialized reference laboratory for further analysis. Also those S. aureus strains exhibiting undeterminable results in susceptibility testing and those being borderline-resistant to oxacillin should be referred for evaluation of the presence of the mecA gene.

In conclusion, based on in vitro susceptibility, 24 (14%) S. aureus strains could not be here definitely classified as resistant or susceptible to methicillin. Yet seven of them were positive for the mecA gene as an indication of genetic resistance to methicillin. Corroborating earlier studies, these results illustrate the difficulty of detecting methicillin resistance/susceptibility based only on susceptibility testing and underscore the importance of confirming methicillin resistance in S. aureus in specialized laboratories.

ACKNOWLEDGEMENTS

We thank Marja-Liisa Lindman, Minna Lamppu, Anna-Liisa Lumiaho, Tuula Randell, Anna-Liisa Manninen and Ritva Scotford for expert technical assistance. The work was supported by a grant from the Sigrid Juselius Foundation.

REFERENCES

1. Tomasz A, Nachman S, Leaf H. Stable classes of phenotypic expression in methicillin-resistant clinical isolates of staphylococci. Antimicrob Agents Chemother 35: 124–129, 1991.
2. Coudron PE, Jones DL, Dalton HP, Archer GL. Evaluation of laboratory tests for detection of methicillin-resistant Staphylococcus aureus and Staphylococcus epidermidis. J Clin Microbiol 24: 764–769, 1986.
3. Archer GL, Pennel E. Detection of methicillin resistance in staphylococci by using a DNA probe. Antimicrob Agents Chemother 34: 1720–1724, 1990.
4. Chambers HF, Sachdeva M. Binding of β-lactam antibiotics to penicillin-binding proteins in methicillin-resistant Staphylococcus aureus. J Infect Dis 161: 1170–1176, 1990.
5. Hartman BJ, Tomasz A. Low-affinity penicillin-binding protein associated with β-lactam resistance in Staphylococcus aureus. J Bacteriol 158: 513–516, 1984.
6. Beck WD, Berger-Bachi B, Kayser FH. Additional DNA in methicillin-resistant Staphylococcus aureus and molecular cloning of mec-specific DNA. J Bacteriol 165: 373–378, 1986.
7. Tonin E, Tomasz A. β-lactam-specific resistant mutants of Staphylococcus aureus. Antimicrob Agents Chemother 30: 577–583, 1986.
8. de Lencastre H, Figueiredo AM, Urban C, Rahal J, Tomasz A. Multiple mechanisms of methicillin resistance and improved methods of detection in clinical isolates of Staphylococcus aureus. Antimicrob Agents Chemother 35: 632–639, 1991.
9. National Committee for Clinical Laboratory Standards. Approved standard M7A2. Methods for dilution antimicrobial susceptibility tests for bacteria that grow aerobically. National Committee for Clinical Laboratory Standards, Villanova, Pa., 1990.
10. Brown DFJ. The E-test challenged with selected strains. Diagn Microbiol Infect Dis 15: 465–468, 1992.
11. Rossi L, Tonin E, Cheng YR, Fontana R. Regulation of penicillin-binding protein activity: description of a methicillin-inducible penicillin-binding protein in Staphylococcus aureus. Antimicrob Agents Chemother 24: 828–831, 1985.
12. Predari SC, Ligozzi M, Fontana R. Genotypic identification of methicillin-resistant coagulase-negative staphylococci by polymerase chain reaction. Antimicrob Agents Chemother 35: 2568–2573, 1991.
13. Song MD, Wachi M, Doi M, Ishino F, Matsuashi M. Evolution of an inducible penicillin-target protein in methicillin-resistant Staphylococcus aureus by gene fusion. FEBS Lett 221: 167–171, 1987.
14. Barg N, Chambers H, Kernodle D. Borderline susceptibility to antistaphylococcal penicillins is not conferred exclusively to the hyperproduction of β-lactamase. Antimicrob Agents Chemother 35: 1975–1979, 1991.
15. McDougal LK, Thornsberry C. The role of β-lactamase in staphylococcal resistance to penicillinase-resistant penicillins and cephalosporins. J Clin Microbiol 23: 832–839, 1986.
16. Tomasz A, Drugeon HB, de Lencastre HM, Jabes D, McDougall L, Bille J. New mechanisms for methicillin resistance in Staphylococcus aureus: clinical isolates that lack the PBP 2a gene and contain normal penicillin-binding proteins with modified penicillin-binding capacity. Antimicrob Agents Chemother 33: 1869–1874, 1989.
17. Thauvin-Eliopoulos C, Rice LB, Eliopoulos GM, Moellering RC Jr. Efficacy of oxacillin and ampicillin-sulbactam combination in experimental endocarditis caused by a beta-lactamase-hyperproducing Staphylococcus aureus. Antimicrob Agents Chemother 34: 728–732, 1990.
18. Brakstad OG, Maeland JA, Tveten Y. Multiplex polymerase chain reaction for detection of genes for Staphylococcus aureus thermonuclease and methicillin resistance and correlation with oxacillin resistance. APMIS 101: 681–688, 1993.
19. Murakami K, Minamide W, Wada K, Nakamura E, Teraoka H, Watanabe S. Identification of methicillin-resistant strains of staphylococci by polymerase chain reaction. J Clin Microbiol 29: 2240–2244, 1991.
20. Unal S, Hoskins J, Flokowitsch JE, Wu CYE, Preston DA, Skatrud PL. Detection of methicillin-resistant staphylococci by using the polymerase chain reaction. J Clin Microbiol 30: 1685–1691, 1992.

Submitted April 18, 1995; accepted July 10, 1995

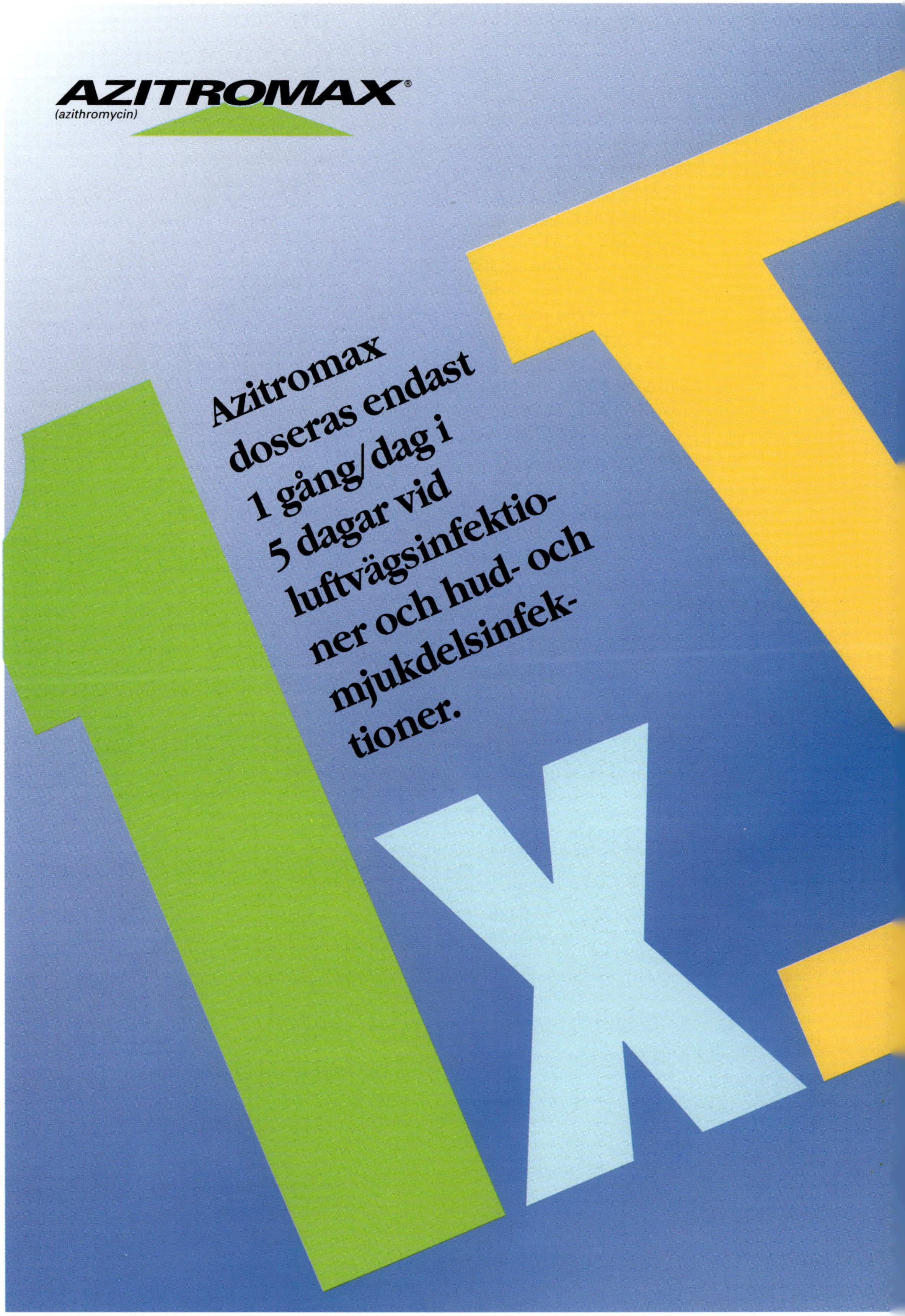
AZITROMAX®
(azithromycin)
Azitromax doseras endast 1 gång/dag i 5 dagar vid luftvägsinfektioner och hud- och mjukdelsinfektioner.

Scand J Infect Dis 27: 483–487, 1995 ORIGINAL ARTICLE

Staphylococcus aureus Endocarditis in Danish Intravenous Drug Users: High Proportion of Left-Sided Endocarditis

METTE FABER[1], NIELS FRIMODT-MØLLER[1], FRANK ESPERSEN[1], PETER SKINHØJ[2] and VIBEKE ROSDAHL[1]

From the [1]Staphylococcus Laboratory, Statens Seruminstitut, and the [2]Department of Infectious Diseases, Rigshospitalet, Copenhagen, Denmark

In a retrospective study covering the years 1982–1989 episodes of Staphylococcus aureus endocarditis in 51 intravenous drug users were studied. Tricuspid involvement dominated (34/51), but the frequency of left-sided involvement (33.3%) was greater than in earlier reports. Involvement of both sides of the heart was not detected, but 27.8% of the left-sided endocarditis cases had multiple pulmonary infiltrates, indicating that some of them might have had a concomitant right-sided endocarditis. The 2 groups were compared: patients with left-sided endocarditis were significantly older and with a longer time of intravenous drug use. The complication rate was the same (44.1%) as was the duration of antibiotic treatment (median 42 days). In total, five patients underwent surgery, two (5.8%) due to right-sided failure and three (29.4%) because of left-sided endocarditis. The mortality of tricuspid endocarditis was low (2.9%), whereas 5 patients (29.4%) with left-sided involvement died. The patients who died were signficantly older and had a shorter duration of symptoms before hospitalization.

M. Faber, MD, Staphylococcus Laboratory, Statens Seruminstitut, Artillerivej 5, DK-2300 Copenhagen S, Denmark

INTRODUCTION

Intravenous drug users (IVDUs) run an increased risk of infections and in particular of endocarditis (1–3). Staphylococcus aureus has been shown to be the main causative organism (2–5). Investigations, mainly in the USA and Sweden, have shown that, in this group of patients, S. aureus predominantly attacks the tricuspid valve; that no underlying cardiac diseases are present; that surgery is rarely necessary; that shorter courses of antibiotic treatment are effective, and that the mortality is low (2–11).

Our clinical impression with endocarditis in Danish IVDUs was that left-sided valve involvement was not uncommon and that antibiotic treatment often had to be continued for more than 4 weeks to achieve clinical cure.

We therefore undertook the present study in order to study S. aureus endocarditis in Danish IVDUs and in particular the distrubution of right- and left-sided endocarditis, the duration of treatment and the clinical outcome.

MATERIALS AND METHODS

Most strains of S. aureus isolated from the blood cultures in Denmark are referred to the Staphylococcus Laboratory, Statens Seruminstitute, Copenhagen, for phage typing. Clinical information is provided from the hospital departments in all but a few cases (12).

Among 6493 S. aureus bacteraemias registered during the period 1982–1989 IVDU was reported in 128 episodes. The hospital departments were requested to remit all medical records including autopsy findings; only the first episode was included if more than one was reported. Nine reports were not available. The final material consisted of 97 reports from 21 departments.

To identify patients with endocarditis the criteria of Durack et al. (13) were used:

1. *Definite endocarditis* defined by pathological criteria.
2. *Definite endocarditis* defined by clinical criteria, using 2 of the following major criteria:
   - —positive blood culture with community-acquired S. aureus in the absence of a primary focus
   - —oscillating intracardiac mass or abscess seen by echocardiography
   - —new valvular regurgitation,

   or 1 major criterion and 3 of the following minor criteria:
   - —predisposition: intravenous drug use
   - —fever (>38°C)
   - —vascular phenomena: arterial embolism, septic pulmonary infarcts, intracranial haemorrhage
   - —immunological phenomena: glomerulonephritis
   - —echocardiogram, consistent with infective endocarditis but not meeting major criteria as noted previously
3. *Rejected.* Firm alternate diagnosis or resolution of manifestations with antibiotic therapy for 4 days or less.

The side of cardiac involvement was determined by direct examination of the heart, by assuming that it corresponded to the side of vegetation of echocardiograms, or to the side of the heart murmur.

Apart for the echocardiograms and X-ray the following data were collected: age, sex, duration of IV drug use, underlying diseases, whether the infection was hospital- or community-acquired, past hospitalization record and the symptoms and clinical findings at admission. The type of drug used was not described frequently enough to permit any conclusive statement.

In addition we recorded the year and the duration of hospitalization, the requirement for surgery, the complications, and the outcome.

Finally we noted the length of antibiotic treatment (including both the parenteral and the oral treatment) appropriate for treating S. aureus infections. Outpatient therapy was only noted if the follow-up control was respected.

The laboratory data were summarized with particular attention to haemoglobin, total leukocyte count, erythrocyte sedimentation rate, and urinanalysis.

 ISSN 0036-5548

Table I. *Diagnostic categorization of 51 cases of Staphylococcus aureus endocarditis*

	Right-sided ($n = 34$)	Left-sided ($n = 17$)	Total ($n = 51$)
Definite pathological criteria			
Autopsy	1	4	5
Surgery	2	2	4
Definite clinical criteria			
Two major criteria	19	5	24
1 major, 3 minor	12	6	18
Total (%)	34 (66.7)	17 (33.3)	51
Rejected	—	—	46

Finally the phage types and the antimicrobial susceptibility were noted.

Statistical analysis

Data were analysed using the chi-square test, Fisher's exact test or the Mann–Whitney rank sum test for independent samples. The data were presented as the medians, including the 10th and 90th percentiles; $p < 0.05$ was considered to be significant.

RESULTS

During the 8-year period investigated, 51/97 patients (52.6%) fulfilled the criteria for endocarditis. An increase in frequency seemed to occur from 1982–1989 (4, 4, 2, 9, 3, 7, 12, and 10 cases per year). The distrubution of endocarditis cases according to the classification is shown in Table I. Nine patients were diagnosed as having definite endocarditis according to pathological criteria. When the clinical criteria were applied, 35 patients were classified as having definite endocarditis. All the cases met one of the major criteria, having positive blood cultures, and 2 of the minor criteria, i.e. IVDU and fever >38°C. Among these 24 patients had a new valvular regurgitation and then fulfilled 2 major criteria, whereas 18 patients were classified by fulfilling 1 major and 3 minor criteria. (Besides the above mentioned minor criteria, valvular vegetations were detected in 9 patients, immunological phenomena in 2 and septic peripheral emboli in 5 patients, respectively). The rejected group consisted of 46 patients.

Table II. *Clinical characteristics of right-sided and left-sided endocarditis in 51 intravenous drug users*

	Right-sided $n = 34$	Left-sided $n = 17$
Median age, years	29.5	32.0[a]
Range	18–44	22–45
Male/female	18/16	13/4
Duration of abuse, years	8.0	16.5[a]
Range	2–19	5–20
Duration of symptoms before hospitalization, days	7.0	4.5
Range	1–20	1–20
Duration of antibiotic treatment, days	42.0	42.0
Range	9–152	16–83
Complication rate, %	44.1	41.2
Surgery (%)	2 (5.8)	3 (17.6)
Mortality (%)	1 (2.9)	5 (29.4)[a]

[a] $p < 0.05$

Apart from the first group, in which a slight and not significant predominance of left-sided endocarditis was seen, endocarditis involving the right-sided valves (33 tricuspid and one both tricuspid and pulmonal) dominated (66.7%).

Among patients with left-sided endocarditis, the vegetations were confined to the aortic valve in 4 patients (2 diagnosed by autopsy and 2 by echocardiocraphy); in the last 13 patients the mitral valves were involved.

Various clinical characteristics are listed in Table II. Patients with left-sided endocarditis were significantly older and with a significantly longer time of IVDU. A slight but not significant preponderance of men was also seen in this group.

The median duration of symptoms was 4.5 days for the left-sided endocarditis and 7.0 days for the right-sided endocarditis, a difference which was not significant. The length of antibiotic treatment did not differ according to side of heart valve infection; both groups were treated for 42 days. The complication rate did not differ between the groups, but the types of complication did: the most common complication in patients with right-sided endocarditis was caused by recurrent septic pulmonary emboli; 3 patients developed pneumothorax, 3 pulmonary abscesses and 1 pleural empyema. Evidence of renal failure developed during hospitalization in 6 patients (3 of these with findings consistent with glomerulonephritis), all of whom required dialysis. Other complications included septic arthritis ($n = 1$) as well as cardiac insufficiency ($n = 3$) and osteomyelitis ($n = 1$). In patients with left-sided involvement all complications were due to metastatic foci: eyes and subcutis ($n = 1$); central nervous system ($n = 2$); spleen ($n = 2$), 1 of whom was splenectomized; kidney ($n = 2$), and intraabdominal abscess ($n = 1$), respectively.

Cardiac surgery was undertaken in 4 cases. Two patients required tricuspid surgery, 1 due to uncontrolled infection and the appearance of Candida albicans in the blood culture besides S. aureus, and the other due to destruction of the valve and haemodynamic failure. Two underwent mitral surgery due to uncontrolled embolization and left ventricular failure. One patient died due to left ventricular failure 5 months after the surgery; the others survived.

The rate of in-hospital mortality was 6/51 (11.8%; 5 male patients with left-sided endocarditis and 1 female with right-sided endocarditis); significantly more patients with left-sided endocarditis died ($p = 0.01$). Three of the 5 patients with aortic involvement died. The patients who died were significantly older than the patients who survived (median 34.5 years, range 31–45, vs. 30 years, range 18–44; $p = 0.002$) and had a significantly shorter duration of symptoms before hospitalization (median 2.5 days, range 1–4, vs. 7 days, range 1–30 $p = 0.02$). One patient died on the day of arrival, in fulminant sepsis; the remaining patients died 6–13 days after arrival, due to cardiac failure and embolic processes in multiple organs, despite relevant antibiotic treatment.

All cases were community-acquired. Regarding underlying diseases, no significant differences were seen between the groups: previous heart diseases were not reported; 7 patients had earlier been hospitalized due to drainage-requiring S. aureus abscesses; 4 patients were infected with HIV and 2 patients were defined to have AIDS. Past viral hepatitis was confirmed by serological tests; 9 caused by hepatitis A virus and 11 by hepatitis B virus.

At presentation, a systolic murmur was noted in 41/51 patients (60.8%). The murmur was more often but not significantly conferred to the right-sided valves.

CNS-involvement, petechiae and splinters were found significantly more frequently in left-sided than in the right-sided endocarditis, whereas pulmonary symptoms (dyspnoea, cough and rales) were significantly more frequent in the right-sided group.

Initial radiographic pulmonary findings consistent with septic emboli were diagnosed in 73.5% of the patients with right-sided endocarditis, but also in 27.8% of the patients with left-sided involvement.

Regarding laboratory data, no significant differences were seen between the 2 groups. The blood leukocyte count was abnormal in 58.7% of the cases, whereas the differential count was abnormal in 82.1%. Haemoglobin values were below normal in 55.3%.

Haematuria as diagnosed by microscopic counting of the red blood cells in urine was found in 15 out of 18 tested (83.3%).

Regarding phage types and antibiotic suspectibility, no significant differences were found for the isolates from IVDUs as compared to all other bacteraemia isolates from the same years. No strain was resistant to methicillin.

DISCUSSION

The association of IVDU and endocarditis is well established (1–8). In this patient population S. aureus predominantly adhere to the tricuspid valve (2, 4, 7). In a Swedish study (7) 33/36 of IVDUs (91%) with S. aureus endocarditis had tricuspid involvement. Levine et al. found approximately the same rate of tricuspid valve involvement in a study in Detroit which included 45 patients (2).

Therefore, the high percentage of left-sided involvement (33.3%) in the present study, exclusively dealing with S. aureus endocarditis, is surprising.

Part of the explanation can depend on different definitions of endocarditis; the clinical diagnosis of infectious endocarditis is difficult and the diagnostic criteria are still debated (13–15).

The triad of IVDU, S. aureus septicaemia and septic pulmonary emboli in the absence of other sources of emboli is considered to be patognomonic (16, 17), and was used as the criteria in the study of Julander et al. (17). However, a risk of overestimating the right-sided involvement is then possible, since foci such as infections in the groin and mycotic aneurysms can be difficult to diagnose (16). Due to improvement of the echocardiographic technique, this investigation is included as a major criterion of endocarditis in the proposed definition of Durack et al. (13). However, the interpretation still offers problems, and depends on the equipment and the skills of the staff. To meet the major criteria of Durack et al., specific echocardiographic findings, such as an oscillating intracardiac mass or intracardiac abscess, are demanded; all other echocardiographic findings are included under minor criteria.

In the present retrospective study, including 21 departments, no homogeneity in the performance of echocardiography could be expected; to ensure the diagnosis of endocarditis we decided to weight the echocardiographic findings in this study as a minor criterion only. Transoesophageal echocardiography has improved sensitivity (18) but was not available at the time of the study.

In this study 6 out of 17 left-sided endocarditis cases were confirmed by autopsy or surgery; the side of the cardiac involvement in the remaining 11 patients was based on heart stethoscopy and the results of the echocardiography. However, even if an involvement of right-sided valves was not demonstrated by the above mentioned investigations, some of the patients might have had a concomitant and non-observed right-sided endocarditis, supported by the fact that a third of these patients had signs of septic emboli in the lungs.

The predominance of the right-sided involvement in S. aureus endocarditis has been explained by the fact that the valves were primed by the continuous injections (2, 6). This point of view is supported by the correlation between age, length of abuse and endocarditis (2). In the present study, patients with left-sided endocarditis were older and had longer duration of IVDU than patients with right-sided involvement. No obvious explanations of the late debut of left-sided endocarditis can be given.

The clinical findings were generally the same as those in previously published studies (2, 5, 7, 20); fever was present in nearly all the patients, and about 60% of the patients presented with heart murmur. Pulmonary manifestations dominated in the right-sided endocarditis, whereas petechiae and CNS involvement were more common findings in the left-sided cases. The leukocyte differential count and the erythrocyte sedimentation rate seem to be the most useful laboratory results.

Therapy for 2 weeks has been shown to offer a high cure rate in patients with right-sided endocarditis (9, 10), whereas the treatment recommendations for left-sided disease follow the same principles as outlined for the general population (19). In the present study, short-term therapy was often planned for the patients with right-sided endocarditis; however, due to prolonged fever and embolic phenomena the treatment had to be extended. In fact, finally, no difference according to side, regarding the duration of treatment was found; both groups were treated for 6 weeks. The antibiotic regimens in USA and Denmark are not comparable, so any conclusions can hardly be drawn regarding optimal length of therapy from these retrospective data. But they may indicate that prolonged fever and complications are not uncommon phenomena even in right-sided endocarditis, which is in agreement with the finding of Hecht & Berger (5).

In a non-addict population S. aureus endocarditis is known to have high morbidity and mortality (6, 20), whereas endocarditis in IVDU population is almost invariably associated with a good prognosis (1, 2, 4–7). The background is only incompletely understood; however, the frequent occurrence of right-sided endocarditis is believed to be essential; even in the case of valve destruction haemodynamic deterioration is a rare complication during right-sided endocarditis. Our study confirms the excellent prognosis of right-sided endocarditis; only 1/34 of the patients with right-sided endocarditis died (2.9%). This study also reaffirms that heart surgery is seldom indicated in tricuspid endocarditis (two patients underwent surgery due to right-sided failure, i.e. 5.8%).

Due to a preponderance of right-sided endocarditis with S. aureus, few data are available on the prognosis of the left-sided disease in IVDUs. Sheagren reported a mortality rate of 20–50% (19), which is in agreement with our findings (29.4%). The presentation of our five patients also corresponds to the description by Sheagren of a fulminant syndrome with a superacute setting, early embolic phenomena, and rapid deterioration of the valve function (19). All the patients had received <14 days antibiotic treatment at the time of death, and 83.3% of these had received <7 days of treatment. This association between outcome and short duration of antimicrobial therapy is in accordance with the findings of Mylotte et al. (21).

The patients who died were significantly older than the patients who survived; the duration of IVDU and age seem to be important risk factors; it is tempting to speculate that a correlation between host response and the extended duration of drug use and age exists.

The indication for surgical intervention in IVDUs with left-sided endocarditis is the same as for non-users; aortic involvement, especially, is more often associated with a fatal outcome (19), thus an early consideration for surgery is recommended. In our study, however, only two patients with left-sided endocarditis underwent surgery. In none of the above mentioned patients with multiorgan failure was surgery considered, because of the rapid progressive deterioration. A more aggressive management of patients of older age, with a long time of IVDU, short duration of symptoms and with aortic involvement seem to be indicated.

REFERENCES

1. Crane LR, Levine DP, Zervos MJ, Cummings G. Bacteremia in narcotic addicts at the Detroit Medical center. I. Microbiology epidemiology, risk factors, and empiric therapy. Rev Infect Dis 8: 364–373, 1986.
2. Levine DP, Crane LR, Zervos MJ. Bacteremia in narcotic addicts at the Detroit Medical Center. II. Infectious endocarditis: a prospective comparative study. Rev Infect Dis 8: 374–396, 1986.
3. Haverkos HW, Lange WR. Serious infections other than human immunodeficiency virus among intravenous drug abusers. J Infect Dis 161: 894–902, 1990.
4. Panidis IP, Kotler MN, Mintz GS, Segal BL, Ross JJ. Right side endocarditis: clinical and echocardiographic features. Amer Heart J 107: 759–764, 1984.
5. Hecht SR, Berger M. Right-sided endocarditis in intravenous drug users. Ann Intern Med 117: 560–566, 1992.
6. Chambers HF, Korzeniowski OM, Sande MA. Staphylococcus aureus endocarditis: clinical manifestations in addicts and non-addicts. Medicine (Baltimore) 62: 170–177, 1983.
7. Julander I. Staphylococcal septicaemia and endocarditis in 80 drug addicts. Scand J Infect Dis Suppl 41: 49–54, 1983.
8. Watanakunakorn C, Burkert T. Infective endocarditis at a large community teaching hospital, 1980–1990. A review of 210 episodes. Medicine 72: 90–102, 1992.
9. Chambers HF, Miller RT, Newman MD. Right-sided Staphylococcus aureus endocarditis in intravenous drug abusers: two week combination therapy. Ann Intern Med 109: 619–624, 1988.
10. Torres-Tortosa M, Cueto M de, Vergara A, Sanchez-Porto A, Perez-Guzman E, Gonzalez-Serrano M, Canueto J. Prospective evaluation of a two week course of intravenous antibiotics in intravenous drug addicts with infective endocarditis. Eur J Clin Microbiol Infect Dis 13: 559–564, 1994.
11. Bayer AS, Blomquist IK, Bello E, Chiu CY, Ward JI, Ginzton LE. Tricuspid valve endocarditis due to Staphylococcus aureus. Correlation of two-dimensional echocardiography with clinical outcome. Chest 93: 247–253, 1988.
12. Rosendal K, Jessen O, Faber V, Bentzon MW. Frequency, phage types and antibiotic resistance of Staphylococcus aureus isolated from blood cultures in Denmark 1975–1981. Scand J Infect Dis Suppl 41: 19–26, 1983.
13. Durack DT, Lukes AS, Bright DK, and the Duke Endocarditis Service. New criteria for diagnosis of infective endocarditis: utilization of specific echocardiographic findings. Amer J Med 96: 200–209, 1994.
14. von Reyn CF, Levy BS, Arbeit RD, Friedland G, Crumpacker CS. Infective endocarditis: an analysis based on strict case definitions. Ann Intern Med 94: 505–518, 1981.
15. Bayer AS, Ward IJ, Ginzton LE, Shapiro SM. Evaluation of new clinical criteria for the diagnosis of infective endocarditis. Amer J Med 96: 211–219, 1994.
16. Bayer AS. Staphylococcal bacteremia and endocarditis. State of the art. Arch Intern Med 142: 1169–1177, 1982.
17. Julander I, Arneborn P, Back E, Hoglund C, Svanbom M. Intravenous drug addiction—staphylococcal septicemia—pulmonary embolism: a triad pathognomonic for tricuspid valve endocarditis? Scand J Infect Dis 15: 257–265, 1983.
18. Birmingham GD, Rahko PS, Ballantyne F. Improved detection of infective endocarditis with transesophageal echocardiography. Am Heart J 123: 774–781, 1991.

19. Sheagren JN. Endocarditis complicating parenteral drug abuse. In: Remington JS, Schwartz MN, eds. Current clinical topics in infectious diseases. Vol 2. New York: McGraw-Hill, 211–233, 1981.
20. Espersen F, Frimodt-Møller N. Staphylococcus aureus endocarditis. A review of 119 cases. Arch Intern Med 146: 1118–1121, 1986.
21. Mylotte JM, McDermott C, Spooner JA. Prospective study of 114 consecutive episodes of Staphyloccoccus aureus bacteremia. Rev Infect Dis 9: 891–907, 1987.

Submitted December 8, 1994; accepted June 18, 1995

Scand J Infect Dis 27: 489–494, 1995 ORIGINAL ARTICLE

Occurrence of Pneumococci with Resistance or Decreased Susceptibility to Penicillin in Southeast Sweden

ERIK KIHLSTRÖM[1] and BENGT NORMANN[2]

From the Departments of [1]Clinical Microbiology, Faculty of Health Sciences, and [2]Infectious Diseases, University Hospital, Linköping, Sweden

The minimal inhibitory concentrations (MICs) of 14 beta-lactam and non-beta-lactam antibiotics were determined for all pneumococci with intermediate susceptibility (I), ($n = 26$) or resistance (R), ($n = 15$) to penicillin G isolated at the Clinical Microbiology Laboratory, University Hospital, Linköping, Sweden during 1994. These isolates accounted for 3% of all pneumococcal isolates. The results were compared with those of 26 penicillin-susceptible isolates. The MICs of all tested beta-lactam antibiotics increased with MICs of penicillin G. The least increase and the lowest MICs of these agents were recorded for cefotaxime and imipenem. 27% of I- and R-strains were multiple-resistant, most often to tetracycline, trimethoprim-sulfametoxazole, erythromycin, chloramphenicol and clindamycin. All strains were susceptible to vancomycin and rifampicin. I-strains belonged to at least 5 different serotypes. However, 12 of the 15 R-strains were serotype 9 and 6 of these were recovered during contact tracing, indicating spread of a single clone within day-care centres.

E. Kihlström, MD, Department of Clinical Microbiology, Faculty of Health Sciences, Linköping University, S-581 85 Linköping, Sweden

INTRODUCTION

The first report on clinical isolates of Streptococcus pneumoniae with decreased susceptibility to penicillin came from Boston, USA in 1965. However, its significance did not appear to be recognized (1). Two years later resistant strains were isolated in Australia (2) and since 1977 multiple-resistant pneumococci have appeared in South Africa (3). In Europe, Spain has experienced a sharp increase in the prevalence of pneumococci with decreased susceptibility to penicillin; from 6% in 1979 to 44% in 1989 (4). Also in other European countries the prevalence of such pneumococci is high, e.g. about 50% of the isolates in Hungary and about 15% in France (5). The Nordic countries have so far been relatively spared. However, in Iceland the prevalence of penicillin-resistant pneumococci increased from the first isolate in December 1988 to 14.5% in the last quarter of 1991. Multiple-resistant serotype 6 isolates have predominated (6). This shows the speed of spreading once a resistant clone has been introduced into a community. In Sweden, penicillin-resistant pneumococi have been rare. During national surveys in 1983 and 1990, 2 and 3%, respectively, of the strains showed intermediate susceptibility to penicillin and in 1990 only one out of 500 tested isolates was fully resistant (7).

During 1994, especially the latter part of that year, we noticed an increasing number of patients infected with pneumococci with decreased sensitivity or resistance to penicillin. Here we report on the antibiotic susceptibility of strains isolated from these patients and the outcome of contact tracing that was introduced during the study period.

MATERIAL AND METHODS

Bacterial strains

All Streptococcus pneumoniae strains resistant or intermediately susceptible to penicillin G isolated at the Clinical Microbiology Laboratory, University Hospital, Linköping, Sweden during 1994 were included. Two isolates could not be recovered viable and were excluded. Initially, they were classified as intermediately susceptible to penicillin G. Isolates were identified as S. pneumoniae on the basis of colony morphology, susceptibility to optochin and positive reaction with specific antisera (Phadebact, Pneumococcus Test, Boule Diagnostics AB, Huddinge, Sweden). Strains were screened for penicillin-susceptibility by disk diffusion using oxacillin (1 μg/disk) on PDM II medium (AB Biodisk, Solna, Sweden) supplemented with 5% defibrinated horse blood and incubated overnight at 37°C in 5% CO_2. Isolates with an inhibition zone of >17 mm were regarded as sensitive. For strains with zones ≤ 17 mm, penicillin resistance was verified by E-test (Biodisk). Breakpoints were defined as: susceptible, Minimal Inhibitory Concentration (MIC) ≤ 0.064 mg/l (S-strains); intermediately susceptible, MIC 0.125–1.0 mg/l (I-strains) and resistant, MIC ≥ 2.0 mg/l (R-strains). By that definition, 15 resistant isolates, all from the nasopharynx, and 26 intermediately susceptible isolates, 22 from the nasopharynx, one each from the eye, middle ear, maxillary sinus and blood, were included. Fourteen of the patients with R-strains and 21 of those with I-strains were below the age of 7. In comparison, 26 consecutive penicillin-susceptible isolates, 24 from the nasopharynx, one each from the middle ear

 ISSN 0036-5548

and a wound in the nose were obtained. Only one isolate per patient was included.

Antimicrobial susceptibility testing

Susceptibility testing was performed once for each isolate against penicillin G, ampicillin, cefuroxime, cefpodoxime, cefotaxime, imipenem, erythromycin, clindamycin, tetracycline, trimethoprim-sulfamethoxazole (TMS), chloramphenicol, vancomycin, rifampicin and ciprofloxacin with E-test and disk diffusion (the latter not against penicillin G). Disks and E-test strips were purchased from Biodisk. Disk diffusion was performed as for oxacillin testing by swabbing plates with a 1:20 dilution of a 0.5 McFarland bacterial suspension. E-tests were done according to the instructions of the supplier; a cotton swab dipped in a 0.5 McFarland suspension in phosphate buffered saline, pH 7.3, was used to inoculate the entire surface of a PDM II agar plate supplemented with 5% defibrinated horse blood.

After allowing the agar surface to dry, the E-test strip was applied and the plate was incubated overnight at 37°C in 5% CO_2. The MIC was read at the intersection between zone of inhibition and concentration scale on the strip. MIC-values were rounded off to the closest higher value used in broth or agar dilution MIC determinations. Breakpoints for susceptibility (S), intermediate susceptibility (I) and resistance (R) for both disk diffusion and E-test MICs were according to the Swedish Reference Group for Antibiotics (SRGA). In order to ensure interassay reproducibility, E-testing of S. pneumoniae ATCC 49619 against penicillin G was included each day during the survey. The variations of MICs from 0.38 to 0.50 mg/l, compared with expected values 0.25–1.0 mg/l, were considered acceptable.

Contact tracing

Contact tracing was introduced during the study period and was done around patients infected with R-strains or with I-strains resistant to another ≥ 4 non-beta-lactam antibiotics. Individuals living in the same household as the infected patient were cultured from the nasopharynx. When an infected child attended a day-care centre, symptomatic children and adults at the centre were cultured. If 1 of these was found to be infected with a penicillin I- or R-strain, all children and personnel, including those without symptoms, were cultured from the nasopharynx. Individuals with respiratory tract symptoms were treated according to in vitro antibiotic sensitivity pattern. The week after completion of treatment, individuals were cultured from the nasopharynx. Infected children were not denied attendance to day-care centres, except those with I- or R- strains resistant to another ≥ 4 non-beta-lactam antibiotics.

RESULTS

Antibiotic susceptibility

During the study period 3% of all S. pneumoniae, i.e. isolates from 43 individuals, identified at our laboratory had decreased susceptibility to penicillin G, i.e. an MIC-value ≥ 0.125 mg/l and 1% was resistant, i.e. had an MIC $\geq$ 2 mg/l.

All R-strains showed no zone of inhibition around the oxacillin disk. Zone of inhibition for I-strains varied from 0 to 12 mm and for S-strains from 22 to 32 mm. Thus, a cut-off zone of 17 mm discriminated between S-strains and I/R-strains.

Resistance of S. pneumoniae strains to antimicrobial agents, according to their susceptibility to penicillin G, is presented in Table I. The highest MIC-value of penicillin G was 4.0 mg/l. With the breakpoints used, all strains resistant to penicillin G were also resistant to cefuroxime and 66.7% to cefpodoxime. No such strain was classified as resistant to ampicillin. However, the distribution of MICs of ampicillin, cefuroxime and cefpodoxime was very similar. The lowest MIC-values of beta-lactam antibiotics were found for cefotaxime and imipenem and no strain was classified as resistant to these agents. The susceptibility to beta-lactams was as expected higher for I-strains than for R-strains and only 2 isolates resistant to cefuroxime were found. MICs of all tested beta-lactam antibiotics increased with MICs of penicillin G (Table II). The highest increase was recorded for cefuroxime and the lowest for imipenem. The MICs of erythromycin, clindamycin, tetracycline, TMS and chloramphenicol increased for penicillin I- and R-strains. A substantial number of strains were resistant to one or more of these 5 agents. However, resistance was more common among I-strains than among R-strains. For the penicillin-sensitive strains only 1 isolate resistant to tetracycline was recovered. Strains intermediately susceptible to penicillin G appeared in 2 populations with respect to sensitivity to tetracycline. Thirteen strains were sensitive to tetracycline (MICs ≤ 0.25 mg/l) and 13 were resistant (MICs ≥ 4.0 mg/l). No strain was found in between. Of the 13 tetracycline-resistant strains, 7 were also resistant to TMS, whereas only 3 of the 13 tetracycline-sensitive were TMS-resistant. Thus, a connection between resistance to tetracycline and TMS is suggested for these isolates. All 67 isolates were sensitive and had low MIC-values for vancomycin and rifampicin. No resistance to ciprofloxacin was found, but most strains had MICs at the S/I breakpoint value.

Six penicillin I- and R-strains were simultaneously resistant to another ≥ 3 non-beta-lactam antibiotics. They included erythromycin, clindamycin, tetracycline, TMS and chloramphenicol. No epidemiological connection could be etablished for 3 serotype 6 isolates with identical antibiograms. Another 5 penicillin I- and R-strains were simultaneously resistant to tetracycline and TMS.

Epidemiology

The contact tracing was introduced in September, 1994 when a patient infected with a resistant strain of S. pneumoniae and with an established contact with a foreign

Table I. *In vitro susceptibility of 67 Streptococcus pneumoniae isolates according to their susceptibility to penicillin G*

Antimicrobial agent	Susceptibility to penicillin G: Sensitive ($n = 26$) MIC$_{50}$[a] mg/l	MIC$_{90}$[a] mg/l	Range mg/l	% resistant[b]	Intermediate susceptible ($n = 26$) MIC$_{50}$[a] mg/l	MIC$_{90}$[a] mg/l	Range mg/l	% resistant[b]	Resistant ($n = 15$) MIC$_{50}$[a] mg/l	MIC$_{90}$[a] mg/l	Range mg/l	% resistant[b]
Penicillin G	0.032	0.064	0.008–0.064	0	0.5	1.0	0.25–1.0	0	2.0	4.0	2.0–4.0	100
Ampicillin	0.032	0.032	≤0.016–0.064	0	0.25	1.0	0.064–1.0	0	4.0	4.0	1.0–4.0	0
Cefuroxime	0.032	0.032	≤0.016–0.064	0	1.0	2.0	0.125–4.0	7.7	4.0	8.0	4.0–8.0	100
Cefpodoxime	0.032	0.064	≤0.016–0.064	0	0.25	2.0	0.064–2.0	0	4.0	4.0	2.0–4.0	66.7
Cefotaxime	0.016	0.032	0.008–0.032	0	0.25	0.5	0.064–1.0	0	1.0	2.0	1.0–2.0	0
Imipenem	0.016	0.032	0.008–0.032	0	0.125	0.125	0.032–0.25	0	0.5	0.5	0.25–0.5	0
Erythromycin	0.125	0.125	0.032–0.25	0	0.125	≥256	0.064–≥256	15.4	0.125	0.125	0.064–≥256	6.7
Clindamycin	0.125	0.25	0.032–0.25	0	0.125	≥256	0.064–≥256	11.5	0.125	0.25	0.064–≥256	6.7
Tetracycline	0.25	0.5	0.125–8.0	3.8	0.25	64	0.125–128	50.0	0.25	32	0.25–64	13.3
TMS[c]	0.25	0.5	0.25–2.0	0	8.0	≥32	0.25–≥32	38.5[d]	16	≥32	8–≥32	33.3[d]
Chloramphenicol	2.0	4.0	1.0–4.0	0	2.0	32	0.5–32	11.5	2.0	16	1.0–321	13.3
Vancomycin	1.0	1.0	0.5–1.0	0	0.5	1.0	0.5–1.0	0	1.0	1.0	0.5–1.0	0
Rifampicin	0.032	0.064	0.008–0.125	0	0.032	0.032	0.008–0.064	0	0.032	0.064	0.032–0.064	0
Ciprofloxacin	1.0	2.0	1.0–2.0	0	1.0	1.0	0.25–2.0	0	1.0	1.0	0.5–1.0	0

[a] MIC$_{50}$ and MIC$_{90}$; concentration of drug that inhibits 50% and 90% of the strains tested, respectively.
[b] According to MIC-breakpoints recommended by SRGA.
[c] Trimethoprim-sulfamethoxazole (1/19).
[d] Per cent of strains that are inhibited by <32 mg/l.

Table II. *Multiples of MIC_{50}-increase of beta-lactam antibiotics according to classification of susceptibility to penicillin G*

Antimicrobial agents	Multiples of MIC_{50}-increase[a] Category of penicillin susceptibility: Intermediate susceptible	Resistant
Penicillin G	15.6	62.5
Ampicillin	7.8	125
Cefuroxime	31.3	125
Cefpodoxime	7.8	125
Cefotaxime	15.6	62.5
Imipenem	7.8	31.3

[a] For each antibiotic the values were calculated as: MIC_{50} in the penicillin G I- or R-category, respectively divided by MIC_{50} in the penicillin S-category.

country with a high prevalence of penicillin-resistant pneumococci was identified.

Case report: A 4-year-old boy with 4 previous episodes of pneumonia was admitted to hospital because of high fever. He had been treated with penicillin V since 4 days without effect. On admittance, pulmonary X-ray confirmed pneumonia. Penicillin was substituted by TMS. Initially, the fever dropped, but relapsed the same day and erythromycin was added. Nasopharyngeal culture yielded growth of S. pneumoniae, serotype 9, resistant to penicillin G (MIC 2.0 mg/l) and to TMS but sensitive to erythromycin. The boy recovered and was discharged from hospital after 6 days. About 2 months before this episode he had been on vacation in Mallorca, Spain. During the vacation he had experienced respiratory symptoms and signs of otitis and was treated with an oral antibiotic mixture, probably a cephalosporin. After the vacation he rejoined his day-care centre group.

After the introduction of our contact tracing programme, tracing was performed around 6 index cases with resistant strains and around 2 cases with multiple-resistant, intermediately susceptible strains. Approximately 100 individuals were screened for the presence of such resistant pneumococci. The first index patient described in the case report did not yield any secondary cases. However, 2–3 months after this case, 5 children infected with penicillin-resistant pneumococci appeared in the same area of Linköping as the first case. Contact tracing around these cases yielded 6 secondary cases in 2 day-care centres. Two of the isolates came from asymptomatic carriers. These 12 penicillin-resistant strains were all isolated from children 6 years or younger attending 5 different day-care centres. All these strains had the same antibiogram and all were serotype 9 (Table III).

Contact tracing around the 2 patients with multiple-resistant I-strains did not yield any secondary cases. Both these patients were infected with multiple-resistant serotype 6 strains. They did not attend the same day-care centre.

Table III. *Antibiotic susceptibility pattern of 12 serotype 9 Streptococcus pneumoniae isolates*

Antimicrobial agents	MIC (mg/l)
Penicillin G	2.0
Ampicillin	4.0
Cefuroxime	4.0
Cefpodoxime	4.0
Cefotaxime	1.0
Imipenem	0.5
Erythromycin	0.125
Clindamycin	0.125
Tetracycline	0.25
TMS[a]	$8-\geq 32$[b]
Chloramphenicol	2.0
Vancomycin	1.0
Rifampicin	0.032
Ciprofloxacin	1.0

[a] Trimethoprim-sulfamethoxazole (1/19).
[b] Three isolates had MICs $\geq$32 mg/l, 8 had MICs 16 mg/l and one had MIC 8 mg/l.

DISCUSSION

Decreased susceptibility of pneumococci to penicillin has been uncommon in Sweden. During a survey in March–June 1994, a national average of 3.4% of isolates had decreased susceptibility to penicillin (8). However, there was great variation from one part of the country to the next. Southern Sweden had the highest prevalence with 16%, an increase compared with the mid-1980s (9). In this area about 10% of isolates were resistant to erythromycin, tetracycline or TMS, figures well above national averages.

In the present study MICs of all tested beta-lactam antibiotics increased with MICs of penicillin G. This has also been observed in other countries (10) and is expected from the mechanism of penicillin-resistance with altered penicillin-binding proteins (11). Distribution of MICs of ampicillin, cefuroxime and cefpodoxime was very similar for pneumococci within the 3 categories of susceptibility. The distribution of MICs of these 3 agents among our strains is similar to that reported from other countries (12, 13). Cefotaxime and imipenem were the beta-lactam antibiotics with highest in vitro activity against penicillin I- and R-strains. Cefotaxime has been used successfully in selected cases of meningitis in adults caused by strains with penicillin MICs as high as 4 mg/l (14). However, failures have been reported and adequate clinical data are lacking for recommendations on its general use in such cases. The same seems to be true for imipenem (15). Pneumococci isolated from cases of meningitis unsuccessfully treated with cefotaxime or ceftriaxone had MICs of 8–32 mg/l for these agents, but were intermediately susceptible to penicillin (MICs 0.25–1 mg/l) (16). This enforces the value of MIC determinations to each beta-lactam antibiotic before its use in therapy.

Twenty-seven % (11/41) of strains intermediately susceptible or resistant to penicillin were multiple-resistant, i.e. resistant to three or more antibiotic classes. No multiple-resistant, penicillin-sensitive strain was identified. Multiple-resistance was most widespread to oral agents used as substitutes for penicillin. Such resistance can be transferred between strains by conjugative transposons, 1 carrying resistance to clindamycin, erythromycin, kanamycin and tetracycline and another resistance to chloramphenicol and tetracycline (17). Penicillin-resistant strains have emerged multiple times and independently of 1 another in diverse geographic areas (18) and acquired multiple-resistance. Thus, the antibiotic sensitivity of penicillin-resistant strains cannot be predicted, but must be determined by in vitro testing. We observed no resistance to vancomycin. Vancomycin has been advocated by some as the agent of choice for treating infections due to penicillin-resistant pneumococci, but failures have occurred (16, 19).

We used the E-test to determine MICs. E-tests to beta-lactam antibiotics have been compared with the reference broth microdilution method for resistant pneumococci and found to be reliable (20). Furthermore, we performed repeated testing of the 14 antimicrobial agents to a S. pneumoniae ATCC 49619 reference strain with E-test and obtained MIC-values within ranges reached by the broth microdilution method. Thus, we consider our MICs to be accurate and comparable to those of other studies. However, disk diffusion was unreliable for SIR classification for some antimicrobials compared with classification obtained by MIC determination with E-test (data not shown). The most frequent discrepancies between E-test and disk diffusion were minor, i.e. an I result instead of an S or R result, for TMS, ciprofloxacin, ampicillin, cefuroxime, cefpodoxime and cefotaxime. Classification of susceptibility to TMS was not reproducible by E-test MIC determinations (Table III). S. pneumoniae species-specific breakpoints and methodological standardizations may resolve this problem.

Our strains intermediately susceptible to penicillin were obviously of diverse clonal origin since they had different antibiograms and belonged within at least 5 different serotypes. The isolates of these strains were also distributed during the whole study year and were from individuals living in different communities in the province of Östergötland. On the contrary, 12 of the 15 penicillin-resistant isolates were serotype 9. Six of these were recovered during contact tracing at 2 day-care centres located close to each other. Of the other 3 resistant strains, 2 were serotype 23 and 1 was not serotyped. Although not proven by genetic analysis, this strongly suggests spread of a single serotype 9 clone. This also means that the antibiotic susceptibility pattern of our penicillin-resistant isolates is less representative because of the predominance of 1 serotype compared with the intermediately susceptible strains.

Acquisition of penicillin- and multiple-resistant pneumococci has been associated with previous antibiotic therapy (19). This applies to our case report. Other risk factors for colonization and infection are age; ≤ 2 years and ≥ 70 years, hospitalization and attendence to day-care centres (19); the latter obvious also in this study. It has been suggested that unless there is evidence of cross-infection with penicillin-resistant strains there is no indication to treat and screen for potential carriers (21). We chose to screen family members and children and adults at day-care centres and treat those who were culture-positive. Only 2 asymptomatic carriers were found. Both were treated with rifampicin. Of the 17 treated patients with I- or R-strains that we followed with a nasopharyngeal culture the week after treatment, all became culture-negative. Two relapsed or were reinfected 3–4 months after the initial episode. Different regimens have been tried to eradicate the carrier state. Erythromycin plus rifampicin was successful in 96% of cases. Multiple-resistant strains were more difficult to eradicate and acquisition of rifampicin-resistance has occurred (15).

In conclusion, our data show the presence of penicillin- and multiple-resistant pneumococci in Sweden and that these strains can spread among individuals. A greater awareness with extended indications for microbiological diagnosis and antimicrobial susceptibility testing and restrictive prescription of antibiotics is needed.

ACKNOWLEDGEMENTS

The skilled technical assistance of Ms Anita Johansson is gratefully acknowledged. We thank the Swedish Institute for Infectious Disease Control for serotyping the pneumococcal isolates.

REFERENCES

1. Kislak JW, Razavi LMB, Daly AK, Finland M. Susceptibility of pneumococci to nine antibiotics. Am J Med Sci 250: 261-268, 1965.
2. Hansman D, Bullen MM. A resistant pneumococcus. Lancet 2: 264–265, 1967.
3. Appelbaum PC, Bhamjee A, Scragg JN, Hallett AF, Bowen AJ, Cooper RC. Streptococcus pneumoniae resistant to penicillin and chloramphenicol. Lancet 2: 995–997, 1977.
4. Fenoll A, Bourgon CM, Muñoz R, Vicioso D, Casal J. Serotype distribution and antimicrobial resistance of Streptococcus pneumoniae isolates causing systemic infections in Spain, 1979-1989. Rev Infect Dis 13: 56–60, 1991.
5. Appelbaum PC. Antimicrobial resistance in Streptococcus pneumoniae: an overview. Clin Infect Dis 15: 77–83, 1992.
6. Kristinsson KG, Hjálmarsdóttir MÁ, Steingrimsson O. Increasing penicillin resistance in pneumococci in Iceland. Lancet 339: 1606–1607, 1992.
7. Olsson-Liljequist B, Burman L, Kallings I, Swedish Respiratory Tract Study Group. Antibiotic susceptibility of upper respiratory tract pathogens in Sweden: a seven year follow-up study including loracarbef. Scand J Infect Dis 24: 485–493, 1992.
8. Olsson-Liljequist B. Antibiotikaresistens hos bakteriella luftvägspatogener i Sverige. Epidaktuellt 1: 3–5, 1995 (in Swedish).
9. Forsgren A, Walder M. Antimicrobial susceptibility of bacterial isolates in south Sweden including a 13-year follow-up study of some respiratory tract pathogens. APMIS 102: 227–235, 1994.

10. Jetté LP, Ringuette L, Dascal A, Lapointe J-R, Turgeon P. Pneumococcal resistance to antimicrobial agents in the province of Québec, Canada. J Clin Microbiol 32: 2572–2575, 1994.
11. Tomasz A. Biochemistry and genetics of penicillin resistance. In: Ferretti JJ, Curtis III R, editors. Streptococcal genetics. Am Soc Microbiol, Washington DC., 87–92, 1987.
12. Sprangler SK, Jacods MR, Appelbaum PC. In vitro susceptibilities of 185 penicillin-susceptible and -resistant pneumococci to WY-49605 (SUN/SY 5555), a new oral penem, compared with those to penicillin G, amoxicillin, amoxicillin-clavulanate, cefixime, cefaclor, cefpodoxime, cefuroxime, and cefdinir. Antimicrob Agents Chemother 38: 2902–2904, 1994.
13. Pankuch GA, Jacobs MR, Appelbaum PC. Susceptibilities of 200 penicillin-susceptible and -resistant pneumococci to piperacillin, piperacillin-tazobactam, ticarcillin, ticarcillin-clavulanate, ampicillin, ampicillin-sulbactam, ceftazidime, and ceftriaxone. Antimicrob Agents Chemother 38: 2905–2907, 1994.
14. Viladrich PF, Gudiol F, Liñares J, Rufi G, Ariza J, Pallares R. Characteristics and antibiotic therapy of adult meningitis due to penicillin-resistant pneumococci. Am J Med 84: 839–846, 1988.
15. Klugman KP. Pneumococcal resistance to antibiotics. Clin Microbiol Rev 3: 171–196, 1990.
16. Jacobs MR. Treatment and diagnosis of infections caused by drug-resistant Streptococcus pneumoniae. Clin Infect Dis 15: 119–127, 1992.
17. Jacoby GA. Prevalence and resistance mechanisms of common bacterial respiratory pathogens. Clin Infect Dis 18: 951–957, 1994.
18. Munoz R, Musser JM, Crain M, Briles DE, Marton A, Parkinson AJ, Sorensen U, Tomasz A. Geographic distribution of penicillin-resistant clones of Streptococcus pneumoniae: characterization by penicillin-binding protein profile, surface protein A typing, and multilocus enzyme analysis. Clin Infect Dis 15: 112–118, 1992.
19. Caputo GM, Appelbaum PC, Liu HH. Infections due to penicillin-resistant pneumococci: clinical, epidemiologic, and microbiologic features. Arch Intern Med 153: 1301–1310, 1993.
20. Krisher KK, Linscott A. Comparison of three commercial MIC systems, E-test, Fastidious Antimicrobial Susceptibility Panel, and FOX Fastidious Panel, for confirmation of penicillin and cephalosporin resistance in Streptococcus pneumoniae. J Clin Microbiol 32: 2242–2245, 1994.
21. Allen KD. Penicillin-resistant pneumococci. J Hosp Infect 17: 3–13, 1991.

Submitted April 20, 1995; accepted July 10, 1995

Scand J Infect Dis 27: 495–498, 1995 ORIGINAL ARTICLE

Enteric Plesiomonas shigelloides Infections in Finnish Patients

HILPI RAUTELIN[1], AULIKKI SIVONEN[1], ARJA KUIKKA[1], OLLI-VEIKKO RENKONEN[1], VILLE VALTONEN[2] and TIMO U. KOSUNEN[1]

From the Departments of [1]Bacteriology and Immunology, and [2]Medicine, Division of Infectious Diseases, University of Helsinki, Helsinki, Finland

Plesiomonas shigelloides was isolated from 20/13,027 stool samples submitted for culture to the Department of Bacteriology and Immunology, University of Helsinki, in 1990. All except 2/20 Plesiomonas-positive patients had diarrhea; 13 patients had acute onset of illness after foreign travel and 5 patients had chronic diarrhea with symptoms lasting ≥2 months. Travel destinations were outside Europe in most cases. In 12 cases Plesiomonas was isolated in pure culture and in 8 cases together with other enteropathogens. All isolates were susceptible to ciprofloxacin, doxycycline, trimethoprim and sulfamethoxazole, gentamicin, cephalexin, cefuroxime, ceftriaxone and cefixime.

H. Rautelin, MD, Department of Bacteriology and Immunology, University of Helsinki, Box 21, FIN-00014 Helsinki, Finland

INTRODUCTION

Plesiomonas shigelloides is a Gram-negative rod which can be isolated from water and from cold-blooded animals such as fish (1), from fecal samples from cats and dogs (1), from human stools and, on rare occasions, from human samples of extraintestinal origin (2, 3). Although Plesiomonas is quite rarely isolated from feces of asymptomatic persons (1) and it has been associated with diarrheal epidemics (4, 5), its role as an enteric pathogen is still controversial (6). Human volunteer studies (7) and animal models (8, 9) of Plesiomonas infection have failed to show enteropathogenicity. Furthermore, in some reports Plesiomonas has been isolated with similar frequencies from persons with and without diarrhea (8, 10).

The present study was undertaken over a 1-year period in Helsinki to investigate the clinical and epidemiological features of patients with Plesiomonas shigelloides isolated from feces.

MATERIAL AND METHODS

Patients

Patients whose stool specimens were submitted to the Department of Bacteriology and Immunology, University of Helsinki, were included in the study if the stool culture yielded P. shigelloides. Questionnaires regarding details of the illness, possible underlying disorders, and foreign travel within 3 months before the illness were sent to Plesiomonas-positive patients. At least 2 follow-up stool specimens were cultured in most cases to study the clearance of Plesiomonas from feces.

Isolation of enteropathogens

Stool samples submitted in Stuart tubes were cultured within 48 h of sampling (mean, 19 h). The samples were inoculated on campylobacter blood-free selective agar (Oxoid, Basingstoke, Hants, UK), on cystine lactose electrolyte-deficient (CLED) agar (Oxoid), xylose lysine deoxycholate (XLD) medium (BBL, Cockeysville, Maryland, USA), yersinia selective agar (Oxoid), and 5% horse blood agar containing 20 mg/l of ampicillin. The plates were incubated at 35°C for 18 h, except for campylobacter agar plates which were incubated at 43°C in an atmosphere of 5% O_2, 10% CO_2, and 85% N_2 for 48 h. For the enrichment of Salmonella species, a sample of feces was inoculated into selenite broth (Oxoid), and subcultured 24 h later on XLD.

Potential Plesiomonas colonies were tested for oxidase and for susceptibility to vibriostatic agent O/129 (2,4-diamino-6,7-diisopropylpteridin) and were further characterized by the API 20 E (Bio Merieux, Marcy-l'Étoile, France).

Determination of minimum inhibitory concentrations (MICs)

The antimicrobial agents studied were doxycycline (Pfizer, New York, USA), ciprofloxacin (Bayer, Leverkusen, Germany), sulfamethoxazole and trimethoprim (Orion, Espoo, Finland) gentamicin (Sigma, St. Louis, Missouri, USA), cephalexin (Sigma), cefuroxime (Glaxo Pharmaceuticals, Greenford, UK), ceftriaxone (F. Hoffman-La Roche, Basle, Switzerland) and cefixime (Orion).

The MICs of these antimicrobials were determined for all 20 isolates by the agar dilution method with Mueller–Hinton agar plates (BBL). Isolate of Escherichia coli ATCC 25922 was included on each plate to serve as a control organism. The plates were incubated for 24 h at 35°C. The MIC was defined as the lowest concentration of the drug that inhibited visible growth completely.

RESULTS

During the 1-year study period, 20 P. shigelloides isolates (from 20 patients) were isolated from 13,027 stool specimens cultured at the Department of Bacteriology and Immunology, University of Helsinki. This gives an isolation rate of 0.2%. The corresponding figures for other enteropathogens isolated during the same period were: Campylobacter sp. 3.6%, Salmonella sp. 3.3%, Aeromonas sp. 1.9%, Yersinia enterocolitica 1.7%, and Shigella sp. 0.4%. In 12 cases P. shigelloides was present in pure culture, and in eight cases it was isolated together with other enteropathogens (Table I). All the plesiomonas isolates were oxidase-positive and susceptible to the vibriostatic

 ISSN 0036-5548

Table I. *Clinical characteristics of 20 Plesiomonas patients*

Age, years	Sex	Underlying disorder	Recent travel	Duration of illness, days chr[a]	Symtoms	Therapy[b]	Mixed infection
14	M	—	Turkey	6	D[c], pain	—	C. jejuni
39	F	—	Africa	14	D, pain	Cipro	
50	F	—	Germany	0	—	—	
21	M	—	Australia	NK	D	—	Salmonella
68	M	NK	—	chr	Arthritis	NK	
26	F	—	Italy	5	D, pain	—	C. jejuni, Salmonella
64	F	—	—	chr	D	—	
72	M	—	—	chr	D	—	Aeromonas
26	F	—	Thailand	18	D	Ery	
30	M	—	Peru	NK	D	—	
20	M	—	Australis	2	D, pain	—	Salmonella
29	M	Crohn's disease	—	chr	D	—	Aeromonas
28	F	—	Turkey	>21	D, pain, fever	Antimicrobial NK	
47	M	—	Far East	4	D, pain	—	
42	M	—	Tunisia	15	D, fever	Ofl	
49	F	—	Ethiopia	33	D bloody, pain	Norfl	
48	M	Crohn's disease	—	chr	D	Cipro	
12	M	—	Russia	11	D, pain, headache, fever	—	C. jejuni
76	F	Addison's disease	—	chr	D, pain	Cipro	
23	F	—	Canary Islands	NK	D, fever	—	C. jejuni

NK = not known.

[a] Duration of illness (in days) for those with acute onset, in ch(onic) cases diarrhea had lasted for months before isolation of Plesiomonas.

[b] Cipro = ciprofloxacin; Ery = erythromycin; Norfl = norfloxacin; Ofl = ofloxacin.

[c] D = Diarrhea.

agent O/129. According to the API 20 E test they all gave excellent identification, and all were susceptible to the antimicrobial agents tested (Table II).

Questionnaires with clinical information were available from 16 patients. Some patient characteristics are presented in Table I. A total of 13 patients (age: mean 29 years; range, 12–49; gender: 7 males), without any underlying disorders, had an acute onset of illness after foreign travel. In 6 of them other enteropathogens were also isolated. Five patients (age: mean, 58 years; range, 29–76; gender: 4 males), 3 of whom had an underlying disorder, had chronic diarrhea with symptoms which had lasted months before the isolation of Plesiomonas.

Table II. *Minimum inhibitory concentrations (MICs) of 8 antimicrobial agents in agar dilutions for 20 Plesiomonas strains*

Antimicrobial agent	MIC, (mg/l)[a] Range	50%	90%
Doxycycline	0.12–2	0.12	1
Ciprofloxacin	0.03	0.03	0.03
Trimethoprim/sulphamethoxazole	0.5/9.5	0.5/9.5	0.5/9.5
Gentamicin	2–4	2	4
Cephalexin	4	4	4
Cefuroxime	0.12	0.12	0.12
Ceftriaxone	0.06	0.06	0.06
Cefixime	0.06	0.06	0.06

[a] 50 and 90%, MICs for 50 and 90% of isolates, respectively.

Watery diarrhea was reported by 11 patients with acute disease, and 1 of them had also experienced bloody stools. For 6 patients, the first symptom was abdominal pain, for 4 it was diarrhea, and for 1 patient it was fever. The symptom reported as the worst was: abdominal pain for 6 patients, diarrhea for 3, fever for 1, and headache for 1 patient. One of the patients had eaten oysters, and 3 further patients had consumed some other seafood. One patient strongly suspected chicken served on an airplane to be the cause of her diarrhea. Nine of 13 patients who had travelled abroad had been swimming outdoors in untreated water.

Follow-up stool cultures were available for 16 patients. In patients with acute onset of illness and who had not received antimicrobials Plesiomonas could not be found from feces taken 7–54 days (mean, 17 days) after the first positive isolation. Two patients excreted Plesiomonas in feces for a longer time. A 72-year-old man had chronic diarrhea without underlying disorders, and he excreted both Plesiomonas and Aeromonas in his feces for at least a month. In the case of another patient, with Crohn's disease and Plesiomonas as the sole enteropathogen, the chronic excretion stopped after administration of ciprofloxacin.

DISCUSSION

The incidence of P. shigelloides-associated diarrhea in the present study was low (0.2%). In other reports, the frequency of Plesiomonas enteritis has also been far from that of Campylobacter and Salmonella (11). Although the role of P. shigelloides as an enteropathogen is still controversial (12), it has been isolated more frequently from diarrheal stools than from normal stools (3). This was also clearly the case in the present study, as all except 2 of our Plesiomonas patients had diarrhea. In our previous study, Plesiomonas could not be found in the feces of 343 asymptomatic persons (13).

Foreign travel, especially in the tropics, has been shown to be a risk factor for Plesiomonas enteritis (11, 14). All our patients with acute onset of illness had travelled abroad before their illness. These patients more often had more exotic travel locations, usually outside of Europe, than previously described for Finnish enteritis patients (15). Furthermore, the only asymptomatic patient in the series had travelled abroad shortly before her illness, although in Europe.

A typical feature for our Plesiomonas patients was that they often had concomitant enteric infections (40%). In a study from the United States the presence of Plesiomonas in mixed infections was almost as high (30%) as in ours (11). Taylor and coworkers also reported a high incidence of polymicrobial enteric infections, including Plesiomonas infections, in Americans in Thailand (16). This could indicate that in the more exotic travel locations outside of Europe, where the incidence of Plesiomonas infections is higher, mixed enteric infections are also more common. Although the number of patients was limited in the present study, the symptoms of patients with Plesiomonas as the sole enteropathogen did not seem to differ from those of patients with several pathogens isolated concomitantly.

All the fecal isolates of Plesiomonas in the present study were susceptible to the antimicrobials tested, including cefixime (Table II). Our results and those of others (17, 18) indicate that several antimicrobials are available for the therapy of Plesiomonas enteritis. In our study, 3 patients with acute onset of illness were treated with antimicrobials effective against Plesiomonas in vitro; however, the timing of the therapy was not known. It has been suggested earlier that Plesiomonas-infected patients treated with antimicrobials have a briefer illness compared to those not treated (11), and good results have been obtained when immunosuppressive Plesiomonas patients with severe symptoms have been treated with antimicrobials (19). One of our patients with chronic diarrhea and long-lasting excretion of Plesiomonas was successfully treated with ciprofloxacin, although a long therapy was needed.

In conclusion, our results indicate that P. shigelloides is a rare cause of bacterial gastroenteritis. However, it may cause diarrhea also in young individuals without any underlying disorders, especially after travel outside of Europe. Plesiomonas may often be found in polymicrobial enteric infections and further studies are needed to verify its relative role in these cases.

ACKNOWLEDGEMENTS

The skilful technical assistance of Ms Sirpa Juvonen is gratefully acknowledged.

REFERENCES

1. Arai T, Ikejima N. A survey of Plesiomonas shigelloides from aquatic environments, domestic animals, pets and humans. J Hyg 84: 203–211, 1980.
2. Brenden RA, Miller MA, Janda JM. Clinical disease spectrum and pathogenic factors associated with Plesiomonas shigelloides infections in humans. Rev Infect Dis 10: 303–316, 1988.
3. Holmberg SD, Farmer JJ III. Aeromonas hydrophila and Plesiomonas shigelloides as causes of intestinal infections. Rev Infect Dis 6: 633–639, 1984.
4. Tsukamoto T, Kinoshita Y. Two epidemics of diarrhoeal disease possibly caused by Plesiomonas shigelloides. J Hyg 80: 275–280, 1978.
5. Rutala WA, Sarubbi Jr. FA, Finch CS, Steinkraus GE. Oyster-associated outbreak of diarrhoeal disease possibly caused by Plesiomonas shigelloides. Lancet 1: 739, 1982.
6. Abbott SL, Kokka RP, Janda JM. Laboratory investigations on the low pathogenic potential of Plesiomonas shigelloides. J Clin Microbiol 29: 148–153, 1991.
7. Herrington DA, Tzipori S, Robins-Browne RM, Tall BD, Levine ML. In vitro and in vivo pathogenicity of Plesiomonas shigelloides. Infect Immun 55: 979–985, 1987.
8. Pitarangsi C, Echeverria P, Whitmire R, Tirapat C, Formal S, Dammin GJ, Tingtalapong M. Enteropathogenicity of Aeromonas hydrophila and Plesiomonas shigelloides: prevalence among individuals with and without diarrhea in Thailand. Infect Immun 35: 666–673, 1982.
9. Penn RG, Giger DK, Knoop FC, Preheim LC. Plesiomonas shigelloides overgrowth in the small intestine. J Clin Microbiol 15: 869–872, 1982.
10. Bhat P, Shanthakumari S, Rajan D. The characterization and significance of Plesiomonas shigelloides and Aeromonas hydrophila isolated from an epidemic of diarrhoea. Indian J Med Res 62: 1051–1060, 1974.
11. Kain KC, Kelly MT. Clinical features, epidemiology, and treatment of Plesiomonas shigelloides diarrhea. J Clin Microbiol 27: 998–1001, 1989.
12. Ljungh Å, Wadström T. Aeromonas and Plesiomonas as possible causes of diarrhoea. Infection 13: 169–173, 1985.
13. Rautelin H, Sivonen A, Kuikka A, Renkonen OV, Valtonen V, Lehti H, Kahanpää A, Kosunen TU. Role of Aeromonas isolated from feces of Finnish patients. Scand J Infect Dis 27: 207–210, 1995.
14. Homberg SD, Wachsmuth IK, Hickman-Brenner FW, Blake PA, Farmer JJ III. Plesiomonas enteric infections in the United States. Ann Intern Med 105: 690–694, 1986.
15. Rautelin HI, Renkonen OV, von Bonsdorff CH, Lähdevirta J, Pitkänen T, Järvinen A, Reinikainen P, Kosunen TU. Prospective study of the etiology of diarrhea in adult outpatients and inpatients. Scand J Gastroenterol 24: 329–333, 1989.
16. Taylor DN, Echeverria P, Blaser MJ, Pitarangsi C, Blacklow N, Cross J, Weniger BG. Polymicrobial aetiology of travellers' diarrhoea. Lancet 1: 381–383, 1985.

17. Reinhardt JF, George WL. Comparative in vitro activities of selected antimicrobial agents against Aeromonas species and Plesiomonas shigelloides. Antimicrob Agents Chemother 27: 643–645, 1985.
18. Clark RB, Lister PD, Arneson-Robert L, Janda MJ. In vitro susceptibilities of Plesiomonas shigelloides to 24 antibiotics and antibiotic-β-lactamse-inhibitor combinations. Antimicrob Agents Chemother 34: 159–160, 1990.
19. Rolston KVI, Hopper RL. Diarrhea due to Plesiomonas shigelloides in cancer patients. J Clin Microbiol 20: 597–598, 1984.

Submitted April 10, 1995; accepted July 6, 1995

Scand J Infect Dis 27: 499–502, 1995 ORIGINAL ARTICLE

Analysis of Restriction Fragment Length Polymorphism and Ribotyping of Multiresistant Stenotrophomonas maltophilia Isolated from Persisting Lung Infection in a Cystic Fibrosis Patient

JÜRG WÜST[1], RENO FREI[2], HULDRYCH GÜNTHARD[3] and MARTIN ALTWEGG[1]

From the [1]Department of Medical Microbiology, University of Zürich, Zürich, the [2]Bacteriology Laboratory, University Hospital Basle, Basle, and the [3]Division of Infectious Diseases, Department of Internal Medicine, University Hospital, Zürich, Switzerland

A cystic fibrosis patient was infected by Stenotrophomonas maltophilia over at least 15 months. The bacteria became increasingly resistant to antimicrobial agents. Determination of restriction fragment length polymorphism and ribotyping showed that resistance was due to changes in that S. maltophilia rather than to infection by another strain.

J. Wüst, Ph.D., Department of Medical Microbiology, University of Zürich, Gloriastrasse 32, CH-8028 Zürich, Switzerland

INTRODUCTION

Stenotrophomonas (formerly Xanthomonas (1)) maltophilia has become an important pathogen in recent years. Colonization and infections have been reported in patients with impaired host defense mechanisms, indwelling catheters, artificial respiration, cystic fibrosis, and cancer (2–5). Because of the inherent resistance of S. maltophilia to many antimicrobial agents, treatment is often difficult (6–8). In cystic fibrosis patients, colonization can become chronic (9).

We report on a patient with cystic fibrosis from whom S. maltophilia could be isolated over a period of at least 15 months. The bacteria became increasingly resistant to antimicrobial agents. Ribotyping and determination of restriction fragment length polymorphism by pulsed-field gel electrophoresis showed that a single S. maltophilia strain colonized the patient during the whole investigation period of 15 months.

CASE REPORT AND METHODS

The 41-year old female patient had suffered since childhood from pulmonary disease related to cystic fibrosis, with recurrent bronchopulmonary exacerbations and various bronchopneumonias. Tracheal secretions obtained at the Cantonal University Hospital in Basle showed chronic colonization by S. maltophilia. The first strain available for investigation was isolated on May 16 1992. Therapy before this date and afterwards included various courses of amoxicillin with clavulanic acid, sulfamethoxazole/trimethoprim, ceftazidime, ceftriaxone, tobramycin and/or ciprofloxacin, resulting in temporary clinical improvement. From May 1992 through November 1992 the patient was in a stable condition, and therefore, she was not hospitalized and no tracheal secretions for microbiological investigations were obtained during this period. From July 1 to 9 1993 she was receiving ceftazidime plus ciprofloxacin before being transferred for a lung transplant to the University Hospital in Zürich. The transplant was performed on July 27 1993. From July 29 to August 2 1993 she received ceftazidime, netilmicin and ciprofloxacin. Due to the increasing resistance of the S. maltophilia to these agents, therapy was switched to chloramphenicol plus amikacin from August 5 to 9 1993. As the combination of piperacillin/tazobactam and amikacin (for both drugs MIC values were in the resistant range when tested alone) exhibited synergism in the checkerboard titration within the therapeutic range, treatment was changed to these antimicrobial agents on August 9 1993. However, production of purulent tracheal secretions continued, though S. maltophilia could no longer be cultivated from August 8 1993 onwards. As polymyxin showed some synergy with amikacin and because sparfloxacin showed borderline activity in vitro, polymyxin by inhalation plus sparfloxacin given orally were added from August 11 1993, after which pus secretion ceased rapidly.

Clinical specimens were cultured aerobically at 37°C with 5% CO_2 on Columbia agar with 5% sheep blood, on Columbia agar with 5% sheep blood, colistin and nalidixic acid (CNA), and on Columbia chocolate agar; MacConkey agar was incubated aerobically without CO_2 (all media were from Becton Dickinson Microbiology Systems, Cockeysville, Maryland, USA). Bacteria were identified according to standard methods (10, 11). API 20NE (API, La-Balme-les-Grottes, France) was used for identification of S. maltophilia. Five independently isolated strains of S. maltophilia (Sm 1–5) were used for comparison.

MIC values were determined by the NCCLS agar dilution test procedure on Mueller–Hinton agar (12). For synergy testing, checkerboard titrations were performed in microtiter plates using volumes of 100 µl per well of cation-adjusted Mueller–Hinton broth (12). Piperacillin/tazobactam was tested at a constant concentration of tazobactam of 4 mg/l (12).

Total genomic DNA was isolated following a standard miniprep procedure as described by Ausubel et al. (13) with the modification that cells were incubated in proteinase K and SDS for 4–6 h. Ribotyping was performed essentially as described by Martinetti & Altwegg (14) using restriction enzyme ClaI (Beohringer Mannheim, Mannheim, Germany).

 ISSN 0036-5548

Table I. *Dates of isolation (month-day-year), preceding antimicrobial therapy, typing results, and MIC values*

Antimicrobial agents used ≤2 days before specimen was taken	AUG[a] SXT CIP ↓	CIP ↓	CAZ CIP ↓	CAZ CIP ↓		SXT ↓				NET CAZ CIP ↓			C AN ↓
Isolate no.	**1[b]**	2	3	**4**	5	**6**	**7**	**8**	**9**	**10**	**11**	**12**	**13**
Date of isolation	**05-16-92**	12-01-92	12-09-92	**12-19-92**	12-19-92	**12-30-92**	**02-22-03**	**03-03-93**	**07-30-93**	**08-01-93**	**08-01-93**	**08-03-93**	**08-06-93**
RFLP type[c]	**I**	II	II	**I**	II	**I**	**I**	**I**	**I**	**I**	**I**	**I**	**I**
rRNA gene patterns with ClaI[c]	**F′**	G	G	**F**	G	**F**	**F″**	**F″**	**F″**	**F**	**F**	**F**	**F**
MIC values by agar dilution, mg/l													
Ceftazidime	**128**	256	512	**128**	512	**64**	**64**	**64**	**128**	**256**	**256**	**512**	**512**
Piperacillin/tazobactam	**1,024**	1,024	1,024	**1,024**	1,024	**128**	**64**	**256**	**1,024**	**1,024**	**1,024**	**1,024**	**1,024**
Ciprofloxacin	**2**	4	4	**2**	16	**16**	**2**	**2**	**2**	**4**	**4**	**4**	**8**
Sparfloxacin	**1**	1	1	**0.5**	4	**1**	**0.5**	**0.5**	**0.5**	**1**	**1**	**2**	**2**
Chloramphenicol	**8**	16	16	**8**	32	**32**	**8**	**8**	**8**	**8**	**8**	**8**	**8**
Colistin	**8**	64	32	**8**	16	**4**	**8**	**4**	**4**	**4**	**4**	**32**	**8**
Amikacin	**256**	128	256	**128**	64	**32**	**128**	**256**	**256**	**512**	**512**	**1,024**	**1,024**
Netilmicin	**64**	128	128	**8**	128	**32**	**64**	**8**	**16**	**512**	**512**	**1,024**	**1,024**

[a] AUG = amoxicillin + clavulanic acid; SXT = sulfamethoxazole/trimethoprim; CIP = ciprofloxacin; CAZ = ceftazidime; NET = netilmicin; C = chloramphenicol; AN = amikacin.
[b] Values of the persisting strain in bold (RFLP type I).
[c] Five independently isolated control strains of S. maltophilia (Sm 1–5) had the RFLP patterns III to VII; their ClaI ribotype patterns were designated A to E.

Restriction fragment length polymorphism (RFLP) was determined by the pulsed-field gel electrophoresis (PFGE) procedure described by Sader et al. (15). In brief, chromosomal DNA was digested by the restriction endonuclease XbaI and ensuing fragments separated by PFGE in a 1% gel at 5 V/cm and 12°C using a CHEF-DR III system (Bio-Rad Laboratories, Richmond, California, USA). The pulse time was ramped from 1 to 40 s over 24 h.

RESULTS AND DISCUSSION

Table I shows the dates of isolation, preceding antimicrobial therapy, results of RFLP and ribotyping as well as the minimum inhibitory (MIC) values of the antimicrobial agents used in treating the patient. Two RFLP types could be found by PFGE (see Fig. 1), type I persisting over the whole period observed, and type II being isolated three times intermittently over the first 7 months. Five epidemiologically unrelated strains were clearly different. Ribotyping (Fig. 2) essentially confirmed these findings. The 3 RFLP type II strains were identical by ribotyping. ClaI patterns of these strains were clearly different from all the rest of the patient's isolates and much more closely related to 2 of the control strains. RFLP type I strains varied slightly in their ribotyping patterns (F, F′, F″). Pattern F′ differed from pattern F in that the smaller of the 2 bands was significantly less intense but reproducibly visible; pattern F″ differed from pattern F by an additional faint band. When compared to controls and strains of RFLP type II of the patient, these patterns were closely related and compatible, with a single strain which exhibited minor changes in rDNA patterns. This view is supported by the fact that the different subtypes were clustered with respect to time of isolation. Variations within a clone detectable by ribotyping do not seem to be very unusual and have been observed before in other organisms (14, 16). Ribotyping seems to be oversensitive in some instances. The frequency of variations may be dependent on the organisms analysed, because in some species patterns have remained constant over long time periods in vivo (17) and over many subcultures in vitro (18). In a recent epidemiology study on S. maltophilia, PFGE yielded reproducible and easily readable patterns (19); therefore, it may be the superior method for typing S. maltophilia.

Endpoint reading of MICs was usually easy. Tailing was encountered with sulfamethoxazole/trimethoprim, for which an endpoint could not be determined over the range 32–512 mg/l. The MICs of antimicrobial agents not shown in the table were: aztreonam, 256 to ≥1,024 mg/l; ceftriaxone, 512 to ≥1,024 mg/l; imipenem, 512 to ≥1,024 mg/l; moxalactam, 4 to 64 mg/l; and gentamicin, 64 to ≥1,024 mg/l (values decreasing or increasing generally in parallel with the other β-lactams and aminoglycosides shown in Table I). An increase in resistance in our isolates was confirmed by testing all strains in parallel simultaneously on the same plates.

Isolate 11 cultured on August 1 1993 was tested in a microtiter checkerboard plate. By this method, the MIC of

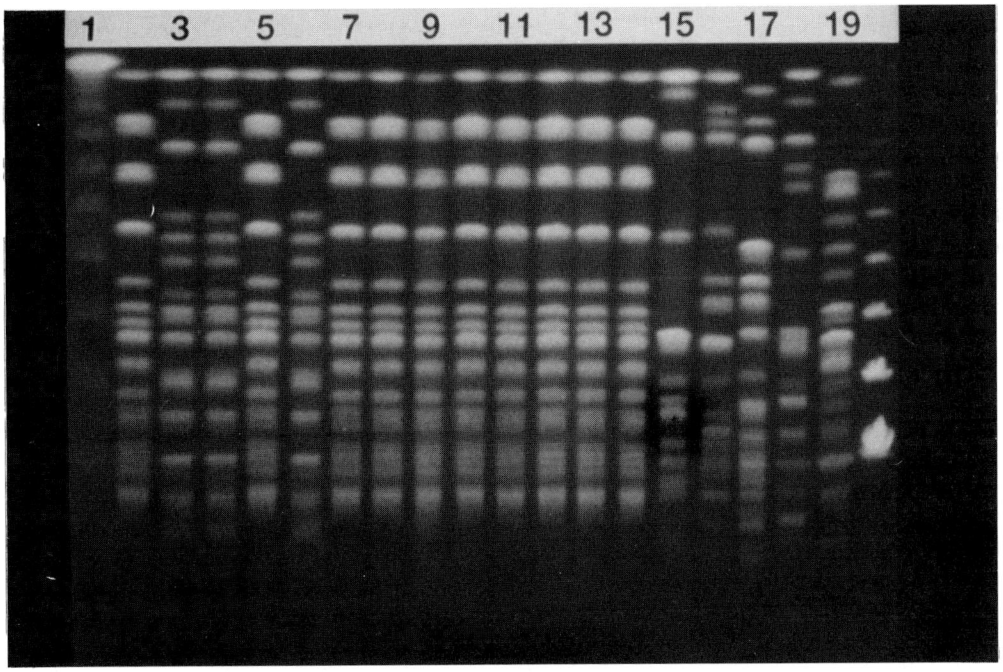

Fig. 1. Restriction fragment length polymorphism analysis of chromosomal DNA of S. maltophilia digested with XbaI. Lanes 1 and 20, 48.5 kb lambda ladder; lanes 3, 4, and 6, patient's isolates of S. maltophilia 2, 3, and 5 (RFLP type II); lanes 2, 5, 7–14, isolates 1, 4, 6–13 (RFLP type I); lanes 15–19, S. maltophilia control strains Sm1–5.

piperacillin/tazobactam alone was 512 mg/l, and of amikacin alone, it was 64 mg/l. In combination, inhibition occurred at 8 mg piperacillin/tazobactam plus 4 mg amikacin per liter with a fractional inhibitory concentration (FIC) index of 0.08 (20). The MIC of sparfloxacin was 0.5 mg/l; no synergism could be observed in combination of sparfloxacin with piperacillin/tazobactam or amikacin. The MIC of colistin was 8 mg/l; in combination with amikacin,

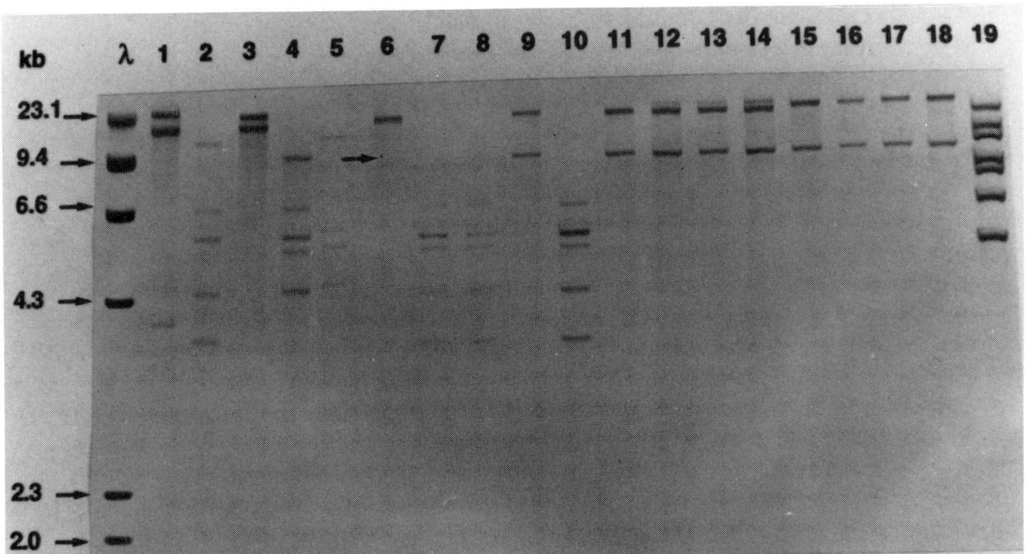

Fig. 2. rDNA patterns of genomic DNA of S. maltophilia digested with ClaI. Lane λ, molecular weight marker lambda DNA digested with HindIII, fragment sizes (in kb) from the top to the bottom are: 23.1, 9.4, 6.6, 4.3, 2.3, 2.0. Lanes 1–5, S. maltophilia control strains Sm 1–5, lanes 7, 8, 10, S. maltophilia isolates 2, 3, and 5 (RFLP type II); lanes 6, 9, 11–18, S. maltophilia isolates 1, 4, 6–13 (RFLP type I) (an arrow in lane 6 depicts a faint band reproducibly visible in the original gels); lane 19, molecular weight marker Serratia fonticola (standard) DNA digested with HindIII, fragment sizes (in kb) from the top to the bottom are: 14.6, 11.8, 10.6, 8.5, 7.9, 6.6, 5.4. Positions of fragments of the molecular weight marker lambda DNA digested with HindIII are indicated at left.

a slight synergism could be demonstrated in vitro (FIC index 0.25).

The data support the hypothesis that most probably a single strain of S. maltophilia permanently colonized the patient, and developed increasing resistance to antimicrobial agents under the selective pressure of antibiotic therapy. Bacteriological eradication of S. maltophilia and clinical success after the lung transplant was achieved with vigorous antimicrobial combination therapy according to in vitro test results. Further studies are needed to determine whether combination therapy can prevent development of resistance and can more effectively eradicate S. maltophilia.

Since both the University Hospitals in Basle and Zürich are separate from children's hospitals, very few patients with cystic fibrosis are treated in these 2 institutions (only adult cystic fibrosis patients or children for cardiopulmonary surgery or neurosurgery). Overall therefore, S. maltophilia is rarely isolated in both microbiology laboratories. Molecular typing of all S. maltophilia isolates ob tained in Basle within a 2-year period showed different types and did not suggest nosocomial transmission.

ACKNOWLEDGEMENT

We thank S. Gilgen, U. Hardegger, E. Huf, and J. Lüthy-Hottenstein, for their skilful technical assistance.

REFERENCES

1. Palleroni NJ, Bradbury JF. Stenotrophomonas, a new bacterial genus for Xanthomonas maltophilia (Hugh 1980) Swings et al. 1983. Int J Syst Bacteriol 43: 606–609, 1993.
2. Elting LS, Khardori N, Bodey GP, Fainstein V. Nosocomial infection caused by Xanthomonas maltophilia: a case–control study of predisposing factors. Infect Control Hosp Epidemiol 11: 134–138, 1990.
3. Hulisz DT, File TM. Predisposing factors and antibiotic use in nosocomial infections caused by Xanthomonas maltophilia. Infect Control Hosp Epidemiol 13: 489–490, 1992.
4. Khardori N, Elting L, Wong E, Schable B, Bodey GP. Nosocomial infections due to Xanthomonas maltophilia (Pseudomonas maltophilia) in patients with cancer. Rev Infect Dis 12: 997–1003, 1990.
5. Marshall WF, Keating MR, Anhalt JP, Steckelberg JM. Xanthomonas maltophilia: an emerging nosocomial pathogen. Mayo Clin Proc 64: 1097–1104, 1989.
6. Khardori N, Reuben A, Rosenbaum B, Rolston K, Bodey P. In vitro susceptibility of Xanthomonas (Pseudomonas) maltophilia to newer antimicrobial agents. Antimicrob Agents Chemother 34: 1609–1610, 1990.
7. Lecso-Bornet M, Pierre J, Sarkis-Karam D, Lubera S, Bergogne-Berezin E. Susceptibility of Xanthomonas maltophilia to six quinolones and study of outer membrane proteins in resistant mutant selected in vitro. Antimicrob Agents Chemother 36: 669–671, 1992.
8. Neu HC, Saha G, Chin NX. Resistance of Xanthomonas maltophilia to antibiotics and the effect of β-lactamase inhibitors. Diagn Microbiol Infect Dis 12: 283–285, 1989.
9. Karpati F, Malmborg A-S, Alfredsson H, Hjelte L, Strandvik B. Bacterial colonisation with Xanthomonas maltophilia – a retrospective study in a cystic fibrosis patient population. Infection 22: 258–263, 1994.
10. Balows A, Hausler WJ, Hermann KL, Isenberg HD, Shadomy HJ, eds. Manual of clinical microbiology, 5th edn. Washington, DC: American Society for Microbiology, 1991.
11. Gilardi GL. Pseudomonas and related genera. In: Balows A, Hausler WJ, Jr, Hermann KL, Isenberg HD, Shadomy HJ, eds. Manual of clinical microbiology, 5th edn. Washington, DC: American Society for Microbiology, 429–441, 1991.
12. National Committee for Clinical Laboratory Standards (NCCLS). Methods for dilution antimicrobial susceptibility tests for bacteria that grow aerobically, 2nd edn. Approved Standard M7-A2. Villanova, Pennsylvania: NCCLS, 1990.
13. Ausubel FM, Brent R, Kingston RE, Moore DD, Seidman JG, Smith JA, Struhl K. Current protocols in molecular biology. Chichester: John Wiley, 1989.
14. Martinetti G, Altwegg M. rRNA gene restriction patterns and plasmid analysis as a tool for typing Salmonella enteritidis. Res Microbiol 141: 1151–1162, 1990.
15. Sader HS, Pignatari AC, Frei R, Hollis RJ, Jones RN. Pulsed-field electrophoresis of restriction-digested genomic DNA and antimicrobial susceptibility of Xanthomonas maltophilia strains from Brazil, Switzerland and the USA. J Antimicrob Chemother 33: 615–618, 1994.
16. Grimont F, Grimont PAD. Ribosomal ribonucleic acid gene restriction patterns as potential taxonomic tools. Ann Inst Pasteur 137 B: 165–175, 1986.
17. Moyer NP, Martinetti G, Lüthy-Hottenstein J, Altwegg M. Value of rRNA gene restriction patterns of Aeromonas spp. for epidemiological investigations. Curr Microbiol 24: 15–21, 1992.
18. Stull TL, LiPuma JJ, Edlind TD. A broad-spectrum probe for molecular epidemiology of bacteria: ribosomal RNA. Res Microbiol 141: 1151–1162, 1988.
19. Laing FPY, Ramotar K, Read RR, Alfieri N, Kureishi A, Henderson EA, Louie TJ. Molecular epidemiology of Xanthomonas maltophilia colonization and infection in the hospital environment. J Clin Microbiol 33: 513–518, 1995.
20. Eliopoulos GM, Moellering RC. Antimicrobial combinations. In: Lorian V, ed. Antibiotics in laboratory medicine, 3rd edn. Baltimore: Williams and Wilkins, 433–492, 1991.

Submitted April 15, 1995; accepted July 5, 1995

Scand J Infect Dis 27: 503–505, 1995 ORIGINAL ARTICLE

Azithromycin for Treatment of Community Acquired Pneumonia Caused by Legionella pneumophila: A Retrospective Study

ILIJA KUZMAN[1], IVAN SOLDO[1], SLAVKO SCHÖNWALD[1] and JOSIP ČULIG[2]

From the [1]University Hospital of Infectious Diseases "Dr Fran Mihaljević" and [2]Pliva Pharmaceutical, Zagreb, Croatia

A clinical, retrospective and non-comparative study was undertaken to assess the clinical efficacy and tolerability of azithromycin in the treatment of community-acquired pneumonia caused by Legionella pneumophila. A total of 16 patients with a serologically confirmed diagnosis of Legionnaires' diseases were included. Azithromycin was administered orally at a total dose of 1.5 g for either 3 or 5 days. All patients were successfully cured; 15 patients became afebrile within 48 h and 1 patient within 96 h after the start of therapy. There were no side-effects requiring discontinuation of the treatment. Further increase of abnormal baseline liver function was recorded in 2 patients and in 1 patient mild, transient eosinophilia. Equal clinical efficacy and tolerability were observed with the 3- and 5-day dosage regimen. These results indicate that azithromycin given at a standard dose of 1.5 g is effective and well tolerated in the treatment of Legionnaires' disease.

I. Kuzman, MD, University Hospital of Infectious Diseases "Dr Fran Mihaljević", Mirogojska 8, HR-10000 Zagreb, Croatia

INTRODUCTION

Legionella pneumophila is a relatively frequent causative pathogen of pneumonia. Numerous clinical investigations in various countries have shown it to be the causative pathogen in 2–10% of community-acquired pneumonias (1–5), and often a cause of nosocomial pneumonias as well (6). There are no reliable clinical, radiological or analytical findings indicating that pneumonia is caused by Legionella spp.

When the clinical diagnosis of pneumonia is established, the etiology is mostly unknown, hence the initial antimicrobial treatment is empirical in the majority of cases. Today, the oral application of macrolides or tetracyclines is recommended as a rational initial treatment for community-acquired pneumonia in previously healthy persons younger than 65 years. Mainly, this refers to pneumonias which manifest clinically in an atypical way and for which Legionella pneumophila is also an important causative pathogen (7).

Numerous investigations and clinical experience traditionally recommend erythromycin as the drug of choice for treatment of Legionnaires' disease. However, therapeutical failures have been recorded (8–10) as well as the appearance of erythromycin-resistant strains (11, 12).

Azithromycin, a novel azalide antibiotic is very active against L. pneumophila. It is superior to erythromycin in vitro as well as in experimental legionellosis (13–15). Although the results of preclinical and pharmacokinetic studies suggest that azithromycin is a promising agent in the treatment of legionellosis, data on clinical efficacy are still limited (10, 16).

We here present our clinical experience with azithromycin in the treatment of community-acquired pneumonia caused by L. pneumophila.

 ISSN 0036-5548

PATIENTS AND METHODS

The study was clinical, non-comparative and retrospective. A total of 16 patients with a serologically confirmed diagnosis of community-acquired pneumonia, caused by L. pneumophila, were included. They were hospitalized as sporadic cases in the University Hospital of Infectious Diseases in Zagreb in the period from 1990–1994. They represent a random choice among 32 patients with serologically confirmed Legionnaires' disease during this period. There was no difference in severity of the disease between them and 16 other patients who were treated with other antibiotics.

Pneumonia was defined as an acute disease accompanied by fever >39.0°C, relevant clinical signs and symptoms and a positive chest X-ray demonstrating the presence of a new infiltrate. A full medical examination was carried out in all patients, including bacteriological assessments of blood, sputum and urine specimens, laboratory testing of hematological and biochemical parameters and a chest X-ray.

No patient had severe chronic cardiac or pulmonary diseases or signs of immunodeficiency. All were males with a mean age of 42.8 years (range 27–60). Out of 16 patients, 12 were smokers.

L. pneumophila, serotype 1, was confirmed in all patients by the Legionella Indirect Fluorescent Antibody (IFA) test (Zeus Scientific, New Jersey, USA) (17), and also in 1 patient by confirmation of antigen in sputum by a direct immunofluorescent method (18). Serological confirmation was based either on a 4-fold rise in titer (from acute to convalescent) or on an acute reciprocal titer of ≥512. In all patients, sputum or blood cultures, as well as serological analyses for the most frequent causative pathogens of atypical pneumonia (Mycoplasma pneumoniae, Chlamydia spp., Coxiella burnetti, influenza A and B viruses, parainfluenza virus, adenoviruses), were negative. Out of 32 patients serologically positive for Legionella pneumophila infection, only 16 were included in the study because they had not received previous antimicrobial therapy effective against L. pneumophila (macrolides, tetracyclines, rifampicin, quinolones, chloramphenicol, co-trimoxazol).

Azithromycin was administered orally at a total dose of 1.5 g, with 11 patients treated for 5 days (first day 500 mg and remaining days 250 mg, once daily) and 5 patients for 3 days (500 mg once daily).

Clinical symptoms and signs, as well as side-effects, were monitored daily. Chest X-rays were done at baseline and were repeated

Table I. *Clinical symptoms and pathological laboratory findings before the start of azithromycin therapy in patients with pneumonia caused by L. pneumophila*

Symptom or laboratory finding	Patients with pathological findings	
	n	%
Fever >40°C	14	88
Headache	15	94
Myalgias	12	75
Diarrhea	8	50
Vomiting	6	38
Hypotension	4	25
Tachypnea/dyspnea	10	63
Neurologic symptoms	4	25
Elevated ESR	16	100
Leukocytosis	8	50
Increased alpha-2 globulin	16	100
Hyponatremia	12	75
Abnormal liver function tests	12	75

after 10–14 days. Hematological and biochemical laboratory analyses were carried out before, 7 and 11–14 days after the start of azithromycin therapy.

The clinical efficacy of azithromycin was evaluated as follows.

1. Very good: resolution of fever within 48 h after the start of treatment with improvement of other signs and symptoms of pneumonia.
2. Good: resolution of fever within 96 h after the start of treatment with improvement of other signs and symptoms of pneumonia.
3. Failure: presence of fever 96 h after the start of treatment or persistence or progression of pneumonic infiltrate on control chest radiograph, or replacement of azithromycin with other antibiotic, or discontinuation of the treatment due to side-effects.

RESULTS

Patients were hospitalized 2–7 days after the appearance of first symptoms (mean 4.7 days) and their hospitalization lasted from 11 to 52 days (mean 20.5 days). All patients had clinical signs and symptoms and laboratory findings indicating the presence of serious infectious disease (Table I). No patient was treated in an intensive care unit. In 11 patients chest X-ray findings were described as interstitial and in 5 as homogeneous alveolar. Pleural effusion was registered in 2 patients and 1 patient had multifocal pneumonia.

Before hospitalization 11/16 patients were treated with beta-lactam antibiotics. Eight of them were treated with penicillins and 3 with cephalosporins. Five patients did not receive any antibiotic prior to azithromycin.

All patients were successfully cured with azithromycin. There were no differences in efficacy (duration of fever) between the 3- or 5-day dosage regimen. After the start of the therapy, 15 patients became afebrile within 48 h and 1 within 96 h. There were no discontinuations of treatment due to clinical failure or side-effects.

Azithromycin was very well tolerated and no side-effects were observed. In 1 patient a transient elevation of the eosinophil count to 11% was registered. In 2 patients with elevated liver aminotransferases at baseline a further 2- and 3-fold elevation was recorded. In both patients the aminotransferase abnormalities resolved spontaneously within the following 2 weeks.

DISCUSSION

Azithromycin is an azalide antibiotic. In comparison with erythromycin, it has a broader antimicrobial spectrum, a longer elimination half-life, better pharmacokinetic properties and it achieves higher tissue concentrations (19). High and prolonged concentrations of azithromycin in pulmonary tissue and alveolar macrophages are also well documented in humans (20, 21).

Pulmonary concentrations of azithromycin are much higher than minimal inhibitory concentrations for various causative pathogens of pneumonia, including L. pneumophila (22, 23). It has been demonstrated in vitro (13, 24) and in vivo (14, 15) that azithromycin has better activity against legionella than erythromycin.

L. pneumophila, as well as other intracellular pathogens, is often not recognized as the causative pathogen when antibiotic therapy is initiated. Therefore, in the majority of cases initial treatment of pneumonia is based on clinical data and is carried out empirically. Since legionellas are relatively frequent causative pathogens, a rational initial therapeutical choice in the treatment of atypical community-acquired pneumonia should include an antibiotic which is clinically effective against Legionella spp.

Azithromycin is equally effective but better tolerated than erythromycin in the treatment of atypical pneumonia caused by Mycoplasma pneumoniae and Chlamydia spp. in adults (25). Similar results have also been achieved in comparison to roxithromycin (26). The 3- and 5-day dosage regimens of azithromycin (total dose of 1.5 g) have both been equally effective and well-tolerated in the treatment of atypical pneumonias (27).

As far as we know, there are only 2 publications regarding the treatment of Legionnaires' disease with azithromycin. In a non-comparative pilot study Myburgh et al. reported successful cure of 8 patients with serologically confirmed L. pneumophila pneumonia. Azithromycin was administered orally, 500 mg once daily for 3 days (16). Dorrell et al. reported a cure in 1 patient treated intravenously with azithromycin after unsuccessful treatment with erythromycin and rifampicin (10).

Our results show that azithromycin, at a total dose of 1.5 g orally, given for 3 or 5 days is clinically very effective in the treatment of Legionnaires' disease. Out of 16 patients, 15 became afebrile within 48 h after the start of azithromycin therapy. We propose that azithromycin is a drug of choice for the initial treatment of atypical community-acquired pneumonia, since it is active against most common causative pathogens including Legionella pneumophila.

Our clinical experience and the results of preclinical pharmacological studies indicate that azithromycin is a useful antibiotic in the treatment of Legionnaires' disease.

REFERENCES

1. Macfarlane JT, Finch RG, Ward MJ, Macrae AD. Hospital study of adult community-acquired pneumonia. Lancet 2: 255–258, 1982.
2. Marrie TD, Durant H, Yates L. Community-acquired pneumonia requiring hospitalization: 5-year prospective study. Rev Infect Dis 11: 586–599, 1989.
3. Walder M, Svanteson B, Ursing J, Cronberg S, Johnsson T, Forsgren A. Incidence of Legionella pneumophila in acute lower respiratory tract infections. Scand J Infect Dis 13: 159–160, 1981.
4. Friis-Møller A, Rechnitzer C, Black FT, Collins MT, Lind K, Aalund O. Prevalence of legionnaires' disease in pneumonia patients admitted to Danish department of infectious diseases. Scand J Infect Dis 18: 321–328, 1986.
5. Fang GD, Fine M, Orloff J. New and emerging etiologies for community-acquired pneumonia with implications for therapy. A prospective multicenter study of 359 cases. Medicine 69: 307–316, 1990.
6. Nguyen MLT, Yu VL. Legionella infection. Clin Chest Med 12: 257–267, 1991.
7. Marrie TJ. Community-acquired pneumonia. Clin Infect Dis 18: 501–515, 1994.
8. Miller AC. Erythromycin in legionnaires' disease: a reappraisal. J Antimicrob Chemother 7: 217–222, 1981.
9. Mercatello A, Frappaz D, Robert D. Failure of erythromycin/rifampicin treatment of Legionella pneumophila. J Infect 10: 282–283, 1985.
10. Dorrell L, Fulton B, Ong ELC. Intravenous azithromycin as salvage therapy in a patient with Legionnaire's disease. Thorax 49: 620–621, 1994.
11. Moffie BG, Mouton RP. Sensitivity and resistance of Legionella pneumophila to some antibiotics and combinations of antibiotics. J Antimicrob Chemother 22: 457–462, 1988.
12. Dowling JN, Mac Devitt DA, Pasculle AW. Isolation and preliminary characterization of erythromycin-resistant variants of Legionella micdadei and Legionella pneumophila. Antimicrob Agents Chemother 27: 272–274, 1985.
13. Arnold B, Ta A, Stout JE, Yu VL. Erythromycin, dirithromycin, azithromycin, clarithromycin, and roxithromycin activity against Legionella by broth dilution and intracellular penetration. Program and Abstracts of the 34th Interscience Conference on Antimicrobial Agents and Chemotherapy, Orlando, Florida, USA, October 4–7, 1994.
14. Fitzgeorge RB, Featherstone ASR, Baskerville A. Efficacy of azithromycin in the treatment of guinea pigs infected with Legionella pneumophila by aerosol. J Antimicrob Chemother 25 (Suppl A): 101–108, 1990.
15. Garcia-de-Lomas J, Millas E, Burgos A, Colomina FJ, Savall F, Simo MJ, Gimeno C. Oral azithromycin in experimental pneumonia by Legionella pneumophila and L. micdadei. Program and abstracts of 33rd Interscience Conference on Antimicrobial Agents and Chemotherapy. New Orleans, Louisiana, October 17–20, 1993, Abstract No. 957.
16. Myburgh J, Nagel GJ, Petschel E. The efficacy and tolerance of three-day course of azithromycin in the treatment of community-acquired pneumonia. J Antimicrob Chemother 31 (Suppl E): 163–169, 1993.
17. Wilkinson HW, Fikes BJ, Cruce DD. Indirect immunofluorescence test for serodiagnosis of legionnaires' disease: evidence for serogroup diversity of legionnaires' disease bacterial antigens and for multiple specificity of human antibodies. J Clin Microbiol 9: 379–383, 1979.
18. Edelstein PH, Meyer RD, Finegold SM. Laboratory diagnosis of legionnaires' disease. Am Rev Respir Dis 121: 317–327, 1980.
19. Ball P. The future role and importance of macrolides. J Hosp Infect 19 (Suppl A): 47–59, 1991.
20. Morris DL, De Souza A, Jones JA, Morgan WE. High and prolonged pulmonary tissue concentrations of azithromycin following a single oral dose. Eur J Clin Microbiol Infect Dis 10: 859–861, 1991.
21. Andrews JM, Ashby JP, Honeybourne D. Persistence of high concentrations of azithromycin in the lung following a single oral dose. Am Rev Resp Dis 141: A598, 1990.
22. Baldwin DR, Wise R, Andrews JM, Ashby JP, Honeybourne D. Azithromycin concentrations at sites of pulmonary infection. Eur Respir J 3: 886–890, 1990.
23. Foulds G, Shepard RM, Johnson RB. The pharmacokinetics of azithromycin in human serum and tissues. J Antimicrob Chemother 25 (Suppl A): 73–82, 1990.
24. Edelstein PH, Edelstein MAC. In vitro activity of azithromycin against clinical isolates of Legionella species. Antimicrob Agents Chemother 35: 180–181, 1991.
25. Schönwald S, Gunjača M, Kolačny-Babić L, Car V, Gošev M. Comparison of azithromycin and erythromycin in the treatment of atypical pneumonias. J Antimicrob Chemother 25 (Suppl): 123–126, 1990.
26. Schönwald S, Baršić B, Klinar I, Gunjača M. Three-day azithromycin compared with ten-day roxithromycin treatment of atypical pneumonia. Scand J Infect Dis 26: 706–710, 1994.
27. Schönwald S, Škerk V, Petričević I, Car V, Majerus-Mišić Lj, Gunjača M. Comparison of 3- and 5-day courses of azithromycin in the treatment of atypical pneumonias. Eur J Clin Microbiol Infect Dis 10: 877–880, 1991.

Submitted May 2, 1995; accepted July 18, 1995

Scand J Infect Dis 27: 507–509, 1995 ORIGINAL ARTICLE

Rapid Diagnosis of Chlamydial Respiratory Infection in Children

SONIA SCHEPETIUK, ROBERT NORTON and TUCKWENG KOK

From the Division of Medical Virology, Institute of Medical and Veterinary Science, Adelaide, South Australia

A study was undertaken to determine the incidence of chlamydial respiratory infection in paediatric patients during a 12-month period by antigen detection. Nasopharyngeal aspirates (NPA) from 514 patients were screened for genus-specific chlamydia antigen using the Pharmacia Chlamydia enzyme immunoassay (EIA) and Kallestad immunofluorescence (IF) assays. EIA screen-positive samples were confirmed by specific blocking antibody. Specimens which were EIA positive or IF positive were cultured for chlamydia. The NPAs from 7 patients were positive in the EIA and IF assays. Four of these patients were culture positive for chlamydia. Our results showed that the incidence of chlamydia respiratory infection by antigen detection was 1.4% or 0.8% if confirmed by culture.

T. Kok, Division of Medical Virology, Institute of Medical and Veterinary Science, Adelaide, SA 5000, South Australia

INTRODUCTION

Chlamydia trachomatis and Chlamydia psittaci have been widely recognized as important respiratory pathogens (1). The former is also the causative agent of trachoma/inclusion conjunctivitis and is a common genital pathogen (2). More recently, Chlamydia pneumoniae (formerly TWAR organism) has been recognized as an important causative agent of atypical pneumonia (3, 4). The signs and symptoms of chlamydial respiratory infection are not pathognomonic. This highlights the importance of laboratory tests which can provide a rapid and specific diagnosis to allow the institution of appropriate chemotherapy (1, 5, 6). The laboratory diagnosis of chlamydial respiratory infection has relied mainly on serodiagnosis, in particular the complement fixation (CF) test. This requires paired sera and is thus not efficient for prompt diagnosis. Culture-confirmed infections have been documented in the absence of marked antibody responses (7). Culture is not efficient for rapid diagnosis, as the organism is fastidious and requires exacting growth conditions (8, 9). More recently, immunoassays (using monoclonal antibodies to detect genus-specific antigen) have been widely used to detect chlamydial antigens in genital specimens (10). However, there have been limited studies relating to the detection of chlamydial antigen in respiratory specimens. Recently, Silis et al. (11) reported the successful detection (by enzyme immunoassay) of chlamydial antigen in sputum samples from adult patients. Rapid antigen detection offers greater efficiency but may lack specificity, unless a confirmatory blocking test is used. This laboratory processes more than 3000 respiratory samples/year, collected from patients generally resident in South Australia, for the presence of seven respiratory viruses and Mycoplasma pneumoniae (12, 13). This study reports the incidence of chlamydia respiratory infection as detected by enzyme immunoassay (EIA) and immunofluorescence (IF) on nasopharyngeal aspirates from a paediatric population.

 ISSN 0036-5548

MATERIALS AND METHODS

Study population

This study population consisted of nasopharyngeal aspirates (NPA) collected during the 12-month period May 1992 to June 1993 from 514 paediatric patients (age 0–15 years) presenting with acute respiratory tract infections. The NPAs were routinely tested for viruses (viz. adenovirus, influenza A and B, parainfluenza 1, 2 and 3 and respiratory syncytial virus) and Mycoplasma pneumoniae by antigen EIA (13) or virus culture (12).

Nasopharyngeal aspirates

The NPAs were collected in Dulbecco's Modified Eagle Medium with 1% foetal bovine serum. The NPAs were spun at 1000 *g*/5 min and half the pellet was resuspended in the Pharmacia EIA diluent buffer for chlamydial antigen detection. The other half was resuspended in PBS for culture and the immunofluorescent (IF) test.

Chlamydial antigen detection (genus specificity) by EIA

Specimens were processed in accordance with the manufacturer's instructions (Pharmacia). All screen-positive specimens were confirmed with the specific blocking antibody from the manufacturer. This kit did not show cross-reactions with a wide range of bacteria (Staphylococcus spp., E. coli, Candida spp., Gardnerella, Neisseria gonorrhoeae, Grp B Streptococcus, Lactobacillus, H. parainfluenzae, Peptostreptococcus anaerobius, Bacteroides fragilis, Acinetobacter spp., Enterococcus faecalis, Enterobacter spp., Proteus mirabilis, Pseudomonas aeruginosa), as well as Herpes simplex virus and cytomegalovirus.

Immunofluorescent test (IF)

The resuspended cell pellet was smeared on a glass slide, air-dried and fixed in cold (−20°C) methanol for 10 min. The cell smear was stained using a genus-specific monoclonal antibody (FITC conjugated, Kallestad). The presence of >2 chlamydia elementary bodies/low power field was regarded as a positive result.

Chlamydia culture

Specimens which were confirmed positive (by the blocking antibody test) for chlamydial antigen using the Pharmacia EIA or IF tests were cultured in HEp-2 cell monolayers (ATCC No: CCL-23) in microwell plates by centrifugation enhancement and DEAE-dextran pretreatment (14). After 4 days the plates were fixed with cold methanol and stained with genus-specific monoclonal antibody (FITC conjugated, Kallestad). All cultures were passaged once.

Table I. *Chlamydia antigen tests by EIA (Pharmacia) and IF (Kallestad) on NPAs from 514 patients*

	EIA positive	EIA negative	Total
IF positive	4	2	6
IF negative	1	507	508
Total	5	509	514

RESULTS

Chlamydia antigen tests by EIA and IF with NPAs

In the group of 514 patients who provided NPAs, 7 were positive in either the EIA or IF assays (Table I). Of these, 4 which were positive in both the EIA and IF assays were stained for C. pneumoniae-specific antigen using specific monoclonal antibody (Washington Research Foundation) (WRF). Two of these showed specific fluorescence staining for C. pneumoniae in the IF test (WRF). In these 2 specimens, the number of brightly fluorescing elementary bodies were much less than those observed when using the genus-specific antibody (Kallestad) – an observation similar to that reported by Sillis et al. (11).

In the group of 7 patients positive for chlamydia by EIA or IF (see Table I), four were culture-positive as detected by immunofluorescence staining of the inoculated cell layers with genus-specific monoclonal antibody (Kallestad). One patient was EIA-positive but IF-negative, as well as culture-negative. Two other specimens were IF-positive but EIA-negative and culture-negative. There were 507 patients whose NPAs were EIA-negative and IF-negative. If direct antigen detection in NPAs by either IF/EIA was used alone, the incidence of chlamydia infection during the 12-month period studied was 1.4% (7/514). However, if positive by another method, such as culture, the incidence was 0.8% (4/514).

The ages of the 7 patients who were chlamydial-antigen-positive (EIA or IF) (Table II) ranged from 2 months to 6 years. Their clinical presentations, fever and cough or pneumonia, were compatible with chlamydial respiratory infection (4, 15). The NPAs which were culture-positive (Table II) were more likely to be from patients (except patient 5) who showed a more severe clinical presentation (i.e. pneumonia) than from those who were culture-negative.

Virus and M. pneumoniae *detection*

Viruses were detected in 207/514 (40%) of the patients and consisted of 148 (29%) respiratory syncytial virus, 30 (6%) influenza A, 19 (4%) parainfluenza, 7 (1%) adenovirus and 3 (0.6%) M. pneumoniae. No virus or M. pneumoniae was dectected in the NPAs from the seven patients who were chlamydia-positive (see Table II).

DISCUSSION

In this study we detected chlamydial-specific antigen in 7/514 patients (1.4%) with acute respiratory infection, from whom NPAs for routine viral and M. pneumoniae diagnosis were obtained. Chlamydial antigen was detected by genus-specific monoclonal antibody by EIA or IF. Although the numbers of chlamydial antigen and culture-positive patients were low, these patients showed clinical symptoms and signs compatible with this type of respiratory infection (4, 15). It may be argued that the provision of serum samples would add to the confirmation of our laboratory diagnoses. This was not attempted, in view of the age of the patients.

The detection of chlamydial antigen and culture of this organism from patients who were in the 2-month to 6-year age group is compatible with the findings of Beem and Saxon (15) and Frommell et al. (16), who isolated C. trachomatis from infants with suspected chlamydial respiratory infection. In 2/7 patients who yielded chlamydial antigen, C. pneumoniae was identified with specific monoclonal antibodies. The pattern of this fluorescence observed was similar to that reported by Sillis et al. (11). In seroprevalence studies of C. pneumoniae, Wang et al. (17) detected C. pneumoniae IgG antibodies in 23.1% of children in the age group 0.5–10 years. Their study and those of Saxon and Beem (15) parallel our findings that infants and children can be infected with different species of chlamydiae.

Table II. *Relation of chlamydia tests (EIA, IF and culture) with the clinical presentation and age of seven patients who provided 10 NPAs*

Patient	Sex	Age	Clinical category	EIA	IF	Cult
1[a]	F	2/12 mths	pneumonia	+/+/+	+/−/+	+/+/−
2[a]	M	4/12 mths	bronchiolitis	+/+	+/+	+/+
3	F	6 yrs	acute LRTI[c]	+	−	−
4	F	2 yrs	fever, cough	−	+	−
5[b]	M	4/12 mths	acute LRTI	+	+	+
6[b]	F	6/12 mths	bronchiolitis	−	+	−
7	F	1 yr	pneumonia	+	+	+

[a] Patients 1 and 2 provided three and two NPAs respectively.
[b] C. pneumoniae positive by IF staining.
[c] LRTI = lower respiratory tract infection.

Although chlamydial pneumonia can be diagnosed by antibody detection (1), this approach requires properly paired acute and convalescent phase sera. If only IgG antibodies are detected this may represent residual maternal antibodies, especially in neonates. With C. pneumoniae infection, Einarsson et al. (18) reported that in their group (*n*, 84–107) of patients aged 0–9 years, only 1 child (3 months of age) showed IgG-specific C. pneumoniae antibodies. In addition, the study by Chirgwin et al. (7) reported that only 3/8 culture-positive patients showed serologic evidence of acute C. pneumoniae infection. Taken together, these studies and ours suggest that rapid antigen detection by EIA or IF offers an alternative and efficient diagnostic approach for suspected chlamydial infection; in particular, those with pneumonia. In conclusion, we have shown that different species of chlamydiae play a small but important part in the aetiology of respiratory disease in South Australia.

ACKNOWLEDGEMENT

The authors thank Pharmacia (Australia) Pty Ltd for their generous gift of EIA kits and Mrs Charli Bayley for typing the manuscript.

REFERENCES

1. Schachter J. Chlamydial infections. N Engl J Med 298: 428–435, 490–549 and 540–549, 1978.
2. Taylor-Robinson D, Thomas BF. The role of Chlamydia trachomatis in genital tract and associated diseases. J Clin Pathol 30: 205–233, 1980.
3. Marrie TJ, Grayston JT, San-Pin W, Kuo CC. Pneumonia associated with TWAR strain of chlamydia. Ann Intern Med 106: 507–511, 1987.
4. Grayston JT, Campbell LA, Kuo CC, Mordhorst CH, Saikku P, Thomas DH, et al. A new respiratory tract pathogen: Chlamydia pneumoniae strain TWAR. J Infect Dis 161: 618–625, 1990.
5. Grayston JT, Wang SP, Kou CC, Campbell LA. Current knowledge on C. pneumoniae strain TWAR, an important cause of pneumonia and other acute respiratory disease. Eur J Clin Microbiol 8: 191–202, 1989.
6. Kou CC, Grayston JT. In vitro susceptibility of Chlamydia sp. strain TWAR. Antimicrob Agents Chemother 32: 257–258, 1988.
7. Chirgwin K, Roblin PM, Gelling M, Hammerschlag MR, Schachter J. Infection with Chlamydia pneumoniae in Brooklyn. J Infect Dis 163 (4): 757–761, 1991.
8. Kuo CC, Wang SP, Wentworth BB, Grayston JT. Primary isolation of TRIC organisms in HeLa 229 cells treated with DEAE-dextran. J Infect Dis 125: 665–668, 1972.
9. Kuo CC, Grayston T. Factors affecting viability and growth in HeLa 229 cells of Chlamydia sp. strain TWAR. J Clin Microbiol 26: 812–815, 1988.
10. Taylor-Robinson D. Laboratory methods for chlamydial infection. J Infect 25: Suppl 1, 61–67, 1992.
11. Sillis M, White P, Caul EO, Paul ID, Treharne JD. The differentiation of Chlamydia species by antigen detection in sputum specimens from patients with community acquired acute respiratory infections. J Infect 25: Suppl 1, 77–86, 1992.
12. Schepetiuk SK, Kok TW. The use of MDCK, MEK and LLC-MK2 cell lines with enayme immunoassay for the isolation of influenza and parainfluenza viruses from clinical specimens. J Virol Methods 42: 241–250, 1993.
13. Kok T-W, Mickan LD, Burrell CJ. Routine diagnosis of seven respiratory viruses and Mycoplasma pneumoniae by enzyme immunoassay. J Virol Meth 50: 87–100, 1994.
14. Kok T-W, Payne LE, Bailey SE, Waddell RG. Urine and the laboratory diagnosis of Chlamydia trachomatis in males. Genitourin Med 69: 51–53, 1993.
15. Beem MO, Saxon EM. Respiratory-tract colonization and a distinctive pneumonia syndrome in infants infected with Chlamydia trachomatis. N Engl J Med 296: 306–310, 1977.
16. Frommell GT, Bruhn FW, Schwartzman JD. Isolation of Chlamydia trachomatis from infant lung tissue. N Engl J Med 296: 1150–1152, 1977.
17. Wang J-H, Liu Y-C, Cheng D-L, Yeng M-Y, Chen Y-S, Chen B-C. Seroprevalence of Chlamydia pneumoniae in Taiwan. Scand J Infect Dis 25: 565–568, 1993.
18. Einarsson S, Sigurdsson HK, Magnusdottir SD, Erlendsdottir H, Briem H, Gudmundsson S. Age-specific prevalence of antibodies against Chlamydia pneumoniae in Iceland. Scand J Infect Dis 26: 393–397, 1994.

Submitted March 3, 1995; accepted July 6, 1995

Scand J Infect Dis 27: 511–514, 1995 ORIGINAL ARTICLE

Cyclospora in Patients with Traveller's Diarrhea

JOAQUIM GASCON[1], MANUEL CORACHAN[1], JOSEP ANTONI BOMBI[2], MARIA EUGENIA VALLS[3] and JOSEP MARIA BORDES[4]

From the [1]Secció Medicina Tropical, Servei Malalties Infeccioses, [2]Servei Anatomia Patológica, [3]Secció Parasitologia, Servei Microbiologia i Parasitologia and the [4]Servei Gastroenterologia, Hospital Clinic of Barcelona, Barcelona, Spain

Following the description in 1986 of a new enteropathogen called Cyanobacteria-like body (CLB), several outbreaks caused by this microorganism have been described. Since then several research teams have agreed to place CLB in the genus Cyclospora and to establish the epidemiological, pathogenical and clinical features of the illness. This paper describes and assesses those features in 20 travellers diagnosed with CLB and reviews the main literature concerning this enteropathogen. CLB was found in 2.8% of all cases of traveller's diarrhea in our series.

J. Gascon MD, Secció Medicina Tropical, Hospital Clinic de Barcelona, c/ Villarroel, 170, E-08036 Barcelona, Spain

INTRODUCTION

In 1986, Soave et al. (1) described a fungal spore or unsporulated coccidian in the feces of immunocompetent travellers to Haiti and Mexico, which was different from other well known coccidians like Cryptosporidium sp or I. belli. Some years later, Hart et al. (2) described a similar organism in the stools of an HIV patient from Puerto Rico. Other authors suggested that this organism, isolated from both immunocompetent and immunosuppressed hosts, was similar to an algae (Cyanobacteria-like body, (CLB)) (3). Ortega et al., in laboratory conditions obtained sporulation and excystation from an oocyst of the CLB, confirmed the presence of typical coccidian organelles and classified this organism in the genus Cyclospora (4).

The organism has been isolated in diarrheal outbreaks in the United States and Nepal (5), characterized by watery diarrhea, fatigue and anorexia. In this paper we present our experience at the travellers' clinic of our hospital and describe the 20 cases of CLB seen to date.

PATIENTS AND METHODS

Patients born in Spain, who attended the travellers' clinic complaining of diarrhea during the period June 1990–December 1994, were included. Diarrhea was defined according to Merson's criteria (6) as the occurrence of ≥ 3 episodes of watery diarrhea within a 24-h period, with or without other symptoms, or as the occurrence of any number of unformed stools accompanied by 1 of the following: abdominal cramps, tenesmus, vomiting, nausea, fever, chills or prostration. All but 1 patient (resident for 2 years in the Dominican Republic) were short-time travellers. Details of 4 patients have been published previously (7).

All the patients with traveller's diarrhea (TD) answered a clinical and epidemiological questionnaire. Routine hematological and biochemical tests were performed, i.e. haemoglobin, haematocrit, platelets, white blood cell, ESR, creatinine, uric acid, transaminases, bilirubin, alcaline-phosphatase, total proteins, calcium, phosphorus, iron and glucose.

The fecal samples were studied by culture methods for bacterial isolates (8) and by optic microscopy methods, directly and after concentration with merthiolate iodine formaldehyde (MIF) for protozoa and helminths. Fecal samples were also studied during treatment, every 4–10 days, and after clinical recovery (weekly or fortnightly), until 2 negative stools and total recovery of symptoms was recorded.

Three cases were also studied by electron microscopy. Two patients underwent an endoscopy examination, including duodenal and jejunal biopsies that were processed for histological and electron microscopy examination. A clinical and parasitological stool examination was performed 2–3 months later in 18 patients.

RESULTS

Patients

From a total of 693 patients with TD, 20 cases (2.8%) of CLB were diagnosed. The patients were 15 males and 5 females between 21 and 70 years. All but 1 were immunocompetent. None of them had a history of gastrointestinal tract illness or of taking antiacid drugs.

Epidemiological data

The travel destinations are shown in Table I. Except for 1 traveller who stayed in the Dominican Republic for 2 years, all the patients were considered as short-trip visitors (7–60 days). Of the patients, 10 stayed in hotels; 4 combined hotels with residence in a local family household or pension, 2 stayed in a pension, and 1 stayed only with a local family. Patients consumed food and drink in small hotels (16), luxury hotels (14), popular restaurants (14), from street stalls (6) and with local families (4).

Only in 1 case (a traveller to Sri Lanka) was it possible to detect a possible source of infection (buffalo milk) 3 days before the initial symptoms. Other possible sources of potential enteropathogens ingested by these travellers were: raw vegetables (14), ice-cubes (10), unpeeled fruits (7), raw fish (6), local beverages (5), raw meat (3), cold coffee (2), ice-cream (1) and open-air water collections (1). Only 2 patients (from India and Gabon) swam in rivers during the trip.

 ISSN 0036-5548

Table I. *Some epidemiological data and characteristics of diarrhea*

Sex	Age, years	Country	Stools/day	Symptom duration, days	Weight loss, kg	Onset[a]	Trip duration, days
M	70	Dominican Republic	5	80	—	3	16
M	47	Dominican Republic	4	60[b]	15	7	15
M	40[c]	Dominican Republic	12	760	15	—	730
M	38	Dominican Republic	4	15	4	17	30
M	38	Mexico	9	20	3	13	7
F	30	Mexico	7	60	5	8	7
F	43	Guatemala	12	30	—	22	18
F	51	India	6	26	—	8	15
M	21	India	2	15	7	55	40
F	34	India	10	120	8	45	60
M	46	India	5	45	—	12	14
M	50	Malaysia	3	12	—	6	11
M	31	Indonesia	8	17	2	12	10
F	29	Indonesia	5	51	—	24	21
M	41	Indonesia	6	30	8	24	21
M	35	Indonesia	2	10	—	28	21
M	39	Indonesia	4	15	10	24	21
M	41	Sri Lanka	8	21	4	15	21
M	29	Turkey	5	23	3	15	15
M	23	Gabon	10	17	4	27	23

[a] Onset of symptoms since first day of trip.
[b] In 3 different episodes.
[c] AIDS patient.

Characteristics of the diarrhea

Diarrhea was watery at onset in all but 1 case. The mean duration of the illness for the immunocompetent patients was 35 days (range 10–120) and in 10 cases it was intermittent. One immunocompetent patient had 3 diarrhoeal episodes during a 2-year–period after a trip to the Dominican Republic. Before consulting us he had travelled only in EEC countries. In the AIDS patient, diarrhea was present for 760 days, and he died 3 months after CLB diagnosis because of salmonellosis and disseminated Kaposi's sarcoma.

Five patients had their first symptoms during the first 8 days of their trip. In Table I the maximum number of stools/days is shown. The main clinical features of these patients were: asthenia (17, 85%), increased bowel movements (16, 80%), loss of weight (12, 60%), dyspeptic symptoms (11, 55%), abdominal cramps (10, 50%), fever (9, 45%), nausea (7, 35%), anorexia (7, 35%), belching (7, 35%) and vomiting (4, 20%). Symptoms vanished in parallel to the disappearance of CLB in the stools. There were no cases of bloody diarrhea or mucus presence in the stools.

Laboratory findings

In all cases optic microscopy revealed spherical hyaline cyst-like formations of 8–9 μm. These were colored red or pink by the Kinyoun stain (acid-fast), and showed shining bluish circles under ultraviolet light. All these findings conformed to Long's diagnostic criteria (3). Our electron microscopic results showed spherical bodies of 4–5 μm with a double coat: a uniform external membrane (70 nm) and an irregular (100 nm) cell wall. The cytoplasm showed glycogen granules: dense bodies limited by a membrane and lighter granules without a membrane. Some specimens had groups of lamellar structures. No nuclei, mitochondria or endoplasmic reticula were seen (Fig. 1).

Ascaris lumbricoides (1 case from the Dominican Rep.), Giardia lamblia (2 cases from Turkey and India) and EPEC (1 case from Indonesia) were also isolated from 4 patients.

Haematologic and biochemical analysis were normal in all cases, but a mild elevation of transaminases was detected in 4 patients (SGOT; 40–63; SGPT; 55–106).

The endoscopic examination of 2 patients showed no macroscopical changes in the duodenal and jejunal mucosae. The biopsies showed a diffuse chronic inflammation of moderate degree, with marked lymphocytic exocytosis and some vacuolization in the surface epithelium. Both cases showed mild to moderately severe partial villi atrophy and crypt hyperplasia. We found no evidence of invasion or inclusion of any organism (virus or others) through optical or electron microscopical techniques. Duodenal fluid aspirates were negative for the organism.

Treatment

Self-medication was used by 7 patients (2 sulfonamide, 2 ciprofloxacin, 1 ampicillin and 2 loperamide) before visiting us. Several antibiotics (mainly spiramycin, ciprofloxacin and metronidazol) were prescribed at our clinic, but without apparent benefit except in 1 patient taking co-trimoxazole. A total of 11 patients received no treatment.

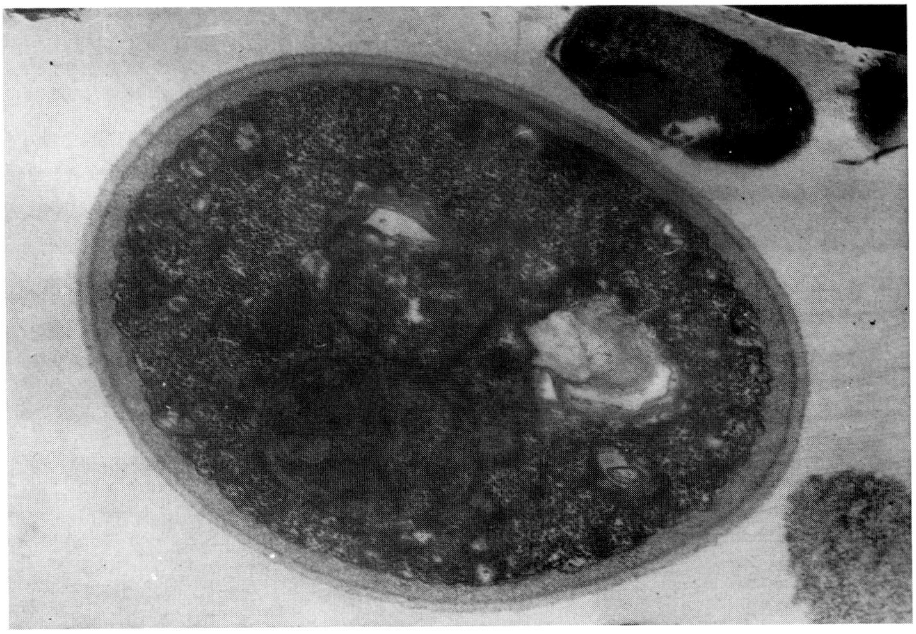

Fig. 1. Irregular internal cell wall (100 nm) with regular membrane (70 nm); abundant glycogen granules.

All patients recovered satisfactorily and stools samples became negative in 18 patients independently of the treatment prescribed. In 2 patients the follow up parasitological data were not recorded.

DISCUSSION

CLB has recently been classified as a coccidium in the Cyclospora family (9). The epidemiological study of Hoge et al. (10) strongly supported the hypothesis that CLB is related to human illness. In our travellers, as with those in Hoge's study, the disappearance of symptoms was correlated to the disappearance of CLB from the stools. CLB represents about 3% of our travellers' diarrhea diagnoses. This is a similar or even higher prevalence compared to other well known pathogens such as salmonella spp. Yersinia enterocolitica or Campylobacter jejuni found in TD patients at our clinic (8). This means that CLB should be suspected and investigated in patients with TD who have compatible clinical and epidemiological features. CLB has been found in travellers coming from Central America and the Caribbean, from South America, Southeast Asia, the Indian subcontinent, Turkey and Gabon.

To our knowledge the patient who came from Gabon is the first CLB case from Central Africa to be diagnosed. Given the importance of AIDS in that region, the significance of CLB as a cause of diarrhea in this area is obvious, because in that case (HIV + CLB) the patients could benefit from co-trimoxazole treatment (11).

The early onset of clinical features during their trip, for some patients, suggests that the incubation period can be very short. This is clearly illustrated in the patient who ingested local buffalo milk. We suspected buffalo milk because it was the only different type of drink or food ingested by the patient compared to his trip companions. (One of them visited us and was clinically asymptomatic with a negative stool.) Transmission seems to occur in most cases through contaminated water (10, 12). The consumption of local drinks (as buffalo milk) contaminated with untreated water should be considered as a risk factor for CLB infection.

The morphologic and staining characteristics of CLB found in feces were similar to those described by other authors (3, 13). A differential diagnosis with Cryptosporidium is obvious and relies mostly in size morphology (CLB being larger) and in the stain distribution within the organism, this being regular in the first and clumpy in the latter. This differentiation is important in view of future management.

In an endoscopic biopsy specimen no tissue organism was detected. The pathogenic mechanism of CLB is unknown. All CLB patients who underwent fibrogastroscopic examination showed histological small bowel pathology in accordance with the clinical presentation. Our results are similar to those found by Connor et al. (14). These results and the fact that, as in other series (10), there was no blood or mucus in the stools, favour a toxin hypothesis as the possible pathogenic mechanism of CLB, as advanced by Connor et al. However, Bendall et al. (15) found intraepithelial coccidia in 2 patients diagnosed as having CLB diarrhea. Pathogenic mechanisms remain a subject for further investigation.

The above pathological findings are compatible with features of tropical sprue and in fact some authors (14) have detected abnormalities in intestinal absorption tests.

The possible role of this enteropathogen in the etiology of tropical sprue also needs further investigation.

The drug response in our series was unconvincing in all cases, except for the patient receiving co-trimoxazole, as it was in the Nepalese study (16). Co-trimoxazole therapy has given good results, in some immunocompetent patients but especially in immunocompromised patients (11, 17). The clinical evaluation of this and other treatments is necessary in order to find a reliable drug that will shorten the duration of clinical symptoms. Even if the illness seems to be self-limited at present, finding an effective treatment could be important for immunodeficient patients. We agree with Chiodini (18) that the existence of asymptomatic carriers can not be excluded, given that 1 of our cases had short intermittent diarrhea episodes for 2 years, and it is certainly an interesting topic for future epidemiological research.

ACKNOWLEDGEMENT

The electron microscopical study was supported by a CIRIT F91 grant.

REFERENCES

1. Soave R, Dubey JP, Ramos LJ, Tummings M. A new intestinal pathogen? Clin Res 34: 533A, 1986.
2. Hart AS, Ridinger MT, Soundarajan R, Peters CS, Swiatlo AL, Kocka FE. Novel organism associated with chronic diarrhoea in AIDS. Lancet 335: 169–170, 1990.
3. Long EG, Ebrahimzadeh A, White EH, Swisher B, Callaway CS. Alga associated with diarrhea in patients with Acquired Immunodeficiency Syndrome and in travellers. J Clin Microbiol 28: 1101–1104, 1990.
4. Ortega YR, Sterling CR, Gilman RH, Cama VA, Diaz F. Cyclospora cayetanensis: A new protozoan pathogen of humans [abstract 289]. Am J Trop Med Hyg 47 (Suppl): 210, 1992.
5. Outbreaks of diarrheal illness associated with Cyanobacteria (blue-green algae)-like bodies in Chicago and Nepal, 1989 and 1990. MMWR 40: 326–327, 1991.
6. Merson MH, Morris GK, Sack DA, Wells JG, Feeley JC, Sack RB, Creech WB, Kapikian AZ, Gangarosa EJ. Traveller's diarrhea in Mexico. A prospective study of physicians and family members attending a congress. N Engl J Med 294: 1299–1305, 1976.
7. Gascon J, Corachán M, Valls ME, Gene A, Bombí JA. Cyanobacteria-like body (CLB) in travellers with diarrhea. Scand J Infect Dis 25: 253–257, 1993.
8. Gascon J, Vila J, Valls ME, Ruiz L, Vidal J, Corachán M, Prats G, Jimenez de Anta MT. Etiology of traveller's diarrhea in Spanish travellers to developing countries. Eur J Epidemiol 9: 217–223, 1993.
9. Ortega YR, Sterling ChR, Gilman RH, Cama VA, Diaz F. Cyclospora species – a new protozoan pathogen of humans. N Engl J Med 328: 1308–1312, 1993.
10. Hoge ChW, Shlim DR, Rajah R, Triplett J, Shear M, Rabold JG, Echevarria P. Epidemiology of diarrhoeal illness associated with coccidian-like organism among travellers and foreign residents in Nepal. Lancet 341: 1175–1179, 1993.
11. Pape JW, Verdier RI, Boncy M, Boncy J, Johnson WD. Cyclospora infection in adults infected with HIV. Ann Intern Med 121: 654–657, 1994.
12. Wurtz RM, Kocka FE, Peters CS, Weldon-Linne CM, Kuritza A, Yingbluth P. Clinical characteristics of seven cases of diarrhea associated with a novel acid-fast organism in the stool. Clin Infect Dis 16: 136–38, 1993.
13. Pollock RCG, Bendall RP. Moody A, Chiodini OL, Churchill DR. Traveller's diarrhoea associated with cyanobacterium-like bodies. Lancet 340: 556–557, 1992.
14. Connor BA, Shlim DR, Scholes JV, Rayburn JL, Reidy J, Rajah R. Pathologic changes in the small bowel in nine patients with diarrhea associated with a coccidia-like body. Ann Intern Med 119: 377–382, 1993.
15. Bendall RP, Lucas S, Moody A, Tovey G, Chiodini PL. Diarrhoea associated with cyanobacterium-like bodies: a new coccidian enteritis of man. Lancet 341: 590–593, 1993.
16. Shlim DR, Cohen MT, Eaton M, Rajah R, Long EG, Ungar BL. An alga-like organism associated with an outbreak of prolonged diarrhea among foreigners in Nepal. Am J Trop Med 45: 383–389, 1991.
17. Madico G, Gilman RH, Miranda E, Cabrera E, Sterling CR. Treatment of cyclospora infections with co-trimoxazole. Lancet 342: 122–123, 1993.
18. Chiodini PL. A "new" parasite: human infection with Cyclospora cayetanensis. Trans Roy Soc Trop Med Hyg 88: 369–371, 1994.

Submitted February 28, 1995; accepted July 4, 1995

Scand J Infect Dis 27: 515–517, 1995 CASE REPORT

Four Fatal Cases of nephropathia epidemica

MATTI VALTONEN[1], MARJUT KAUPPILA[2], PIRKKO KOTILAINEN[2], JUHANI LÄHDEVIRTA[3], CARL-MARCUS SVARTBÄCK[5], OLLI KOSUNEN[6], JARKKO NURMINEN[7], HANNU SARKKINEN and MARKUS BRUMMER-KORVENKONTIO[8]

From the Department of [1]Medicine, Helsinki University Central Hospital, Helsinki, Departments of [2]Medicine and [4]Pathology, Turku University Central Hospital, Turku, [3]Aurora Hospital, Helsinki, Department of [5]Pathology, Kuopio University, Kuopio, Departments of [6]Medicine and [7]Microbiology, Pohjois-Karjala Central Hospital, Joensuu, and the Department of [8]Virology, Helsinki University, Helsinki, Finland

Four serologically confirmed fatal cases of nephropathia epidemica (NE), the mild form of hemorrhagic fever with renal syndrome (HFRS) are described. All the patients had disseminated intravascular coagulation. Autopsies revealed hemorrhage and necrotic areas of their pituitary glands, myocarditis, venous congestion and hemorrhage of the kidneys as well as pulmonary edema and hemorrhage of the lungs in all patients. This report provides new evidence that NE can be a fatal disease.

M. Valtonen, MD, Department of Medicine, Helsinki University Central Hospital, Haartmaninkatu 4, FIN-00290 Helsinki, Finland

INTRODUCTION

Nephropathia epidemica (NE), the mild form of hemorrhagic fever with renal syndrome (HFRS), is an endemic disease in Finland (1070 serologically diagnosed cases in 1994) as in the other Scandinavian countries (1–5). It is caused by a hantavirus, called the Puumala virus, which belongs to the hantavirus genus of the family Bunyaviridae. NE is serologically related to the severe form of HFRS, Korean hemorrhagic fever, caused by the Hantaan virus, which is endemic in Asia (6). A newly recognized and characterized hantavirus causes the recently discovered disease hantavirus pulmonary syndrome (HPS), which is quite distinct from HFRS and NE with severe, non-cardiac pulmonary edema and shock (7, 8).

NE is characterized by sudden fever, headache, myopia, oliguria, myalgia, nausea, vomiting, back and abdominal pain. Rare manifestations are myopericarditis, meningoencephalitis and hypopituitarism. Laboratory findings in NE are thrombocytopenia, leukocytosis, azotemia, proteinuria and hematuria (1–5). NE usually has a favorable outcome (1–5), only sporadic fatal cases have been reported from Sweden (9), Finland (10, 11) and Yugoslavia (12). However, in a series of 126 patients with NE all of them recovered (5). We now describe fatal Finnish cases of NE (including 2 cases reported previously in Finnish (10)).

MATERIALS AND METHODS

The diagnosis of NE was serologically confirmed by means of an IgG avidity (functional affinity) assay with Puumala virus as the antigen in an indirect fluorescent antibody test (13). The avidity of IgG was calculated as the ratio of IgG titers without urea/with urea. According to this method high (≥ 32) titer ratios (low avidity) are diagnostic of acute NE. By contrast, low (≤ 4) ratios (high avidity) rule out NE during the previous month (13).

CASE REPORTS

Case 1

A previously healthy 37-year-old man living in the central part of Finland presented on December 23, 1984 with a high fever of 40.0°C and back pain. The next day he started to have abdominal pain and diarrhea. On December 25 he received indomethacin for symptomatic relief and was referred to a hospital. On admission the patient was critically ill and oliguric. The pulse rate was 173, respiratory rate 32/min and systolic blood pressure was 70 mmHg. Hemoglobin (Hb) was 106 g/l, and the white blood cell (WBC) count was 34.8×10^9/l with 20% band neutrophils, 16% segmented neutrophils, 2% myeolocytes, 2% metamyelocytes, 39% lymphocytes, 8% atypical lymphocytes, 2% plasma cells, 5% eosinophils, 1% basophils and 5% monocytes, the platelet count was 20×10^9/l (normal range $140–320 \times 10^9$/l) and serum creatinine was 536 mM (normal, <115 mM). Urinalysis showed proteinuria and hematuria. Laboratory data revealed disseminated intravascular coagulation (DIC)

The patient was given fluid therapy and cefotaxime and was intubated. He was referred to the University Central Hospital, where he received fresh frozen plasma, thrombocytes, fresh blood, albumin and dopamine. The patient died the next day after less than 5 days of illness.

The autopsy revealed blood in the peritoneal cavity as a sign of bleeding, and strong venous congestion and hemorrhage both in the pituitary gland and the kidneys. In the liver there were also focal hemorrhages and necrotic areas. The autopsy findings supported the diagnosis of NE as a hemorrhagic fever with renal syndrome. The serological diagnosis of NE was made from the sample on the 5th day after the start of the disease. The Puumala antibody titre was 160 with a low IgG avidity titer ratio (≥ 32).

Case 2

A previously healthy 44-year-old man living in south western area of Finland presented on December 8, 1988, with a high fever of 40.0°C, headache, abdominal pain and severe myalgia. He received phenoxymethylpenicillin the same day. He began to lose vision 2 days later and was referred to a hospital. On admission the patient was critically ill and oliguric. His pulse rate was 130 and systolic blood pressure was 85 mmHg. Hb was 206 g/l, WBC count

 ISSN 0036-5548

25.3×10^9/l, platelet count 9×10^9/l, C-reactive protein (CRP) 74 mg/l (normal, <5 mg/l), and serum creatinine was 253 μmol/l. Laboratory data revealed DIC. Urinalysis showed proteinuria and hematuria.

The patient was given fluid therapy, red blood cells, thrombocytes, dopamine, cefuroxime and was intubated. No dialysis or plasmapheresis was performed. The patient died 5 days after the onset of fever.

The autopsy revealed blood in the peritoneal cavity and in the gastrointestinal tract. It also revealed hemorrhage of both the kidneys, stasis of the liver and edema of the brain. Microscopic examination showed venous congestion and hemorrhage in both kidneys. There were hemorrhages and necrotic areas in the pituitary gland and the gastrointestinal tract. Myocarditis was also seen. On the 4th day of illness, the Puumala antibody titer was 80 (<20 against Hantaan virus) and the IgG avidity was weak (≥32).

Case 3

A previously healthy 46-year-old man from the eastern part of Finland presented on April 8, 1989 with a high fever of 40.0°C and headache. The next day he started to vomit and to lose his vision, and was referred to a hospital on April 10. On admission the patient was critically ill and oliguric. Pulse rate was 113, and blood pressure was 126/32 mmHg, subsequently falling to 30 mmHg. Hb was 206 g/l, WBC count 31.1×10^9/l, platelet count 18×10^9/l, serum creatinine 298 μM, and CRP 61 mg/l. Laboratory data revealed DIC, urinalysis showed proteinuria and hematuria.

The patient was given fluid therapy, dopamine, noradrenaline, benzylpenicillin and netilmicin, and he was intubated. No dialysis or plasmapheresis was performed. He died of cardiac arrest the same evening, less than 3 days after the onset of fever. Autopsy revealed hemorrhage in both kidneys, myocarditis, stasis and inflammatory cells in the liver, DIC and brain edema. Autopsy findings supported the diagnosis of NE as a hemorrhagic fever with renal syndrome. On the 3rd day the Puumala antibody titer was 40 (<20 against Hantaan virus), and the avidity was weak.

Case 4

A 58-year-old woman with over 10 years' history of rheumatoid arthritis (RA) was admitted to a hospital on October 25, 1991, because of a high fever of 39°C with diarrhoea for 5 days. The RA had been inactive and stable for years with prednisolone 5 mg/day and acetosalicyclic acid. On admission the patient was critically ill and oliguric. The pulse rate was 120 and blood pressure was 90/50 mmHg. Hb was 198 g/l, and the WBC count was 24.0×10^9/l, with 11% band neutrophils, 67% segmented neutrophils, 1% myelocytes, 12% lymphocytes, 6% monocytes and 3% atypical lymphocytes, and the platelet count was 16×10^9/l, serum creatinine 182 mM, subsequently rising to 250 mM and CRP was 70 mg/l. Laboratory data revealed DIC. Urinalysis showed proteinuria and hematuria.

Fluid therapy and ceftriaxone were started. The patient was referred to the University Central Hospital, where she was given thrombocytes, fresh frozen plasma, dobutamine, dopamine, cefotaxime, ciprofloxacin, and was intubated. After 40 h of treatment the first ultrafiltration and hemodialysis were carried out. They were repeated 24 h later. On the next day, however, she again became hypotonic, developed ventricular fibrillation and died 7 days after the start of symptoms.

The autopsy revealed necrosis and hemorrhage of the pituitary gland and venous congestion, hemorrhage and necrosis in both kidneys. Hemorrhage was seen also in the endomyocardium. On the 6th day after the start of the symptoms and signs of the disease the Puumala antibody titer was 160 with low IgG avidity titer ratio (≥64) and on the 8th day it was 640 (avidity titer ratio 256).

DISCUSSION

The clinical symptoms of our 4 patients were consistent with the early phase of NE (1–5). The onset was sudden with high fever, severe headache, myalgia, abdominal pain, and visual disturbances. Three of the 4 patients were previously healthy, middle-aged men, and all 4 patients lived in the countryside, thus being exposed to bank voles (2). Also, the laboratory data, such as leukocytosis, severe thrombocytopenia, DIC, azotemia, proteinuria and hematuria, were in accordance with earlier published reports on NE (1, 3, 5). The clinical presentation in these cases, however, was exceptionally severe. All the patients were critically ill, already with low blood pressure on admission, developed anuria, and died within a short time. In this respect, the disease resembled its relative, Korean hemorrhagic fever, which is associated with 5–10% mortality. More recent reports suggest the rate to be below 5% with good supportive therapy.

The autopsy findings also supported the diagnosis of NE as a hemorrhagic fever with renal syndrome. The macroscopic and microscopic findings of the hemorrhagic kidneys of all four patients were in agreement with the renal biopsy findings in NE (3). Furthermore, the findings in the pituitary glands of 3 out of the four patients were in agreement with the autopsy findings in Korean hemorrhagic fever (14, 15). It is noteworthy that autopsies revealed pulmonary odema and hemorrhage of the lungs in all our patients, as in patients with HPS. All 4 patients also had signs of venous congestion and edema in other organs (liver, kidneys, gastrointestinal tract and brains).

Capillary leakage in the pathogenesis of a hantaviral disease should be taken into account in the treatment of seriously ill NE, HFRS and HPS patients (8, 14, 15). Clinical experience has shown that administration of large volumes of saline and dextrose solutions may cause severe leakage of the fluid into the extracellular space, and thereby enhance circulatory shock and even cause fatal cerebral edema. Therefore, in order to prevent iatrogenic damage, intravascular volume expanders are considered to be preferable to ordinary electrolyte solutions in the intravenous fluid therapy of these patients (14). If the normal water balance cannot be maintained, dehydration is considered preferable to overhydration (14). Treatment of the hypotensive phase may also require administration of pressor or inotropic agents (8). Ribavirin has been shown to reduce the mortality in HFRS (16). Since June 1993 this antiviral drug has been available in the USA for patients with HPS, through an open-label trial (26). Newly isolated American hantaviruses are susceptible to ribavirin in cell culture as is the Hantaan virus. The role of ribavirin in the treatment of HPS and NE remains to be defined. However, at the moment we would recommend ribavirin to be given to early in severe cases of these infections, based on the favorable results in HFRS.

REFERENCES

1. Lähdevirta J. Nephropathia epidemica in Finland: a clinical, histological and epidemiological study. Ann Clin Res 3, (Suppl 8): 1–154, 1971.
2. Settergren B. Nephropathia epidemica (hemorrhagic fever with renal syndrome) in Scandinavia. Rev Inf Dis 13: 736–744, 1991.
3. Settergren B, Juto P, Trollfors B, Wadell G, Norrby SR. Clinical characteristics of Nephropathia epidemica in Sweden: prospective study of 74 cases. Rev Infect Dis 11: 921–927, 1989.
4. Lähdevirta J. Clinical features of HFRS in Scandinavia as compared with East Asia. Scand J Infect Dis Suppl 36: 93–95, 1982.
5. Mustonen J, Brummer-Korvenkontio M, Hedman K, Pasternack A, Pietilä K, Vaheri A. Nephropathia epidemica in Finland: a retrospective study of 126 cases. Scand J Infect Dis 26: 7–13, 1994.
6. Lee HW, van der Groen G. Hemorrhagic fever with renal syndrome. Progr Med Virol 36: 62–102, 1989.
7. Hughes JM, Petersen CJ, Cohen ML, Mahy BWJ. Hantavirus pulmonary syndrome: an emerging infectious disease. Science 262: 850–851, 1993.
8. Duchin JS, Koster FT, Peters CJ, Simpson GL, Tempest B, Zaki SR, Ksiazek TG, Rollin PE, Nichol S, Umland ET, Moolenaar RL, Reef SE, Nolte KB, Gallaher MM, Butler JC, Breiman RF, the Hantavirus Study Group. Hantavirus pulmonary syndrome: a clinical description of 17 patients with a newly recognized disease. N Engl J Med 330: 949–955, 1994.
9. Linderholm M, Settergren B, Ahlm C, Burman L-Å, Träff S, Bäcklund U, Juto P. A Swedish fatal case of Nephropathia epidemica. Scand J Infect Dis 23: 501–502, 1991.
10. Kauppila M, Kotilainen P, Lähdevirta J, Svartbäck C-M, Kosunen O, Nurminen J, Sarkkinen H, Salonen E-M, Brummer-Korvenkontio M. Ensimmäiset serologiseti varmistetut myyräkuumekuolemat. Duodecim 106: 1103–1106, 1990.
11. Forslund T, Saltevo JS, Anttinen J, Auvinen S, Brummer-Korvenkontio M, Korhonen A, Poutiainen M. Complications of nephropathia epidemica: three cases. J Intern Med 232: 87–90, 1992.
12. Diglisic G, Xiao S-Y, Gligic A, Obradovic M, Sstojanovic R, Velimirovic D, Lukac V, Rossi CA, LeDuc JW. Isolation of a Puumala-like virus from Mus musculus captured in Yugoslavia and its association with severe hemorrhagic fever with renal syndrome. J Infect Dis 169: 204–207, 1994.
13. Hedman K, Vaheri A, Brummer-Korvenkontio M. Rapid diagnosis of hantavirus disease with an IgG-avidity assay. Lancet 338: 1353–1356, 1991.
14. Chun CH. Korean hemorrhagic fever (Hantaan virus infection). In: Lee HW, Dairymple JM. Manual of hemorrhagic fever with renal syndrome. Seoul: WHO Collaborating Center for Virus Reference and Research Institute for Viral Diseases, Korea University: 21–29, 1989.
15. Gosgriff TM. Mechanisms of disease in hantavirus infection: pathophysiology of hemorrhagic fever with renal syndrome. Rev Infect Dis 13: 97–107, 1991.16.
16. Butler JC, Peters CJ. Hantaviruses and hantavirus pulmonary syndrome. Clin Infect Dis 19: 398–395, 1994.

Submitted February 7, 1995; accepted May 23, 1995

Severe Psittacosis during Pregnancy and Suppression of Antibody Response with Early Therapy

RIAD KHATIB[a], MUTHAYIPALAYAM C. THIRUMOORTHI[b], BRIAN KELLY[c] and KEVIN J. GRADY[a]

From the Departments of Obstetrics and Gynecology[c], Medicine[a] and Pediatrics[b], St John Hospital and Medical Center, Detroit, Michigan, USA

A cluster of 3 cases of psittacosis occurred among members of one family. The initial case was a pregnant woman who presented with extensive multilobar infiltrates and severe respiratory distress necessitating mechanical ventilation. Her respiratory failure worsened during 36 h of erythromycin therapy. Improvement coincided with the termination of pregnancy and the initiation of doxycycline treatment. The remaining patients developed milder illness. Serologic assessment of the affected subjects suggests that early treatment may suppress antibody response.

R. Khatib, MD, Medical Education Office, St John Hospital and Medical Center, 22101 Moross Road, Detroit, Michigan 48236, USA

INTRODUCTION

Psittacosis, a multi-system disease caused by Chlamydia psittaci, varies in severity from asymptomatic infection to severe illness with appreciable morbidity and mortality (1–4). A few cases have been reported in pregnant women, but whether infection is more severe during pregnancy is unknown (5). This infection is usually diagnosed by a compatible clinical illness and a diagnostic change in antibody titer (6–8). Although demonstration of the presence of the organism by culture, antigen detection, or polymerase chain reaction is also diagnostic, these methods are not readily available (7, 9). Once the diagnosis is considered, treatment results in a favorable outcome. Effective drugs include tetracycline or its analogues (which are the treatment of choice), erythromycin and the quinolones. Despite the availability of these agents, treatment of severe psittacosis in pregnancy may present a challenge. Although erythromycin is safe, this drug has not been adequately evaluated in severe and life-threatening disease (7, 10). We describe an outbreak of psittacosis among 3 family members, one of whom was a pregnant woman who developed severe pneumonia and respiratory failure necessitating mechanical ventilation. Additionally, our findings suggest that early treatment may suppress antibody response.

DESCRIPTION OF THE OUTBREAK

The outbreak occurred in a family with 2 parents and 7 children who were between 2 and 14 years of age. Most of them had symptoms suggestive of an upper respiratory tract infection about a month prior to the outbreak. These symptoms resolved within a few days.

The family had purchased 3 8-week old birds, a Quaker parrot and 2 Jenay Conures, 18 days before the onset of illness in the mother. The parrot was noted to be sick and died 3 days after the patient became ill. The other 2 birds appeared well at the time. The mother hand-fed these birds and frequently cleaned up their droppings.

Case 1

The mother, who was 31 weeks pregnant, developed severe back ache, which was most pronounced in the neck, headache and fever, over 24 h, followed by dry cough and pleuritic chest pain. Her headache and chest pain worsened over the next day and she became nauseated. During physical examination she was noted to be in respiratory distress.

Her respiratory rate was 20/min, pulse rate 125/min, BP 115/64 mmHg and temperature 39°C. The neck was supple but movement in all directions was painful. The lungs were clear and the rest of the examination was unremarkable. Her laboratory tests showed a white blood cell count of 10.7×10^9/l with a normal differential count, a hemoglobin of 10.7×10^1 g/l and a platelet count of 186×10^9/l. A chest X-ray showed patchy infiltrates in both upper lobes and in left lower lobe.

She was started on erythromycin (2 g/day intravenously) for presumed atypical pneumonia, and O_2 (3 l/min) was supplemented because of the apparent dyspnea. Over the next day, she remained febrile (maximum temperature 39.5°C), the pulmonary infiltrates became more extensive, the respiratory rate increased to 40/min and the dyspnea worsened (O_2 saturation was 93% despite supplementation). At this point she was intubated and placed on mechanical ventilation. Thereupon, because of concerns about the patient's condition due to the rapid progression of her pneumonic process and about the effect of suboptimal oxygenation on the fetus, we elected to terminate the pregnancy prematurely by Caesarean section, 36 h after her admission and 6 h after intubation.

After the termination of pregnancy, doxycycline was started at 100 mg twice daily intravenously, and erythromycin was discontinued the following day. Her condition slowly improved. She defervesced over the next 72 h, her pulmonary infiltrates slowly resolved and she was extubated 4 days after the operation. Doxycycline therapy was continued orally for a total of 14 days. Acute and convalescent sera showed serologic conversion to Chlamydia psittaci (Table I). Antibody testing was performed at a reference commercial laboratory (Associated Regional and University Pathologists, Salt Lake City, Utah) by a complement fixing method utilizing Chlamydia psittaci specific antigen.

Table I. *Chlamydia psittaci (CPs) and Mycoplasma pneumoniae (MPn) antibody among family members*

Family member	Age, years	Sex	Contact with birds	Symptoms	Antibody titer		
					MPn IgM	MPn IgG	CPs
SB (case 1)	31	F	+	+	Not done	Not done	<1:8, 1:32[a]
BB (case 2)	33	M	+	+	<1:16	+	1:8, 1:6[b],
MK (case 3)	14	F	+	+	<1:16	−	<1:8, <1:8[b]
EB	13	M	−	−	<1:16	+	<1:8[c]
RB	8	F	−	−	<1:16	+	<1:8[c]
JH	6	F	−	−	<1:16	−	<1:8[c]
RH	5	F	−	−	<1:16	+	<1:8[c]
CH	3	F	−	−	<1:16	+	<1:8[c]
TH	2	M	−	−	<1:16	+	<1:8[c]

[a] Days 8 and 24 after the onset of illness

[b] Days 28 and 84 after the onset of illness.

[c] Random titer drawn at day 28 after the onset of illness in case 2.

The newborn baby was well at the time of delivery but he was given a 10-day course of erythromycin. He was tested for the presence of Chlamydia psittaci antibody at the age of 5 weeks and was seronegative.

Case 2 and 3

Eight and 10 days, respectively, after the onset of illness in case 1, the husband (case 2) and the oldest child (case 3) became ill. Both developed fever, headache, and nonproductive cough and case 3 experienced pleuritic chest pain. Both were found to have a patchy pulmonary infiltrate localized to a single lobe. They were promptly started on doxycycline and improved remarkably within a few days. Two serum samples each drawn from these demonstrated a nondiagnostic low titer of antibody to Chlamydia psittaci in case 2 and remained nonreactive in case 3 (Table I). Both patients had hand-fed the birds and cleaned up their droppings after the mother became ill.

None of the other children fed the birds or cleaned their droppings. All these children remained well and without detectable antibodies to Chlamydia psittaci.

The entire family, except the mother, were also checked for IgM and IgG antibodies to Mycoplasma pneumoniae (performed at a reference commercial laboratory). None of them were found to have IgM antibodies but IgG antibodies were detected in case 2 and in 5 asymptomatic children.

We were unable to obtain a postmorten examination of the dead bird. However, one of the remaining birds became ill 2 weeks after the parrot died. It was examined at a veterinarian clinic and the diagnosis of psittacosis was confirmed by demonstrating the presence of Chlamydia psittaci antigen in the bird's cloaca. Both birds were treated with tetracycline at the clinic and the ill bird improved.

DISCUSSION

Psittacosis is a rare zoonotic infection with an average of 200 cases reported each year (1). The actual incidence might be higher as some cases go undiagnosed or are not always reported (10). The pathogenesis and the manifestations are well characterized and response to tetracycline therapy is usually favorable. Erythromycin is also effective but tetracycline remains the drug of choice (10).

The clinical characteristics of our outbreak suggest that close contact with the implicated source is necessary for effective transmission, as all of the affected subjects hand-fed the birds or cleaned up their droppings frequently. Our findings also indicate that psittacosis may be more severe in pregnancy. The illness of the pregnant woman was much worse than that of the other family members, and resulted in rapid development of respiratory failure necessitating mechanical ventilation. Whether her symptoms were more severe because of a higher inoculum due to prolonged and repetitive exposures to the implicated source, or because of the pregnancy, or whether early treatment of the other family members impeded the development of severe disease remains uncertain.

As to treatment, the initial deterioration of our pregnant patient despite beginning erythromycin treatment was disturbing. Although erythromycin is considered effective in psittacosis, most of documentated experience has been in mild to moderate infections (7, 10). It has not been adequately evaluated in severe disease. Therefore, we elected to change therapy to doxycycline immediately after the termination of pregnancy and she improved rapidly. Whether her lack of improvement during the short period of erythromycin therapy reflects suboptimal treatment, or if it is due to the severe illness that could have eventually improved with erythromycin treatment remains uncertain. We suspect that her improvement was due to the termination of pregnancy and not because of changing therapy. However, failure of erythromycin could not be excluded. In fact, similar concerns had been raised in a recent review of severe psittacosis reported from the Netherlands (11).

The diagnosis of psittacosis in this outbreak is based on the development of illness among two of the implicated birds, the confirmation of the presence of Chlamydia psittaci in one of these birds, the onset of illness after the acquisition of the birds with an appropriate incubation period, the compatible clinical manifestations in the affected family members, and the diagnostic rise in antibody titer to Chlamydia psittaci in one of the affected patients. The presence of IgG antibody to Mycoplasma pneumoniae in some family members probably reflects an old exposure which could have been the preceding respiratory illness. The lack of serologic response to Chlamydia psittaci in cases 2 and 3 is interesting. Although their illness might have been caused by another respiratory pathogen, coincidental to the onset of psittacosis in case 1, this probability seems unlikely. This view is based on the resemblance in manifestations between all three cases and the onset of illness, after close contact during hand-feeding the birds and cleaning up their droppings, with an appropriate incubation period. Additionally, the presence of a low antibody titer to an uncommon agent such as Chlamydia psittaci, although nondiagnostic, tends to incriminate Chlamydia psittaci in the illness. We believe that early treatment may have been the cause of the blunted serologic response. However, careful assessment of the effect of early therapy in patients whose infection is documented by culture, by detection of the antigen or by polymerase chain reaction is necessary to substantiate this view.

REFERENCES

1. Kirchner JT, Boyarsky SA. Chlamydia psittaci. An uncommon cause of community-acquired pneumonia. Arch Fam Med 2: 997–1001, 1993
2. Schlossberg D, Delgado J, Moore MM, Wishner A, Mohn J. An epidemic of avian and human psittacosis. Arch Intern Med 153: 2594–2596, 1993.
3. Hinton DG, Shipley A, Galvin JW, Harkin JT, Brunton RA. Chlamydiosis in workers at a duck farm and processing plant. Austr Veterin J 70: 174–176, 1993.
4. Morrison WM, Huchison RB, Thomason J, Harrington JH, Herd GW. An outbreak of psittacosis. J Infect 22: 71–75, 1991.
5. Villemonteix P, Ducroz B, Rouffineau J, Plocoste V, Castets M, Magnin G. Pregnancy complicated by severe Chlamydia psittaci infection acquired from a goat flock: a case report. Eur J Obstet Gynecol Reprod Biol 37: 91–94, 1990.
6. Hedberg K, White KE, Hedberg CW, Brandriet J, Osterholm MT, MacDonald KL. Persistence of Chlamydia complement-fixation antibody titer after an outbreak of psittacosis. J Infect Dis 167: 502–503, 1993.
7. Oehme A, Musholt PB, Dreesbach K. Chlamydiae as pathogens – an overview of diagnostic techniques, clinical features, and therapy of human infections. Klin Wochenschr 69: 463–473, 1991.
8. Wreghitt T. Chlamydial infection of the respiratory tract. Communic Dis Rep CDR Review 3: R119–124, 1993.
9. Tony CY, Sillis M. Detection of Chlamydia pneumoniae and Chlamydia psittaci in sputum by PCR. J Clin Pathol 46: 313–317, 1993.
10. Hammers-Berggren S, Granath F, Julander I, Kalin M. Erythromycin for treatment of ornithosis. Scand J Infect Dis 23: 159–162, 1991.
11. Verweij PE, Meis JFG, Eijk R, Melchers WJG, Galama JMD. Severe human psittacosis requiring artificial ventilation: case report and review. Clin Infect Dis 20: 440–442, 1995.

Submitted March 27, 1995; accepted July 5, 1995

Scand J Infect Dis 27: 523–525, 1995

Disseminated Cytomegalovirus Infection in an Immunocompetent Adult Successfully Treated with Ganciclovir

JOAQUIN LÓPEZ-CONTRERAS[1], JOSEP RIS[1], PERE DOMINGO[1], MIREIA PUIG[1], NURIA RABELLA[2], and JOAN NOLLA[1]

From the Departments of [1]Internal Medicine and [2]Microbiology, Hospital de la Santa Creu i Sant Pau, Universitat Autonoma de Barcelona, Barcelona, Spain

We report the case of a previously healthy man who suffered a disseminated cytomegalovirus infection. He presented with prolonged fever, weight loss of 8 kg, anicteric hepatitis, upper digestive tract bleeding from gastric ulcers, acute polyneuritis and bilateral retinitis. Immunodeficiency was not detected either during admission or during a 3-year follow-up period. The patient was treated with ganciclovir (5 mg/kg BID) during 4 weeks with a favourable clinical outcome. To our knowledge, this is the first reported case with such characteristics.

J. López-Contreras, MD, Department of Internal Medicine, Hospital de la Santa Creu i Sant Pau, Avinguda Sant Antoni Maria Claret, 167, E-08025 Barcelona, Spain

INTRODUCTION

Cytomegalovirus (CMV) infection in the immunocompetent host is usually asymptomatic, but may present as self-limiting fever (1). Fever of the unknown origin (FUO), hepatitis, gastric ulcers, polyneuritis and retinitis have been associated with CMV infection in immunocompromised patients (1–6). These syndromes, always as isolated events, have only rarely been reported to affect normal hosts (1, 7, 8).

We report a case of primary CMV infection in a normal host. It was characterized by its extreme severity and by multiorganic involvement, similar to the typical presentation in immunocompromised patients. To our knowledge, such a clinical presentation has not been previously reported.

CASE REPORT

A 62-year-old man was admitted to hospital with a 6-week history of high fever and weight loss of 8 kg. Ten days before admission, he noted paraesthesia in his hands and feet. White blood cell and differential counts were 13 700 leukocytes/μl with 80% neutrophils and 16% lymphocytes. Two urine analyses showed microhaematuria. Blood and urine cultures were negative. A chest X-ray, abdominal ultrasonogram and intravenous pyelogram were normal. Past medical history was unremarkable, except for gouty arthritis. He had never received corticosteroid or immunosuppressive therapy or blood transfusions.

Physical examination on admission revealed a severely ill patient with high fever (39.9°C). Findings of interest were: liver and spleen enlargement, a small soft left supraclavicular lymphadenopathy, and hypoaesthesia of the sole of the right foot. Fundoscopic examination was normal. White blood cell count was 24 900/μl, with 8% band forms, 78% neutrophils, 2% eosinophils, no basophils and 9% lymphocytes. Haemoglobin was 91 g/l, mean corpuscular volume 93 fl, and platelet count 479 000/μl. Erythrocyte sedimentation rate was 134 mm. AST value was 310 U/l (normal 11–28), ALT 344 U/l (12–41), alkaline phosphatase 407 U/l (95–235), and GGPT 137 U/l (13–54). Total and conjugated bilirrubin were normal. Total proteins were 74.2 g/l (69–74), albumin 22.9 g/l (41–49), γ-globulin 27.09 g/l (8.2–14), α_1-globulin 5.54 g/l (1–32), α_2-globulin 7.41 g/l (3.8–7), and β-globulin 7.87 g/l (5–9.7).

Rheumatoid factor and antinuclear, anti-DNA, anti-thyroglobulin, antimicrosomal, anti-mitochondrial, and antineutrophil antibodies were all negative, and CH_{50} was normal. Thyroid function tests, total and prostatic acid phosphatases, prostatic specific antigen, carcino-embryogenic antigen, and α-fetoprotein were normal, as was cerebrospinal fluid examination. Chest, paranasal sinuses and bone serial X-rays were all normal. A thoraco-abdominal CT-scan showed localized bronchiectasis in the anterior segment of the right upper lobe, hepatosplenomegaly, and a few slightly enlarged retroperitoneal lymph nodes. Mesenteric and renal arteriograms were normal. Electromyography showed an axonal mononeuropathy affecting the tibial nerve below the knee. Colonoscopy was normal. Three urine cytologies were negative for malignant cells. A bone marrow biopsy showed reactive changes without granulomas. Findings in hepatic biopsy included preserved architecture, slight periportal fibrosis, inflammatory infiltrate in portal areas, and slight steatosis.

A complement fixation test for anti-CMV antibodies was positive at a titre of 1:256. Specific anti-CMV IgM antibody by indirect immunofluorescence assay (IFA) was negative. Blood, urine, cerebrospinal fluid, bone marrow and liver biopsy cultures were negative for bacteria, mycobacteria, viruses and fungi. Examination and culture of stool for ova and parasites was negative. The search for early CMV antigen by indirect immunofluorescence technique in blood, urine, liver and bone marrow biopsy specimens was also negative. Serological tests to rule out other causes of FUO were performed (see Table I).

Four days after admission, the patient had an upper digestive tract hemorrhage, and endoscopy revealed 4 gastric ulcers. Biopsies showed a chronic inflammatory infiltrate. Human fibroblast cultures of biopsy specimens were positive for CMV, and cultures for bacteria were negative. A second fundoscopy revealed white-yellowish peripheric exudate in both eyes, and a preretinal hemorrhage in the right eye. Treatment with ganciclovir 300 mg every 12 h was started. An immunological screening was performed to rule out immunodeficiency (see Table II).

Table I. *Infectious diseases that may present with FUO and that were ruled out by serological methods*

Serological tests	
Salmonella thyphi	Negative
Brucella	Negative
Coxiella burnetti	Negative
Syphilis	Negative
Toxoplasma	Negative
Epstein-Barr virus	Negative
Hepatitis A virus (IgM)	Negative
Hepatitis B virus (Anti-HBc IgM)	Negative
Hepatitis C virus	Negative
HIV type 1	Negative
HIV type 2	Negative
HIV-1 antigen	Negative

A subjective improvement of general status was observed a few days after ganciclovir was initiated. At the 4th week of treatment, fever was no longer detected, the patient had gained 2 kg, and no active lesions were found at fundoscopic examination. Skin tests were repeated 2 months after discharge, and were positive to 5/7 antigens. He recovered his normal weight 4 months after treatment. An electromyographic study was repeated at that time, and did not show any changes with respect to the previous study. The hypoaestesia of the right sole disappeared 18 months after discharge. Three years later he is asymptomatic. Laboratory data since discharge have been normal. Immunological status and HIV serologies have been reassessed twice during follow-up and have been normal or negative. Complement-fixation titres against CMV decreased to 1 : 128 during this time. Urine cultures have remained negative for CMV during the follow-up period.

DISCUSSION

The diagnosis of CMV infection is made on the basis of a consistent clinical presentation together with either a 4-fold elevation of the anti-CMV antibody titre or the recovery of CMV from a biopsy specimen or organic fluid culture together with a high anti-CMV antibody titre (7). Our patient clearly fulfils the latter conditions. Specific IgM anti-CMV antibodies were negative and the typical 4-fold rise of anti-CMV antibody titre measured by a complement fixation test was not detected as both were performed late in the illness.

Because of the overwhelming nature of the clinical presentation we believe that CMV disease in the patient reported was a primary infection. To our knowledge no case of clinically evident reactivation of CMV infection has been described in immunocompetent individuals, although it is a well-known complication in immunosuppressed patients (5, 6). Serologic tests do not always allow differentiation between primary and reactivated cases, as occurred in our patient.

Table II. *Immunological screening*

Test	Patient values	Normal values
Serum inmunoelectrophoresis	No monoclonal bands	
Urine immunoelectrophoresis	No monoclonal bands	
Serum IgG	2710 mg/100 ml	600–1800 mg/100 ml
Serum IgM	369 mg/100 ml	60–300 mg/100 ml
Serum IgA	498 mg/100 ml	50–150 mg/100 ml
Serum B_{12} and its carriers	Normal	
Urinary cortisol	127.9 nmol/24 h	50–280 nmol/24 h
Anti HIV-1 antibodies (WB)	Negative	
Anti-HIV-2 antibodies	Negative	
HIV-1 antigen	Negative	
T-lymphocytes count	3094/mm^3 (91%)	1000–2000/mm^3 (84–93%)
CD4 lymphocytes count	1836/mm^3 (54%)	600–1200/mm^3 (35–45%)
CD8 lymphocytes count	850/mm^3 (25%)	500–1000/mm^3 (30–40%)
B-lymphocytes count	135/mm^3 (4%)	100–400/mm^3 (7–16%)
Lymphocyte-transformation tests against:		
Phytohemaglutinin	79%	
Concanavalin	95%	
Pokeweed mitogen	114%	
Intradermal skin tests for:		
Candida	Negative	
Proteus	Negative	
Trycophyton	Negative	
Streptococcus	Negative	
Tetanus toxoid	Negative	
Diphteria	Negative	
Tuberculin	Negative	

CMV-associated ulcers have been described in many different sites of the gastrointestinal tract (1). The role of CMV in ulcer pathogenesis has not yet been established, and it may represent only a non-pathogenic bystander of pre-existent ulcers. However, the detection of CMV in the absence of other microorganisms, the improvement of gastrointestinal lesions with specific anti-CMV therapy and their recurrence when this treatment is discontinued in immunocompromised patients, suggest a true pathogenic role of CMV (1, 9). In the present case, CMV was cultured from gastric biopsy specimens. Furthermore, the patient had no previous history of peptic disease, and neither the endoscopic nor the pathologic appearance of the ulcers suggested acute gastric musosal lesions.

Liver function tests are almost always abnormal in symptomatic cases of CMV primary infection (7). A chronic inflammatory infiltrate in portal areas together with a preserved hepatic architecture, as seen in our patient's liver biopsy, are the most frequent findings in CMV anicteric hepatitis (10–12).

On admission, our patient had paraesthesia in the hands and feet, and both neurological examination and electromyogram showed only a tibial nerve mononeuropathy. CMV-associated mononeuropathy is an uncommon complication of primary CMV infection (7, 13, 14) and involvement of the tibial nerve has not been reported previously. Furthermore, tibial mononeuropathy is usually associated with mechanical nerve compression, and although we did not identify any circumstance that precluded such an etiology it cannot be completely ruled out. In spite of the above-mentioned considerations and the absence of objective findings, we consider that the patient had a CMV-associated peripheral polyneuritis, as symptoms resolved only after ganciclovir therapy, and because a lack of objective findings is fairly common in polyneuritis.

CMV retinitis is accepted as a marker of severe immunodeficiency, and is a frequent complication in HIV-infected patients and transplant recipients. Only one well-documented case of CMV retinitis in a non-immunocompromised adult has been reported to date, but the patient had been transfused 14 days prior to development of ocular lesions (8). Three other possible cases of CMV retinitis have been described previously (15–17). Nevertheless, immunodeficiency was not completely excluded in two of them (15, 16). Diagnosis was established from immunohistochemical techniques in the third case, even though the clinical and pathologic findings were not suggestive of CMV retinitis (17). Our patient had characteristic clinical and fundoscopic findings of CMV retinitis, and the retinal involvement played a key role in establishing the diagnosis of CMV infection. Improvement of the lesions was seen only after anti-CMV therapy was initiated.

As far as we know, ganciclovir has not been used in the immunocompetent host, because of the benign and self-limiting nature of CMV infection in such patients. Ganciclovir therapy was administered in our patient because of the overwhelming nature of the infection. Although we cannot be certain that the patient may have recovered without treatment, the fact is that after 9 weeks of continuous worsening, the patient only began to improve after anti-CMV treatment was started. Moreover, we feel that ganciclovir therapy was decisive in avoiding ocular sequelae.

Previous reports on immunocompromised patients (18), as well as this report, suggest that treatment with ganciclovir or foscarnet is advisable in cases of severe CMV infection if irreversible sequelae are to be avoided.

REFERENCES

1. Goodgame RW. Gastrointestinal cytomegalovirus disease. Ann Intern Med 119: 924–935, 1993.
2. Pollard RB, Egbert PR, Gallagher JG, Merigan TC. Cytomegalovirus retinitis in immunosuppressed hosts. I. Natural history and effects of treatment with adenine arabinoside. Ann Intern Med 93: 655–664, 1980.
3. Bloom JN, Palestine AG. The diagnosis of cytomegalovirus retinitis. Ann Intern Med 109: 963–969, 1988.
4. Kim YS, Hollander H. Polyradiculopathy due to cytomegalovirus: report of two cases in which improvement occurred after prolonged therapy and review of the literature. Clin Infect Dis 17: 32–37, 1993.
5. Rubin RH. Impact of cytomegalovirus infection on organ transplant recipients. Rev Infect Dis 12 (Suppl 7): S754–S766, 1990.
6. Schooley RT. Cytomegalovirus infection in the setting of infection with human immunodeficiency virus. Rev Infect Dis 12 (Suppl 7): S811–S819, 1990.
7. Cohen JI, Corey GR. Cytomegalovirus infection in the normal host. Medicine 64: 100–114, 1985.
8. England AC, Miller SA, Maki DG. Ocular findings of acute cytomegalovirus infection in an immunologically competent adult. N Engl J Med 307: 94–95, 1982.
9. Munckhof WJ, Richards MJ. Cytometalovirus-associated gastric ulcer. Ann Intern Med 117: 877, 1992.
10. Klemola E, Kääriäinen L, von Essen R, Haltia K, Koivuniemi A, von Bonsdorff CH. Further studies on cytomegalovirus mononucleosis in previously healthy individuals. Acta Med Scand 182: 311–322, 1967.
11. Spiller RC, Lovell D, Silk DBA. Adult acquired cytomegalovirus infection with gastric and duodenal ulceration. Gut 29: 1109–1111, 1988.
12. Shusterman NH, Frauenhoffer C, Kinsey MD. Fatal massive hepatic necrosis in cytomegalovirus mononucleosis. Ann Intern Med 88: 810–812, 1978.
13. Duchowmy M, Caplan L, Siber G. Cytomegalovirus infection of the adult nervous system. Ann Neurol 5: 458–461, 1979.
14. Sundkvist T. Cytomegalovirus infection complicated by neuralgic amyotrophy. N Engl J Med 308: 461, 1983.
15. Foerster HW. Pathology of granulomatous uveitis. Surv Ophthalmol 4: 296–299, 1959.
16. Chawla HB, Ford MJ, Munro JF, Scorgie RE, Watson AR. Ocular involvement in cytomegalovirus infection in a previously healthy adult. Br Med J 2: 281–282, 1976.
17. Freeman WR, Stern WH, Gross JG, Taylor PB, Nadel AJ, Wiley CA. Pathologic observations made by retinal biopsy. Retina 10: 195–204, 1990.
18. Balfour Jr HH. Management of cytomegalovirus disease with antiviral drugs. Rev Infect Dis 12 Suppl 7: S849–S859, 1990.

Submitted March 31, 1995; accepted July 7, 1995

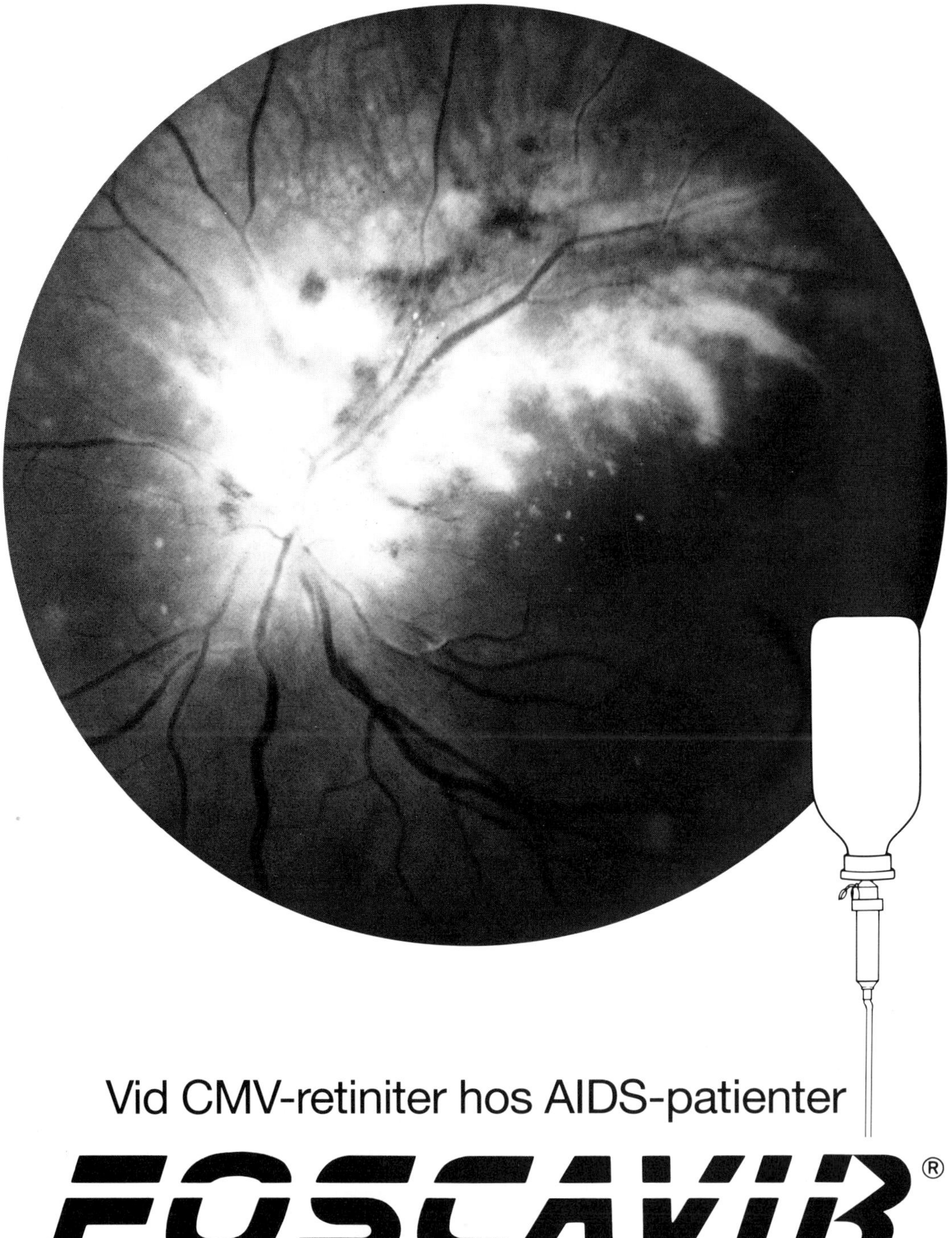

Scand J Infect Dis 27: 527–528, 1995 CASE REPORT

Fatal Rickettsial Meningitis in Hong Kong: A Need for Rapid Laboratory Diagnosis

ROBERT P. YOUNG[1], MARGARET IP[2] and DAVID C. J. BASSETT[2]

From the Departments of [1]Medicine and [2]Microbiology, Chinese University of Hong Kong, Prince of Wales Hospital, Shatin, Hong Kong

A 22-year-old Chinese male, investigated elsewhere for fever and myalgia, was transferred to our hospital drowsy, unresponsive to commands and with a petechial rash. Partially treated meningococcal meningitis was suspected and high-dose antibiotics were immediately started. Rising Weil-Felix titres occurred too late for anti-rickettsial therapy to prevent a fatal outcome. Subsequent specific serology showed rising titres against Rickettsia conori. The desirability of more rapid and reliable methods of laboratory diagnosis of rickettsial infection is evident.

R. P. Young, MD, Department of Medicine, Chinese University of Hong Kong, Prince of Wales Hospital, Shatin, Hong Kong

INTRODUCTION

In Hong Kong, the aetiological diagnosis of central nervous system infections in adults is complicated by the prevalent misuse of antimicrobial drugs. Partially treated pyogenic meningitis frequently figures in the differential diagnosis of patients with fever, neurological symptoms and indeterminate cerebrospinal fluid findings. The relative importance of the various causative agents of adult meningitis in Hong Kong is very different from that seen in Western countries (1), and the range of possible causes includes Gram-negative bacilli (1), Mycobacterium tuberculosis (2), Streptococcus suis (3), Angiostrongylus cantonesis (4), and Rickettsia species (5), in addition to the 3 classical pathogens Neisseria meningitidis, Haemophilus influenzae and Streptococcus pneumoniae. Failure to make a microbiological diagnosis may indeed be due to prior use of antimicrobials, but this cannot be taken as the true cause in any particular case. The fatal case of rickettsial spotted fever we describe illustrates 1 of the many guises of that infection, shows the need for appropriate empirical treatment and the great importance of full aetiological investigations.

CASE REPORT

A 22-year-old Chinese male engineer was admitted to our hospital with suspected encephalomeningitis with multi-organ involvement. He had been well up until 2 days prior to his admission to a nearby private hospital. At that time he complained of fever and myalgia and was admitted for investigation. Physical examination was normal and initial investigations revealed the following: ESR = 8, WBC = 5.3×10^9/l (normal differential), platelet count of 46×19^9/l, moderate elevation of the liver transaminases with low albumin and gross elevation of creatinine kinase. Chest X-ray was normal. Blood and urine cultures were both negative.

The patient was started empirically on intravenous ceftriaxone 500 mg × 4/day 2 days after admission. Electromyographic studies were reported "as consistent with a myopathic process" and a muscle biopsy was subsequently found to be non-specific. On day 4 of his admission the patient developed a rash which started on the neck and spread to the hands, face, limbs and trunk. The rash consisted of multiple discrete non-itchy macular papules. At this time, a mild headache and photophobia were reported. Physical examination revealed no focus of infection or neurological abnormality. Computerized tomography (CT) of the brain and lumbar puncture were not performed. Ultrasonography of the abdomen showed mild hepatosplenomegaly. Rheumatoid factor was negative. The liver function was deteriorating with increasing transaminases and bilrubin. In the absence of a focus of infection, an aggressive form of autoimmune hepatitis or connective tissue disease was suspected and intravenous methylprednisolone 500 mg daily was started. Two days later, the patient became drowsy and confused and was transferred to our hospital due to financial constraints.

On examination the patient was drowsy and unresponsive to questions or commands with a Glasgow coma scale of 9/15 (E3V2M4). He was covered in a speckled haemorrhagic macular rash over the entire body. No eschar was evident. He had a tachycardia of 110, tachypnoeic with RR 20/min and temperature of 36.4°C. He was mildly jaundiced, with no pallor. There was a palpable axillary lymph node of 1.5 cm but no other lymphadenopathy. Examination of the cardiorespiratory system was normal. The abdomen was tender with generalized guarding but no rebound tenderness. He had mild neck stiffness and the pupils were sluggish to direct light bilaterally. Fundi were difficult to assess due to apparent photophobia. Tone and reflexes were increased in all four limbs and plantar reflexes were down-going bilaterally. An immediate blood glucose estimate was normal and the patient underwent an emergency CT brain scan which was reported as normal. A lumbar puncture was performed. The opening pressure was 23 cm of H_2O and xanthochromic CSF showed 65 red cells/μ, 1 white cell/μl. Gram stain, India ink and Ziehl-Neelsen stains were all negative. The CSF protein was 1.13 g/l and the CSF glucose was 44% of the plasma value. There was a peripheral blood leukocytosis of 17×10^9/l with 94% neutrophilia. Microbiological investigations are detailed below.

The patient was suspected to have a partially treated bacterial (most likely meningococcal) meningitis and was started on high-dose intravenous benzylpenicillin and ceftazidine. Ten hours after admission the patient's condition deteriorated with decreased consciousness, unequal pupils, fixed dilated on the right and initially brief focal seizures followed by a generalized convulsion. The patient was then admitted to the intensive care unit for sedation and intubation. Repeat CT scan of the brain showed early features of cerebral oedema with reduced sulci and symmetrically narrowed ventricles. Despite intravenous mannitol, 24 h after admission, the patient's condition deteriorated further with bilateral fixed dilated pupils, hypotension and deteriorating renal function. The patient was supported with dobutamine and noradrenaline infusions but his condition remained poor and on day 4 of his admission to our hospital he was declared clinically brain dead. On day 8 cerebral angiography confirmed brain death status.

 ISSN 0036-5548

Serial samples of serum were taken from this patient. Weil-Felix tests showed a marked rise of OX2 (1/40 to 1/1280), minimal rise in OX19 (1/40 to 1/160) and OXK (1/20) between days 8 and 15 of his illness (days 1 to 7 of his admission). Specific antibodies (IgG, IgM) to Rickettsia rickettsiae, R. typhi and R. tsutsugamushi assayed by immunofluorescence tests, were all negative. The sera were therefore sent to CAMR (Centre for Applied Microbiology and Research), Porton Down, U.K. for confirmation of the serial rise of spotted fever group antibody from 1/160 to >1/2560 using antigens of R. conori.

In addition, sepsis screening included blood and urine cultures, blood films to exclude malaria, serological tests for Salmonella typhi (Widal), brucella and mycoplasma. Viral serology for varicella zoster, herpes simplex 1 and 2, measles and enteroviruses were all negative.

DISCUSSION

This patient represented an unusual case of meningitis in Hong Kong. In retrospect, the clinical picture resembled classical Rocky Mountain spotted fever-like illness, with an abrupt onset of fever and myalgia, followed by headache, a maculo-papular rash which became petechial and meningo-encephalitis. No history of tick bite was elicited and there was no eschar. There was no history of recent travel. His occupation was that of an engineer and involved maintenance of satellite dishes on the mountains in the countryside. Infection with the spotted fever (SF) group of rickettsias is not included among the notifiable diseases in Hong Kong and there is insufficient epidemiological data to determine the local prevalence of spotted fever. However, there have been several documented cases of such disease (reviewed in ref. 6), one of which also presented with signs of meningism. Experience with SF is limited and the species implicated in this region is far from established and we have not attempted to isolate the rickettsia from the patient. The previous cases were confirmed using the antigens to R. sibirica which is known to be present in the northern provinces of China (7). R. conori infection extends across continents from the Mediterranean, Africa to India and may also be the aetiologic agent in Southeastern Asia. In recent years, SF has also been described in Japan (8), Thailand (9) and Australia (10).

Empirical therapy in meningitis is based on the local knowledge of the most likely pathogen with regard to the patient's age and immune status. In Hong Kong, the epidemiological pattern of bacterial meningitis differs significantly from those of Western countries. The 3 classical meningeal pathogens; N. meningitidis, H. influenzae and S. pneumoniae together account for 80% and 75% of all bacteria causing meningitis in the USA and the UK respectively (11, 12). However, in Hong Kong, these are relatively much less common (12) and from our departmental data account for <5% of all bacterial isolates from CSF in 1993 and 1994. In contrast, gram-negative bacilli account for a much higher proportion, in the order of 30% (1). Other unusual causes were also prevalent with meningitis due to Streptococcus suis in those with an occupational risk (3). The numbers of tick-borne rickettsiosis causing meningitis or meningoencephalitis in Hong Kong are unknown except for the previously reported case in 1988 (5).

The laboratory diagnosis of rickettsial diseases in Hong Kong is currently based on the Weil-Felix (WF) reaction. Although commercial tests employing rickettsial antigens are available, the limited knowledge and availability of suitable antigens for this locality may prove a problem in confirming a case of SF. Management of such a case of SF is based on the clinical suspicion of the disease and the serial rise in OX2 or OX19 titres. Immunofluorescent detection of the rickettsial antigens on skin biopsy (13) or the use of polymerase chain reaction (14) may be alternative means of early diagnosis in the future.

The use of adjunctive dexamethasone for treatment of children with bacterial meningitis has been shown to be beneficial (11), but for adults, the benefits are less certain. In this case, the fatality was partly attributed to failure to establish the diagnosis of rickettsial spotted fever early, with resultant delay in instituting appropriate treatment.

REFERENCES

1. Kay R. Clinics in neurology: the treatment of bacterial meningitis: a reappraisal. J Hong Kong Med Ass 39: 185–186, 1987.
2. Teoh R, Humphries MJ, Hoare RD, O'Mahony GO. Clinical correlation of CT changes in 64 Chinese patients with tuberculous meningitis. N Neurol 236: 48–51, 1989.
3. Chau PY, Huang CY, Kay R. Streptococcus suis meningitis. Med J Aust 1: 414–417, 1983.
4. Ko RC, Chan SW, Chan KW, Lam K, Farrington M, Wong HW, Yuen P. Four documented cases of eosinophilic meningoencephalitis due to Angiostrongylus cantonesis in Hong Kong. Trans Soc Trop Med Hyg 81: 807–810, 1987.
5. Woo ML, Leung JWC, French GL. Rickettsial infection presenting as culture-negative meningitis. Postgrad Med J 64: 614–616, 1988.
6. Bassett DCJ, Ho KC, Tam JSL, Lam LY, Cheng AFB. The laboratory diagnosis of rickettsial diseases in Hong Kong. J Trop Med Hyg 95: 327–330, 1992.
7. Wang JC, Walker DH. Identification of spotted fever group Rickettsiae from human and tick sources in the People's Republic of China. J Infect Dis 156: 665–669, 1987.
8. Uchida T, Uchiyama T, Kumano K, Walker DH. Rickettsia japonica sp. nov., the etiological agent of spotted fever group rickettsiosis in Japan. Int J Syst Bacteriol 42: 303–305, 1992.
9. Sirisanthana T, Pinyopornpanit V, Sirisanthana V, Strickman D, Kelly DJ, Dasch GA. First cases of spotted fever group rickettsiosis in Thailand. Am J Trop Med Hyg 50: 682–686, 1994.
10. Walker DH. Rickettsiosis of the spotted fever group around the world. J Dermatol 16: 169–177, 1989.
11. Quagliarello VJ, Scheld VM. New perspectives on bacterial meningitis. Clin Infect Dis 17: 603–610, 1993.
12. French GL, Cheng AFB, Duthie R, Cockram C. Septicaemia in Hong Kong. J Antimicrob Chemother 25 Suppl C: 115–125, 1990.
13. Walker DH, Cain BG, Olmstead PM. Laboratory diagnosis of Rocky Mountain Spotted Fever by immunofluorescent demonstration of Rickettsia rickettsii in cutaneous lesions. Am J Clin Pathol 69: 619–623, 1978.
14. Sexton DJ, Kanj SS, Wilson K, Corey G, Hegarty BC, Levy MG, Breitschwerdt EB. The use of a polymerase chain reaction as a diagnostic test for Rocky Mountain Spotted Fever. Am J Trop Med Hyg 50: 59–63, 1994.

Submitted May 12, 1995; accepted July 11, 1995

Scand J Infect Dis 27: 529–532, 1995 CASE REPORT

Protracted and Recurrent Methicillin-resistant Staphylococcus aureus Bacteremia Despite Defervescence with Vancomycin Therapy

RIAD KHATIB, KATHLEEN M. RIEDERER, MARILYN HELD and HIND ALJUNDI

From the Department of Medicine, St John Hospital and Medical Center, Detroit, Michigan, USA

Methicillin-resistant Staphylococcus aureus (MRSA) bacteremia persisted for 46 days in a 63-year-old patient and recurred over 98 days in a 79-year-old patient, despite vancomycin therapy. Although the fever resolved, patient 1 developed a spinal epidural abscess 38 days after beginning therapy and patient 2 sustained multiple relapses. A time–kill study demonstrated a reduced vancomycin killing rate in both isolates when compared to the killing rate of a control MRSA strain. The bacteremia persisted after increasing the vancomycin dose to achieve trough levels of 15–20 μg; it cleared after adding gentamicin. These cases illustrate that MRSA bacteremia may persist during vancomycin therapy despite resolution of fever and may lead to delayed complications, and that adding gentamicin may be necessary for ultimate clearance of the bacteremia.

R. Khatib, MD, Medical Education Office, St John Hospital, 22101 Moross Rd., Detroit, Michigan 48236, USA

INTRODUCTION

Persistence of bacteremia is well recognized in clinical and experimental Staphylococcus aureus endocarditis (1), particularly in cases with methicillin-resistant strains (2). It is usually detected during evaluation of patients with persistent fever in the initial phase of therapy. Although it may be associated with continuous fever and increased morbidity, the bacteremia eventually clears without attributable complication (1–4). We describe 2 cases of methicillin-resistant S. aureus (MRSA) bacteremia, one with a protracted course and one with multiple relapses despite conventional vancomycin therapy. Despite defervescence, blood cultures remained positive in both patients until gentamicin was added. Both isolates displayed a reduced vancomycin killing rate.

CASE REPORT (Fig. 1)

A 63-year-old white morbidly obese male with sleep apnea developed MRSA bacteremia 3 weeks after insertion of a permanent pacemaker. The vancomycin minimal inhibitory concentration (MIC) was 0.8 μg. He was started on vancomycin (trough levels were 3.9–5.4 μg/ml and peak levels were 23.5–26 μg/ml) followed by the addition of rifampin (600 mg/day, orally) 3 days afterward. The pacemaker was removed 11 days after starting therapy. (Gram stain and culture of the pacemaker did not reveal any organisms). He slowly improved, but all 17 blood cultures obtained in the initial 21 days of therapy remained positive.

At this point the vancomycin dose was increased (new trough levels were 15–20 μg/ml). Thereafter, bacteremia became intermittent (2/10 blood cultures were positive over the next 27 days; the last positive culture was detected on day 48 after beginning therapy) and he became afebrile. A transesophageal echocardiogram failed to show echocardiographic abnormalities and computed tomography of the abdomen demonstrated normal spleen.

Despite the apparent improvement and the partial clearance of bacteremia, he manifested severe back ache 38 days after starting vancomycin. He was found to have vertebral osteomyelitis and an epidural abscess at level T4, that necessitated laminectomy and surgical drainage of the abscess from which MRSA was recovered. Thereupon, rifampin was discontinued and gentamicin was added to achieve a peak level of 3 μg/ml. All ensuing blood cultures were sterile. He received a total of 78 days of intravenous therapy followed by 3 months of trimethoprim/sulfamethoxazole orally. Subsequently, he remained afebrile and without recurrence of bacteremia during 1 year of follow up.

CASE REPORT 2 (Fig. 1)

A 79-year-old diabetic white female with a chronic osteomyelitis of the right foot and with a permanent pacemaker for over 10 years developed MRSA bacteremia (a total of 6 positive blood cultures over a 3-day period). The vancomycin MIC was 1.6 μg. Vancomycin therapy was initiated (trough levels were 10.6–16.5 μg/ml), and rifampin was added (600 mg/day orally) a few days later. She defervesced over a few days and therapy was continuous for a total of 42 days. The patient declined removal of the pacemaker. She was readmitted with lower gastrointestinal bleeding, 8 weeks after discharge. The patient was afebrile but 2 blood cultures, obtained because of unexplained leukocytosis, were positive for MRSA.

Subsequent management consisted of restarting vancomycin at the previous dose, below-knee amputation for the non-healing osteomyelitis, followed by the removal of the pacemaker, from which MRSA was recovered. A transthoracic echocardiogram failed to show abnormal findings. Vancomycin was continued for 4 weeks after the removal of pacemaker; blood cultures were not repeated during treatment as the patient was afebrile.

At 4 weeks after finishing therapy, fever recurred and MRSA was recovered from 4/4 new blood cultures. The patient was restarted on vancomycin and she defervesced quickly but 9/10 blood cultures that were obtained over the next 22 days remained positive. At this point the vancomycin dose was increased (the new trough levels were 15–20 μg/ml) and gentamicin was added a few days later (the peak level was 3 μg/ml).

Combined therapy was continued for a total of 42 days after which the patient remained well and free of bacteremia over a 9-month period.

 ISSN 0036-5548

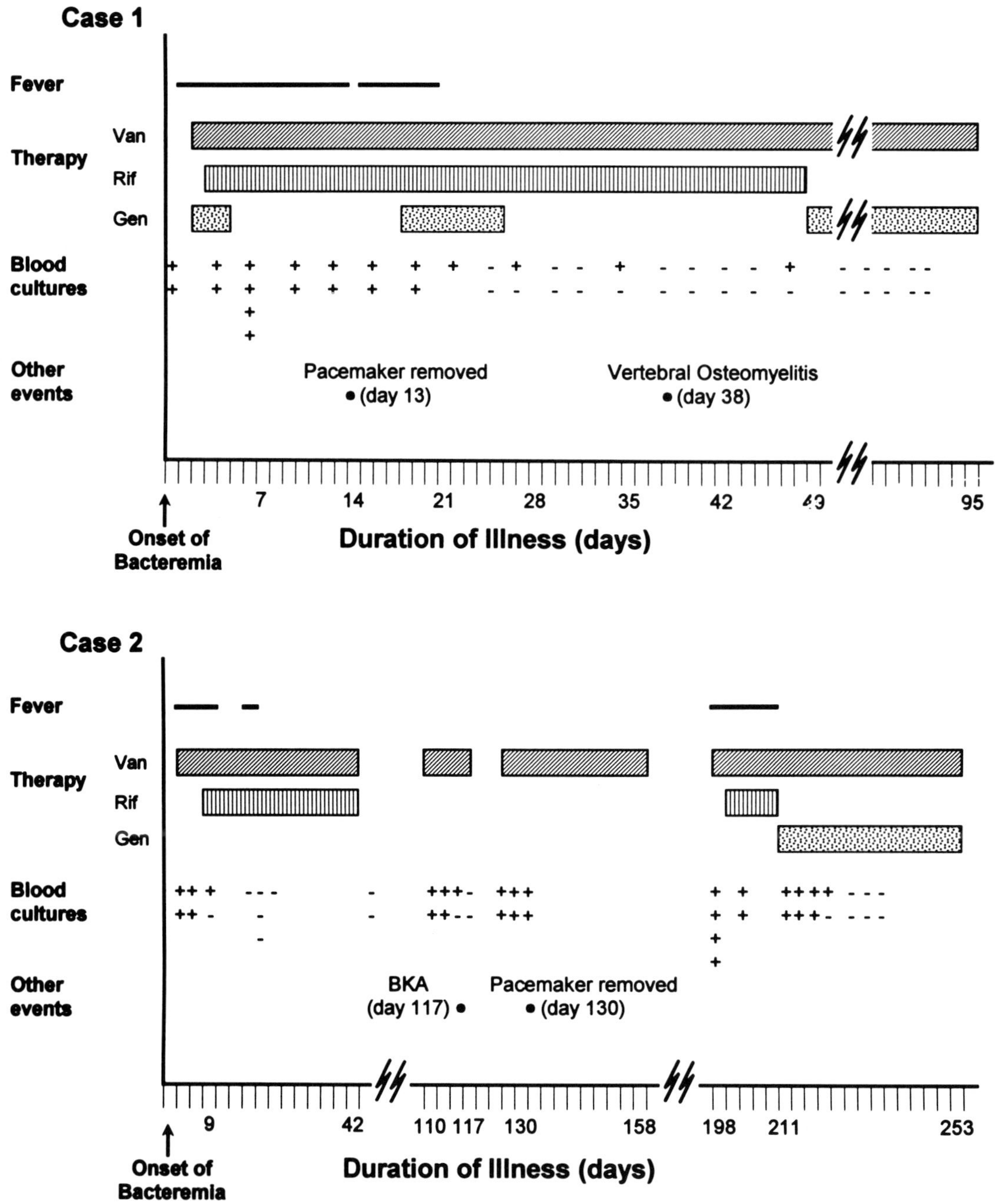

Fig. 1. Protracted course of vancomycin-tolerant MRSA bacteremia: persistent bacteremia despite defervescence during vancomycin therapy. Case 1: a patient with epidural abscess that developed 38 days after beginning therapy. Case 2: a patient with multiple relapses despite vancomycin therapy. Van, vancomycin; Rif, rifampin; Gen, gentamicin.

MATERIALS AND METHODS

Organism identification and susceptibility

Blood isolates were identified as catalase-positive and coagulase-positive by StaphAurex latex agglutination (Murex Diagnostics, Dartford, England) according to the manufacturer's instructions. The methicillin resistance was determined by spot inoculating a 0.5 McFarland suspension of organism onto BBL MRSA Screen Agar (Becton Dickinson Microbiology Products, Cockeysville, Maryland, USA), containing 6.0 mg oxacillin, and observing growth after a 24-h incubation at 35°C in ambient air. The MICs of various antibiotics were determined by the Vitek automated system, utilizing Gram-Positive Susceptibility Cards.

Time–kill studies

Time–kill studies for both isolates and for a MRSA strain used in our laboratory for control purposes (vancomycin MIC = 0.8 μg) were performed utilizing the macrobroth dilution procedure (5) with vancomycin at 2 and 10 μg/ml, and gentamicin at 1 and 5 μg/ml.

Briefly, the surface of 10–20 isolated colonies was touched, inoculated into Mueller–Hinton broth (Difco Laboratories,

Detroit, Michigan, USA), incubated with agitation and adjusted to 0.5 McFarland turbidity in logarithmic growth phase. All the organisms were diluted to an inoculum size of 5×10^5 CFU/ml, and each isolate was inoculated into an individual antibiotic suspension. The tubes were incubated at 35°C in ambient air for 24 h. The colony count was determined by serial 10-fold dilutions of each suspension at times zero, 4 h, 8 h, and 24 h; 10 µl was subcultured to TSA with 5% sheep blood and examined at 24 and 48 h. Colonies were counted at the 48-h end point and plotted as $\log_{10}$ CFU/ml vs. time.

RESULTS

The killing rate of the control strain with vancomycin and gentamicin (at high and low concentrations) was complete after a 4-h incubation. In contrast, the killing rates with vancomycin were low at 4 and 8 h for both isolates; the killing rate for gentamicin was low for both isolates at the low but not at the high concentration (Fig. 2).

DISCUSSION

Infections with S. aureus are generally considered acute although chronic and relapsing disease are well described (6). Additionally, persistence of bacteremia despite appropriate therapy is well recognized in S. aureus endocarditis (1, 2). This persistence is generally ignored because it eventually clears without attributable complications (2).

However, our first case illustrates that bacteremia may persist after defervescence and that it may lead to delayed complication. The basis for this persistence remains obscure. In some cases, the presence of small colony variants has been proposed as a possible reason for persistence, particularly in cases with osteomyelitis (6). We were unable to detect such colonies in either of our cases.

Our findings show that the isolates of both our patients displayed reduced killing rates of vancomycin and to a lesser degree of gentamicin. These in vitro results seem to correspond to the in vivo performance of vancomycin in both cases. Although both patients defervesced, their blood cultures stayed positive. The first patient remained bacteremic for 46 days and developed a distant site of infection 38 days after initiation of therapy. The second patient relapsed despite 4 weeks of treatment with vancomycin after removal of the pacemaker, and she remained bacteremic for 22 additional days after restarting therapy. In both cases, bacteremia persisted despite high vancomycin levels; it cleared after gentamicin was added.

There are several possible explanations for the inadequate response to vancomycin therapy in our cases. For example, delaying the removal of the pacemaker could have resulted in higher than usual bacterial inoculum which could have impeded vancomycin efficacy. In support of this hypothesis, vancomycin activity appears to be influenced by inoculum and by dose (7, 8). Furthermore, Chuard et al. have demonstrated that the MIC of vancomycin as well as that of other antibiotics, was much higher among isolates

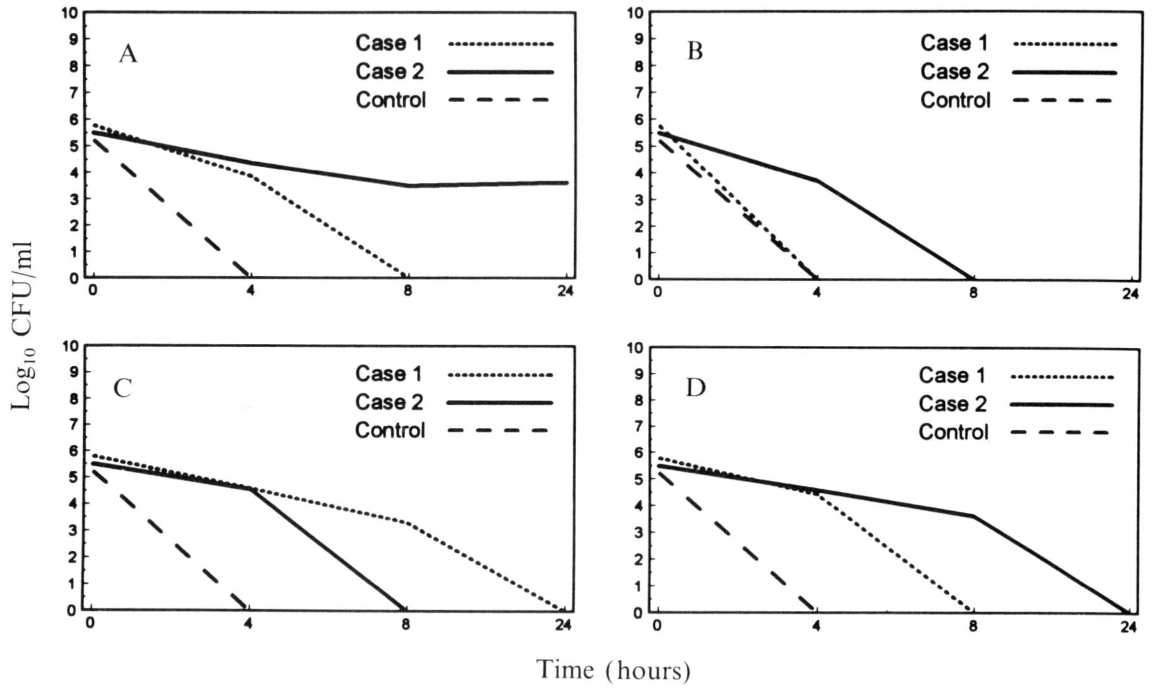

Fig. 2. Time–kill study of MRSA. A, with gentamicin at 1 µg/ml; B, with gentamicin at 5 µg/ml; C, with vancomycin at 2 µg/ml; D, with vancomycin at 10 µg/ml. The results show decreased killing rates for both isolated with vancomycin at high and low concentrations, and with gentamicin at low concentration, when compared to a control MRSA strain.

recovered from infected foreign bodies (9). It is also possible that suboptimal concentrations of vancomycin could have been the cause of the inadequate response, especially in our first case. These possibilities appear to be unlikely as bacteremia persisted long after the foreign body was removed and after increasing the vancomycin dose; clearance of the bacteremia coincided with the addition of gentamicin. We believe that the reduced killing rate, as compared to the killing rate of the control strain, is the most likely explanation for the slow response to therapy.

Whatever the mechanism may be, our cases illustrate that MRSA bacteremia may persist in the absence of fever and may lead to delayed complications long after initiating vancomycin therapy is initiated. In these cases, combining a high dose of vancomycin with gentamicin may expedite clearance of the bacteremia and may reduce the likelihood of delayed complications.

ACKNOWLEDGEMENT

This work was supported by funds from the St John Hospital and Medical Center.

REFERENCES

1. Reyman MT, Holley HP Jr, Cobbs CG. Persistent bacteremia in staphylococcal endocarditis. Am J Med 65: 729–737, 1978.
2. Levine DP, Fromm BS, Reddy BR. Slow response to vancomycin or vancomycin plus rifampin in methicillin-resistant Staphylococcus aureus endocarditis. Ann Intern Med 115: 674–680, 1991.
3. Rajashekaraiah JR, Rice T, Rao VS, Marsh D, Ramakrishna B, Kallick CA. Clinical significance of tolerance of Staphylococcus aureus in patients with endocarditis. Ann Intern Med 93: 796–801, 1980.
4. Denny AE, Peterson LR, Gerding DN, Hall WH. Serious staphylococcal infections with strains tolerant to bactericidal antibiotics. Arch Intern Med 139: 1026–1031, 1979.
5. Stratton CW, Cooksey RC. Susceptibility tests: special tests. In: Balows A, Hausler WJ Jr, Herrmann KL, Isenberg HD, Shadomy HJ, eds. Manual of clinical microbiology, 5th edn. Washington: American Society for Microbiology. 1153–1162, 1991.
6. Proctor RA, van Langevelde P, Kristjansson M, Maslo NJ, Arbeit RD. Persistent and relapsing infections associated with small-colony varients of Staphylococcus aureus. Clin Infect Dis: 20: 95–102, 1995.
7. Cantoni L, Clauser MP, Bille J. Comparative efficacy of daptomycin vancomycin, and cloxacillin for the treatment of Staphylococcus aureus endocarditis in rats and the role of test conditions in this determination. Antimicrob Agents Chemother 34: 2348–2353, 1990.
8. Gopal V, Bisno AL, Silverblatt FJ. Failure of vancomycin treatment in Staphylococcus aureus endocarditis. In vivo and in vitro observation. J Am Med Assoc 236: 1604–1606, 1976.
9. Chuard C, Lucet J-C, Rohner P, Herrmann M, Auckenthaler R, Waldvogel FA, Lew DP. Resistance of Staphylococcus aureus recovered from infected foreign body in vivo to killing by antimicrobials. J Infect Dis 163: 1369–1373, 1991.

Submitted February 13, 1995; accepted May 17, 1995

Scand J Infect Dis 27: 533–535, 1995 CASE REPORT

Low Levels of Cytokines and Endotoxin in a Fatal Case of Myocardial Depression and Septic Shock Due to Yersinia pseudotuberculosis

MATTI VALTONEN[1], JYRI LOMMI[1], SINIKKA POHJOLA-SINTONEN[1], PÄIVI LJUNGBERG[3], MARJA HYNNINEN[2], and MARTTI VAARA[3]

From the Departments of [1]Medicine and [2]Anesthesia, Helsinki University Central Hospital, and [3]Bacteriology and Immunology, University of Helsinki, Helsinki, Finland

We present a fatal case of Yersinia pseudotuberculosis sepsis with global cardiac dysfunction and shock, where the plasma levels of endotoxin, TNF-α and interleukin IL-1-β were undetectable, IL-6 was low and IL-10 was increased 3 h before death.

M. Valtonen, MD, Department of Medicine, Helsinki University Central Hospital, Haartmaninkatu 4, FIN-00290 Helsinki, Finland

INTRODUCTION

Yersinia pseudotuberculosis is an uncommon cause of sepsis and cardiac shock (1–5). The pathogenic mechanisms underlying the cardiovascular dysfunction of septic shock are complex (6, 7). Bacterial components (including endotoxin) induce a host to produce cytokines such as tumor necrosis factor-α (TNF-α) and interleukin-6 (IL-6) (8). They have been shown to cause myocardial depression, which can be blocked by nitric oxide (NO) synthase inhibitors. Thus, cytokines may induce overproduction of nitric oxide in the cardiovascular system accompanied by vasodilation and loss of cardiac contractile function (9–11). We present a case of acute fatal cardiac failure caused by Yersinia pseudotuberculosis sepsis. However, the plasma levels of cytokines (except interleukin-10 (IL-10)) and endotoxin were low 3 h before death.

CASE REPORT

A 57-year-old man with adult onset diabetes mellitus was admitted to hospital with a history of 2 days' fever and dyspnea. One day before admission a general practitioner had prescribed him penicillin V for pharyngitis. He used isophan insulin (8 units) and oral glibenclamide (3.5 mg) daily for diabetes. He had no history of diabetic complications or heart disease and he did not use alcohol regularly.

On physical examination the temperature was 39.5°C and he had respiratory distress with auscultatory wet rales and rhonchi on breathing covering the heart sounds. Blood pressure was 150/110 mmHg and heart rate 150 beats/min. The jugular veins were distended. There was no lymphadenopathy and the spleen and the liver were not enlarged.

Laboratory data showed WBC of 52.0×10^9/l (normal 4.0–10.0×10^9/l) with 1% myelocytes, 30% band neutrophils, 49% segmented neutrophils, 18% lymphocytes, 2% monocytes and 2% erythoblasts. Serum C-reactive protein level was 246 mg/l (normal < 5 mg/l); serum aspartate aminotransferase was 267 U/l (normal 10–50 U/l) and serum creatinine phosphokinase was 525 U/l (normal < 270 U/l) with MB fraction 10 U/l. Blood hemoglobin, platelet count and serum electrolytes were within normal limits.

The chest X-ray showed an enlarged heart and pulmonary edema. Electrocardiography (ECG) revealed sinustachycardia and a < 1 mm ST-segment depression on the chest leads V5–V6. Nitro infusion was started as well as oxygen with a continuous positive airway pressure. Transthoracic echocardiography showed dilation of both ventricles but no pericardial fluid. The end-diastolic diameter on the left ventricle was 57 mm. The systolic function of the left ventricle was globally decreased, the ejection fraction being less than 20%. A mild mitral regurgitation was seen. Transesophageal echocardiography (TEE) did not reveal severe valvular dysfunction or other specific causes for systolic dysfunction.

The patient developed cardiac shock and ventricular tachycardia after TEE. Despite intensive treatment and ventilatory support the patient died within 1 h. Blood cultures taken on admission 3 h before death yielded Yersinia pseudotuberculosis. Blood samples concomitantly with the blood cultures showed undetectable levels of plasma endotoxin (< 12.5 pg/ml), IL-1β (< 3.9 pg/ml) and TNF-α (< 15.7 pg/ml), a low level of IL-6 (190 pg/ml) and an increased level of IL-10 (43 pg/ml). An autopsy performed 17 h after death revealed an enlarged heart and dilated ventricles. The myocardium, valves and coronary arteries appeared normal. Microscopical investigation of the myocardium failed to show inflammatory changes. The liver was enlarged and full of small (about 5 mm diameter) septic abscesses containing small Gram-negative rods on microscopic examination.

Plasma levels of endotoxin and cytokines were quantified in duplicate samples using commerically available test systems: for endotoxin (Coatest® Endotoxin, Chromogenix), for TNF-α, IL-1β and IL-6 (Quantikine TM, Research and Diagnostic Systems, Minneapolis, USA) and for IL-10 (Pharmingen, San Diego, USA). The detection limits of assays for endotoxin TNF-α, IL-1β, IL-6 were 12.5 pg/ml, 15.7 pg/ml, 3.9 pg/ml, 3.9 pg/ml and 12.5 pg/ml, respectively. The positive controls included in the kits performed appropriately.

DISCUSSION

Yersinia pseudotuberculosis accounted for about 10% of yersinia infections in a series of 334 patients in Finland.

 ISSN 0036-5548

The most typical symptoms included fever, abdominal pain, diarrhea and erythema nodosum (1). Yersinia pseudotuberculosis sepsis is a rarity. An analysis of Yersinia bacteremias in Denmark over a period of 13 years revealed only one Y. pseudotuberculosis septicemia (2). Septic Y. pseudotuberculosis infection affects elderly, particularly males, and may be associated with alcholism, cirrhosis, diabetes mellitus and hemochromatosis. The mortality rate 75, is high (3–5).

The pathogensis underlying cardiovascular dysfunction of septic shock is complex (6, 7). Paradoxically, the patients surviving a septic shock often have an initial ejection fraction less than 40%, compared to the non-survivors who have an initial ejection fraction over 40% (7). The initial ejection fraction of our patient was less than 20%. Microorganism-elaborated exotoxins, endotoxins from the cell wall of Gram-negative bacteria, and host defense systems, including complement, kinin and coagulation cascades, as well as cytokines, generate an acute inflammatory response (6, 8). Elevated plasma endotoxin, TNF-α, IL-1β and especially interleukin-6 levels have been shown to correlate with mortality in patients with sepsis syndrome (12, 13). The appearance and disappearance of cytokines from the circulation depends on the bacterial species, and on the immune response of the host (8).

Our patient had a clearly increased IL-10 level, and a slightly elevated plasma IL-6 level, but undetectable endotoxin, TNF-α and IL-1β levels. The samples were taken at the same time as Y. pseudotuberculosis positive blood cultures, i.e. 3 h before death. Thus, free endotoxin, TNF-α and IL-1β were probably not acting as factors depressing myocardial function in this patient. On the other hand endotoxin concentrations do not correlate reliably, unfortunately, to the disease severity (8). Furthermore, pre-existing high plasma levels of pro-inflammatory cytokines cannot be ruled out, as well as high local tissue concentrations. IL-10 downregulates TNF-α and IL-1β production (14), and could explain the low levels of TNF-α and IL-1β and the increased level IL-10. In a recent study, patients with septic shock had significantly higher IL-10 levels (58 pg/ml) than septicaemic patients without shock (11 pg/ml) (14). On the other hand, increased IL-10 levels reduce mortality in experimental endotoxemia (15, 16). High IL-6 levels (median, 189 ng/ml) have been shown to correlate with septic shock and death, whereas levels of less than 3.0 ng/ml correlate with survival (13). In another study, a median IL-6 level of 197 pg/ml was determined for healthy controls (12). It seems therefore unlikely that an IL-6 level of 190 pg/ml could have been responsible for the myocardial dysfunction and heart failure. However, it is evident from the high CRP level that an IL-6 response must have been present before admission.

Nitric oxide synthase induction is a potential mechanism for myocardial depression in sepsis. Animal studies suggest that cytokines can induce sustained nitric oxide production for at least 18 h by upregulating transcription of inducible NO synthase (iNOs) (9, 16). Myocardial depression due to NOS induction might thus be seen after the peak and subsequent normalization of cytokine levels. A failure to detect late circulating cytokine levels in patients with several hours of disease does not necessarily rule out earlier activation of iNOS.

In a pilot study, administration of anti-TNF antibody has been shown to improve left ventricular function in patients with septic shock (17). Blocking TNF alone might not be sufficient to prevent the development of cardiac shock because of the synergy among various cytokines and cell fragments; therefore, cocktails of monoclonal antibodies against cytokines have been suggested (8), as well as NO synthase inhibitors (11).

More studies are thus needed to resolve the role of circulating cytokines, NO and possibly other, yet unknown, mediators of myocardial depression in the pathogensis of septic shock.

REFERENCES

1. Ahvonen P. Human yersiniosis in Finland. Ann Clin Res 4: 39–48, 1972.
2. Arpi M, Jensen KT, Frederiksen W. Yesinia enterocolitica bacteremia: an analysis of thirty-six patients in Denmark and a review of the literature. Contrib Microbiol Immunol 12: 260–264, 1991.
3. Yamashiro KM, Goldman RH, Harris D, Uyeda CT. Pasteurella pseudotuberculosis. Acute sepsis with survival. Arch Intern Med 128: 605–608, 1971.
4. Macaulay JD, Wilson JAC, Abbott JD, Mair NS. Fatal case of Pasteurella pseudotuberculosis infection associates with hepatic cirrhosis. Br Med J 2: 553–554, 1967.
5. Butler T. Yersinia species. In: Mandell GL, Douglas RG, Bennett JE, eds. Principle and practice of infectious diseases. 4th ed. New York: Churchill Livingstone, 2070–2078, 1995.
6. Parillo JE. Pathogenetic mechanisms of septic shock. N Engl J Med 328: 1471–1477, 1993.
7. Parker MM, Shelhamer JH, Bacharach SL, Green MV, Natanson Ch, Frederick TM, Damske BA, Parillo JE. Profound but reversible myocardial depression in patients with septic shock. Ann Intern Med 100: 483–490, 1984.
8. Glauser MP, Heumann D, Baumgartner JD, Cohen J. Pathogenesis and potential strategies for prevention and treatment of septic shock: an update. Clin Infect Dis 18: S205–S216, 1994.
9. Schulz R, Nava E, Moncada S. Induction and potential biological relevance of a Ca^{+}-independent nitric oxide synthase in the myocardium. Br J. Pharmacol 105: 575–580, 1992.
10. Finkel MS, Oddis CV, Jacob TD, Watkins SC, Hattler BG, Simmons RL. Negative inotropic effects of cytokines on the heart mediated by nitric oxide. Science 257: 387–389, 1992.
11. Petros A, Bennett D, Vallance P. Effect of nitric oxide synthesis inhibitors on hypotension in patients with septic shock. Lancet 338: 1557–1558, 1991.
12. Casey LC, Balk RA, Bone RC. Plasma cytokine and endotoxin levels correlate with survival in patients with the sepsis syndrome. Ann Intern Med 119: 771–778, 1993.
13. Waage A, Brandtzaeg P, Halstensen A, Kierulf P, Espevik T. The complex of cytokines in serum from patients with meningococcal septic shock. Association between interleukin 6, interleukin 1, and fatal outcome. J Exp Med 169: 333–338, 1989.

14. Marchant A, Devière J, Byl B, De Groote D, Vincent J-L, Goldman M. Interleukin-10 production during septicaemia. Lancet 343: 707–708, 1994.
15. Howard M, Muchamuel T, Andrade S, Menon S. Interleukin 10 protects mice from lethal endotoxemia. J Exp Med 177: 1205–1208, 1993.
16. Gérard C, Bruyns C, Marchant A, Abramowicz D, Vandenabeele P, Delvaux A, Fiers W, Goldman M, Velu T. Interleukin 10 reduces the release of tumor necrosis factor and prevents lethality in experimental endotoxemia. J Exp Med 177: 547–550, 1993.
17. Vincent J-L, Bakker J, Marecaux G, Schandene L, Kahn RJ, Dupont E: Administration of anti-TNF antibody improves left ventricular function in septic shock patients. Chest 101: 810–815, 1992.

Submitted February 16, 1995; accepted June 16, 1995

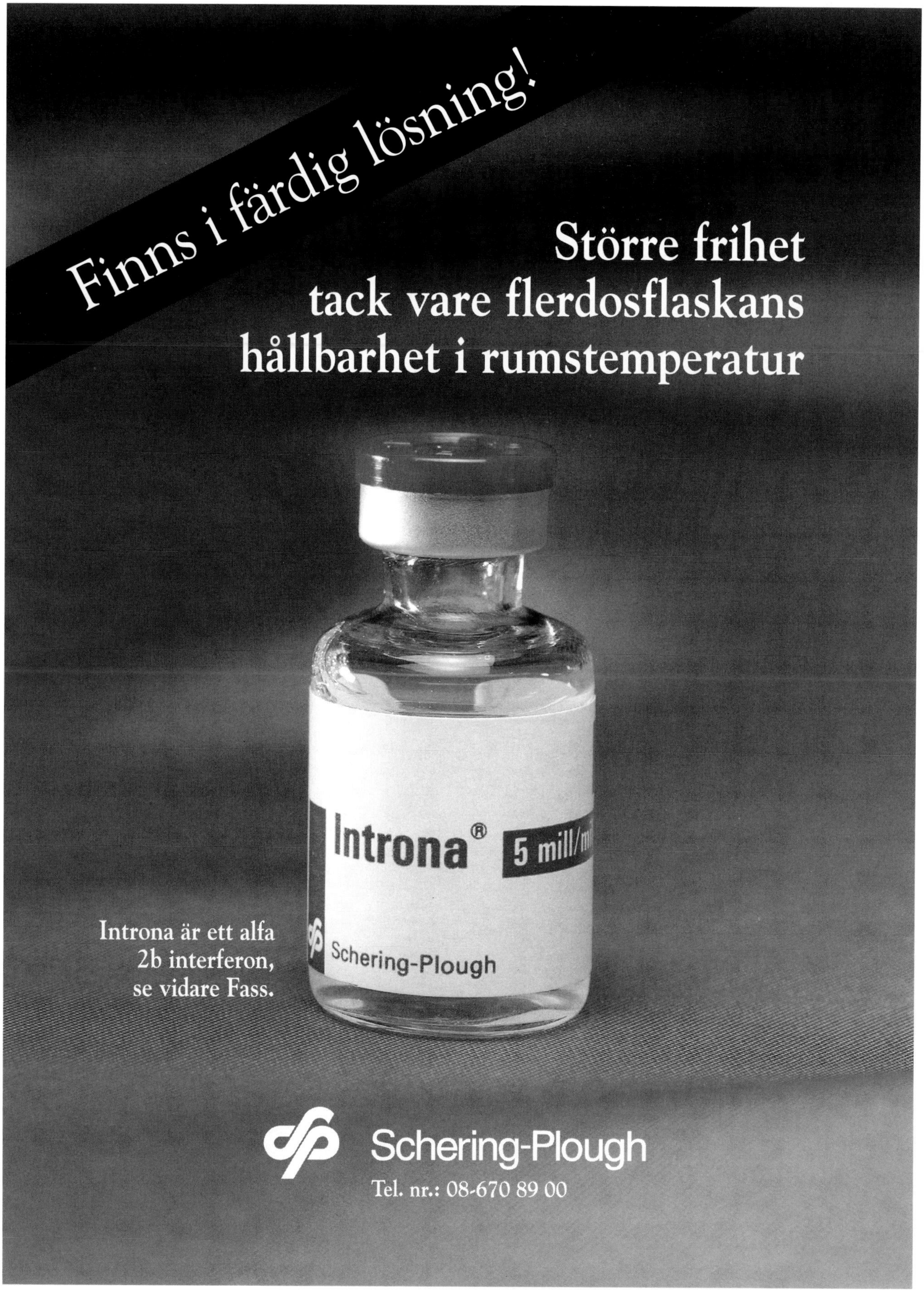
Finns i färdig lösning!
Större frihet
tack vare flerdosflaskans
hållbarhet i rumstemperatur
Introna®
Schering-Plough
Introna är ett alfa
2b interferon,
se vidare Fass.
Schering-Plough
Tel. nr.: 08-670 89 00

Scand J Infect Dis 27: 537–539, 1995 SHORT COMMUNICATION

Rapid Diagnosis of Bacterial Meningitis by a Seminested PCR Strategy

PER OLCÉN[1], PÄR-GUNNAR LANTZ[2], ANDERS BÄCKMAN[1] and PETER RÅDSTRÖM[2]

From the Departments of [1]Clinical Microbiology and Immunology, Örebro Medical Center Hospital, Örebro, and [2]Applied Microbiology, Lund Institute of Technology, Lund University, Lund, Sweden

A polymerase chain reaction (PCR) based diagnostic assay has been developed for the simultaneous detection in cerebrospinal fluid (CSF) of Neisseria meningitidis, Haemophilus influenzae, Streptococcus pneumoniae, Streptococcus agalactiae, Listeria monocytogenes and bacteria in general. In the present communication we describe the design of primers for S. pneumoniae, S. agalactiae, and L. monocytogenes, and a general PCR protocol for the assay. The diagnostic outcome is presented for a small collection of CSF specimens including 2 samples from patients with culture-negative purulent meningitis.

P. Olcén, MD, Department of Clinical Microbiology and Immunology, Örebro Medical Center Hospital, S-701 85 Örebro, Sweden

INTRODUCTION

Bacterial meningitis is a life-threatening and CNS-damaging infection. Rapid and accurate diagnosis is therefore of fundamental importance for effective treatment. Culture and direct microscopic examination of cerebrospinal fluid (CSF) form the basis for routine etiological diagnosis. However, these methods have well known shortcomings.

Microscopy lacks specificity and requires a high concentration of bacteria in CSF ($\geq 10^5$/ml) for a positive result. Culture is time-consuming and false-negative results are sometimes obtained due to prior antibiotic treatment for example, a situation that has become more prevalent as early treatment has been stressed (1).

Specific and rapid etiological/diagnostic methods such as immunoelectro-osmophoresis, coagglutination, latex agglutination, direct immunofluorescence and EIA/ELISA have been developed for antigens in CSF (2–5). However, some obstacles exist with these immunological methods, such as the following.

1. A bacterial concentration of 10^3–10^4 CFU/ml is required for a positive reaction.
2. High quality reagents for Neisseria meningitidis serogroup B have been difficult to produce.
3. Haemophilus influenzae of other than serotype b have not been included.
4. All types of Streptococcus pneumoniae have been difficult to cover;
5. Other meningitidis-causing bacteria, such as Listeria monocytogenes, have not been included.

In order to overcome some of these difficulties, a 2-step polymerase chain reaction (PCR) assay for the simultaneous detection of N. meningitidis, H. influenzae and streptococci, as well as eubacteria in general has been developed (6). In the present study the strategy has been further developed to include L. monocytogenes and to specifically identify S. pneumoniae and group B streptococci. In the first PCR step (I in Fig. 1), primers specific for eubacteria are used. The amplicon is then used as a template in the second PCR step, IIa and IIb.

MATERIAL AND METHODS

The first step of the PCR assay (see I in Fig. 1) was performed as previously described (6). Briefly, the universal primers u3 and ru8 were used in 50 µl of UV-radiated reaction mixture with 10 µl of CSF boiled in a waterbath for 30 min. The second step consisted either of amplification with primers for N. meningitidis (NM), H. influenzae (HI) and streptococci (STREP) together with ru8 (see IIa in Fig. 1) as previously described (6), or amplification with primers for S. pneumoniae (5′-GCT GTG GCT TAA CCA TAG TAG-3′), group B streptococci (5′-ACC GGC CTA GAG ATA GGC-3′) and L. monocytogenes (5′-GGA GCT AAT CCC ATA AAA CTA-′3) together with ru8 (see IIb in Fig. 1). The primers designated SP, GBS and LM, respectively, were constructed from published nucleotide sequences (6, 7).

The amplicon from step one was diluted 1:500 in double-distilled, deionized and UV-treated water. The second amplifications, IIa and IIb, were run in 50 µl with 2 µl and 5 µl samples from respective dilution. The reaction mixtures contained 1 × PCR buffer (Boehringer Mannheim, Germany), 1.25 U of Taq DNA polymerase (Boehringer Mannheim), 0.5 µmol/l of each primer and 0.2 mmol/l of dATP, dCTP, dGTP and dTTP respectively.

The first amplification was run under the following conditions: heat denaturation at 94°C for 6 min; 28 cycles with heat denaturation at 94°C for 1 min; primer annealing at 54°C for 1 min and DNA extension at 72°C for 2 min. Finally, the samples were maintained at 72°C for 7 min to complete the synthesis of all strands.

The second amplifications were run under conditions similar to those described for the first amplification, but for 25 cycles with annealing at 55°C for IIa, and at 60°C for IIb. All the reactions were performed in a thermocycler (DNA thermal cycler, Perkin Elmer Cetus). PCR products from the first and second steps were analysed in a 2% agarose gel electrophoresis in 1 × TAE buffer with ethidium bromide and visualized by UV irradiation (8).

 ISSN 0036-5548

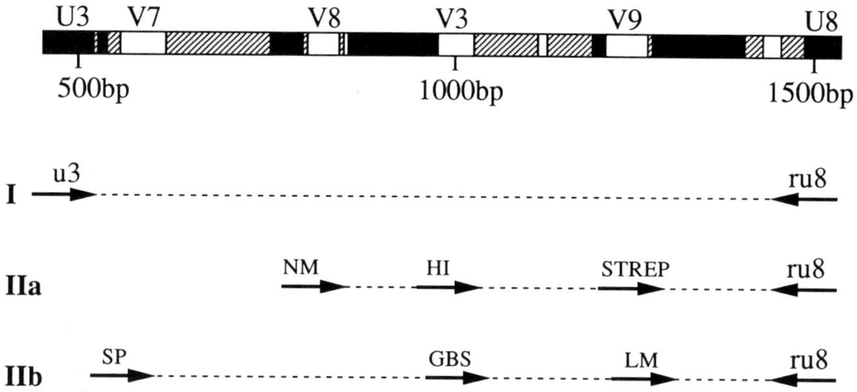

Fig. 1. Binding sites for individual PCR primers on the universal (U, black) and variable (V, white) parts of the 16 S rRNA gene (500–1,500 bp) of the bacterial genome. Hatched zones are semivariable. The different PCR steps used in the assay are designated I, IIa and IIb. In PCR step I the u3 and ru8 primers produce a 1,030 bp fragment from bacterial DNA. A dilution of this was used in the following PCR steps. PCR step IIa produced 3 different fragments: 710 bp with NM primer for N. meningitidis, 540 bp with HI-primer for H. influenzae and 300 bp with STREP primer for streptococci. PCR step IIb produced three different fragments: 937 bp with SP primer for S. pneumoniae, 544 bp with GBS primer for group B streptococci and 265 bp with LM primer for L. monocytogenes.

RESULTS

Five strains each of S. pneumoniae, group B streptococci and for L. monocytogenes gave the expected PCR products of 937 bp, 544 bp and 265 bp.

CSF from patients with acute meningitidis and positive culture of S. pneumoniae ($n = 5$), group B streptococci ($n = 3$) and L. monocytogenes ($n = 3$) in CSF or blood, collected from 1983 to 1994 and stored at −20°C or −70°C, were tested. All CSFs with S. pneumoniae were positive, 2/3 CSFs with group B streptococci were positive and 1/3 CSFs with L. monocytogenes was positive. The cultured bacteria from the 3 PCR-negative CSFs were subjected to the assay, and PCR products with the expected sizes were seen in all the 3 isolates. The false-negative PCR results may be due to PCR inhibitory substances and/or a low concentration of the bacteria in the original CFS

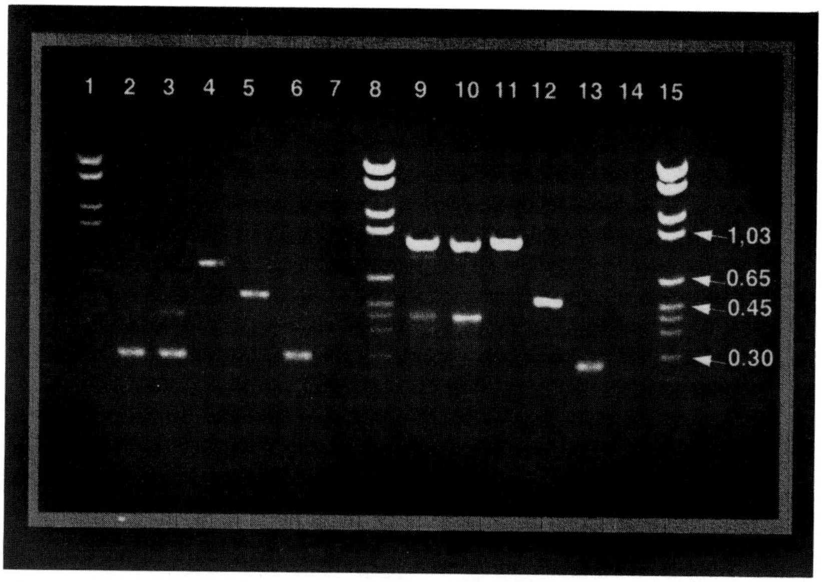

Fig. 2. The PCR products were run on agarose gel in ethidium bromide and visualized with UV light. Lanes 1, 8 and 15 are molecular size standards, in kilobasepairs and arrows indicate the corresponding DNA band. Lanes 2–7 are PCR products from step IIa and lanes 9–14 from step IIb. PCR products from culture-negative cerebrospinal fluid samples from patient 9499-14 are seen in lane 2 and 9, and from patient 9499-15 in lane 3 and 10. These DNA bands correspond to streptococcal DNA in IIa (300 bp) and S. pneumoniae DNA in IIb (937 bp). The other lanes show the PCR products from boiled bacterial dilutions: lane 4, N. meningitidis (710 bp); lane 5, H. influenzae (540 bp); lanes 6 and 11, S. pneumoniae (300 bp and 937 bp, respectively); lane 12, S. agalactiae (544 bp); lane 13, L. monocytogenes (265 bp). Lanes 7 and 14 are negative PCR results with sterile water.

sample. These results emphasize the need for rapid and convenient preparation methods before PCR can be used as a general detection method in clinical microbiology.

The assay was then tested on CSF from 2 patients with suspected acute bacterial meningitidis. The first patient was a previously healthy 68-year-old man, treated with oral penicillin for pneumonia on an outpatient basis. Within less than 24 h he was admitted with a clinical status suggesting meningitis and cefotaxime was promptly administrated i.v. before a computerized tomography of the scull was performed, which was normal. A lumbar puncture was then carried out and gave a cloudy CSF with $1{,}600 \times 10^6$ leucocytes/l (65% polymorphonuclear cells) and glucose of 1.3 mmol/l (blood 7.5). Microscopy and culture were both negative. Fig. 2 shows the results from the PCR assay. A general bacterial amplicon of 1,030 bp was obtained from the first reaction. The second reactions, IIa and IIb, showed a streptococcal product of 300 bp and a specific S. pneumoniae product of 937 bp. The patient was treated in the intensive care unit for 4 days with artificial ventilation and i.v. antibiotics. He was released from hospital after 11 days in a fair general condition and without evident sequelae.

The second patient was a 1.5-year-old previously healthy boy who was admitted to hospital with high grade fever and lethargy without signs of meningitis. Invasive bacterial infection could not be ruled out and i.v. cefuroxime treatment was started. Due to deterioration, a lumbar puncture was performed. The CSF had $2{,}700 \times 10^6$ leucocytes/l (67% polymorphonuclear cells) and glucose 1.0 (blood 7.3). Culture of CSF was negative and microscopy not conclusive. The PCR assay gave a specific amplicon for S. pneumoniae (Fig. 2). After 12 days of hospitalization the patient was released, without evident sequelae, for later follow-up.

DISCUSSION

The present seminested PCR of CSF for bacteria as such, and specifically for N. meningitidis, H. influenzae, S. pneumoniae, group B streptococcus and L. monocytogenes, is a further improvement in the set of available rapid and specific diagnostic methods. Indications for investigation with the PCR assay could be when the culture of CSF is negative and the antigen test results are negative or inconclusive. Since the antigen assays require larger volumes of CSF, a seminested PCR (10 μl of CSF) might actually be the only analysis that can be conducted when small sample volumes are available. With the present composition of primers, most N. meningitidis, H. influenzae, S. pneumoniae, group B streptococci and L. monocytogenes, irrespective of group/type, are detected. However, extended systematically conducted studies must be performed to learn about limitations as well as about the possibilities for improving sample preparation and primer design and, circumventing inhibitors.

REFERENCES

1. Cartwright K, Strang J, Gossain S, Begg N. Early treatment of meningococcal disease. Br Med J 305: 774, 1992.
2. Olcén P, Danielsson D, Kjellander J. The use of protein A-containing staphylococci sensitized with anti-meningococcal antibodies for grouping Neisseria meningitidis and demonstration of meningococcal antigen in CSF. Acta Pathol Microbiol Scand B 83: 387–396, 1975.
3. Olcén P. Serological methods for rapid diagnosis of Haemophilus influenzae, Neisseria meningitidis, and Streptococcus pneumoniae in cerebrospinal fluid: a comparison of co-agglutination, immunofluorescence and immunoelectroosmophoresis. Scand J Infect Dis 10: 283–289, 1978.
4. Salih MAM, Ahmed HS, Hofvander Y, Danielsson D, Olcén P. Rapid diagnosis of bacterial meningitis by an enzyme immunoassay of cerebrospinal fluid. Epidemiol Infect 103: 301–310, 1989.
5. Nato F, Mazie JC, Fournier JM, Slizewicz B, Sagon N, Guibourdenche M, Postic D, Riou JY. Production of polyclonal and monoclonal antibodies against group A, B, C capsular polysaccharides of Neisseria meningitidis and preparation of latex reagents. J Clin Microbiol 29: 1447–1452, 1991.
6. Rådström P, Bäckman A, Qian N, Kragsbjerg P, Påhlson C, Olcén P. Detection of bacterial DNA in cerebrospinal fluid by an assay for simultaneous detection of Neisseria meningitidis, Haemophilus influenzae, and streptococci using a seminested PCR strategy. J Clin Microbiol 32: 2738–2744, 1994.
7. Collins MDS, Wallbanks S, Lane DJ, Shah J, Nietupski R, Smida J, Dorsch M, Stackebrandt E. Phylogenetic analysis of the genus Listeria based on reverse transcriptase sequencing of 16S rRNA. Int J Syst Bacteriol 41: 240–246, 1991.
8. Sambrook I, Fritsch EF, Maniatis T. Molecular cloning. A laboratory manual. Cold Spring Harbour: Cold Spring Harbour Laboratory Press, 1989.

Submitted February 9, 1995; accepted June 6, 1995

Ref

1 Guerra J G et al. Imipenem/cilastatin VS, gentamicin/clindamycin for the treatment of moderate to severe infections in hospitalized patients. Rev Infect Dis 1985; 7:463–470

2 Heseltine PNR et al. Imipenem therapy for perforated gangrenous appendicitis. Surg Gynecol Obstet 1986; 162: 43–48

3 Gonzenbach H R, Simmen HP, Amgwerd R. Imipenem (N–F–Thienamycin) versus netilmicin plus clindamycin:A controlled and randomized comparison in intra abdominal infections. Ann Surg 1987; 205(3): 271–275

Scandinavian Journal of

INFECTIOUS DISEASES

Vol. 27, no. 6, 1995
pp. 541–656

SCANDINAVIAN
UNIVERSITY PRESS

Oslo - Copenhagen -
Stockholm - Boston

Scand J Infect Dis 27: 543–546, 1995 ORIGINAL ARTICLE

Hepatitis E Virus Infections in Patients with Acute Hepatitis non-A–D in Sweden

P. J. HUGO JOHANSSON[1], ISA K. MUSHAHWAR[2], GUNNAR NORKRANS[3], OLA WEILAND[4] and ERIK NORDENFELT[5]

From the [1]Department of Medical Microbiology, Section of Virology, University of Lund, Lund, Sweden, [2]Experimental Biology Research, Abbott Laboratories, North Chicago, Illinois, USA, Departments of [3]Infectious Diseases, Östra Hospital, University of Göteborg, Göteborg, [4]Infectious Diseases, Karolinska Institute, Huddinge Hospital, Huddinge, and [5]Virology, Swedish Institute for Infections Disease Control, Stockholm, Sweden

A total of 12 patients previously treated for acute hepatitis of unknown aetiology were retrospectively found to be anti-hepatitis E virus (HEV) IgG-positive. Four patients were anti-HEV IgM- and IgG-positive consistent with an acute HEV infection. All 4 had travelled to or were immigrants from HEV-endemic countries. One anti-HEV IgM-negative patient seroconverted from anti-HEV IgG-negative to positive and 3 from anti-HEV IgG-positive to negative in 2 consecutive serum samples. Of the remaining 4 patients without anti-HEV IgM, 3 had a history of recent travel to an HEV-endemic country. Most patients were young adults and all but 1 recovered from the hepatitis. One patient with a fulminant hepatitis was anti-HEV IgG-positive when tested 4 months after a journey to Turkey. She died from her fulminant hepatitis shortly after admission. All the other patients but 1 normalized their serum liver enzymes within 1–2 months after the onset of disease.

P. J. H. Johansson, MD, Department of Medical Microbiology, Virology Section, Sölvegatan 23, S-223 62, Lund, Sweden

INTRODUCTION

Hepatitis E virus (HEV) infection is an enterically transmitted hepatitis that occurs mostly in large outbreaks in developing countries (1). The role of HEV as a cause of acute sporadic hepatitis in developed countries has not been extensively studied because of the lack of commercially available specific serological tests. The recent cloning and sequencing of HEV (2) has made it possible to develop anti-HEV tests for detection of HEV antibodies (3). We have retrospectively tested sera from patients treated for acute non-A, non-B, non-C hepatitis at Swedish hospitals for the presence of HEV antibodies in order to study the existence of HEV infections among these patients.

PATIENTS AND METHODS

Patients

Patients with verified clinical and biochemical acute viral hepatitis, who tested negative for markers indicating acute hepatitis A, B, C and D and from whom stored frozen sera were available, were selected for retrospective anti-HEV testing by ELISA. The patients were from 3 University hospitals (University hospital of Lund, Lund, Östra hospital, Göteborg and Huddinge hospital, Stockholm) in Sweden. The sera were collected between 1982 and 1992 in Stockholm, 1979 to 1989 in Lund and 1982 to 1985 in Göteborg.

The diagnosis of hepatitis was based on clinical and biochemical findings (elevated alanine aminotransferase (s-ALT) of more than 10 times the upper normal limit). Liver biopsy or autopsy was performed only in patients with a fulminant hepatitis or with a prolonged course (> 6 months) of elevated s-ALT.

Besides exclusion of acute hepatitis A, B, C and D infection, patients with recent infections with cytomegalovirus and Epstein–Barr virus, or with liver injury due to hepatotoxic drugs, biliary disease or autoimmune disease, or with liver disease secondary to diseases with involvement of other organs, were excluded from the study.

Patients reactive in anti-HEV tests were further studied with regard to clinical and epidemiological findings, as the purpose of the study was to see whether HEV infections were present or not in Sweden and whether the infection was imported or not.

Anti-HEV tests

Anti-HEV IgG and IgM antibodies in human samples were detected by ELISA, as described (3). All the reactive samples were analysed in several supplementary ELISA procedures utilizing synthetic HEV peptides, and Western blots using recombinant HEV proteins (4). Specimens with a positive result in ≥1 supplementary assays were considered positive.

RESULTS

A total of 12 patients treated for acute non-A, non-B, non-C hepatitis reacted with recombinant and synthetic HEV peptides (Table I). Of these patients, 4 were anti-HEV IgM- and IgG-positive, and 7 were anti-HEV IgG-positive but IgM-negative. Of the 8 IgM-negative patients, 1 (patient 7 in Table 1) had and initially borderline positive anti-HEV IgG ELISA test, later proven to be negative. He was included due to positive supplementary tests indicating HEV. Another IgM-negative patient seroconverted from anti-HEV IgG-negative to positive 15–24 days after the onset of disease (patient 6) and 3 patients converted from anti-HEV IgG-positive to negative on 2 consecutive serum samples taken 4–10 month apart (patients 7, 8 and 9).

The details of age, sex, peak serum liver enzyme values and recent travel abroad of the 12 patients are shown in Table II. Most patients were young adults, and only 3 were middle-aged (37, 40 and 59 years old). All the patients had a significant rise in their s-ALT levels consistent with acute hepatitis.

Table I. *Results of anti-HEV testing on HEV enzyme-linked immunoassay (ELISA) and HEV Western blot (WB) of sera from patients with acute non-A, non-B, non-C hepatitis*

Patient no.	Time of sample, days after onset of disease	Anti-HEV test results					
		IgM[a]	IgG[a]	IgG spB3-2[b]	IgG spB4-2[b]	WB[c]	Final IgG result
1	3	+	+	+	−	+	+
	25	+	+	+	+	+	+
2	11	+	+	+	ND[d]	ND	+
3	1	+	+	+	+	ND	+
4	3	+	+	+	+	ND	+
5	?[e]	−	+	+	−	ND	+
6	15	−	−	−	−	−	−
	24	−	+	+	+	−	+
7	17	−	+[f]	+	−	+	+
	193	−	−	−	−	+	−
8	6	−	+	−	−	+	+
	305	−	−	−	−	−	−
9	8	−	+	−	−	+	+
	127	−	−	−	−	+	−
10	17	−	+	+	−	−	+
	74	−	+	+	−	−	+
11	24	−	+	+	+	−	+
	55	−	+	+	+	−	+
12	10	−	+	+	ND	+	+
	106	−	+	+	ND	+	+

[a] Antibodies against recombinant HEV peptides SG-3 and/or 8-5 in HEV ELISA.
[b] Antibodies against synthetic HEV peptides spB3-2 and spB4-2 in HEV ELISA.
[c] Antibodies against HEV peptides in Western blot.
[d] ND, not done
[e] Unable to determine onset of disease.
[f] Borderline positive.

The 4 patients with anti-HEV IgM reactivity had a history of recent travel to, or were immigrants from, HEV-endemic countries. One had emigrated from Bangladesh 4 weeks before the onset of disease (patient 2), and another (patient 3) had emigrated from India to Sweden 7 years earlier, but had returned from a visit to India 5 weeks before the onset of hepatitis. Another 2 patients, travelling in Asia (Malaysia, Singapore, Laos, Vietnam, Thailand, Indonesia, India) (patient 4), and travelling in Israel (patient 1), had taken gammaglobulin prophylaxis. The onset of their hepatitis episodes occurred 2 and 4 weeks, respectively, after the end of their journey.

Four patients (patient 5, 9, 11 and 12) without HEV IgM also had a history of recent travel abroad. One of these patients (patient 5) had a fulminant hepatitis on admission when she presented with ascites and icterus 4 months after returning from a journey to Turkey. The onset of her liver disease cannot be established exactly. She died from her fulminant hepatitis within 1 week after admission and at autopsy a massive liver necrosis was seen.

All the other patients recovered and all but 1 (patient 8) had normalized their s-ALT levels 1–2 months after the onset of their disease. Patient 8 did not normalize his serum bilirubin and ALT level until 2 years after the onset of disease. Due to the prolonged course in this patient, liver biopsy was performed 11 months after onset, and showed mild acute hepatitis.

DISCUSSION

Enterically transmitted HEV infection is responsible for major epidemic ourbreaks in developing countries (1). Sporadic HEV infections in developed countries have not been extensively studied, mainly because of the lack of specific serological tests. The recent cloning and sequencing of HEV, a single-stranded, positive sense RNA virus of about 7.5 kb, has made it possible to develop tests for detection of HEV antibodies. We utilized assays with recombinant and synthetic HEV peptides as well as Western blots for detection of HEV antibodies (4). Specimens with a

Table II. *Age, sex, peak values of s-bilirubin (normal upper limit <20 μmol/l), s-alkaline phosphate (s-ALP, <4.6 μkat/l), alanine aminotransaminase (s-ALT, <0.7 μkat/l), aspartic aminotransaminase (s-AST, <0.7 μkat/l), and travel destination, in patients with an acute non-A, non-B, non-C hepatitis and antibodies against HEV*

			Peak serum liver enzyme values				
Patient no.	Age, years	Sex	s-Bilirubin	s-ALP	s-ALT	s-AST	Travel abroad
1	19	F	340	10.0	106	104	Israel[a]
2	22	M	120	11.0	18	19	Bangladesh[b]
3	27	F	363	12.0	56	39	India[c]
4	29	F	241	11.7	9	12	Asia[d]
5[e]	59	F	138	9.0	21	36	Turkey[f]
6	22	F	250	7.0	21	7	No
7	37	M	86	6.2	54	28	No
8	30	M	192[g]	9.3	57[g]	31[g]	No
9	40	M	84	8.1	47	15	Germany[h]
10	22	F	73	7.6	8	3	No
11	19	M	79	7.7	38	17	India[i]
12	25	F	61	8.0	42	26	Asia[j]

[a] Travel from Israel 4 weeks before onset of disease.
[b] Immigrant from Bangladesh 4 weeks before onset of disease.
[c] Previous immigrant from India, now travel from India 5 weeks before onset of disease.
[d] Travel from Asia (Malaysia, Singapore, Laos, Vietnam, Thailand, Indonesia, India) 2 weeks before onset of disease.
[e] Ad mortem in fulminant hepatitis.
[f] Travel from Turkey 4 months before admission to hospital.
[g] Not normalized 6 months after onset of disease.
[h] Travel from Germany before onset of disease.
[i] Travel from India 6 weeks before onset of disease.
[j] Travel from Asia (Japan, Hong Kong, Bangkok and India) 5 days before onset of disease.

positive result in ≥1 supplementary assays were considered positive.

A total of 12 patients treated for acute non-A, non-B, non-C hepatitis in Swedish hospitals tested positive for the presence of HEV IgG antibodies. Of these, 4 had an additional IgM response confirming a recent HEV infection. All 4 had a history of recent travel to or were immigrants from an HEV-endemic country. HEV infection occurred in 2 patients despite prophylaxis with gammaglobulin. The start of their hepatitis was within 40 days after they left the HEV-endemic areas which is well within the proposed incubation period of HEV (5). This supports previous reports that the majority of HEV infections in industrialized countries derive from immigrants and travellers from endemic countries (6–9). In Sweden, 8 other cases of acute hepatitis E infection during 1991 and 1993 have recently been diagnosed, all infected abroad (Dr Lars Magnius, personal communication). A report from Norway also describes 3 young patients with acute HEV infections, all with a history of recent travel to endemic areas (9).

Of our patents, only 3/12 were older than 30 years of age, well in line with the reported predominance of young adults as the major incidence group (10). All patients were icteric with makedly increased serum ALT levels. The increase of serum ALP levels in our patients was not pronounced, a feature earlier reported to be characteristic of HEV infections (10). Apart from 1 patient with elevated liver enzymes for 2 years, no sign of persistent liver infection was seen.

Whether the 8 patients without an IgM response had an acute HEV infection is more difficult to decide. Of these 3 patients had recently been travelling in HEV-endemic countries, and the patient with a fulminant hepatitis had travelled to Turkey 4 months prior to admission to hospital. She presented with ascites and icterus and died shortly after admission due to liver failure. Fulminant hepatitis with high mortality occurs in HEV infections, especially among pregnant woman (11, 12). Our patient may have had an acute HEV infection but lost her IgM antibodies before admission as HEV IgM is known to revert to negative about 3 months after onset of infection (9, 16).

Four other patients without recent travel abroad had a discrepancy between their acute and convalescent sera; one seroconverted from negative to positive HEV IgG without an IgM response, and 3 lost the HEV IgG antibodies in the convalescent serum taken 4–10 months after the onset of disease. Although IgG antibodies are believed to remain for several years (16), a decrease or negative anti-HEV IgG result during the convalescent phase can sometimes be seen (16). An acute HEV infection in these patients cannot therefore, be ruled out.

For the remaining anti-HEV IgG-positive but IgM-negative patients, the anti-HEV response could be a relic of a past HEV infection without connection to their present hepatitis. Unfortunately, we do not know whether these patients had a previous history of travel in an endemic area. If so, it could not be excluded that they had then obtained HEV IgG antibodies that persisted until their present hepatitis.

For some patients, discrepancies in results were seen between the various HEV tests. This can be explained by differences in sensitivity and specificity for tests utilizing synthetic or recombinant HEV peptides (3, 4). The interpretation of serological results can therefore sometimes be difficult with these first-generation tests, because of the lack of a commercially available confirmatory assay.

The prevalence of HEV antibodies in the Swedish population is not known, but for European countries like the Netherlands it is around 0.4% among healthy blood donors (7). There are indications that not all HEV infections in industrialized countries are connected with a recent visit to a HEV-endemic country (7, 16). HEV is believed to be a largely waterborne infection, transmitted by the faecal–oral route and with a very limited secondary person-to-person transmission (5). The means of transmission and the frequency of HEV in patients with sporadic hepatitis, in non-endemic areas without a history of travel in an endemic country, is at present not known.

ACKNOWLEDGEMENTS

We thank Miss Monica Öberg for her skilful technical assistance. This work was supported by grants from the Medical Faculty, University of Lund, and the Swedish Medical Research Council grant number B93-16x-02865.

REFERENCES

1. Bradley BW. Hepatitis E: epidemiology, aetiology and molecular biology. Med Virol 2: 19–28, 1992.
2. Tam AW, Smith MM, Guerra ME, Huang CC, Bradley DW, Fry KE, Reyes GR. Hepatitis E virus (HEV): molecular cloning and sequencing of the full-length viral genome. Virology 185: 120–131, 1991.
3. Dawson GJ, Chau KH, Cabal CM, Yarbough PO, Reyes GR, Mushahwar IK. Solid-phase enzyme-linked immuonsorbent assay for hepatitis E virus IgG and IgM antibodies utilizing recombinant antigens and synthetic peptides. J Virol Methods 38: 175–186, 1992.
4. Dawson G, Paul D, Gutierrez R, Pilot-Matias T, Chau K, Kyrk C, Buijk S, Knigge M, Heynen C, Leung T, Cabal C, Mushahwar IK. Recombinant antigens and synthetic peptides for serodiagnosis of hepatitis E virus infection. In: Nishioka K, Suzuki H, Mishiro S, Oda T, eds. Viral hepatitis and liver disease. Tokyo: Springer-Verlag, 371–374, 1994.
5. Velasquez O, Stetler HC, Avila C, Ornelas G, Alvarez C, Hadler SC, Bradley DW, Sepulveda J. Epidemic transmission of enterically transmitted non-A, non-B hepatitis in Mexico, 1986–1987. JAMA 263: 3281–3285, 1990.
6. de Cock KM, Bradley DW, Sandford NL, Govindarajan S, Maynard JE, Redeker AG. Epidemic non-A, non-B hepatitis in patients from Pakistan. Ann Intern Med 106: 227–230, 1987.
7. Zaaijer HL, Kok M, Lelie PN, Timmerman RJ, Chau K, van der Pal J. Hepatitis E in The Netherlands: imported and endemic. Lancet 341: 826, 1993.
8. Jardi R, Buti M, Rodriguez-Frias F, Esteban R. Hepatitis E infections in acute sporadic hepatitis in Spain. Lancet 341: 1355–1356, 1993.
9. Skaug K, Hagen IJ, von der Lippe B. Three cases of acute hepatitis E virus infection imported into Norway. Scand J Infect Dis 26: 137–139, 1994.
10. Khuroo MS. Study of an epidemic non-A/non-B hepatitis. Possibility of another human hepatitis virus distinct from post-transfusion non-A, non-B type. Am J Med 68: 818–824, 1980.
11. Bradley DW. Enterically-transmitted non-A, non-B hepatitis. Br Med Bull 46: 422–461, 1990.
12. Tsega E, Hansson BG, Nordenfelt E, Krawczinsky K. Acute sporadic viral hepatitis in Ethiopia: causes, risk factors and effects on pregnancy. Clin Infect Dis 14: 961–965, 1992.
13. Purdy MA, Tam AW, Huang C-C, Yarbough PO, Reyes GR. Hepatitis E virus: a non-enveloped member of the "alpha-like" RNA virus supergroup? Semin Virol 4: 319–326, 1993.
14. Favorov MO, Fields HA, Purdy MA, Yashina TL, Aleksandrov AG, Alter MJ, Yarasheva DM, Bradley DW, Margolis HS. Serologic identification of hepatitis E virus infections in epidemic and endemic settings. J Med Virol 36: 246–250, 1992.
15. Goldsmith R, Yaroug PO, Reyes GR, Fry KE, Gabor KA, Kamel M, Zakaria S, Amer S, Gaffar Y. Enzyme-linked immunosorbent assay for diagnosis of acute sporadic hepatitis E in Egyptian children. Lancet 339: 328–331, 1992.
16. Skidmore SJ, Yarbough PO, Gabor KA, Tam AW, Reyes GR. Imported hepatitis E in UK. Lancet 337: 1541, 1991.

Submitted April 21, 1995; accepted September 8, 1995

Scand J Infect Dis 27: 547–550, 1995 ORIGINAL ARTICLE

HTLV Infections Among Swedish Intravenous Drug Users in 1992

SÖREN ANDERSSON[1], AUD KROOK[2], KERSTIN KÄLL[3,4], INGER JULANDER[2], RIGMOR THORSTENSSON[1] and GUNNEL BIBERFELD[1]

From the Departments of [1]Immunology, Swedish Institute for Infectious Disease Control, and [3]Psychiatry, St Göran's Hospital, Stockholm, and [2]Infectious Diseases, Huddinge Hospital, Huddinge and [4]Social Medicine, Kronan Health Institute, Sundbyberg; all at the Karolinska Institute, Stockholm, Sweden

Serum samples collected in 1992 from 1158 intravenous drug users (IVDUs) in Stockholm, Sweden, were tested retrospectively for antibodies to human T-lymphotropic virus type I and II (HTLV-I and II). The overall prevalence rate of HTLV infections was 2.4% (28/1158). A majority of the HTLV infections were caused by HTLV-II (27/28). A significant association between HTLV-II and HIV-1 seropositivity was found, the prevalence of HTLV-II infection being 11.4% (11/96) in HIV-seropositive individuals compared with 1.5% (16/1062) in HIV-seronegative persons ($p < 0.001$). All the HTLV-infected individuals were of Scandinavian origin. No significant differences in age and sex distribution were observed in HTLV-infected persons compared to seronegative individuals. This study confirms that HTLV-II infection is present in the Swedish IVDU population and the findings provide baseline information for future epidemiological studies.

S. Andersson, MD, Department of Immunology, Swedish Institute for Infectious Disease Control, S-105 21 Stockholm, Sweden

INTRODUCTION

Human T-lymphotropic virus type I (HTLV-I) is associated with adult T-cell leukaemia/lymphoma (ATLL), tropic spastic paraparesis (TSP) (1), and possibly with other disease manifestations such as polymyositis (2), uveitis (3) and Sjögren's syndrome (4). The closely related HTLV-II has not unequivocally been connected to any disease or symptoms, although case reports are accumulating that suggest a possible relationship between HTLV-II infection and, for instance a TSP-like disease and leukaemia (5, 6).

HTLV-I is found globally with high endemic foci in south-western Japan, Melanesia/Papua New Guinea, the Caribbean and certain areas of Latin America and Africa (1, 7). The epidemiology of HTLV-II is less well known but HTLV-II infection has been demonstrated among intravenous drug users (IVDUs) in the USA, Spain, Italy, France and Norway (1, 8–11) and in native Indian populations in North and South America (12, 13). Occasional cases of HTLV-II have also been found in Africa (14–16). Recent investigations have revealed the existence of HTLV-II among IVDUs in Sweden also (17, 18). Two subtypes of HTLV-II, HTLV-II_a and -II_b, have been identified, both of which are prevalent among IVDUs in the USA (19).

In order to assess the prevalence rate of HTLV among Swedish IVDUs we carried out a retrospective survey of IVDUs in Stockholm from 1992. The results confirm that HTLV-II infection is prevalent among Swedish IVDUs, with a prevalence rate of 2.3%, whereas HTLV-I is virtually absent.

MATERIAL AND METHODS

Patients and sera

Samples were collected from 2 main sources. The first was specimens sent to the Swedish Institute for Infectious Disease Control for HIV testing, including sera mainly from previously HIV-uninfected or persons not tested for HIV ($n = 1067$). The samples were obtained through a project set up for IVDUs under the auspices of the Departments of Social Medicine and Psychiatry, Karolinska Institute, Stockholm, situated at the remand prison, Stockholm. Samples were also collected at a clinic for IVDUs at Sabbatsbergs Hospital, Stockholm, and a few samples were obtained at various jails outside Stockholm. The second main source was specimens from HIV-infected IVDUs ($n = 91$), obtained at the Department of Infectious Diseases, Huddinge University Hospital, Stockholm.

A total of 1158 frozen serum samples, taken during 1992, from IVDUs in the county of Stockholm were included, constituting nearly 27% of the estimated total number of 4300 IVDUs in the Stockholm area (i.e. the county of Stockholm including the municipality) (20). The specimens were tested retrospectively and anonymously. Data on age, sex and country of origin were obtained.

Serological tests

All samples were screened with an ELISA for HTLV-I/II antibodies, either Diagnostic Biotechnology HTLV-I/II ELISA (Diagnostic Biotechnology, Science Park, Singapore) or Abbott HTLV-I EIA 2.0 (Abbott Laboratories, Diagnostic Division, Wilmington, Illinois, USA). ELISA reactive specimens were tested by a Western blot (WB) assay (Diagnostic Biotechnology HTLV-blot 2.3; Diagnostic Biotechnology, Science Park, Singapore), incorporating recombinant proteins corresponding to parts of gp 21 (common for HTLV-I and -II) and gp 46 (2 separate proteins for discrimination between HTLV-I and HTLV-II). Only samples with at least 2 env-bands, either recombinant or native, and one gag-band were considered as positive. All other samples showing bands on the WB but not fulfilling the criteria for seropositivity were designated as indeterminate.

HIV results were obtained from the records. The majority of the samples had been tested at the Department of Immunology, Swedish Institute for Infectious Disease Control, using ELISA for screening (Behring Enzygnost anti HIV-1/HIV-2; Behringwerke, Marburg, Germany and/or Wellcozyme HIV-1 + 2; Murex Diagnostics, Dartford, UK) and WB for confirmation (Diagnostic Biotechnology HIV-blot 2.2). The samples from Huddinge University Hospital had been HIV tested at the Department of Virology,

Table I. *HTLV seroprevalence in Swedish IVDUs, 1992*

	No. tested	HTLV-I	HTLV-II
HIV-negative	1,062	1 (0.09%)	16 (1.5%)[a]
HIV-positive	96 (8.3%)	0	11 (11.4%)[a]
Total	1,158	1 (0.09%)	27 (2.3%)

[a] For HTLV-II/HIV-positive vs. HTLV-II/HIV-negative, $p < 0.001$.

the Central Microbiology Laboratory of Stockholm County Council with Abbott second generation EIA (Abbott Laboratories) and confirmed with WB as above. The criteria recommended by the WHO with at least two env-bands for seropositivity had been applied (21).

Statistics

The chi-square test with Yates' correction was used for significance testing.

RESULTS

A total of 28 persons (2.4%) with serologically confirmed HTLV infection were found among the 1158 IVDUs tested (Table I). One individual was seropositive for HTLV-I, the rest for HTLV-II (2.3%). The prevalence of HIV infection was 8.3% (96/1158). A significant association between HTLV-II and HIV infection was found: the prevalence of HTLV-II infection was 11.4% among HIV-infected whereas 1.5% of HIV-seronegative persons were HTLV-II seropositive ($p < 0.001$) (Table I). An indeterminate WB pattern was seen in 14/1158 (1.2%) samples.

The mean age of the IVDUs tested was 34.1 years (women 30.4 and men 35.1 years) (Table II). Of the HTLV-II-infected persons, 75% (21/28) were men but the sex-specific prevalence rates did not differ as a majority (78%) of the persons tested were men (Table II). The mean age of the HTLV-II-infected individuals was slightly higher as compared to the HTLV-seronegative persons (Table II). There was no significant difference in age and sex distribution between HIV-1/HTLV-II double infected persons compared to HTLV-II-infected only individuals (data not shown). All the HTLV-I/II-infected individuals were of Swedish or Scandinavian origin.

The HTLV-I-infected person was a 54-year-old HIV-seronegative man.

DISCUSSION

We have performed a retrospective seroepidemiological survey of HTLV infections among IVDUs in Stockholm 1992. The prevalence rate of HTLV-II was 2.3% and a significant association between HIV-1 and HTLV-II infection was observed. Only one HTLV-I seropositive specimen was found.

It is well established that HTLV-II is prevalent among IVDUs in several European countries and the USA. The occurrence of HTLV-II among Swedish IVDUs has also been reported. In a study of a selected group of IVDUs, treated at the Roslagstull Infectious Diseases Hospital in Stockholm during 1990–1992, 10 out of 134 individuals (7.5%) were HTLV-II seropositive (18). The HTLV-II seroprevalence rate in samples from HIV-infected individuals was 15.6% and among HIV-negative samples it was 3.4% (the HIV seroprevalence was 33.6% or 45/134). The higher overall prevalences found in the previous study, compared to the findings presented here, are probably due to differences in sample selection. The difference in HTLV prevalence between HIV-infected persons in the previous study (18) and our study is not significant. Our study has also confirmed that previously HIV-uninfected or not HIV-tested IVDUs in a group mainly outside the hospital environment carry HTLV, albeit at a significantly lower prevalence rate. The findings mark the importance of how the material in seroepidemiological studies is selected.

The HIV seroprevalence in our material was 8.3%. According to available statistics at the Department of Epidemiology, Swedish Institute for Infectious Disease Control, the Division of Infectious Diseases Epidemiology at the Stockholm County Council and surveys carried out in the IVDU project at the remand prison (22), the figure corresponds well with the estimated HIV prevalence rate in the whole group of IVDUs. The HIV prevalence among IVDUs known to the Social Welfare Committees in the municipality of Stockholm was 14% in 1992 (23). This excludes the rest of the county of Stockholm where the HIV prevalence is considered to be lower.

In a previous study including 100 serum samples of IVDUs from Stockholm collected in 1988–1989, no case of HTLV infection was found (24). If not caused by a sampling bias it indicates that HTLV-II was uncommon in the Swedish IVDU population before 1989. In order to further

Table II. *Age and sex distribution of Swedish IVDUs tested for HTLV-infection*

	Tested			HTLV-II-positive		
	n	%	Mean age (range), years	*n*	%	Mean age (range), years
Women	228	(19.7)	30.4 (17–61)	5	(2.2)	33.2 (28–37)
Men	903	(78.0)	35.1 (17–61)	21	(2.3)	39.6 (29–50)
Not known	27	(2.3)	32.0 (20–61)	1	(3.7)	40.0
Total	1,158		34.1 (17–61)	27	(2.3)	38.3 (28–50)

characterize the epidemic of HTLV-II among Swedish IVDUs a prospective study has been started during 1994. The study will address issues regarding epidemiological correlates, the origin of the epidemic, virus subtypes involved and possible clinical manifestations.

In HTLV-I endemic areas the prevalence rates are usually higher in women and increase with age (25). Although the HTLV-infected persons were slightly older than the seronegative individuals there was no significant age and sex trend in our study. In HTLV-I-endemic areas the majority of HTLV carriers have been infected through the heterosexual route or in early childhood by vertical transmission. Apart from possible differences in transmission dynamics for HTLV-II, it can be assumed that the transmission pattern among IVDUs is different and, thus, the age- and sex-specific prevalence rates will differ, compared to what is observed in general populations in endemic areas.

The reasons for the comparatively high prevalence rates of HTLV-II and not HTLV-I among IVDUs, shown in several countries, are not well understood. This may only reflect that HTLV-II was introduced before HTLV-I in certain areas and population groups. It can also be speculated that HTLV-II has a higher transmission rate than HTLV-I through the intravenous route. It may be noted that in IVDUs in the USA both subtypes of HTLV-II (HTLV-II_a and -II_b) are prevalent as well as HTLV-I (6, 19). Further research is needed in order to clarify the reasons for the differences in the distribution of the HTLVs in various population groups.

In conclusion, this study has confirmed the existence of HTLV-II among IVDUs in Stockholm. In contrast, HTLV-I seems to be rare. The data provide baseline information for future epidemiological studies.

ACKNOWLEDGEMENTS

We thank associate professor Anders Sönnerborg, the Department of Virology, the Central Microbiology Laboratory of Stockholm County Council, for providing some of the HIV results; Dr Ulla Pettersson, Sabbatsbergs hospital for providing specimens and Elizabeth Ericsson-Ståhle and Helen Linder for skilful technical assistance.

REFERENCES

1. Centers for Disease Control. Position paper. Recommendations for counselling persons infected with human T-lymphotropic virus, type I and II. Ann Intern Med 6: 448–454, 1993.
2. Morgan OS, Rogers-Johnson P, Mora C, Char G. HTLV-I and polymyositis in Jamaica. Lancet 2: 1184–1187, 1989.
3. Mochizuki M, Watanabe T, Yamaguchi K, Takatsuki K, Yoshimura K, Shirao M, Nakashima S, Mori S, Araki S, Miyata N. HTLV-I uveitis: a distinct clinical entity caused by HTLV-I. Jpn J Cancer Res 83: 236–239, 1992.
4. Terada K, Katamine S, Eguchi K, Moriuchi R, Kita M, Shimada H, Yamashita I, Iwata K, Tsuji Y, Nagataki S, Miyamoto T. Prevalence of serum and salivary antibodies to HTLV-1 in Sjögren's syndrome. Lancet 344: 1116–1119, 1994.
5. Murphy EL. HTLV-II related disease. Lancet 341: 888, 1993.
6. Weiss SH. The evolving epidemiology of human T lymphotropic virus type II. J Infect Dis 169: 1080–1083, 1994.
7. World Health Organization. Virus diseases – human T-cell lymphotropic virus-1 (HTLV-1). Wkly Epidemiol Rec 67: 213–217, 1992.
8. Soriano V, Calderon E, Esparza B, Cilla G, Aguilera A, Gutierrez M, Tor J, Pujol E, Merino F, Perez-Trallero E, Leal M, Gonzalez-Lahoz J. HTLV-I/II infections in Spain. Int J Epidemiol 22: 716–719, 1993.
9. Zella D, Mori L, Sala M. HTLV-II infection in Italian drug abusers. Lancet 2: 575–576, 1990.
10. Vignoli C, Zandotti C, De Lamballerie X, Tamalet C, Gastaut JA, De Micco P. Prevalence of HTLV-II in HIV-1 infected drug addicts in Marseille. Eur J Epidemiol 9: 351–352, 1993.
11. Flø RW, Holm Samdal H, Kalland K-H, The Oslo HIV Cohort Study Group, Nielsen A, Haukenes G. Diagnosis of infection with human T-lymphotropic virus type II (HTLV-II) in Norwegian HIV infected individuals. Clin Diagn Virol 1: 143–152, 1993.
12. Levine PH, Jacobson S, Elliott R, Cavallero A, Colclough G, Dorry C, Stephson C, Knigge RM, Drummond J, Nishimura M, Taylor ME, Wiktor S, Shaw GM. HTLV-II infections in Florida Indians. AIDS Res Hum Retroviruses 9: 123–127, 1993.
13. Fujiyama C, Fujiyoshi T, Miura T, Yashiki S, Matsumoto D, Zaninovic V, Blanco O, Harrington Jr W, Byrnes JJ, Hayami M, Tajima K, Sonoda S. A new endemic focus of human T lymphotropic virus type II carriers among Orinoco natives in Colombia. J Infect Dis 168: 1075–1077, 1993.
14. Delaporte E, Louwagie J, Peeters M, Montplaisir N, d'Auriol L, Ville Y, Bedjabaga L, Larouze B, Van der Groen G, Piot P. Evidence of HTLV-II infection in Central Africa. AIDS 5: 771–772, 1991.
15. Igarashi T, Yamashita M, Miura T, Osei-Kwasi M, Aysi NK, Shiraki H, Kurimura T, Hayami M. Isolation and genomic analysis of human T lymphotropic virus type II from Ghana. AIDS Res Hum Retroviruses 9: 1039–1042, 1993.
16. Gessain A, Tuppin P, Kazanji M, Cosnefroy J-Y, Georges-Courbot M-C, Georges AJ, de Thé G. A distinct molecular variant of HTLV-IIB in Gabon, Central Africa. AIDS Res Hum Retroviruses 10: 753–755, 1994.
17. Andersson S, Biberfeld G, Thorstensson R, Linglöf T. HTLV-II upptäckt bland intravenösa missbrukare i Sverige. Epid-aktuellt, Smittskyddsinstitutet 10: 3, 1993. [In Swedish]
18. Krook A, Blomberg J. HTLV-II among injecting drug users in Stockholm. Scand J Infect Dis 26: 129–132, 1994.
19. Hall WW, Takahashi H, Liu C, Kaplan MH, Scheewind O, Ijichi S, Nagashima K, Gallo RC. Multiple isolates and characteristics of human T-cell leukemia virus type II. J Virol 66: 2456–2463, 1992.
20. Olsson O, Byqvist S, Gomér G. Det tunga narkotikamissbrukets omfattning i Stockholms län 1992. Centralförbundet för alkohol- och narkotikaupplysning (CAN), Stockholm, 1993. [In Swedish]
21. World Health Organization Global Programme on AIDS. Proposed WHO criteria for interpretation of results from Western blot assay for HIV-1, HIV-2 and HTLV-I/HTLV-II. Wkly Epidemiol Rec 37: 281–283, 1990.
22. Käll K, Olin R. Unchanged annual incidence of HIV infection among iv drug abusers; five-year follow-up among drug abusers at the remand prison in Stockholm. Läkartidningen 89: 2837–2840, 1992. [In Swedish with summary in English]

23. Ågren G, Anderzon K, Berglund E, Dundar A. Narkotika i Stockholm. Socialtjänsten i Stockholm, FoU-byrån, 1993. [In Swedish]
24. Blomberg J, Moestrup T, Frimand J, Hansson B-G, Krogsgaard K, Grillner L, Nordenfelt E. HTLV-I and -II in intravenous drug users from Sweden and Denmark. Scand J Infect Dis 26: 23–26, 1994.
25. Blattner WA. Epidemiology of HTLV-I and associated diseases. In: Blattner WA, ed. Human retrovirology: HTLV. New York: Raven Press, 251–265, 1990.

Submitted March 8, 1995; accepted August 18, 1995

Scand J Infect Dis 27: 551–557, 1995

ORIGINAL ARTICLE

Parvovirus B19 Infection – Persistence and Genetic Variation

JONATHAN R. KERR[1], MARTIN D. CURRAN[2], JOHN E. MOORE[1] and PHILIP G. MURPHY[1]

From the Departments of [1]Bacteriology and [2]Tissue Typing, Belfast City Hospital, Lisburn Road, Belfast, Northern Ireland

53 patients with acute B19 infection were studied; symptoms at acute infection were rash and arthralgia ($n = 26$), rash ($n = 7$), arthralgia ($n = 16$), aplastic crisis ($n = 3$), and intrauterine fetal death ($n = 1$). These patients were followed for 26–85 months (mean 57 months) and re-assessed for persistent symptoms, anti-B19 antibodies, and B19 DNA. At follow-up, 7 individuals were positive for serum B19 DNA, compared with none of the controls (2-tailed p value = 0.016). All 7 of those persistently infected were women, 3 of whom had symptoms; 1 had a chronic haemolytic anaemia (initial presentation was aplastic crisis); 1 had persistent arthralgia in both knees (initial presentation was bilateral knee arthralgia); and 1 had arthralgia in one knee and chronic fatigue syndrome (initial presentation was bilateral arthralgia in knees and shoulders). For the 7 persistently infected patients, serum from the time of diagnosis of acute B19 infection was available for 4, all of which contained B19 DNA. With single-stranded conformational polymorphism (SSCP) assay of these 11 PCR products, identical SSCP types were demonstrated in 5 of 7 follow-up isolates. In 2 of the 4 cases for which both acute and follow-up PCR product was available, the SSCP type of the follow-up product was different from that of the acute product. Two B19 virus types were demonstrated in one patient (with persistent arthralgia and chronic fatigue syndrome) at follow-up assessment.

J. Kerr, MD, Bacteriology, Belfast City Hospital, Lisburn Road, Belfast BT9 7AB, Northern Ireland

INTRODUCTION

Human Parvovirus B19 is the aetiologic agent of erythema infectiosum (EI) and transient aplastic crisis (TAC) in patients with haemolytic anaemia, and has been associated with fetal death, acute and chronic arthritis, chronic anaemia in immunocompromised patients, congenital red cell aplasia and vasculitis syndromes (1). Persistent B19 infection has been associated with a lack of humoral responsiveness to the unique region of B19 viral protein 1 (VP1), occurs in various groups of immunocompromised patients including congenital immunodeficiency syndromes, AIDS, lymproliferative disorders, and transplant patients, and is manifested as pure red cell aplasia (PRCA) (2). Persistent B19 infection has also been reported in patients in which no immune defect has been demonstrated. In the present study, we assessed the incidence of persistent B19 infection in 53 patients without a known immune defect.

MATERIALS AND METHODS

Test patients

53 patients testing positive for serum anti-B19 IgM between 1987 and 1992 were studied. The definition of a case of B19 infection was a positive test for serum anti-B19 IgM. Each of these 53 patients was re-assessed in August 1994. The period of follow-up ranged from 26–85 months with a mean of 57 months (**Test sera**). Of the 53 patients for whom follow-up assessment was successful, serum samples from the time of initial B19 infection was available for 33 (**Presentation sera**).

Control patients

A control group was included as a comparison for both the serum anti-B19 IgG and serum B19 DNA results of the Test patients. 53 sera from 53 age- (to within 3 years) and sex-matched control patients were tested; these were patients whose sera tested negative for serological evidence of one of a variety of viral and bacterial diseases, and whose symptoms did not include rash or arthralgia (**Control sera**).

IgM capture Radioimmunoassay (MACRIA)

From January 1987 to June 1989, serum anti-B19 IgM was routinely detected in serum at initial B19 infection at the Regional Virus Laboratory by MACRIA, provided by Dr Bernard Cohen, Central Public Health Laboratory, Colindale, London (3).

IgM capture Enzymeimmunoassay (MACEIA)

From July 1989 to 1992, serum anti-B19 IgM was routinely detected in serum at initial B19 infection at the Regional virus Laboratory by MACEIA (4).

Serum anti-B19 fluorescent antibody test (FAT)

SF9 insect cells infected with recombinant Autographica California Nuclear Polyhedrosis Virus containing a plasmid encoding the B19 VP1 nucleotide sequence were used to prepare immunofluorescence slides (5). For IgG determination, 25 µl of a 1 : 50 dilution of each serum, was added to immunofluorescence slide wells and incubated for 30 min at 37°C in a humidified chamber. After washing in PBS, 25 µl of goat anti-human IgG FITC conjugate (Sigma) at its working dilution of 1 : 30 in PBS was applied for 30 min at 37°C. After a further wash in PBS, the slides were mounted and viewed using a fluorescence microscope (Zeiss). Results were recorded in a semi-quantitative fashion depending on intensity of fluorescence as follows; trace (+/−), present (+), strong (++), very strong (+++).

For IgM determination, serum was diluted 1 : 10 in GullSORB (Gull Laboratories, Utah, USA) and allowed to stand at room temperature for 15 min, to precipitate competing specific IgG and rheumatoid factor (RF). 20 µl of this was then added to immunofluorescence slide wells. From this point, the test was conducted as above, except that the conjugate used was goat anti-human IgM FITC (Sigma) at its working dilution of 1 : 50 in PBS. For each test run, known negative and positive serum controls were included.

 ISSN 0036-5548

PCR assay

DNA was obtained from serum by phenol/chloroform extraction (6). A newly developed nested PCR assay was employed (7). In the first reaction, primers P11 and P66, corresponding to nucleotides 1355–1374 and 1703–1723, respectively, of B19 genomic DNA (8), were used for 35 cycles to amplify a 369bp fragment. Extracted DNA (10 µl) was added to the PCR mixture containing 10 mM Tris (pH 8.3); 2.0 mM $MgCl_2$; 50 mM KCl; 200 µM each dATP, dCTP, dGTP, dTTP; 0.5 µM (each) oligonucleotide primer and 2.5 U of Taq polymerase (Perkin-Elmer-Cetus, Norwalk, CT, USA) in a total volume of 100 µl. Amplifications were carried out on a thermal cycler (Gene Amp PCR 9600 System, Perkin-Elmer-Cetus, Norwalk, CT, USA) for 35 cycles of 94°C (45 s); 55°C (60 s); 72°C (60 s). In the second amplification, 1 µl of PCR product was added to reaction mixture (above) containing primers P1 and P6 for a further 25 cycles. Primers P1 and P6, correspond to nucleotides 1399–1422 and 1659–1682, respectively, of B19 genomic DNA, and amplify a 284-bp fragment. Amplified product was electrophoresed on 1.4% (w/v) agarose (Metaphor, FMC, USA) incorporating ethidium bromide, and examined under UV light.

Assay of the sensitivity of the PCR assay

To assay the sensitivity of the PCR reaction, viraemic serum from an asymptomatic blood donor was used. The titre of B19 virus in this serum had previously been estimated by EM to contain 10^{11} virus particles per ml (4). Fourteen 10-fold dilutions of viraemic serum were made in sterile distilled water and the DNA from each of these, including the neat serum, was extracted. These DNAs were then subjected to nested PCR assay as above.

SSCP assay

2 µl of PCR product was mixed with 11 µl deionised formamide dye including 1 mM EDTA and 0.25% bromophenol blue dye, heated to 90°C for 2–3 min. and immediately transferred to ice. The mixture was applied to a Mutation Detection Enhancement acrylamide gel (20 × 40 × 0.4 cm) (AT Biochem, Malvern, PA, USA) in a well of 10 mm width and subjected to electrophoresis in 90 mM Tris-borate, pH 8.3/4 mM EDTA at a constant power of 20 W for 5 h at 23°C in a Sequi-Gen, vertical gel electrophoresis apparatus (Bio-Rad). After electrophoresis, the glass plates were separated using a plastic wedge; the gel remained strongly attached to the short glass plate due to pre-treatment with binding solution. The gel was then stained by a silver staining technique (Promega Corporation, Madison, WI, USA) while still attached to the glass plate and viewed on a light box.

Statistics

Results were examined for significance using McNemar's test.

RESULTS

Clinical aspects

Of the 53 patients, the female to male ratio was 7.5 : 1. The patients ages ranged from 5–49 years with a mean of 31 years. 12 patients were managed in hospital while 41 patients were managed in the community. The period of follow-up ranged from 26–85 months with a mean of 57 months. Table I shows the clinical information on this group of 53 patients; symptoms of acute B19 infection, joints affected by arthralgia if present, duration of symptoms from the time of acute B19 infection, all symptoms present during the follow-up period, and joints affected by arthralgia if present during the follow-up period.

Symptoms at the time of acute B19 infection were rash and arthralgia ($n = 26$), rash ($n = 7$), arthralgia ($n = 16$), TAC ($n = 3$), and intrauterine death ($n = 1$). One patient with rash and arthralgia had a history of hereditary spherocytosis but did not suffer TAC. One and 2 patients with arthralgia also had lymphadenopathy and localised muscle weakness, respectively. There were a total of 42 patients with arthralgia. Particular joints affected were the fingers, wrists, elbows, shoulders, hips, knees, and ankles. Of patients with arthralgia ($n = 42$), the knee was affected in 39 cases; in 24 cases it was the only joint affected. Five patients had generalised arthralgia, involving more than 5 of the above joints. In all cases of acute B19 infection, the arthralgia affected joints in a symmetrical pattern.

At the follow-up assessment, the total duration of clinical symptoms after the initial acute B19 infection was determined. Of the 7 patients whose acute symptoms consisted of rash alone, all showed disease resolution within 1 month; none had relapsed by the time of follow-up. Of the 42 patients with arthralgia (with or without rash), 19 cases had symptoms which resolved within 1 month and the remaining 23 cases had symptoms persisting for longer. Of these 23 with persistent arthralgia, in 3 cases the symptoms had resolved within 1 year and in 20 cases symptoms persisted for 4–7 years; in 11 of these, symptoms were present constantly; in the remaining 9 cases, symptoms were intermittent. The pattern of joint involvement at the time of follow-up in those patients with persistent arthralgia tended to be different from that at the time of initial presentation. However, in all patients with persistent arthralgia, arthralgia was part of the initial presentation. In 2 cases with persistent arthralgia for >1 year, a rash was also present with the arthralgia (patient numbers 12 and 17). Patient number 48, who had persistent arthralgia for more than 1 year in her knees, elbows and shoulders, had been diagnosed as having rheumatoid arthritis and was attending a rheumatology clinic. This patient had no symptoms prior to B19 infection.

In 2 cases with persistent arthralgia, chronic fatigue was also present (patient numbers 27 and 51); this was marked in both cases. In patient number 51, a 22-year-old girl at university (at follow-up), the clinical impact of this was that she could no longer play energetic sport (due to both general tiredness and pain in her knee and shoulder), stay up late at night, or study for more than 1 h at a time (due to poor concentration); this was a significant change for her as she had remarkable energy prior to acute B19 infection in March 1989. In patient number 27, a 49-year-old professional man (at follow-up), long-standing extreme tiredness necessitated early retirement and loss of a successful business. This man subsequently became clinically depressed.

Three patients had TAC at acute B19 infection. Of these, 2 were asymptomatic at follow-up and one (patient 50) had a chronic undiagnosed haemolytic anaemia which necessitated occasional blood transfusion.

Table I. *Symptoms in 53 B19-infected persons at onset of infection and at follow-up assessment*

Patient number	Symptoms at onset[a]	Joints affected at onset[b]	Duration of symptoms[c] (months)	Symptoms at follow-up[a]	Joints affected at follow-up[b]
1	R. A	FWE	<1	–	–
2	R, A	Gen	64; i	A	H (R)
3	R, A	FK	6	–	–
4	R, A	S	85; i	A	S (R)
5	AC, HS	–	<1	–	–
6	R, A	K	<1	–	–
7	R, A	K	<1	–	–
8	R, A	Gen	<1	–	–
9	R, A	Gen	64; i	A	K (R)
10	R, A	KES	60	A	KES
11	A	K	<1	–	–
12	R, A	Gen	67	R, A	Gen
13	R	–	<1	–	–
14	R	–	<1	–	–
15	R, A	KF	63; i	A	KF
16	A	K	<1	–	–
17	R, A	K	60; i	R, A	Gen
18	R, A	Gen	59	A	Gen
19	A	KAF	73; i	A	KAF
20	R, A	K	<1	–	–
21	IUD	–	–	–	–
22	A	K	47	A	KF
23	A, W	K	4	–	–
24	R	–	<1	–	–
25	A	KW	3	–	–
26	R, A	K	<1	–	–
27	A, W	FTHK	51	A, CF	FTH
28	AC, HS	–	<1	–	–
29	R, A, HS	K	<1	–	–
30	R, A	K	<1	–	–
31	R, A	KF	48; i	A	F
32	R, A	KAF	<1	–	–
33	R, A	K	<1	–	–
34	R, A	KAF	66	A	F
35	R	–	<1	–	–
36	R	–	<1	–	–
37	R, A	K	<1	–	–
38	A	K	61	A	K
39	A	K	<1	–	–
40	A	K	61	A	K
41	R	–	<1	–	–
42	A	KAF	59	A	KAF
43	R, A	K	<1	–	–
44	R, A	K	52; i	A	KWF
45	R, A	K	<1	–	–
46	R	–	<1	–	–
47	A	K	<1	–	–
48	A	K	48; i	A	KES (ra)
49	A	K	<1	–	–
50	AC	–	26	CHA	–
51	A	KS	65	A, CF	KS
52	R, A	K	<1	–	–
53	A, L	S	51	A	S (R)

[a] R = rash; A = arthralgia; AC = aplastic crisis; HS = hereditary spherocytosis; IUD = intra-uterine death; W = localised muscle weakness; CHA = Chronic haemolytic anaemia; L = lymphadenopathy; CF = chronic fatigue.

[b] F = fingers; W = wrists; E = elbows; K = knees; S = shoulders; A = ankles; H = hips; Gen = generalised polyarthropathy; R = right side; ps = diagnosed and treated as psoriasis; ra = diagnosed and treated as rheumatoid arthritis.

[c] i = intermittent symptoms.

Table II. *Results of serum testing for anti-B19 IgG and B19 DNA in 53 B19-infected patients at onset and at follow-up*

Patient number	Onset interval[a] (days)	B19 DNA at onset	Follow-up interval (months)	B19 DNA at follow-up	IgG at follow-up
1	11	−	66	−	+
2	–	+	64	−	+/−
3	6	+	50	−	++
4	7	−	85	−	+
5	–	+	70	−	+
6	–	−	64	−	++
7	–	+	64	−	++
8	4	NT	64	−	++
9	–	+	64	−	+++
10	10	NT	60	−	+
11	–	NT	67	−	+
12	–	NT	67	−	+
13	–	+	64	−	++
14	20	+	63	−	+/−
15	–	+	63	−	+
16	7	−	65	−	+
17	–	NT	60	−	+
18	30	+	59	−	+++
19	4	NT	73	−	+
20	2	+	55	−	+
21	–	+	50	−	+
22	14	+	47	−	++
23	24	+	61	−	++
24	5	NT	55	+	+/−
25	–	NT	53	−	+
26	–	NT	53	−	+
27	16	+	51	−	+
28	9	+	51	−	++
29	–	NT	50	−	+
30	5	NT	49	−	+
31	10	+	48	−	+
32	–	+	47	−	+
33	16	NT	42	−	+
34	43	+	66	−	++
35	1	NT	29	−	+
36	2	+	63	−	++
37	3	NT	62	−	++
38	36	NT	61	−	+
39	60	+	61	+	+/−
40	–	+	61	+	++
41	6	+	60	+	++
42	2	+	59	−	++
43	–	+	52	−	+
44	13	+	52	−	++
45	–	NT	52	−	+
46	7	NT	50	+	+
47	20	NT	49	−	+
48	–	NT	48	−	+++
49	1	+	29	−	++
50	–	+	26	+	+
51	–	NT	65	+	+
52	15	+	63	−	+/−
53	23	+	51	−	+/−

[a] Interval between symptom onset and serum sampling.
NT = not tested.

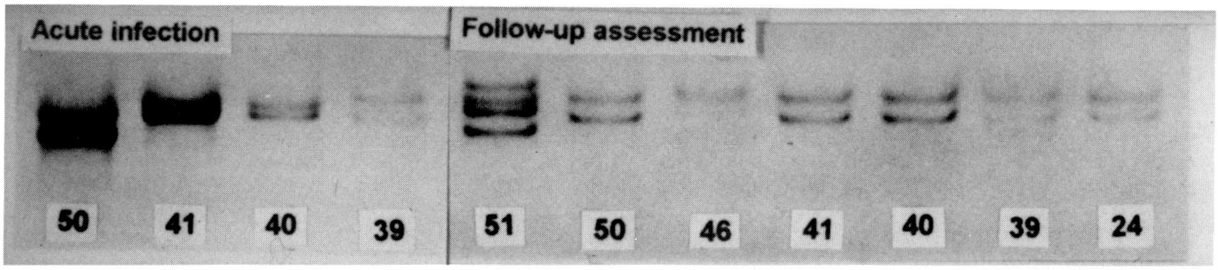

Fig. 1. SSCP analysis of PCR products from the serum of 7 patients with persistent B19 infection. Each specimen showed double-stranded DNA of 284 bp (nt 1399 to nt 1682) on conventional agarose gel electrophoresis. PCR products were denatured at 90°C in formamide and subjected to electrophoresis in a Mutation Detection Enhancement acrylamide gel (AT Biochem) in 90 mM Tris-borate, pH 8.3/4 mM EDTA at a constant power of 20 W for 5 h at 23°C in a vertical gel electrophoresis apparatus (Bio-Rad). The gel was stained by a silver staining method (Promega), and viewed and photographed on a light box.

Serum anti-B19 antibody testing

Among the Test patients, in 32 cases the interval between symptom onset at presentation and the date of blood sampling was known; this ranged from 1–60 days with a mean of 13.5 days (Table II). All 53 patients were serum anti-B19 IgM (MACRIA or MACEIA) positive at initial B19 infection (the sole criterion used to diagnose acute B19 infection). Of 33 Presentation sera, 32 were tested for anti-B19 IgG (FAT). In 29 of these this test was positive; in the 3 cases in which serum at presentation was anti-B19 IgG negative, the interval between onset of symptoms and serum sampling was only 1–2 days. All Test and Control sera were negative for anti-B19 IgM. All 53 Test Sera were positive for anti-B19 IgG (Table II) compared with 45 of 53 Control sera; a significant difference (2-tailed p value = 0.008).

PCR

Results of PCR for serum B19 DNA are shown in Table II. 29 of 33 Presentation sera (B19-infected patients at presentation) were positive for B19 DNA. Of the Test sera (B19-infected patients at follow-up), 7 were positive for B19 DNA, compared with none of 53 age and sex-matched control patients; a significant difference (2-tailed p value = 0.016). All 7 patients with persistent infection were women. Patients 24, 41 and 46 presented at ages 10, 54 and 22 years, respectively, with self-limiting erthyema infectiosum and were asymptomatic at follow-up. Patient 39 presented at age 49 with self-limiting arthralgia in both knees and was asymptomatic at follow-up. Patient 40 presented at age 29 with arthralgia in both knees which persisted until follow-up. Patient 50 presented at age 29 with aplastic crisis, which resolved but subsequently developed an undiagnosed persistent mild haemolytic anaemia present throughout the follow-up period. Patient 51 presented at age 17 with arthralgia in both knees and shoulders which persisted in one knee and one shoulder; chronic fatigue was also present throughout the follow-up period.

Single-stranded conformational polymorphism (SSCP) assay

For the 7 persistently infected patients, serum from the time of diagnosis of acute B19 infection was available for 4, all of which contained B19 DNA. With SSCP assay of these 11 PCR products (shown in Fig. 1), identical SSCP types were observed in 5 of 7 follow-up isolates. In 2 of the 4 cases for which both acute and follow-up PCR product was available, the SSCP type of the follow-up product was different from that of the acute product. In addition, SSCP demonstrated 2 B19 virus types co-existing in patient number 51 at follow-up assessment.

DISCUSSION

Viraemic serum, estimated to contain 10^{11} viral particles/ml by electron microscopy (4), was used to assess the sensitivity of the PCR assay. As viraemic serum in the acute stage of infection has been reported to contain a titre of approximately 10^{11}–10^{14} viral particles per ml (9, 10), and the present PCR assay detected viral genome to a dilution of 10^{-13}, the sensitivity of the PCR was of the order of 10–100 particles per ml. This level of sensitivity is similar to that in other PCR assays for B19 genome detection (11, 12).

Electrophoretic mobility of a DNA molecule in a gel is sensitive to both its size and shape. In non-denaturing conditions, single-stranded DNA has a folded structure that is determined by intramolecular interactions and, therefore, by its sequence. In SSCP analysis, a mutated sequence is detected as a change of mobility in polyacrylamide gel electrophoresis caused by its altered folded structure. It may seem that only a limited number of sequence changes can cause a detectable structural change of the molecule. However, it has been found that because of its high resolving power, polyacrylamide gel electrophoresis can distinguish most conformational changes caused by subtle sequence differences such as one base substitution in a several hundred base fragment (13). A previous study of

50 parvovirus strains confirmed the sensitivity of the method, in which no nucleotide substitutions were detected that did not affect electrophoretic mobility (7).

In 2 of the 4 cases for which both acute and follow-up PCR product was available, the SSCP type of the follow-up product was different from that of the acute product. In 5 of 7 B19 isolates detected at follow-up assessment, the SSCP type was identical; this would seem to suggest an advantage to the virus of this particular type. Regarding the particular region studied, we observed 2 B19 DNA types co-existing in one patient (patient number 51; Fig. 1). This is a phenomenon which has not so far been demonstrated for B19, however, nucleotide sequence analysis of Aleutian mink disease parvovirus shows that multiple virus types are present in infected minks (14). SSCP analysis, by virtue of its ability to separate different single-stranded conformational types (which may differ from each other by only a single base mutation), may be used to screen for the presence of more than one species within a PCR product population, which appears as a single molecular weight band on conventional agarose gel electrophoresis. It is noteworthy that this phenomenon occured in a follow-up specimen of serum and not an acute sample, either in the present study or previously (7). Despite persistent B19 infection in 7 patients at follow-up, these persons were serum anti-B19 IgM negative; we are unable to explain this, however, this phenomenon has previously been documented in persistent B19 infection in AIDS patients (15).

This group of 53 B19-infected patients was generated by requests for serological virus diagnosis in patients in whom symptoms were severe enough for medical consultation, a request for serological virus diagnosis, and hospital management in some cases (23%) and does not therefore represent a typical group of B19-infected persons. This is reflected in the mean age in these patients of 31 years, and a high female : male ratio of 7.5 : 1. B19 infection most commonly occurs in children, and is thought to occur with equal frequency in male and female. The high female : male ratio seen in these patients at follow-up probably reflects the high incidence of arthralgia at onset of B19 infection in this group (79%), as B19 arthralgia is more common in women (16). The severity and high incidence of disease (38%) and B19 persistence (13.2%) at follow-up may be related to the severity of acute illness in this group, a finding that is in contrast with the accepted sequence of events following acute parvovirus B19 infection in immunocompetent individuals; a short incubation, viraemia, bone marrow infection, development of specific antibody, and viral clearance (17, 18). These persons may not, therefore, be immunocompetent.

One patient at follow-up fulfilled the American Rheumatism Association (ARA) criteria for a diagnosis of RA (19). Although B19 is known to cause chronic arthropathy (20), its role in the aetiology of RA is doubtful (12, 21). In view of 2 B19 virus types co-existing in a 22-year-old girl (patient 51) with chronic fatigue syndrome and persistent arthralgia, the pathogenetic role of B19 in chronic fatigue syndrome merits further investigation.

B19 non-structural protein is required for replication (22) and DNA sequence changes in this region may possibly modify viral replication and allow persistent infection. Sequence analysis is in progress to determine the nature and relevance of the substitutions detected. In conclusion, B19 persistence may be more common than was previously thought; the 13.2% incidence of serum PCR positivity demonstrated in the present study at follow-up assessment challenges presently held views of B19 persistence and, if confirmed in other studies, will lead to a new understanding of how this virus might cause chronic disease. Perhaps because of the limited number of epitopes presented by the limited B19 genome (5.6 kb) to the immune system, the congenital immunodeficiency states associated with persistent infection may be clinically subtle with susceptibility largely restricted to parvovirus B19, and possibly also relatively common.

ACKNOWLEDGEMENTS

The authors thank Dr PV Coyle, Regional Virus Laboratory, Royal Victoria Hospital, Belfast, for serum anti-B19 serological testing and positive control serum for PCR, and Dr CC Patterson, Department of Medical Statistics, Royal Victoria Hospital, Belfast, for statistical advice.

REFERENCES

1. Brown KE, Young NS, Liu JM. Molecular, cellular and clinical aspects of parvovirus B19 infection. Crit Rev Oncol Hematol 16: 1–31, 1994.
2. Kurtzman GJ, Cohen BJ, Field AM, Oseas R, Blease RM, Young NS. Immune response to B19 parvovirus and an antibody defect in persistent viral infection. J Clin Invest 84: 1114–1123, 1989.
3. Cohen BJ, Mortimer PP, Pereira MS. Diagnostic assays with monoclonal antibodies for the human serum parvovirus-like virus (SPLV). J Hyg Camb 91: 113–130, 1983.
4. O'Neill HJ, Coyle PV. Two anti-parvovirus B19 IgM capture assays incorporating a mouse monoclonal antibody specific for B19 viral capsid proteins VP1 and VP2. Arch Virol 123: 125–134, 1992.
5. Kerr JR, O'Neill HJ, Deleys R, Wright C, Coyle PV. Design and production of a target-specific monoclonal antibody to parvovirus B19 capsid proteins. J Immunol Meth 180: 101–106, 1995.
6. Sambrook J, Maniatis T, Fritsch EF. Molecular cloning: A laboratory manual 2nd edn. New York: Cold Spring Harbor Laboratory, 1989.
7. Kerr JR, Curran MD, Moore JE, Erdman DD, Coyle PV, Nunoue T, Middleton D, Ferguson WP. Genetic diversity in the non-structural gene of parvovirus B19 detected by single-stranded conformational polymorphism assay (SSCP) and partial nucleotide sequencing. J Virol Meth 53: 213–222, 1995.
8. Shade RO, Blundell MC, Cotmore SF, Tattersall P, Astell CR. Nucleotide sequence and genome organisation of human parvovirus B19 isolated from the serum of a child aplastic crisis. J Virol 58: 921–936, 1986.
9. Anderson MJ, Davies LR, Hodgson J, et al. Occurrence of infection with a parvovirus-like agent in children with sickle

cell anaemia during a two-year period. J Clin Pathol 35: 744–749, 1982.
10. Clewley JP. Detection of human parvovirus using a molecularly cloned probe. J Med Virol 15: 173–181, 1985.
11. Saal JG, Steidle M, Einsele H, Muller CA, Fritz P, Zacher J. Persistence of B19 parvovirus in synovial membranes of patients with rheumatoid arthritis. Rheumatol Int 12: 147–151, 1992.
12. Nikkari S, Luukkainen R, Mottonen T, Meurman O, Hannonen P, Skurnik M, Toivanen P. Does parvovirus B19 have a role in rheumatoid arthritis? Ann Rheum Dis 53: 106–111, 1994.
13. Hayashi K. PCR-SSCP: A simple and sensitive method for detection of mutations in the genomic DNA. PCR Methods Appl 1: 34–38, 1991.
14. Gottschalck E, Alexandersen S, Cohen A, Poulsen LA, Bloom ME, Aasted B. Nucleotide sequence analysis of aleutian mink disease parvovirus shows that multiple virus types are present in infected mink. J Virol 65: 4378–4386, 1991.
15. Naides SJ, Howard EJ, Swack NS, True CA, Stapleton JT. Parvovirus B19 infection in human immunodeficiency virus type-1-infected persons failing or intolerant to zidovuding therapy. J Infect Dis 168: 101–105, 1993.
16. Woolf AD, Campion GV, Chishick A, Wise S, Cohen BJ, Klouda PT, Caul O, Dieppe PA. Clinical manifestations of human parvovirus B19 in adults. Arch Intern Med 149: 1153–1156, 1989.
17. Anderson MJ, Higgins PG, Davis LR, William JS, Jones SE, Kidd IM, Pattison JR, Tyrell DAJ. Experimental parvoviral infection in humans. J Infect Dis 152: 257–265, 1985.
18. Potter CG, Potter AC, Hatton CSR, Chapel HM, Anderson MJ, Pattison JR, Tyrrell DAJ, Higgins PG, Willman JS, Parry HF, Cotes PM. Variation of erythroid and myeloid precursors in the marrow and peripheral blood of volunteer subjects infected with human parvovirus (B19). J Clin Invest 79: 1486–1492, 1987.
19. Arnett FC, Edworthy SM, Bloch DA, McShane DJ, Fries JF, Cooper NS, Healey LA, Kaplan SR, Liang MH, Luthra HS, Medsger TA, Mitchell DM, Neustadt DH, Pinals RS, Schaller JG, Sharp JT, Wilder RL, Hunder GG. The American Rheumatism Association 1987 revised criteria for the classification of rheumatoid arthritis. Arthritis Rheum 31: 315–324, 1988.
20. Naides SJ. Parvovirus B19 infection. Rheum Dis Clin North Am 19: 457–475, 1992.
21. Kerr JR, Cartron JP, Curran MD, Moore JE, Elliot JRM, Mollan RAB. A study of the role of parvovirus B19 in rheumatoid arthritis. Br J Rheumatol 1995 (in press).
22. Ozawa K, Young N. Characterisation of capsid and non-capsid proteins of B19 parvovirus propagated in human erythroid bone marrow cell cultures. J Virol 61: 2627–2630, 1987.

Submitted May 15, 1995; accepted August 10, 1995

Scand J Infect Dis 27: 559–561, 1995 ORIGINAL ARTICLE

Quantitation of Human Cytomegalovirus (HCMV) DNA in Cerebrospinal Fluid by Competitive PCR in AIDS Patients with Different HCMV Central Nervous System Diseases

MIKA SHINKAI and STEPHEN A. SPECTOR

From the Department of Pediatrics and Center for Molecular Genetics, University of California, San Diego, La Jolla, CA, USA

The current study was designed to quantitate human cytomegalovirus (HCMV) DNA in cerebrospinal fluid (CSF) of persons with AIDS with specific HCMV-related CNS disease. DNA present in CSF obtained from AIDS patients was initially detected by a qualitative PCR procedure and then quantitated using a competitive PCR assay. In a group of 21 AIDS patients with HCMV-related CNS disease, 12 patients with HCMV polyradiculopathy had a mean ± SEM of 11,982 ± 4,480 copies/μl in their CSF compared to 1,747 ± 929 for 9 patients with HCMV encephalitis $p = 0.017$). Of the 14 patients with >1,000 copies/μl of HCMV DNA in CSF, 11(79%) had HCMV polyradiculopathy including all 3 with >10,000 copies/μl. Ganciclovir treatment of 3 patients with HCMV-related CNS disease was associated with a decline in HCMV DNA detectable within CSF. These data indicate that quantities of HCMV DNA in CSF are higher in persons with HCMV-related polyradiculopathy than encephalitis, and that quantitation of HCMV DNA can be useful in monitoring antiviral therapy.

S. Spector, MD, University of California, San Diego, Clinical Sciences Building, 9500 Gilman Drive, La Jolla, California 92093-0672, USA

INTRODUCTION

Human cytomegalovirus (HCMV) is a common pathogen of the central nervous system (CNS) in persons with AIDS. We and others have previously demonstrated the utility of the PCR of HCMV DNA in cerebrospinal fluid (CSF) for the diagnosis of HCMV-related CNS disease (1–3). Recently, we have developed a quantitative competitive PCR (QC-PCR) assay for HCMV DNA in plasma, and have demonstrated that high quantities of plasma HCMV DNA are found in AIDS patients at highest risk for development of HCMV disease (4). In this study, we report the application of this QC-PCR assay to CSF specimens obtained from AIDS patients with CNS disease.

MATERIALS AND METHODS

CSF QC-PCR, competitor DNA and standard curves

CSF PCR for HCMV was performed by using oligonucleotide primers from the EcoRI fragment D region of HCMV strain AD169 (1, 5). A constant quantity (1,000 copies) of DNA fragments of the same length and sequence as the target genomic DNA (except for a 20-nt insertion in the middle) was used as competitor for quantitative PCR (6). A standard curve was constructed from the data obtained by quantitative analysis of the ratio between PCR products of competitor and wild type DNA in a set of samples containing a known amount of fragment D DNA ranging from 6×10^4 copies to 6 copies. The standard curve was calculated using a least squares analysis and was used to quantitate the amount of wild type template (152 bp) in unknown samples by using the ratio of the 152 bp to the 172 bp PCR products (7). We have found this assay to have high intra- and interassay reproducibility and to be useful in monitoring plasma samples of persons with AIDS (unpublished data).

Patient population and clinical specimens

A total of 25 PCR positive CSF specimens was obtained from 21 persons with AIDS and HCMV-related CNS disease. Ten, 1 or 0.1 μl of CSF were used for the QC-PCR assay. CSF specimens were stored at −20°C until assayed.

RESULTS

QC-PCR of HCMV DNA Present in CSF from AIDS patients with HCMV-related CNS disease

In our initial studies, we were interested in determining the quantity of HCMV DNA present in persons with AIDS and HCMV-related CNS disease. For each assay, HCMV DNA was quantitated from a standard curve with the dynamic range from 6 to 10,000 copies. To quantitate DNA copy number in the clinical specimens, the ratio of the CSF sample and competitor PCR products was compared to the standard curve. In the group of 21 AIDS patients with HCMV-related CNS disease, the 12 patients with HCMV polyradiculopathy had a mean ± SEM of 11,982 ± 4,480 copies/μl in their CSF compared to 1,747 ± 929 for the 9 patients with HCMV encephalitis ($p = 0.017$). Of 14 patients with greater than 1,000 copies/μl of HCMV DNA in CSF, 11(79%) had HCMV polyradiculopathy. Thus, of the 12 patients with polyradiculopathy, 11(92%) had greater than 1,000 copies, while one patient had less than 100 copies in CSF. Of the 9 individuals with HCMV encephalitis,

 ISSN 0036-5548

Table I. *Quantitative HCMV CSF PCR and clinical diagnosis of HCMV-related CNS disease*

	Polyradiculopathy ($n = 12$)	Encephalitis[a] ($n = 9$)
Mean DNA copies/μl	11,982*	1,747*
±SEM	4,480	929
Median DNA copies/μl	4,632	612
Range DNA copies/μl	1–48,240	1–8,048
DNA copies/μl	Polyradiculopathy ($n = 12$)	Encephalitis[a] ($n = 9$)
>10,000	3	0
1,000–10,000	8	3
100–1,000	0	3
<100	1	3

* $p = 0.017$ (Mann-Whitney Rank test); [a] one patient was diagnosed from autopsy specimen.

3(33%) had greater than 1,000 copies/μl, 3(33%) had between 100 and 1,000 copies/μl and 3(33%) had less than 100 copies/μl (Table I).

QC-PCR can be used to monitor HCMV DNA load during treatment of HCMV-related CNS disease

Three patients with HCMV-related CNS disease had a second specimen obtained while receiving treatment. Fig. 1 shows the HCMV DNA copy number/μl in CSF specimens from the 3 individuals diagnosed with either HCMV encephalitis or polyradiculopathy. In each patient, a marked decline in HCMV DNA was detected after 1 to 3 weeks of intravenous ganciclovir therapy. Patient no. 1, who was diagnosed with HCMV encephalitis, had the greatest quantity of HCMV DNA present in his CSF of any patient with HCMV encephalitis, demonstrated a decrease in HCMV DNA copies/μl from 8,048 to 118 following 3 weeks of treatment. Patients nos 2 and 3, were diagnosed with HCMV polyradiculopathy. Whereas Patient 2, who received 17 days of treatment, demonstrated a decrease in HCMV DNA copies/μl from 3,666 to 121, patient 3, after 7 days of therapy demonstrated a decline from 25,245 to 6,001 copies/μl during treatment. Thus, following intravenous ganciclovir 5 mg/kg twice daily, patients experienced a decline in HCMV DNA copy number in their CSF which ranged from a 4-fold decline at 7 days to an ~70-fold decline after 3 weeks of treatment.

DISCUSSION

In the current study, we have applied a quantitative competitive PCR procedure for HCMV to determine the relative abundance of HCMV DNA present in AIDS patients with HCMV-related polyradiculopathy or encephalitis. Our findings indicate that persons with HCMV disease have high amounts of DNA within their CSF and that patients with the polyradiculopathy syndrome have 3- to 8-fold

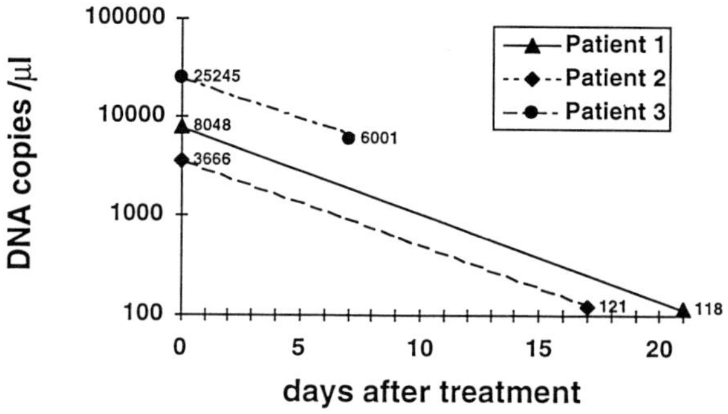

Fig. 1. HCMV DNA copies in CSF specimens before and during treatment with ganciclovir in 3 patients with AIDS and HCMV-related CNS disease. Week 0 indicates the time HCMV-related CNS disease was diagnosed.

greater quantities of DNA in their CSF than AIDS patients with encephalitis. It is likely that because the polyradiculopathy syndrome involves nerves roots adjacent to the spinal cord that the proximity of this syndrome to CSF may lead to the high quantities of HCMV DNA present in affected patients. Additionally, these data are consistent with culture results which indicate that HCMV can be cultured from CSF in 30% to 50% of persons with polyradiculopathy while such cultures are rarely positive in persons with AIDS encephalitis (1–3, 8, 9).

Our findings have also demonstrated that quantitation of HCMV DNA can be useful for monitoring patients receiving antiviral treatment for HCMV-related CNS disease. In the three patients followed with repeat quantitation of HCMV DNA within their CSF from 7 to 21 days on ganciclovir therapy, each demonstrated a decline in the amount of HCMV DNA within their CSF.

In summary, our findings indicate that AIDS patients with HCMV-related CNS disease have high quantities of HCMV DNA in their CSF, and that patients with polyradiculopathy have the greatest quantities of detectable viral DNA. Additionally, quantitation of HCMV DNA in CSF can be a useful marker for monitoring the antiviral effectiveness of therapies of HCMV-related CNS disease.

ACKNOWLEDGEMENT

This research was supported by Public Health Service grants MH-45294 from the National Institute of Mental Health, and AI-27670, AI-27563, AI-28270 and the UCSD CFAR AI-36214 from the National Institute of Allergy and Infectious Diseases.

REFERENCES

1. Wolf DG, Spector SA. Diagnosis of human cytomegalovirus central nervous system disease in AIDS patients by DNA amplification from cerebrospinal fluid. J Infect Dis 166: 1412–5, 1992.
2. Cinque P, Vago L, Brytting M, Castagna A, Accordini A, Sundqvist V-A, Zanchetta N, Monforte AD, Wahren B, Lazzario A, Linde A. Cytomegalovirus infection of the central nervous system in patients with AIDS: Diagnosis by DNA amplification from cerebrospinal fluid. J Infect Dis 166: 1408–11, 1992.

3. Gozlan J, Salord J, Roullet E, Baudrimont M, Caburet F, Picard O, Meyohas M-C, Duvivier C, Jacomet C, Petit J-C. Rapid detection of cytomegalovirus DNA in cerebrospinal fluid of AIDS patients with neurologic disorders. J Infect Dis 166: 1416–21, 1992.
4. Shinkai M, Spector SA, ACTG 181 protocol team. Quantitation of Human Cytomegalovirus (CMV) DNA in Plasma by a Competitive PCR Assay Identifies AIDS Patients at Highest Risk for CMV Disease. In: 34th Interscience Conference on Antimicrobial Agents and Chemotherapy. Orlando, Florida: 1994.
5. Spector SA, Merrill R, Wolf D, Dankner WM. Detection of human cytomegalovirus in plasma of AIDS patients during acute visceral disease by DNA amplification. J Clin Microbiol 30: 2359–65, 1992.
6. Diviacco S, Norio P, Zentilin L, Menzo S, Clementi M, Biamonti G, Riva S, Falaschi A, Giacca M. A novel procedure for quantitative polymerase chain reaction by coamplification of competitive templates. Gene 122: 313–20, 1992.
7. Zachar V, Thomas RA, Goustin AS. Absolute quantification of target DNA: a simple competitive PCR for efficient analysis of multiple samples. Nucleic Acids Res 21: 2017–8, 1993.
8. Vinters HV, Kwos MK, Ho HW, Anders KH, Tomiyasu U, Wolfson WL, Robert F. Cytomegalovirus in the nervous system of patients with the acquired immune deficiency syndrome. Brain 112: 245–68, 1989.
9. Morgello S, Cho ES, Nielson S, Devinsky O, Petito C. Cytomegalovirus encephalitis in patients with acquired immunodeficiency syndrome: an autopsy study of 30 cases and a review of literature. Hum Pathol 18: 289–97, 1987.

Submitted June 8, 1995; accepted October 23, 1995

Claforan®
cefotaxim

Vältolererad
Välbalanserad G^+ och G^- effekt

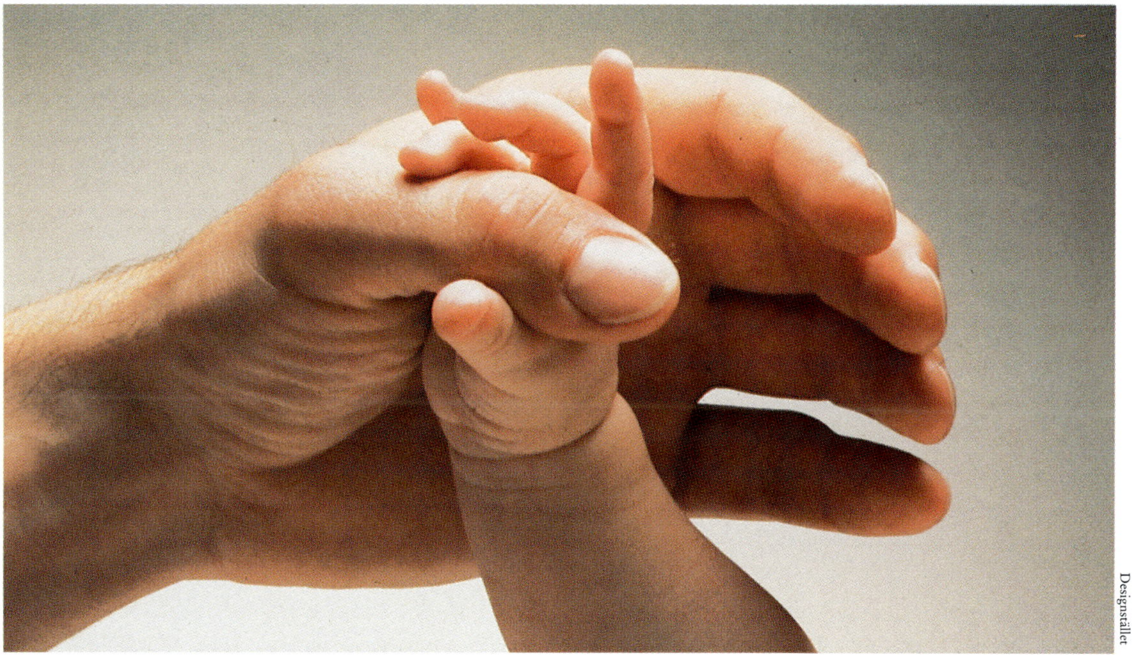

Designstället

Rätt behandling redan från början

Efter 14 års användning över hela världen och mer än 20 miljoner behandlade patienter är Claforan en säker och tillförlitlig 3:e generationens cefalosporin för parenteral behandling av allvarliga infektioner.[1] Claforan tolereras väl i alla åldrar och har liten gastrointestinal påverkan.[2,3]

Ref:
1. Todd et al. Drugs 1990; 40 (4): 608–651.
2. Neu et al. J Clin Pharmacol 1990; 30: 396–403.
3. Guggenbichler et al. Infection 1985; 13 (suppl. 1): 137–139.

Indikationer: Allvarliga infektioner t ex septikemi, meningit, övre urinvägsinfektioner, och nedre luftvägsinfektioner hos nedgångna patienter. Gonorré orsakad av penicillin-resistenta gonokocker. Profylax vid kolorektal kirurgi i kombination med lämpligt anaerob-medel.
Normal dos: 1 g x 2.
Förpackningar: Injektionssubstans 0,5 g, 1 g, 2 g och infusionssubstans 2 g.
För fullständig information se FASS.

Svenska Hoechst AB
Läkemedelsdivisionen
Box 42026, 126 12 Stockholm
Telefon 08-775 70 00

Hoechst

Scand J Infect Dis 27: 563–568, 1995 ORIGINAL ARTICLE

Staphylococcus aureus Bacteremia: a 14-year Nationwide Study in Hematological Patients with Malignant Disease or Agranulocytosis

ROBERT SKOV[1], ADAM GOTTSCHAU[2], PETER SKINHØJ[3], NIELS FRIMODT-MØLLER[4], VIBEKE T. ROSDAHL[3] and FRANK ESPERSEN[3]

From the [1]Staphylococcus Laboratory, and the Departments of [2]Biostatistics and [4]Clinical Microbiology, Statens Seruminstitut and the [3]Department of Infectious Diseases, Rigshospitalet, Copenhagen, Denmark

This retrospective nationwide study of 756 cases of S. aureus bacteremia in hematological patients, between 1977–1990, confirms that S. aureus bacteremia is disproportionately prevalent among, and a major cause of morbidity and mortality in, hematological patients. The case mortality rate attributable to S. aureus bacteremia (44%) was significantly higher than the rate (29%) found in patients without hematological disease. A decreasing mortality was, however, observed from the first to the last part of the study period (53 and 37% respectively). A logistic regression analysis showed that mortality was further dependent on age, the type of hematological disease and origin of infection/primary focus of infection. Analysis of clinical features confirmed that in comparison with other patients, S. aureus bacteremia in hematological patients more often was hospital-acquired, acquired without known portal of infection/primary focus of infection and much less frequently resulted in osteomyelitis or endocarditis. From phage typing and antibiotic susceptibility patterns no specific types of S. aureus were associated with hematological patients.

R. Skov, MD, Department of Clinical Microbiology, Aalborg Hospital, Hobrovej 18–22, Box 365, DK-9100 Aalborg, Denmark

INTRODUCTION

A change in the spectrum of bacteria causing septicemia in hematological and cancer patients, towards Gram-positive predominance, has been reported from many centres during the last 15 years (1–6). This increase has mostly been due to infections caused by coagulase-negative staphylococci and streptococci (1, 2, 5–7). However, infections, especially bacteremia due to Staphylococcus aureus, are still major causes of morbidity and mortality in these patients (3, 8). In Denmark S. aureus accounts for 8–17% of all bacteremias in major hematological institutions in 1990 (9), which equals what has been reported from other hematological departments (4, 6, 7, 10). The fact that a reference laboratory exists in Denmark to which nearly all strains of S. aureus isolated from blood are referred for phage typing, has made it possible to perform a nationwide study of S. aureus bacteremia in hematological patients between 1977–1990, including a total of 756 patients.

The purpose of this study is to report the incidence, clinical characteristics and outcome of S. aureus bacteremia in these patients and compare these cases with cases of S. aureus bacteremia in other patients.

MATERIAL AND METHODS

Since 1957 a central, nationwide registration of S. aureus infections has been carried out in Denmark at the Staphylococcus Laboratory, Statens Seruminstitut. More than 95% of S. aureus strains isolated from blood cultures in this period have been referred to this department for phage typing and registration of bacteriological and clinical data. The clinical data were obtained by chart review. The charts from the different departments were requested and obtained at least 3–6 months after the actual episode, which gives some accuracy to the hematological diagnosis and presence of secondary foci (see below).

Bacteriology

The strains were phage typed according to the method of Blair & Williams (11), using the present international set of phages. The susceptibility to penicillin, streptomycin, tetracycline, erythromycin, chloramphenicol, gentamicin and methicillin was determined by a 20-h prediffusion method (12, 13) in the first part of the study period, and by a disc diffusion method with Neosensitabs (Rosco, Taastrup, Denmark) in the second part. All isolates were stored as either freeze-dried or at −80°C.

Clinical data

Clinical data were obtained in all but a few cases and included: age and sex of the patient; predisposing conditions (e.g. hematological disease); the acquisition of the infection (hospital- or community-acquired); presumed portal of entry of the infection/primary focus of infection (e.g. skin, lungs, postoperative wound infection, catheter-related infection, miscellaneous or unknown); presence of secondary foci (e.g. endocarditis and/or osteomyelitis), and mortality. The latter was defined as death caused by and/or with S. aureus bacteremia as it can be difficult exactly to determine the cause of death in these patients.

In the present study all data from the period 1977–1990 were reviewed. Cases of S. aureus bacteremia in patients with malignant hematological disease or hematological agranulocytosis, defined as myelodysplastic disease, anaemia aplastica and primary agranulocytosis were selected for further study. (Patients with, for example, agranulocytosis due to chemotherapy of cancers etc. were not included, as the data from these patients was not accurately registered in the period). In addition the hospital and department where the patients were treated was recorded, and the type of hematological disease was noted, categorized into the following groups: acute myelocytic leukemia (AML); acute lymphatic leukemia (ALL); chronic lymphatic leukemia (CLL), including 4 cases of hairy cell leukemia; myeloproliferative diseases (MPD) (chronic myelocytic leukemia, myelofibrosis and polycythemia vera); multiple myeloma (MM); malignant lymphoma (ML) (Hodgkin disease and non-Hodgkin lymphoma); agranulocytosis (myelodysplastic disease, anaemia aplastica and primary agranulocytosis), and unclassified leukemia (UCL).

Statistical methods

Hematological and non-hematological patients were compared with respect to age, sex, site of acquisition, portal of entry/primary focus of infection, manifestations of secondary foci, phage type distribution and antibiotic resistance pattern of the infecting strains and mortality using the chi-square test. The effect on mortality in hematological patients of: time of isolation (1977–1983, 1984–1990); age (≤ 50, > 50), sex; portal of entry/primary infection (unknown, cathether, pulmonary infection and others (skin, $n = 48$, wounds, $n = 21$) and miscellaneous ($n = 10$); diagnosis (AGR, AML, CLL, ALL, MPD, MM, ML, UCL); resistance to penicillin (resistant, susceptible), and site of acquisition (hospital, community, unknown) was investigated by logistic regression using SAS software (SAS Institute, Cary, North Carolina, USA).

RESULTS

Phage types and antibiotic resistance

A total of 10 493 episodes of S. aureus bacteremia was recorded during the 14-year study period. Of these cases 756 (7.2%) were from patients with hematological malignancies or agranulocytosis (HMA). The overall phage type distribution as well as the antibiotic resistance pattern showed no difference when infecting strains from patients with HMA were compared to the remaining 9737 cases with S. aureus bacteremia (data not shown). A total of 14.1% of strains found among hematological patients were susceptible to all antibiotics tested; 80.3% were resistant only to penicillin, while 5.6% of the strains showed other patterns of resistance, including 0.4% (representing 3 strains) that were resistant to methicillin.

Table I. *Underlying hematological diseases in 756 patients with S. aureus bacteremia in Denmark, 1977–1990*

Diagnosis	n	(%)	Disease incidence, cases/10^5/year[a], (%)
Acute myelocytic leukemia	157	(21)	4.45 (2.65)
Multiple myeloma	133	(18)	5.65 (2.7)
Malignant lymphoma	124	(16)	12.65 (8.55)
Chronic lymphatic leukemia[b]	97	(13)	5.95 (2.8)[c]
Acute lymphoblastic leukemia	87	(12)	1.5 (1.85)
Agranulocytosis[d]	79	(10)	No information
Myeloproliferative diseases[e]	61	(8)	1.6 (0.9)[f]
Unclassified leukemia	18	(2)	No information

[a] Crude incidence of cancer in Denmark (14).
[b] Including hairy cell leukemia.
[c] Chronic lymphatic leukemia only.
[d] Primary agranulocytosis, anemia aplastica and myelodysplastic syndrome.
[e] Chronic myelocytic leukemia, polycytemia vera and myelofibrosis.
[f] Chronic myelocytic leukemia only.

Clinical data

The distribution of the underlying hematological diseases together with the reported national figures on incidence rates for these diagnosis groups are listed in Table I. Detailed data of prevalence rates (e.g. patient year at risk) were not available. AML was the most frequent diagnosis followed by MM, ML, CLL, ALL, AGR, and MPD (Table I). In 18 cases (2%) no definite diagnosis was established (UCL).

The age distribution (Fig. 1) was biphasic with a minor peak in the age group 11–20 years and a major peak in the age group 61–80 years. Although the median age and the range was nearly identical for HMA and non-HMA patients, the age distribution was significantly different, especially among younger patients, when tested using the chi-square test (Table II and Fig. 1). The male/female ratio was 1.4:1.

Comparisons of different clinical and bacteriological parameters between HMA and non-HMA cases are listed in Table II. Hospital-acquired cases were more common among HMA patients (67%) than non-HMA patients (60%). Also, absence of identifiable portal of entry/primary focus of infection (69 vs. 50%) was more common in HMA patients. Intravenous catheter-related infections were more common, whereas skin, postoperative wound infections and miscellaneous infections were less common, compared with non-HMA patients (Table II). Secondary foci were found in only 6 episodes, 4 cases of endocarditis and 2 cases of osteomyelitis which is a 10-fold lower frequency than that found in non-HMA patients (Table II). The total mortality among HMA patients was 44%, in contrast to 29% among non-HMA patients (Table II).

Mortality

The mortality rate for selected parameters is shown in Table III. A decrease in mortality from 53 to 37% between

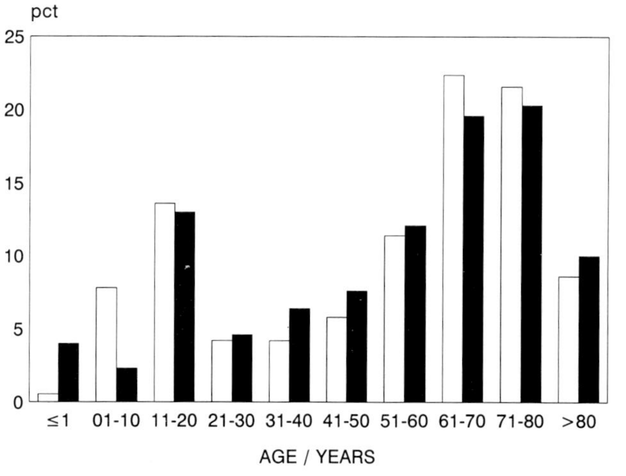

Fig. 1. Age distribution of patients with S. aureus bacteremia in Denmark. ■ Hematological (HMA) patients; □ non-hematological (non-HMA) patients.

Table II. *Comparison of S. aureus bacteremia in patients with hematological malignancy (HMA) with other cases of S. aureus bacteremia (non-HMA) in Denmark 1977–1990*[a]

Characteristics	HMA	non-HMA	*p*
Age distribution			
median	70	70	<0.001[b]
range	0–92	0–100	
Male/female ratio	1.4:1	1.5:1	n.s.[c]
Source, *n* (%)			
Hospital	507 (67)	5869 (60)	<0.0001
Community	133 (18)	2570 (26)	<0.0001
Unknown	116 (15)	1298 (13)	n.s.
Portal of entry, *n* (%)			
Lungs	91 (12)	1102 (11)	n.s.
Skin	48 (5)	880 (9)	<0.05
Postoperative wounds	21 (3)	1057 (11)	<0.0001
Intravenous device	65 (9)	651 (7)	<0.05
Miscellaneous	10 (1)	722 (7)	<0.0001
Unknown	521 (69)	4908 (50)	<0.0001
Secondary foci, *n* (%)			
Endocarditis	4 (0.5)	551 (6)	<0.0001
Osteomyelitis	2 (0.3)	779 (8)	<0.0001
Mortality	330 (44)	2797 (29)	0.05

[a] Analysed by chi-square test.
[b] $\chi^2 = 122$, 9 degrees of freedom.
[c] n.s., not significant.

the first and the last period of the study was observed. For non-HMA patients the mortality decreased from 32 to 26%.

Age more than 50 years and a pulmonary portal of entry/primary focus of infection were both associated with a mortality rate greater than 50%, whereas intravenous catheter-associated infection had a much lower mortality (12%).

When divided according to diagnosis the highest mortality (78%) was found in patients with UCL; MM, MPD and CLL were also associated with a mortality greater than 50%. Patients with ALL had the lowest mortality (22%).

The sex, site of acquisition and penicillin-susceptibility pattern of the infective strain did not influence the mortality (Table III). Also, the phage type of the infecting strain did not have any influence on mortality (data not shown).

Logistic regression analysis of the above parameters revealed that infection during the period 1977–1983, age > 50 years and pulmonary portal of entry were all independently correlated to an adverse outcome, whereas intravenous catheter-associated infection had a significantly better prognosis (Table III).

DISCUSSION

Although S. aureus bacteremia continues to be a major problem in HMA patients, few papers focusing on this topic have been published (15–20). The present study concentrated on the impact of different clinical and epidemiological parameters on mortality, and on whether the decline in mortality observed among all cases of S. aureus bacteremia was also present among HMA patients.

The fact that HMA patients comprise less than 0.2% of the population (21), but account for 7% of all S. aureus bacteremia illustrates that these patients are a group at high risk. The observation that most cases of S. aureus bacteremia in this study were found among patients older than 50 years, is similar to what has been reported previously (22, 23). The high incidence of S. aureus bacteremia found in children reflects the incidence of ALL in this age group. The slight preponderance of S. aureus bacteremia in males among HMA patients corresponds to the difference between the sexes in the incidence of hematological diseases (14). The same phenomenon has, however, previously been observed among non-HMA patients, the reason for this being unknown (24). The absence of an identifiable portal of entry/primary focus of infection was, in this study, both significantly more common in HMA patients as compared to non-HMA patients, but also higher than in the 11–42% found in previous studies of S. aureus bacteremia in HMA patients (17, 18, 20). The difference between HMA and non-HMA patients was expected, and can at least partially be explained by these patients being immunocompromised and thereby having a reduced ability to produce clinical signs of infection. The very low frequency of secondary foci observed in this study, and in other studies of HMA patients (15–19), has been explained by the thrombocytopenic state of these patients, the close observation for signs of infection and early institution of broad spectrum antibiotic therapy when infections appear (15).

The overall mortality attributable to S. aureus bacteremia of 44% among HMA patients was significantly higher than the 29% found among non-HMA patients. Whereas the mortality of non-HMA patients was comparable to other studies of S. aureus bacteremia in unselected patients (22, 23), the mortality was considerably higher in HMA patients as compared to other studies of S. aureus bacteremia in hematological or cancer patients (10, 17–20, 25–27). The very high overall mortality in this study might partly be due to the high median age (70 years), which is considerably higher than what has been reported in most studies of both immunodeficient patients and unselected patients (1, 4, 7, 8, 17, 28–30). However, the fact that this is a nationwide study may also play a role. The mortality rate found in this study is comparable to that reported in patients with Gram-negative bacteremia (1, 8, 31). Univariate analysis and logistic regression analysis of the mortality data revealed that mortality significantly and independently decreased from 53% in the first 7 years to 37% in the last 7 years. The considerable general improvement in mortality in the latter period, which was even better than that seen for all cases of S. aureus bacteremia, is probably due to the improvements in the treatment of hematological malignan-

Table III. *Mortality among 756 hematological patients (HMA)*

Parameter	No. of episodes	Mortality *n* (%)	Odds ratio of death[a]	95% confidence limits
Period				
1977–1983	314	166 (53)	1.00	—
1984–1990	442	164 (37)	0.61	0.44–0.86
Age, years				
≤50	228	43 (19)	1.00	—
>50	528	287 (54)	4.58	2.89–7.27
Diagnosis[b]				
AGR	79	31 (39)	1.28	0.68–2.39
AML	157	57 (36)	1.00	—
CLL	97	50 (52)	1.53	0.86–2.72
ALL	87	19 (22)	1.33	0.65–2.72
MPD	61	33 (54)	2.44	1.25–4.78
MM	133	79 (59)	2.00	1.17–3.41
ML	124	47 (38)	1.17	0.68–2.01
UCL	18	14 (78)	8.92	2.20–36.20
Acquisition site				
Hospital	507	230 (45)	1	—
Community	133	56 (42)	0.68	0.44–1.06
Unknown	116	44 (38)	0.91	0.56–1.49
Sex				
Male	437	194 (44)	1	—
Female	319	136 (43)	0.92	0.66–1.29
Penecillin resistance				
Sensitive	109	45 (41)	1	—
Resistant	647	285 (44)	1.18	0.74–1.86
Portal of entry				
Unknown	521	231 (44)	1.00	—
Catheter	65	8 (12)	0.12	0.05–0.28
Skin, PWI, miscellaneous	79	30 (38)	0.62	0.36–1.07
Lungs	91	61 (67)	1.88	1.13–3.15

[a] Estimated by logistic regression analysis.

[b] Abbreviations: AGR, agranulocytosis; AML, acute myelocytic leukemia; CLL, chronic lymphatic leukemia; ALL, acute lymphatic leukemia; MPD, myeloproliferative diseases; MM, multiple myeloma; ML, malignant lymphoma; UCL, unclassified leukemia; PWI, postoperative wound infection.

cies and supportive care achieved during this period, as both empirical and specific antistaphylococcal treatment has remained unchanged on the whole during the study period. A specific anti-staphylococcal agent is seldom included in initial empirical therapy in Denmark. However these regimens often include an aminoglycoside and a beta-lactam antibiotic with some antistaphylococcal activity.

The observation that age above 50 years was associated with much higher mortality has been found previously (23, 30). Among the different diagnoses, ALL was associated with the lowest mortality; logistic regression analysis showed that this in part was a reflection of the large proportion of younger patients with this disease. UCL, MM, MPD and CLL were associated with mortalities of more than 50%, and except for CLL these diagnoses were independently associated with an adverse outcome when compared to AML patients. A pulmonary portal of entry/primary focus of infection was independently associated with very high mortality, whereas intravenous catheter-associated infection was associated with a low mortality, as compared to cases without an identifiable portal of entry. Both observations fit well with previous findings (23, 32).

Major differences, with regard to resistance- and phage-type patterns, between S. aureus strains isolated from hospital-acquired and community-acquired infections have previously been recorded in Denmark (24, 33). However, this has changed and today these strains have nearly identical resistance- and phage-type patterns (34). Also, epidemic outbreaks with resistant staphylococci seem to have disappeared in Denmark (35, 36). This may also have importance for patients with hematological malignancies and should be investigated.

In conclusion this study confirms that S. aureus bacteremia still is a major cause of morbidity and mortality among hematological patients, with a mortality that equals that reported in patients with Gram-negative bacteremia. This raises the question of whether an antistaphylococcal agent should be added to the empirical antibiotic treatment used in these patients.

ACKNOWLEDGEMENT

Parts of this study were supported by the Danish Medical Research Council, grant no. 12-1618.

REFERENCES

1. Johansson PJH, Sternby E, Ursing B. Septicemia in granulocytopenic patients: A shift in bacterial etiology. Scand J Infect Dis 24: 357–360, 1992.
2. Fredlund H, Björeman M, Kjellander J, Sjöberg L, Bjorne L, Öhlin AL. A 10-year survey of clinically significant blood culture isolates and antibiotic susceptibilities from adult patients with hematological diseases at a major Swedish hospital. Scand J Infect Dis 22: 381–391, 1990.
3. European Organisation for Research and Treatment of Cancer (EORTC) International Antimicrobial Therapy Cooperative Group. Gram-positive bacteraemia in granulocytopenic cancer patients. Eur J Cancer 26: 569–574, 1990.
4. Rubio M, Palau L, Romero Vivas J, del Potro E, Diaz-Mediavilla J, Alvarez A, Martinez R, Picazo JJ. Predominance of Gram-positive microorganisms as a cause of septicemia in patients with hematological malignancies. Infect Control Hosp Epidemiol 15: 101–104, 1994.
5. Coullioud D, Van der Auwera P, Viot M, Lasset C, CEMIC (French-Belgian Study Club of Infectious Diseases in Cancer). Prospective multicentric study of the etiology of 1051 bacteremic episodes in 782 cancer patients. Support Care Cancer 1: 34–46, 1993.
6. Kiehn TE, Armstrong D. Changes in the spectrum of organisms causing bacteremia and fungemia in immunocompromised patients due to venous access devices. Eur J Clin Microbiol Infect Dis 9: 869–872, 1990.
7. European Organisation for Research and Treatment of Cancer (EORTC) International Antimicrobial Therapy Cooperative Group, National Cancer Institute of Canada. Vancomycin added to empirical combination antibiotic therapy for fever in granulocytopenic cancer patients. J Infect Dis 163: 951–958, 1991.
8. Whimbey E, Kiehn TE, Brannon P, Blevins A, Armstrong D. Bacteremia and fungemia in patients with neoplastic disease. Am J Med 82: 723–729, 1987.
9. Arpi M, Victor MA, Møller JK, Jønsson V, Mørk Hansen M, Peterslund NA, Bruun B. Changing etiology of bacteremia in patients with hematological malignancies in Denmark. Scand J Infect Dis 26: 157–162, 1994.
10. Günther G, Björkholm M, Björklind A, Engervall P, Stiernstedt G. Septicemia in patients with hematological disorders and neutropenia. Scand J Infect Dis 23: 589–598, 1991.
11. Blair JE, Williams REO. Phage typing of staphylococci. Bull WHO 24: 771–784, 1961.
12. Thomsen VF. Correlation of the plate-dilution method to the agar diffusion method (disc and tablet methods) with a special view to the importance of pre-diffusion. Acta Pathol Microbiol Scand 54: 107–120, 1962.
13. Thomsen VF. The relation between inoculum and zone size in sensitivity tests by the agar diffusion method, with a special view to the importance of prediffusion. Acta Pathol Microbiol Scand 61: 303–316, 1964.
14. Clemmensen IH, Storm HH. Kræft i Danmark. København: Kræftens Bekæmpelse, 1–97, 1993.
15. Espersen F, Frimodt-Møller N, Rosdahl VT, Jessen O, Faber V, Rosendal K. Staphylococcus aureus bacteremia in patients with hematological malignancies and/or agranulocytosis. Acta Med Scand 222: 465–470, 1987.
16. Grossi M, Green DM. Staphylococcus aureus bacteremia in children and adolescents with acute lymphoblastic leukemia. Oncology 40: 321–325, 1983.
17. Sotman SB, Schimpff SC, Young VM. Staphylococcus aureus bacteremia in patients with acute leukemia. Am J Med 69: 814–818, 1980.
18. Miser JS, Miser AW. Staphylococcus aureus sepsis in childhood malignancy. Am J Dis Child 134: 831–833, 1980.
19. Ladish S, Pizzo PA. Staphylococcus aureus sepsis in children with cancer. Pediatrics 61: 231–234, 1978.
20. Funada H, Yoneyama H, Machi T, Matsuda T. Staphylococcus aureus bacteremia in patients with hematologic disorders. Kansenshogaku Zasshi 66: 1436–1443, 1992.
21. Tulinius H, Storm HH, Pukkala E, Andersen A, Ericsson J. Cancer in the Nordic countries 1981–86. APMIS S 100: 1992.
22. Gransden WR, Eykin SJ, Phillips I. Staphylococcus aureus bacteremia: 400 episodes in St Thomas's Hospital. Br Med J 288: 300–303, 1984.
23. Mylotte JM, McDermott C, Spooner JA. Prospective study of 114 consecutive episodes of Staphylococcus aureus bacteremia. Rev Infect Dis 9: 891–907, 1987.
24. Jessen O, Rosendal K, Bülow P, Faber V, Eriksen KR. Changing staphylococci and staphylococcal infection. A ten years' study of bacteria and cases of bacteremia. N Engl J Med 281: 627–635, 1969.
25. Hovgaard D, Skinhøj P, Bangsborg J, Bruun B, Hansen MM, Nissen NI. Bacteremia and candidemia in hematological malignancies: Clinical findings. Scand J Infect Dis 20: 495–501, 1988.
26. Hedström SÅ, Christensson B. Staphylococcus aureus septicaemia and endocarditis at the University Hospital in Lund 1976–1980. Scand J Infect Dis Suppl 41: 38–46, 1983.
27. Singer C, Kaplan MH, Armstrong D. Bacteremia and fungemia complicating neoplastic disease: a study of 364 cases. Am J Med 62: 731–742, 1977.
28. Leyland MJ, Bayston KF, Cohen J, Warren R, Newland AC, Bint AJ, Cefai C, White DG, Murray SA, Bareford D, Deaney NB. A comparative study of imipenem versus piperacillin plus gentamicin in the initial management of febrile neutropenic patients with haematological malignancies. J Antimicrob Chemother 30: 843–854, 1992.
29. Nolan CM, Beaty HN. Staphylococcus aureus bacteremia. Am J Med 60: 495–500, 1976.
30. Shah M, Watanakunakorn C. Changing patterns of Staphylococcus aureus bacteremia. Am J Med Sci 278: 115–121, 1979.
31. European Organisation for Research and Treatment of Cancer (EORTC) International Antimicrobial Therapy Cooperative Group. Ceftazidime combined with a short or long course of amikacin for empirical treatment therapy of gram-negative bacteremia in cancer patients with granulocytopenia. N Engl J Med 317: 1692–1698, 1987.
32. Iannini PB, Crossley K. Therapy of Staphylococcus aureus bacteremia associated with a removable focus of infection. Ann Intern Med 84: 558–560, 1976.
33. Rosendal K, Jessen O, Bentzon MW, Bülow P. Antibiotic policy and spread of Staphylococcus aureus strains in Danish hospitals, 1969–1974. Acta Pathol Microbiol Immunol Scand [B] 85: 143–152, 1977.
34. Espersen F, Rosdahl VT, Frimodt-Møller N, Skinhøj P. Epi-

demiology of Staphylococcus aureus bacteremia in Denmark. J Chemother 6: 219–225, 1994.

35. Rosdahl VT, Knudsen AM. The decline of methicillin resistance among Danish Staphylococcus aureus strains. Infect Control Hosp Epidemiol 12: 82–88, 1991.

36. Westh H, Jarløv JO, Kjersem H, Rosdahl VT. The disappearance of multiresistant Staphylococcus aureus in Denmark: Changes in strains of the 83A complex between 1969 and 1989. Clin Infect Dis 14: 1186–1194, 1992

Submitted March 31, 1995; accepted August 17, 1995

Scand J Infect Dis 27: 569–573, 1995 ORIGINAL ARTICLE

Staphylococcus aureus Meningitis: a Review of 28 Consecutive Community-Acquired Cases

AXEL LERCHE[1], NIELS RASMUSSEN[2], JOHAN H. WANDALL[3], and VILHELM A. BOHR[4]

From the Departments of [1]Infectious Diseases and [2]Otolaryngology, Head and Neck Surgery, Rigshospitalet, and [3]Medicine B, Infectious Diseases Unit, Frederiksberg Hospital, Copenhagen, Denmark, and [4]Laboratory of Molecular Genetics, National Institute on Aging, National Institutes of Health, Baltimore, USA

From 1966 to 1989 a total of 1,830 cases of bacterial meningitis were recorded at the Department of Infectious Diseases, Rigshospitalet, Denmark. Staphylococcus aureus meningitis accounted for 44 (2.4%) of these cases. Among these, 28 cases were classified as community-acquired S. aureus meningitis. The mortality rate for these cases was 43%. A retrospective study of clinical features and parameters in these community-acquired cases showed the following conditions to be associated with a high mortality risk: advanced age, an underlying condition requiring artificial ventilation, cardiovascular disease and immune deficiencies. At admission, more than 75% of the patients had fever, nuchal rigidity and decreased consciousness. In 57% of cases the focus for the S. aureus infection was endocarditis, pneumonia or skin infections. All the patients had complications due to the meningitis, the major one being insufficient respiration. Autopsy performed in 9 of the 12 fatalities showed endocarditis in 5, pneumonia in 4, and pyelonephritis in 2. All of the brains examined at autopsy showed cerebral and subarachnoid hemorrhage.

A. Lerche, MD, Department of Medicine B, Frederiksberg Hospital, Ndr. Fasanvej, DK-2000 Copenhagen F, Denmark

INTRODUCTION

Staphylococcus aureus (S. aureus) meningitis is an uncommon severe illness, that accounts for 1–9% of bacterial meningitis cases (1–4). Recent studies have shown that within this disease entity there are considerable differences between the hospital-acquired and the community-acquired form (4–8).

The hospital-acquired (nosocomial) form is the mildest and the most common of the two. It is primarily observed as an occasional complication to neurosurgical procedures, the presence of medical devices, or to certain skin infections (5–7). Hospital acquired S. aureus meningitis is generally associated with a favourable prognosis and has a relatively low mortality rate (5–7).

In contrast, community-acquired S. aureus meningitis (CASAM), has a mortality rate of 50–60% (5–9), but only one previous investigation has dealt with the frequency of complications (6). No previous study has described autopsy findings after CASAM. Since CASAM represents a severe form of bacterial meningitis, we have studied a consecutive series of such patients in an attempt to disclose underlying and/or associated conditions. In this retrospective study the clinical presentation, laboratory findings, predisposing conditions, complications and mortality rates among 28 cases of CASAM hospitalized in the years 1966 to 1989 were reviewed.

MATERIALS AND METHODS

Patients

Records from patients admitted to the Department of Infectious Disease, Rigshospital, Denmark, between 1 January 1966 and 31 December 1989 were reviewed. A total of 1,830 cases of bacterial meningitis were diagnosed in this period, and 44 cases were diagnosed as having S. aureus meningitis. This diagnosis was based on the following criteria: (i) characteristic clinical findings; (ii) CSF leukocyte concentration $> 50 \times 10^6$/l with $> 80\%$ neutrophils, and (iii) bacterial cultures of CSF showing staphylococci on microscopy. In cases with a negative CSF culture a positive blood culture with staphylococci and CSF pleocytosis was considered indicative of S. aureus as the etiologic agent.

In guidelines provided by the Centers for Disease Control (CDC), USA (10), a community-acquired infection is defined as being present of incubating at the time of admission, and not related to present or previous hospitalization. Based on this definition, 28 patients in our material had CASAM.

The remaining 16 cases were classified as nosocomially acquired (11), and were not included in this study. The majority of the nosocomial cases occurring during this period were diagnosed and treated in other departments of the hospital.

Medical data from each patient were recorded on standardized charts. The data included information on age, sex, CSF and blood cultures, clinical history, the mode of admission, predisposing conditions, the source of infection and its port of entry, the presence of other hematogenous foci (such as endocarditis, urinary tract infections, arthritis or osteomyelitis), physical findings, laboratory findings, antibiotic treatment, the start of initial treatment or the start of specific treatment, complications such as shock, need for mechanical ventilation, and the registration of evident sequelae on discharge or within 3 months after discharge. When registering mortality we included a period of 6 months after hospitalization, and deaths from causes that were clearly related to the meningitis were included in our numbers. Examples of sequelae included hemiplegia, intellectual dysfunction and epileptic fits. Autopsy records were available in 9 cases, and in 5 of those a brain autopsy was present.

Treatment

In the period from 1966 to 1989 two standard antibiotic regimens for the initial treatment of bacterial meningitis were used. A total of 10 patients received the 1966 regimen of penicillin, sulfadiazin and streptomycin (2), whereas 14 patients received the 1977 regimen consisting of ampicillin and gentamycin (12). In addition, 2 patients received a cephalosporin, 1 received penicillin alone, and 1 patient was initially treated with penicillinase-resistant penicillin.

After the diagnosis of S. aureus was established, 1 patient died before penicillinase-resistant penicillin was installed. The remaining 27 patients all received penicillinase-resistant penicillin (methicillin), in combination with fusidic acid (18 cases), with rifampicin (2 cases), or with both fusidic acid and rifampicin (3 cases). None of the isolated S. aureus strains were resistant to methicillin, and 75% of the patients were infected by S. aureus resistant to penicillin.

Corticosteroids (dexamethasone at 0.2 mg/kg daily for about 4 days) were, in some cases, given at the time of the antistaphylococcal treatment, in cases of incipient incarceration of the brain or in otherwise critically ill patients.

From 1966 to 1974 the indications for artificial ventilation were obstruction of the airways or respiratory arrest often followed by cardiovascular collapse. These indications were expanded in 1975 to include serious cerebral symptoms of incipient cerebral herniation, severe agitation, coma, stupor or $Pa\text{CO}_2$ of > 3.5 kPa, and/or clinical signs of respiratory insufficiency, such as cyanosis (2, 13).

Statistical methods

The Mann–Whitney U-test and Fisher's exact test were applied. A p value < 0.05 was considered to be significant.

RESULTS

Characteristics of survivors and fatalities

In Table I, the patients who died from and those who survived CASAM are compared with reference to a number of parameters. A total of 28 patients were diagnosed as having CASAM between 1966 and 1989, 12 between 1966 and 1976, and 16 patients between 1977 and 1989. The fatal cases were older than the survivors. There was no difference in gender distribution between these groups. A known predisposing condition was more often seen in patients who died than in those who survived ($p < 0.01$), while a known focus of infection or treatment with corticosteroid during initial antibiotic therapy had no influence on survival. The duration from the appearance of symptoms until admission to hospital was on average 2.8 days, and was similar for the fatal cases and survivors. The average duration of hospital stay was 68 days (range 31–172) for survivors, and 30 days (range 2–174) for those who succumbed (Table I). Of the patients, 75% had decreased consciousness on admission. However, 14% of the patients had received relaxants prior to admission, and thus could not be evaluated for consciousness. Three patients (11%) were alert but suffered from fever and severe headache. Upon admission or during the first 48 h, 25% of the patients had seizures, and 55% of the latter died or had severe neurological sequelae.

Table I. *Characteristics of community-acquired S. aureus meningitis; comparison between survivors and fatal cases*

	Fatal cases $n = 12$	Survivors $n = 16$
No. of patients, 1966–1976	4	8
No. of patients, 1977–1989	8	8
Age, years, median (range)	60.5 (32–84)[a]	46 (14–80)[a]
Male/female ratio	6/6	9/7
Predisposing conditions		
Known	10[b]	4[b]
Unknown	2	12
Focus of infection		
Known	8	8
Unknown	4	8
Decreased consciousness at admission	8[c]	13
Corticosteroid treatment	5	8
Median time (range) between symptoms of meningitis and admission to hospital	2 (0–3)	3 (0–5)
Hospital treatment median time (range), days	30 (2–174)	68 (31–172)

[a] The age of patients who died tended to be higher, but not significantly so ($p = 0.07$).
[b] More frequent $p < 0.05$ among patients who died.
[c] 4 patients received relaxants and are not included.

Table II. *Foci of infection and predisposing conditions in S. aureus meningitis*

	Fatal cases, n	Survivors, n
Focus of infection		
Unknown	4	8
Endocarditis	4	3
Pneumonia	2	4
Skin lesion	1	5
Urinary infection	2	1
Head injury	1	0
Predisposing conditions		
Unknown	2	12
Heart valve disease	4	2
Alcohol/drug abuse	2	2
Immunodeficiency	0	4
Urinary infections	2	0

Clinical findings and causes for hospital transfer

The classical triad of fever, nuchal rigidity and decreased consciousness were observed in more than two-thirds of the patients. On admission, 27 patients had fever, 3 had no cerebral effects and 7 patients presented without neck stiffness (4 of these had received relaxants). One patient presented without fever, nuchal rigidity or decreased consciousness. This patient was in preshock at admission, and later died. At admission 13 patients had insufficient respiration. Petechiae were observed in 10 patients.

Some 27 (96%) were transferred from other wards or hospitals, primarily because of suspected meningitis (78%), insufficient ventilation (48%), shock (15%), convulsions (4%), complicated infections (11%), or a combination of the aforementioned reasons. Among patients who later

Table III. *Microbiological findings in cerebrospinal fluid and blood in 28 patients without community-acquired meningitis (no. of fatal cases in parentheses)*

		CSF culture, *n*		
	Total	Positive	Negative	Not done
		20 (10)	1 (1)	7 (2)
Blood culture				
Positive	22 (9)	14 (7)	1 (0)	7 (2)
Negative	4 (2)	4 (2)	0	0
Not done	2 (1)	2 (1)	0	0
CSF microscopy				
Positive	18 (6)	14 (6)	0	4
Negative	4 (1)	3 (1)	1 (0)	0
Not done	6 (5)	3 (3)	0	3 (2)

died, insufficient respiration (67%) and shock (67%) were common causes of transferral. Only one patient was admitted directly from home.

Foci and predisposing conditions

Table II shows details of the suspected foci of infection. A probable focus for the hematogenous spreading to the meninges of S. aureus was found in 57% of the patients. A quarter of the patients had endocarditis, and other causes were pneumonia, skin infections and urinary tract infections. At least two possible foci of entrance were found in 5 patients. More than half of the patients with endocarditis or uninary tract infections died. One-third of the patients with unknown foci had a fatal outcome.

Predisposing conditions were found in 50% of the cases (Table II) with heart valve diseases, diabetes mellitus, urinary tract infections, or drug or alcohol abuse occurring in 83% of the fatal cases. Two patients had had bacterial meningitis 20 years earlier, caused by M. tuberculosis and S. pneumoniae, respectively. Another 2 patients had two or more predisposing conditions (diabetes mellitus and heart valve disease, urinary tract disease and diabetes mellitus), and both died.

Cerebrospinal fluid findings and results of blood cultures

CSF samples were obtained in all 28 patients with CASAM. The median value for the white cell count in CSF was 1,376 × 10^3 cells/ml (range (70–9,480) × 10^3). The median value for the fraction of neutrophils was 91% (range 75–99). The median value for CSF protein concentration was 1.2 g/l (range 0.4–37.9). The median value for the CSF glucose/blood glucose ratio was 0.48 (range 0.10–0.81). There were no significant differences in CSF findings between fatal cases and survivors.

For 8 patients there was a negative or no culture sampling from CSF (Table III); however a positive microscopy was found in 4 of these patients. All the cases with a negative or no CSF culture had positive blood culture for S. aureus. Of the 8 patients, 4 had received antibiotics prior to the lumbar puncture. S. aureus was also cultured from sputum in 4 patients, from skin in 6 and from urine in 3 patients.

Table IV. *Major complications and special treatment of patients with community-acquired meningitis*

	Fatal cases (%) $n = 12$	Survivors (%) $n = 16$
Complications		
Shock	5 (42)	2 (13)
Pneumonia	1 (8)	4 (25)
Insufficient kidney function	3 (25)	2 (13)
Prolonged duration of fever[a]	—	2 (13)
Convulsions	3 (25)	4 (25)
Disseminated intravascular coagulation	1 (8)	1 (6)
Cerebral herniation	3 (25)	—
Special treatment		
Assisted ventilation	9 (75)	6 (38)
Rehabilitation	2 (17)	5 (31)
Heart valve operation	1 (8)	2 (13)

[a] Fever with unknown cause for more than 8 days of relevant treatment.

Complications during treatment

Complications during hospitalization are shown in Table IV. The rate of complications was highest among patients with fatal outcome. The major complications were: insufficient kidney function, shock and cerebral herniation. Among the surviving patients, 69% had insufficient kidney function, convulsions, pneumonia or shock. Pneumonia was a common complication and led to a long rehabilitation period. Artificial ventilation was used in patients with insufficiency caused by shock (5 cases), pneumonia (6 cases), seizures (2 cases) or incipient herniation (2 cases). Of the patients who needed artificial ventilation, 60% died.

Treatment and outcome

The median duration from initial symptoms to the onset of antibiotic treatment was 5 days (range 2–8), and the time

Table V. *Neurological sequelae in 16 patients surviving community-acquired S. aureus meningitis 1966–1989*

Neurological sequelae	No. of patients	%
Hemiparesis	1	6
Facial palsy	1	6
Dementia	1	6
Seizures	2	12
Dizziness	3	18
Headache	1	6
Hearing deficits	2	12
Total	7	44

from the first symptoms of the disease to admission was 3 days (range 0–5 days) on average. There was no apparent difference between survivors and non-survivors regarding these parameters. After the diagnosis of CASAM, 4 patients were treated with a penicillinase-resistant penicillin alone, and 2 of these died. A total of 21 patients were given fusidic acid in addition to penicillinase-resistant penicillin, and 7 of these died.

Patients infected with penicillin-sensitive S. aureus tended to have a better prognosis than those with a penicillin-resistant strain (45 vs. 29%; NS).

Of the patients 46% were given corticosteroids; these patients did not differ with respect to mortality or neurological sequelae from those not treated with steroids (Table I). Half of the patients received artificial ventilation (Table IV). During 1966–1976, 5 patients were on assisted ventilation, and 4 of these died. During 1977–1989, 10 patients were on assisted ventilation, and 5 of them died. Two factors were associated with an increased mortality: the presence of predisposing disease, and respirator treatment (Table IV). Furthermore, patients with a fatal outcome showed a trend towards higher age (average 60.5 years) compared to survivors (average 46 years), (Table I), $p = 0.07$.

The neurological sequelae were evaluated 3 and 6 months after the onset of meningitis in 14 patients. The 2 remaining patients were out of the country, but had been discharged having shown no sequelae. Of the 16 surviving patients, 7 had neurological sequelae (Table V), and in 3 of them these were severe. The recorded sequeale were: hemiparesis, facial palsy, dementia, recurrent convulsions, dizziness, headache and hearing deficits, and 3 patients had 2 or more of these neurological sequelae. There was no obvious age association with the presence of sequelae.

Autopsy findings

Autopsy was performed in 75% of the fatal cases, and brain autopsy in 5 patients (42% of the fatal cases) who died within a few weeks after the onset of meningitis (Table VI). Cerebral and subarachnoid hemorrhage, meningoencephalitis and cerebral edema were the major findings. All these patients had clinical symptoms compatible with cerebral herniation.

A cerebral abscess was suspected in 1 patient with endocarditis, but an intracerebral hemorrhage was found at autopsy. No other patients had a brain abscess.

DISCUSSION

Very few investigations of community-acquired S. aureus meningitis (CASAM) have been reported. The current investigation represents, to our knowledge, the second largest reported series of CASAM. In our study of bacterial meningitis, there were 19 cases of S. aureus meningitis in 875 patients during the period 1966–1976, corresponding to a frequency of 2.2%. In the period 1977–1989 there were 25 cases of S. aureus among 1,036 patients with bacterial meningitis, a frequency of 2.6%. This may suggest that the relative incidence of S. aureus meningitis is increasing, but the difference is not statistically significant (chi-square test, $p = 0.64$).

Table VI. *Autopsy results in 9 patients with community-acquired S. aureus meningitis*

Major autopsy diagnosis ($n = 9$)	
(Brain not included)	
Endocarditis	5
Aortic valve stenosis	3
Pneumonia	4
Arteriosclerosis	6
Pulmonary edema	7
Chronic pyelonephritis with acute exacerbation	2
Renal infarction	3
Myocardial infarction	1
Brain autopsy ($n = 5$)	
Cerebral hemorrhage	5
Subarachnoid hemorrhage	5
Cerebral edema	4
Meningoencephalitis	5
Cerebral hemorrhagic infarction	1
Cerebral thrombosis	1

The patients with CASAM were of a relatively advanced age and had a short history of symptoms before admission to hospital, as also reported by others (5, 7, 8). At admission most patients (not already treated with artificial ventilation) had decreased consciousness, and in most cases fever and nuchal rigidity. This is in accordance with previous reports (5–9). These symptoms, as well as the laboratory results (cell count, protein level or glucose concentration in CSF) were as previously reported for patients with this type of bacterial meningitis (2, 3, 14). In a recent review of 493 episodes of acute bacterial meningitis (14), advanced age and impaired consciousness at admission increased the relative risk of death 3–4-fold. Since almost all our patients not only had these signs at admission, but in addition displayed other signs and symptoms associated with a poor prognosis, a high fatality rate was to be expected. However, as seen in Table VII our fatality rate compares favorably with that of other series.

Treatment and surveillance were carried out by trained personnel in specialized departments, and this may account for the low mortality rate in our series (5, 7, 8). The mean time from start of symptoms to appropriate therapy was about 5 days, which is much longer than for other common types of acute bacterial meningitis (2, 14). We could not detect an improved outcome among patients with a relatively short incubation time, an observation also noted by Jensen et al. (7).

A high proportion of the patients with CASAM were admitted with impaired consciousness, and 25% had seizures at admission or during the hospitalization, indicating cerebral edema. The brain autopsy findings in 5 patients

Table VII. *Mortality from community-acquired S. aureus meningitis in the present and 3 previous studies*

Source	Number of patients	Age, mean (range), years	Mortality (%)	Bacteremia rate (%)
Present study	28	52 (15–84)	12/28 (43)	22/28 (79)
Jensen et al. 1993 (7)[a]	43	67 (0.1–85)	24/43 (56)	35/43 (81)
Gordon et al. 1985 (8)	10	57 (31–85)	3/10 (30)	10/10 (100)
Fong & Ranelli 1984 (5)	15	47 (1–83)	9/15 (60)	9/15 (60)
Total	96	56 (0.1–85)	48/95 (50)	76/96 (79)

[a] These 43 cases were classified as hematogenous meningitis; 84% of these were community-acquired, but they had not been stratified and identified.

(who died within 2 weeks from the start of their symptoms) showed severe edema, inflammation of the meninges, and cerebral and subarachnoid hemorrhage. In an attempt to curtail the inflammatory response in the brain and lower the intracranial pressure, corticosteroids have been used (15, 16). In this series low-dose steroid therapy did not have any effect on mortality or neurological sequelae.

In patients with bacterial meningitis of unknown etiology, clinical examination may disclose heart disease, pneumonia, a skin abscess or a wound. If there is a history of predisposing conditions, such as diabetes, heart valve disease, drug or alcohol abuse, or a reduced immune response, the standard initial meningitis regimen could be supplemented with antistaphylococcal therapy, i.e. a third-generation cephalosporin. Standard antibiotic regimens with ampicillin and aminoglycoid or penicillin, streptomycin and sulphadiazin have a limited bactericidal effect on S. aureus. In accordance with other studies (7), we found that patients infected with penicillin-sensitive S. aureus strains had a trend towards better survival than those infected with a penicillin-resistant strain.

Jensen et al. (7) reported a beneficial effect of fusidic acid. As the vast majority of our patients received a combination of fusidic acid and penicillinase-resistant penicillin, we could no evaluate the effect of fusidic acid alone. However, the mortality in our patients was 43% against 56% in their study, supporting a possible role of fusidic acid in the treatment of CASAM. Nevertheless, the morbidity and mortality of CASAM may have increased over the last 30 years. Prospective studies involving new antibiotics or more targeted molecular therapy are thus warranted.

ACKNOWLEDGEMENT

We thank Professor Peter Skinhøj for critical comments.

REFERENCES

1. Eigler JOC, Wellman WE, Rooke ED, Keith HM, Svein HJ. Bacterial meningitis, I: general review (294 cases). Mayo Clin Proc 36: 357–365, 1961.
2. Bohr V, Hansen B, Jessen O, Johnsen O, Kjersem H, Kristensen HS, Nyboe J, Rasmussen N. Eight hundred and seventy five cases of bacterial meningitis. Part one of a three part series. Clinical data, prognosis and the role of specialized hospital departments. J Infect 7: 21–30, 1983.
3. Geiseler PJ, Nelson KE, Levin S, Reddi KT, Moses VK. Community acquired purulent meningitis. A review of 1,316 cases during the antibiotic area 1954–1976. Rev Infect Dis 2: 725–745, 1980.
4. Roberts FJ, Smith JA, Wagner KR. Staphylococcus aureus meningitis: 26 years experience of Vancouver General Hospital. Can Med Assoc J 128: 1418–1420, 1983.
5. Fong IW, Ranelli P. Staphylococcus aureus meningitis. Quart J Med 53: 289–299, 1984.
6. Schlesinger LS, Ross SC, Schaberg DR. Staphylococcus aureus meningitis: a broad-based epidemiologic study. Medicine (Baltimore) 66: 148–156, 1987.
7. Jensen AG, Espersen F, Skinhøj P, Rosdahl VT, Frimodt-Møller N. Staphylococcus aureus meningitis. Arch Intern Med 153: 1902–1908, 1993.
8. Gordon JJ, Harter HD, Phair JP. Meningitis due to Staphylococcus aureus. Am J Med 78: 965–970, 1985.
9. Kim JH, Van der Horst C, Mulrow CD, Corey GR. Staphylococcus aureus meningitis: review of 28 cases. Rev Infect Dis 11: 698–706, 1989.
10. Valenti WM, Chiarello LA. Overview of hospital infection control and nosocomial infections. In: Mandell 545–558, 1990.
11. Garner JS, Jarvis WR, Emori TG, Horan TC, Hughes JM. CDC definitions for nosocomial infections. Am J Infect Control 16: 128–140, 1988 [Erratum Am J Infect Control 16: 177, 1988.]
12 Jessen O, Kristensen HS. Treatment of bacterial meningitis. Ugeskr Læg 141: 1–4, 1979.
13. Rasmussen N, Hansen B, Bohr V, Kristensen HS. Artificial ventilation and prognostic factors in bacterial meningitis. Infection 16: 158–162, 1988.
14. Durand ML, Calderwood SB, Weber DJ, Miller SI, Southwick FS, Caviness VS, Swartz MN. Acute bacterial meningitis in adults. A review of 493 episodes. N. Engl J Med 382: 21–28, 1993.
15. Igarashi M, Gilmartin RC, Gerald B, Wilburn F, Jabbour JT. Cerebral arteritis and bacterial meningitis. Arch Neurol 41: 531–535, 1984.
16. Schaad UB, Lips U, Gnehm, HE, Blumberg A, Heinzer I, Wedgwood. J. Swiss Meningitis Study Group. Dexamethasone therapy for bacterial meningitis in children. Lancet 342: 457–461, 1993.

Submitted April 19, 1995; accepted September 10, 1995

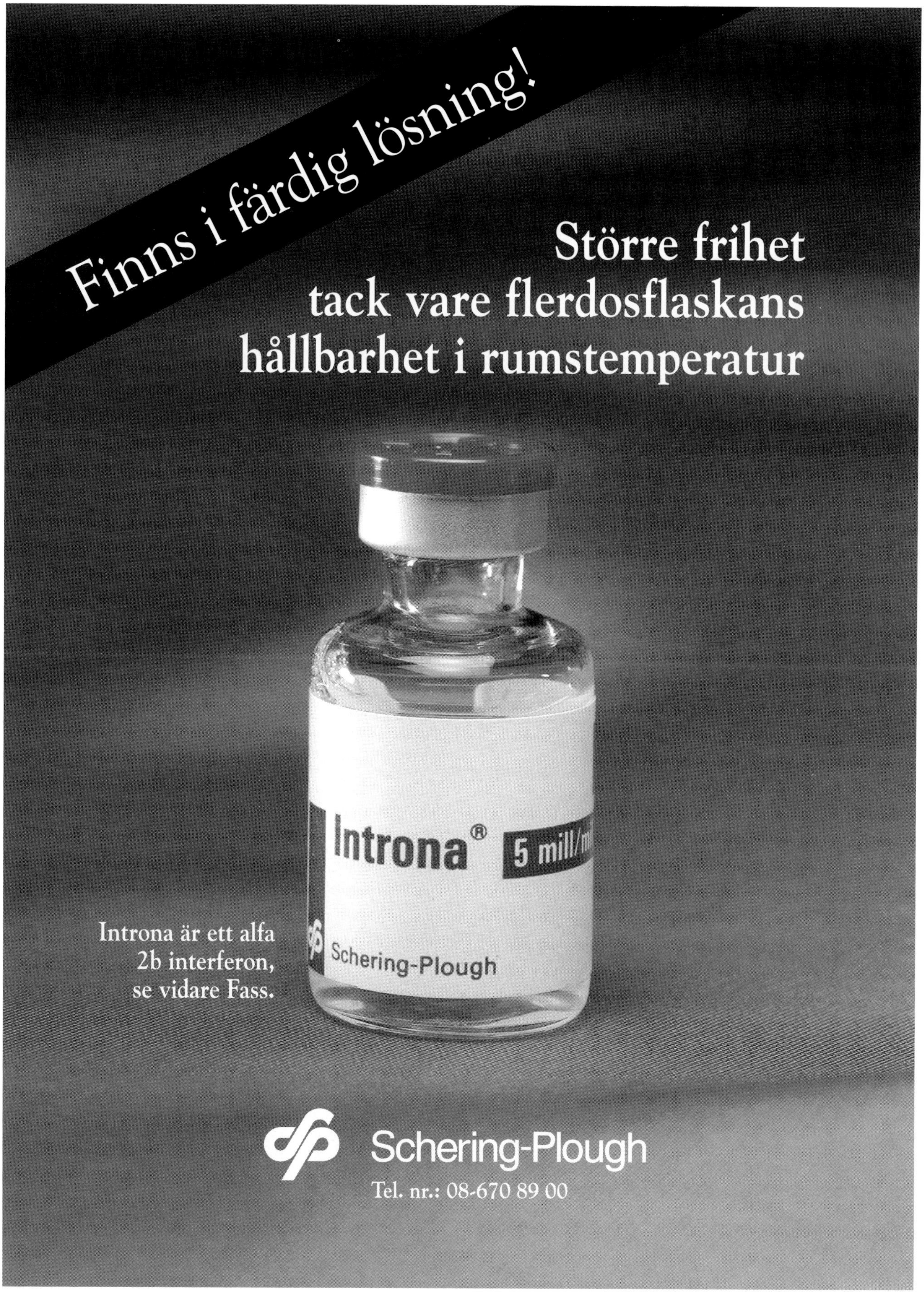
Finns i färdig lösning!
Större frihet
tack vare flerdosflaskans
hållbarhet i rumstemperatur
Introna®
Schering-Plough
Introna är ett alfa
2b interferon,
se vidare Fass.
Schering-Plough
Tel. nr.: 08-670 89 00

Scand J Infect Dis 27: 575–580, 1995 ORIGINAL ARTICLE

Molecular Epidemiology of Staphylococcus epidermidis Isolates in a Hematological Unit during a 4-month Survey

OUTI LYYTIKÄINEN[1,2], VILLE VALTONEN[1], AULIKKI SIVONEN[3], RIITTA RYHÄNEN[4] and JAANA VUOPIO-VARKILA[4]

From the [1]Department of Medicine, Division of Infectious Diseases, Helsinki University Central Hospital, the [3]Department of Bacteriology and Immunology, University of Helsinki and the Departments of [2]Infection Epidemiology and [4]Special Bacterial Pathogens, National Public Health Institute, Helsinki, Finland

In order to study the strain variety, clonal stability and epidemiology of Staphylococcus epidermidis, isolates from all bacterial cultures taken when clinically indicated in 2 wards of the hematological unit of Helsinki University Hospital, during a 4-month period, were characterized by 3 typing methods: antibiogram, plasmid profile and ribotype. A total of 141 distinct S. epidermidis colonies, from 28 blood cultures and 37 cultures from other sources in 32 patients were studied. Plasmid profiles and ribopatterns revealed 47 different strains of which 16 were bacteremic. One of these strains caused bacteremia in 4 different patients over a 3-month period and it was isolated from blood on 7 different sampling occasions. The occurrence of this clone was constant; it was usually found in both of 2 blood culture bottles inoculated (6/7 pairs) and dominated among the 17 distinct S. epidermidis colonies studied from the positive bottles (94% of the total). The clones causing bacteremias in the 2 wards were distinct. These findings indicate that certain clones of S. epidermidis can predominate in hematological wards and that nosocomial transmission of S. epidermidis strains may occur among patients, particularly within the same ward.

O. Lyytikäinen, MD, Department of Medicine, Division of Infectious Diseases, Helsinki University Central Hospital, Haartmaninkatu 4, FIN-00290 Helsinki, Finland

INTRODUCTION

Staphylococcus epidermidis is a major causative agent of bacteremia in neutropenic patients with permanent indwelling venous catheters (1, 2). Although these infections have previously been regarded as mainly endogenous in origin, there is growing evidence that nosocomial transmission also occurs (3–6). As bacterial flora from the skin may contaminate blood cultures, a repetitive isolation of the same strain has traditionally been taken as proof of true infection (7). Molecular typing methods now provide a new tool for studying the epidemiology of S. epidermidis infections and the relatedness of different S. epidermidis isolates (8–13).

S. epidermidis predominates among bacteremias of adult acute leukemic patients in our hematological unit. The aim of the present study was to define the molecular epidemiology of S. epidermidis isolates in 2 different hematological wards. The focus was on evaluating the strain varieties among different patients and on the clonal stability of strains. All bacterial cultures positive for S. epidermidis obtained from these wards during a 4-month period were subjected to typing with various methods (antimicrobial susceptibility pattern, plasmid profiling and ribotyping).

MATERIALS AND METHODS

Setting

Helsinki University Central Hospital is a tertiary care teaching hospital. The hematological unit for adults consists of 2 wards located on different floors; ward A with 12 beds and ward B with 16 beds, both including several isolation rooms equipped with high efficiency particulate air (HEPA) filters for the incoming air. Severely neutropenic patients ($<0.50 \times 10^9/l$) are treated in single rooms with reverse isolation with an emphasis on hand-washing and disinfection practice. The wards have their own nursing staff but doctors are shared. Movement of patients between the wards seldom occurs.

Bone marrow transplantation (BMT) patients, treated on ward A, receive daily oral trimethoprim sulfamethoxazole as prophylaxis against bacterial infections during their neutropenic period, but no other prophylaxis is used. Long-term indwelling catheters, inserted with vancomycin prophylaxis, are routinely used during treatment. Vancomycin is not used as a first-line empirical antibiotic for neutropenic patients with fever. No routine surveillance cultures are performed.

Bacterial cultures and description of patients

Between October 28 1992 and February 28 1993, all bacterial cultures, excluding urine cultures, positive for S. epidermidis from wards A and B, taken when clinically indicated, were included in this study. Blood samples were taken by venipuncture (not through catheters).

The positive cultures ($n = 65$) were obtained from 32 different patients (ward A, 21; ward B, 11) of whom 12 were bone marrow recipients. Of the patients, 17 had acute leukemia, 6 had non-Hodgkin lymphoma, 5 chronic myelogenous leukemia and the remaining 4 various malignant hematological diseases.

Identification and storage of bacteria

S. epidermidis isolates were identified by standard laboratory methods at the Department of Bacteriology and Immunology, University of Helsinki and the primary isolation plates were then sent to the Staphylococcus Reference Laboratory at the National Public Health Institute in Helsinki for further studies.

A total of 1–4 representative colonies were collected from each agar plate for identification and typing. Confirmation of species identification was based on the production of acid from sugars (arabinose, lactose, maltose, mannitol, fructose, ribose, sucrose, trehalose, xylitol and xylose) and using API STAPH or ID 32 STAPH (Bio Mérieux, Marcy-l'Étoile, France) tests.

The isolates were then stored in skim milk at − 70°C.

Antimicrobial susceptibility

This was basically determined as recommended by the National Committee for Clinical Laboratory Standards; however, Neo-Sensitabs discs (A/S Rosco, Taastrup, Denmark) and Mueller–Hinton II medium were used.

The antibiotics tested for were oxacillin, penicillin, ampicillin, cephalothin, cefuroxime, erythromycin, clindamycin, tetracyline, chloramphenicol, rifampin, trimethoprim sulfamethoxazole, fusidic acid, gentamicin, tobramycin, vancomycin and ciprofloxacin. Resistance to methicillin was assayed with 1 μg oxacillin discs after incubation for 24 h at 30°C.

Plasmid profiling

Samples of 1.5 ml of grown brain–heart infusion (BHI) broth bacterial culture (overnight at 37°C) were collected by centrifugation in Eppendorf tubes. Plasmid DNA was isolated by standard small-scale techniques (14), and separated by electrophoresis in 0.7% agarose gels at 25V for 18 h.

The plasmid types were determined by visual comparison of ethidium bromide-stained and photographed gels and differentiated by identifying the number and size of the plasmids. A difference of 1 band was considered as discriminatory. A lambda EcoRI/HindIII DNA marker (Promega, Madison, Wisconsin, USA) was used as a molecular weight standard.

Ribotyping

Genomic DNA was purified as described by Pither et al. (15), digested with EcoRI and HindIII endonucleases (Boehringer Mannheim, Mannheim, Germany) according to the manufacturer's instructions and separated by electrophoresis in 0.7% agarose gels, using 75V for 4.5 h. DNA fragments were stained with ethidium bromide, photographed and transferred to a positively charged nylon membrane as described earlier (16).

DNA fragments were hybridized with the plasmid pKK3535, which consists of the cloning vector pBR322 and the rrn rRNA operon of the E. coli chromosome (17). E. coli DH5α carrying plasmid pKK3535 (17), which was provided by M. Saarela (Institute of Dentistry, University of Helsinki) and used for hybridization, was grown in Luria broth supplemented with 50 μg of ampicillin/ml. Plasmid DNA was isolated from E. coli DH5α by standard techniques (14). Preparation of the labelled pKK3535 probe, hybridization and detection were performed as described earlier (16). Ribotype patterns were determined by visual comparison and were designated by a capital letter for the EcoRI patterns, and a lower case letter for the HindIII patterns. A one-band difference in hybridization pattern was considered sufficient to define different ribotype. A lambda EcoRI/HindIII DNA marker (Promega) was used as a molecular weight standard.

Table I. *Plasmid types and ribotypes of 141 S. epidermidis isolates from 65 cultures yielding S. epidermidis taken in 2 hematological wards*

	Ward A ($n = 89$)	Ward B ($n = 52$)	No. of isolates ($n = 141$)
Plasmid type			
Plasmidless		1	1
1	39	3	42
2		4	4
3	12	1	13
4		3	2
5		8	8
6		3	3
7	1	3	4
8	4	2	6
9	1	1	2
10	2	1	3
11	4		4
12	3		3
13	2	2	4
14	2	2	4
15	4		4
16		6	6
17	2		2
18	2		2
19	2		2
20		3	3
21	2		2
22		2	2
23		2	2
Sporadic	7	5	12
No. of types	22	21	35
Ribotype[a]			
A:a	31	9	40
N:f	16	7	23
C:c	20		20
Q:q	3	17	20
T:a	9		9
E:a		7	7
Y:u		7	7
V:t	3		3
X:v		2	2
Z:h	2		2
AA:s	2		2
BB:r	2		2
Sporadic	1	3	4
No of types	10	9	16

[a] Ribotypes were coded by a capital letter for the EcoRI pattern and a lower case letter for the HindIII pattern.

RESULTS

A total of 65 cultures yielding S. epidermidis were studied. 28 blood cultures (ward A 19, and ward B 9) and 37 cultures from other sources (ward A 21, and ward B 16) (catheter tip or opening, 8; skin or mucous membrane, 12; bronchoalveolar lavage fluid or sputum, 9; feces, 4; post-mortem specimen, 4). A total of 1–4 representative colonies were studied from each agar plate or blood culture bottle (blood cultures, mean 2.4; other cultures, mean 2.0). The total number of distinct S. epidermidis colonies studied was 141: 68 colonies from blood cultures and 73 from other sources.

Most of the patients with a positive blood culture had an indwelling central venous catheter (13/14) and were severely neutropenic at the time of S. epidermidis bacteremia (11/14).

Table II. *Subdivision of S. epidermidis isolates from 28 blood cultures yielding S. epidermidis taken in 2 hematological wards by plasmid profiling and ribotyping*[a]

	Plasmid type (No. of isolates)												
Ribotype	1	2	3	4	5	6	8	13	17	18	19	Sporadic	Total
Ward A													
A:a	17											1	18
N:f			1									1	2
C:c	15												15
T:a			7										7
Z:h										2			2
AA:s											2		2
BB:r									2				2
Total	32	0	8	0	0	0	0	0	2	2	2	2	48
Ward B													
A:a							1	2					3
N:f						3	1						4
Q:q		4		2	7								13
Total	0	4	0	2	7	3	2	2	0	0	0	0	20

[a] See footnote Table I.

Antibiograms

Of all 141 isolates studied, 94% were multiresistant, i.e. resistant to methicillin and to at least 2 antibiotic classes other than beta-lactams (ward A 91%, and ward B 100%). Resistance to ciprofloxacin was as high as 78% (ward A 82%, and ward B 71%).

Plasmid types

A total of 35 different plasmid patterns were observed (Table I). There was a clear predominance of 2 patterns, type 1 (30%) and type 3 (9%), mostly in ward A. Eight plasmid patterns were common to both wards. There was only 1 strain without detectable plasmids.

Ribotypes

A total of 16 different rRNA hybridization patterns were identified after EcoRI digestion and 10 patterns after HindIII digestion of genomic DNA. When combining these results 16 ribotypes were observed (Table I). The most common ribotypes were A:a (28%), N:f (16%) and Q:q (14%) found in both wards, and C:c (22%) and T:a (10%) found predominantly in ward A.

Clonality of isolates

When ribotype results were combined with those of plasmid analysis, 47 different clones were identified (ward A $n = 28$, and ward B $n = 23$), of which 16 caused bacteremia; none of the bacteremic clones were common to the 2 wards and 3 (A:a1, C:c1 and T:a3) predominated in ward A (Table II).

Genotype A:a1. This was found in 7 different patients of whom 6 were from ward A. Bacteremia due to clone A:a1 occurred in 4 patients of ward A (I, II, IV, V) (Table III). It was isolated from 7 different blood cultures and usually from both blood culture bottles (6/7). With one exception (A:a sporadic) multiple colonies studied from the same blood culture were of the same clone i.e. A:a. In addition, A:a1 was found in a skin lesion and a catheter opening in 2 patients without bacteremic episodes (Table III). In ward B clone A:a1 was isolated from 2 postmortem specimens from 1 patient.

Clone C:c1. This was obtained from 2 patients in ward A causing bacteremia in one of them and being isolated twice from 2 blood culture bottles and from a catheter tip (Table III). In addition, it was found from the catheter of 1 patient with bacteremia caused by clone A:a1.

Clone T:a3. This clone was found in 2 different patients in ward A. It caused 2 episodes of bacteremia in 1 patient with a 3 month interval, and the same clone was also isolated from feces 1 month before the first bacteremic episode (Table III).

(A:a1, A:a13, N:f8 and N:f14). These 4 clones were found in both wards. Clones A:a13 and N:f8 caused bacteremia in ward B, but were isolated from sources other than blood in ward A, i.e. skin lesions and sputum. Clone N:f14 was found in ward A from a catheter and in ward B from bronchoalveolar lavage fluid.

DISCUSSION

During the last decade, mainly due to improved empirical antibiotic regimens directed against Gram-negative organisms and the increased use of indwelling venous access devices, increasing rates of S. epidermidis bacteremia in neutropenic hoses have been noted (18). In the present

Table III. *Isolation of the predominant S. epidermidis clones in Ward A*

Patient	Source	Date	Time	Clone	No of colonies with identical pattern[a]	Other pattern[a]
I	Blood	28.10.92	11.05	A:a1	2/2	
II	Blood	13.11.92	7.55	A:a1	2/2	
	Blood	13.11.92	9.25	A:a1	2/2	
	Blood	13.11.92	15.40	A:a1	2/2	
III	Feces	29.10.92		T:a3	2/3	N:f9
	Blood	1.12.92	19.20	T:a3	2/2	
	Blood	1.12.92	19.50	T:a3	2/2	
	Blood	23.2.93	23.30	T:a3	2/2	
IV	Blood	21.1.93	18.30	A:a1	2/2	
V	Catheter	22.1.94		C:c1	1/2	C:c7
	Blood	1.2.93	17.40	A:a1	3/4	A:a sporadic
	Blood	1.2.93	18.30	A:a1	4/4	
VI	Blood	19.2.93	20.40	C:c1	4/4	
	Blood	19.2.93	21.10	C:c1	4/4	
	Blood	22.2.93	18.00	C:c1	1/2	T:a3
	Blood	26.2.93	22.10	C:c1	2/2	
	Blood	27.2.93	13.30	C:c1	2/2	
	Blood	27.2.93	14.00	C:c1	2/2	
	Catheter	28.2.92		C:c1	2/3	C:c sporadic
VII	Catheter	11.12.92		A:a1	2/2	
VIII	Skin	27.1.93		A:a1	2/2	

[a] 1–4 representative colonies from each agar plate or blood culture bottle were studied.

study, we defined the strain variation and clonal stability of strains in bacterial cultures positive for S. epidermidis taken in 2 wards of a hematological unit, in the absence of a recognized outbreak. Of all 47 strains identified, 16 caused bacteremia. Bacteremic strains differed between the 2 wards; one such strain in ward A was isolated on a total of 7 different sampling occasions form 6 different patients, 4 of whom suffered from bacteremia. This predominant strain was usually obtained from both blood culture bottles, and dominated among the distinct clonies studied from each blood culture. These findings suggest that certain clones of S. epidermidis can predominate, especially among immunosuppressed patients, and that exogenous sources may be important in development of bacteremias due to S. epidermidis among these patients.

Birnbaum et al. have summarized several studies of nosocomial coagulase-negative (CN) staphylococci (CN) infections in the absence of recognized outbreaks, and suggested that fewer than 10% of endemic CN staphylococcal infections may be explained by transmission between patients (19). None of the studies were performed in hematological units. Thore et al. found that in an orthopedic ward the drug-resistant nosocomial CN staphylococci strains, which rapidly colonized the new patients, occurred equally often among staff as among the previously admitted patients (20). The persistence of distinct strains of S. epidermidis, as evidence of nosocomial transmission, has been shown to occur in neonatal intensive care units (21, 22, 16). During a 1 week survey in a bone marrow transplant unit a few ciprofloxacin-resistant S. epidermidis strains were found to be widely spread in the air and to contaminate the clothes of staff (6). The colonized patients were thought to be the main source of environmental contamination and it was speculated that strain transmission occurred via hospital personnel or directly. No bacteremias occurred during the study period. Only 2 studies on nosocomial cross-infection in hematological units during outbreaks have been published. Both were caused by ciprofloxacin-resistant CN staphylococci soon after the introdution of the drug as part of empirical treatment and prophylaxis (4, 5).

Bacteremias due to S. epidermidis in neutropenic patients are mostly of unknown origin (18). Systemic antibiotic administration has been shown to promote colonization with antibiotic-resistant CN staphylococci (23, 24). Mucosal damage of the alimentary tract and concurrent colonization of mucous membranes have also been shown to be risk factors for S. epidermidis infection (3, 25). Moreover, central venous catheters are routinely used in hematological units. Thus, catheters are often incriminated as a possible route or source of S. epidermidis bacteremias (18). The diagnosis of catheter-related bacteremia is difficult, especially in neutropenic hosts, because of the lack of inflammatory signs. Even with immunocompetent hosts, only half of patients with catheter infection exhibit local signs fo infection (18). There is increasing evidence that beside the skin insertion site, especially for the long-term catheters, the exogenous colonization of the catheter hub and the intraluminal migration of bacteria correlate to catheter-related sepsis (26–29). Organisms may be introduced into the hub from the hands of staff and multiple manipulations of the hub increase the risk of infection. In our study, all 4 patients with bacteremia due to the predominant S. epidermidis clone had a long-term catheter.

Repeated isolation of organisms with identical markers if felt to be indicative of infection (7, 30). In addition, a small study using multilocus enzyme electrophoresis as a typing method has demonstrated that repeated isolation of the same CN staphylococcus strain during the course of catheter-related sepsis was due to ongoing bacteremia, rather than culture contamination (29). In another study, the isolation of the same CN staphylococcus strain from both blood bottles has been evaluated, where 82% (9/11) pairs had the same plasmid profie but a large part of the isolates studied were not biotypable (31). As we have previously demonstrated, the ribotyping and plasmid profile analysis as used here work well in the subtyping of S. epidermidis strains when used in combination (16). We found that a certain clone dominated in repeated blood samples; in both of 2 blood culture bottles and among multiple colonies from each blood culture.

In conclusion, our results indicate that transmission of S. epidermidis strains may occur between patients in a BMT unit despite protective isolation measures, although the routes of transmission and the role of catheters are still unknown.

REFERENCES

1. Ehni WF, Reller LB, Ellison RT III. Bacteremia in granulocytopenic patients in a tertiary care general hospital. Rev Infect Dis 13: 613–619, 1991.
2. Rubio M, Palau L, Vivas R, del Potro E, Diaz-Mediavilla J, Alvarez A, Martinez R, Picazo JJ. Predominance of gram-positive microorganisms as a cause fo septicemia in patients with hematological malignancies. Infect Control Hosp Epidemiol 15: 101–104, 1994.
3. Wade JC, Schimpff SC, Newman KA, Wiernik PH. Staphylococcus epidermidis: an increasing cause of infection in patients with granulocytopenia. Ann Intern Med 97: 503–508, 1982.
4. Oppenheim BA, Hartley JW, Lee W, Burnie JP. Outbreak of coagulase-negative staphylococcus highly resistant to ciprofloxacin in a leukaemia unit. Br Med J 299: 294–297, 1989.
5. Kotilainen P, Nikoskelainen J, Huovinen P. Emergence of ciprofloxacin-resistant coagualase-negative staphylococcal skin flora in immunocompromised patients receiving ciprofloxacin. J Infect Dis 161: 41–44, 1990.
6. Hedin G, Hambraeus A. Multiply antibiotic-resistant Staphylococcus epidermidis in patients, staff and environment – a one-week survey in a bone marrow transplant unit. J Hosp Infect 17: 95–106, 1991.
7. Archer GL, Karchmer AW, Vishniavsky N, Johnston JL. Plasmid-pattern analysis for the differentiation of infecting from noninfecting Staphylococcus epidermidis. J Infect Dis 149: 913–920, 1984.
8. Parisi JT, Hect DW. Plasmid profiles in epidemiologic studies of infections by Staphylococcus epidermidis. J Infect Dis 141: 637–643, 1980.
9. Renaud F, Freney J, Etienne J, Bes M, Brun Y, Barsotti O, Andre S, Fleurette J. Restriction endonuclease analysis of Staphylococcus epidermidis DNA may be a useful epidemiological marker. J Clin Microbiol 26: 1729–1734, 1988.
10. De Buyser M–L, Morvan A, Grimont F, El Sohl N. Characterization of staphylococcal species by ribosomal RNA gene restriction patterns. J Gen Microbiol 135: 989–999, 1989.
11. Bialkowska-Hobrzanska H, Harry V, Jaskot D, Hammerberg O. Typing of coagulase-negative staphylococci by Southern hybridization of chromosmal DNA fingerprints using a ribosomal RNA probe. Eur J Clin Microbiol Infect Dis 9: 588–594, 1990.
12. Izard NC, Hächler H, Grehn M, Kayser FH. Ribotyping of coagulase-negative staphylococci with special emphasis on intraspecific typing of Staphylococcus epidermidis. J Clin Microbiol 30: 817–823, 1992.
13. Goering RV, Winters MA. Rapid method for epidemiological evaluation of gram-positive cocci by field inversion gel electrophoresis. J Clin Microbiol 30: 577–580, 1992.
14. Sambrook J, Fritsch EF, Maniatis T. Molecular cloning: a laboratory manual, 2nd edn. Cold Spring Harbor, New York: Cold Spring Harbour Laboratory Press, 1.34–9, 1989.
15. Pither DG, Saunders NA, Owen RJ. Rapid extraction of bacterial genomic DNA with guanidium thiocyanate. Lett Appl Microbiol 8: 151–156, 1989.
16. Lyytikäinen O, Saxen H, Ryhänen R, Vaara M, Vuopio-Varkila J. Persistence of a multiresistant clone of Staphylocuccus epidermidis in a neonatal intensive care unit for a four-year period. Clin Infect Dis 20: 24–29, 1995.
17. Brosius J, Ullrich A, Raker MA, Gray A, Dull TJ, Gutell RR, Noller HF. Construction and fine mapping of recombinant plasmids containing the rrnB ribosomal RNA operon of E. coli. Plasmid 6: 112–118, 1981.
18. Rupp ME, Archer GL. Coagulase-negative staphylococci: pathogens associated with medical progress. Clin Infect Dis 19: 231–245, 1994.
19. Birnabum D, Kelly M, Chow AW. Epidemiologic typing systems for coagulase-negative staphylococci. Infect Control Hosp Epidemiol 12: 319–326, 1991.
20. Thore M, Kühn I, Löfdahl S, Burman LG. Drug-resistant coagulase-negative skin staphylococci: evaluation of four marker systems and epidemiology in an orthopaedic ward. Epidemiol Infect 105: 95–105, 1990.
21. Carlos CC, Ringertz S, Rylander M, Huovinen P, Faxelius G. Nosocomial Staphylococcus epidermidis septicaemia among very low birth weight neonates in an intensive care unit. J Hosp Infect 19: 201–207, 1991.
22. Huebner J, Pier GB, Maslow JN, Muller E, Shiro H, Parent M, Kropec A, Arbeit RD, Goldmann DA. Endemic nosocomial transmission of Staphylococcus epidermidis bacteremia isolates in a neonatal intensive care unit over 10 years. J Infect Dis 169: 526–531, 1994.
23. Archer GL, Tenebaum MJ. Antibiotic-resistant, Staphylococcus epidermidis in patients undergoing cardiac surgery. Antimicrob Agents Chemother 17: 269–272, 1980.
24. Archer GL, Armstrong BC. Alteration of staphylococcal flora in cardiac surgery patients receiving antibiotic prophylaxis. J Infect Dis 147: 642–649, 1983.

25. Herwaldt LA, Hollis RJ, Boyken LD, Phaller MA. Molecular epidemiology of coagulase-negative staphylococci isolated from immunocompromised patients. Infect Control Hosp Epidemiol 13: 86–92, 1992.
26. Linares J, Sitges-Serra A, Garau J, Perez JG, Martin R. Pathogenesis of catheter sepsis: a prospective study with quantitative and semiquantitative cultures of catheter hub and segments. J Clin Microbiol 21: 357–360, 1985.
27. Sitges-Serra A, Puig P, Linares J, Perez JL, Farrero N, Jaurrieta E, Garau J. Hub colonization as the initial step in an outbreak of catheter-related sepsis due to coagulase negative staphylococci during parenteral nutrition. J Parenter Enteral Nutr 8: 668–672, 1984.
28. Sitges-Serra A, Linares J, Prez JL, Jaurrieta E, Lorente L. A randomized trial on the effect of tubing changes on hub contamination and catheter sepsis during parenteral nutrition. J Parenter Enteral Nutr 9: 322–325, 1985.
29. Tan TQ, Musser JM, Shulman RJ, Mason EO, Mahoney DH Jr, Kaplan SL. Molecular epidemiology of coagulase-negative staphylococcus blood isolates from neonates with persistent bacteremia and children with central venous catheter infections. J Infect Dis 169: 1393–1397, 1994.
30. Valentine CR, Yandle SH, Marsik FJ, Ebright JR, Dawson MS. Evaluation of the variety of plasmid profiles in Staphylococcus epidermidis isolates from hospital patients and staff. Infect Control Hosp Epidemiol 9: 441–446, 1988.
31. Ringberg H, Thoren A, Bredberg A. Evaluation of coagulase-negative staphylococci in blood cultures. A prospective clinical and microbiological study. Scand J Infect Dis 23: 315–323, 1991.

Submitted March 30, 1995; accepted August 31, 1995

Scand J Infect Dis 27: 581–584, 1995 ORIGINAL ARTICLE

Corynebacterium CDC Group JK (Corynebacterium jeikeium) Sepsis in Haematological Patients: A Report of Three Cases and a Systematic Literature Review

HANS VAN DER LELIE[1], MAURINE LEVERSTEIN-VAN HALL[2], MARC MERTENS[1], HENK C. T. VAN ZAANEN[1], RIEN H. J. VAN OERS[1], BER L. M. THOMAS[1], ALBERT E. G. Kr. VON DEM BORNE[1] and ED J. KUIJPER[2]

From the Department of [1]Internal Medicine, Division of Haematology, and [2]Medical Microbiology, Academic Medical Centre, University of Amsterdam, Amsterdam, The Netherlands

We describe 3 patients with Corynebacterium jeikeium sepsis in neutropenic phase during treatment for acute myeloid leukaemia. Fever was the first symptom. All had a central venous catheter which was removed. Two patients developed subcutaneous nodules containing pus when the neutrophil count recovered; 1 had intracutaneous and pulmonary lesions. They were treated with vancomycin and recovered when the neutrophil count started to rise. A review of 80 neutropenic patients with C. jeikeium sepsis reported in the literature, together with our 3 cases indicates that risk factors for infection are the presence of a central venous catheter, being an adult male or postmenopausal female, profound and prolonged neutropenia and exposure to multiple antibiotics. Skin lesions are reported in 48% and pulmonary lesions in 36% of the patients. The overall mortality is 34% but in patients with recovery of the bone marrow only 5%. Therefore haematopoietic growth factors should be considered in neutropenic patients with C. jeikeium infection.

H. van der Lelie, MD, Academic Medical Centre, University of Amsterdam, Department of Internal Medicine, Division of Haematology, Box 22700, NL-1100 DE Amsterdam, The Netherlands

INTRODUCTION

In 1976 Hande et al. (1) described severe sepsis with a new species of corynebacterium, highly resistant to multiple antibiotics in 3 haematological patients with profound neutropenia and in a patient with a ventricular CSF shunt. Additional cases were described in haematological patients with severe neutropenia (2) and patients undergoing allogenic bone marrow transplantation (3). In 1979 this pathogen was further characterized by the CDC in Atlanta and designated as group JK (4), after Johnson and Kaye, who had earlier reported serious infections with corynebacteriae (5). Later this was changed to corynebacterium jeikeium (6). After the first reports an increasing number of other cases had been published (7–16). We describe 3 new patients and by reviewing the cases published sofar give a further clinical characterization of this serious infection.

CASE REPORTS

Patient 1, a 71-year-old female was admitted in 1987 with a newly diagnosed AML type M1. After introduction of a central venous catheter (CVC), she started treatment with mitoxantrone and cytarabine. As infection prophylaxis she received ciprofloxacin and ketoconazole. She was nursed in a single room with simple reversed isolation. The clinical course was uneventful until 19 days after the start of the chemotherapy, when she developed a temperature of 39.9°C. Blood pressure was normal and physical examination revealed no abnormalities. There were no pulmonary symptons and the chest X-ray was normal. The neutrophil count at that time was $0.1 \times 10^9/l$. Blood cultures revealed growth of C. jeikeium, which was also isolated from a subcutaneous nodule of 2×2 cm that became apparent 2 days after the beginning of the fever. She was treated with vancomycin 500 mg q.i.d. for 10 days. C. jeikeium could not be isolated from the CVC, removed after 5 days of treatment with vancomycin. There were no local signs of infection at the entry side of the CVC. One week after the start of the fever she had bone marrow recovery and a complete remission was documented by bone marrow examination. At this time she started to develop multiple subcutaneous nodules on her shoulder, back, groin, forehead, buttocks and knee, all about 2×2 cm. There were little or no local signs of inflammation and the nodules were not painful. During the next 2 weeks 12 nodules were drained. They contained pus, but no micro-organisms were detected in the Gram stain and cultures remained sterile. Because of persisting fever and the development of the nodules the treatment with vancomycin was resumed and continued until 6 weeks after the first signs of the infection. Ten and 18 days after discontinuation of treatment with vancomycin 2 final nodules were drained, which also appeared to be sterile. Relapses of the AML after 0.5, 1.5 and 2 years were treated with intensive chemotherapy without infectious complications. After the last relapse no complete remission could be obtained and she died of leukaemia.

Patient 2, a 55-year-old man was admitted in 1992 with a newly diagnosed AML M6. After introduction of a CVC he started treatment with daunorubicin and cytarabin. As infection prophylaxis he received oral amphotericin B and ciprofloxacin and intravenous penicillin G, the latter to prevent streptococcal infection. He was nursed in a single room with simple reversed isolation. On

 ISSN 0036-5548

Table I. *Characteristics of Corynebacterium jeikeium sepsis in haematological patients*

Author, year	n	Male	Skin lesions	Pulmonary lesions	Infection related mortality	Mortality in patients with BM recovery
Hande, 1976	3	3	2/3	3/3	3/3	0/3
Pearson, 1977	12	9	3/12	3/12	4/12	nd
Stamm, 1979	32	26	nd	nd	10/32	2/24[a]
Hoffman, 1983	1	1	0/1	0/1	1/1	0/1
Downie, 1984	1	0	nd	nd	1/1	0/1
Riebel, 1986	5	2	nd	nd	3/5	nd
Guarino, 1987	1	1	1/1	1/1	0/1	0/1
Jerdan, 1987	1	1	1/1	0/1	0/1	0/1
Telander, 1988	2	0	1/2	0/2	2/2	0/2
Dan, 1988	1	1	1/1	0/1	0/1	0/1
Waters, 1989	1	0	0/1	1/1	1/1	0/1
Rozdzinski, 1991	19	13	nd	nd	3/19	nd
Orrett, 1993	1	0	nd	nd	0/1	0/1
Present study	3	2	3/3	1/3	0/3	0/3
Pooled	83	59 (71%)	12/25 (48%)	9/25 (36%)	28/83 (34%)	2/39 (5%)

nd: no details given; [a] no details for the other 8 patients; only 3 patients (4%) were younger than 16 years of age; a CVC was present in 64 of 65 patients where this information was given. All patients had low neutrophil counts (usually below 0.5×10^9/l).

day 13 after the start of the chemotherapy he started to develop fever till 38.9°C. At physical examination there were no abnormalities, the blood pressure and the chest X-ray were normal. The neutrophil count at that time was 0.1×10^9/l. Blood cultures were positive for C. jeikeium and he was treated with vancomycin q.i.d. The tip of the CVC, which was removed after 6 days of treatment with vancomycin was sterile. There were no clinical signs of infection at the entry side of the CVC. Ten days after the first symptoms of infection there was bone marrow recovery and the temperature normalised. At that time a subcutaneous nodule of 2 × 2 cm became apparent on his shoulder. It was not painful and there were no local signs of infection. Yet, at drainage it contained pus and culture yielded C. jeikeium despite 15 days treatment with vancomycin. For that reason rifampicin was added to the treatment for 14 days. An echocardiogram showed no valvular abnormalities. No new nodules developed. Three weeks after the first signs of infection the vancomycin was stopped and the patient was discharged and treated as an out patient for 3 more weeks with once daily 200 mg teicoplanin. Thereafter he received 2 intensive chemotherapy cycles as consolidation, without infectious complications, despite persistent colonization with C. jeikeium in the axilla and groin. During the neutropenic phases he received vancomycin prophylactically.

Patient 3, a 53-year-old man was admitted in 1994 with a newly diagnosed AML M5. On admission he had pulmonary infiltrates and Staphyloccus aureus was cultured from his sputum. He was successfully treated with flucloxacillin. After placement of a CVC he was treated with daunorubicin and cytarabin. As infection prophylaxis he received oral amphotericin B and ciprofloxacin; flucloxacillin was replaced by cephalotin as prophylaxis against further Gram positive infections. He was nursed in a single room with simple reverse isolation. 19 days after the start of the chemotherapy he developed temperature of 40.2°C. Vancomycin q.i.d. was given instead of cephalotin after blood cultures had been taken. Initially there was no response to this treatment. He started to develop multiple sub- and intracutaneous nodules. Furthermore he became progressively dyspnoic with multiple nodular infiltrates on the chest X-ray. The CVC was removed. Blood cultures and the tip of the CVC showed growth of C. jeikeium. Eight days after the beginning of the fever all symptoms started to clear, concomitantly with recovery of the bone marrow. He appeared to be in complete remission. He received a cycle of consolidation chemotherapy, using vancomycin as prophylaxis. There were no infectious complications, despite the fact of persistent positive surveillance cultures for C. jeikeium taken from groin and axilla.

Microbiological characterization

Blood cultures from the 3 patients contained Gram-positive coccobacillary rods resembling streptococci. Subcultures onto non-serum containing media and all anaerobic subcultures remained negative, whereas slow growing, non-haemolytic grey colonies with a glistening metallic sheen were visible on blood agar plates after 3 days of incubation at 37°C in a CO_2 rich environment. The bacteria were identified as C. jeikeium on the basis of its inability to reduce nitrate, to hydrolyse esculin, to ferment sucrose, mannitol, and xylose and on the basis of its capacity to ferment glucose and maltose (17). Using a disk-diffusion assay, all isolates were resistant to penicillin, cephalotin, gentamicin erythromycin, lincomycin, ciprofloxacin and susceptible to vancomycin, fusidic acid, tetracyclin and rifampicin.

Systematic literature review

By a CDROM Medline literature search from 1976 till 1995 we selected all clinical studies on sepsis by C. jeikeium in haematological patients. Descriptions of 80 patients were found of which 63 came from 3 studies (2, 3, 15). Recorded were age, sex, neutrophil count, underlying disease, presence of a CVC and skin and pulmonary lesions, infection related mortality, overall and in relation to bone marrow recovery. Detailed information on all items could not be found from all patients. Results including data from our patients are summarised in Table I. 71% of the patients were male and only 4% below the age of 16. In great majority they had severe neutropenia and nearly all had been treated with intensive chemotherapy. 38 patients underwent a bone marrow transplantation. The others were treated for acute leukaemia or CML blast crisis (39 patients), lymphoma (4 patients) and multiple myeloma or aplastic anaemia (each 1 patient). In 98% of patients where this information was given, a CVC was present. Skin lesions were described in 48%, pulmonary lesions in 36%. Infection related mortality was high: 34%, however in patients who had recovery of their bone marrow this was only 5%.

DISCUSSION

Serious infections caused by C. jeikeium are found in haematologic patients with severe neutropenia (1–3, 7–16), patients with prosthetic heart valve endocarditis (18, 19), infected ventricular CSF shunts (1, 9, 20–22), CAPD patients with peritonitis (9, 23, 24) and patients with major traumata and surgery with complications (9, 25). We describe 3 new cases of sepsis by C. jeikeium in patients with severe neutropenia after treatment with intensive chemotherapy for AML. Fever was the first symptom in all 3 and all had a very low neutrophil count. The first 2 patients developed subcutaneous nodules concomitantly with, and probably related to neutrophil recovery. The other patient had intracutaneous lesions. Skin lesions are reported in almost half of the neutropenic patients with C. jeikeium sepsis, but not in the other patient categories with this infection (18–25). Local skin infections may also occur at sites where the skin is disrupted as for instance after a bone marrow biopsy (13). Pulmonary lesions as in one of our patients are reported in about one third. The mortality rate of the infection in neutropenic patients is high. Bone marrow recovery appears to be very important for a favourable outcome. Yet, C. jeikeium per se seems not to be a very aggressive pathogen: in patients with infected ventricular CSF shunts and CAPD peritonitis there was no mortality and in most the infection could be easily treated (20–24).

C. jeikeium appears to exist as part of the normal skin flora of both patients and healthy persons. Colonization of the skin was found in 20–51% of hospitalized patients (3, 12, 26–29), 20% in chronic care institutions (29) and 0%–36% of hospital workers (3, 12, 27, 28). During an outbreak of C. jeikeium infection, in 4 out of 13 nurses and doctors handwashings were found positive for C. jeikeium (27). Transmission from patient to patient and spread through healthcare workers were held responsible for this outbreak. A strict hygiene program has been shown to substantially reduce the number of colonizations and infections with C. jeikeium (30). The reduced sensitivity of C. jeikeium to antiseptics such as cetrimide, propamide and ethidium bromide when compared to other coryneforms, is probably also of influence for nosocomial spread in hospitals (31). With restriction endonuclease analysis of bacterial DNA it has been found that strains obtained from different patients were heterogeneous, whereas in individual patients the same strain could be demonstrated over prolonged periods of time (32). This suggests that patient to patient transmission does not occur. However using a ribosomal RNA gene probe Pitcher et al. come to opposite findings (33). Our 3 patients were isolated cases of C. jeikeium infection.

Body sites most commonly positive in case of colonization are the groin, axilla and rectum (3, 26, 29). Colonization is predominantly found in adult men and postmenopausal women. This might be related to the skin sebum production under influence of sex hormones and the lipid requirement for growth of C. jeikeium (3). Infection in children is rare.

Risk factors for colonization further are neutropenia, prolonged hospital stay and exposure to multiple antibiotics (3, 27). However there are also patients who are already colonized on admission (3, 26). Apparently only a very small number of colonized patients develops sepsis. Our patients 2 and 3 remained colonized during their next cycles of chemotherapy without infection. The most important risk factor for infection in colonized patients is the presence of a device such as a CVC, ventricular CSF shunt, CAPD catheter or prosthetic heart valve. 98% of the neutropenic patients from whom the information was available had a CVC inserted. Further risk factors are the same as for colonization: being an adult male or postmenopausal female, prolonged and severe neutropenia and exposure to multiple antibiotics.

The diagnosis in neutropenic patients is made by culturing C. jeikeium from the blood. The characterization with biochemical reactions and antibiotic susceptibility patterns in 1979 (4), resulted in a practical phenotypical identification, despite a considerable genomic diversity at the species level (34). Antimicrobial susceptibilities cannot be used as a major criterion for the identification of C. jeikeium. Other multiple resistant coryneforms have been found and not all C. jeikeium strains are multiple resistant.

Vancomycin is the treatment of choice. It is not known whether combination with rifampicin (in case the micro-organism is sensitive) as we did in our second patient, offers an advantage. Usually it is advised to remove the CVC immediately. Because bone marrow recovery is so important for a favourable outcome the use of haematopoietic growth factors should be considered. There are no firm data on how long to continue treatment. In any case treatment should be continued until bone marrow recovery.

The only proven effective way to prevent colonization and subsequent infection with C. jeikeium, are hygienic measures such as careful handwashing and the use of povidone-iodine impregnated scrub sponges (30). Though in vitro a good bactericidal activity of ciprofloxacin on C. jeikeium has been found (35), it did not prevent the infection in our 3 patients, who all had received ciprofloxacin prophylactically.

C. jeikeium is not susceptible to the commonly used local antibiotic mupirocin (36). In cases of an outbreak prophylactic vancomycin in colonized patients can be considered, but is today a less attractive option because of an increasing number of reports on vancomycin resistant enterococci causing serious infection.

REFERENCES

1. Hande KR, Witebski FG, Brown MS, Schulman CB, Anderson SE, Levine AS, MacLowry JD, Chabner BA. Sepsis with a new species of Corynebacterium. Ann Int Med 85: 423–426, 1976.
2. Pearson TA, Braine HG, Rathbun HK. Corynebacterium sepsis in oncology patients. JAMA 238: 1737–1740, 1977.
3. Stamm WE, Tompkins LS, Wagner KF, Counts GW, Thomas ED, Meyers JD. Infections due to Corynebacterium species in marrow transplant patients. Ann Int Med 91: 167–173, 1979.
4. Riley PS, Hollis DG, Utter GB, Weaver RE, Baker CN. Characterization and identification of 95 diphtheroid (group JK) cultures isolated from clinical specimens. J Clin Microbiol 9: 418–424, 1979.
5. Johnson WD, Kaye D. Serious infections caused by diphtheroids. Ann NY Acad Sci 174: 568–576, 1970.
6. Jackman PJH, Pitcher DG, Pelczynska S, Borman P. Classification of corynbacteria associated with endocarditis (group JK) as Corynebacterium jeikeium sp. nov. Syst Appl Microbiol 9: 83–90, 1987.
7. Hoffmann S, Ersgaard H, Justesen T, Friis H. Fatal meningitis with group JK Corynebacterium in a leucopenic patient. Eur J Clin Microbiol 2: 213–215, 1983.
8. Downie GW, Gill DS. Infection in an immunocompromised patient caused by 'group JK' Corynebacterium. J Infect 8: 262–263, 1984.
9. Riebel W, Frantz N, Adelstein D, Spagnuolo PJ. Corynebacterium JK: a cause of nosocomial device-related infection. Rev Infect Dis 8: 42–49, 1986.
10. Guarino MJ, Qazi R, Woll JE, Rubins J. Septicemia, rash, and pulmonary infiltrates secondary to corynebacterium group JK infection. Am J Med 82: 132–134, 1987.
11. Jerdan MS, Shapiro RS, Smith NB, Virshup DM, Hood AF. Cutaneous manifestations of Corynebacterium JK sepsis. J Am Acad Dermatol 16: 444–447, 1987.
12 Telander B, Lerner R, Palmbald J, Ringertz O. Corynebacterium group JK in a haematological ward: infections, colonization and environmental contamination. Scand J Infect Dis 20: 55–61, 1988.
13. Dan M, Somer I, Knobel B, Gutman R. Cutaneous manifestations of infection with Corynebacterium group JK. Rev Infect Dis 10: 1204–1207, 1988.
14. Waters BL. Pathology of culture proven JK corynebacterium pneumonia. An autopsy case report. Am J Clin Pathol 91: 616–619, 1989.
15. Rozdzinski E, Kern W, Schmeiser T, Kurrle E. Corynebacterium jeikeium bacteremia at a tertiary care centre. Infection 19: 201–204, 1991.
16. Orrett FA, Fosi-Mbantenkhu JM. Corynebacterium jeikeium infection in Trinidad. J Hosp Infect 24: 327–329, 1993.
17. Krech T, Hollis DG. Corynebacterium and related organisms. In: Balows A, Hausler WJ, Herrmann KL, Isenberg HD, Shadomy HJ eds. Manual of clinical microbiology, fifth ed. ASM, Washington DC, 277–286, 1991.
18. Van Scoy RE, Cohen SN, Geraci JE, Washington JA. Coryneform bacterial endocarditis. Difficulties in diagnosis and treatment, presentation of three cases and a review of the literature. Mayo Clin Proc 52: 216–219, 1977.
19. Murray BE, Karchmer AW, Moellering RC. Diphteroid prosthetic valve endocarditis. A study of clinical features and infecting organisms. Am J Med 69: 838–847, 1980.
20. Allen KD, Green HT. Infections due to a 'Group JK' corynebacterium. J Infect 13: 41–44, 1986.
21. Morrison VA, Weishel EL, Luikart SD. Corynebacterium JK: a new pathogen in ventriculostomy infection. J Neurooncol 11: 65–69, 1991.
22. Greene KA, Clark RJ, Zambramski JM. Ventricular CSF shunt infections associated with Corynebacterium jeikeium: report of three cases and review. Clin Infect Dis 16: 139–141, 1993.
23. Pierard D, Lauwers S, Mouton MC, Sennesael J, Verbeelen D. Group JK corynebacterium peritonitis in a patient undergoing continuous ambulatory peritoneal dialysis. J Clin Microbiol 18: 1011–1014, 1983.
24. Altwegg M, Zaruba K, Von Graevenitz A. Corynebacterium group JK peritonitis in patients on continuous ambulatory peritoneal dialysis. Klin Wochenschrift 62: 793–794, 1984.
25. Wirsing von König CH, Drechsler HJ, Wichmann S, Finger H. Corynebakterien der JK-Gruppe als Sepsiserreger. Klin Wochenschrift 60: 263–264, 1982.
26. Gill VJ, Manning C, Lamson M, Woltering P, Pizzo PA. Antibiotic-resistant group JK bacteria in hospitals. J Clin Microbiol 13: 472–477, 1981.
27. Quinn JP, Arnow PM, Weil D, Rosenbluth J. Outbreak of JK diphtheroid infections associated with envioromental contamination. J Clin Microbiol 19: 668–671, 1984.
28. Wichmann S, Wirsing von König CH, Becker-Boost E, Finger H. Group JK corynebacteria in skin flora of healthy persons and patients. Eur J Clin Microbiol 4: 502–504, 1985.
29. Soriano F, Rodriguez-Tudela JL, Fernández-Roblas R, Aguado JM, Santamaria M. Skin colonization by corynebacterium groups D2 and JK in hospitalized patients. J Clin Microbiol 26: 1878–1880, 1988.
30. Eagan JA, Blevins A, Armstrong D. Prevention of skin colonization and subsequent bacteremia with CDC-JK organisms in patients with cancer. Cancer Practice 1: 325–328, 1993.
31. Lewis R Antiseptic resistance in JK and other coryneforms. J Hosp Infect 11: 150–154, 1988.
32. Khabaz RF, Kaper JB, Moody MR, Schimpff SC, Tenney JH. Molecular epidemiology of group JK Corynebacterium on a cancer ward: lack of evidence for patient-to-patient transmission. J Infect Dis 154: 95–99, 1986.
33. Pitcher D, Johnson A, Allerberger F, Woodford N, George R. An investigation of nosocomial infection with Corynebacterium jeikeium in surgical patients using a ribosomal RNA gene probe. Eur J Clin Microbiol Infect Dis 9: 643–648, 1990.
34. Riegel P, De Briel D, Prévost G, Jehl F, Monteil H. Genomic diversity among Corynebacterium jeikeium strains and comparison with biochemical characteristics and antimicrobial susceptibilities. J Clin Microbiol 32: 1860–1865, 1994.
35. Venezio FR, Tatarowicz W, Divincenzo CA, O'Keefe JP. Activity of ciprofloxacin against multiply resistant strains of Pseudomonas aeruginosa, Staphylococcus epidermidis, and group JK corynebacteria. Antimicrob Agents Chemother 30: 940–941, 1986.
36. Dealler SF. In-vitro activity of LY 146032 daptomycin and other agents against JK diphtheroids. J Antimicrob Chemoth 21: 807–808, 1988.

Submitted July 3, 1995; accepted September 12, 1995

Scand J Infect Dis 27: 585–588, 1995 ORIGINAL ARTICLE

Restriction Fragment Length Polymorphisms (RFLP) of Cholera Toxin Genes in Vibrio cholerae O139 Recovered from Patients in Thailand, India and Bangladesh

ANDERS DALSGAARD[1], ORALAK SERICHANTALERGS[2] and PETER ECHEVERRIA[2]

From the [1]Department of Veterinary Microbiology, The Royal Veterinary and Agricultural University, Frederiksberg, Denmark, and the [2]Armed Forces Research Institute of Medical Sciences, Bangkok, Thailand

Since its first appearance in 1992, Vibrio cholerae O139 has caused large epidemics of a cholera-like disease in India and Bangladesh and has subsequently spread to several neighboring countries. We characterized and compared 56 V. cholerae O139 isolates recovered from patients in Thailand, India and Bangladesh by analyzing restriction fragment length polymorphisms (RFLP) of their *ctx* genes. The strains comprised 9 different *BglI* cleavage patterns of *ctx* genes (CT genotypes) and contained 1–4 gene copies. A total of 6 different CT genotypes were found among the 52 Thai isolates studied whereas the 2 Indian isolates and 1 isolate from Bangladesh all showed unique CT genotypes. The molecular analysis of *ctx* genes appeared superior to ribotyping for subspecies differentiation of O139 strains since ribotyping revealed 3 different *BglI* ribotypes. In addition, no correlation was found between the two methods. The molecular analysis of virulence determinants such as ctx genes in combination with other molecular techniques appears to be promising for the study of genetic changes within V. cholerae O139.

A. Dalsgaard, DVM, Department of Veterinary Microbiology, The Royal Veterinary and Agricultural University, DK-1870 Frederiksberg C, Denmark

INTRODUCTION

In October 1992, and outbreak of a cholera-like disease caused by a non-O1 strain of Vibrio cholerae occurred in Madras, India and subsequently spread rapidly throughout India (1) and Bangladesh (2). The new non-O1 strain of V. cholerae has been designated V. cholerae O139 synonym Bengal (3), and in 1993 this strain was identified for the first time in Thailand (4).

Like V. cholerae serogroup O1 strains, O139 isolates can cause an acute secretory diarrhea and, unlike most other V. cholerae non-O1 strains, produce cholera toxin (CT) (5–7). As reported for V. cholerae O1 biotype E1 Tor, serogroup O139 strains have *ctx* (cholera toxin), *zot* (zonula occludens toxin) (8), *ace* (accessory cholera enterotoxin) (9), and RS1 (repeated sequences) (10) elements organized in virulence gene complexes (11). Molecular techniques have been applied to differentiate V. cholerae O139 strains with varying degree of success. Faruque et al. (12) compared the restriction fragment length polymorphisms (RFLP) of *ctx*A and rRNA genes of 29 V. cholerae O139 isolates from Bangladesh and India and found that the isolates comprised 2 cholera toxin genotypes and that they all belonged to a single ribotype. Pulsed field gel electrophoresis (PFGE) of *Not*I-digested DNA of 9 V. cholerae O139 strains, isolated in India, revealed identical profiles, as did Southern blot hybridization of *Not*I-digested DNA with a cholera toxin probe (13). We recently found 4 different *Bgl*I ribotypes among 49 V. cholerae O139 strains isolated in Bangladesh, India and Thailand (14). In short, previously applied molecular techniques have proved only limited discrimination between V. cholerae O139 strains. Therefore, additional methods are needed for successful monitoring of the spread of V. cholerae O139.

The objective of the study was to characterize and compare 56 V. cholerae O139 isolates recovered from patients in Thailand, India, and Bangladesh by analyzing RFLPs of their *ctx* genes. In addition, the RFLPs were compared to *Bgl*I ribotypes peviously reported.

MATERIALS AND METHODS

A total of 56 O139 V. cholerae isolates recovered from patients in Thailand (52 isolates), Inida (2 isolates), and Bangladesh (2 isolates), were studied (Table I). The characterization and identification of all the V. cholerae O139 isolates have been described previously (14). All the strains were shown to contain sequences for the O139 virulence gene complex in colony hybridization studies, except strains NG 288/36 and NG 653/36 which did agglutinate in O139 specific antisera.

The RFLPs of the *ctx* genes were studied by Southern blot analysis of *Bgl*I-digested chromosomal DNA with a radioactive CT probe. *Bgl*I has previously been successfully used in Southern blot analysis of O139 isolates from Bangladesh and India (12). The CT probe consisted of a 950 base-pair fragment of an *Xba*I/*Hind*II digest of plasmid DNA isolated from E. coli MS 371 pJM17 (15), and was labelled with 10^6 cpm of α-^{32}P by the random priming method (16). Prehybridization and hybridization reactions were performed under stringent hybridization conditions essentially as described by Hanchalay et al. (17). Nylon membranes (Hybond-N+, Amersham, UK) were autoradiographed using Kodak X-OMAT film (Kodak, Rochester, NY). CT genotypes were given arbitrary numbers based on differences in the numbers and electrophoretic mobilities of fragments generated in the Southern blot analysis.

Studies were repeated for 18 isolates using new DNA extracts. In addition, all isolates included in Fig. 1 were studied following 9

Table *1. Cholera toxin genotypes and BglI ribotypes of 56 V. cholerae O139 isolates*

Isolate	Country	Ribotype[a]	CT genotype[a]
IPD 694	Thailand	3	1
NG 492/36	Thailand	1	1
NG 493/36	Thailand	1	1
VC 4220/36	Thailand	1	1
ADC 1221/9	Thailand	1	1
ADC 1243/9	Thailand	1	1
ADC 1125/9	Thailand	1	1
ADC 1551/8	Thailand	1	1
NG 465/36	Thailand	2	1
SPH 895	Thailand	1	2
ADC 1221/9	Thailand	1	2
ADC 1243	Thailand	1	2
NG 469/36	Thailand	1	2
NG 482/36	Thailand	1	2
NG 483/36	Thailand	1	2
NG 487/36	Thailand	1	2
NG 488/36	Thailand	1	2
NG 489/36	Thailand	1	2
NG 481/36	Thailand	3	2
NIH 178	Thailand	3	2
NG 486/36	Thailand	1	2
A 4450	Bangladesh	1	2
NG 368/36	Thailand	3	2
ADC 711/9	Thailand	1	2
ADC 753/9	Thailand	1	2
ADC 910/9	Thailand	1	2
ADC 987/9	Thailand	1	2
ADC 995/9	Thailand	1	2
ADC 1095/9	Thailand	1	2
ADC 1115/9	Thailand	1	2
ADC 1207/9	Thailand	1	2
ADC 573/9	Thailand	1	2
ADC 856/9	Thailand	2	2
NG 377/36	Thailand	3	3
NG 392/36	Thailand	3	3
NG 408/36	Thailand	3	3
V 39	Thailand	3	3
ADC 2039/6	Thailand	3	3
ADC 978/6	Thailand	3	3
ADC 700/7	Thailand	3	3
ADC 498/7	Thailand	3	3
ADC 1/7	Thailand	3	3
IPD 935	Thailand	3	3
ADC 820/7	Thailand	3	3
ADC 225/8	Thailand	3	4
IPD 60	Thailand	3	4
ADC 373/9	Thailand	1	4
AD 2441	Thailand	3	4
IPD 58	Thailand	3	5
IPD 145	Thailand	3	5
MO10	India	1	6
MO45	India	1	7
IPD 440	Thailand	1	8
A-1-1841	Bangladesh	1	9
NG 288/36	Thailand	4	[b]
NG 653/36	Thailand	7	[b]

[a] Ribotypes and CT (cholera toxin) genotypes were established on *BglI* restriction patterns.

[b] No hybridization with the CT probe.

months' storage at −70°C and 5 subsequent subcultures of the isolates on tryptic soy agar (Difco, Detroit, Michigan, USA).

RESULTS

Southern blot analysis of *BglI*-digested chromosomal DNA revealed 9 different cleavage patterns of the *ctx* genes among the 56 V. cholerae O139 isolates studied. V. cholerae O139 strains NG 288/36 and NG 653/36 did not contain sequences which hybridized with the CT probe. The restriction patterns consisted of 1–4 fragments ranging from 3.2 to 12.0 kb in size. Examples of the different cleavage patterns and a schematic presentation of all the patterns are shown in Figs 1 and 2, respectively. A total of 6 different CT genotypes were present among 52 Thai isolates which previously have been shown to comprise 3 different ribotypes. Strains belonging to ribotype 3, which was previously found to be unique for Thai isolates compared to ribotypes of strains from India and Bangladesh, could be further differentiated into 5 different CT genotypes. The 2 Indian strains, MO10, and MO45, represented 2 unique genotypes 6 and 7, respectively, and strain A-1-1841 from Bangladesh belonged to a unique genotype 9. Strain A 4450 from Bangladesh belonged to genotype 2 which also contained 23 of the Thai isolates. Ribotyping showed the presence of 3 different patterns among the 54 isolates containing the virulence gene complex whereas molecular analysis of *ctx* genes exhibited 9 different CT genotypes (Table I). Strains of ribotype 1 belonged to one of 6 CT genotypes (CT types 1, 2, 4, 6, 7, 8, or 9, respectively) whereas CT genotype 2 was found among ribotypes 1, 2, and 3 strains. Hence no correlation was shown between *BglI* ribotypes and CT genotypes. Strains NG 288/36 and NG 653/36 both exhibited unique ribotypes. Furthermore, there was no correlation between CT genotypes and the origin of the Thai isolates.

Repeated studies of 18 isolates and all the isolates included in Fig. 1 showed no variation in the distribution of fragments. However, isolates belonging to CT genotype 1 showed an additional fragment of 6.4 kb in size, whereas isolates belonging to CT genotypes 3 and 4 all showed a double fragment of sizes 7.1 kb and 7.4 kb, respectively. These variations were apparently associated with variations in DNA concentrations, the amount of ^{32}P-labelled CT probe used, and the exposure time of nylon membranes to the Kodak X-OMAT film.

DISCUSSION

The copy number and organization of *ctx* genes within V. cholerae O139 have been disputed in recent reports. Using an oligonucleotide probe against *ctx*, in Southern blot analysis of DNA from 12 O139 isolates from patients in Bangladesh and India, Iida et al. (18) found 5 *PstI* RFLP patterns among 11 isolates containing 2 *ctx* copies and 1 isolate containing 1 copy, respectively. Das et al. (19)

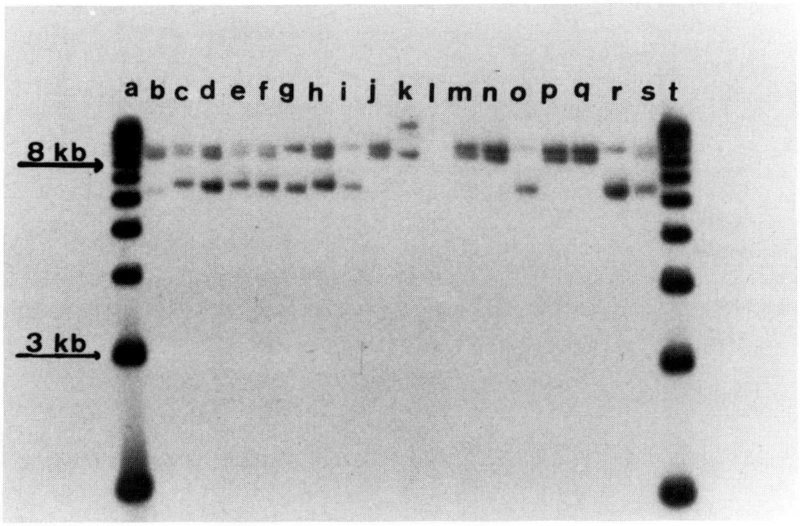

Fig. 1. Examples of Southern blot analysis of chromosomal DNA from V. cholerae O139 digested with *BglI* and hybridized with a CT probe. Lanes: a, 1 Kb DNA ladder; b, strain ADC 1/7, CT genotype 3; c, strain ADC 498/7, type 3; d, strain ADC 700/7 type 3; e, strain ADC 987/6, type 3; f, strain ADC 2039/6, type 3; g, strain AD 2441, type 4; h, strain IPD 935, type 3; i, strain ADC 373/9, type 4; j, strain ADC 1551/8, type 1; k, strain A-1-1841, type 9; l, strain NG 653/36, no CT genotype; m, strain NG 465/36, type 1; n, strain ADC 1125/9, type 1; o, strain IPD 60, type 4; p, strain ADC 1243/9, type 1; q, strain ADC 1221/9, type 1; r, strain ADC 225/8, type 4; s, strain ADC 820/7, type 3; t, 1 Kb DNA ladder.

concluded that O139 carries at least 10 *ctx* copies. Southern blot hybridization of *NotI*-digested genomic DNA, with *ctx* as probe, of 9 V. cholerae O139 isolates from different parts of India, revealed that most O139 strains contained 2 copies of *ctx* in tandem and exhibited no RFLP (13). In addition, Popovic et al. (20) found 2 *BglI* ribotypes and 4 very similar *NotI* PFGE patterns among 20 isolates from Bangladesh and India. Based on the data presented here, RFLP of *ctx* genes, using restriction enzyme *BglI*, was superior to ribotyping for subspecies differentiation of V. cholerae O139, since molecular analysis of *ctx* genes revealed 9 different CT genotypes whereas ribotyping showed 3 different *BglI* ribotypes only. Studies of 4 strains from Bangladesh and India presented 3 unique CT genotypes which were not seen among any of the Thai strains. Cholera toxin genotypes were demonstrated to be stable after prolonged culture. However, in repeated studies, the CT genotype patterns showed some variation in band intensity.

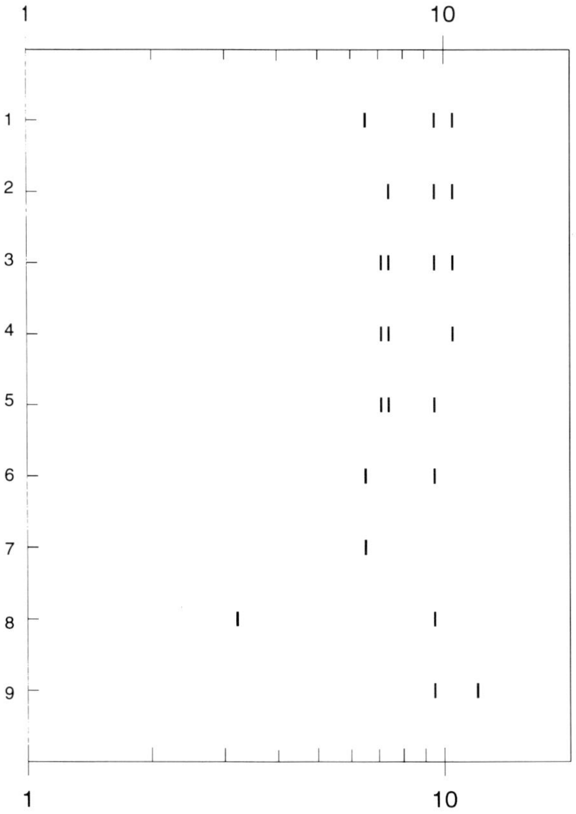

Fig. 2. Schematic presentation of 9 cholera toxin genotypes (CT genotypes) shown among 56 V. cholerae O139 strains by Southern blot hybridization of *BglI*-digested chromosomal DNA with a cholera toxin probe. CT genotype designations are indicated at the far left and molecular sizes are shown by numbers at the top and at the bottom.

Wachsmuth et al. (21) suggested that the origin of toxigenic US Gulf Coast V. cholerae O1 biotype El Tor strains was due to the transformation of a non-toxigenic V. cholerae strain by the acquisition of toxin genes. Thus, our previous description of 2 O139 strains, NG 288/36 and NG 653/36, which did not contain the virulence gene complex is interesting and should be studied further.

The results of the present study provide further evidence that V. cholerae O139 strains exhibit genetic polymorphisms and are not strictly clonal in origin (12). It is likely that the differences in CT genotypes and *BglI* ribotypes among V. cholerae O139 isolates in Thailand reflect random mutations that have occurred as the epidemic has spread. The Thai strains included in this study were isolated less than 1 year after serogroup O139 was first identified in Thailand (4). Olsvik et al. (22) reported that sequence conservation among *ctx* genes from different strains of V. cholerae O1 is relatively high. The molecular analysis of virulence determinants in combination with ribotyping, PFGE, and (PCR) polymerase chain reactions appears to be promising for the study of the molecular epidemiology of V. cholerae O139. We are currently applying the PFGE technique to study the genetic polymorphisms of O139.

ACKNOWLEDGEMENTS

We are grateful for the technical assistance of Chittima Pitarangsi, Apichai Srijan, and Pranee Ratarasarn of the Armed Forces Research Institute of Medical Sciences, Bangkok. In Denmark, the technical assistance of Mr Lasse Smidt is greatly appreciated. This study was supported by the Plasmid Foundation and by a grant to A. Dalsgaard from the Danish Council for Development Research, Danida (Danish International Development Assistance), Fellowship no. 104.8/553.

REFERENCES

1. Ramamurthy T, Garg S, Sharma R, Bhatacharya SK, Nair GB, Shimada T, Takeda T, Karasawa T, Kurazanu H, Pal A, Takeda Y. Emergence of novel strain of Vibrio cholerae with epidemic potential in southern and eastern India. Lancet 341: 703–704, 1993.
2. Richardson S. A disease in resurgence. Science 260: 832, 1993.
3. Shimada T, Nair GB, Deb BC, Albert MJ, Sack RB. Outbreak of Vibrio cholerae non-O1 in India and Bangladesh. Lancet 341: 1347, 1993.
4. Chongsa-nguan M, Chaicumpa W, Moolasart P, Kandhasingha P, Shimada T, Kurazanu H, Takeda Y. Vibrio cholerae O139 Bengal in Bangkok. Lancet 342: 430–431, 1993.
5. Albert MJ, Siddique AK, Islam MS, Faruque ASG, Ansaruzzaman M, Faruque SM, Sack RB. Large outbreak of clinical cholera due to Vibrio cholerae non-O1 in Bangladesh. Lancet 341: 704–705, 1993.
6. Mandal BK. Epidemic cholera due to a novel strain of V. cholerae non-O1 – the beginning of a new pandemic? J Infect 27: 115–117, 1993.
7. Janda JM, Powers C, Bryant RG, Abbott SL. Current perspective on the epidemiology and pathogenesis of clinically significant Vibrio spp. Clin Microbiol Rev 1: 245–267, 1988.
8. Baudry BA, Fasano A, Ketley J, Kaper JB. Cloning of a gene (*zot*) encoding a new toxin produced by Vibrio cholerae. Infect Immun 60: 428–434, 1992.
9. Trucksis M, Galen JE, Michalski J, Fasano A, Kaper JB. Accessory cholera enterotoxin (Ace), the third toxin of a Vibrio cholerae virulence cassette. Proc Natl Acad Sci USA 90: 5267–5271, 1993.
10. Goldberg I, Mekalanos J. Effect of a *rec*A mutation on cholera toxin gene amplification and deletion events. J Bacteriol 165: 723–731, 1986.
11. Johnson JA, Albert MJ, Panigrahi P, Wright AC, Joseph A, Comstock L, Trucksis M, Michalski J, Johnson RJ, Kaper JB, Morris JG. Non-O1 Vibrio cholerae (O139 synom. Bengal) from the India/Bangladesh epidemic are encapsulated [abstract]. 29th Joint Conference Cholera Related Diarrheal Dis, 1993.
12. Faruque SM, Abdul Alim RM, Roy SK, Khan R, Nair GB, Sack RB, Albert MJ. Molecular analysis of rRNA and cholera toxin genes carried by the new epidemic strain of toxigenic Vibrio cholerae O139 synonym Bengal. J Clin Microbiol 32: 1050–1053, 1994.
13. Bhadra RK, Choudhury SR, Das J. Vibrio cholerae O139 El Tor biotype. Lancet 343: 728, 1994.
14. Echeverria P, Hoge CW, Bodhidatta L, Serichantalergs O, Dalsgaard A, Eampokalap B, Perrault J, Pazzaglia G, O'Hanley P, English C. Molecular characterization of Vibrio cholerae O139 isolates from Asia. Am J Trop Med Hyg 52: 124–127, 1995.
15. Mekalanos J. Duplication and amplification of toxin genes in Vibrio cholerae. Cell 35: 253–263, 1983.
16. Sambrook J, Fritsch EF, Maniatis T. Molecular cloning: a laboratory manual. Cold Spring Harbor, New York: Cold Spring Harbor Laboratory, 1989.
17. Hanchalay S, Seriwatana J, Echeverria P, Holmgren J, Tirapat C, Moseley SL, Taylor DN. Non-O1 Vibrio cholerae in Thailand: homology with cloned cholera toxin genes. J Clin Microbiol 21: 288–289, 1985.
18. Iida T, Shrestha J, Yamamoto K, Honda T [letter]. Lancet 342: 926, 1993.
19. Das B, Ghosh RK, Sharma C, Vasin N, Ghosh A. Tandem repeats of cholera toxin gene in Vibrio cholerae O139. Lancet 342: 1174, 1993.
20. Popovic T, Fields PI, Olsvik Ö, Wells JG, Evins GM, Cameron DN, Wachsmuth RB, Stack RB, Albert JM, Balakrish N, Feeley JC [abstract]. 29th Joint Conference Cholera and Related Diarrheal Dis, 1993.
21. Wachsmuth IK, Evins GM, Fields PI, Olsvik Ö, Popovic T, Bopp CA, Wells JG, Carrillo C, Blake PA. The molecular epidemiology of cholera in Latin America. J Infect Dis 167; 621–626, 1993.
22. Olsvik Ö, Wahlberg J, Petterson B, Uhlén M, Popovic T, Wachsmuth IK, Fields PI. Use of automated sequencing of polymerase chain reaction-generated amplicons to identify three types of cholera toxin subunit B in Vibrio cholerae O1 strains. J Clin Microbiol 31: 22–25, 1993.

Submitted November 16, 1994; accepted August 25, 1995

Scand J Infect Dis 27: 589–593, 1995

ORIGINAL ARTICLE

Campylobacter jejuni/coli and Enterotoxigenic Eschericia coli (ETEC) in Faeces from Children and Adults in Tanzania

GUN-BRITT LINDBLOM[1], CHRISTINA ÅHRÉN[2], JOHN CHANGALUCHA[3], REVERIANUS GABONE[3], BERTIL KAIJSER[1], LARS-ÅKE NILSSON[2], EVA SJÖGREN[1], ANN-MARI SVENNERHOLM[2] and MANSUET TEMU[3]

From the Departments of [1]Clinical Bacteriology and [2]Medical Microbiology and Immunology, University of Göteborg, Göteborg, Sweden, and [3]National Institute for Medical Research, Mwanza Centre, Mwanza, Tanzania

The occurrence of Campylobacter and enterotoxigenic E. coli (ETEC) was studied in faecal samples from Tanzanian children (< 5 years of age), adolescents and adults (only Campylobacter) with and without diarrhoea. The Campylobacter strains isolated were tested for subspecies, enterotoxigenicity and serotype. Out of 394 children with diarrhoea 18% were infected with Campylobacter and 20% with ETEC. In 278 samples tested for Campylobacter and 136 tested for ETEC from asymptomatic children the corresponding numbers were 12 and 5%, respectively. In children < 18 months with diarrhoea Campylobacter was noted in 22% and ETEC in 18%, whereas the figures were 11 and 4% respectively in asymptomatic children. In the age group 18 months to 5 years Campylobacter was demonstrated in 2% of the children with diarrhoea and 27% had ETEC, while the figures were 15 and 8% for asymptomatic children. Among adults the prevalence of Campylobacter-positive samples was 1% both for symptomatic and asymptomatic individuals. There were no seasonal differences in the prevalences of both Campylobacter and ETEC either in the symptomatic or the asymptomatic group. Campylobacter jejuni was the dominating Campylobacter species among both symptomatic and asymptomatic individuals. C. jejuni strains from patients with diarrhoea were significantly more often enterotoxigenic than were C. coli strains. The serotype pattern regarding Campylobacter was in general similar for symptomatic and asymptomatic individuals. We conclude that Campylobacter and ETEC are common causes of bacterial diarrhoea in Tanzanian children, and that Campylobacter infections are more important in children younger than 18 months, than in older ones.

G.-B. Lindblom, MD, Department of Clinical Bacteriology, Göteborg University, Guldhedsgatan 10 A, S-413 46 Göteborg, Sweden

INTRODUCTION

Diarrhoeal diseases are among the leading causes of childhood morbidity and mortality in developing countries. Annually, at least 750 million of diarrhoeal episodes, with a calculated mortality of 4–5 million children, occur in these countries and it has been estimated that children spend 15–20% of their first 2 years of life being sick from diarrhoea (1). Furthermore, diarrhoeal diseases are often accompanied by other infections, e.g. measles, malaria, pneumonia and other acute respiratory infections.

In Tanzania, the annual reports of the Mwanza municipal hospital indicate that, diarrhoeal diseases are responsible for up to 40% of new attendances at the clinic and mortality among these patients has been reported to be as high as 18–20%. Diarrhoeal diseases have been ranked third after malaria and measles as the most important causes of morbidity in children below the age of 5 years. Data obtained from maternal and health clinics in endemic areas also indicate seasonal variations in the incidence and severity of diarrhoeal disease of childhood. Differences have been observed during the dry and wet seasons, with marked increases of diarrhoea during the transitional periods between dry and wet seasons (Annual Report of Bugando Medical Centre 1990).

In developing countries, the 2 most common bacterial agents causing diarrhoea are Campylobacter and enterotoxigenic Escherichia coli (ETEC) (2–4). Very little is known about the prevalence of Campylobacter and ETEC in children in Tanzania. In order to apply control measures rationally, knowledge of the infectious agents and their clinical significance is necessary.

The purpose of this study was to survey, in Mwanza municipality, Tanzania, during different seasons, the prevalence of the enteropathogens Campylobacter and ETEC, in faeces from children under the age of 5 with and without diarrhoea, as well as in adolescents and adults with and without diarrhoea.

MATERIAL AND METHODS

Children

Rectal swabs were collected from children < 5 years of age attending the diarrhoeal diseases control (DDC) clinic or the child health clinic in Mwanza. Mwanza is the second largest city in Tanzania, situated on the southern shore of Lake Victoria. The sampling was done both during the rainy and the dry seansons.

Samples were obtained from 394 children with diarrhoea in March–April and September–October 1990. The control group consisted of 278 children attending the child health clinic and who had not had any diarrhoeal episodes for at least 6 weeks before sampling. Samples were obtained from 136 of these children during the rainy season March–April 1990 and from 142 during the dry season, September–October 1993. The latter group was analysed only for Campylobacter.

On 1 occasion 2 rectal swabs were collected from each child. One swab was put into Stuart transport medium for transportation to Göteborg, Sweden, where cultivation for ETEC, was done. The second swab was used for cultivation of Campylobacter at the National Institute for Medical Research in Mwanza.

Adolescents and adults

This group was tested for Campylobacter only. Faeces samples were collected during the dry seasons of 1993 from 82 patients (age range 10–62 years) attending the Sekou Toure Hospital, Mwanza, because of diarrhoea.

In addition, samples were obtained from 247 individuals without diarrhoea (10–47 years of age) on 2 different occasions, i.e. from 118 teachers and pupils in schools on Kome Island during the rainy season March–April 1990, and from 129 individuals attending the students and pupils clinic, Mwanza during the dry seasons of 1993.

On Kome, an island of Lake Victoria, 70 km west of Mwanza, sampling was done with 1 rectal swab per person and at the students and pupils clinic faeces samples were collected.

Campylobacter

For identification of Campylobacter, a rectal swab or a loopful of faeces was inoculated directly onto Campylobacter blood-free selective (BFS) agar, containing i.a. 1 mg cefoperazone and 100 mg cycloheximide/l medium, before transferring the swab or the faeces into Campylobacter enrichment broth (5).

The BFS agar plates were incubated in candle jars at 42°C for 48–72 h and the enrichment tubes were incubated for 24 h before subcultivation onto BFS agar plates. Identification of Campylobacter was done by the oxidase reaction, Gram staining, and hippurate hydrolysis test. All Campylobacter strains were further analysed at the Department of Clinical Bacteriology, Göteborg, Sweden.

Chinese hamster ovary (CHO) cells were used to detect the presence of enterotoxin using supernatants after cultivation of Campylobacter strains grown overnight in Gc-medium (OXOID). A total of 100 CHO cells were observed, and elongation of >50% of the cells was considered to be evidence for toxin production. All samples were tested in duplicate, and positive and negative controls were always included (6).

Serotyping of Campylobacter was done by slide agglutination with whole live bacteria based on heat-labile (HL) antigenic factors. Serotyping was performed for HL antigens 1–22 and 36, excluding numbers 3, 14, and 15. By means of the HL antisera used, it had been possible to type 90% of strains from Swedish, Mexican and Kuwaiti patients (7, 8, 9). The definition of a non-typable strain, adapted in this study, was a strain which was not typable with the HL antisera used.

ETEC

For identification of ETEC, rectal swabs were inoculated immediately upon arrival in Sweden on blood agar and incubated overnight at 37°C. A total of 6 representative colonies with the appearance of Gram-negative rods were selected from the blood agar plates, and each of these was analysed simultaneously for the production of heat-labile enterotoxin (LT) by GM1-ELISA (10) and for heat-stable enterotoxin (ST) by an ST-GM1ELISA inhibition method (11), by direct culture in microplates as described (12). Toxin-positive colonies were subsequently subjected to biochemical typing according to standard procedures.

Statistics

The statistical significance of differences between groups was tested using the χ^2 test with Yates' correction.

RESULTS

Children

Out of 394 children of <5 years with diarrhoea (symptomatic group) 18% ($n = 70$) were positive for Campylobacter and 20% ($n = 78$) were positive for ETEC (Table I). Mixed infections with Campylobacter and ETEC were registered in 15 cases. In 306 children of <18 months with diarrhoea, Campylobacter was noted in 22% and ETEC in 18%, whereas the figures were 11 and 4% in asymptomatic children of the same age (Fig. 1, Table I).

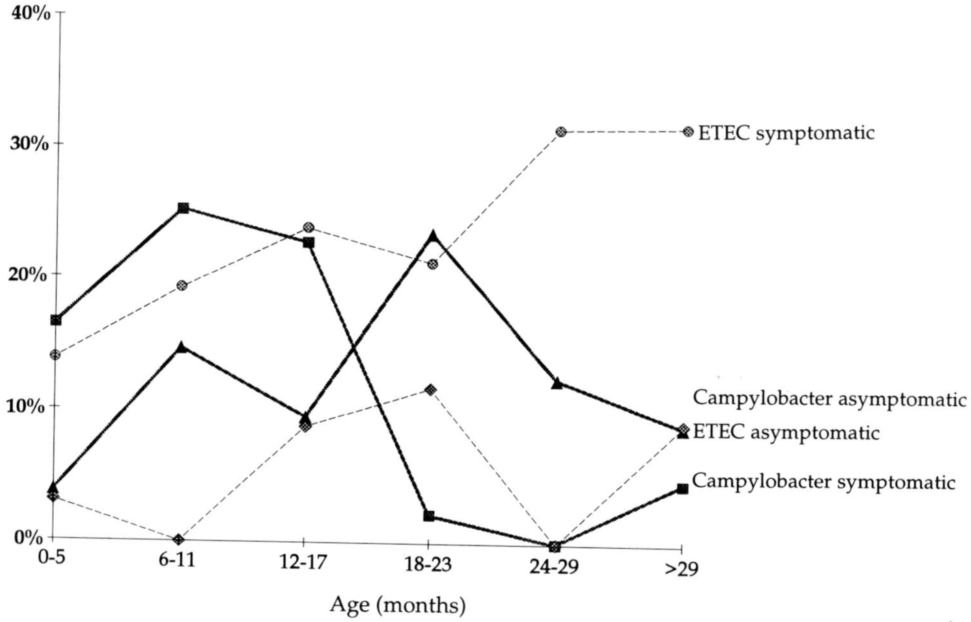

Fig. 1. Age-specific prevalence of Campylobacter and enterotoxigenic Escherichia coli (ETEC) in children with and without diarrhoea.

Table I. *Percentage prevalence of Campylobacter (Camp) and enterotoxigenic Escherichia coli (ETEC) in children <5 years of age, with and without diarrhoea, according to season and age group. (Numbers in parentheses)*

Age	Season		
	Rainy	Dry	Total
With diarrhoea			
0–17 months			
Camp	28 (30/108)	20 (38/198)	22 (68/306)[a]
ETEC	16 (17/108)	19 (37/198)	18 (54/306)[b]
18 months–5 years			
Camp	2 (1/41)	2 (1/47)	2 (2/88)[a,c]
ETEC	27 (11/41)	28 (13/47)	27 (24/88)[b]
Total (0–5 years)			
Camp	21 (31/149)	16 (39/245)	18 (70/394)
ETEC	19 (28/149)	20 (50/245)	20 (78/394)
Without diarrhoea			
0–17 months			
Camp	9 (9/100)	13 (13/99)	11 (22/199)
ETEC	4 (4/100)	ND[d]	4 (4/100)
18 months–5 years			
Camp	19 (7/36)	12 (5/43)	15 (12/79)[c]
ETEC	8 (3/36)	ND	8 (3/36)
Total (0–5 years)			
Camp	12 (16/136)	13 (18/142)	12 (34/278)
ETEC	5 (7/136)	ND	5 (7/136)

[a] $\chi^2 = 18.6$, $p < 0.001$.
[b] $\chi^2 = 3.99$, $p < 0.05$.
[c] $\chi^2 = 9.0$, $p < 0.01$; Camplylobacter more prevalent among asymptomatic than among symptomatic children >18 months of age.
[d] ND = not done.

In 88 symptomatic children, of the age group 18 months to 5 years, Campylobacter was seen in 2% whereas ETEC was found in 27%. The corresponding figures for asymptomatic individuals were 15 and 8%.

Among all children without diarrhoea 12% were positive for Campylobacter and 5% for ETEC (Table I). No mixed infections were found. There were no significant differences with regard to season between the prevalences of Campylobacter and ETEC, either for symptomatic or asymptomatic individuals. (Table I).

Out of 70 Campylobacter-positive samples in the symptomatic group we were able to test 65 strains for subspecies classification and 58 strains for enterotoxigenicity. In the asymptomatic group 16/34 of the isolated Campylobacter strains were tested regarding subspecies and 15 for enterotoxigenicity (Table II). Campylobacter jejuni was the dominating species in both the symptomatic and the asymptomatic group, at 80 and 94% respectively. In symptomatic children, C. jejuni strains were significantly more often enterotoxigenic than C. coli strains ($\chi^2 = 5.43$; $p < 0.02$) (Table II).

Table II. *Campylobacter jejuni and Campylobacter coli strains from Tanzanian children (<5 years of age), with and without diarrhoea, with regard to subspecies (%) and production of enterotoxin (%). (Numbers in parentheses)*

	Symptomatic	Asymptomatic
Subspecies, %		
C. jejuni	80 (52/65)	94 (15/16)
C. coli	20 (13/65)	6 (1/16)
Enterotoxigenicity, %		
C. jejuni	84 (38/45)[a]	93 (13/14)
C. coli	54 (7/13)[a]	100 (1/1)
Total	78 (45/48)	94 (14/15)

[a] $\chi^2 = 5.43$; $p < 0.02$.

Campylobacter heat-labile (HL) antigen was identified in 53 strains from symptomatic and in 14 strains from asymptomatic individuals. The serotype pattern was in general similar for both groups, HL1 and HL11 being most prevalent in both.

Adolescents and adults

These persons were investigated only for the presence of Campylobacter. One 21-year-old woman, out of 82 patients with diarrhoea, was positive for Campylobacter. Among the 247 individuals without diarrhoea, 3 schoolchildren from Kome were positive for Campylobacter.

DISCUSSION

Campylobacter has been shown to be as common as ETEC and rotavirus in children with diarrhoea in developing countries (2–4). The dominating sources of Campylobacter infection are wild or domestic animals, especially chicken (13, 14) and transmission to man may occur either directly or indirectly through, for instance, unpasteurized milk (15) or water (16). In developing countries campylobacteriosis has been considered as a disease of young children (4, 17) while in industrialized countries it is a disease affecting mainly adults (18). Some investigators have noticed that Campylobacter is as common in faeces from symptomatic children as from asymptomatic ones but they have found a difference among those under the age of 18 months (3, 19, 20). The results of the present study confirm these observations, showing that young children are more often infected with Campylobacter jejuni/coli than older ones. Campylobacter infections seem to be especially important under the age of 18 months. The reason for this has been claimed to be that in developing countries repeated infections in young children induce immunity (21). This is in agreement with previous findings in chicken slaughterhouse workers (22). A comparison between persons who were recently employed at a chicken slaughterhouse and persons who had been employed for many years were performed. It was found that workers suffered from repeated episodes of diarrhoea during their first period of employment. Those who had been employed for many years had significantly higher levels of Campylobacter antibodies and fewer episodes of diarrhoea. The induced immunity did not, however, protect against symptomless colonization of Campylobacter (22). However, in the present study among adolescents and adults, only 1% were colonized with Campylobacter.

The significance of Campylobacter antibodies for immunity against the disease is not clear (23). It might well be that serum antibodies reveal ongoing or passed infection while locally produced secretory IgA antibodies on the gut mucous membranes may represent a protective immunity factor. Furthermore, it is not known which antigens are important for induction of immunity. Several candidates have however been suggested, such as major outer membrane proteins and the flagellar (heat-labile) antigen.

The results of the present study might indicate that the HL antigens are not important protective antigens, since there was a similar prevalence of the most commonly occurring HL antigens on strains from children with diarrhoea as compared with strains from children without diarrhoea.

In the present investigation the significance of ETEC as a cause of diarrhoea was verified. Up to the age of 18 months the prevalence figures for Campylobacter and ETEC are more or less the same for children with diarrhoea, while there is a significant difference after this age; Campylobacter decreases significantly and ETEC increases significantly. The prevalence of Campylobacter strains isolated from children without diarrhoea is completely different, Campylobacter colonization increases up to the age of 24 months, thereafter there is a slow decrease.

Enterotoxin-producing Campylobacter strains were found in a high proportion from the symptomatic as well as from the asymptomatic group. The dominant species in both groups was Campylobacter jejuni. In an earlier study we have found Campylobacter jejuni strains from adults with diarrhoea to be enterotoxigenic significantly more often than were C. coli strains (24). These findings are in concordance with the results of the present study. Similar results were also found in a study of Algerian children (25).

Diarrhoea caused by C. jejuni and C. coli is common in young children in developing countries. The mechanism for disease is a combination of adherence to the mucous membranes, invasion and toxin production. After a number of diarrhoeal episodes immunity may protect against disease but not against colonization.

We conclude that Campylobacter and ETEC are common causes of diarrhoea in Tanzania, and that Campylobacter infections are more important in children younger than 18 months than in older ones.

ACKNOWLEDGEMENTS

This investigation was supported by grants (8673)(16X-09084) from the Swedish Medical Research Council, by grant (472) from the Swedish Council for Forestry and Agricultural Research and by grant from the Swedish Agency for Research Cooperation with Developing Countries (SAREC).

Many thanks are due to Mary-Louise Shu Shu, Kerstin Andersson and Maria Johansson for laboratory work and to Ms Anne-Bell Ek, for typing the manuscript.

REFERENCES

1. Programme for Control of Diarrhoeal Diseases. V programme report 1984–85. WHO/CDD 16: 61–63, 1986.
2. Cravioto A, Reyeyes RE, Ortega R, Fernandez G, Hernandez R, Lopez D. A prospective study of diarrhoeal disease in a cohort of rural Mexican children. Incidence and isolation of pathogens during first 2 years of life. Epidemiol Infect 101: 124–134, 1988.
3. Steele AD, Geyer A, Alexander JJ, Crewe-Brown HH, Fripp PJ. Enteropathogens isolated from children with gastroenteritis at Ga-Rankuwa Hospital, South Africa. Ann Trop Paediatr 8: 262–267, 1988.
4. Khalil K, Lindblom GB, Mazhar K, Khan SR, Kaijser B. Early child health in Lahore, Pakistan, VIII Microbiol Acta Paediatr 390 Suppl: 87–94, 1993.
5. Chan FTH, Mackenzie AMR, Fuite LA. Modified bloodfree selective and enrichment media for the isolation of thermophilic campylobacters. In: Kaijser B, Falsen E, eds. Camp. IV. Göteborg, Sweden. Abstr. No. 34, 1987.
6. Lindblom GB, Sjögren E, Kaijser B. Enterotoxin production and serogroups of Campylobacter jejuni and Campylobacter coli from patients with diarrhoea and from healthy laying hens. J Clin Microbiol 27: 1272–1276, 1989.
7. Kaijser B, Sjögren E. Campylobacter strains in Sweden. Serotyping and Correlation to clinical symptoms. APMIS 93: 315–322, 1985.
8. Sjögren E, Ruiz-Palacios G, Kaijser B. Campylobacter jejuni isolations from Mexican and Swedish patients, with repeated symptomatic and/or asymptomatic diarrhoea episodes. Epidemiol Infect 102: 47–57, 1989.
9. Sjögren E, Johny M, Kaijser B. The serotype distribution of Campylobacter in patients with diarrhoea in Kuwait. FEMS Microbiol Lett 57: 237–240, 1989.
10. Svennerholm AM, Wiklud G. Rapid GM1-enzyme-linked immunosorbent assay with visual reading for identification of Escherichia coli heat-labile enterotoxin. J Clin Microbiol 17: 596–600, 1983.
11. Svennerholm AM, Wikström M, Lindblad M, Holmgren J. Monoclonal antibodies against Escherichia coli heat-stable toxin and their use in a diagnostic ST ganglioside GM1-enzyme-linked immunosorbent assay. J Clin Microbiol 24: 585–590, 1986.
12. Åhrén CM, Jertborn M, Herclik L, Kaijser B, Svennerholm AM. Infection with bacterial enteropathogens in Swedish travellers to South-East Asia – a prospective study. Epidemiol Infect 105: 325–333, 1990.
13. Lindblom GB, Sjögren E, Kaijser B. Natural colonization in chicken raised under different environmental conditions. J Hyg 96: 385–391, 1985.
14. Khalil K, Lindblom GB, Mazhar K, Sjögren E, Kaijser B. Frequency and enterotoxigenicity of Campylobacter jejuni and C. Coli in domestic animals in Pakistan as compared to Sweden. J Trop Med Hyg 96: 35–40, 1993.
15. Schmid GP, Shaefer RE, Plikaitis BD, Shaefer JR, Bryner JH, Wintermeyer LA, Kaufmann AF. A one-year study of endemic campylobacteriosis in a Mid-western city: association with consumption of raw milk. J Infect Dis 156: 218–222, 1987.

16. Mentzing LO. Waterborne outbreaks of Campylobacter enteritis in Central Sweden. Lancet 2: 352–354, 1981.
17. Mölbak K, Höjlyng N. High prevalence of Campylobacter excretors among Liberian children related to environmental conditions. Epidemiol Infect 100: 227–237, 1988.
18. Kaijser B. Campylobacter jejuni/coli. APMIS 96: 283–288, 1988.
19. Ringertz S, Rockhill RC, Ringertz O, Sutomo A. Campylobacter fetus subsp. jejuni as a cause of gastroenteritis in Jakarta, Indonesia. J Clin Microbiol 12: 538–540, 1980.
20. Haq JA, Rahman KM. Camplylobacter jejuni as a cause of acute diarrhoea in children: a study at an urban hospital in Bangladesh. J Trop Med Hyg 94: 50–54, 1991.
21. Blaser MJ, Black RE; Duncan DJ, Amer J. Campylobacter jejuni-specific antibodies are elevated in healthy Bangladeshi children. J Clin Microbiol 21: 164–167, 1985.
22. Christenson B, Ringer A, Blücher C, Billaudelle H, Gundtoft KN, Eriksson G, Böttiger M. An out-break of Campylobacter enteritis among the staff of a poultry abattoir in Sweden. Scand J Infect Dis 15: 167–172, 1983.
23. Svedhem Å, Gunnarsson H, Kaijser B. Diffusion-in-gel enzyme-linked immunosorbent assay for routine detection of IgG and IgM antibodies to Campylobacter jejuni. J Infect Dis 148: 82–92, 1983.
24. Lindblom GB, Johny M, Khalil K, Mazhar K, Ruiz-Palacios GM, Kaijser B. Enterotoxigenicity and frequency of Campylobacter jejuni, C. coli and C. laridis in human and animal isolates from different countries. FEMS Microbiol Lett 66: 163–168, 1990.
25. Belbouri A, Megraud F. Enterotoxin-like activity produced by Campylobacter jejuni and C. coli isolated from patients and healthy controls in Algeria. FEMS Microbiol Lett 51: 25–28, 1988.

Submitted April 12, 1995; accepted September 6, 1995

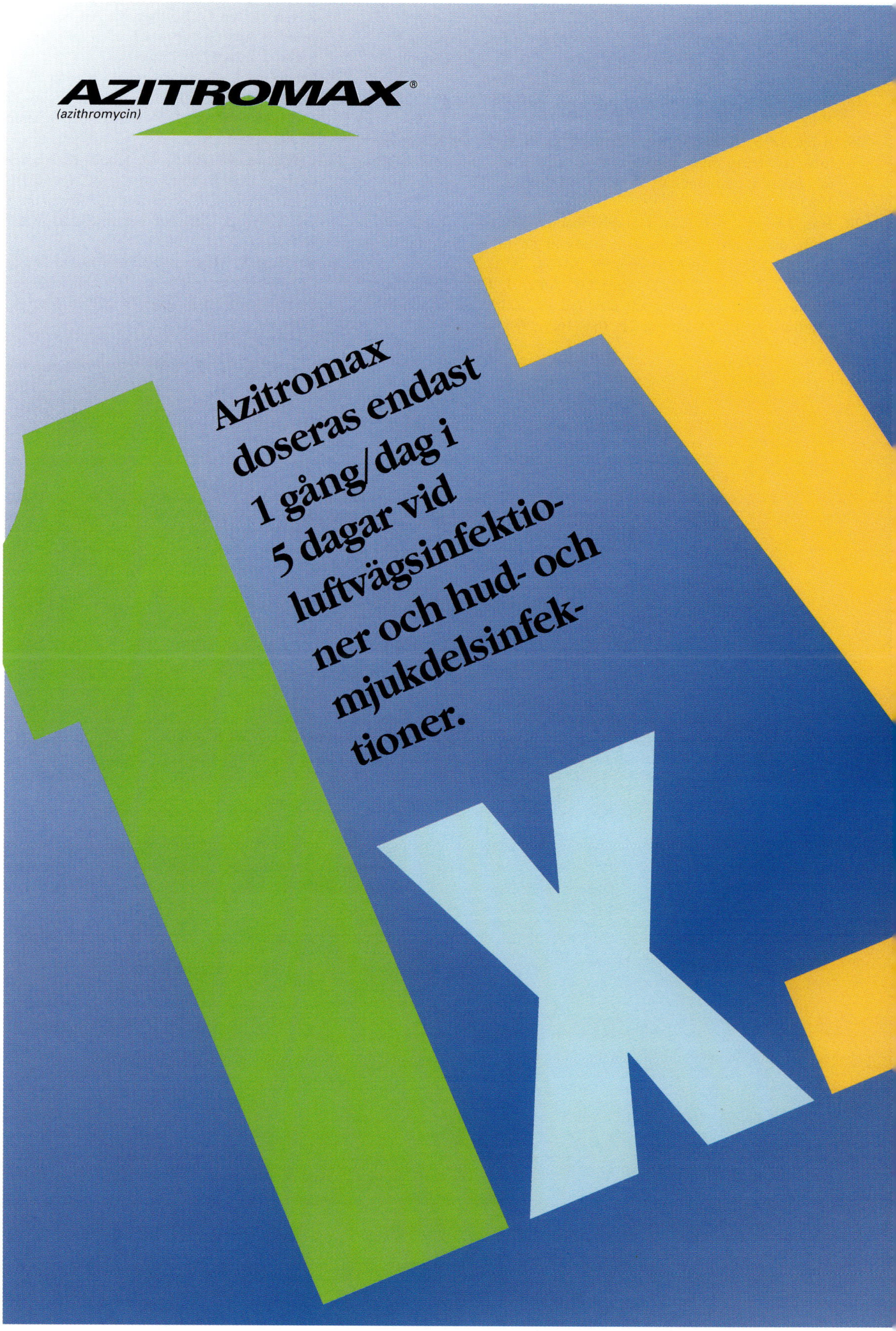
AZITROMAX®
(azithromycin)
Azitromax doseras endast 1 gång/dag i 5 dagar vid luftvägsinfektioner och hud- och mjukdelsinfektioner.

Scand J Infect Dis 27: 597–601, 1995

Prevalence of Borrelia burgdorferi sensu lato Infection in Ixodes ricinus in Sweden

ROLF GUSTAFSON[1], THOMAS G. T. JAENSON[2], ANN GARDULF[3], HANS MEJLON[2] and BO SVENUNGSSON[1]

From the Department of Immunology, Microbiology, Pathology and Infectious Diseases, Division of [1]Infectious Diseases and [3]Clinical Immunology, Karolinska Institute, Huddinge Hospital, Huddinge, and the [2]Department of Zoology, Section of Entomology and Zoological Museum, University of Uppsala, Uppsala, Sweden

Between 1988–1991, a total of 3,141 Ixodes ricinus ticks, 2,740 adults and 401 nymphs, was collected from different localities in 23 of the 25 provinces of Sweden. The ticks were identified, dissected and examined for the presence of Borrelia spirochetes. Indirect immunofluorescence was performed, using an antiserum obtained from rabbits, immunized with sonicated, whole Borrelia burgdorferi spirochetes isolated from Swedish Ixodes ricinus ticks. Borrelia-positive I. ricinus were found in all 23 provinces. The prevalence of infection in adults ranged from 3% in Jämtland to 23% in Södermanland. In nymphs, the infection prevalence ranged from 0% in 9 provinces to 15% in Södermanland. A significantly greater proportion of the adult ticks were found to be positive for Borrelia in the southern and central parts of Sweden as compared to the northern part (Norrland). No significant difference in prevalence could be demonstrated between the western and eastern parts of Sweden. On average, 10% of the nymphs and 15% of the adult I. ricinus were positive for Borrelia. Of 41 non-I. ricinus ticks, none was positive for Borrelia. This study shows that Borrelia burgdorferi sensu lato is present throughout the distributional area of I. ricinus in Sweden. This should lead to increased awareness of signs and symptoms compatible with Lyme borreliosis in persons living in or visiting areas where I. ricinus is present.

R. Gustafson, MD, Department of Immunology, Microbiology, Pathology and Infectious Diseases, Division of Infectious Diseases, Huddinge Hospital, S-141 86 Huddinge, Sweden

INTRODUCTION

The medically most important and abundant tick species in Sweden, as well as in most other parts of Europe, is the wood tick Ixodes ricinus (1–3). All of its active stages (larva, nymph, adult) need a blood meal from a vertebrate host before entering the next stage of the life cycle (4). In the climatic conditions of northern Europe, the developmental cycle from egg to adult tick usually takes 3 years (4). Blood hosts for larval I. ricinus include lizards, birds and small, medium-sized and large mammals, whereas nymphs and adult ticks usually engorge successfully only on medium-sized and large mammals (1, 2).

I. ricinus is most abundant in the southern and central parts of Sweden, especially in coastal and archipelago areas, but it is also common in some localities along the coast of northern Sweden (Norrland) (2, 5).

The most important human pathogens transmitted by I. ricinus are Borrelia burgdorferi sensu lato, causing Lyme borreliosis (LB), and the tick-borne encephalitis (TBE) virus. More than 2,000 cases of human LB and between 50 and 80 cases of TBE are estimated to occur in Sweden each year.

Information concerning the prevalence of Borrelia spirochetes in tick populations is an essential part of epidemiological surveys of LB. We have earlier found that approximately 30% of ticks collected in the surroundings of Stockholm, are positive for Borrelia spirochetes (6). However, in residents of this area, only 1 in 70 tick bites noted was estimated to result in LB with clinical symptoms (7). The aim of the present study was to investigate the prevalence of Borrelia infection in ticks in different parts of Sweden.

MATERIALS AND METHODS

During the 3-year period 1988–1991, a total of 3,141 I. ricinus ticks (2,740 adults and 401 nymphs), and 41 ticks belonging to other species (Haemaphysalis punctata, Rhipicephalus sanguineus and Ixodes hexagonus), were obtained from 188 different localities in 23 provinces of Sweden, from Skåne in the south to Norrbotten in the north (Table I). Most ticks were collected by dragging a white flannel cloth (1 × 1 m in size) over vegetation. The cloth was checked at regular intervals, and attached ticks were put in moist plastic tubes and kept in a refrigerator until further investigation. Some of the ticks were collected in various regions of Sweden by persons who were aware of the present study. Many of these ticks had been found on dogs, cats or humans and were blood-filled. These ticks were mailed to the laboratory. Only live ticks were used for the study.

All ticks were examined and identified, using a binocular microscope, within 1 month after collection. After dissection, the body content of each tick was suspended in a drop of phosphate-buffered saline (PBS, 0.05 mol/l, pH 7.2) on a glass slide for indirect immunofluorescence.

A Borrelia antiserum was obtained from rabbits, immunized by means of 6-monthly intravenous injections with sonicated, whole, Borrelia burgdorferi s. l. spirochetes isolated from Swedish I. ricinus ticks (strain STG 25) (courtesy of Dr Mats Karlsson, Stockholm). A fluorescein-isothiocyanate-conjugated (FITC) sheep anti-rabbit immunoglobulin (obtained from the National Bacteriological Laboratory, Stockholm, Sweden; Molar F/P ratio, 3.1), was used as conjugate. The working dilutions used, determined by titration, were 1/80 for the antiserum and 1/10 for the conjugate. The method has previously been described in detail (8).

Slides were examined at 400× under a Leitz Orthoplan fluorescence microscope for the presence of Borrelia spirochetes. The

 ISSN 0036-5548

Table I. *The infection prevalence (%) of Borrelia nymphal and adult I. ricinus ticks in Sweden*

Province	No. of localities sampled	Nymphal ticks: No. examined, Unfed	Nymphal ticks: No. examined, Fed	Nymphal ticks: Infection prevalence, %, Unfed	Nymphal ticks: Infection prevalence, %, Fed	Adult ticks: No. examined, Unfed	Adult ticks: No. examined, Fed	Adult ticks: Infection prevalence, %, Unfed	Adult ticks: Infection prevalence, %, Fed
Skåne	14	0	0	—	—	107	12	15	17
Blekinge	6	46	0	13	—	88	2	17	—
Halland	10	14	0	7	—	67	10	15	20
Småland	14	5	0	—	—	99	15	16	13
Öland	6	2	0	—	—	122	4	16	—
Gotland	8	77	0	10	—	156	6	18	—
Östergötland	10	5	0	—	—	165	0	13	—
Västergötland	15	32	0	6	—	173	13	13	15
Bohuslän	11	63	0	10	—	293	5	17	—
Dalsland	4	4	0	—	—	93	0	10	—
Närke	7	9	0	—	—	86	1	13	—
Södermanland	10	71	0	15	—	342	4	23	—
Uppland	16	55	4	13	0	351	21	18	29
Västmanland	10	5	0	—	—	130	9	12	—
Värmland	12	3	0	—	—	85	9	9	—
Dalarna	10	1	0	—	—	64	13	6	8
Gästrikland	6	2	0	—	—	70	11	7	9
Hälsingland	3	3	0	—	—	23	4	4	0
Medelpad	4	0	0	—	—	22	6	5	0
Jämtland	4	0	0	—	—	34	2	3	0
Ångermanland	4	0	0	—	—	5	9	—	—
Västerbotten	3	0	0	—	—	2	6	—	0
Norrbotten	1	0	0	—	—	0	1	—	—
Total	188	397	4	10		2,577	163	15	16

fluorescence was scored as positive only when it was strong with brilliant margins. Each slide was examined for some 10 min before it was considered to be negative. I. ricinus spirochete strain STG 25, cultured in modified Kelly's medium (9, 10), was used as a positive control.

All microscopic examinations were made by one person (R.G.). All the samples were coded, without the examiners having any knowledge of the stage of development and geographic origin of the ticks. Differences between groups were compared by contingency table analysis.

RESULTS

I. ricinus was collected in 23 out of the 25 provinces in Sweden. No I. ricinus was obtained from Härjedalen or Lappland.

The percentages of I. ricinus positive for Borrelia amongst those examined from the different provinces, are given in Table I. With the exception of Norrbotten, ticks had been collected from at least 3 localities in each province. The number of ticks obtained from the northern provinces was, however, limited.

The southernmost locality where I. ricinus was present was Ystad in Skåne and the northernmost one was Vittjärv, a few kilometers north-east of Boden in Norrbotten. The distance between these places is about 1,280 kilometers. Borrelia-positive ticks were found at both these localities. The proportions of Borrelia-positive, unfed, adult I. ricinus ranged from 3% in Jämtland to 23% in Södermanland. A comparison of the infection prevalences in ticks from southern (Götaland) and central (Svealand) Sweden with that in ticks from northern Sweden (Norrland) showed a significantly higher proportion of Borrelia-positive adult ticks in the southern and central parts ($p < 0.001$). No significant difference in the proportion of Borrelia-positive I. ricinus adults and nymphs was seen between the western (Halland, Västergötland and Bohuslän) and eastern provinces of Sweden (Östergötland, Södermanland and Uppland). Out of all I. ricinus ticks examined, 15% of the adults and 10% of the nymphs were positive for Borrelia.

The majority of the ticks investigated were unfed when collected. However, 169/3,141 of the ticks (5%) were in some state of engorgement (having been found on dogs, cats, roe deer, moose, cattle or humans).

Besides I. ricinus, 3 other tick species were found: H. punctata (30 adults from Stora Karlsö, Gotland), R. sanguineus (4 adults and 2 nymphs from dogs in Gotland and Uppland) and I. hexagonus (5 adults from Halland and Västmanland). No Borrelia spirochetes were discovered in any of these 41 non-I. ricinus ticks.

DISCUSSION

I. ricinus is known to be found in many parts of Sweden, as illustrated in this study. It was thus collected from 23 out of the 25 Swedish provinces. Several factors such as climate, vegetation and access to hosts for feeding and reproduction, are important in the provision of suitable conditions for I. ricinus (4). It is especially abundant in the coastal areas in southern and central Sweden, whereas its presence and abundance seems to be substantially lower in northern Sweden (Norrland). This is demonstrated by the low number of ticks collected in the northern provinces in the present study despite determined efforts. Adverse climatic conditions are probably the main reasons for the sparseness of ticks in northern Sweden. Moreover, the proportion of ticks positive for Borrelia was significantly lower in the northern provinces, which is in accordance with the relatively few number of human cases of LB reported from northern Sweden.

Previously published reports concerning the infection prevalence in Swedish I. ricinus, are shown in Table II. These data are in agreement with those of the present study, with a relatively high infection prevalence in southern Sweden (e.g. at Aspö) but relatively low in northern Sweden (e.g. at Norrbyskär). The data in Table II also show that the nymphs, in general, are less commonly infected than the adults, whereas the larvae are usually not infected at all. The infection prevalences recorded in other parts of Europe (17, 18) conform, in general, to the prevalences recorded in Sweden.

B. burgdorferi can be transmitted transovarially from the adult female tick to her offspring. However, this mode of transmission seems to be of minor importance in maintaining circulation of the spirochete in nature (19). More important is the role of Borrelia-infected mammals, in acting as spirochete reservoirs and hosts for bloodsucking ticks (12). Among the most important reservoirs are shrews, rodents and hares (12).

In Sweden, it has been speculated that the number of human cases of LB has increased as a consequence of a drastic increase in the roe deer population (14). From an estimated number of 2,000 roe deer in 1863 (20), there seems at present to be > 1 million roe deer in Sweden (14). Roe deer do not seem to be a competent reservoir for B. burgdorferi, but serve as an important blood source for all stages of I. ricinus (14). Thus, in areas where deer are now abundant the density of I. ricinus may have increased. As a consequence, the circulation of B. burgdorferi s. l. may have become more effective, leading to greater number of infected ticks.

In a recent study (11), the seasonal risk of human LB infection in different vegetation types in southern Sweden was estimated. It was found that the prevalence of Borrelia infection among nymphal ticks differed significantly between years and sampling sites. Infection prevalence was

Table II. *Published records of the prevalence of Borrelia infection in I. ricinus in Sweden*

Stage	Locality	Infection prevalence, %	No. of ticks examined	Method of examination	Reference
Unfed larvae	Torö[a]	0	336	PCM	11
Unfed larvae	Kungshamn-Morga[b]	0	85	PCM	11
Unfed larvae	Bogesund[b]	0	191	PCM	12
Unfed nymphs	Aspö[c]	17	92	IIF	13
Unfed nymphs	Torö[a]	10 (2–15)	955	PCM	11
Unfed nymphs	Bogesund[b]	9 (8–12)	396	PCM	14
Unfed nymphs	Kungshamn-Morga[b]	0–38	450	PCM	11
Unfed nymphs	Kungshamn-Morga[b]	13	126	PCM	11
Unfed nymphs	Kungshamn-Morga[b]	9	324	PCM	11
Unfed nymphs	Norrbyskär[d]	2	42	PCM	5
Unfed adults	Aspö[c]	26	57	IIF	13
Unfed males	Torö[a]	15	55	PCM	11
Unfed males	Torö[a]	29	35	PCM	11
Unfed males	Kungshamn-Morga[b]	15	26	PCM	11
Unfed females	Kungshamn-Morga[b]	26	23	PCM	11
Nymphs and adults	Gotland	6	18	Culture	15
Nymphs and adults	Lisö[a]	21	47	PCM	15
Nymphs and adults	Ekerö[b]	13	67	PCM	15
Nymphs and adults	Stockholm	9	64	Dark-field microscopy	16
Unfed adults	Norrbyskär[d]	13	8	PCM	5

[a] Södermanland; [b] Uppland; [c] Blekinge; [d] Ångermanland.
PCM, phase contrast microscopy; IIF, indirect immunofluorescence.

greater in adult ticks than in nymphs but was similar in female and male ticks. In the present study, we also recorded that adult I. ricinus are infected with Borrelia more often than are nymphs. This should be the result if most larvae feed on reservoir-competent small mammals and a significant proportion of the nymphs also feed on reservoir-competent mammals, e.g. hares.

The reasons for the lower percentages of Borrelia-positive ticks in the northern provinces can only be speculated upon. A low density of ticks may be one reason why a circulation of Borrelia spirochetes high enough to produce and maintain a high prevalence is not obtained.

The ticks in this study were collected during a 3-year period. It is most likely that the proportion and number of Borrelia-carrying ticks vary from one year to another (11), due to changes in climatic factors and in the abundance of reservoir-competent hosts. Therefore, comparisons between samples collected from different provinces over a period of years should be made with caution.

Several species of ticks belonging to the I. ricinus complex have been shown to be competent vectors of B. burgdorferi. I. hexagonus, which rarely feeds on humans, is also a competent vector of B. burgdorferi (21). Borrelia spirochetes have also been detected in H. punctata (22). However, there is no evidence that the latter species or R. sanguineus are competent vectors of B. burgdorferi s. l. In this study, no spirochetes were detected in any of the non-I. ricinus ticks investigated which, however, were only few in number.

Different techniques can be used for the detection of Borrelia spirochetes in ticks, such as the polymerase chain reaction (PCR) (23), cultivation (9, 10), dark-field (16) or phase-contrast microscopy (5, 11, 12, 14), as well as direct (24) or indirect immunofluorescence (15). In the present study, we used indirect immunofluorescence, since we had previously found this method to be rapid, reliable and simple for measuring the infection prevalence in ticks (6). The antiserum used was obtained from rabbits immunized with a sonicated, whole cell antigen. This crude antigen could be expected to stimulate production of polyclonal antibodies with affinity to several different epitopes. Such a polyclonal antiserum may give rise to false-positive reactions. However, the morphological characteristics of spirochetes make them relatively easy to differentiate from other microorganisms. Since no other spirochetes have been isolated from I. ricinus in Sweden we believe that the spirochetes recorded in this study belong to B. burgdorferi s. l. (25, 26).

The main conclusion of the present study is that B. burgdorferi s. l. seems to be present in practically all populations of I. ricinus in Sweden. This should lead to increased awareness of signs and symptoms compatible with LB in persons living in or visiting areas where I. ricinus ticks are present.

ACKNOWLEDGEMENTS

We would like to thank Dr Mats Karlsson, Department of Infectious Diseases, Danderyds Hospital, Stockholm, Sweden, for kindly providing the Borrelia antiserum.

This study was supported by grants from the Karolinska Institute, Stockholm, Sweden, by the Stockholm County Council to R.G. and from the Swedish Natural Science Research Council and Magnus Bergvalls Stiftelse to T.G.T.J.

REFERENCES

1. Arthur DR. British ticks. London: Butterworths, 1963.
2. Jaenson TGT, Tälleklint L, Lundqvist L, Olsén B, Chirico J, Mejlon H. Geographical distribution, host associations and vector roles of ticks (Acari: Ixodidae, Argasidae) in Sweden. J Med Entomol 31: 240–256, 1994.
3. Grist N. Ticks are topical. J Infect 24: 117–121, 1992.
4. Balashov YS. Bloodsucking ticks (Ixodoidea) – vectors of disease of man and animals [English translation]. Misc Publ Entomol Soc Am 8: 163–376, 1972.
5. Jaenson TGT, Bergström S, Burman N, Chirico J, Jonsson M. Spiroketinfekterade fästingar (Ixodes ricinus) – risk för angrepp även i Norrland [Spirochete-infected ticks (Ixodes ricinus) – risk of infection even in Northern Sweden]. Läkartidningen 86: 2584, 1989.
6. Gustafson R, Gardulf A, Svenungsson B. Comparison of culture, indirect immunofluorescence and dark-field microscopy for detection of spirochetes from Ixodes ricinus ticks. Eur J Clin Microbiol Infect Dis 8: 570–572, 1989.
7. Gustafson R, Svenungsson B, Forsgren M, Gardulf A, Granström M. Two-year survey of the incidence of Lyme borreliosis and tick-borne encephalitis in a high-risk population in Sweden. Eur J Clin Microbiol Infect Dis 11: 894–900, 1992.
8. Svenungsson B, Lindberg AA. Synthetic disaccharide-protein antigens for production of specific 04 and 09 antisera for immunofluorescence diagnosis of Salmonella. Med Microbiol Immunol 163: 1–11, 1977.
9. Steere AC, Grodzicky RI, Kornblatt AN, Craft JE, Barbour AG, Burgdorfer W, Schmid GP, Johnson E, Malawista SE. The spirochetal etiology of Lyme disease. N Engl J Med 308: 733–742, 1983.
10. Stiernstedt G, Eriksson G, Enfors W, Jörbeck H, Svenungsson B, Sköldenberg B, Granström M. Erythema chronicum migrans in Sweden: clinical manifestations and antibodies to Ixodes ricinus spirochete measured by indirect immunofluorescence and enzyme-linked immunosorbent assay. Scand J Infect Dis 18: 217–224, 1986.
11. Mejlon H, Jaenson TGT. Seasonal prevalence of Borrelia burgdorferi in Ixodes ricinus in different vegetation type in Sweden. Scand J Infect Dis 25: 449–456, 1993.
12. Tälleklint L, Jaenson TGT. Maintenance by hares of European Borrelia burgdorferi in ecosystems without rodents. J Med Entomol 30: 273–276, 1993.
13. Berglund J, Eitrem R. Tick-borne borreliosis in the archipelago of Southern Sweden. Scand J Infect Dis 25: 67–72, 1993.
14. Jaenson TGT, Tälleklint L. Incompetence of roe deer as reservoirs of the Lyme borreliosis spirochete. J Med Entomol 29: 813–817, 1992.
15. Stiernstedt G. Tick-borne Borrelia infection in Sweden. Scand J Infect Dis Suppl 45: 1–69, 1985.
16. Åsbrink E, Hederstedt B, Hovmark A. The spirochetal etiology of erythema chronicum migrans Afzelius. Acta Dermatol Venereol 64: 291–295, 1984.

17. Stanek G, Pletschette M, Flamm H, Hirschl AM, Aberer E, Kristoferitsch W, Schmutzhard E. European Lyme borreliosis. Ann NY Acad Sci 539: 274–282, 1988.
18. Gern L, Burgdorfer W, Aeschlimann A, Krampitz HE. The ecology of Lyme borreliosis in Europe. In: Weber K, Burgdorfer W, eds. Aspects of Lyme borreliosis. Berlin: Springer Verlag, 59–69, 1993.
19. Jaenson TGT. The epidemiology of Lyme borreliosis. Parasitol Today 7: 39–45, 1991.
20. Bjärvall A, Ullström S, Däggdjur. Alla Europas arter [Mammals. All species in Europe]. Stockholm: Wahlström and Widstrand, 1985.
21. Gern L, Toutoungi LN, Hu CM, Aeschlimann A. Ixodes (Pholeoixodes) hexagonus, an efficient vector of Borrelia burgdorferi in the laboratory. Med Vet Entomol 5: 431–435, 1991.
22. Marquez FJ, Constan MC. Infection d'Ixodes ricinus (L., 1758) et Haemaphysalis punctata Canestrini et Fanzago, 1877 (Acarina, Ixodidae) par Borrelia burgdorferi dans le nord de la péninsule Ibérique (pays Basque Espagnol et Navarre). Bull Soc Françe, Parasitol 8: 323–330, 1990.
23. Bergström S, Olsén B, Burman N, Gothefors L, Jaenson TGT, Jonsson M, Mejlon HA. Molecular characterization of Borrelia burgdorferi isolated from Ixodes ricinus in northern Sweden. Scand J Infect Dis Suppl 45: 1985.
24. Piesman J, Mather TN, Donahue JG, Levine J, Campbell JD, Karakashian SJ, Spielman A. Comparative prevalence of Babesia microti and Borrelia burgdorferi in populations of Ixodes dammini in eastern Massachusetts. Acta Trop 43: 263–270, 1986.
25. Baranton G, Postic D, Saint Giron I, Boerlin P, Piffaretti J-C, Assous M, Grimont PAD. Delineation of Borrelia burgdorferi sensu stricto, Borrelia garinii sp nov, and group VS461 associated with Lyme borreliosis. Int J Syst Bacteriol 42: 378–383, 1992.
26. Canica MM, Nako F, du Merle L, Mazie JC, Baranton G, Postic D. Monoclonal antibodies for identification of Borrelia afzelii sp. nov. associated with late cutaneous manifestations of Lyme borreliosis. Scand J Infect Dis 25: 441–448, 1993.

Submitted January 31, 1995; accepted October 16, 1995

Scand J Infect Dis 27: 603–611, 1995 ORIGINAL ARTICLE

Dipslide Culture in Colonic Surgery: A Tool for Assessment of Surgical Performance and a Guide to Antibiotic Use

BERNDT E. B. CLAESSON[1], STEN FILIPSSON[2] and DAN E. W. HOLMLUND[3]

Department of [1]Clinical Microbiology and [3]Surgery Kärnsjukhuset, Skövde, and [2]Department of Surgery, Bassjukhuset, Lidköping, Sweden

We evaluated a bacterial culture system for the assessment of surgical performance during colorectal operations, and for assessing the impact of selective postoperative antibiotics in contaminated cases. Surgically related infections were recorded and their risk factors were estimated, using univariate and multivariate methods, in 1079 patients undergoing elective colorectal operations. (Study period 1 was prospective, controlled and randomized, and study period 2 was prospective and open). All the patients were given metronidazole, 1 g i.v., at induction of anaesthesia and 12 h postoperatively. The number of colony-forming units (CFU) on an intraoperative dipslide culture was classified as 0, 1–4 or ⩾5 ($n = 591$, 183 and 305). Patients with ⩾5 CFU were randomized to receive either no further antibiotics or cefuroxime (1.5 g, i.v. every 8 h for 2 days) during the first study period (30 months). During the second period (84 months), all patients with ⩾5 CFU were to be given cefuroxime. Increasing age ($p = 0.014$), postoperative transfusion of packed red blood cells ($p < 0.001$), and high bacterial numbers ($p < 0.001$) were independently associated with infection. Surgeon-related rates of operative bacterial contamination varied between 12 and 50% ($p < 0.001$). In patients given only metronidazole, the likelihood of infection rose as the density of bacteria in the wound increased according to a sigmoid dose–response curve (5.1, 9.8 and 47.5% with CFU 0, 1–4 and ⩾5, respectively). In the category with ⩾5 CFU, 265 patients were treated with cefuroxime and 23 (8.7%) subsequently had infections of 40 patients with ⩾5 CFU who did not receive cefuroxime postoperatively, 19 developed infections ($p < 0.001$, relative risk 5.47; 95% confidence interval 3.29–9.10). In conclusion, dipslide culture can identify patients at high risk of infection after colonic operations. It can be used to assess surgical performance. The addition of postoperative antibiotic cover for aerobic bacteria, detected by the dipslide, reduced the risk of infection more than 5-fold and almost eliminated the risk of contamination.

B. Claesson, MD, Department of Clinical Microbiology, Kärnsjukhuset, S-541 85 Skövde, Sweden

INTRODUCTION

This current study was planned in the early 1980s because we wanted to reduce the unacceptably high incidence of wound infection after colonic surgery. Our standard prophylactic regimen, metronidazole 1 g i.v. given 30 min before and 12 h after the operation, gave an infection rate of 18%. Metronidazole eradicated the anaerobes, but most of the infected wounds grew Enterobacteriaceae species. We decided to combine metronidazole with cefuroxime, a second-generation cephalosporin with a potent effect on the coliform flora. Because of its wide spectrum of activity, we were concerned that cefuroxime would disturb the normal gut flora and cause problems of resistance. Ideally, the drug should be given only to those patients who needed it (more than 80% of the patients apparently did not), but we had no method of selecting the patients at risk before the operation.

A simple culture technique to detect contamination of the wound with bacteria of bowel origin showed promising results in a pilot study, but results were not available until the day after the operation. At this stage, antimicrobial drugs could not be expected to be effective (1), but the efficacy of a mixed strategy, i.e. a regimen directed against anaerobic bacteria given just before the operation and another directed against aerobic bacteria 24 h later, had not been tried. We decided to try this approach in a subset of patients with a contamination proved by culture. We also wanted to assess the role of the surgeon in causing endogenous wound contamination, and relate this to other potential risk factors of infection.

The current series was divided into 2 periods because of a change in study design. Some of the results from the first period, which concerns one-fifth of the total series, have been reported previously (2–4). We included the first period in this final report, because it is part of a consecutive series and offers an interesting assessment of outcome when moving from a controlled trial into an audit of clinical practice.

PATIENTS AND METHODS

Study design

Period 1. All patients were given metronidazole (Elyzol®), 1 g i.v., at induction of anaesthesia and 12 h postoperatively. At the end of the operation, after standard saline irrigation of the abdominal cavity, residual lavage fluid was sampled with a dipslide to measure bacterial densities. The degree of contamination was judged 18 h later from the dipslide colony count of Enterobacteriaceae or Staphylococcus aureus. Three categories were recognized: 0 CFU (colony-forming units), 1–4 CFU and ⩾5 CFU. Additional antibiotics were considered only in the last category. Patients with ⩾5 CFU in their peritoneal fluid were randomized, from a block of 10 sealed envelopes with 5 in each arm to receive no more antibiotic or to receive cefuroxime (Zinacef®), 1.5 g i.v., every 8 h for 2 days, starting 24 h postoperatively. The results of the culture

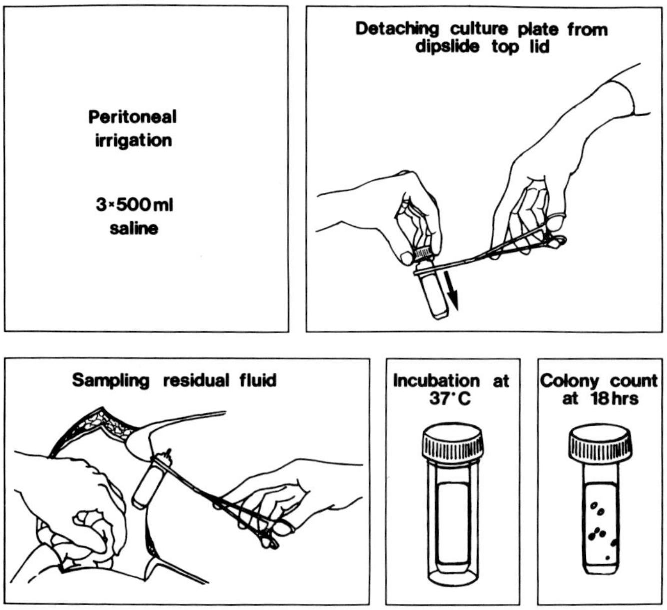

Fig. 1. Dipslide sampling and culture.

were known only to a research technician who told the ward staff which patients were to receive cefuroxime. Although allocation to cefuroxime obviously implied ⩾5 CFU, the staff were unaware of the results in the other cases.

Period 2. The routines were as during period 1, except that cultures were run in the normal routine, results reported to the staff within 24 h, and all patients with ⩾5 CFU were to be given cefuroxime.

Registration of complications

Surgically related infections included primary local wound infection (5), perineal infection, fistula, intra-abdominal abscess, peritonitis, clinically overt anastomotic leakage confirmed at reoperation or by imaging (radiography or ultrasound), and septicaemia (spiking fever with a growth of intestinal bacteria in the blood culture but no urinary tract infection or pneumonia).

A ward nurse inspected wounds and was responsible for bacteriological sampling if any signs of infection appeared. At discharge, each patient received written instructions to contact the hospital immediately for sampling if there was even a slight suspicion of a wound complication in the postoperative period. A surgeon updated the record sheets at the end of the hospital stay and at a check-up 4 weeks postoperatively. A hospital infection epidemiologist reviewed all medical charts and made a final evaluation.

The record sheets and the culture results were statistically analysed by an independent consultant.

The study was approved by the local research committee.

Patients and surgical routines

Patients who were to undergo a planned colorectal operation in 2 surgical departments (Kärnsjukhuset, Skövde and Bassjukhuset, Lidköping) were eligible for inclusion. During the first study period we excluded patients according to previously formulated criteria: closure of colostomy, antimicrobial medication within the week before surgery, serum creatinine >200 µmol/l, hypersensitivity to beta-lactam antibiotics, or signs of infection before the operation. Three patients were withdrawn because of incorrect protocol and 2 because infection was recognized at surgery; none of these patients developed postoperative infections. During the second period, closure of colostomy and infection recognized at surgery were the only exclusion criteria; no patients were withdrawn. Patients receiving postoperative antimicrobial medication for non-surgical infections were eligible for analysis. In total, 1079 patients (238 in the first series and 841 in the second series) were finally included.

Cancer of the colon or rectum was the most common diagnosis ($n = 692$), followed by inflammatory bowel disorders, i.e. Crohn's disease (138), ulcerative colitis (26), diverticulosis (82), volvulus (24) and miscellaneous (117). The latter category included: carcinoid, chronic obstipation, colonic stenosis, endometriosis, familial polyposis, fistula, lipoma, lymphoma, malignant melanoma, non-specific colitis, rectal prolapse, polyp, and villous adenoma.

A low-residue diet (Biosorbin®) was given for 48 h before operation. Mechanical preparation of the bowel was by saline enema and an oral laxative (Toilax®, 5 mg × 2) 2 days preoperatively. Antimicrobial agents were not used for bowel preparation. Each patient had a whole body wash with 4% chlorhexidine (Hibiscrub®) on the evening before operation. The abdominal area was washed with an alcoholic solution of 0.5% chlorhexidine before incision. Blood was transfused either as packed red blood cells or as plasma.

The surgical routines were unchanged in the study period. Vicryl® 000 (Ethicon) was used for suture of anastomoses, Vicryl 0 or 00 for closure of the deep abdominal layers, and Ethilon® for the skin. Whenever possible, low anterior resections were done with an EEA stapling device. Before abdominal wound closure, the peritoneal cavity was washed 3 times with warm saline (0.85% NaCl); 500 ml was used for each washing. The lavage fluid was allowed to stand for a few seconds before being removed by suction. The number of operations by each surgeon ranged from 1 to 176, and 44 surgeons participated.

Bacteriological sampling and culture methods

The peritoneal fluid was sampled with a Uricult® dipslide (Orion Diagnostica, Trosa, Sweden). After the third washout, the sterile dipslide was detached from its top lid with forceps and dipped in the residual fluid lodged in the pelvis (Fig. 1). The slide was then put into the original container and transported to the local laboratory for incubation within 10 min. The dipslide cultures were incubated aerobically at 37°C for 18 h. The number of CFU on the CLED agar side was recorded. Control experiments to determine the amount of fluid cultured with the dipslide were carried out. E coli

Table I. *Septic complications and mortality in the various groups of contamination*

	No. of complications			
Type of complication	0 CFU $n = 591$	1–4 CFU $n = 183$	≥5 CFU $n = 40$	≥5 CFU + cefuroxime $n = 265$
Local wound infection	15	14	11	9
Perineal infection	8	2	2	1
Intra-abdominal abscess	4	1	2	6
Peritonitis	0	1	0	2
Anastomotic leak	3	4	5	8
Fistula	2	1	1	0
Septicaemia	2	1	2	2
Mortality	6	2	2	9
Total no. of infections	34	24	23	28
Total no. of patients with infections	30	18	19	23

strain ATCC 25922 was cultured in Müller–Hinton broth overnight and diluted 10^{-3}, 10^{-4} and 10^{-5} in saline. Aliquots were added to saline–blood suspensions to a final volume of 200 ml, mimicking the haemoglobin concentrations found in irrigation fluids obtained at operation (0, 6, and 12 g/l). The suspensions were mixed with a magnetic stirrer. From each of 24 suspensions, 100 µl was streaked onto each of 5 blood agar plates; 10–25 dipslides were then dipped in the same suspensions. Colony counts of blood agar plates and the dipslide CLED agar side were done after overnight incubation.

Infected wounds were sampled with cotton swabs and transported to the laboratory in a modified Stuart's medium. Specimens from deep foci were collected with a syringe and transported in sealed CO_2-gassed bottles. At least 3 blood cultures were taken when septicaemia was suspected. Methods of susceptibility testing and identification of aerobic and anaerobic bacteria have been described previously (2, 3).

Analysis of risk factors

The following risk factors were recorded: age, sex, preoperative hospital stay, serum albumin and haemoglobin concentrations, body mass index (kg/m²), type and duration of operation, visible faecal contamination as judged by the surgeon, use of abdominal drains, transfusion of plasma and of packed red blood cells within 5 days of the operation, diagnosis, the degree of bacterial contamination (dipslide colony count), and cefuroxime medication postoperatively.

Statistical analysis

Fisher's exact test and the test for trend in contingency tables were used to compare infection rates among the various contamination groups. The results were expressed as relative risks and odds ratios with 95% confidence intervals. Risk factors for surgical infection were initially assessed with univariate analyses using Pitman's test which includes Fisher's permutation test and Fisher's exact test (6). Factors that correlated significantly with infection ($p < 0.05$), were then subjected to stepwise logistic analysis. This technique was used with the aim of identifying those variables whose correlation with infection could not be explained by their correlation with other variables (Mantel's test). The probability of infection was assumed to be a function of the form:

$$1/[1 + \exp(-Ax_1 - Bx_2 - Cx_3 - \text{constant})],$$

where A, B, C, were estimated by the likelihood method.

Variables which could not be assigned to a natural order of risk, for example diagnosis, surgeon, and operative procedure, were not included in the multivariate analysis. Instead, the chi-square test was used to compare the observed and expected number of infections based on the logistic regression analysis. Only 2-sided tests were used.

RESULTS

Clinical outcome

There were a total of 109 infections in 90 patients (Table I). The median duration of development of infection after operation was 7 days. The results from 2 study periods were similar (Table II). Further analysis was therefore based on the entire study population. In the 0-CFU group, assigned relative risk 1.0, there were 30 cases of infection

Table II. *Infection rates in the various groups of contamination during the 2 study periods*

	Period 1		Period 2		Total			
No. of CFU	Patients	Infected cases (%)	Patients	Infected cases (%)	Patients	Infected cases (%)	Relative risk (95% CI)	Odds ratio (95% CI)
0	133	9 (6.8)	458	21 (4.6)	591	30 (5.1)	1.00	
1–4	34	3 (8.8)	149	15 (10.1)	183	18 (9.8)	1.94 (1.11–3.39)	2.04 (1.04–3.89)
≥5	35	15 (42.9)	5[a]	4 (80.0)	40	19 (47.5)	9.36 (5.81–15.08)	16.92 (7.65–36.8)
≥5 (addition of cefuroxime)	36	4 (11.1)	229	19 (8.3)	265	23 (8.7)	1.71 (1.01–2.89)	1.78 (0.96–3.24)

[a] The addition of cefuroxime was missed in these 5 patients (2 patients in 1985 and 1 in each of the years 1989, 1990, and 1991).

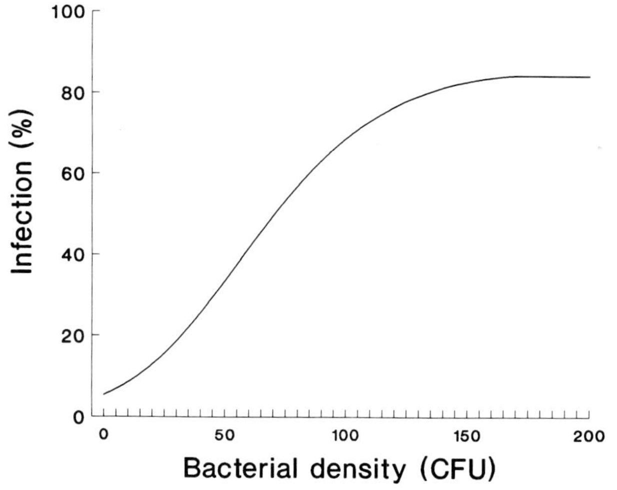

Fig. 2. Probability of infection, as a function of the number of CFU by the dipslide method, in patients not given cefuroxime postoperatively ($n = 814$). The graph was estimated according to the equation: $P(x) = 1/[1 + \exp(-\{\alpha + \beta x + \sigma x^2\})]$, where x is the number of CFU and $\alpha = -2.864$, $\beta = 0.05037$ and $\sigma = -0.0001398$.

among 591 patients (5.1%). In the 1–4-CFU group there were 18 cases of infection among 183 patients (9.8%) ($p = 0.037$; relative risk 1.94; 95% confidence interval 1.11–3.39). In the ⩾5-CFU group with no cefuroxime treatment, there were 19 cases of infection among 40 patients (47.5%) ($p < 0.001$; relative risk 9.36; 95% confidence interval 5.81–15.08). The incidence of infections in the groups without cefuroxime rose with the dipslide bacterial count ($p < 0.001$). The association between the density of bacteria in the operative wound and the probability of infection was described by a sigmoid dose–response curve (Fig. 2).

There were 23 cases of infection among 265 patients (8.7%) in the ⩾5-CFU group given cefuroxime postoperatively (Table II). When cefuroxime was not given to patients with ⩾5 CFU, there was a high risk of infection ($p < 0.001$; relative risk 5.47; 95% confidence interval 3.29–9.10). The overall infection rate in clinical practice was 7% during the second study period.

There were 19 deaths within 30 days of the operation (1.8%). The causes of death were: anastomotic dehiscence with peritonitis or septic shock, or both ($n = 3$); suspected septic shock ($n = 1$); pneumonia ($n = 3$); septicaemia and stroke ($n = 1$); circulatory disorders of the heart, lung or brain ($n = 9$), asthma ($n = 1$), and advanced cancer ($n = 1$). Of 8 cases in whom the cause of death was an infection, 7 had ⩾5 CFU on the dipslide (Table I).

In vitro control of dipslides

The relationship between the streak plate (x CFU/ml) and the dipslide methods (y CFU) was described (Fig. 3) by a first-degree equation:

$$y = 0.022x - 0.12 \pm 0.97 \text{ (SD)}; \quad r = 0.99.$$

One CFU on the dipslide corresponded to about 50 CFU/ml.

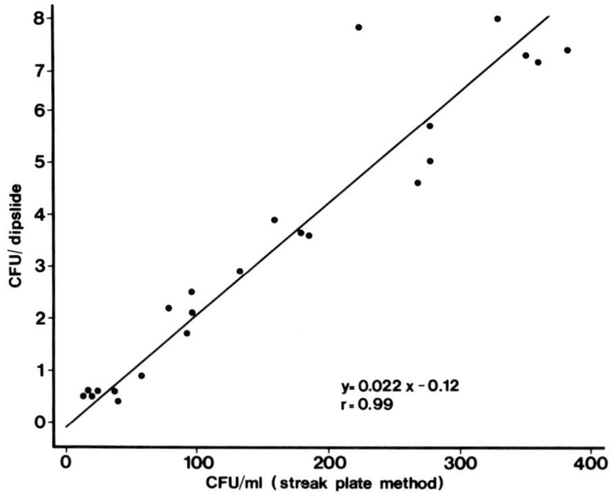

Fig. 3. Colony count of E. coli determined with dipslide and streak plate methods in saline-blood suspensions. Each point represents the mean of 5 streak plates and 10–25 dipslides.

Bacteriology

There was a predominance of enteric bacteria among the 622 stains isolated from operative dipslide cultures. Enterobacteriaceae sp. and enterococci constituted 88%, staphylococci 8%, non-fermentative Gram-negative rods 3%, and streptococci 1%. The most common species isolated was Escherichia coli ($n = 453$).

Cultures were available from 75 infections. The type of bacteria in cultures from postoperative infections differed markedly between the 0-CFU group (53 strains) and the other groups with ⩾1 CFU (72 strains); the respective incidences were: Enterobacteriaceae 31 and 66%, enterococci 2 and 11%, streptococci 18 and 10%, staphylococci 17 and 11%, non-fermentative Gram-negative rods 6 and 1% and anaerobes 26 and 1%.

The same type of aerobic organism was isolated from cultures taken during and after the operation in 28/30 (34) local wound infections available for culture, 5/7 (9) intra-abdominal abscesses, 3/3 (3) cases of peritonitis, 8/8 (17) anastomotic leaks and 1/1 (2) fistula; agreement in 92% of cases. (The figures in parenthesis represent the total number of each infection type in patients with ⩾1 CFU on the dipslide.) Similarity between the 2 cultures was, however seen in only 1/4 (5) perineal wounds and 1/5 (5) cases of septicaemia. The following species were cultured from both the operation and the postoperative infection: Escherichia coli ($n = 42$), Klebsiella pneumoniae ($n = 1$), Pseudomonas aeruginosa ($n = 1$), Enterococcus faecalis ($n = 1$), and Staphylococcus aureus ($n = 2$).

Of the strains of Enterobacteriaceae isolated during the operation, 5/518 (1%) were resistant to cefuroxime (MIC ⩾ 16 μg/ml); i.e. Klebsiella pneumoniae ($n = 3$) and Enterobacter sp. ($n = 2$). These strains were not associated with postoperative infection. Resistance to cefuroxime in postoperative infections was noted in all 4 groups: Entero-

Table III. *Univariate analysis of potential risk factors. Figures are number of patients unless otherwise stated*

Risk factor	Infection	No infection	*p*
Age, years			
Mean	67.2	62.9	0.007
Range	17–86	11–92	
Sex			
Male	53	474	0.0596
Female	37	515	
Mean preoperative hospital stay, days	5.4	5.4	>0.30
Mean body mass index, kg/m^2	25.2	24.2	0.046
Mean haemoglobin, g/l	127	128	>0.30
Mean serum albumin, g/l	36.9	38.1	0.036
Mean operative time, min	156	129	<0.001
No. of transfused units (means)			
Preoperative plasma	0	0.05	>0.30
Preoperative packed cells	0.14	0.13	>0.30
Intraoperative plasma	1.36	1.09	0.14
Intraoperative packed cells	1.69	0.79	<0.001
Postoperative plasma	1.02	0.36	<0.001
Postoperative packed cells	0.78	0.34	<0.001
Transfusion			
Yes	76	567	<0.001
No	14	422	
Faecal contamination			
Yes	9	87	>0.30
No	81	902	
Abdominal drains			
Yes	13	39	<0.001
No	77	950	
Cefuroxime			
Yes	23	242	<0.001
No	19	21	
Bacterial contamination			
<5 CFU	48	726	<0.001
≥5 CFU	19	21	
Diagnosis			
Cancer colon and rectum	78	614	<0.001
Crohn's disease	1	137	<0.001
Ulcerative colitis	3	23	>0.30
Diverticulosis	2	80	0.049
Volvolus	0	24	0.24
Miscellaneous	6	111	0.26
Surgical procedure			
Ileocaecal resection	5	116	0.09
Right hemicolectomy	13	196	>0.30
Transversum resection	1	35	>0.30
Left hemicolectomy	10	42	0.02
Sigmoid resection	13	228	0.07
Anterior resection	10	60	0.12
Abdominoperineal resection	17	94	0.01
Proctocolectomy	4	22	>0.30
Resection of anastomosis	1	36	>0.30
Anterior resection with stoma	12	64	0.04
Subtotal colectomy	3	28	>0.30
Enterotomy	0	37	0.08
Hartmann's operation	1	31	>0.30

bacter cloacae ($n = 4$), Klebsiella pneumoniae ($n = 2$), Citrobacter freundii ($n = 1$), and Providencia rettgeri ($n = 1$). There were no cases of Clostridium difficile-associated colitis in the study.

Risk factors

Univariate analysis of risk factors showed that high age, low serum albumin concentration, high body mass index, long operation, use of abdominal drains, degree of bacterial

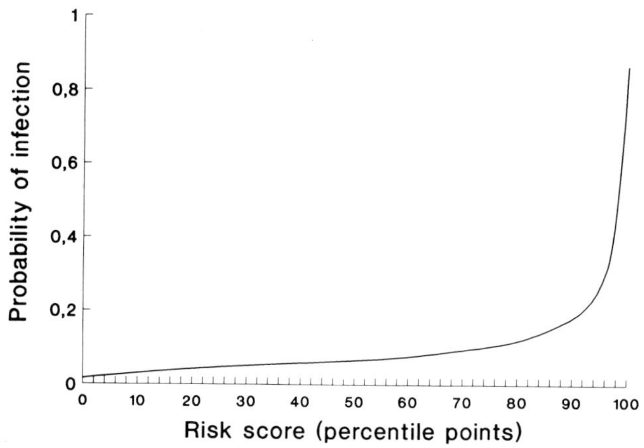

Fig. 4. Probability of infection plotted against the percentile points of risk based on the logistic regression analysis of the 4 significant variables (age, number of units of packed red blood cells given postoperatively, cefuroxime, and log (CFU + 1). The 50th percentile indicates the point at which the risk which exceeds that of half the patients and falls below that of the other half (the median).

contamination, not giving cefuroxime postoperatively, and transfusion within 5 days of operation were associated with infection (Table III). The incidence of infection rose with the number of units of packed red blood cells given intra- or postoperatively and of plasma given postoperatively.

Cancer was the most common diagnosis in the infected group and Crohn's disease the most uncommon. The following operations were most likely to be associated with infection: left hemicolectomy, abdominoperineal resection, and anterior resection with stoma. Preoperative hospital stay, haemoglobin concentration, sex, and visible faecal contamination during the operation, did not correlate with infection.

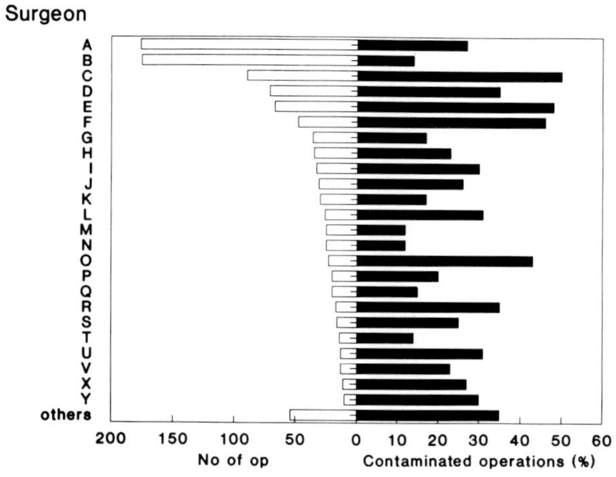

Fig. 5. The incidence of contaminated operations ($\geqslant 5$ CFU) for individual surgeons who did $\geqslant 10$ operations. The last bar represents all operations done by surgeons who did < 10 operations during the study period.

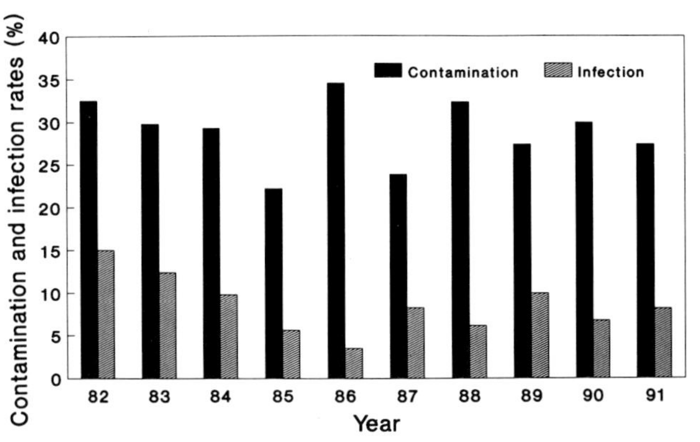

Fig. 6. Overall contamination and infection rates for each year. Changes in feedback reporting of culture results to the surgeons were made at the end of 1984 and 1986.

Multivariate analysis showed that greater age ($p = 0.014$), transfusion of packed red blood cells (PRC) after operation ($p < 0.001$) and bacterial contamination ($p < 0.001$) correlated positively with infection. Cefuroxime given postoperatively correlated negatively with infection ($p < 0.001$). A comparison between observed infections and a corrected estimate based on the logistic analysis showed that the operative procedure and the diagnosis did not contribute independently to infection.

The probability of infection was estimated as a function of the 4 significant variables:

$$1/[1 + \exp\{-(-4.15) - (0.019 \times \text{age}) - (0.372 \times \text{no. of units of PRC}) - (-1.84 \times \text{cefuroxime (yes} = 1, \text{no} = 0)) - 0.586 \times \log(\text{CFU} + 1)\}]$$

The probability of infection was plotted against the percentile points of risk (Fig. 4). The graph shows that the 4 significant variables identified a subgroup of patients with a high risk of infection.

Analysis of individual surgeons

Infection rates in operations by surgeons who did $\geqslant 25$ operations varied from 3.0 to 23.1%. When the actual figures were compared with a corrected estimate based on the four significant risk factors, no single surgeon did significantly better or worse than the rest. There was, however, more than a 4-fold difference in the rate of contaminated operations among individual surgeons (range 12–50%; chi-square = 73.08; 14 d.f.; $p < 0.001$) (Fig. 5).

Audit of contamination rate

The annual contamination rate ($\geqslant 5$ CFU) during the first study period (1982–June 1984) was 29–32% (Fig. 6). At that time, the surgeons were not aware of their results. During the second study period all results of dipslide cultures were reported to the surgeons within 24 h of the operation. In 1985, the first year of rapid feedback reporting, there was a reduction in the contamination rate to 22%. In 1986, however, there was an increase to 34%, the highest recording ever. At the end of that year, the surgeons were given a data sheet of their collected individual results. The following year, the rate dropped again to 24% but rose to 32% in 1988. During the last 3 years the rate of contamination has settled at 27–30%. Annual infection rates during study period 2 varied between 4 and 10% (Fig. 6).

DISCUSSION

This is the final report of the Skaraborg colon study; 10 years' experience of a new strategy for prophylaxis based on the assessment of operative bacterial contamination. The study design permitted a blinded evaluation of postoperative infections in relation to the density of aerobic bacteria. All patients were given prophylaxis against anaerobic bacteria with metronidazole. During the first study period (30 months) patients with a high density of aerobic bacteria (30%) were randomized to receive either a brief course of cefuroxime postoperatively, or no additional antibiotic. The improvement in outcome among patients given supplementary antibiotics during the first period, as previously reported (3), was confirmed in a large open evaluation of clinical practice during the second study period (84 months). The infection rate in contaminated patients was reduced from 47.5% to 8.7%, a more than 5-fold reduction, by giving cefuroxime postoperatively ($p < 0.001$). The infection rate in the group with no contamination was 5.1%. The addition of selective postoperative antibiotic cover of aerobic contaminants thus almost eliminated this risk factor.

The results from the audit of the second period include 5 cases in whom cefuroxime medication was missed by the ward or ICU staff, and 4 of these patients developed postoperative infections. These patients would be withdrawn in a controlled clinical trial situation such as study period 1. The audit analysis reflects the clinical situation more accurately. The most striking result was, however, the close resemblance in outcome, despite the different approaches in study design, when each of the different groups of contamination from the first period was compared with its corresponding group in the second period. The overall incidence in surgically related infections dropped from 18 to 7% (annual range 4–10) during the study. This result compares favourably with other controlled studies in which metronidazole plus cefuroxime has been given as preoperative prophylaxis (7–9).

Cultures from postoperative infections in patients with confirmed contamination grew bacteria of enteric origin with a heavy predominance of E. coli. During the entire study, resistance to cefuroxime was low in strains of Enterobacteriaceae from the peritoneal cavity and from postoperative infections. No single case of Clostridium difficile associated colitis was recorded. Our concern about problems of resistance and ecological disturbances by cefuroxime was not verified.

Our experience, with metronidazole given preoperatively for protection against anaerobes and cefuroxime postoperatively for aerobic cover, is an extension of Burke's concept of a very limited period of effective prophylactic action (1). Apart from obvious differences in the density of the inoculum, the type of micro-organisms involved, and the time between bacterial seeding and recognizable infection between colorectal surgery in man and the experimental animal model used by Burke, little attention has previously been paid to the timing of antimicrobials for prophylaxis of mixed aerobic and anaerobic infections.

Ingham et al. (10) showed that Bacteroides fragilis impaired the phagocytosis of facultative aerobic bacteria. Tofte et al. (11) proposed that B fragilis exerted this effect by competition for serum opsonins, a hypothesis supported by subsequent studies. Ingham et al. (12) suggested that the enhanced bactericidal effect of metronidazole on B fragilis in the presence of E. coli resulted from oxygen depletion of the medium by E. coli, which optimized the milieu for metronidazole which is active only under reduced conditions. A 2-phase strategy of treating a mixed anaerobic and aerobic flora (B. fragils and E. coli) with metronidazole and cefuroxime was studied in a cell culture model with oxygen tension comparable to that in surgical wounds in the immediate postoperative period (13). Anaerobic bacteria were killed more effectively when the initiation of cefuroxime treatment was delayed until 6 h after the start of the metronidazole. In the present study the percentage of anaerobic strains in septic wounds was much lower in patients who had intraoperative growth of coliforms (1%) than in patients who did not (26%). This finding corroborates well with Ingham's study (12) and our experience from the cell culture model (13).

To explain the beneficial results of postoperative cefuroxime in the current study, we postulated that a mixed aerobic (E. coli) and anaerobic (B. fragilis) wound inoculum is subject to the following process. During the first 24 h metronidazole effectively kills B. fragilis, partly through a promotor effect elicited by E. coli. Meanwhile the host defence is allowed to combat E. coli without the interference of B. fragilis. The addition of cefuroxime 24 h after the operation gives the necessary assistance to neutrophils to eradicate E. coli. The dynamics of this system suggest that there may be advantages in killing aerobic and anaerobic bacteria in 2 phases when metronidazole is used as the antianaerobic agent.

A recent audit of clinical practice with a large case mix, showed that antibiotics given postoperatively offer less protection against infection than those given before operation (14). The reasons for giving antibiotics postoperatively were not reported. According to Pettigrew et al. (15), the surgeon's opinion immediately after the operation about the risk of complications is a strong indicator of outcome.

It may well be therefore that the surgeons in the audit (14) selectively chose to give antimicrobials postoperatively to patients at high risk of infection.

The current study, which mainly involved "clean-contaminated" wounds, showed that there are large differences in risk within this particular category. Of 3 significant risk factors, 2 were related to the management of the patient. Bacterial contamination proved on culture, transfusion of packed red blood cells after operation, and increased age, were highly discriminatory risk factors on logistic regression analysis. The corresponding factors in the previous analysis during the first study period were bacterial contamination, increased age and operations with decompressive colostomy (4). The slight difference in identified risk factors may be attributed to the fact that blood transfusion was added to the present analysis, a factor which recently has been recognized as an important factor (16).

Animal studies favour the concept that blood transfusion causes immune suppression that increases susceptibility to infection. The specific component of blood that is responsible has not been identified. The use of whole blood in clincial practice makes it difficult to address this question in patients. In the current study, blood was transfused either as packed red cells or as plasma, but not as whole blood. An interesting finding was that postoperative transfusion of packed red blood cells was the only transfusion factor that was independently associated with surgical infection. In a recent study of septic patients, systemic oxygen uptake decreased and splanchnic ischaemia developed after transfusion of old packed red blood cells (17). Further studies are needed to establish whether transfusion of red blood cells exerts a detrimental effect on the microcirculation of the surgical wound tissues and on resistance to infection.

The degree of contamination as judged by the number of CFU on a dipslide was the strongest indicator of infection. The probability of infection was a function of the number of CFU according to a sigmoid dose–response curve, which means that the culture method detects clinically important differences in the degree of contamination. In vitro control of the dipslide showed an excellent correlation with the streak plate method. Despite its simplicity, the dipslide thus adds a quantitative dimension to the well known predictive criterion of wound bacteria for the outcome (18).

Raahave showed, with velvet pad sampling, that the distribution of bacteria in the wound is not uniform (19). Areas of high density are adjacent to areas of low density. This random distribution is a challenge in the surveillance of wound contamination, as it is practically impossible to sample all surfaces. In addition, the pressure applied during sampling is also crucial but difficult to standardize. The standardized irrigation and sampling manoeuvre used in the present study made it possible to assess the vast peritoneal surface under a constant pressure (gravity). Another attractive feature of the dipslide culture was that the same type of micro-organism was recovered postoperatively in 92% of cases with local wound infection, fistula, intra-abdominal abscess, diffuse peritonitis, and anastomotic leaks. Lower rates have been reported for other sampling methods.

The study showed that visible faecal contamination is not a significant risk factor for infection, and there was no correlation between visible contamination and that shown on culture (4). The conclusions are that bacterial contamination occurs without the surgeon's knowledge and that soilage with visible faecal matter is easy to control and therefore not always associated with detectable bacterial contamination.

It is disappointing that the annual contamination rate of about 30% did not improve consistently. The recording of obvious fluctuations from one year to another after changes in the system of feedback reporting to the surgeons suggests, however, that contamination is partly controllable. The strong correlation between the number of bacteria and infection may be that the dipslide culture recording is not only a result of the magnitude of bacterial contamination. It can be regarded as a summation of the dynamics between management factors, including surgical performance on the one hand, and host parasite interaction on the other.

Surgeon-related infection rates varied 8-fold (3.0–23.1%). When the figures were compared with a corrected estimate based on the logistic regression, no single surgeon did significantly better or worse than colleagues. The difference among surgeons could therefore be explained by a highly significant difference in contamination rate, shown to be the most important risk factor (12–50%, $p < 0.001$).

ACKNOWLEDGEMENTS

The study was presented in part at the Fifth Annual Meeting of the Surgical Infection Society-Europe (Joint meeting with SIS-North America), Santiago de Compostela, Spain, June 1992. The study was supported by a grant from The Skaraborg Institute of Public Health.

REFERENCES

1. Burke JF. The effective period of preventive antibiotic action in experimental incisions and dermal lesions. Surgery 50: 160–168, 1961.
2. Claesson BEB, Holmlund DEW. Dip slide culture of intraoperative peritoneal irrigation fluid for prediction of septic complication in elective colorectal surgery. J Clin Microbiol 24: 922–928, 1986.
3. Claesson BEB, Filipsson S, Holmlund DEW, Mätzsch TW, Wählby L. Selective cefuroxime prophylazis following colorectal surgery based on intra-operative dipslide culture. Br J Surg 73: 953–957, 1986.
4. Claesson BEB, Holmlund DEW, Predictors of intraoperative bacterial contamination and postoperative infection in elective colorectal surgery. J Hosp Infect 11: 127–135, 1988.
5. Pollock AV. Surgical wound sepsis. Lancet 2: 1283–1286, 1979.
6. Bradley JW. Distribution-free statistical tests. London: Prentice-Hall, 1968.

7. Mitchell NJ, Evans DS, Pollock D. Single dose metronidazole with and without cefuroxime in elective colorectal surgery. Br J Surg 70: 668–669, 1983.
8. Cunliffe WJ, Carr N, Schofield PF. Prophylactic metronidazole with and without cefuroxime in elective colorectal surgery. J Roy Coll Surg Edinb 30: 123–125, 1985.
9. Mittermayer H, Gross C, Brücke P. Prophylaxis with single dose cefuroxime/metronidazole versus metronidazole alone in elective colorectal surgery. Res Clin Forum 5: 109–117, 1983.
10. Ingham HR, Sisson PR, Tharagonnet D, Selkon JB, Codd AA. Inhibition of phagocytosis in vitro by obligate anaerobes. Lancet 2: 1252–1254, 1977.
11. Tofte RW, Peterson PK, Schmeling D, Bracke J, Kim Y, Quie PG. Opsonization of four Bacteroides species; the role of the classical complement pathway and immunoglobulin. Infect Immun 27: 784–792, 1980.
12. Ingham HR, Sisson PR, Eisenstadt RL, Sprott MS, Byrne PO, Selkon JB. Enhancement of activity of metronidazole by Escherichia coli under suboptimal anaerobic conditions. J Antimicrob Chemother 8: 475–479, 1981.
13. Claesson BEB, Gotthardsson IH. A tissue culture model for study of growth promotion and antimicrobial susceptibility in Bacteroides fragilis. J Antimicrob Chemother 21: 17–26, 1988.
14. Classen DC, Evans RS, Pestotnik SL, Horn SD, Menlove RL, Burke JP. The timing of prophylactic administration of antibiotics and the risk of surgical-wound infection. N Engl J Med 326: 281–286, 1992.
15. Pettigrew RA, Burns HJG, Carter DC. Evaluating surgical risk: the importance of technical factors in determining outcome. Br J Surg 74: 791–794, 1987.
16. Tartter PI. Blood transfusion and infectious complications following colorectal cancer surgery. Br J Surg 75: 789–792, 1988.
17. Marik PE, Sibbald WJ. Effect of stored-blood transfusion on oxygen delivery in patients with sepsis. J Am Med Assoc 269: 3024–3029, 1993.
18. Davidson AIG, Clarke C, Smith G. Postoperative wound infection: a computor analysis. Br J Surg 58: 333–337, 1971.
19. Raahave D. Effect of plastic skin and wound drapes on the density of bacteria in operation wounds. Br J Surg 63: 421–426, 1976.

Submitted March 3, 1995; accepted August 16, 1995

Scand J Infect Dis 27: 613–617, 1995 ORIGINAL ARTICLE

Fluconazole Compared with Itraconazole in the Treatment of Esophageal Candidiasis in AIDS Patients: A Double-blind, Randomized, Controlled Clinical Study

GIUSEPPE BARBARO[2], GIORGIO BARBARINI[1] and GABRIELLA DI LORENZO[2]

From the [1]Department of Emergency Medicine, University of Rome "La Sapienza", and the [2]Department of Infectious Diseases IRCCS Policlinico S. Matteo, University of Pavia, Italy

The aim of this study was to assess the role and the therapeutic efficacy of 2 azole antifungal drugs, fluconazole and itraconazole, in the treatment of endoscopically diagnosed Candida esophagitis in patients with acquired immunodeficiency syndrome (AIDS). The study involved 123 human immunodeficiency virus (HIV)-positive patients (70 males and 53 females, mean age 27 years) at their first episode of esophageal candidiasis diagnosed by endoscopy. The patients were randomized in a double-blind design to receive either fluconazole (100 mb b.i.d. per os) or itraconazole (100 mg b.i.d. per os). In order to evaluate the efficacy of treatment, clinical examinations were performed every week up to the end of follow-up (2 months); endoscopic examination was performed at baseline, at the end of treatment (3 weeks) and at the end of follow-up. At the end of the treatment, cure, as judged by endoscopy, was observed in 74% of fluconazole-treated patients and in 47.2% of itraconazole-treated patients ($p < 0.01$); at the end of follow-up, cure was observed endoscopically in 71.7% of fluconazole-treated patients and in 43.2% of the itraconazole-treated patients ($p < 0.05$). As regards clinical cure, no statistically significant difference was observed between the groups, at the end of pharmacological treatment and at the end of follow-up. The results of this study demonstrate that both fluconazole and itraconazole are efficacious in the treatment of Candida esophagitis in AIDS patients; fluconazole is associated with higher rate of endoscopic cure than is itraconazole.

G. Barbaro, MD, Viale Anicio Gallo n.63, I-00174, Rome, Italy

INTRODUCTION

Esophageal candidiasis is one of the most common mycotic opportunistic infections in acquired immunodeficiency syndrome (AIDS) patients, with the mean incidence of 15–20%. In 3–10% of cases candida esophagitis represents the first opportunistic infection, and may precede the outbreak of more severe infections in more than 50% of cases (1). The most clinically important species is C. albicans (80% of cases). Other species reported are: C. tropicalis, C. pseudotropicalis, C. krusei, C. parapsilosis, C. glabrata (15–20% of cases) (1).

Contrasting opinions exist about the pharmacological treatment of esophageal candidiasis in human immunodeficiency virus (HIV)-positive patients. A number of agents have been used to treat candida esophagitis, including topical medications such as nystatin, clotrimazole and miconazole, oral compounds such as ketoconazole and 5-flucytosine and intravenous agents such as amphotericin B. Nevertheless, little information is actually available regarding the response of candida esophagitis to antifungal therapy (2–6).

The aim of this study was to assess, using a double-blind controlled design, the role, therapeutic efficacy and safety of use of 2 azole antifungal drugs, fluconazole and itraconazole, in the treatment of endoscopically diagnosed esophageal candidiasis in AIDS patients.

MATERIALS AND METHODS

Patient selection criteria and mycological assessment

HIV-positive patients without a previous history of candida esophagitis and with mild-to-moderate symptoms of odynophagia, dysphagia or retrosternal pain, not compromising swallowing and nutritional capacity, were eligible for the study, if upper gastrointestinal endoscopy revealed white plaques or exudate consistent with a diagnosis of candida infection, and if pseudohyphae were identified on brushing and/or biopsy of esophageal mucosa. Patients in the following categories were excluded from study:

- Under 18 years of age
- with evidence of non-candidal systemic fungal infection
- who had received previous therapy with antifungal drugs
- with a history of allergy to imidazoles
- who had received therapy with antiretroviral and/or immunomodulant drugs and/or with anticoagulants, rifampin, ansamycin, cyclosporin A, with medications that raise gastric pH (H_2-receptor blocking agents, antacids, omeprazole), myelotoxic, cytotoxic, nephrotoxic or experimental drugs
- who had used illicit drugs in the last 6 months
- who were pregnant or lactating
- with total white blood cell count (WBC) $<2500/mm^3$, and with neutrophil granulocyte count (NGC) $<1000/mm^3$
- with a hemoglobin value (Hb) $< 10 g/dl$
- with transaminase and bilirubin levels >3 times the normal values, and/or with prothrombin time >5s over control
- with levels of creatininemia >2 times normal values
- with serious acute infection
- with serious diseases not specifically related to HIV infection (cardiomyopathies, diabetes, hypertension, epilepsy, psychopathy, neoplastic diseases)

 ISSN 0036-5548

- with a life expectancy <3 months
- those not able to provide informed consent.

Mycological assessment was made by culture of endoscopic brushing and/or bioptic samples of esophageal mucosa on Sabouraud 4% glucose agar. After 48–72 h at 37°C, yeast colonies were isolated and identfied. For identification of the various Candida species, germ tube formation in bovine serum, and the presence of chlamydospores and pseudomycelia on Tween-rice agar were tested. Finally, the yeasts were characterized by means of an API20C or ATB 32C system (Mérieux, Lyon, France).

Endoscopic examination was carried out using an Olympus GIF Q-IT20 instrument. Endoscopic lesions were graded on a scale of 0–III by a modification of Kodsi et al endoscopic classification of Candida esophagitis (7):

- grade 0, normal esophageal mucosa;
- grade I, individual raised plaques, each ≤2 mm in size
- grade II, individual raised plaques >2 mm in size
- grade III, confluent plaques combined or not with ulceration and/or increased friability of mucosa.

Clinical symptoms were graded on a scale of 0–III by modification of a clinical classification proposed by Barbaro & Di Lorenzo in a previous study (6):

- grade 0, absence of symptoms
- grade I, symptoms of mild entity
- grade II, symptoms of moderate entity not compromising (grade IIa) or compromising (grade IIb) the swallowing function
- grade III, symptoms of severe entity, not compromising (grade IIIa) or compromising (grade IIIb) the swallowing function.

No other opportunistic infection of the esophagus was detected.

Randomization

The patients selected for the study were randomized using a double-blind method, and assigned to receive identical capsules of fluconazole (100 mb b.i.d. per os) or itraconazole (100 mg b.i.d. per os), according to a computer-generated randomization schedule kept by an independent investigator. Doses could be doubled at week 1 or 2 if no symptomatic improvement occurred during the preceding week. The capsules given to the patients in the 2 randomized groups were provided by the Department of Clinical Pharmacology of the University of Pavia.

Compliance

Compliance with the prescribed therapy was verified during the clinical follow-up of the patients selected for the study by counting the remaining capsules at each visit. Patients were considered compliant if they took at least 75% of the prescribed dosage of the drug during the entire study.

Clinical evaluation and follow-up

In order to evaluate the efficacy of the drug treatment, clinical examination and routine hematochemical tests were performed at baseline and every week up to the end of follow-up (2 months); endoscopic examination was performed at baseline, at the end of treatment (3 weeks) and at the end of follow-up.

Endoscopic cure (grade 0 according to Kodsi et al.) was considered as the complete disappearance of visible candidiasis in the patients of both groups at the end of pharmacological treatment. The endoscopic lesions observed at the end of treatment and at the end of follow-up were graded according to the modified scale of Kodsi et al. already mentioned. Clinical cure (Barbaro & Di Lorenzo grade 0) was considered as the resolution of symptoms as compared with baseline. Clinical symptoms reported by patients at the end of pharmacological treatment and at the end of follow-up were graded according the modified scale of Barbaro and Di Lorenzo, mentioned above.

Table I. *Patient characteristics at baseline in the 2 study groups*

Characteristics	Fluconazole ($n=62$)	Itraconazole ($n=61$)
Male	36	33
Female	26	28
Mean age, years	28	27
Drug addiction	45	43
Homosexual	15	13
Heterosexual	2	5
T cells CD4+, cells/mm^3, mean value	66	68
Endoscopic grade I esophagitis	4	2
Endoscopic grade II esophagitis	58	59
Clinical symptoms grade I	6	3
Clinical symptoms grade IIa	56	58

p = n.s. for comparison of each characteristic between fluconazole and itraconazole group.

Reduction of drug dosage and interruption of pharmacological treatment

The drug dosage in the groups of study could be reduced in the presence of the following conditions: anaemia (Hb <8 g/dl); granulocytopenia (NGC <750/mm^3) and leucopenia (WBC <1500/mm^3); serious alterations of liver and kidney function or symptoms of intolerance to pharmacological therapy not requiring the interruption of the treatment.

The pharmacological treatment could be interrupted in the presence of: progressive myeloinhibition (Hb <7g/dl; WBC <1000/mm^3; NGC <500/mm^3); serious relapsing infections; serious toxic effects; the need to begin treatments interfering with antifungal therapy; manifestation of severe intolerance to pharmacological treatment, or serious and progressive compromise of clinical conditions.

Statistical analysis

The sample size was estimated on the basis of a mean expected rate of positive response of 80% in the patients of both groups (5, 6). Assuming a mean difference of 20% in the expected response between the treatment groups (5) and a test power of 80% ($\alpha = 0.05$; $\theta = 0.20$, one-tailed test), with a 90% compliance of selected patients, a sample size of 120 patients was determined.

As nominal scales were used, the data, regarding endoscopic and clinical responses and the incidence of side-effects in the 2 study groups, were evaluated using the chi-square test for 2 × 2 tables with Yates' correction (8). The risk ratio for endoscopic and clinical responses in the 2 treatment groups (percentage response observed in fluconazole-treated patients/percentage response observed in itraconazole-treated patients) with 95% confidence intervals (95% CI) was also calculated (8). The Kaplan-Meier method was used for the evaluation of the probability of cure (grade 0 Kodsi et al., and grade 0 Barbaro et al.), regarding both endoscopic and clinical responses in the patients of the different study groups.

The patients lost to follow up and those withdrew from the study were censored in this analysis.

The 95% CI, for the probabilities of cure were computed using normal approximations of the estimates of probabilities and their variances (8).

Informed consent

The research was carried out in accordance with the Helsinki Declaration. The study protocol was explained to all the patients

Table II. *Endoscopic assessment of esophageal candidiasis and clinical response in the 2 study groups at the end of pharmacological treatment*

Endoscopic and clinical grades	Fluconazole[a] ($n = 54$)	Itraconazole[b] $n = 53$)	Risk ratio (95% confidence interval (CI))	p value
Endoscopic grade 0	40	25	1.57 (1.38–2.26)	< 0.01
Endoscopic grade I	10	17	0.58 (0.27–0.77)	n.s.
Endoscopic grade II	3	11	0.27 (– 0.044–0.49)	n.s.
Clinical grade 0	42	40	1.03 (0.87–1.13)	n.s.
Clinical grade I	11	10	1.07 (0.51–1.15)	n.s.
Clinical grade IIa	1	3	0.33 (– 0.48–0.70)	n.s.

[a] 8 patients withdrew from the trial because of side-effects.
[b] 7 patients withdrew because of side-effects; 1 patient withdrew because of intolerance to continued drug treatment.

selected. All the patients selected for the study provided informed consent.

RESULTS

Study population and withdrawal from the trial

A total of 123 patients (70 males and 53 females, mean age 27 ± 5 years) fulfilled the selection criteria and entered the trial. In 114 patients (92.7%) Candida albicans was responsible for esophagitis, and in the other 9 patients Candida tropicalis (4 patients (3.3%)) and Candida glabrata (5 patients (4%)) were responsible. Baseline patient characteristics in the 2 treatment groups are shown in Table I. Of the patients 62 (58 patients with Candida albicans, 3 patients with Candida glabrata and 1 patient with Candida tropicalis esophagitis) were randomized to receive fluconazole, and 61 patients (56 patients with Candida albicans, 3 patients with Candida tropicalis and 2 patients with Candida glabrata esophagitis) were randomized to receive itraconazole. In the fluconazole group 8 patients withdrew, after 2 weeks of treatment, because of side-effects. In the itraconazole-group, 7 patients after 1 week and 5 after 2 weeks of treatment (p = n.s.) because of side effects withdrew from the study. A patient in the itraconazole-group withdrew because of intolerance to the drug therapy, and 1 patient in the fluconazole group and 2 in the itraconazole group were lost to follow-up after the 3 weeks of treatment.

The drug dose was doubled in 6 patients treated with fluconazole (4 patients at week 2, and 2 patients at week 3) and in 8 patients given itraconazole (5 patients at week 2 and 3 patients at week 3) (p = n.s.).

Endoscopic and clinical response at the end of drug treatment

The endoscopic assessments of esophageal candidiasis and the clinical responses observed at the end of treatment in the 2 study groups are shown in Table II.

Endoscopic cure was observed in 40/54 patients (74%) in the fluconazole group and in 25/53 patients (47.2%) in the itraconazole group (risk ratio, 1.57; 95% CI, 1.38–2.26; $p < 0.01$).

Clinical cure was observed in 42/54 patients (77.8%) in the fluconazole goup and in 40/53 patients (75.5%) in the itraconazole group (risk ratio, 1.03; 95% CI, 0.87–1.13; p = n.s.)

Endoscopic and clinical response at the end of follow-up

The endoscopic assessment of esophageal candidiasis and the clinical response observed at the end of follow-up in the 2 study groups are shown in Table III.

Endoscopic cure was observed in 38/53 patients (71.7%) in the fluconazole group and in 22/51 patients (43.2%) in the itraconazole group (risk ratio, 1.66; 95% CI, 1.19–2.35; $p < 0.05$).

Table III. *Endoscopic assessment of esophageal candidiasis and clinical response to pharmacological treatment in the 2 study groups at the end of follow-up*

Endoscopic and clinical grades	Fluconazole[a] ($n = 53$)	Itraconazole[b] ($n = 51$	Risk ratio (95% CI)	p value
Endoscopic grade 0	38	22	1.66 (1.19–2.35)	< 0.05
Endoscopic grade I	12	25	0.48 (0.24–0.64)	< 0.05
Endoscopic grade II	3	4	0.72 (– 0.36–0.95)	n.s.
Clinical grade 0	40	38	1.01 (0.85–1.09)	n.s.
Clinical grade I	11	12	0.88 (0.45–0.98)	n.s.
Clinical grade IIa	2	1	1.94 (1.38–2.73)	n.s.

[a] 1 patient lost to follow up.
[b] 2 patients lost to follow up.

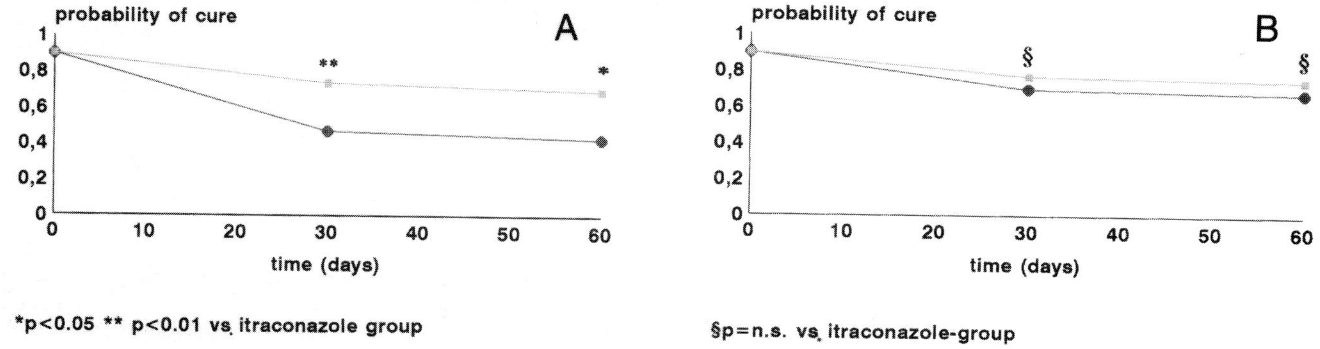

Fig. 1. Probability of cure as assessed by A endoscopic response, and B clinical response in the patients of the 2 study groups. At day 30 the probability of endoscopic cure (grade 0, Kodsi et al.) was 74% in the fluconazole group compared with 47% in the itraconazole group ($\Delta = 27\%$; 95% confidence interval (CI), 0.085–0.455, $p < 0.01$). At day 60 the probability of endoscopic cure was 70% in the fluconazole group compared with 43% in the itraconazole group ($\Delta = 27\%$; 95% CI, 0.080–0.460; $p < 0.05$), At day 30 the probability of clinical cure (grade 0, Barbaro & Di Lorenzo) was 77% in the fluconazole group compared with 75% in the itraconazole group ($\Delta = 2\%$; 95% CI, −0.142–0.182; p = n.s.). At day 60 the probability of clinical cure was 75% in the fluconazole group compared with 74% in the itraconazole group ($\Delta = 1\%$; 95% CI, −0.158–0.178; p = n.s.). ■ = Fluconazole, ● = itraconazole.

Clinical cure was observed in 40/53 patients (75.5%) in the fluconazole group and in 38/51 patients (74.5%) in the itraconazole group (risk ratio, 1.01; 95% CI, 0.85–1.09; p = n.s.)

Probability of cure

The probability of cure as evaluated by endoscopic response and clinical response over time in the patients in the 2 groups is shown in Fig 1.

Side-effects and compliance

The most commonly reported side-effects were epigastric pain (7 patients in the fluconazole group and 5 in the itraconazole group), nausea (9 and 6 patients respectively), diarrhea (4 and 3 patients respectively), and skin rash (4 patients in the itraconazole group). No modification of hematochemical test values was noticed at the end of the follow up in the patients of both study groups, as compared with baseline.

In the fluconazole-group compliance was 87% compared with 86% in itraconazole-group (p = n.s.).

DISCUSSION

Fluconazole and itraconazole are azole antifungal drugs which can be applied in the treatment of topical and systemic mycoses (9). They inhibit 14-α-demethylation of lanosterol in fungi by binding to one of the cytochrome P-450 enzymes. This leads to accumulation of 14-α-methylsterol and reduced concentrations of ergosterol, a steroid essential for a normal fungal cytoplasmic membrane (5, 9).

Despite its marked structural similarity to ketoconazole, itraconazole differs in several respects. Peak blood levels are lower than with ketoconazole, but tissue levels are higher; the terminal elimination half-life of itraconazole is significantly longer than that of ketoconazole (24–42 compared with 7–10 h and similar to that of fluconazole (22–31 h) (9). Antifungal activity is better in both susceptibility testing and in vitro systems measuring the inhibition of Candida albicans cytochrome P-450 (9). The presence of a triazole ring in fluconazole results in greater polarity and water solubility with a reduced protein binding (11%). On the other hand, as with ketoconazole, about 99% of serum itraconazole is protein-bound (9). Both fluconazole and itraconazole have shown therapeutic activity in the treatment of fungal infections in HIV-positive patients (4, 5, 9–12).

In our study, fluconazole demonstrates a greater therapeutic efficacy than itraconazole in the treatment of esophageal candidiasis in AIDS patients, with a complete remission of clinical symptomatology in 75.5% of patients (compared with 74.5% of itraconazole-treated patients) and of endoscopic lesions in 71.7% of patients (compared with 43.2% of itraconazole-treated patients). Comparison of clinical and endoscopic responses showed that 95% of fluconazole-treated patients with a clinical cure also had an endoscopic cure, whereas only 57.9% of itraconazole-treated patients with resolution of symptoms also had an endoscopic cure.

Therefore, symptoms of Candida esophagitis may resolve despite continuing endoscopically demonstrable gross involvement of the esophageal mucosa (5, 6). According to our experience, a spontaneous remission of clinical symptomatology can be observed up to 30% of patients without resolution of endoscopic lesions (6). On the other hand, some investigators have noted that approximately 10–20% of HIV-positive patients who have esophageal symptoms have no evidence of esophageal abnormalities at endoscopy (3, 13), In our experience, no evidence of endoscopic lesions was observed in 15% of HIV-positive patients with esophageal symptoms (6). The subjective evaluation of clinical symptomatology compared with objective evaluation of endoscopic lesions may explain, in part, the discrepancy between clinical and endoscopic findings (5, 6).

The rates of clinical and endoscopic responses in the fluconazole-treated group reported in our study are in agreement with those reported in other controlled clinical and endoscopic studies (5). However, in the itraconazole-treated group, while the rate of clinical response is in agreement with that reported in other clinical studies (4, 11, 12), the rate of endoscopic response is lower, although few trials (4) and preliminary reports (11, 12) have been published on this topic. It must be emphasized that in these clinical studies only small sized samples have been used for endoscopic evaluation of the therapeutic efficacy of itraconazole. Thus in analysing the reported results, it is difficult to draw any specific conclusion because of high beta-type errors. Furthermore, in those trials the selection criteria for patients were different from ours and thus the results cannot be compared because of the interference of several (clinical and pharmacological) factors.

The shortness of the follow-up period represents the principal limitation of our study, but the accurate selection of the patients and the evaluation of clinical and endoscopic responses according to quantitative parameters, with a 80% statistical power, characterize our study compared with other clinical and endoscopic trials regarding the treatment of Candida esophagitis in AIDS patients (2, 4).

A possible explanation for the difference in therapeutic response to fluconazole and itraconazole may be related to a greater bioavailability of fluconazole for a significantly reduced protein binding, to a higher peak plasma concentration (10.2 μg/ml of fluconazole vs. 0.2–0.4 μg/ml of itraconazole) and to a more consistent oral absorption of fluconazole (gastric pH-independent) (9, 14, 15). The absorption of itraconazole, like that of ketoconazole, may be impaired in AIDS patients as a result of reduced gastric acid secretion (16); pharmacokinetics studies have demonstrated that the absorption of oral itraconazole is reduced by approximately 50% in AIDS patients compared with healthy volunteers (17). While it has been demonstrated that fluconazole has greater activity in vivo against Candida species than does ketoconazole, possibly greater activity of fluconazole in vivo compared with itraconazole can be assumed, but is still to be ascertained (14, 15).

In summary, both fluconazole and itraconazole present good therapeutic effect in terms of clinical response with a significant compliance level, especially in short-term treatment of Candida esophagitis in AIDS patients. Treatment with fluconazole is associated with higher rates of endoscopic and clinical cure than itraconazole, with a statistically significant difference as regards endoscopic cure.

ACKNOWLEDGEMENTS

The Authors thank Dr Pierangela Alcini, of the Department of Clinical Pharmacology of the University of Pavia, for her collaboration in providing the pharmacological material used in the study.

REFERENCES

1. Rondanelli EG. AIDS. Clinical and laboratory atlas. Pavia: Edizioni Medico-Scientifiche, 86–91, 1989.
2. Deschamps MM, Pape JW, Verdier RI, DeHovitz J, Thomas F, Johnson WD Jr. Treatment of Candida esophagitis in AIDS patients. Am J Gastroenterol 83: 20–21, 1988.
3. Connoly GM Hawkins D, Harcourt-Webster JN, Parson PA, Husain OA, Gazzard BG. Oesophageal symptoms, their causes, treatment and prognosis in patients with the acquired immunodeficiency syndrome. Gut 30: 1033–1039, 1989.
4. Smith DE, Midgley J, Allan M, Connonly GM, Gazzard BG. Itraconazole vs. ketakonazole in the treatment of oral and oesophageal candidosis in patients infected with HIV. AIDS 5: 1367–1371, 1991.
5. Laine L, Dretler RH, Conteas CN et al. Fluconazole compared with ketoconazole for the treatment of Candida esophagitis in AIDS. A randomized trial. Ann Intern Med 117: 655–660, 1992.
6. Barbaro G, Di Lorenzo G. Fluconazole vs. flucytosine in the treatment of esophageal candidiasis in AIDS patients: a double-blind, placebo-controlled study [abstract]. Proceedings of 3rd United European Digestive Week; 1994 June 25–29, Oslo. 34–35.
7. Kodsi BE, Wicremesinghe PC, Kozinn PJ, Iswara K, Goldberg PK. Candida esophagitis. A prospective study of 27 cases. Gastroenterology 71: 715–719, 1976.
8. Armitage P, Berry G. Statistical methods in medical research, 2nd edn. Oxford: Blackwell Scientific, 1987.
9. Bennett JE. Antifungal agents. In: Mandell GL, Douglas RG Jr, Bennett JE, eds. Principles and practice of infectious diseases, 3rd edn. New York: Churchill Livingstone, 361–370, 1990.
10. Just-Nubling G, Gentschew G, Dohle M, Bottinger C. Helm EB, Stille W. Fluconazole in the treatment of oropharingeal candidosis in HIV-positive patients. Mycoses 33: 435–440, 1990.
11. Phillips P, Fetchick R, Weisman I, et al. Tolerance and efficacy of itraconazole in treatment of systemic mycoses. Prelimary results. Rev Infect Dis 9 Suppl 1: S87–S93, 1987.
12. Grant SM, Clissold SP. Itraconazole: a review of its pharmacodynamic and pharmacokinetics properties, and therapeutic potential in superficial and systemic mycoses. Drugs 39: 877–916, 1990.
13. Bonacini M, Young T, Laine L. The causes of esophageal symptoms in human immunodeficiency virus infection. A prospective study of 110 patients. Arch Intern Med 115: 1567–1572, 1991.
14. Saag MS, Dismukes WE. Azole antifungal agents: emphasis on new triazoles. Antimicrob Agents Chemother 32: 1–8, 1988.
15. Como JA, Dismukes WE. Oral azole drugs as systemic antifungal therapy. N Engl J Med 330: 263–272, 1994.
16. Lake-Bakaar G, Tom W, Lake Bakaar D, et al. Gastropathy and ketoconazole malabsorption in the acquired immunodeficiency syndrome (AIDS). Ann Intern Med 109: 471–473, 1988.
17. Smith D, Woestenborghs R, Heykants J, Gazzard B. The pharmacokinetics of oral itraconazole in AIDS patients. Proceedings of the 7th International Conference on AIDS; 1991 June 16–21; Florence. 225A.

Submitted January 13, 1995; accepted September 6, 1995

Scand J Infect Dis 27: 619–622, 1995 ORIGINAL ARTICLE

Pneumonia in Mechanically Ventilated Children

ITZHAK BROOK

From the Department of Pediatrics, Georgetown University School of Medicine, Washington DC, USA

The quantitative aerobic and anaerobic microbiology of bronchial aspirates, obtained using protective brush catheters, from 10 children with ventilator-associated pneumonia, is presented. Aerobic or faculative organisms only were isolated in 1 child, anaerobic bacteria only in 3, and aerobic mixed with anaerobic bacteria in 6. There were 10 aerobic or faculative and 17 anaerobic isolates. The predominant aerobes were Pseudomonas aeruginosa (2 isolates) and Klebsiella sp. (2). The predominant anaerobes were pigmented Prevotella and Porphyromonas species (5), Peptostreptococcus sp. (4), Fusobacterium sp. and B. fragilis group (2). A total of 10 beta-lactamase-producing aerobic and anaerobic bacteria were isolated in 8 patients. All patients except 1 responded to antimicrobial therapy directed against the recovered isolates. These data highlight the polymicrobial aerobic–anaerobic flora isolated from pulmonary specimens of patients with ventilator-associated pneumonia.

I. Brook, MD, Box 70412, Chevy Chase, MD 20813-0412, USA

INTRODUCTION

Ventilator-associated pneumonia (VAP) is one of the most common complications in intubated children. The establishment of the bacterial etiology of respiratory infection in mechanically ventilated adults has been determined to be best based upon quantitative cultures of bronchial specimens obtained with protective brush catheters (PBC) (1–5).

Although mechanical ventilation is frequently used in children, no studies were found where the methods used could identify the aerobic as well as the anaerobic microbiology of the pneumonia associated with this procedure. This study describes the author's personal experience in evaluating the aerobic and anaerobic microbiology of ventilator-associated pneumonia in children.

PATIENTS AND METHODS

A total of 10 children who developed VAP, and whose pulmonary aspirates were studied for aerobic and anaerobic bacteria, were included in the study. The patients were seen and treated by the author between 1976 and 1986 at the University of California Medical Center (2 patients) and the University of Southern California Medical Center in Los Angeles (1 patient), California; at the Fairview State Hospital in Costa Mesa, California (4 patients); Children's Hospital National Medical Center (2 patients), and the South-East Medical Center (1 patient), Washington, DC.

The patients' ages ranged from 6 to 16 years (average 10) and 6 were males. Each patient received mechanical ventilation via a nasotracheal or tracheal tube connected to a ventilator. The patients included had been hospitalized for >72 h and had an endotracheal tube in place for >48 h.

For each patient studied, the chart was reviewed for the following parameters: age; sex; date of intubation or tracheostomy; duration of mechanical ventilation; previous pulmonary infections, and antibiotics received prior to the day of sampling. Samplings were performed because of the diagnosis of nosocomial pneumonia.

The diagnosis of ventilator-associated pneumonia required all 5 of the following criteria during or within 48 h of sampling:

1 purulent sputum with a Gram stain showing >25 leukocytes and <10 squamous epithelial cells/high power field;
2 a respiratory or nosocomial pathogen isolated from sputum cultures and/or bacteria seen on Gram-stained smears of the sputum;
3 a peripheral leukocyte count of $>15{,}000/\mu l$;
4 fever $>38°C$, and
5 a new and persistent infiltrate on chest X-ray.

Collection and processing of specimens

Following careful endotracheal suctioning, the protected specimen brush (PSB) was inserted 10–25 cm into the airway via the endotracheal tube, until it could not be advanced further, then it was retracted a few centimeters. The brush was then advanced 2–3 cm beyond the tip of the outer sheath, extruding the plug. The brush was retracted into the outer sheath, and the entire unit was removed from the patient. The outside of the catheter was cleaned with 70% alcohol and a 1 cm portion of the inner sheath was cut off. The brush was then readvanced, cut off with a sterile clippers, and placed into a sterile specimen container with 1 ml of prereduced sterile saline.

Specimens were transported immediately to the microbiology laboratory for Gram staining and quantitative cultures. Following 30 s of vigorous agitation using a vortex mixer, 2 serial 100-fold dilutions of the samples were prepared to give final concentrations of 10^{-2} and 10^{-4}. Gram stains were obtained on aliquots from the original 1 ml sample. Aliquots of 0.1 ml of the undiluted specimens and the 2 dilutions were taken for aerobic and anaerobic bacterial cultures. The results were obtained in colony-forming units/ml of the original 1 ml dilution (cfu/ml). A positive culture was determined as the recovery of $\geq 10^5$ cfu/ml of a potential pathogen. Organisms that were recovered in quantities $<10^5$ cfu/ml were considered as contaminants.

Specimens were inoculated onto 5% sheep blood, chocolate and MacConkey's agar plates for aerobic and facultative organisms. These plates were incubated at 37°C aerobically (MacConkey) or in 5% CO_2 (5% sheep blood and chocolate), and were examined at 24 and 48 h.

Table I. *Microbiology and clinical features of 10 children with VAP*

Patient no.	Age, years	Sex	Underlying condition	Culture results, cfu/ml: Aerobic bacteria	Culture results, cfu/ml: Anaerobic bacteria	Duration of ventilation prior to culture, days	Antibiotic: Prior to culture	Antibiotic: After culture	Outcome
1	6	F	Coma	K. pneumoniae[a] (4×10^6) P. aeruginosa[a] (6×10^5)	Peptostreptococcus (9×10^5)	10	None	Ampicillin + gentamicin	Died
2	8	M	Encephalitis	P. mirabilis (3×10^5)	P. intermedia[a] (7×10^5) F. nucleatum (5×10^5)	25	None	Clindamycin + gentamicin	Improved
3	12	M	Head trauma	H. influenzae type B[a,b] (7×10^5)	P. asaccharolytica (10^6) P. micros (3×10^7)	13	None	Chloramphenicol + penicillin	Recovered
4	16	F	Drug overdose	—	F. nucleatum[a] (6×10^5) P. asaccharolytica (3×10^6)	5	None	Ticarcillin-clavulanate	Recovered
5	9	F	Brain tumor	E. coli (7×10^6) S. mitis (6×10^5)	B. fragilis[a] (10^6) Veillonella sp. (2×10^5)	6	None	Clindamycin + gentamicin	Improved
6	7	M	Head trauma	—	Bacteroides sp. (2×10^6) Bifidobacterium sp. (6×10^5)	9	Penicillin	Clindamycin + gentamicin	Recovered
7	8	F	Brain damage (postencephalitis)	S. aureus[a] (1.6×10^6) Microaerophilic streptococcus (7×10^7)	—	84	Ampicillin Gentamicin	Vancomycin	Improved
8	7	M	Drowning	P. aeruginosa[a] (10^7)	B. vulgatus[a] (9×10^5) P. micros (5×10^6)	10	Amoxicillin	Clindamycin + amikacin	Recovered
9	12	M	Drowning	K. oxytoca (2×10^5)	P. oralis (6×10^6) P. intermedia[a] (4×10^6)	8	Cefazolin	Ticarcillin-clavulanate	Recovered
10	13	M	Brain abscess	—	F. nucleatum[b] (4×10^6) Peptostreptococcus sp. (2×10^5)	6	Metronidazole Methicillin	Clindamycin	Improved

[a] beta-lactamase producing bacteria.
[b] also recovered from the blood.

For anaerobes the material was plated onto prereduced vitamin K_1-enriched Brucella blood agar, an anaerobic blood agar plate containing kanamycin and vancomycin, an anaerobic blood plate containing phenylethyl alcohol and an enriched thioglycolate broth (containing hemin and vitamin K_1) (6). The anaerobic plates and thioglycolate broth were incubated in GasPak® jars (BBL, Cockeysville, Maryland, USA) and were examined at 48 and 96 h.

Venous blood for blood cultures was obtained from 8 of the patients.

Anaerobes were identified by techniques described previously (6). Aerobic bacteria and their antimicrobial susceptibility were determined by conventional methods (7). Beta-lactamase activity was determined on all organisms, with the use of the chromogenic cephalosporin analog 87/312 method (8).

RESULTS

Microbiology

Aerobic or facultative organisms only were isolated from 1 patient (Table I, no. 7), anaerobic bacteria only in 3 (nos. 4, 6 and 10), and mixed aerobic–anaerobic infection in 6. There were totals of 10 aerobic or facultative (1.0/patient) and 17 anaerobic bacteria (1.7/patient). The predominant aerobic bacteria were Pseudomonas aeruginosa (2 isolates), Klebsiella sp. (2), and the predominant anaerobic bacteria were pigmented Prevotella and Porphyromonas species (5), Peptostreptococcus sp. (4), Fusobacterium sp. (3), and Bacteroides fragilis group (2). Gram stain preparation of the aspirates showed some organisms that were compatible with those isolated in 8/10 cases. Organisms similar to those isolated from the endotracheal culture were also recovered from the blood of 2 patients (nos. 3 and 10).

A total of 10 beta-lactamase-producing organisms were recovered from 8 patients (Table I). These included all the 2 isolates each of P. aeruginosa, and B. fragilis group, and 2/5 pigmented Prevotella and Porphyromonas, 1/3 Fusobacterium sp. and the single isolates of Staphylococcus aureus, H. influenzae and Klebsiella pneumoniae.

Clinical findings

Underlying conditions were drowning (2), head trauma (2), and 1 each of coma, encephalitis, brain tumor, brain abscess, drug overdose, and brain damage (postencephalitis) (Table I).

The duration of mechanical ventilation prior to culture varied from 5 to 84 days (average 17.5 days). Antimicrobials were administered prior to collection of specimen in 5 of the patients (cases 6–10), and to all 10 afterward. The choice of antimicrobials was based on culture and susceptibility results and clinical judgement. The antimicrobials given after cultures were obtained were clindamycin (in 5), aminoglycoside (5), ticarcillin-clavulanic acid (2), and chloramphenicol, penicillin, and vancomycin (1 each).

Outcome

All but 1 patient responded to the antimicrobial therapy that was also accompanied by respiratory therapy. Complete recovery was observed in 5 patients. All of the latter patients did not require prolonged mechanical ventilation and were respirator-free within 10 days to 3 weeks. Improvement only occurred in 4 cases (nos. 2, 5, 7 and 10), whose underlying condition was serious and required prolonged mechanical ventilation.

DISCUSSION

This retrospective study demonstrates that polymicrobial aerobic–anaerobic flora can be recovered from properly collected endotracheal aspirates of patients with VAP. The isolation of Gram-negative aerobic and facultative bacteria such as P. aeruginosa and Enterobacteraceae conforms with the results obtained in adults. However, anaerobic bacteria were rarely isolated in adults (1–5) and strict anaerobic organisms had not been previously recovered in children with VAP.

The recovery of anaerobic bacteria in significant numbers ($> 10^5$ cfu/ml) in tracheal aspirates is not surprising as they are part of the normal oropharyngeal flora, where they reach 10^{10} organisms/ml of saliva, outnumbering aerobic bacteria in a ratio of 10 to 1 (9). Anaerobes, primarily of the oral flora, have been isolated in children with upper and lower respiratory tract infections, including aspiration pneumonia (10), lung abscess (11), bacterial tracheitis (12), and wounds (13) following tracheotomy.

Following intubation, patients may be prone to develop infections with aerobic and anaerobic oral flora bacteria. This susceptibility is due to their inability to spontaneously clear their secretions as they become dependent on mechanical suctioning.

The data presented suggest that anaerobic bacteria participate in the inflammatory process that develops in VAP. The recovery of these organisms as the only isolates in the sputum in 3 of the children, and in the blood in 1 child, underscores their importance. It is therefore advisable that properly collected pulmonary aspirates from patients with VAP are routinely processed for the recovery of both aerobic and anaerobic bacteria.

When anaerobic bacteria are isolated from pulmonary aspirates, antimicrobials directed against them can facilitate the patients' recovery (14, 15). Many of the anaerobic bacteria recovered from patients with respiratory tract infections are resistant to beta-lactam antibiotics through the production of beta-lactamase (16). Over 40% of the isolates of Prevotella and Porphyromonas sp. (previously Bacteroides melaninogenicus group) and Fusobacterium sp., resist beta-lactam antibiotics through the production of beta-lactamase, and are also not inhibited by erythromycin (17). The recovery of these organisms requires the administration of appropriate antimicrobial agents such as clindamycin, lincomycin, chloramphenicol, metronidazole, cefoxitin, the combination of a penicillin and a beta-lactamase inhibitor or imipenen. Agents that are effective against S. aureus (i.e. beta-lactam-resistant penicillins) and H. influenzae (second and third generation cephalosporins) are generally not effective against beta-lactamase-producing anaerobes. The choice of antibiotic and the addition of therapy effective against aerobic and facultative Gram-positive (i.e. S. aureus) or Gram-negative (i.e. P. aeruginosa) bacteria should be based on the results of Gram-staining, the bacterial culture and clinical judgement.

This study has not included all the children who had VAP during the period studied, but only those who were adequately cultured for aerobic and anaerobic bacteria. The goal of this report has not been to provide data on the prevalence of VAP, but to alert physicians to the polymicrobial nature of the pneumonia.

Prospective studies to further explore the importance of anaerobic bacteria in VAP in children and adults, and the effect of antimicrobial therapy directed at these bacteria on the clinical outcome, are warranted.

ACKNOWLEDGEMENTS

The author acknowledges the laboratory support of D. Citron, L. Calhoun, P. Yocum, and J. Perry and the secretarial support of Sarah Thorpe.

REFERENCES

1. Baughman RP, Thorpe JE, Staneck J, Rashkin M, Frame PT. Use of the protected specimen brush in patient with endotracheal or tracheostomy tubes. Chest 91: 233–236, 1987.
2. Pollock HM, Hawkins EL, Bonner JR, Sparkman T, Bass JB Jr. Diagnosis of bacterial pulmonary infections with quantitative protected catheter cultures obtained during bronchoscopy. J Clin Microbiol 17: 255–259, 1983.
3. Chastre J, Viau F, Brun P, Pierre J, Dauge M-C, Bouchama A, Akesbi A, Gibert C. Prospective evaluation of the protected specimen brush for the diagnosis of pulmonary infections in ventilated patients. Am Rev Respir Dis 130: 924–929, 1984.
4. Fagon J-Y, Chastre J, Hance AJ, Guiguet M, Trouillet J-L, Domart Y, Pierre J, Gibert C. Detection of nosocomial lung infection in ventilated patients. Am Rev Respir Dis 138: 110–116, 1988.
5. Lambert RS, Vereen LE, George RB. Comparison of tracheal aspirates and protected brush catheter specimens for identifying pathogenic bacteria in mechanically ventilated patients. Am J Med Sci 297: 377–382, 1989.
6. Sutter VL, Citron DM, Edelstein MAC, Finegold SM. Wadsworth anaerobic bacteriology manual. 4th edn. Belmont, CA: Star Publication Co., 1985.
7. Lennette EH, Ballows A, Hausler W Jr, Shadomy HJ. Manual of clinical microbiology, 4th edn. Washington DC: American Society for Microbiology, 1985.
8. O'Callaghan CH, Morris A, Kirby SM, Shingler AH. Novel method for detection of beta-lactamase by using a chromogenic cephalosporin substrate. Antimicrob Agents Chemother 1: 283–288, 1972.
9. Rosebury T. Microorganisms indigenous to man. New York: McGraw-Hill, 1962.
10. Brook I, Finegold SM. Bacteriology of aspiration pneumonia in children. Pediatrics 65: 1115–1119, 1980.
11. Brook I, Finegold SM. Bacteriology and therapy of lung abscess in children. J Pediatr 94: 10–12, 1979.
12. Brook I. Bacterial colonization, tracheobronchitis and pneumonia, following tracheostomy and long-term intubation in pediatric patients. Chest 76: 420–425, 1979.
13. Brook I. Microbiological studies of tracheostomy site wounds. Eur J Respir Dis 71: 380–383, 1987.
14. Levison ME, Mangura CT, Lorbert B. Clindamycin compared with penicillin for the treatment of lung abscess. Ann Intern Med 98: 446–471, 1983.
15. Gudiol F, Manresa F, Pallares R, Oorca J, Rufi G, Boadu J, Ariza X, Cusanova A, Viladrich PF. Clindamycin vs. penicillin for anaerobic lung infection: high rate of penicillin failures associated with penicillin-resistant Bacteroides melaninogenicus. Arch Intern Med 150: 2525–2529, 1990.
16. Brook I. Beta-lactamase-producing bacteria in head and neck infection. Laryngoscope 98: 428–431, 1988.
17. Sutter VL, Finegold SM. Susceptibility of anaerobic bacteria to 23 antimicrobial agents. Antimicrob Agents Chemother 10: 736–752, 1976.

Submitted March 28, 1995; accepted August 16, 1995

Scand J Infect Dis 27: 623–625, 1995

Chronic Ulcerating Acyclovir-Resistant Varicella Zoster Lesions in an AIDS Patient

PETER BERNHARD and NIELS OBEL

From the Department of Infectious Diseases, Rigshospitalet, Copenhagen, Denmark

We describe a 28-year-old HIV-infected woman with AIDS, defined by cerebral toxoplasmosis and a CD4-count of less than 10×10^6 cells/L, who, after several eruptions of genital herpes and typical dermatomal herpes zoster, all successfully treated with acyclovir, developed chronic cutaneous ulcerating lesions on a finger and on the tibia. The lesions were found to contain varicella zoster virus antigen but repeated treatment courses with acyclovir were unsuccessful. After a course of intravenous foscarnet the lesions resolved. They recurred after discontinuation of foscarnet but finally responded to a second course of treatment.

P. Bernhard, MD, Department of Infectious Diseases, Rigshospitalet, Tagensvej 20, DK-2200 Copenhagen, Denmark

INTRODUCTION

Uncommon manifestations of common pathogens as well as increased frequency of common diseases are well known in HIV-infected patients. Common manifestations of varicella zoster virus include primary infection (varicella or chicken pox) and recrudescence of the latent varicella zoster virus infection, herpes zoster or shingles. The latter is recognised with increased frequency in HIV-infected patients. Varicella zoster virus also causes a number of atypical manifestations in patients with AIDS. Severe chicken pox (1), frequent, severe, prolonged or disseminated outbreaks of zoster (2, 3), various forms of spinal, cerebal or meningeal affections (4, 5), debilitating retinopathy (6), periodontal destruction or palatogingivostomatitis (7), and chronic verrucous hyperkeratotic papules (8–10) have been reported in HIV-infected patients. Resistance of varicella zoster virus to acyclovir is well established in HIV-infected patients and is often associated with prolonged or frequent treatment with acyclovir (11–13). The patient with AIDS, described in this report, developed repeated chronic ulcerations on the fingers which could be ascribed to acyclovir-resistant varicella zoster virus infection.

CASE REPORT

A 28-year-old HIV-infected woman was referred to our clinic in April 1992. At the same time she received an AIDS diagnosis, due to cerebral toxoplasmosis confirmed by CT scanning. The CD4 count was essentially zero. The HIV infection was presumed to have been heterosexually acquired more than 5 years previously. The patient had repeated episodes of genital herpes simplex and extensive oral candidiasis.

During the following 22 months she had 4 seperate attacks of typical herpes zoster located to dermatome Th V. The attacks were successfully treated with oral acyclovir 800 mg × 5 daily for 7–10 days. After the 3rd herpes zoster eruption she was started on oral acyclovir 400 mg × 2 for prophylaxis.

In February 1994, shortly after the 4th zoster attack, the patient presented with a painful ulcer on her right forefinger and vesicular and partly confluent elements on her right hand. At the time of presentation the condition was already improving subsequent to the start of oral acyclovir treatment a few days previously because of a dermatomal herpes zoster eruption.

In May 1994 the ulcer recurred on the right forefinger with periodic secretion of pus. Despite soaking in soap-water b.i.d., treatment with silver sulphadiazine ointment daily, and administration of oral ciprofloxacin 500 mg × 3, netilmycin 300 mg × 1 combined with cefuroxim 1.5 g × 3 and parenteral vancomycin 1 g × 2, the ulcer increased in size and tenderness. Repeated cultures from the finger revealed only Staphylococcus epidermidis and blood cultures were negative. X-ray and bone scintigraphy showed no evidence of osteomyelitis. Repeated ELISA tests for herpes simplex virus were negative. In October 1994 varicella zoster virus antigen was detected by the ELISA test (Statens Seruminstitut, Denmark) in a scraping specimen from the ulcer on the forefinger. Although the patient had been on prophylatic treatment with oral acyclovir 400 mg × 2, as a consequence of the positive varicella zoster virus test the dose was inscreased to oral acyclovir 800 mg × 5 for 10 days without clinical effect. A repeated ELISA test for varicella zoster virus antigen was positive, whereupon the treatment was changed to intravenous foscarnet 60 mg/kg (3,000 mg) t.i.d. for 9 days, with remarkable clinical effect, the ulcer on the right forefinger healing for the first time in 9 months. The patient was at this time discharged in good condition with an increased dosage of oral acyclovir, 400 mg × 3, for prophylaxis.

In March 1995 the patient had a recurrence of the right forefinger ulcer (Fig. 1) and also presented with a 2 × 2 cm red, painful and swollen ulcer on the right lower leg. Scrapings from both ulcers revealed varicella zoster virus antigen and simultaneous examination for herpes simplex viurs antigen was negative. Varicella zoster virus could not be cultured from the ulcers. The patient was again treated with intravenous foscarnet 60 mg/kg (3,000 mg) t.i.d. for 16 days this time. After a few days of treatment there was again a remarkable improvement, and at the end of treatment both lesions had improved considerably. The patient was discharged on oral prophylaxis with famciclovir 250 mg t.i.d., and 2 months later there was no recurrence of the lesions.

DISCUSSION

Smith et al. (14) have followed the cutaneous manifestations of 912 HIV-1-infected patients over a period of 42 months, and found very high frequencies of cutaneous diseases. Asteatosis and seborrhoeic dermatitis were the most frequently described dermatological complaints. Cuta-

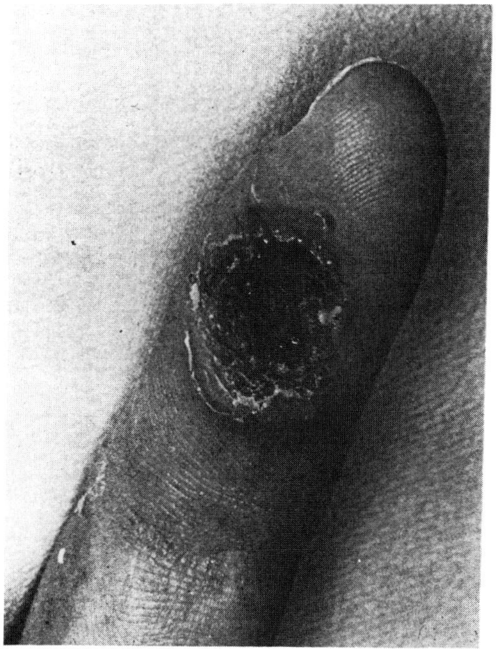

Fig. 1. A chronic ulcer on the right forefinger of an AIDS patient caused by an acyclovir-resistant varicella zoster strain.

neous manifestations associated with an advanced stage of HIV included drug eruptions, seborrhoeic dermatitis, oral candidiasis, oral hairy leukoplakia, molluscum contagiosum, and herpes zoster. Herpes zoster was found to occur in 6% of the patients but 15% reported a history of herpes zoster, compared to a normal occurrence in a non-HIV-infected population of 0.34%. Atypical manifestations of varicella zoster virus often present as verrucous hyperkeratotic skin lesions (8–10, 12, 13, 15–17) that may be solitary, multiple, or even disseminated. Many of the reported cases have been associated with acyclovir resistance (10, 12, 13, 16, 17).

Chronic atypical ulcerative cutaneous lesions caused by varicella zoster virus like those we described have been reported only rarely. Gilson et al. (18) described 3 cases that all responded to acyclovir therapy. Janier et al. reported one case of disseminated multiple ulcerative lesions resistant to acyclovir (19).

We describe a case of 2 widely separated chronic ulcerative cutaneous lesions caused by varicella zoster virus. Our patient had previously had genital herpes and recurrent dermatomal herpes zoster, and was successfully treated with acyclovir for these conditions. The atypical lesions, after responding to acyclovir treatment initially, later failed to respond to acyclovir. As in a number of other reported cases of acyclovir-resistant varicella zoster virus infection, our patient responded well to intravenous treatment with foscarnet (10, 16, 17). We were unable to culture varicella zoster virus from one scraping sample, which is consistent with findings reported by Gilson et al., who recommend repeated cultures (13).

The viral resistance mechanism is based on altered or deficient viral thymidine kinase activity (11, 12, 17), probably by selection through subtherapeutic serum levels of acyclovir during tretment or prophylaxis. Inadequate and irregular drug administration, and reduced bioavailability due to diarrhoea or malabsorption, conditions that are common in AIDS patients, may contribute to this phenomenon. Foscarnet does not require thymidine kinase for its action and seems quite effective against acyclovir-resistant varicella zoster strains. We started prophylaxis with famciclovir, and so far the lesions seem to be controlled. However, the period of follow-up is only a few months, and we cannot draw conclusions at this time as to the efficacy of this drug as compared to acyclovir.

We conclude that in the absence of an obvious etiology for chronic cutaneous ulcers in HIV patients with low CD4 counts, varicella zoster virus should be considered. In the literature it is reported that atypical manifestations of zoster are often, but not always, preceded by recurrent classic zoster lesions and prophylactic acyclovir treatment. Furthermore, viral resistance to acyclovir seems to occur frequently in atypical manifestations, and treatment with an alternative drug such as foscarnet is required.

REFERENCES

1. Perronne C, Lazanas M, Leport C, Simon F, Salmon D, Dallot A, Vildé JL. Varicella in patients with the human immunodeficiency virus. Arch Dermatol 126: 1033–1036, 1990.
2. Gulick RM. Heath-Chiozzi M, Crumpacker CS. Varicella zoster virus disease in patients with human immunodeficiency virus infection. Arch Dermatol 126: 1086–1088, 1990.
3. Cohen PR, Beltrani VP, Grossman ME. Disseminated herpes zoster in patients with acquired immunodeficiency syndrome. Am J Med 84: 1076–1080, 1988.
4. Gray F, Bélec L. Lescs MC, Chrétien F, Ciardi A, Hassine D, Flament-Saillour M, de Truchis P, Clair B, Scaravilli F. Varicella zoster virus infection of the central nervous system in the acquired immune deficiency syndrome. Brain 117: 987–999, 1994.
5. Gómez-Tortosa E. Gadea I, Gegúndez MI, Esteban A, Rábano J, Fernández-Guerrero ML, Soriano F. Development of myelopathy before a Herpes zoster rash in a patient with AIDS. Clin Infect Dis 18: 810–812, 1994.
6. Johnston WH, Holland GN, Engstrom RE, Rimmer S. Recurrance of presumed varicella zoster virus retinopathy in patients with acquired immunodeficiency syndrome. Am J Ophthalmol 116: 42–50, 1993.
7. Moskow BS, Hernandez G. Aggressive periodontal destruction and herpes zoster in a suspected AIDS patient. J Parodontol 10: 359–369, 1991.
8. Grossman MC, Grossman ME. Chronic hyperkeratotic herpes zoster and human immunodeficiency virus infection. J Am Acad Dermatol 28: 306–308, 1993.
9. LeBoit PE, Límová M, Yen TS, Palefsky JM, White CR Jr, Berger TG. Chronic verrucous varicella zoster virus infection in patients with the acquired immunodeficiency syndrome (AIDS). Histologic and molecular biologic findings. Am J Dermatopathol 14: 1–7, 1992.

10. Lokke Jensen B, Weisman K, Mathiesen L, Klem Thomsen H. Atypical varicella zoster infection in AIDS. Acta Dermatol Venereol 73: 123–125, 1993.
11. Jacobson MA, Berger TG, Fikrig S, Becherer P, Moohr JW, Stanat SC, Biron KK. Acyclovir-resistant varicella zoster virus infection after chronic oral acyclovir therapy in patients with the acquired immunodeficiency syndrome (AIDS). Ann Intern Med 112: 187–191, 1990.
12. Linnemann CC Jr, Biron KK, Hoppenjans WG, Solinger AM. Emergence of acyclovir-resistant varicella zoster virus in an AIDS patient on prolonged acyclovir therapy. AIDS 4: 577–579, 1990.
13. Lyall EG, Ogilvie MM, Smith NM, Burns S. Acyclovir-resistant varicella zoster and HIV infection. Arch Dis Child 70: 133–135, 1994.
14. Smith KJ, Skelton HJ, Yeager J, Ledsky R, McCarthy W, Baxter D, Wagner KF. Cutaneous findings in HIV-1-positive patients: a 42–month prospective study. Military Medical Consortium for the Advancement of Retroviral Research. J Am Acad Dermatol 31: 746–754, 1994.
15. Disler RS, Dover JS. Chronic localized herpes zoster in the acquired immunodeficiency syndrome. Arch Dermatol 126: 1105–1106, 1990.
16. Hoppenjans WB, Bibler MR, Orme RL, Solinger AM. Prolonged cutaneous herpes zoster in acquired immunodeficiency syndrome. Arch Dermatol 126: 1048–1050, 1990.
17. Safrin S, Berger TG, Gilson I, Wolfe PR. Wofsy CB, Mills J, Biron KK. Foscarnet therapy in five patients with AIDS and acyclovir-resistant varicella zoster virus infection. Ann Intern Med 115: 19–21, 1991.
18. Gilson IH, Barnett JH, Conant MA, Laskin OL, Williams J, Jones PG. Disseminated ecthymatous herpes varicella-zoster virus infection in patients with acquired immunodeficiency syndrome. J Am Acad Dermatol 20: 637–642, 1989.
19. Janier M, Hillion B, Baccard M, Morinet F, Scieux C, Perol Y, Civatte J. Chronic varicella zoster infection in acquired immunodeficiency syndrome. J Am Acad Dermatol 18: 584–585, 1988.

Submitted June 30, 1995; accepted August 30, 1995

Scand J Infect Dis 27: 627–629, 1995

Liver Failure due to Disseminated HSV-1 Infection in a Newborn Twin

FRANK T. HUFERT[1], THOMAS DIEBOLD[3], BEATE ERMISCH[2], DOROTHEE VON LAER[1], URSULA MEYER-KÖNIG[1] and DIETER NEUMANN-HAEFELIN[1]

From the Departments of [1]Virology, Institut für Medizinische Mikrobiologie und Hygiene, and [2]Childpathology, Institut für Pathologie Universität Freiburg, and [3]Universitätskinderklinik Freiburg, Freiburg, Germany

Most cases of neonatal herpes simplex virus (HSV) infection result from contact with maternal genital tract secretions and are caused by infections with HSV type 2. We report on a fatal HSV-1 infection in a newborn twin presenting with liver failure. The infection was acquired by single contact with an aunt. The route of transmission was proven by PCR followed by restriction endonuclease fingerprinting and DNA sequencing. This report demonstrates that liver failure may be an early and single symptom in life-threatening neonatal HSV-1 infection.

F. Hufert, MD, Abteilung Virologie, Institut für Medizinische Mikrobiologie & Hygiene, Universität Freiburg, Hermann-Herder-Straße 11, D-79104 Freiburg, Germany

INTRODUCTION

Disseminated herpes simplex virus infection with symptoms of severe liver failure has been described (1) but occurs much less often than mucocutaneous or central nervous system HSV disease. The majority of cases have been infected by contact with HSV-2 containing maternal genital secretion. We report a newborn twin who presented with liver failure and had been infected postnatally with HSV-1 by his aunt. To our knowledge this is the first report of a postnatally acquired HSV-1 infection in a twin presenting with liver failure.

CASE REPORT

A 2710 g female twin and her male brother were delivered by caesarean section because of fetal distress at week 38 of pregnancy. The pregnancy of the 27-year-old white second gravida was uneventful. The Apgar scores of the patient were 10/10 (1 min/5 min) and the umbilical cord blood pH was normal. Physical examination at birth was normal. There was no maternal history of genital or oral herpes, but post partum the infants were kissed by family members (father, aunt) who both had episodes of recurrent herpes labialis. On the 3rd day of life the female infant developed fever, vomiting, jaundice, and was admitted to hospital on day 4. The baby was dehydrated and had signs of circular centralization and of hypersensitivity and a temperature of 39°C. Laboratory data revealed a leucopenia (6.3×10^9/l) with different cell count of 38% band forms, 40% polymorphonuclear cells, 14% monocytes, and 7% lymphocytes. The hemoglobin and further laboratory investigations (glucose, liver enzymes, CRP, bilirubin, sodium, potassium and creatinine) were normal with the exception of ammonia (184 µmol). In the urine, enterococci and non-coagulase positive staphylococci were detected (10^6/ml). Blood cultures were negative. X-ray of chest and abdomen and ultrasound of the head were negative. The clinical diagnosis of septicemia was established and treatment started with piperacillin and tobramycin. On day 5 fever decreased and clinical symptoms improved. On day 7 the condition deteriorated and liver failure with hemorrhagic diathesis appeared (ALAT 5.68 µkat/l, ASAT 33.2 µkat/l, ammonia 134 µmol, Quick and PTT: under the limit of detection) which was treated with fresh frozen plasma, AT III and heparin. On day 9 she developed anuria. On day 10 the first herpetic skin lesions appeared. Treatment with acyclovir and immunoglobulin was initiated. The patient developed multiple bleeding from all puncture sites. The patient was treated with artificial ventilation, fresh frozen plasma, transfusions, bicarbonate, hemofiltration and plasmapheresis. Nevertheless her condition deteriorated, and she died on day 14 because of a profuse gastrointestinal bleeding. Autopsy was performed the next day.

METHODS

Microbiological surveillance and virus isolation

Assays for the detection of IgG and IgM antibodies specific to HBV, HAV, rubella virus (Sorin, Düsseldorf, Germany), HCV (Ortho Diagnostics Systems, Raritan, USA), HCMV (Medac, Hamburg, Germany), and HSV (Behringwerke, Marburg, Germany) were performed using ELISA tests. Complement fixation tests were carried out to detect antibodies to HSV and mycoplasma antigens. Immunofluorescence assays were used to test for IgG and IgM response to HSV and EBV (VCA, EBNA).

Blister fluid and post mortem biopsies were obtained for viral isolation using human diploid fibroblasts and green monkey kidney (GMK) cells. 24 h after inocculation cytopathic changes typical of HSV appeared and the supernatant was subcultivated with BJAB cells (EBV negative Burkitt lymphoma cell line) for 24 h. Virus typing was performed by immunofluorescence using BJAB cytospins and monoclonal antibodies specific for HSV-1 and HSV-2 (Micro Trak HSV-1/HSV-2 culture confirmation/typing test, Syva, Palo Alto, USA).

DNA isolation, polymerase chain reaction, restriction endonuclease fingerprinting and DNA sequencing

DNA was extracted from tissue samples using TurboGen DNA purification kit (Invitogen, San Diego Ca, USA). DNA from plasma and feces were adsorbed on silica particles as described by Boom et al. (2).

PCR was performed using primers (HS13/14) from the UL 42 region of HSV-1. Amplified DNA was detected by Southern blotting following hybridization as reported elsewhere (3). For restriction endonuclease fingerprinting, a 500 bp fragment of the HSV-1 thymidine kinase (TK) gene was amplified using culture supernatant, and the fragment was digested using Alu I, Kpn I and Rsa I

 ISSN 0036-5548

Table I. *Detection of HSV-1 by PCR and virus isolation*

Sample	PCR	Virus isolation
Bone marrow[a]	+	+
Brain[a]	+	+
Liver[a]	+	+
Lymphe node[a]	+	+
Skin efflorescence[a]	+	+
Lung[a]	negative	negative
Adrenal glands[a]	+	+
Spleen[a]	+	+
Blister fluid[c]	+	+
Serum[b]	+	negative
Feces[b]	+	negative

[a] Samples obtained at autopsy, 12 h after death.
[b] Samples obtained at day 7 of life (day 4 after onset of disease), investigated retrospectively.
[c] Sample obtained at day 10 of life (day 7 after onset of disease).

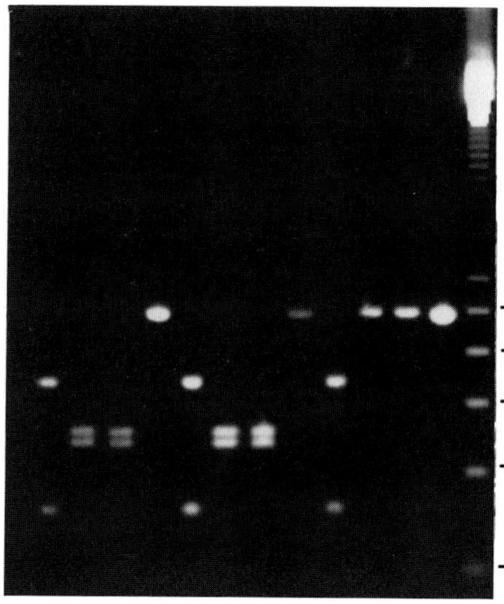

Fig. 1. Typing of HSV isolates. HSV isolates from the newborn female twin child, her aunt and father analyzed by PCR and subsequent restriction fragment polymorphism. A 500 bp fragment of the TK gene was amplified from tissue culture supernatant of the isolates obtained from the child, aunt and father. The amplified DNA fragment was digested with Alu I, Kpn I and Rsa I. Lane 1–4: HSV isolate of the child; lane 1: Alu 1 restriction, lane 2: Kpn I restriction, lane 3: Rsa I restriction, lane 4: no restriction; lane 5–8: HSV isolate of the aunt; lane 5: Alu 1 restriction, lane 6: Kpn I restriction, lane 7: Rsa I restriction, lane 8: no restriction; lane 9–12: HSV isolate of the father; lane 9: Alu 1 restriction, lane 10: Kpn I restriction, lane 11: Rsa I restriction; lane 12: no restriction. Lane 13: molecular weight marker.

as previously described (4). The differences of restriction patterns were confirmed by DNA sequencing. The TK gene amplification product was cloned in pCR II vector (Invitrogen, San Diego, Ca, USA). The cloned plasmid was then transformed in E. coli strain INVaF and the DNA sequence of the insert was determined using Sequenase^{TM} DNA sequencing kit (USB, Cleveland, Ohio).

RESULTS

Autopsy revealed that the patient had died of a profuse bleeding from the distal esophagus with mucosal detachment. Histopathological investigations showed multiple disseminated hemorrhagic foci of necroses in liver, esophagus, small intestine, spleen, kidney, and adrenal glands. In the brain, bleeding into the subarachnoid space, edema, and hypoxic neuron damage could be demonstrated. The stomach showed hemorrhagic infiltration, and edema of the myocardium was found. There was a pneumonia of the right basal lobe with bacterial colonization of necrotic tissue. Necrotic organs lacked inflammatory infiltration by macrophages, lymphocytes and granulocytes. Granulocytes and bacteria were only found in the lung. At autopsy, tissue biopsies were taken from bone marrow, brain, liver, lymph node, skin lesion, lung, adrenal and spleen. Virus isolation and PCR for HSV DNA were performed. HSV-1 was isolated from all samples except the lungs. The data are summarized in Table I. The first skin lesions appeared on day 10, and HSV-1 was isolated from blister fluid. Retrospectively, HSV-1 DNA could be detected by PCR in serum at day 7 and in feces at day 4. However, no virus could be isolated from these samples. No rotaviral antigen was detected in feces. Serological investigation excluded HBV, HAV, HCV, rubella virus, EBV, CMV and mycoplasma infection. The twins and their mother were HSV-seronegative at birth. A serological follow-up showed that mother and the male healthy twin were both still HSV-seronegative 2 months later. Father and aunt were HSV-seropositive and both had herpes labialis at the time of birth. Both had a close contact (kissing) with the patient. In addition, HSV-1 was isolated 4 months later from the relative labial blister fluid. A 500 bp part of the TK gene was amplified by PCR using the isolates obtained from patient, aunt, and father. The PCR products were compared by restriction fragment length polymorphism analysis using Alu I, Kpn I and Rsa I digestion. The isolates from patient and aunt had identical restriction patterns, whereas the isolate from the father was different (Fig. 1). Differences in DNA sequence of the 500 bp fragment was confirmed by DNA sequencing after cloning in pCR II vector (data not shown). Thus, restriction fragment length polymorphism analysis and DNA sequencing clearly showed that the child was infected by the aunt.

DISCUSSION

As described previously (1) for HSV-2 and rarely for HSV-1, this report demonstrates that generalized HSV infection in neonates can present with the major symptom of liver failure. In such cases the clinical diagnosis of disseminated HSV infection may be missed, especially when skin lesions are absent or appear late after onset of disease. In our patient, the first clinical diagnosis was septicemia with liver failure. As maternal risk factors of HSV infection were absent, antiviral therapy was initiated late, after herpetic skin lesions had appeared, and therefore failed to prevent the tissue damage caused by HSV. The diagnosis of disseminated HSV infection was clearly established by PCR and virus isolation using ex vivo blister fluid and samples from different tissues obtained at autopsy. Histopathological investigations showed the typical pattern of necrosis in liver, adrenal glands, and other tissues, but cellular infiltration was lacking (5, 6). Histopathology failed to detect typical intranuclear inclusion bodies which often provide the etiological diagnosis. However, this phenomenon may eventually be missing (7) due to antiviral treatment. Although the lung showed necrotic zones, HSV-1 was not detected in this organ. It was the only organ showing bacterial and cellular infiltration, which was most likely due to pneumonia after artificial hyperventilation. Surprisingly, the male twin was not infected.

The clinical suspicion of neonatal HSV infection can be confirmed by virus isolation and PCR from skin vesicles, oropharyngeal swaps, CSF, urine, plasma, and stool (8). Since only 30%–50% of HSV-infected newborns develop skin lesions, the clinician cannot rely on the presence of skin vesicles. In certain cases, biopsy from brain or liver may be needed to prove the diagnosis intra vitam. In our case, HSV DNA could retrospectively be demonstrated by PCR in a plasma sample obtained on day 4 after onset of disease. In contrast, the virus could not be isolated from this plasma sample. This confirms that PCR is the most powerful tool in the early diagnosis of HSV infection as described for encephalitis cases (9, 10). Samples taken at the onset of clinical symptoms should be investigated primarily by PCR to further prove the diagnostic value of PCR in the early detection of disseminated neonatal HSV infection. Furthermore, this case demonstrates that transmission can be traced efficiently by PCR followed by restriction endonuclease fingerprinting and DNA sequencing.

Rapid diagnosis of HSV infection is the major difficulty. Therefore, antiviral treatment has to be started with the onset of symptoms and may be discontinued upon negative PCR results. Aciclovir is the first choice for neonates (11, 12).

The clinical outcome depends also on the type of virus and on immune host factors poorly understood so far. Mothers with recurrent infections provide antibodies to the fetus that are likely to inhibit at least viral dissemination after perinatal transmission (13). However, humoral immunity is not totally protective. This may be due to different amounts of neutralizing antibodies in the maternal blood (13, 14). Cellular immunity has been considered to be important in the host defense against HSV. In neonates, however, the generation of functional T cells is restricted due to delayed blastogenic response (13).

In conclusion, severe neonatal HSV-1 infection must also be considered if maternal risk factors (serology, genital lesions) are absent. In babies of HSV-seronegative mothers, every postnatal contact with sources of potential HSV must be avoided.

ACKNOWLEDGMENTS

We thank Bernd Rädle and Susanne Dollweth for excellent technical assistance and Otto Haller for critical reading of the manuscript.

REFERENCES

1. Benador N, Mannhardt W, Schranz D, Braegger C, Fanconi S, Hassam S, Talebzadeh V, Cox J, Suter S. Three cases of neonatal herpes simplex virus infection presenting as fulminant hepatitis. Eur J Pediatr 149: 555–559, 1990.
2. Boom R, Sol CJ, Salimans MM, Jansen CL, Wertheim van Dillen PM, van der Noordaa J. Rapid and simple method for purification of nucleic acids. J Clin Microbiol 28: 495–503, 1990.
3. Puchhammer Stockl E, Popow Kraupp T, Heinz FX, Mandl CW, Kunz C. Detection of varicella-zoster virus DNA by polymerase chain reaction in the cerebrospinal fluid of patients suffering from neurological complications associated with chicken pox or herpes zoster. J Clin Microbiol 29: 1513–1516, 1991.
4. Vogel J-U, Weber B, Doerr HW. Typing and strain differentiation of clinical herpes simplex virus type 1 and 2 isolates by polymerase chain reaction and subsequent restriction fragment length polymorphism analysis. Int J Med Microbiol 281: 502–512, 1994.
5. Stocker JT, Dehner PL. Congenital and acquired systemic infectious diseases. In: Stocker JT and Dehner LP, eds. Pediatric pathology. Philadelphia: J.B. Lippincott Company, 212–213, 1992.
6. Kaschula ROC. Congenital and neonatal herpes simplex viral infections. In Colin LB, ed. Paediatric pathology. 2nd edn. London: Springer Verlag, 666–729, 1989.
7. Robbins SL, Cotran RS, Kuman V. Pathologic basis of disease. Philadelphia: W.B. Saunders Company, 284–285, 1984.
8. Brann AW, Hall RT, Harper RG, Little GA, Maisels MJ, McCracken GH, Poland RL, Sunshine P, Whittinghill JA. Perinatal herpes simplex virus infection. Pediatrics 66: 147–148, 1980.
9. Puchhammer Stockl E, Popow Kraupp T, Heinz FX, Mandl CW, Kunz C. Establishment of PCR for the early diagnosis of herpes simplex encephalitis. J Med Virol 32: 77–82, 1990.
10. Troendle Atkins J, Demmler GJ, Buffone GJ. Rapid diagnosis of herpes simplex virus encephalitis by using the polymerase chain reaction. J Pediatr 123: 376–380, 1993.
11. Arvin AM, Johnson RT, Whitley RT, Nelson JD, McCracken GHJ. Consensus: management of the patient with herpes simplex encephalitis. Pediatr Infect Dis J 6: 2–5, 1987.
12. Sköldenberg B, Forsgren M, Alestig K, Bergstrom T, Burman L, Dahlqvist E, Forkman A, Fryden A, Lovgren K, Norlin K, et al. Acyclovir versus vidarabine in herpes simplex encephalitis. Randomised multicentre study in consecutive Swedish patients. Lancet 2: 707–711, 1984.
13. Prober CG, Sullender WM, Yasukawa LL, Au DS, Yeager AS, Arvin AM. Low risk of herpes simplex virus infections in neonates exposed to the virus at the time of vaginal delivery to mothers with recurrent genital herpes simplex virus infections. N Engl J Med 316: 240–244, 1987.
14. Yeager AS, Arvin AM. Reasons for the absence of a history of recurrent genital infections in mothers of neonates infected with herpes simplex virus. Pediatrics 73: 188–193, 1984.

Submitted April 18, 1995; accepted August 10, 1995

Scand J Infect Dis 27: 631–633, 1995 CASE REPORT

Parvovirus B19 Infection Associated with Encephalitis in a Patient Suffering from Malignant Lymphoma

ERIK D. HEEGAARD[1], NIELS A. PETERSLUND[2] and ALLAN HORNSLETH[1]

From the Departments of [1]Virology, Institute of Medical Microbiology and Immunology, University of Copenhagen, and [2]Hematology, Aarhus Amtssygehus, Denmark

A parvovirus B19 infection was established in a 58-year-old woman undergoing treatment for malignant lymphoma. Clinically, the patient displayed a variety of neurologic symptoms that could not readily be explained by the mere presence of lymphoblastic cells within the central nervous system. This is the first time parvovirus B19 DNA has been detected in the cerebrospinal fluid of a patient suffering from encephalitis.

E. D. Heegaard, MD, c/o Allan Hornsleth, Department of Virology, Institute of Medical Microbiology and Immunology, Panum Institute Bldg. 24.2, Blegdamsvej 3 C, DK-2200 Copenhagen N, Denmark

INTRODUCTION

The discovery of human parvovirus B19 in 1975 and subsequent studies of its effects in humans have identified this virus as the causative agent of a broad range of diseases (1).

These include:
– diseases found in normal hosts (asymptomatic disease, erythema infectiosum, arthropathy, hydrops fetalis),
– hematologic diseases (aplastic crisis, chronic anemia, idiopathic thrombocytopenic purpura, transient erythroblastopenia of childhood, Diamond–Blackfan anemia);
– a heterogeneous group of diseases, in which the etiologic role of the parvovirus is less clear and sometimes putative (neurologic and rheumatologic disease, vascular and myocardial syndromes).

Only a few reports on neurologic involvement have been published. These include descriptions of encephalitis and encephalopathy in association with the erythema infectiosum reported before the advent of specific virologic techniques (2, 3). More recently, 3 additional cases of encephalopathy (4–6), a few cases of aseptic meningitis (7–9), and a case of unclassified neurologic involvement (10) have been published, where specific immunoglobulins and/or B19 DNA in blood and cerebrospinal fluid (CSF) were detected. Fatal encephalitis associated with parvovirus B19 has never been reported. Finally, a small number of cases linking parvovirus with numbness and tingling of fingers as well as with neuralgic amyotrophy have been observed (11–14). Parvovirus B19 DNA has been detected in a variety of tissues and fluids, but only very rarely has CSF been examined. At present, only limited knowledge is available concerning the finding of parvovirus B19 DNA and specific immunoglobulins in the CSF, and concerning the possible clinical implications.

We present a patient suffering from malignant lymphoma who died from what appeared to be acute encephalitis. The only potentially pathogenic infectious agent detectable in the cerebrospinal fluid was parvovirus B19.

CASE REPORT

A previously healthy 58-year-old woman was admitted to hospital (day 1) due to fever and abdominal pain mainly located below the left costal margin. A diagnosis of malignant B-cell lymphoma, stage 4, was established. The patient received treatment with cyclophosphamide, prednisolone and vincristine 5 times (days: 14, 38, 59, 90 and 111). A renewed CT scan (day 113) showed normalization of all areas previously involved.

On day 95 a week-long period of slight fever, universal soreness and general malaise occurred. No rash was observed.

Before consolidating CHOP treatments could be instituted the patient suddenly developed an almost total loss of vision in the left eye over a period of 10 days (commencing day 130). She also experienced impaired coordination of the lower extremities. Computerized tomography (day 138) and magnetic resonance (MR) (day 145) scans of the brain showed no abnormalities. Opthalmologic evaluation (days 138, 181 and 197) indicated that the visionary defects were due to neuritis. Lymphoblastic involvement of the central nervous system was revealed when the CSF was examined (day 146).

The patient received intrathecal infusion of methotrexate, hydrocortisone and cytarabine twice weekly from day 147.

During the ensuing 10 days the patient exhibited further neurologic impairments including reduced vision in the right eye, peripheral tingling and lack of coordination of the tongue and facial muscles. A renewed examination of the CSF on day 160 showed no abnormalities. At this time the patient experienced a marked bilateral improvement in her vision.

The patient had spells of aphasia and increasing difficulty in coordinating the right arm and the left leg 2 weeks later. These symptoms subsided within 10 days.

At the same time (day 182) an MR scan revealed diffuse thickening of the meninges at various locations. The CSF was repeatedly free of lymphoblastic cells.

A renewed set of neurologic symptoms presented themselves 10 days later. These consisted of vertigo attacks, headache, numbness of a part of the face and palsy in some of the cranial motor nerves. These symptoms improved gradually over 1 week.

 ISSN 0036-5548

Table I. *Laboratory findings in a 58-year-old woman undergoing treatment for malignant lymphoma*

	Day					
	1	132	146	158	172	199
Hemoglobin, mmol/l	7.6	8.2	8.0	6.7	5.5	8.4
Neutrocytes, 10^9/l	10.6	4	4.6	1.1	7.2	23.5
Lymphocytes, 10^9/l	25	0.6	0.5	0.1	0.3	0.5
Platelets, 10^9/l	159	354	313	213	1160	261
Cerebrospinal fluid (lymphoblasts)	ND	ND	Yes	No	No	No
Bone marrow (lymphoblasts)	Yes	No	ND	ND	No	ND

ND, not done.

Finally, and fatally, an overt clinical picture of encephalitis was shown from day 199. This consisted of increasingly severe headache, moderate stiffness of the neck, palsy in eye muscles and left-sided extremities, generalized convulsions and an increasingly depressed level of consciousness leading to coma and death (day 204). A request for autopsy was denied.

Laboratory findings

The laboratory findings are shown in Table I. The number of reticulocytes was not measured.

Microbiologic examinations

Serologic titers showed no acute infection by toxoplasmosis, Epstein–Barr virus, cytomegalovirus, varicella zoster virus, herpes virus 6, human immunodeficiency virus 1 and 2, treponema pallidum, or by hepatitis virus A, B or C. Titers for herpes virus 6 and cytomegalovirus in the CSF were negative. Cultures of the blood and the CSF were repeatedly negative for cytomegalovirus, herpes simplex virus, mycobacteria, and other bacteria.

In the final stages of the disease, investigation for the presence of parvovirus B19 infection was carried out on a variety of stored samples. (see Table II). In the blood, parvovirus B19-specific IgM and IgG were detected in samples collected at an interval of more than 40 days (days 146 and 188). Examination for the presence of parvovirus B19 DNA by the PCR technique (15) could only be carried out in the later sample (day 188) and was negative for both the VP 1 and NS 1 regions of the B19 genome. A search of the bone marrow for parvovirus B19 DNA (day 174) was also negative.

The CSF (day 188) contained parvovirus B19-specific IgG but no IgM. Finally, an examination of the CSF (day 199) for parvovirus B19 DNA was repeatedly positive for both the VP 1 and NS 1 regions. No additional material was available for investigation.

Serum from a patient, chronically infected by parvovirus B19, served as a positive control (15).

Table II. *Detection of parvovirus B19 DNA and specific immunoglobulins*

	Day				
	146	174	188		199
	Blood	Bone marrow	Blood	CSF	CSF
B19 DNA	ND	Negative	Negative	ND	Positive
IgM	Positive	ND	Positive	Negative	ND
IgG	Positive	ND	Positive	Positive	ND

ND, not done; CSF, cerebrospinal fluid.

DISCUSSION

Reports concerning neurologic involvement by parvovirus B19 have mainly concerned cases of aseptic meningitis and encephalopathy, most of which have been benign and self-limiting. One patient suffering from seizures received successful immunoglobulin therapy (5). The detection of parvovirus B19-specific IgM (7) and parvovirus B19 DNA (6, 8–10) in the CSF seems to be a very rare event reported in only 5 patients.

There are at least two intriguing aspects to this case. First, how did parvovirus B19 infect the central nervous system, and second what role, if any, did it play in the course of the disease and the fatal outcome.

Prior to the appearance of the neurologic symptoms the patient had been responding satisfactorily to the treatment given. Clinically, the patient then displayed a puzzling array of symptoms which could not readily be explained by the mere presence of lymphoblastic cells within the central nervous system. Undoubtedly, the spread of lymphoblastic cells within the central nervous system had adverse effects. Nevertheless, the symptoms varied and seemed partly reversible and eventually did not match the general clinical presentation of lymphoblastic involvement of the central nervous system. The malignant cells could no longer be observed in the CSF after 13 days of intrathecal medical treatment but still the symptoms progressed. This prompted a search for an infectious agent, possibly working in conjunction with the previously observed lymphoblastic cells to produce the observed symptoms.

On day 95 of her illness the patient suffered from malaise, general soreness and low grade fever. This was interpreted, at the time, as an unclassified viral disease, most probably influenza. It is possible, however, that this episode marks the initial infection by parvovirus B19, and corresponds well with findings of specific IgM in the serum during the following 3 months. The presence of IgM may also explain why no parvovirus B19 DNA could be detected in serum or the bone marrow. It is still unclear, however, how parvovirus B19 spread to the central nervous system in this patient and managed to escape eradication by the specific immunoglobulins even after 3 months of disease.

The chemotherapy involved in treating the malignant lymphoma may have facilitated the survival of the virus by inducing an impaired immune response. Such long-term disease is a well-known aspect of parvovirus B19 infections among immunocompromised hosts and patients suffering from various malignant diseases (1). Recently, such chronic infections have also been observed in presumably immunologically healthy individuals (16–18).

Considering the marked tropism of parvovirus B19 for erythrogenic precursors and the fact that no virus could be detected in the bone marrow, the site of viral replication in this case remains obscure. One report tells of parvovirus B19 DNA being detected in the blood for 37 weeks following an acute infection with meningitis in an immunocompetent patient (9). Unfortunately, the bone marrow was never tested and the CSF was tested only at the onset of disease so this case (9) does not shed light on the pathogenesis in our patient.

In retrospect, it is arguable to what extent the different symptoms can be ascribed to the spread of malignant cells or parvovirus B19 to the central nervous system. Had the diagnosis of parvovirus B19 been made earlier, it might have been appropriate to administer immunoglobulins to help eradicate the virus, even though the outlook in this case, considering the underlying malignant disease, would make the prospect of success of such therapy dubious.

To the best of our knowledge this is the first time parvovirus B19 DNA has been detected in the CSF in a lethal case of encephalitis. This may be a coincidental finding, as discussed above, but with an increased awareness and the advent of the PCR technique, more information elucidating these issues can be expected.

REFERENCES

1. Heegaard ED, Hornsleth A. Parvovirus: the expanding spectrum of disease. Acta Pediatr 84: 109–117, 1995.
2. Balfour HH, Schiff GM, Bloom JE. Encephalitis associated with erythma infectiosum. J Pediatr 77(1): 133–136, 1970.
3. Hall CB, Homer FA. Encephalopathy with erythema infectiosum. Am J Dis Child 131: 65–67, 1977.
4. Zerbini M, Musiani M, Venturoli S, Gallinella G, Gibellini D, Gentilomi G, La Placa M. Different syndromes associated with B19 parvovirus viraemia in paediatric patients: report of four cases. Eur J Pediatr 151: 815–817, 1992.
5. Nigro G, D'Eufemia P, Zerbini M, Krzysztofiak A, Finocchiaro R, Giardini O. Parvovirus B19 infection in a hypogammaglobulinemic infant with neurologic disorders and anemia: successful immunoglobulin therapy. Pediatr Inf Dis J 13: 1019–1021, 1994.
6. Watanabe T, Satoh M, Oda Y. Human parvovirus B19 encephalopathy. Arch Dis Child 70: 71, 1994.
7. Tsuji A, Uchida N, Asamura S, Matsunaga Y, Yamazaki S. Aseptic meningitis with erythema infectiosum. Eur J Pediatr 149: 449–450, 1990.
8. Okumura A, Ichikawa T. Aseptic meningitis caused by human parvovirus B19. Arch Dis Child 68: 784–785, 1993.
9. Cassinotti P, Schultze D, Schlageter P, Chevili S, Siegl G. Persistent human parvovirus B19 infection following an acute infection with meningitis in an immunocompetent patient. Eur J Clin Microbiol Infect Dis 12: 701–704, 1993.
10. Yoto Y, Kudoh T, Asanuma H, Numazaki K, Tsutsumi Y, Nakata S, Chiba S. Transient disturbance of consciousness and hepatic dysfunction associated with human parvovirus B19 infection. Lancet 344: 624–625, 1994.
11. Faden H, Gary GW, Korman M. Numbness and tingling of fingers associated with parvovirus B19 infection. J Infect Dis 161: 354–355, 1990.
12. Pellas F, Olivares JP, Zandotti C, Delarque A. Neuralgic amyotrophy after parvovirus B19 infection. Lancet 342: 503–504, 1993.
13. Denning DW, Amos A, Rudge P, Cohen BJ. Neuralgic amyotrophy due to parvovirus infection. J Neurol Neurosurg Psychiatr 50: 641–642, 1987.
14. Walsh KJ, Armstrong RD, Turner AM. Brachial plexus neuropathy associated with human parvovirus infection. Br Med J 296: 896, 1988.
15. Hornsleth A, Carlsen KM, Christensen LS, Gundestrup M, Heegaard ED, Myhre J. Estimation of serum concentration of parvovirus B19 DNA by PCR in patients with chronic anaemia. Res Virol 145: 379–386, 1994.
16. Faden H, gary GW, Anderson LJ. Chronic parvovirus infection in a presumably immunologically healthy woman. Clin Inf Dis 15: 595–597, 1992.
17. Murray JC, Greisik MV, Leger F, McClain KL. B19 parvovirus induced anemia in a normal child. Am J Ped hematol Oncol 15: 420–423, 1993.
18. Kerr JR, Curran MD, Moore JE, Coyle PV, Ferguson WP. Persistent parvovirus B19 infection. Lancet 345: 1118, 1995.

Submitted July 24, 1995; accepted September 26, 1995

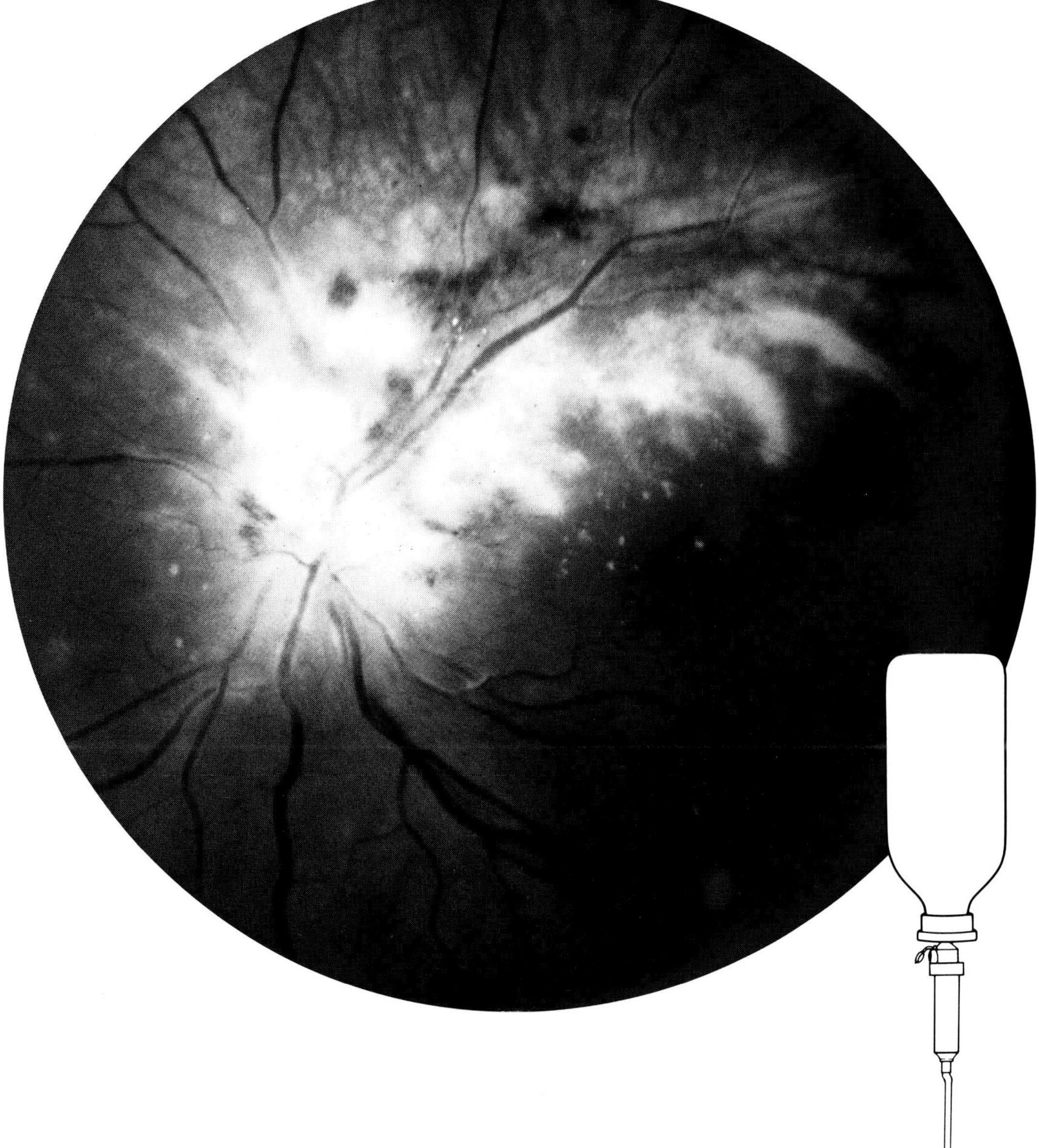

Scand J Infect Dis 27: 635–636, 1995 CASE REPORT

Total Knee Arthroplasty Complicated by Corynebacterium jeikeium Infection

SULHİYE YILDIZ[1], H. YUSUF YILDIZ[2], İLKER ÇETİN[2] and D. HAKAN UÇAR[2]

From the [1]Department of Pharmaceutical Microbiology, Faculty of Pharmacy, and the [2]Department of Orthopaedic Surgery and Traumatology, İbn-i Sina Hospital, School of Medicine, Ankara University, Ankara, Turkey

Corynebacterium jeikeium is a slow-growing multiresistant micro-organism. It causes serious opportunistic infections in patients with long hospital stays who receive broad-spectrum antibiotics. It can be isolated from blood and other sites in neutropenic, immunosuppressed bone marrow recipients and in patients with indwelling catheters. Cases of infection related to bone and joint replacements are rare. This case is the first where Corynebacterium jeikeium has been isolated from an infected knee following total knee arthroplasty.

S. Yıldız, PhD, Department of Pharmaceutical Microbiology, Ankara University, Faculty of Pharmacy, Tandoğan 06100, Ankara, Turkey

INTRODUCTION

Johnson & Kaye (1) first described serious infections, in 52 cases, caused by coryneforms other than Corynebacterium diphtheriae. In 1976, Hande et al. (2) reported 4 cases of sepsis due to "a new species" of Corynebacterium. Riley et al. (3) collected 95 strains of multiresistant coryneforms 3 years later, and reported their characteristics. These organisms have been designated as Corynebacterium JK (group JK) by the Centers for Disease Control, Atlanta.

C. jeikeium has been defined as non-sporulating, non-capsulate, non-mobile, non-haemolytic, obligate aerob, Gram-positive coccobacilli (3, 5, 6).

CASE REPORT

Our 67-year-old female patient had been treated by total knee replacement for right gonarthrosis in 1988 at an institute other than ours, in Ankara. She had stayed at the hospital for 2 months (1 month each pre- and postoperatively). She had intermittent pain beginning 2 months postoperatively and her pain became continuous after 6 months.

She had disabling pain and 0–65 degrees range of motion (ROM) in her right knee when she came to our Department in September 1991. Loosening could barely be observed in the X-rays. Revision total knee arthroplasty was performed in October 1991, 15 days after she was admitted to the hospital. There was no growth in cultures from the specimens taken during surgery. The patient was discharged from the hospital 10 days after the operation.

She reported relapsing pain in the right knee in follow-up visits. When her pain became more intense, her knee was aspirated 4 times with an interval of 10–12 days beginning from May 1994. From the second and fourth aspirates, there was growth at the 4th day on aerobic, 37°C incubation on Tryptone Soy Broth (Oxoid) enriched with 1% Tween 80 and 1% yeast extract. A pure culture was obtained after 72 h when bacteria were subcultured on sheep's blood agar. The colonies were < 0.5 mm, gray-white and without haemolysis. Gram stain showed Gram-positive coccobacilli, identified as Corynebacterium jeikeium on the basis of biochemical test results. Antimicrobial susceptibility testing by disk diffusion on plates prepared by adding 5% sheep blood to Müller–Hinton Agar (Oxoid) (11), showed the micro-organism to be sensitive to tetracycline and vancomycin but resistant to benzyl penicillin mezlocillin, imipenem, chloramphenicol, ofloxacin, ciprofloxacin, pefloxacin, enoxacin, trimethoprim-sulphametoxazole, gentamicin, tobramycin, erythromycin, sulbactam-ampicillin, amoxycillin-clavulanic acid, cephradine, cefuroxime, cefoperazone and cefotaxime.

The patient was readmitted to hospital with the aim of 2-stage reimplantation. She had no fever, and a leucocyte count of 8,200/μl. On physical examination, there was a 0–45 degrees ROM and a positive patellar shock test. The patellar button was grossly loose and there was a thin, global radiolucency around the bone–cement interface of both the tibial and femoral components on X-ray.

During the operation only the patellar button was removed and a thorough debridement and lavage was done. The same micro-organism grew from 3/5 specimens taken during surgery. Postoperatively the patient was treated by i.v. vancomycin (5 weeks) and oral tetracyclin (8 weeks).

The patient has "little or no" pain and a 0–55 degrees ROM at the 7th postoperative month.

DISCUSSION

C. jeikeium can be found among the normal flora of the skin and mucous membranes (8–10), but may become an opportunistic pathogen in patients with prosthetic valves, in immunosuppressed neutropenic patients with haematologic malignancies, or in bone marrow transplant recipients who have indwelling catheters or breaks in mucocutaneous barriers (7, 11). Cases of endocarditis, peritonitis, sepsis, meningitis and liver abscess due to C. jeikeium have been reported in these at-risk patients (2, 4, 12–14). Only 4 cases of C. jeikeium infection localized to the bone and joint system have been reported up to date (15–17): 1 at the mandible of a young male, 1 after elective intramedullary fixation of a closed tibia fracture and 2 following total hip arthroplasties.

Two clues made us think that our patient had probably acquired the infection at the first operation: her pain had begun approximately 2 months postoperatively, and the gross radiolucency around all 3 components. However, there was no growth in samples taken during the revision. This might be due to the unsuitability of routine laboratory

 ISSN 0036-5548

culture media for C. jeikeium and the relatively short incubation period. As no organisms could be isolated, ceftriaxone in preventive dosage and duration was administered after the revision procedure. Because C. jeikeium is uniformly resistant to penicillin and susceptible to vancomycin, and mostly resistant to other antibacterials (3, 6), we believe that the administered ceftriaxone was not suitable for eradicating the infection.

C. jeikeium was isolated from the knee joint aspirates before and from the samples taken during the last operation. This confirmed the diagnosis and enabled us to choose the appropriate antibiotics.

Including our case, among the 5 patients where C. jeikeium now has been identified as the infecting organism in the bone and joint system, 4 have been operated more than once. Multiple surgery is associated with longer hospitalizations and longer duration of antibiotic administration, and this prepares the basis for C. jeikeium colonization, especially in the perineum, groin and axilla, and therefore for infection. It has been demonstrated that colonization of C. jeikeium cannot be eliminated by systemic administration of vancomycin (9) and that it may last for weeks, even months (8). People at risk should be investigated for C. jeikeium colonization preoperatively. If this organism is detected, effective antiseptics in appropriate concentrations or routine bathing with an antimicrobial soap may reduce levels of resistant skin flora, and lessen the risk of infection (9).

In contrast to the other cases, there was no drainage or abscess formation in our patient. She only had minimal local temperature rise and anterior knee pain.

In conclusion, if clinical and radiological findings suggest the presence of a postoperative infection in patients at risk, but an organism cannot be isolated in the routine cultures, it must be kept in mind that C. jeikeium might be the cause. In situations such as these, the use of suitable enriched media and lengthening the incubation period might give more chance of detecting the infecting organism, if there is any.

REFERENCES

1. Johnson WD, Kaye D. Serious infections caused by diphtheroids. Ann N Y Acad Sci 174: 568–576, 1970.
2. Hande KR, Witebsky FG, Brown MS, Schulman CB, Anderson SE, Levine AS, MacLowry JD, Chabner BA. Sepsis with a new species of Corynebacterium. Ann Intern Med 85: 423–426, 1976.
3. Riley PS, Hollis DG, Utter GB, Weaver RE, Baker CN. Characterization and identification of 95 diphtheroid (group JK) cultures isolated from clinical specimens. J Clin Microbiol 9: 418–424, 1979.
4. Jackman PJH, Pitcher DG, Pelczynska S, Borman P. Classification of corynebacterium associated with endocarditis (group JK) as Corynebacterium jeikeium sp. nov. System Appl Microbiol 9: 83–90, 1987.
5. Bayston R, Higgins J. Biochemical and cultural characteristics of "JK" coryneforms. J Clin Pathol 39: 654–660, 1986.
6. Riegel P, DeBriel D, Prevost G, Jehl F, Monteil H. Genomic diversity with biochemical characteristics and antimicrobial susceptibilities. J Clin Microbiol 32: 1860–1865, 1994.
7. Wichmann S, Wirsing von Koenig CH, Becker-Boost E, Finger H. Isolation of Corynebacterium group JK from clinical specimens with a semiselective medium. J Clin Microbiol 19: 204–206, 1984.
8. Gill VJ, Manning C, Lamson M, Woltering P, Pizzo PA. Antibiotic-resistant group JK bacteria in hospitals. J Clin Microbiol 13: 472–477, 1981.
9. Larson EL, McGinley KJ, Leyden JJ, Cooley ME, Talbot GH. Skin colonization with antibiotic-resistant (JK group) and antibiotic-sensitive lipophilic diphtheroids in hospitalized and normal adults. J Infect Dis 153: 701–706, 1986.
10. Soriano F, Rodriguez-Tudela JL, Fernandez-Roblas R, Aguado JM, Santamaria M. Skin colonization by Corynebacterium groups D2 and JK in hospitalized patients. J Clin Microbiol 26: 1878–1880, 1988.
11. Riebel W, Frantz N, Adelstein D, Spagnuolo PJ. Corynebacterium JK: a cause of nosocomial device-related infection. Rev Infect Dis 8: 42–49, 1986.
12. Fosi-Mbantenkhu J, Orett FA. Predisposition of Corynebacterium jeikeium infection in acute lymphoblastic leukemia: a report of two cases in Trinidad. Med Pediatr Oncol 22: 350–354, 1994.
13. Johnson A, Hulse P, Oppenheim BA. Corynebacterium jeikeium meningitis and transverse myelitis in a neutropenic patient. Eur J Clin Microbiol Infect Dis 11: 473–474, 1992.
14. Turett GS, Fazal BA, Johnston BE, Telzak EE. Liver abscess due to Corynebacterium jeikeium in a patient with AIDS. Clin Infect Dis 17: 514–515, 1993.
15. Farnam J, Griffin JE, Schow CE, Mader JT, Grant JA. Recurrent diffuse osteomyelitis involving the mandible. Oral Surg Oral Med Oral Pathol 57: 374–378, 1984.
16. Claeys G, Vershchraegen G, DeSmet L, Verdonk R, Claessens H. Corynebacterium JK (Johnson–Kay strain) infection of a Küntscher-nailed tibial fracture. Clin Orthop 202: 227–229, 1986.
17. Weller TMA, Smith PM, Crook DW. Corynebacterium jeikeium osteomyelitis following total hip joint replacement. J Infect 29: 113–114, 1994.

Submitted April 20, 1995; accepted August 28, 1995

Scand J Infect Dis 27: 637–639, 1995 CASE REPORT

Corynebacterium afermentans Subsp. lipophilum: Multiple Abscess Formation in Brain and Liver

ROELF S. DYKHUIZEN[1], GRAHAM DOUGLAS[1], JAMIE WEIR[2] and IAN M. GOULD[3]

From the [1]Infection Unit, and the Departments of [2]Radiology, and [3]Medical Microbiology, Aberdeen Royal Infirmary, Aberdeen, Scotland

Corynebacterium afermentans, a species recently identified, has previously been isolated from human blood cultures. We report the case of a previously healthy 39-year-old man who developed a brain abscess and a liver abscess due to Corynebacterium afermentans subsp. lipophilum. The liver abscess penetrated through the diaphragm to cause pleural effusion and periostitis of the ribs. We believe this is the first reported case of disseminated infection with abscess formation due to this organism.

R. S. Dyhuizen, MD, Infection Unit, Aberdeen Royal Infirmary, Forresterhill, Aberdeen, AB9 2ZB, Scotland, UK

INTRODUCTION

Coryneform bacteria are recognized pathogens in patients who are immunocompromised or where prosthetic implants have become contaminated (1). During the last few years there has been an increasing number of reports describing infections caused by these organisms. This is partly because of the increasing number of patients who are immunosuppressed and with prosthetic implants, and partly because of greater awareness among clinical microbiologists of coryneforms as potential pathogens. Liver abscess due to Corynebacterium jeikeium (2), and brain abscess due to Corynebacterium haemolyticum (3, 4) have been described.

The newly defined species Corynebacterium afermentans subsp. afermentans and Corynebacterium afermentans subsp. lipophilum (former CDC coryneform group ANF-1) were, although retrieved from blood cultures, initially believed to be non-pathogenic. However, recently a case of prosthetic valve endocarditis was demonstrated to be caused by Corynebacterium afermentans subsp. lipophilum (5), and in this report we describe the first case of abscess formation by this organism in an immunocompetent patient.

CASE REPORT

A 39-year-old man was admitted to hospital with a 3-month history of general malaise, weight loss, night sweats and a cough. He was a heavy smoker but did not admit to alcohol or drug abuse. On examination he was febrile, unwell, and unkempt. There was advanced dental caries. A small area on the right hemithorax appeared erythematous, pustular, indurated and tender. Dullness on percussion and inspiratory crackles were noted at the right base.

Chest radiograph showed consolidation with subsegmental collapse at the right base. The white cell count was 18.4×10^9/l, with 15.8×10^9/l neutrophils. Liver function tests showed albumin 22 g/l, aspartate aminotransferase 26 U/l, alkaline phosphatase 269 U/l, γ-glutamyl transferase 108 U/l, and creatinine phosphokinase 282 U/l.

Treatment was started with intravenous ampicillin 500 mg t.d.s., flucloxacillin 500 mg q.d.s. and metronidazole 500 mg t.d.s. Three days later, the patient developed a grand mal seizure followed by flaccid paresis of the left arm. Computer tomography (CT) scan of the head revealed an area of focal oedema in the right parietal lobe in which a rounded lesion showed moderate wall enhancement after contrast. Small areas of contrast enhancement were seen in the right internal capsule and in the right frontal lobe. 15 ml of pus was aspirated from the parietal lesion under strict aseptic technique. Irregular Gram-positive non-acid fast rods ($0.5 \times 1-1.5$ μm) were observed on microscopy. Metachromatic granules were present. There was some crossing of individual organisms but no true branching. CT scan of the chest showed pleural thickening posteriorly and inferiorly, with marked thickening of the diaphragm and anterolateral chest wall associated with localized periostitis. Ultrasound of the abdomen demonstrated an abscess in the right lobe of the liver and aspiration revealed irregular Gram-positive rods, identical to those obtained from the brain abscess.

After brain and liver abscess aspiration, antimicrobial therapy was changed to benzylpenicillin 3 MU q.d.s., cefotaxime 2 g t.d.s. and metronidazole 500 mg t.d.s. A reducing course of dexamethasone was given. Antimicrobial therapy was continued for 8 weeks and there was complete resolution of neurological, pulmonary and liver abnormalities.

Profuse growth of Corynebacterium spp. was obtained from the brain abscess after 48 h of incubation both aerobically and anaerobically, which was sensitive to penicillin, cefotaxime, erythromycin, gentamycin, vancomycin, ciprofloxacin, teicoplanin and resistant to trimethoprim, clindamycin and metronidazole. Further identification was performed by the National Collection of Type Cultures, London, UK. The colonies on SBA plates were non-haemolytic, <0.5 mm in diameter and had a glassy grayish appearance. The organism showed the biochemical testing pattern of Corynebacterium aftermentans subsp. lipophilum (Table I).

No growth was obtained from the liver abscess and neither specimen yielded any other organism even after extended (10 days) incubation and enrichment in cooked meat broth.

DISCUSSION

Coryneform bacteria include both aerobic and anaerobic non-spore-forming, non-acid-fast, pleomorphic, Gram-positive bacilli. In 1993 corynebacterium afermentans as a new

 ISSN 0036-5548

Table I. *Characteristics and biochemical testing pattern of the micro-organism (strain no. 31/94) isolated from the brain abscess (+ = present, − = absent)*

Morphology		*Characteristics*		*Fermentation*	
Shape	Rods	Growth on		Arabinose	−
Colour	Grey	MRS	−	Fructose	−
Opacity	Translucent	Tellurite	+	Galactose	−
Staining	Easy; Gram +ve	Blood agar	+	Glucose	−
Size	0.5 × 1–1.5 μm	Growth 37°C		Glycerol	−
Sides	Parallel	Aerobic	+	Lactose	−
Ends	Rounded	Anaerobic	+	Maltose	−
Axis	Straight	Catalase	+	Mannitol	−
Regularity	Monomorphic	Oxidase	−	Mannose	−
Arrangement	Singly and in clusters	Tween 20–80 growth and hydrolysis	+	Raffinose	−
Consistency	Butyrous	Methyl red	−	Salicin	−
Emulsifiability	Easy	VP	−	Sorbitol	−
Suspension	Uniform	ONPG	−	Starch	−
		Haemolysis	−	Sucrose	−
		Hydrolysis		Trehalose	−
		Urea	−	Xylose	−
		Aesculin	−	Glucose ammonium salt sugar	−
		Starch	−		
		Casein	−		
		Gelatin	−		
		Arginine	−		
		Tyrosine growth	+		
		Tyrosine hydrolysis	−		

species, containing 2 subspecies: C. afermentans subsp. afermentans and C. afermentans subsp. lipophilum, was proposed by Riegel et al. (6). The new species was defined on the basis of rRNA gene restriction patterns and DNA–DNA relatedness studies from 11 strains of Corynebacterium group absolute nonfermenter-1 (CDC group ANF-1), as first described in 1981 at the Centers for Disease Control by Hollis & Weaver (7). Corynebacterium group ANF-1 had been isolated from blood cultures, but until Sewell et al. (5) showed it to be the aetiological agent in a case of prosthetic valve endocarditis, no disease due to the organism had been reported.

Our patient presented with abscess formation in the brain and the liver. The liver abscess penetrated through the diaphragm to cause pleural thickening, pleural effusion and periostitis of the ribs with erythema and induration of the overlying skin. Chronic suppurative infection and abscess formation, with spread to contiguous tissues without regard for normal anatomical barriers, is considered to be characteristic of actinomycosis. The spectrum of pulmonary consolidation, pleural thickening, periostitis and chest wall involvement, is highly suggestive of this infection. Ascending infection from the liver into the right lung base and haematogenous spread to produce a brain abscess are well recognized (8). Actinomyces organisms are frequently found in dental caries and at gingival margins in persons, like our patient, with poor oral hygiene. However, the presence of metachromatic granules, and the absence of branching or sulphur granules on microscopy indicated rather infection by a coryneform and this was confirmed during further identification (Table I). Coryneforms are commensals of skin and mucous membranes, and perhaps the patient's poor dentition allowed the organism to disseminate via the bloodstream.

The significance of the isolation of coryneforms from clinical specimens depends on patient data such as immune status, intravenous drug abuse, alcoholism, the presence of prosthetic implants or pre-existing heart disease, and on laboratory data such as scanty or profuse growth, numbers of positive cultures and risk of contamination. In our patient the immune status was apparently normal, and he denied alcohol or drug abuse. Profuse growth from the brain abscess was observed within 48 h. The liver abscess revealed no growth, which is not surprising after 4 days of antimicrobial therapy which would stunt growth in an aspirate obtained from an organ as well perfused as the liver, as opposed to the brain.

Corynebacterium afermentans subsp. lipophilum seems to have significant pathogenic potential even in apparently immunocompetent patients who are not implanted with prostheses.

ACKNOWLEDGEMENTS

We would like to thank Dr H. Malnick of the Central Public Health Laboratory, Colindale Avenue, London, for the identification of the micro-organism.

REFERENCES

1. Coyle MB, Lipsky BA. Coryneform bacteria in infectious diseases: clinical and laboratory aspects. Clin Microbiol Rev 3: 227–246, 1990.
2. Turett GS, Fazal BA, Johnston BE, Telzak EE. Liver abscess due to corynebacterium jeikeium in a patient with AIDS. Clin Infect Dis 17: 514–515, 1993.
3. Washington JA, Martin WJ, Spiekerman RE. Brian abscess with Corynebacterium haemolyticum: report of a case. Am J Clin Path 56: 212–215, 1971.
4. Altmann G, Bogokovsky B. Brain absces due to Corynebacterium haemolyticum. Lancet 321: 378–379, 1973.
5. Sewell DL, Coyle MB, Funke G. Prosthetic valve endocarditis caused by Corynebacterium afermentans subsp. lipophilum (CDC coryneform group ANF-1). J Clin Microbiol 33: 759–761, 1995.
6. Riegel P, De Briel D, Prévost G, Jehl F, Monteil H, Minck R. Taxonomic study of Corynebacterium group ANF-1 strains: proposal of Corynebacterium afermentans sp. nov. containing the subspecies C. afermentans subsp. afermentans subsp. nov. and C. afermentans subsp. lipophilum subsp. nov. Int J Syst Bacteriol 43: 287–292, 1993.
7. Hollis DG, Weaver RA. Gram-positive organisms: a guide to identification. Atlanta, Georgia: Special Bacteriology Section, Centers for Disease Control, 1981.
8. Brown JR. Human actinomycosis. A study of 181 subjects. Hum Pathol 4: 319–330, 1073.

Submitted May 15, 1995; accepted July 11, 1995

Scand J Infect Dis 27: 641–642, 1995 CASE REPORT

A Case of Brucella melitensis Endocarditis Successfully Treated by a Combination of Surgical Resection and Antibiotics

R. SCHVARCZ[1], J. SVEDENHAG[2] and K. RÅDEGRAN[3]

From the Departments of [1]Infectious Diseases and [2]Clinical Physiology, Huddinge University Hospital, Huddinge, and the [3]Department of Thoracic Surgery, Karolinska University Hospital, Solna, Sweden

Endocarditis is a rare complication of brucellosis, often fatal, and the treatment is controversial. We present a case of Brucella melitensis endocarditis successfully treated by a combination of surgical resection and antibiotics.

R. Schvarcz, MD, Department of Infectious Diseases, I 73, Huddinge University Hospital, S-141 86 Huddinge, Sweden

INTRODUCTION

Human brucellosis is endemic in many parts of the world, but occurs in Sweden only as imported cases. It can run a complicated course with focal manifestations, e.g. spondylitis and meningitis (1). Endocarditis is also a well recognized complication of brucellosis. Although rare, with an incidence of <1% in cases of brucellosis, it is important since it is often fatal and responsible for the majority of deaths from this infection (1, 2). We report a case of Brucella melitensis endocarditis successfully treated by a combination of surgical resection and antibiotics.

CASE REPORT

A 48-year-old male of Turkish origin, who had lived in Sweden since 1987, presented at the department of infectious diseases on 18 October 1993, with a history of fever for 2 months.

As a teenager he had suffered a "rheumatic" disease which was cured by treatment with "injections". Apart from that, he had previously been healthy and did not take any regular medications. During June–July 1993 he had visited his family in Turkey.

His current symptoms consisted of fever, chills, general weakness, loss of appetite and loss of weight, (7 kg) over 2 months. In the last few weeks he had also had diffuse pain in the legs. He had been put on treatment with norfloxacin, 200 twice daily, 10 days before admission because of a suspected urinary tract infection, but he had not improved.

On admission the patient was febrile with a temperature of 38.5°C, and had a grade II systolic murmur but no signs of cardiac failure. C-reactive protein in serum (CRP) was moderately raised 81 mg/l (reference value <10), and he had a slight anaemia, (haemoglobin was 118 g/l). The white cell count and a chest X-ray were normal.

The patient was hospitalized. On suspicion of subacute bacterial endocarditis, parenteral therapy with benzyl penicillin (3 g × 4) and netilmicin (120 mg × 2) was given after cultures from blood and urine. He responded well to treatment, with normalization of temperature in 3 days and an improvement in his general condition. A biplanar transoesophageal echocardiography (TEE) performed 2 days after admission revealed the presence of a large (8 × 22 mm) oscillating vegetation on the mitral valve (Fig. 1) and

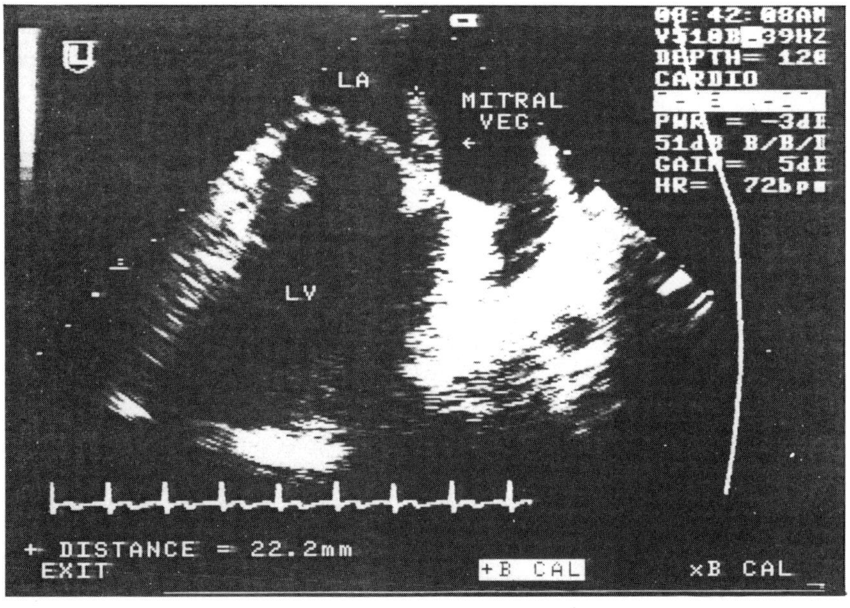

Fig. 1. Transoesophageal echocardiogram, longitudinal plane. A large vegetation is seen on the anterior mitral leaflet. The length of the vegetation (22 mm) is indicated by markers (+). LA, left atrium. LV, left ventricle.

 ISSN 0036-5548

small mitral and aortic regurgitations. After 7 days the blood cultures drawn at admission yielded growth of B. melitensis, sensitive to rifampicin, doxycycline, trimethoprim-sulfamethoxazole, aminoglycoside and chloramphenicol. At this point the patient recalled having drunk unpasteurized goat's milk once at a neighbour's farm during his summer visit to Turkey. The therapy was changed. Netilmicin was continued with the addition of oral rifampicin (900 mg/d) and doxycycline (200 mg/d). Because of the apparent risk of embolization, surgery was performed with excision of the vegetation on the eighth day of hospitalization. During operation it was also noted that the mitral valve had changes consistent with a previous rheumatic fever, but not to the extent that valve replacement was necessary. B melitensis was isolated from the excised vegetation. Serology with ELISA showed raised antibody levels against brucella of both IgG and IgM classes.

After surgery, the patient made an uneventful recovery. His temperature remained normal, he improved steadily and he was discharged from hospital after 4 weeks. Netilmicin was withdrawn after 4 weeks because of a slight temporary raise in serum creatinine level. Oral treatment with doxycycline and rifampicin was continued for a total of 6 months. Regular clinical check-ups during 15 months showed a good general condition and repeatedly normal CRP values. Serological tests showed markedly declining antibody titres. TEE performed 1, 6 and 15 months after the onset of disease showed only a minimal stationary high density vegetation on the mitral valve and small mitral and aortic regurgitations.

DISCUSSION

Our patient's illness had an insidious onset and other symptoms similar to those also seen in cases of subacute endocarditis caused by viridans streptococci. Apart from the epidemiological information it was not possible to distinguish clinically between the 2 conditions. As a teenager, the patient had probably acquired a lesion of the mitral valve from rheumatic fever, predisposing him towards endocarditis. It is most probable that he acquired brucellosis when he drank unpasteurized goat's milk, since this is one of the major routes of transmission in countries where B. melitensis infection is endemic (1).

Uncomplicated brucellosis in adults is usually treated with a combination of doxycycline and rifampicin for 1 month (3). The treatment of brucella endocarditis, however, remains controversial (1–5). Without treatment the prognosis is poor, but even with antibiotics the risk of recurrence after cessation of therapy is high, probably due to the intracellular nature of brucella (1–4). In a review of the literature, Jacobs et al. concluded that brucella endocarditis is usually fatal if treated by antibiotics alone (2). There are, however, cases cured by medical treatment alone (5). To avoid recurrence, it has been suggested that antibiotic treatment should be given for prolonged periods of time and that to reach optimal efficacy it should consist of a combination of drugs (1–3). Trimethoprim-sulfamethoxazole or rifampicin should be added to the classical combination of doxycycline and aminoglycoside (2). The treatment should be given in high doses for at least 2 months, but possibly for even longer periods. Because of the high risk of recurrence and the poor prognosis with antibiotic treatment alone, there are authors who advocate a combined approach with valve replacement and antibiotic treatment (1–4). Our patient neither had haemodynamic complications nor treatment failure that made valve replacement necessary, and apparently the treatment given, i.e. excision of the vegetation without valve replacement, combined with antibiotic treatment for 6 months, was successful.

This case shows the importance of getting a correct epidemiological history. In patients coming from countries where brucellosis is endemic, brucella should be considered as one of the aetiological possibilities if endocarditis is suspected. Hence, appropriate cultures should be taken, and if the suspicion is great, the initial antibiotic regimen should be adjusted to cover this possibility.

REFERENCES

1. Young EJ. Human brucellosis. Rev Infect Dis 5: 821–842, 1983.
2. Jacobs F, Abramowicz D, Vereerstraeten P, Le Clerc JL, Zech F, Thys JP. Brucella endocarditis: The role of combined medical and surgical treatment. Rev Infect Dis 12: 740–744, 1990.
3. Hall WH. Modern chemotherapy for brucellosis in humans. Rev Infect Dis 12: 1060–1099, 1990.
4. Platt P, Gray J, Carson P. Brucella endocarditis – a successfully treated case. J Infect 2: 275–278, 1980.
5. Cisneros JM, Pachón J, Cuello JA, Martinez A. Brucella endocarditis cured by medical treatment. J Infect Dis 160: 907, 1989.
6. Acocella G, Bertrand A, Beytout J, Durrande JB, Garcia Rodriguez J-A, Kosmidis J, Micoud M, Rey M, Rodriguez Zapata M, Roux J, Stahl J-P. Comparison of three different regimens in the treatment of acute brucellosis: a multicenter multinational study. J Antimicrob Chemother 23: 433–439, 1989.

Submitted June 21, 1995; accepted September 8, 1995

Scand J Infect Dis 27: 643–644, 1995 CASE REPORT

Overwhelming Myocarditis due to Fusarium oxysporum following Bone Marrow Transplantation

ISMAEL MOHAMMEDI[1], BERTRAND GACHOT[1], MARGUERITE GROSSIN[2], CLAUDIE MARCHE[2], MICHEL WOLFF[1] and FRANÇOIS VACHON[1]

From the [1]Clinique de Réanimation des Maladies Infectieuses and the [2]Service d'Anatomie et de Cytologie Pathologiques, Bichat-Claude Bernard Hospital, Paris, France

Disseminated infection by Fusarium is being increasingly reported in immunocompromised patients. We report the first case of Fusarium oxysporum disseminated infection with well-documented fungal myocarditis. Despite antifungal therapy and hematologic recovery, the patient died in cardiogenic shock, myocardial involvement clearly contributing to the fatal outcome.

B. Gachot, MD, PhD, Clinique de Réanimation des Maladies Infectieuses, Hôpital Bichat-Claude Bernard, 46, rue Henri Huchard, F-75018 Paris, France

INTRODUCTION

Invasive fungal infections are a major cause of morbidity and mortality in immunosuppressed patients, and the incidence of these life-threatening complications is increasing. Fungi previously considered to be contaminants are now emerging as significant pathogens. Fusarium species belong to this category. We report a case of disseminated fusariosis that is unique in terms of its specific myocardial involvement.

CASE REPORT

The patient was a 49-year-old man, with no past medical history, in whom a diagnosis of idiopathic aplastic anemia was made in November 1992. While he was granulocytopenic, he received empiric broad-spectrum antibiotics and amphotericin B for febrile episodes without documented infection.

In March 1993, he developed multiple non-pruriginous, painful, purpuric skin nodules (each 0.2–1.5 cm in diameter) on the arms, legs and thorax. Culture of a skin biopsy specimen grew Fusarium species, later identified as F. oxysporum. The same fungus was subsequently isolated from a blood culture. The dose of amphotericin B was increased to 1.5 mg/kg/day and itraconazole (600 mg per os daily) was added on the basis of in vitro antifungal susceptibility testing. The minimal inhibitory concentrations (MICs) of antifungal drugs were determined using a microtiter method on casitone liquid (1) and were 0.18 and 0.09 mg/l respectively, for amphotericin B and itraconazole.

The patient underwent allogenic bone marrow transplantation after preparation consisting of cyclophosphamide and total-body irradiation. Multiple cultures of blood collected shortly before and after bone marrow transplantation grew F. oxysporum, despite antifungal therapy, until the patient again had a neutrophil count $> 500/\mu l$ (13 days after transplantation).

A week later, diffuse pulmonary infiltrates appeared on the chest radiograph, and the patient was empirically given ganciclovir and trimethoprim-sulfamethoxazole between day 21 and 31, in addition to other antibiotics. Profound neutropenia occurred and resolved slowly after discontinuation of both drugs (day 43). During this time, a urine culture grew F. oxysporum.

On day 47, the patient was given mechanical ventilation for respiratory failure and was subsequently admitted to the intensive care unit. Hemodynamic status was normal at this time. Arterial blood gas analysis showed pH 7.33, Pa_{CO_2} 34 mmHg, Pa_{O_2} 298 mmHg with 100% FiO_2. The leukocyte count was 4,400/μl, with 90% neutrophils. The chest radiograph revealed bilateral interstitial infiltrates. Two-dimensional echocardiography was considered normal.

Despite therapy, fungemia continued, with new skin nodules, 3 positive blood cultures (days 48 and 50), and a skin biopsy growing F. oxysporum. All catheters were removed, and were negative for bacteria and fungi on culture.

On day 51, the patient's clinical status declined, with hypotension persisting despite fluid administration. The electrocardiogram and cardiac enzyme activities were normal. Septic shock was suspected and a pulmonary artery catheter was inserted. Initial measures revealed a high pulmonary wedge pressure (27 mmHg), low cardiac index ($1.37\ l/min/m^2$), and systemic vascular resistance of 1400 dynes $s/cm^5\ m^2$.

A diagnosis of fulminant myocarditis was considered. Despite increasing doses of dobutamine and epinephrine combined with maximal antifungal therapy, the patient remained in shock and died 5 days after ICU admission. Blood drawn on the day of death yielded F. oxysporum.

Autopsy revealed multiorgan granulomas. Fungal hyphae were detected microscopically in skin, lungs, kidneys, esophagus and heart (Fig. 1). Tissue samples grew F. oxysporum.

DISCUSSION

Disseminated infection by Fusarium is restricted to the immunocompromised host. Many predisposing factors have been identified, including the use of intensive chemotherapy regimens, previous exposure to antimicrobial agents, and the depth and duration of granulocytopenia. The authors of a recent review (2) analysed 41 reported cases. Since then, another 4 cases have been reported (3, 4). The majority of patients had skin lesions. Other sites of involvement were relatively common (sinuses, oropharynx), or less so (central venous catheters, kidneys, lungs, eyes and urine). Heart involvement appears to be unusual and is always diagnosed postmortem (5–7). To our knowledge, the case we report is the first of Fusarium myocardial

 ISSN 0036-5548

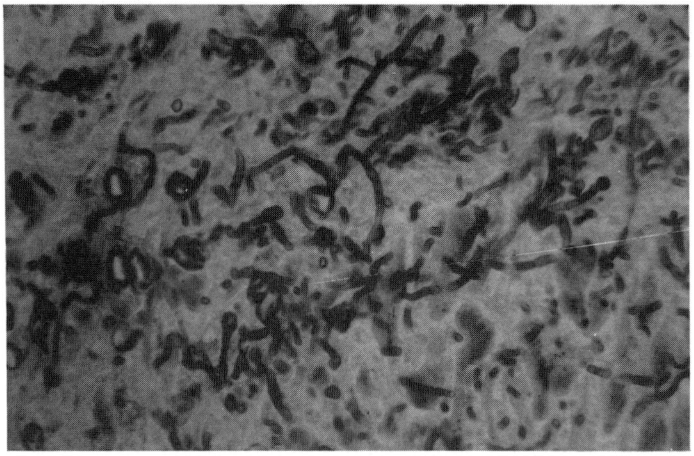

Fig. 1. Septate filaments of Fusarium oxysporum in the myocardium (Grocott silver stain; magnification ×40).

involvement clinically suspected prior to death and documented both by culture and histopathological examination postmortem.

Most patients with disseminated infection by Fusarium species and persistent neutropenia die despite antifungal therapy (2, 8). In the case we describe, fungemia persisted despite hematologic recovery, and catheter-related infection and endocarditis were ruled out. Multiple skin lesions were the consequence rather than the cause of dissemination, and there was no other fungal focus of infection accessible to surgery; this latter approach has been recommended in order to prevent dissemination from a localized cutaneous lesion (9). In addition, the isolates appeared susceptible in vitro to both amphotericin B and itraconazole. However, correlations between in vitro susceptibility and clinical responses are questionable, owing to the lack of standardized test methods (10). Kiehn et al. (11) isolated Fusarium strains which were sensitive to amphotericin B by the broth dilution method with yeast nitrogen broth, but resistant when tested in Sabouraud glucose broth. Despite evidence of multiple abscesses at autopsy, our patient died of cardiogenic rather than septic shock. This suggests that long-term antifungal therapy might have controlled the infection if fatal heart failure had not occurred.

ACKNOWLEDGEMENT

The authors thank Professor B. Dupont for antifungal susceptibility testing of the strain.

REFERENCES

1. Regli P, Ferrari H, Goudard M, Buffard Y. Intérêt du milieu Casitone pour l'étude de la sensibilité in vitro des champignons levuriformes aux antifongiques dérivés de l'imidazole. Bull Soc Franç Mycol Med 11: 359–362, 1982.
2. Gamis AS, Gudnason T, Giebink GS, Ramsay NKC. Disseminated infection with Fusarium in recipients of bone marrow transplants. Rev Infect Dis 13: 1077–1088, 1991.
3. Ammari LK, Puck JM, McGowan KL. Catheter-related Fusarium solani fungemia and pulmonary infection in a patient with leukemia in remission. Clin Infect Dis 16: 148–150, 1993.
4. Mardiak J, Danisovicova A, Trupl J, Sloboda J, Jesenska Z, Krcmery V. Three cases of fatal infection due to Fusarium solani in patients with cancer. Clin Infect Dis 17: 930–932, 1993.
5. Abramowsky CR, Quinn D, Bradford WD, Conant NF. Systemic infection by Fusarium in a burned child. J Pediatr 84: 561–564, 1974.
6. Young NA, Kwon-Chung KJ, Kubota TT, Jennings AE, Fisher RI. Disseminated infection by Fusarium moniliforme during treatment for malignant lymphoma. J Clin Microbiol 7: 589–594, 1978.
7. Anaissie E, Kantarjian H, Ro J, et al. The emerging role of Fusarium infections in patients with cancer. Medicine 67: 77–83, 1988.
8. Richardson SE, Bannatyne RM, Summerbell RC, Milliken J, Gold R, Weitzman SS. Disseminated fusarial infection in the immunocompromised host. Rev Infect Dis 10: 1171–1181, 1988.
9. Ellis ME, Clink H, Younge D, Hainau B. Successful combined surgical and medical treatment of Fusarium infection after bone marrow transplantation. Scand J Infect Dis 26: 225–228, 1994.
10. Sheehan DJ, Espinel-Ingroff A, Moore LS, Weeb CD. Antifungal susceptibility testing of yeasts: a brief overview. Clin Infect Dis 17: S494–S500, 1993.
11. Kiehn TE, Nelson PE, Bernard EM, Edwards FF, Koziner B, Armstrong D. Catheter-associated fungemia caused by Fusarium chlamydosporum in a patient with lymphocytic lymphoma. J Clin Microbiol 21: 501–504, 1985.

Submitted June 6, 1995; accepted August 28, 1995

Scand J Infect Dis 27: 645–646, 1995 CASE REPORT

Acute Clonorchiasis

MARGARET IP[1], NANCY LEUNG[2] and AUGUSTINE F. CHENG[1]

From the Departments of [1]Microbiology and [2]Medicine, Chinese University of Hong Kong, Prince of Wales Hospital, Shatin, Hong Kong.

A 42-year-old Chinese woman developed 3 weeks of swinging fever, rash, malaise, and discomfort at the right upper quadrant of the abdomen. Acute Clonorchis sinensis infection eventually became evident and the patient responded to praziquantel. Although acute infestation is usually asymptomatic, occasional cases suffer severe symptoms and present difficulties in clinical diagnosis. Clonorchiasis is endemic in South East Asia. With the increasing popularity of travel to these countries and the global migration of Asians, physicians need to be aware of the condition. Treatment with praziquantel is effective and prevents the serious sequelae of chronic infection.

M. Ip, MD, Department of Microbiology, Chinese University of Hong Kong, Prince of Wales Hospital, Shatin, Hong Kong

INTRODUCTION

Infection with the oriental liver fluke, Clonorchis sinensis, is endemic in the Far East and is common in Hong Kong and mainland China (1). Man becomes infected by ingestion of the cysts present in the flesh of raw or partially-cooked freshwater fish. It is estimated that 19 million people are infected (1) and it is the most common intestinal parasite isolated in Hong Kong (2). Although acute infestation is very often subclinical, severe acute infections due to heavy infestation may result in considerable morbidity. The present case illustrates an unusually severe presentation of acute infection by Clonorchis sinensis which might easily mimic acute hepatitis, cholecystitis or as a case of pyrexia of unknown origin.

CASE REPORT

A previously healthy 42-year old female factory worker was admitted with 2 weeks' history of fever, nausea, vomiting and intermittent watery diarrhoea. She also had symptoms of malaise, anorexia, myalgia and developed a generalized maculopapular rash. Five days prior to admission, she had discomfort at the right upper quadrant of the abdomen, and a persisting fever with rigors. On examination, she had a temperature of 37.5°C, was not icteric, and had generalized non-tender lymphadenopathy. She had a tender liver palpable 4 cm below the costal margin. There were no chest signs and other systems examinations were unremarkable. A presumptive diagnosis of acute cholecystitis or hepatitis was made.

Investigations showed a leucocytosis (18.9×10^9/L) with marked lymphocytosis (55%) and eosinophilia (11%). The eosinophilia rose to 26% and persisted for the next 2 weeks. The alanine aminotransferase was 401 U/l (<58 U/l), alkaline phosphatase 210 U/l (30–80 IU/l), total bilirubin 12 μmol/l (0–15 μmol/l) and albumin 32 g/l (36–48 g/l). Renal function showed urea 2.1 mmol/l (3.4–8.9 mmol/l), creatinine 73 μmol/l (44–107 μmol/l), sodium 133 mmol/l (134–145 mmol/l) and potassium 3.7 mmol/l (3.5–5.1 mmol/l). Ultrasonography demonstrated a distended, thick-walled gallbladder. There was mild hepatosplenomegaly with small amount of ascites. The common bile duct and intrahepatic ducts were normal and no calculi were seen. ERCP was performed and showed no ductal stones nor cholestasis. Bile was not sent for microscopy. Screening for infectious mononucleosis was negative, as was that for malaria parasites. Repeated blood, urine, and throat cultures were all negative. Serology for hepatitis A and B, mycoplasma, brucella, leptospira, Q fever, chlamydia, rickettsial disease and Salmonella typhi and paratyphi A, B and C were all negative. Viral serology including influenza A and B, adenovirus, CMV and enteroviruses were also all negative.

The patient was put on empirical treatment for acute cholecystitis with ampicillin, cefuroxime and metronidazole. The high swinging fever fluctuated between 37–40°C and persisted despite 7 days of antibiotics and she continued to have localized right upper quadrant tenderness although the rash was disappearing and the lymphadenopathy less prominent. She also complained of further watery diarrhoea which then revealed numerous Clonorchis sinensis ova on repeated stool examinations. The patient was given a course of praziquantel at 75 mg/kg body weight divided into 3 doses by oral route. She improved, her fever settled within 24 hours of treatment and was discharged home. At follow up, she remained well; her blood picture and liver enzymes returned to normal 4 weeks after discharge from hospital.

DISCUSSION

This case illustrates the clinical picture of severe, acute infection with Clonorchis sinensis as described by Koenigstein (3). The initial symptoms were due to invasion of the biliary passages by adolescercariae which matured into adult flukes, and after about 3 their ova appeared in faeces. Significant eosinophilia seen in this case was typical of an acute infection and not a feature in chronic infections. It is unusual for severe, acute infections to occur, especially in the Chinese who probably have some immunity to the fluke from previous exposure. In this patient, the severity may have been associated with exposure to a heavy fluke burden. This was reflected by the large numbers of ova seen in stool which is an uncommon feature in those harbouring few clonorchis. Acute infection is usually self-limited but in this case, the patient remained ill and symptoms persisted until specific treatment was instituted. Response to treatment with praziquantel was prompt with the relief of symptoms and complete recovery of liver function and eradication of infection.

The diagnosis of hepatic clonorchiasis was made by demonstration of ova in stool but this was not possible until the flukes had matured and started to shed ova.

Repeated examinations were therefore required. Examination of bile or duodenal aspirate for ova and flukes is also helpful for an early diagnosis of the infection (4). Ultrasonography is useful, showing diffuse dilatation of the small intrahepatic bile ducts but without changes in the large intra and extrahepatic ducts (5). In our patient, retrospective examination of the ERCP films revealed the presence of irregularities and elliptical appearances in the small intrahepatic ducts compatible with a diagnosis of fluke infestation, suggesting that the diagnosis can easily be missed if not clinically suspected.

The source of infection was not elicited in this case, but in Hong Kong and southern parts of China, the range of local culinary habits is wide. A popular dish being fish congee, where boiling congee is poured over raw slices of carp or other freshwater fish. Fish may be eaten pickled in vinegar, raw in 'sashimi' (covered in soybean paste) and in 'sushi' which are popular Korean and Japanese cuisines. The cysts can withstand a temperature of 50–70°C for 15 minutes (1). Humans and animals are the natural reservoir hosts, and the cysts are found in many species of freshwater fish in faecally contaminated lakes and rivers. Suitable snail hosts of the species; Parafossarulus manchouricus and Bithynia fuchsiana [1] are present in large numbers in the southern Chinese provinces. In Fujian province of China, freshwater shrimps were also incriminated as sources of infection in children. The infection rate is generally between 1 and 10%, but in some provinces the rate is above 30% (6). The incidence is highest in the age group 30–50 years, when people are exposed to a more varied diet. In Hong Kong, clonorchiasis has remained the commonest parasitic infection diagnosed. The infection rate ranged between 11–17.7% (2) in the past and in 1992, a retrospective survey on 8590 stool samples revealed the presence of Clonorchis sinensis ova in 5.3% (2). Our data on examination of 5200 stool specimens revealed the presence of Clonorchis sinensis ova in 4.6%, constituting 55% of all the intestinal parasites detected. Control measures to reduce infestation by thorough cooking of fish and health education are difficult to implement, especially when it involves changing the local culinary practice.

Clonorchiasis in Chinese patients is usually mild and of a chronic nature; with vague symptoms of irregular appetite, fullness of the abdomen, and diarrhoea (3). The flukes have a long life span and can persist within the biliary trees for decades. Infected patients present late in the chronic stage with complications of recurrent pyogenic cholangitis (7), pancreatitis (8), cholangio-carcinoma and hepatocellular carcinoma (9). Among Chinese immigrants in the United States and Canada, an infestation rate has been estimated at 15.5% (1). Sun (1) also reported two cases of clonorchiasis in American residents who contracted the infection through visits to endemic areas. Treatment with praziquantel is effective and prevents the development of complications associated with chronic infection. With increased migration and travelling, and with the increasing popularity of consumption of raw fish in 'sushi' and 'sashimi', physicians need to be aware of the manifestations of Clonorchis sinensis infection. It will not be surprising that the incidence and endemicity of clonorchiasis is under recognized.

REFERENCES

1. Manson-Bahr PEC, Bell DR. Manson's Tropical Diseases 19th edn. London: Bailliere Tindall, 496–502, 1987.
2. Kam KM. Intestinal parasites in Hong Kong. J Trop Med & Hygiene 97: 117–120, 1994.
3. Koenigstein RP. Observations on the epidemiology of infections with Clonorchis sinensis. Trans R Soc Trop Med Hyg 42: 503–506, 1949.
4. Hartley JPR, Douglas AP. A case of clonorchiasis in England. BMJ 3; 5983: 575, 1975.
5. Lim JH, Ko YT, Lee DH, Kim SY. Clonorchiasis: sonographic findings in 59 proved cases. AJR Am J Roentgenol 152: 761–764, 1989.
6. Liu YS, Du WP, Wu YM, Chen YG, Zheng KY, Shi JM, Hu XZ, Li GY, You CF, Wu ZX. Application of dot-immunogold-silver staining in the diagnosis of clonorchiasis. J Trop Med Hyg 98: 151–154, 1995.
7. Fung J. Liver fluke infestation and cholangio-hepatitis. Br J Surg 48: 404–415, 1961.
8. Chan PH, Teoh TB. The pathology of Clonorchis sinensis infestation of the pancreas. J Pathol Bacteriol 93: 185–189, 1967.
9. Hou PC. Relationship between primary carcinoma of liver and infestation with Clonorchis sinensis. J Pathol Bacteriol 72: 239–246, 1956.
10. Seah SK. Intestinal parasites in Chinese immigrants in a Canadian city. J Trop Med Hyg 76: 291–293, 1973.
11. Sun T. Clonorchiasis: A report of four cases and discussion of unusual manifestations. Am J Trop Med Hyg 29: 1223–1227, 1980.

Submitted August 21, 1995; accepted October 23, 1995

LIST OF AUTHORS

For Å and Ä see A, for Ö and Ø see O

Abbeele van den K. 89
Abdi Y. 149
Admoni O. 139
Åhrén C. 589
Albay A. 425
Albrecht H. 71
Aljundi H. 529
Altwegg M. 499
Al-Eissa Y. A. 339
Al-Kassab A. 183
Ämmälä P. 265
Ammassari A. 235
Andersen H.-K. 245
Andersen L. P. D. 347
Andersen P. L. 191
Andersson S. 547
Andersson-Ellström A. 315
Antinori A. 235
Antonelli M. 381
Antonius J. 157
Antony S.J. 401, 411
Arasteh K. 71
Arpi M. 245
Aygen B. 135
Azher Q. 183

Babu P.-G. 105
Backer V. 351
Bäckman A. 537
Bader G. 279
Bagg J. 149
Bakir M. 135
Banatvala N. 149
Banke S. 463
Barbarini G. 613
Barbaro G. 613
Barreto L. 279
Bassett D. C. J. 527
Baysallar M. 425
Bazarbashi M. 157
Ben R.-J. 415
Bergmann K.-C. 369
Bernacchia R. 441
Bernhard P. 623
Biberfeld G. 547
Bienzle U. 331
Blatter M. 279
Bobrowska E. 15
Bobrowski M. 15
Bohr V. A. 569
Boiron P. 23
Bombi J. A. 511
Bongaerts G. 83
Bordes J. M. 511
Born P. 419
Borne von dem A. E. G. Kr. 581
Borrelli S. 303
Bouchama A. 157
Bouchaud O. 96
Braconier J. H. 111, 325

Brancart F. 358
Brandt L. 191
Brolös O. 191
Brook I. 619
Brummer-Korvenkontio M. 515
Bruno A.-M. 463
Bruun B. 419

Cabellos C. 93
Cabié A. 96
Calangu S. 135
Carlson P. 17
Carlsson M. 463
Carlström A. 457
Cayazzo M. 385
Çetin I. 635
Cetinkaya F. 241
Changalucha J. 589
Chen A.-C. 289
Chen C.-T. 289
Chen M. 319
Cheng A. F. 645
Cheng K.-C. 295
Chevret S. 201
Chiodo F. 405
Chiu C.-H. 75
Chryssanthou E. 391, 421
Cilla G. 344
Cinar E. 425
Claesson B. E. B. 603
Clausen N. 153
Clement J. 453
Clements L. 149
Cobeljic M. 427
Codeluppi M. 173
Colebunders R. 89
Coll-Seck A. M. 9
Colson P. 453
Conti G. 381
Coppens L. 409
Corachán M. 511
Corbella X. 93
Corona R. 441
Coulaud J.-P. 96
Coursaget P. 9
Crausman R. S. 77
Cronberg S. 463
Culig J. 503
Curran M. D. 551
Dalsgaard A. 585
Davies J. 149
De Vol E. B. 157
Diebold T. 627
Doedens R. A. 399
Doganay M. 135
Doganci L. 69, 425
Domingo P. 95, 523
Douglas G. 637
Driesel G. 331
Duberg A.-S. 449

Dykhuizen R. S. 637
D'Amelio R. 12
D'Andrea L. 173

Eastwood B. 279
Echeverria P. 585
Eerola E. 45, 475
Ekdal K. 111
Ellis M. E. 157
Elmrud H. 463
Elowsson S. 463
Ende van den J. 89
Engman K. 325
Engstrand L. 119
Enogat N. 9
Eriksson B. M. 435
Ermisch B. 627
Esbjörner E. 63
Espersen F. 483, 563

Faber M. 483
Falck G. 179
Farina C. 23
Feldman R. A. 149
Fernandez-Viladrich P. 93, 165
Ferraro P. 441
Ferrer I. 165
Filipsson S. 603
Finnish Study Group..., 52
Fisher M. 297
Forsgren M. 3
Forssman L. 315
Frederiksen W. 145, 153
Frei R. 499
Friland A. 19
Frimodt-Møller N. 483, 563
Fuentes-Martinez F. 469

Gabone R. 589
Gachot B. 643
Gajdos P. 201
Galanti C. 441
Gardulf A. 597
Garpenholt Ö. 63
Gascon J. 511
Gasparetto A. 381
George R. C. 291
Gharbi Y. 9
Gnarpe H. 179
Gnarpe J. 179
Goglio A. 23
Golan A. 139
Golden R. 297
Gomez-Lus Centelles M. L. 469
González de Etxabarri S. 177
Gottschau A. 19, 253, 563
Gould I. M. 637
Grady K. J. 519
Graham J. C. 171

Grahn E. 221
Griffis J. C. 211
Grillner L. 435
Groeneveld P. H. P. 453
Grosse G. 71
Grossin M. 643
Grzesczuk A. 15
Guaraldi G. 173
Guasparini R. 279
Gudiol F. 165
Gün H. 69, 425
Günthard H. 499
Gürses N. 241
Gustafson R. 303, 597
Gutiérrez A. 177

Haas D. W. 411
Habte-Gabr E. 183
Halperin S. A. 279
Hammarström L. 303
Hansen H. L. 191
Hansson L.-O. 32
Hansson-Westerberg J. 187
Hardie J. M. 149
Hauben E. 89
Haznedaroğlu T. 425
Hedlund J. 32, 457
Hedman K. 265
Hedvall G. 273
Heegaard E. D. 631
Heise W. 71
Held M. 529
Henning C. 221
Herbert A.-M. 149
Heremans T. 89
Heresi G. 385
Hermodsson S. 99
Hertramps E. 385
Herva E. 57
Heyman L. 179
Hiilesmaa V. 265
Hökeberg I. 435
Holm S. E. 125
Holm S. 221
Holmberg H. 375
Holmdahl T. 81
Holmlund D. E. W. 603
Hornsleth A. 631
Horowitz I. 139
Hsieh J.-M. 295
Huang Y.-C. 75
Hufert F. T. 627
Hugosson S. 63
Humphreys G. 279
Huovinen P. 45, 52, 57, 475
Hur T. 295
Hynninen M. 533
Hyvärinen J. 475

Ip M. 527, 645
Isacson J. 273

Ishida T. 105
Islek I. 241
Izquierdo J. 469

Jaenson T. G. T. 597
Jahnson L. 421
Jalouk J. 381
Jarlöv J. O. 419
Järvinen H. 475
Jennings C. A. 77
Jensen B. N. 217, 351
Johansson P. J. H. 543
John T. J. 105
Johnson A. P. 291
Jonasson J. 303
Jones I. 375
Jönsson E. 195
Josefsson K. 463
Julander I. 547

Kahanpää A. 207
Kaijser B. 187, 589
Kalayci A. G. 241
Kalin M. 457
Käll K. 547
Kastally R. 9
Katila M.-L. 57
Kato H. 85
Kauppila M. 515
Keene G. S. 291
Kelly B. 519
Kenes Y. 139
Kerr J. R. 551
Keyserling H. 279
Khatib R. 519, 529
Khougeer F. 157
Khuong M.-A. 96
Kihlström E. 489
Kimpen J. L. L. 399
Kok T. W. 507
Kolmos H. J. 253, 363
Kontiainen S. 17, 57
Korman D. 409
Koskela P. 265
Koskiniemi M. 265
Kosunen O. 515
Kosunen T. U. 207, 495
Kotilainen P. 475, 515
Krarup E. 445
Krarup H. B. 445
Kristensen B. 153
Krook A. 547
Kuijper E. J. 83, 581
Kuikka A. 207, 495
Kuzman I. 503
Kwappenberg K. M. C. 453

Lähdevirta J. 515
Landsaat P. M. 83
Lantz P.-G. 537
Lappalainen M. 265
Larsen S. O. 245
Lauritsen A. 431
Lebech M. 259
Leboulleux D. 9
Lee C. 211
Lee H.-S. 415
Lehti H. 207
Lehtonen O.-P. 475
Lelie van der H. 83
Lelie van der J. 581
Lepsanovic Z. 427
Lerche A. 363, 569
Leung N. 645
Leverstein-Van Hall M. 581
Lidman K. 3
Liesnard C. 358
Liitmatainen O. 57
Lin T.-Y. 75
Lindberg A. A. 303
Lindblom G.-B. 187, 589
Lindh G. 319
Lindholm A.-C. 463
Lindholm A. 99
Lindquist B. 63
Linglöf T. O. 299
Linko L. 475
Linzalone A. 235
Liu C.-C. 289
Ljungberg P. 533
Logar J. 163
Lomberg H. 221
Lommi J. 533
Lopez-Contreras J. 523
Lorenzo Di G. 613
Lundgren J. D. 363
Lund-Tønnesen S. 397
Lustman F. 409
Lyytikäinen O. 575
L'Age M. 71

Main J. 297
Makimura K. 85
Malm E. 99
Manfredi R. 405
Manicardi G. 173
Manninen R. 45
Månsson A. 195
Marasca G. 235
Marche C. 643
Marck van E. 89
Marimon J. M. 344
Marinacci G. 405
Martino P. 381
Martín-Caminero M. M. 469
Maruoka T. 85
Matherin P. 401
Matheron S. 96
Mathiesen L. R. 217, 363
Matricardi P. M. 12
Mattsson L. 319
Mazzoni A. 405
McBride M. O. 297
McKendrick M. W. 171
Medd L. 279
Mejlon H. 597
Mele A. 12, 441
Melhus Å. 81
Mertens M. 581
Mertsola J. 39
Meyer-König U. 627
Miedema C. J. 399
Mills E. 279
Mirelis B. 95
Mohammedi I. 643
Moine P. 201
Moiraghi A. 441
Mongiardo N. 173
Montelius H. 463
Montes M. 344
Moonens F. 358
Moore J. E. 551
Morace G. 235
Moss P. J. 171
Motohiro T. 85
Mueller W. F. 183
Müller R. 331
Müns G. 369
Murphy J. R. 385
Murphy P. G. 551
Murri R. 235
Mushahwar I. K. 543
Mussini C. 173

Nagai K. 85
Nanetti A. 405
Ndao M.-A. 9
Nelsing S. 217, 351, 445
Neringer R. 463
Nesadoss J. 105
Neumann-Haefelin D. 627
Nevalainen T. 39
Nielsen B. 245
Nielsen H. 347
Nielsen J. O. 217, 363, 445
Nielsen T. L. 217, 445
Nikoskelainen J. 39
Nilsson L.-Å. 589
Nisini R. 12
Nissinen A. 52, 57
Nolla J. 523
Norda R. 449
Nordenfelt E. 195, 543
Norgren M. 125
Norkrans G. 99, 319, 543
Normann B. 489
Norrby-Teglund A. 125
Northern Italy Collabora . . . 23
Norton R. 507
Novaco F. 441
Novak-Antolic Z. 163
Nurminen J. 515

Obel N. 623
Öberg B. 431
Ode B. 463
Oers van M. H. J. 581
Oetomo S. B. 399
Oh H. M. L. 79
Oinonen S. 57
Olcén P. 63, 449, 537
Olding-Stenkvist E. 435
Olesen B. 253
Olivares M. 385
Ørskov F. 253
Ørskov I. 253
Örtqvist Å. 32, 457
Österlund A. 119, 131
O'Driscoll J. C. 291

Palepou M.-F. 291
Palumbo F. 441
Pauksens K. 125
Paulsen O. 325
Perez J. L. 165
Pérez-Trallero E. 344
Pericas R. 95
Persson K. 195
Petersen E. 259
Peterslund N. A. 153, 631
Petrini B. 391, 421
Pizarro F. 385
Pluss W. T. 77
Podzamczer D. 165
Pohjola-Sintonen S. 533
Prats G. 95
Prieto J. 469
Prokopowicz D. 15
Provost F. 23
Puig M. 95, 523
Pulkki K. 39

Rabella N. 523
Rådegran K. 641
Rådström P. 537
Rahlenbeck S. I. 29
Rapicetta M. 12
Raponi G. M. 381
Rasmussen N. 569
Rautelin H. 207, 495
Reichard O. 3
Reisinger K. 279
Reñe R. 165
Renkonen O.-V. 17, 207, 495
Renneberg J. 245
Riederer K. M. 529
Rienzo B. De. 173
Rintala E. 39
Ris J. 523
Roberts E. A. 279
Rosa G. 381
Rosdahl V. T. 19, 483, 563
Rosthøj S. 153
Rubinstein I. 369
Rufi G. 93
Ryhänen R. 575

Saimot A. G. 96
Sakata Y. 85
Salazar A. 165
Samuelson A. 303
San Joaquin V. H. 211
Sangfelt P. 3
Santamaría J. M. 177
Santin M. 165
Sarkkinen H. 515
Savolainen S. 229
Schepetiuk S. K. 507
Schifroni G. 139
Schønheyder H. C. 19, 145, 153
Schönwald S. 503
Schreier E. 331
Schvarcz R. 319, 641

Sears C. L. 211
Seboxa T. 29
Seppälä H. 52
Serichantalergs O. 585
Serruys E. 358
Shepherd J. P. 149
Shev S. 99
Shinkai M. 559
Silfverdal S.-A. 63
Sintonen H. 265
Sivonen A. 17, 207, 475, 495, 575
Sjögren E. 187, 589
Sjöholm A. G. 111
Skinhøj P. 217, 483, 563
Skinner C. J. 297
Skörde J. 71
Skøt J. 363, 445
Skov R. 563
Smith C. I. E. 303
Söderquist B. 375
Söderqvist A. 229
Søgaard P. 145
Soldo I. 503
Sönnerborg A. 319, 449
Spector S. A. 559
Spence D. 157
Squadrini F. 173
Staley H. 221
Stark K. 331
Stekel A. 385
Stellbrink H.-J. 71
Stenlund G. 463
Stratton C. 401
Stroffolini T. 12
Sundqvist K.-G. 375
Svanteson B. 463
Svartbäck C.-M. 515
Svedenhag J. 641
Svennerholm A.-M. 589
Svennerholm B. 315
Svenungsson B. 597
Sydow C. von 229
Sydow M. von 3
Sztern B. 409

Takala A. K. 57
Tanyüksel M. 69
Taranger J. 273
Tay L. 79
Teira R. 177
Temu M. 589
Teramo K. 265
The French Study Group... 201
The Fungal Study Group 157
Thirumoorthi M. C. 519
Thomas L. L. M. 581
Thorén A. 463
Thorstensson R. 547
Tjernberg I. 81
Tominaga K. 85
Torssander J. 391
Tosti M. E. 12, 441
Trematerra M. 12
Trenti F. 173
Trollfors B. 273
Truedsson L. 111
Tsumura N. 85
Tuesta J. L. Diaz de 344
Tufvesson G. 435
Turgut H. 135

Uçar D. H. 635
Uysal S. 241

Vaara M. 533
Vachon F. 643
Vadillo M. 93
Valls M. E. 511
Valtonen M. 515, 533
Valtonen V. 207, 495, 575
Varona M. 177
Velimirovic S. 427
Vercken J. B. 201
Verstraeten T. 89
Vikerfors T. 63, 375, 421
Villano U. 12
Visakorpi R. 17
Von Laer D. 627
Vooren J. P. Van 358
Vuopio-Varkila J. 475, 575

Wahl M. 319
Walder M. 463
Wallmark E. 463
Walter T. 385
Wandall J. H. 569
Wang J.-Y. 289
Wantzin P. 445
Weiland O. 319, 543
Weinbren M. J. 291
Weir J. 637
Wejstål R. 319
Werner B. 63
Widell A. 99, 319, 325
Wirth D. 331
Wolff M. 643
Wretlind B. 457
Wüst J. 499

Yagupsky P. 139
Yamada S. 85
Yamada T. 85
Yamaguchi H. 85
Yao W.-J. 289
Yildiz H. Y. 635
Yildiz S. 635
Young R. P. 527
Young T. 415

Zaanen van H. C. T. 581
Zackrisson G. 273
Zore A. 163
Zweygberg Wirgart B. 435

ACKNOWLEDGEMENTS

The Editors of Scandinavian Journal of Infectious Diseases wish to express their sincere gratitude to the following persons outside the Editorial Board who have acted as referees during the past year. The standard of the journal depends to a very large extent on the skill and interest of these reviewers.

Alestig K.
Andersson J.
Arneborn P.
Aronsson B.
Aust-Kettis A.

Berglund O.
Bernander S.
Björkman A.
Bjune G.
Bohlin A.-B.
Bolinder C.
Boman G.
Braconier J. H.
Britton S.
Brorson J.-E.
Burman L. G.
Bäck E.

Cars O.
Christenson B.

Dornbusch K.

Eitrem R.
Eklund A.
Ekvall E.
Elvin K.
Engstrand L.
Engvall P.
Eriksson M.
Evengård B.
Ewald U.

Forsgren M.

Gårdlund B.
Glimåker M.
Gnarpe H.
Gothefors L.
Granström M.

Hagberg L.
Hallander H.
Hambraeus A.
Hammarström L.
Hansson B. G.
Hedin G.
Hedström S.-Å.
Hellgren U.
Heurlin N.
Hjelm E.
Hofvander Y.
Hovi T.

Iversen J.

Kalin M.
Kamme C.
Karlsson-Parra A.
Kollberg H.
Källenius G.
Kroogsgaard K.

Lappalainen M.
Larsen F. P.
Lebech M.
Lebens M.
Lidman C.
Linde A.
Lindhart B. Ø.
Lindquist L.
Ljung Å.
Ljungberg B.
Ljungman P.
Ljungström I.
Lumio J.
Lundholm M.

Mattsson L.
Möllby R.

Niklasson B.
Nilsson-Ehle I.
Nord C. E.
Nordenfelt E.
Norkrans G.
Nyrén O.
Nyström B.

Odenholt I.
Olcén P.
Olsson-Liljequist B.
Palmblad J.
Peltola H.
Persson K.
Petrini B.
Philipson A.
Prellner K.
Påhlson C.

Ripa T.
Rombo L.
Rynnel B.

Saikku P.
Saiku P.
Sandberg T.
Sandström E.
Schrumpf E.
Schvarcz R.
Schwan A.
Settergren B.
Sjölin J.
Stiernstedt G.
Stintzing G.
Strömberg A.
Struve J.
Svanborg-Eden C.
Svedmyr A.
Svenungsson B.
Sönnerborg A.

Taube A.
Trollfors B.

Uhnoo I.

Wadell G.
Walder M.
Wejstål R.
Wiström J.
Wretlind B.

Ånsehn S.

Örtqvist Å.
Österlund A.
Örskov Lindhardt B.